FOURTH EDITION

HYPERTENSION PRIMER

THE ESSENTIALS OF HIGH BLOOD PRESSURE

HYPERTENSION PRIMER

Editors

Joseph L. Izzo, Jr., MD
Professor of Medicine, Pharmacology,
and Toxicology
State University of New York at Buffalo
Clinical Director, Department of Medicine
Erie County Medical Center
Buffalo, New York

Domenic A. Sica, MD
Professor of Medicine and Pharmacology
Chairman, Clinical Pharmacology
and Hypertension
Department of Medicine
Virginia Commonwealth University Health System
Richmond, Virginia

Henry R. Black, MD
Clinical Professor of Internal Medicine
New York University School of Medicine
Director, Hypertension Research
New York, New York

From the Council on High Blood Pressure Research
American Heart Association

Acquisitions Editor: Frances DeStefano
Managing Editor: Chris Potash
Project Manager: Cindy Oberle
Senior Manufacturing Manager: Ben Rivera
Marketing Manager: Kimberly Schonberger
Creative Director: Doug Smock
Production Services: Laserwords Private Limited, Chennai, India

© 2008 American Heart Association, Dallas, Texas

Format, Design, and Index © 2008
LIPPINCOTT WILLIAMS & WILKINS
530 Walnut Street
Philadelphia, PA 19106 USA
LWW.com

First Edition © 1998 Williams & Wilkins

Library of Congress Cataloging-in-Publication Data

Hypertension primer : the essentials of high blood pressure : basic science, population science, and clinical management / editors, Joseph L. Izzo Jr., Domenic A. Sica, Henry R. Black.—4th ed.
   p. ; cm.
"From the Council on High Blood Pressure, American Heart Association."
Includes bibliographical references and index.
ISBN 978-0-7817-8205-0
1. Hypertension. I. Izzo, Joseph L. II. Sica, Domenic A. III. Black, Henry R. (Henry Richard), 1942- IV. Council for High Blood Pressure Research (American Heart Association)
[DNLM: 1. Hypertension. WG 340 H99654 2008]
RC685.H8H923 2008
616.1′32—dc22
           2007037803

10 9 8 7 6 5 4 3 2

To my wonderful identical twin sons, Allan and Andrew, for the personal inspiration they provide and the important life lesson they have taught me: our genes are not necessarily more important than how we interact with our environment

JLI

To my wife Jennifer, who always provided the reason to go on, and to Mike, Chris, and Steve for their never ending support

DAS

To the people I love: my wife and perfect partner, Benita; my children, Dana and Matt; my granddaughter, Sabrina; my daughter-in-law, Becky; and to Emily and Josh, the newest members of my family: for their support and inspiration these many years. And also to my colleagues and their patients: I hope they will benefit from our efforts

HRB

CONTENTS

Preface   xvii
Contributing Authors   xix

PART A ■ BASIC SCIENCE

SECTION I ■ ION TRANSPORT AND SIGNAL TRANSDUCTION

Chapter 1   Signal Transduction: Receptors   1
             Greti Aguilera, MD

Chapter 2   Guanine Nucleotide Binding Proteins   4
             James C. Garrison, PhD

Chapter 3   Cyclic Nucleotides and Their Regulation   8
             Stanko S. Stojilkovic, PhD

Chapter 4   Signal Transduction: Inositol Phospholipids and Inositol Phosphates   12
             Tamas Balla, MD, PhD

Chapter 5   Protein Phosphorylation   16
             George W. Booz, PhD and Kenneth M. Baker, MD

Chapter 6   Intracellular pH and Cell Volume   21
             Bradford C. Berk, MD, PhD

Chapter 7   Cellular Potassium Transport   24
             Jason X.-J. Yuan, MD, PhD and Mordecai P. Blaustein, MD

Chapter 8   Calcium Transport and Calmodulin   27
             David J. Triggle, PhD, DSc (Hon.)

Chapter 9   Reactive Oxygen Species and Mediators of Oxidative Stress   30
             Rhian M. Touyz, MD, PhD

Chapter 10   Vascular Smooth Muscle Contraction and Relaxation   34
             Rita C. Tostes, PhD, Romulo Leite, PhD and R. Clinton Webb, PhD

SECTION II ■ VASOACTIVE SUBSTANCES

Chapter 11   Catecholamine Synthesis, Release, Reuptake, and Metabolism   37
             David S. Goldstein, MD, PhD and Graeme Eisenhofer, PhD

Chapter 12   Adrenergic and Dopaminergic Receptors and Actions   39
             Kathleen H. Berecek, PhD and Robert M. Carey, MD, MACP

Chapter 13   Prorenin and Renin   44
             William H. Beierwaltes, PhD

Chapter 14   Angiotensinogen   47
Morton P. Printz, PhD

Chapter 15   Angiotensin I–Converting Enzyme and Neprilysin (Neutral Endopeptidase)   49
Randal A. Skidgel, PhD and Ervin G. Erdös, MD

Chapter 16   Angiotensin Formation and Degradation   52
Carlos M. Ferrario, MD and Mark C. Chappell, PhD

Chapter 17   Angiotensins: Actions and Receptors   54
Theodore L. Goodfriend, MD

Chapter 18   Tissue Renin-Angiotensin Systems   59
Nancy J. Brown, MD

Chapter 19   Adrenal Steroid Synthesis and Regulation   61
Celso E. Gomez-Sanchez, MD

Chapter 20   Mineralocorticoid Receptors   64
Tae-Yon Chun, PhD and J. Howard Pratt, MD

Chapter 21   Endothelin   66
Ernesto L. Schiffrin, MD, PhD, FRSC, FRCPC, FACP

Chapter 22   Vasopressin and Neuropeptide Y   70
Allen W. Cowley, Jr., PhD and Mieczyslaw Michalkiewicz, DVM, PhD

Chapter 23   Calcitonin Gene–Related Peptides and Adrenomedullin-Derived Peptides   73
Donald J. DiPette, MD and Scott Supowit, PhD

Chapter 24   Acetylcholine, γ-Aminobutyric Acid, Serotonin, Adenosine, and Endogenous Ouabain   75
John M. Hamlyn, PhD

Chapter 25   Vascular and Renal Nitric Oxide   78
Leopoldo Raij, MD

Chapter 26   Kinins   82
Oscar A. Carretero, MD and Nour-Eddine Rhaleb, PhD

Chapter 27   Endogenous Natriuretic Peptides   85
Willis K. Samson, PhD and Domenic A. Sica, MD

Chapter 28   Vasoactive Growth Factors   88
Carrie A. Northcott, PhD and Stephanie W. Watts, PhD

Chapter 29   Plasminogen Activation and the Renin-Angiotensin System   91
Douglas E. Vaughan, MD

Chapter 30   Prostaglandins and P450 Metabolites   94
Alberto Nasjletti, MD and John C. McGiff, MD

Chapter 31   Lipoxygenase Products   97
Michael D. Williams, MD and Jerry L. Nadler, MD

Chapter 32   Peroxisome Proliferator–Activated Receptors   100
Sanjeev A. Francis, MD and Jorge Plutzky, MD

Chapter 33   Endocannabinoids   103
George Kunos, MD, PhD, FAHA and Pál Pacher, MD, PhD, FAHA

Chapter 34   Active Products of Adipocytes   107
Nathaniel Winer, MD

Chapter 35   Leptin   110
              William G. Haynes, MD

Chapter 36   Adiponectin   113
              Willa A. Hsueh, MD and Rajendra K. Tangirala, PhD

SECTION III ■ VASOREGULATORY SYSTEMS

Chapter 37   Central Nervous System in Arterial Pressure Regulation   116
              J. Michael Wyss, PhD

Chapter 38   Arterial Baroreflexes   120
              Mark W. Chapleau, PhD

Chapter 39   Cardiopulmonary Baroreflexes   123
              Mark E. Dunlap, MD

Chapter 40   Renal Sympathetic Nerves and Extracellular Fluid Volume Regulation 126
              Edward J. Johns, BSc, PhD, DSc

Chapter 41   Systemic Hemodynamics and Regional Blood Flow Regulation   129
              Thomas G. Coleman, PhD and John E. Hall, PhD

Chapter 42   Local Autoregulation of Tissue Blood Flow   132
              Robert L. Hester, PhD and John E. Hall, PhD

Chapter 43   Respiration and Blood Pressure   136
              Gianfranco Parati, MD, FAHA, FESC, Joseph L. Izzo, Jr., MD
              and Benjamin Gavish, PhD

Chapter 44   Pulsatile Blood Flow and Shear Stress   139
              Michel E. Safar, MD and Gary F. Mitchell, MD

SECTION IV ■ PATHOPHYSIOLOGY OF PRIMARY AND SECONDARY HYPERTENSION

Chapter 45   Aging, Arterial Function, and Systolic Hypertension   144
              Stanley S. Franklin, MD, FACP, FACC and Gary F. Mitchell, MD

Chapter 46   Obesity-Related Hypertension   149
              Efrain Reisin, MD

Chapter 47   Insulin Actions and Insulin Resistance   151
              Adam Whaley-Connell, DO, MSPH, Samy I. McFarlane, MD, MPH and
              James R. Sowers, MD, ASCI

Chapter 48   Polycystic Ovary Syndrome   154
              Caren G. Solomon, MD and Ellen W. Seely, MD

Chapter 49   Salt Sensitivity   156
              Fernando Elijovich, MD and Cheryl L. Laffer, MD, PhD

Chapter 50   Pathophysiology of Renal Parenchymal Hypertension   159
              Vito M. Campese, MD and Jeanie Park, MD

Chapter 51   Pathophysiology of Renovascular Hypertension   162
              L. Gabriel Navar, PhD and David W. Ploth, MD

Chapter 52   Coarctation of the Aorta   166
              Albert P. Rocchini, MD

Chapter 53   Hypertension Caused by Thyroid and Parathyroid Abnormalities,
              Acromegaly, and Androgens   168
              Yoram Shenker, MD

Chapter 54   Pathophysiology of Preeclampsia   171
              Ellen W. Seely, MD and Marshall D. Lindheimer, MD

Chapter 55   Pathophysiology of Sleep Apnea   174
              Barbara J. Morgan, PhD

Chapter 56   Blood Pressure Variability and Reactivity   177
              Joseph L. Izzo, Jr., MD

Chapter 57   Experimental Models of Hypertension   181
              Ralph E. Watson, MD, FACP and Donald J. DiPette, MD

SECTION V ■ MECHANISMS OF TARGET ORGAN DAMAGE

Chapter 58   Aging, Hypertension, and the Heart   184
              Edward G. Lakatta, MD and Samer S. Najjar, MD

Chapter 59   Pathogenesis of Hypertensive Left Ventricular Hypertrophy
              and Diastolic Dysfunction   188
              Edward D. Frohlich, MD

Chapter 60   Pathogenesis of Chronic Heart Failure   191
              Thierry H. Le Jemtel, MD and Pierre V. Ennezat, MD

Chapter 61   Mechanisms of Vascular Remodeling   195
              Gary L. Baumbach, MD

Chapter 62   Microvascular Regulation and Dysregulation   198
              Andrew S. Greene, PhD

Chapter 63   Oxidative Stress and Hypertension   201
              David G. Harrison, MD and Kathy K. Griendling, PhD

Chapter 64   Endothelial Function and Cardiovascular Disease   204
              Julian P.J. Halcox, MA, MD, FRCP and Arshed A. Quyyumi, MD, FACC,
              FRCP

Chapter 65   Atherogenesis and Coronary Artery Disease   209
              Thomas D. Giles, MD

Chapter 66   Pathogenesis of Stroke   214
              J. David Spence, BA, MBA, MD, FRCPC, FAHA

Chapter 67   Pathogenesis of Acute Hypertensive Encephalopathy   217
              Donald D. Heistad, MD, Frank M. Faraci, PhD
              and William T. Talman, MD

Chapter 68   Pathogenesis of Mild Cognitive Impairment and Dementia   219
              Linda A. Hershey, MD, PhD

Chapter 69   Pathogenesis of Nephrosclerosis and Chronic Kidney Disease   222
              Sharon Anderson, MD

Chapter 70   The Eye in Hypertension   226
              Robert N. Frank, MD

SECTION VI ■ BASIC GENETICS

Chapter 71   Genetics of Hypertension   229
              Alan B. Weder, MD

Chapter 72   Monogenic Determinants of Blood Pressure   232
              Robert G. Dluhy, MD

Chapter 73   Heritability of Hypertension and Target Organ Damage   236
              Donna K. Arnett, PhD, MSPH

PART B ■ POPULATION SCIENCE

SECTION I ■ CARDIOVASCULAR RISK IN POPULATIONS
AND INDIVIDUALS

Chapter 74   Geographic Patterns of Hypertension: A Global Perspective   239
Richard S. Cooper, MD and Bamidele Tayo, PhD

Chapter 75   Geographic Patterns of Hypertension in the United States   241
George A. Mensah, MD

Chapter 76   Cardiovascular Risk Factors and Hypertension   244
William B. Kannel, MD, MPH and Peter W.F. Wilson, MD

Chapter 77   Ischemic Heart Disease Risk   249
Donald M. Lloyd-Jones, MD, ScM

Chapter 78   Left Ventricular Hypertrophy and Cardiovascular Disease Risk   254
Daniel Levy, MD

Chapter 79   Cerebrovascular Risk   257
Philip A. Wolf, MD

Chapter 80   Renal Risk   261
Luis M. Ruilope, MD and Joseph L. Izzo, Jr., MD

Chapter 81   Peripheral Arterial Disease and Hypertension   265
Emile R. Mohler III, MD, MS and Michael H. Criqui, MD, MPH

SECTION II ■ HYPERTENSION IN SPECIAL POPULATIONS

Chapter 82   Gender and Blood Pressure   269
Eduardo Pimenta, MD and Suzanne Oparil, MD

Chapter 83   Blood Pressure in Children   273
Bruce Z. Morgenstern, MD and Alan R. Sinaiko, MD

Chapter 84   Ethnicity and Socioeconomic Status in Hypertension   276
*John M. Flack, MD, MPH, Samar A. Nasser, PA-C, MPH
and Shannon M. O'Connor, BS*

Chapter 85   Hypertension in Blacks   279
Keith C. Ferdinand, MD

Chapter 86   Hypertension Among Hispanics in the United States   281
*Carlos J. Crespo, DrPH, MS, FACSM and Mario R. Garcia-Palmieri, MD,
FACC*

Chapter 87   Hypertension in South Asians   284
Prakash C. Deedwania, MD and Rajeev Gupta, MD, PhD

Chapter 88   Hypertension in East Asians and Native Hawaiians   287
Khiet C. Hoang, MD and Nathan D. Wong, PhD, MPH

SECTION III ■ LIFESTYLE FACTORS AND BLOOD PRESSURE

Chapter 89   Stress, White Coat Hypertension, and Masked Hypertension   289
Thomas G. Pickering, MD, DPhil

Chapter 90   Obesity, Body Fat Distribution, and Insulin Resistance: Clinical
Relevance   292
Steven M. Haffner, MD and Henry R. Black, MD

Chapter 91   Physical Activity and Blood Pressure   295
Denise G. Simons-Morton, MD, PhD

Chapter 92   Dietary Patterns and Blood Pressure   297
Frank M. Sacks, MD

Chapter 93   Salt and Blood Pressure   301
Myron H. Weinberger, MD

Chapter 94   Potassium and Blood Pressure   304
Paul K. Whelton, MD, MS

Chapter 95   Blood Pressure Effects of Dietary Calcium, Magnesium Intake,
and Heavy Metal Exposure   307
Lawrence J. Appel, MD, MPH and Ana Navas-Acien, MD, PhD

Chapter 96   Alcohol Use and Blood Pressure   310
William C. Cushman, MD

SECTION IV ■ PREVENTION AND CONTROL

Chapter 97   Trends in Blood Pressure Control and Mortality   314
Thomas J. Thom, BA and Edward J. Roccella, PhD, MPH

Chapter 98   Prevention of Hypertension   318
Jeffrey A. Cutler, MD, MPH and Jeremiah Stamler, MD

Chapter 99   Community-Based Management Programs   322
Daniel T. Lackland, DrPH and Brent M. Egan, MD

Chapter 100   Antihypertensive Treatment Trials: Outcomes   325
William J. Elliott, MD, PhD

Chapter 101   Antihypertensive Treatment Trials: Quality of Life   329
Richard H. Grimm, Jr., MD, PhD and Carrie L. Schleis, MA

Chapter 102   Economic Considerations in Hypertension Management   331
William J. Elliott, MD, PhD

PART C ■ CLINICAL MANAGEMENT

SECTION I ■ GENERAL DIAGNOSTIC ASPECTS

Chapter 103   Blood Pressure Measurement   335
Carlene M. Grim, MSN, SpDN and Clarence E. Grim, MS, MD

Chapter 104   Ambulatory and Home Blood Pressure Monitoring   339
William B. White, MD

Chapter 105   Initial Workup of Adults with Hypertension   343
Joseph L. Izzo, Jr., MD, Domenic A. Sica, MD and Henry R. Black, MD

Chapter 106   Resistant Hypertension   348
Norman M. Kaplan, MD and Domenic A. Sica, MD

Chapter 107   Defining the Syndrome of Hypertension   351
Joseph L. Izzo, Jr., MD, Thomas D. Giles, MD and Barry J. Materson, MD

SECTION II ■ EVALUATION OF TARGET ORGANS

Chapter 108   Evaluation of Electrolyte Abnormalites in Hypertension   356
John W. Graves, MD, FACP, FACC

Chapter 109   Basic Cardiac Evaluation: Physical Examination, Electrocardiogram,
Chest Radiograph, and Stress Testing   359
Clarence Shub, MD and Andrew J. Luisi, Jr., MD

Chapter 110	Cardiac Imaging *Clarence Shub, MD*	363
Chapter 111	Evaluation of Heart Failure *Kirkwood F. Adams, Jr., MD*	367
Chapter 112	Evaluation of Arterial Stiffness and Central Systolic Pressure *Joseph L. Izzo, Jr., MD*	370
Chapter 113	Evaluation of the Peripheral Circulation *Jeffrey W. Olin, DO*	374
Chapter 114	Neurologic Evaluation in Hypertension *Stephen J. Phillips, MBBS, FRCPC*	379
Chapter 115	Evaluation of Chronic Kidney Disease *Michael A. Moore, MD, FACP, FAHA and Domenic A. Sica, MD*	382
Chapter 116	Evaluation of Renovascular Disease *Stephen C. Textor, MD*	387
Chapter 117	Evaluation of Aortocarotid Baroreflexes *Addison A. Taylor, MD, PhD and Naveed Iqbal, MD*	391

SECTION III ■ PRINCIPLES OF MANAGEMENT

Chapter 118	Evolution of American, European, and British Hypertension Guidelines *Henry R. Black, MD, Bryan Williams, MD and Joseph L. Izzo, Jr., MD*	395
Chapter 119	Office Management of Hypertension *Joseph L. Izzo, Jr., MD, Henry R. Black, MD and Domenic A. Sica, MD*	401
Chapter 120	Lifestyle Modifications *Theodore A. Kotchen, MD and Jane Morley Kotchen, MD, MPH*	406
Chapter 121	Exercise Therapy *Denise G. Simons-Morton, MD, PhD*	410
Chapter 122	Patient Education *Daniel W. Jones, MD*	412
Chapter 123	Adherence to Antihypertensive Therapy *Cheryl R. Dennison, ANP, PhD and Nancy Houston Miller, RN*	413
Chapter 124	Barriers to Blood Pressure Control *David J. Hyman, MD and Valory N. Pavlik, PhD*	418
Chapter 125	Hypertension Consultations *Lawrence R. Krakoff, MD*	421
Chapter 126	Nonphysician Providers and the Management of Hypertension *Barry L. Carter, PharmD*	424
Chapter 127	Hypertension Recordkeeping and Electronic Management Systems *Mary K. Goldstein, MD, MS and Brian B. Hoffman, MD*	428

SECTION IV ■ ANTIHYPERTENSIVE DRUGS

Chapter 128	Antihypertensive Drugs: Pharmacologic Principles and Dosing Effects *Joseph L. Izzo, Jr., MD and Domenic A. Sica, MD*	432
Chapter 129	Drug Combinations *Alan H. Gradman, MD*	435
Chapter 130	Thiazide and Loop Diuretics *Domenic A. Sica, MD*	439

Chapter 131   **Aldosterone Blockers and Potassium-Sparing Diuretics**   443
Murray Epstein, MD, FACP

Chapter 132   **β-Adrenergic Blockers**   446
William H. Frishman, MD and Domenic A. Sica, MD

Chapter 133   **α-Adrenoceptor Antagonists**   450
James L. Pool, MD

Chapter 134   **Central and Peripheral Sympatholytics**   453
Barry J. Materson, MD

Chapter 135   **Renin Inhibitors**   455
Norman K. Hollenberg, MD, PhD

Chapter 136   **Angiotensin-Converting Enzyme Inhibitors**   457
Domenic A. Sica, MD

Chapter 137   **Angiotensin Receptor Blockers**   461
Michael A. Weber, MD

Chapter 138   **Calcium Antagonists**   465
Matthew R. Weir, MD

Chapter 139   **Direct Arterial Dilators**   469
C. Venkata S. Ram, MD, FACC, MACP and Andrew Fenves, MD, FACP

Chapter 140   **Nitrates, Dopamine Agonists, Potassium Channel Openers, and Serotonin-Related Agents**   472
Alexander M. M. Shepherd, MD, PhD

Chapter 141   **Vasopressin Inhibitors**   474
Haralambos Gavras, MD, FRCP and Irene Gavras, MD

Chapter 142   **Endothelin Antagonists**   476
William J. Elliott, MD, PhD

Chapter 143   **Antihypertensive Effects of Nonantihypertensive Drugs**   478
Ross D. Feldman, MD

Chapter 144   **Blood Pressure–Raising Effects of Anti-inflammatory Drugs, Angiogenesis Inhibitors, and Cholesterol-Ester-Transfer Protein Inhibitors**   480
Raymond R. Townsend, MD

SECTION V ■ MANAGING HYPERTENSION IN SPECIAL POPULATIONS

Chapter 145   **Treatment of Prehypertension**   483
Henry R. Black, MD and Joseph L. Izzo, Jr., MD

Chapter 146   **Treatment of the Elderly Hypertensive: Systolic Hypertension**   485
Jan N. Basile, MD

Chapter 147   **Treatment of Hypertensive Urgencies and Emergencies**   489
Donald G. Vidt, MD

Chapter 148   **Treatment of Hypertension in Minorities**   493
Mahboob Rahman, MD, MS and Jackson T. Wright, Jr., MD, PhD

Chapter 149   **Treatment of Hypertensive Patients with Ischemic Heart Disease**   496
Clive Rosendorff, MD, PhD, FRCP

Chapter 150   **Management of Hypertensive Patients with Left Ventricular Hypertrophy and Diastolic Dysfunction**   501
Richard B. Devereux, MD

Chapter 151   **Treatment of Hypertensive Patients with Left Ventricular Systolic Dysfunction**   505
John B. Kostis, MD

Chapter 152   **Treatment of Hypertensive Patients with Peripheral Arterial Disease**   509
Jeffrey W. Olin, DO

Chapter 153   Treatment of Hypertensive Patients with Cerebrovascular Disease   512
Robert D. Brown, Jr., MD, MPH

Chapter 154   Treatment of Orthostatic Disorders and Baroreflex Failure   515
David Robertson, MD

Chapter 155   Sexual Dysfunction and Hypertension   519
L. Michael Prisant, MD, FAHA, FACC, FACP

Chapter 156   Treatment of Hypertension with Chronic Renal Insufficiency
or Albuminuria   522
Atul R. Chugh, MD and George L. Bakris, MD

Chapter 157   Treatment of the Obese Hypertensive Patient   526
Xavier Pi-Sunyer, MD, MPH

Chapter 158   Treatment of Hypertensive Patients with Abnormal Blood Glucose   529
Guido Lastra, MD, Samy I. McFarlane, MD, MPH and James R. Sowers,
MD

Chapter 159   Dyslipidemia Management in Hypertensives   532
Peter P. Toth, MD, PhD

Chapter 160   Treatment of Pregnant Hypertensive Patients   536
Sandra J. Taler, MD

Chapter 161   Treatment of Hypertensive Children and Adolescents   540
Bonita Falkner, MD

Chapter 162   Management of Hypertension and Psychiatric Disorders   545
Steven L. Dubovsky, MD

Chapter 163   Hypertension in Athletes   550
John J. Leddy, MD, FACSM

Chapter 164   Perioperative Management of Hypertension   553
John D. Bisognano, MD, PhD and Michael W. Fong, MD

SECTION VI ■ MANAGEMENT OF SECONDARY HYPERTENSION

Chapter 165   Management of Sleep Apnea   556
Virend K. Somers, MD, PhD and Sean M. Caples, DO

Chapter 166   Management of Drug-Induced and Iatrogenic Hypertension   560
Ehud Grossman, MD, Franz H. Messerli, MD, FACC
and Domenic A. Sica, MD

Chapter 167   Management of Hyperaldosteronism and Hypercortisolism   564
David A. Calhoun, MD

Chapter 168   Treatment of Renovascular Hypertension   568
Joseph V. Nally, Jr., MD

Chapter 169   Management of Pheochromocytoma   571
William F. Young, Jr., MD, MSc and Sheldon G. Sheps, MD

Chapter 170   Management of Thyroid and Parathyroid Disorders   574
William F. Young, Jr., MD, MSc

Chapter 171   Management of Post-transplant Hypertension   576
Vincent J. Canzanello, MD

Conflict of Interest Table   579
Index   593

■ PREFACE

The primary goal of the *Hypertension Primer* remains the provision of the highest level of expert opinion to the greatest number of learners in a concise, information-dense format. The *Primer* provides the entire spectrum of "science-based" information in its comprehensive subject treatment, which spans the best available information from molecular science to clinical trials to therapeutic recommendations. The unique synthesis provided by our eminent contributors is the quintessential value of the Hypertension Primer. The editors wish to thank all of the distinguished contributors for their outstanding contributions and for their participation in the rigorous new peer review system that was employed. Secondary goals of the project remain the support for other educational programs sponsored by the Council for High Blood Pressure Research, most notably the Hypertension Summer School.

The 4th Edition of the *Hypertension Primer* embodies state-of-the-art knowledge in our field and remains a showcase for the individual efforts and contributions of the members of the Council for High Blood Pressure Research of the American Heart Association. In the 4th Edition, a greater number of international contributors are found, indicating the growing awareness of the *Primer* on a worldwide basis. Our contributor list continues to evolve, in part because of the untimely death of authors from prior editions, including our good friends and colleagues Lawrence Resnick and Ray Gifford, whom we miss greatly.

The editors' responsibilities have changed from previous editions in order to conform to the expectations of the American Heart Association and the current publisher. The editors have attempted in all cases to respect the opinions of the individual contributors. They have also put forth their best efforts to achieve consensus among the several authors who wrote chapters on diverse aspects of a particular topic under the familiar "superheadings" of basic, population, and clinical science. From past experience it is clear that this consistency has made the *Primer* such a highly effective educational tool. Great emphasis has been placed on the Clinical Science section of the 4th Edition in the hopes that the enormous amount of clinical expertise contained in this part of the book will directly improve clinical practice.

The 4th Edition would not have been possible without an unrestricted educational grant from Novartis Pharmaceuticals. We believe that the *Primer* embodies the aspects of cooperation and collaboration among not-for-profit, for-profit, and academic institutions and individual clinicians and scientists. Specific acknowledgments must include Ms. Nancy Lurker, Mr. Joseph McHale, and Mr. Kishane Davis of Novartis Pharmaceuticals and to Heather Goodell of the American Heart Association. As has been the case since the 1st edition, the work would not have been able to be completed were it not for the tireless efforts of Julie Kostyo, our external Project Manager. Finally, the editors also wish to thank our readers and to re-extend our long-standing invitation to provide any feedback that will make the *Primer* more accurate, "user-friendly," and practically relevant. At the end, we remain dedicated to providing a meaningful scientific and practice-based foundation for anyone interested in the most important of all cardiovascular, cerebrovascular, and renal risk factors: hypertension.

Joseph L. Izzo, Jr., MD
Domenic A. Sica, MD
Henry R. Black, MD

Kirkwood F. Adams, Jr., MD
Associate Professor of Medicine and Radiology
Director, Heart Failure Program
University of North Carolina at Chapel Hill
Chapel Hill, North Carolina

Greti Aguilera, MD
Chief, Section on Endocrine Physiology
Developmental Endocrinology Branch
National Institute of Child Health and Human Development
National Institutes of Health
   Bethesda, Maryland

Sharon Anderson, MD
Professor and Vice Chair
Division of Nephrology and Hypertension
Department of Medicine
Oregon Health and Science University
Portland, Oregon

Lawrence J. Appel, MD, MPH
Professor of Medicine, Epidemiology, and International Health
Johns Hopkins Hospital
Baltimore, Maryland

Donna K. Arnett, PhD, MSPH
Professor and Chair
Department of Epidemiology
University of Alabama, School of Public Health
Birmingham, Alabama

Kenneth M. Baker, MD
Professor and Director, Division of Molecular Cardiology
Vice Chair of Research, Department of Medicine
Texas A&M University Health Science Centre
Temple, Texas

George L. Bakris, MD
Professor of Medicine
Director, Hypertension Center
University of Chicago Pritzker School of Medicine
Chicago, Illinois

Tamas Balla, MD, PhD
Senior Investigator
Head, Section on Molecular Signal Transduction
National Institute of Child Health and Human Development
National Institutes of Health
Bethesda, Maryland

Jan N. Basile, MD
Professor of Medicine
Medical University of South Carolina
Director, Primary Care Service Line
Ralph H. Johnson VA Medical Center
Charleston, South Carolina

Gary L. Baumbach, MD
Professor, Department of Pathology
University of Iowa Carver College of Medicine
University of Iowa Hospitals and Clinics
Iowa City, Iowa

William H. Beierwaltes, PhD
Professor, Department of Medicine
Senior Research Scientist, Hypertension and Vascular Research
   Division
Henry Ford Hospital
Detroit, Michigan

Kathleen H. Berecek, PhD
Professor of Physiology and Biophysics
University of Alabama at Birmingham
University Hospital
Birmingham, Alabama

Bradford C. Berk, MD, PhD
Professor of Medicine
Vice President for Health Sciences
University of Rochester Medical Center
Rochester, Minnesota

John D. Bisognano, MD, PhD
Associate Professor of Medicine
Director of Outpatient Cardiology Services
University of Rochester Medical Center
Strong Memorial Hospital
Rochester, New York

Henry R. Black, MD
Clinical Professor of Internal Medicine
New York University School of Medicine
Director of Hypertension Research
New York, New York

Mordecai P. Blaustein, MD
Professor of Physiology and Medicine
University of Maryland, School of Medicine
Director, Maryland Center for Heart, Hypertension and Kidney
   Disease
Baltimore, Maryland

George W. Booz, PhD
Assistant Professor of Molecular Cardiology and Medicine
Texas A&M Health Science Center College of Medicine
Temple, Texas

Robert D. Brown, Jr., MD, MPH
Professor of Neurology
Mayo Clinic College of Medicine
Chair, Department of Neurology
Mayo Clinic
Rochester, Minnesota

Nancy J. Brown, MD
Associate Dean
Clinical and Translational Scientist Development
Robert H. Williams Professor of Medicine
Professor of Pharmacology
Vanderbilt University School of Medicine
Nashville, Tennessee

David A. Calhoun, MD
Professor of Medicine
Vascular Biology and Hypertension Program
University of Alabama at Birmingham
Birmingham, Alabama

Vito M. Campese, MD
Professor of Medicine
Division of Physiology and Biophysics
University of Southern California, Keck School of Medicine
Chief, Division of Nephrology and Hypertension Center
Los Angeles, California

Vincent J. Canzanello, MD
Associate Professor of Medicine
Mayo Clinic College of Medicine
Rochester, Minnesota

Sean M. Caples, DO
Consultant, Department of Pulmonary & Critical Care Medicine
Sleep Disorders Center
Mayo Clinic
Rochester, Minnesota

Robert M. Carey, MD, MACP
Harrison Distinguished Professor of Medicine
Department of Medicine
University of Virginia
Charlottesville, Virginia

Oscar A. Carretero, MD
Division Head
Hypertension and Vascular Research
Henry Ford Health Systems
Detroit, Michigan

Barry L. Carter, PharmD
Professor, College of Pharmacy
Professor, Family Medicine
Family Medicine
University of Iowa
Iowa City, Iowa

Mark W. Chapleau, PhD
Professor, Departments of Internal Medicine and Molecular
Physiology & Biophysics
University of Iowa Roy J. and Lucille A. Carver College
of Medicine
Research Health Science Specialist
Veterans Affairs Medical Center
Iowa City, Iowa

Mark C. Chappell, PhD
Associate Professor
Hypertension and Vascular Disease Center
Department of Physiology and Pharmacology
Wake Forest University School of Medicine
Winston-Salem, North Carolina

Atul R. Chugh, MD
Fellow in Hypertension, Department of Medicine
University of Chicago Pritzker School of Medicine
University of Chicago Hospitals
Chicago, Illinois

Tae-Yon Chun, PhD
Research Assistant Professor of Medicine
Indiana University School of Medicine
Indianapolis, Indiana

Thomas G. Coleman, PhD
Professor Emeritus
Department of Physiology & Biophysics
University of Mississippi Medical Center
Jackson, Mississippi

Richard S. Cooper, MD
Professor and Chair
Preventive Medicine and Epidemiology
Loyola University School of Medicine
Maywood, Illinois

Allen W. Cowley, Jr., PhD
Professor and Chairman
Department of Physiology
Medical College of Wisconsin
Milwaukee, Wisconsin

Carlos J. Crespo, DrPH, MS, FACSM
Professor and Director
School of Community Health
Portland State University
Portland, Oregon

Michael H. Criqui, MD, MPH
Professor, Department of Family and Preventive Medicine
University of California, San Diego
La Jolla, California

William C. Cushman, MD
Professor, Department of Preventive Medicine and Medicine
University of Tennessee Health Science Center
Chief, Preventive Medicine Section
Veterans Affairs Medical Center
Memphis, Tennessee

Jeffrey A. Cutler, MD, MPH
Consultant
Division of Prevention and Population Sciences
   and Division of Cardiovascular Diseases
National Heart Lung and Blood Institute
Bethesda, Maryland

Prakash C. Deedwania, MD
Professor, Department of Medicine
Chief, Cardiology Division
University of California, San Francisco, School of Medicine
Fresno, California

Cheryl R. Dennison, ANP, PhD
Assistant Professor, School of Nursing
Johns Hopkins University
Baltimore, Maryland

Richard B. Devereux, MD
Professor, Department of Medicine
Weill Medical College of Cornell University
New York Presbyterian Hospital
New York, New York

Donald J. DiPette, MD
Vice President for Medical Affairs and Dean
Health Sciences Distinguished Professor
School of Medicine
University of South Carolina
Columbia, South Carolina

Robert G. Dluhy, MD
Professor, Department of Medicine
Harvard Medical School
Program Director, Fellowship in Endocrinology
Fellowship in Endocrinology
Brigham and Women's Hospital
Boston, Massachusetts

Steven L. Dubovsky, MD
Professor and Chair
Department of Psychiatry
State University of New York at Buffalo
Buffalo, New York

Mark E. Dunlap, MD
Associate Professor, Departments of Medicine, Physiology and
   Biophysics
Case Western Reserve University
Director, Heart Failure Section
The Heart and Vascular Center
MetroHealth Medical Center
Cleveland, Ohio

Brent M. Egan, MD
Professor of Medicine and Pharmacology
Head, Hypertension Section
Division of General Medicine
Medical University of South Carolina
Charleston, South Carolina

Graeme Eisenhofer, PhD
Professor and Chief Division of Clinical Neurochemistry
Department of Clinical Chemistry and Laboratory Medicine
Department of Medicine
University of Dresden
Germany

Fernando Elijovich, MD
Professor & Chief, Division of General Internal Medicine
Department of Medicine
Texas A&M Health Science Center College of Medicine
Scott & White Memorial Hospital & Clinic
Temple, Texas

William J. Elliott, MD, PhD
Professor of Preventive Medicine, Internal Medicine and
   Pharmacology
Department of Preventive Medicine
Rush Medical College
Chicago Illinois

Pierre V. Ennezat, MD
Médecin des Hôpitaux
Soins Intensifs Cardiologiques
Centre Hospitalier Régional et Universitaire
Lille, France

Murray Epstein, MD, FACP
Professor of Medicine
University of Miami School of Medicine
Miami, Florida

Ervin G. Erdös, MD
Professor, Department of Pharmacology
University of Illinois College of Medicine
Chicago, Illinois

Bonita Falkner, MD
Professor, Department of Medicine and Pediatrics
Thomas Jefferson University
Philadelphia, Pennsylvania

Frank M. Faraci, PhD
Professor of Internal Medicine
University of Iowa College of Medicine
Iowa City, Iowa

Ross D. Feldman, MD
R.W. Gunton Professor of Therapeutics
Departments of Medicine and Physiology & Pharmacology
University of Western Ontario
Deputy Scientific Director
Robarts Research Institute
London, Ontario

Andrew Fenves, MD, FACP
Dallas Nephrology Associates
Baylor University Medical Center
University of Texas Southwestern Medical Center at Dallas
Dallas, Texas

Keith C. Ferdinand, MD
Clinical Professor
Cardiology Division
Emory University
Atlanta, Georgia

Carlos M. Ferrario, MD
Professor and Director
Hypertension & Vascular Research Center
Wake Forest University School Of Medicine
Winston-Salem, North Carolina

John M. Flack, MD, MPH
Professor, Interim Chairman and Chief
Department of Internal Medicine
Division of Translational Research and Clinical Epidemiology
Wayne State University
Specialist in Chief, Detroit Medical Center
Detroit, Michigan

Michael W. Fong, MD
Senior Instructor of Medicine
Department of Medicine, Cardiology Division
University of Rochester
Strong Memorial Hospital
Rochester, New York

Sanjeev A. Francis, MD
Fellow in Cardiovascular Medicine
Harvard Medical School
Brigham and Women's Hospital
Boston, Massachusetts

Robert N. Frank, MD
The Robert S. Jampel Professor of Ophthalmology
    and Professor of Anatomy/Cell Biology
The Kresge Eye Institute
Department of Opthamology
Wayne State University School of Medicine
Detroit, Michigan

Stanley S. Franklin, MD, FACP, FACC
Clinical Professor of Medicine
Department of Medicine
University Of California Irvine Medical Sciences
Irvine, California

William H. Frishman, MD
Chairman and Professor, Department of Medicine
New York Medical College
Director of Medicine
Westchester Medical Center
Valhalla, New York

Edward D. Frohlich, MD
Alton Ochsner Distinguished Scientist
Hypertension
Ochsner Clinic Foundation
New Orleans, Louisiana

Mario R. Garcia-Palmieri, MD, FACC
Head, Section of Cardiology
Department of Medicine
School of Medicine University of Puerto Rico
San Juan, Puerto Rico

James C. Garrison, PhD
Professor and Chairman, Department of Pharmacology
University of Virginia Medical School
Charlottesville, Virginia

Benjamin Gavish, PhD
InterCure Ltd.
Communication Park
Israel

Haralambos Gavras, MD, FRCP
Professor, Department of Medicine
Boston University School of Medicine
Chief, Hypertension and Atherosclerosis Section
Boston Medical Center
Boston, Massachusetts

Irene Gavras, MD
Professor of Medicine
Boston University School of Medicine
Hypertension and Atherosclerosis Section
Boston Medical Center
Boston, Massachusetts

Thomas D. Giles, MD
Professor of Medicine
Cardiology/Internal Medicine
Tulane University School of Medicine
New Orleans, Louisiana

David S. Goldstein, MD, PhD
Chief, Clinical Neurocardiology Section
National Institute of Neurological Disorders and Stroke
Bethesda, Maryland

Mary K. Goldstein, MD, MS
Acting Director
Geriatrics Research Education and Clinical Center
VA Palo Alto Health Care System
Professor, Department of Medicine
Stanford University
Stanford, California

Celso E. Gomez-Sanchez, MD
Professor of Medicine, Endocrinology
The University of Mississippi Medical Center
G.V. (Sonny) Montgomery VA Medical Center
Jackson, Mississippi

Theodore L. Goodfriend, MD
Professor Emeritus, Departments of Medicine and Pharmacology
University of Wisconsin, Veterans Hospital
Associate Chief of Staff, Research Service
William S. Middleton Memorial Veterans Hospital
Madison, Wisconsin

Alan H. Gradman, MD
Professor, Department of Medicine
Temple University School of Medicine
Philadelphia, Pennsylvania;
Chief, Division of Cardiovascular Diseases
Division of Cardiovascular Diseases
The Western Pennsylvania Hospital
Pittsburgh, Pennsylvania

John W. Graves, MD, FACP, FACC
Associate Professor of Medicine
Division of Nephrology and Hypertension
Mayo Clinic College of Medicine
Rochester, Minnesota

Andrew S. Greene, PhD
Professor of Physiology
Director, Biotechnology and Bioengineering
Medical College of Wisconsin
Milwaukee, Wisconsin

Kathy K. Griendling, PhD
Professor
Department of Medicine
Emory University
Atlanta, Georgia

Carlene M. Grim, MSN, SpDN
President
Shared Care Research and Education Consulting Inc
Milwaukee, Wisconsin

Clarence E. Grim, MS, MD
Senior Consultant to Shared Care Research and Consulting, Inc.
Clinical Professor
Department of Internal Medicine and Epidemiology
Medical College Wisconsin
Clinical Professor, Department of Nursing
University of Wisconsin
Milwaukee, Wisconsin

Richard H. Grimm, Jr., MD, PhD
Professor, Department of Cardiology and Epidemiology
University of Minnesota
Section Head, Clinical Epidemiology
Hennepin County Medical Center
Minneapolis, Minnesota

Ehud Grossman, MD
Professor of Medicine, Vice Dean for Acacemic Promotions
Sackler Faculty of Medicine
Tel Aviv University
Head, Internal Medicine and Hypertension Unit
The Chaim Sheba Medical Center
Tel-Hashomer, Israel

Rajeev Gupta, MD, PhD
Professor, Department of Medicine
Mahatma Gandhi National Institute of Medical Sciences
Senior Consultant and Director Academics and Research
Fortis Escorts Hospital
Jaipur, India

Steven M. Haffner, MD
Professor, Department of Medicine
University of Texas Health Science Center at San Antonio
San Antonio, Texas

Julian P.J. Halcox, MA, MD, FRCP
Professor, Department of Cardiology
Cardiff University
Wales Heart Research Institute
University Hospital of Wales
Cardiff, Wales

John E. Hall, PhD
Arthur C. Guyton Professor and Chair
Department of Physiology & Biophysics
Associate Vice Chancellor of Research
University of Mississippi Medical Center
Jackson, Mississippi

John M. Hamlyn, PhD
Professor, Department of Physiology
University of Maryland Baltimore
Baltimore, Maryland

David G. Harrison, MD
Professor, Department of Medicine
Emory University
Atlanta, Georgia

William G. Haynes, MD
Professor
Department of Internal Medicine
Director, General Clinical Research Center
Carver College of Medicine
University of Iowa
Iowa City, Iowa

Donald D. Heistad, MD
Zahn Professor
Departments of Internal Medicine and Pharmacology
University of Iowa College of Medicine
University of Iowa Health Care
Iowa City, Iowa

Linda A. Hershey, MD, PhD
Professor, Department of Neurology and Pharmacology
State University of New York at Buffalo, School of Medicine
Chief, Department of Neurology Service
VA WNY Healthcare System
Buffalo, New York

Robert L. Hester, PhD
Professor, Department of Physiology and Biophysics
Department of Physiology & Biophysics
University of Mississippi Medical Center
Jackson, Mississippi

Khiet C. Hoang, MD
Fellow, Department of Cardiology
University of California Irvine
Irvine, California

Brian B. Hoffman, MD
Professor, Department of Medicine
Harvard Medical School
Chief, Department of Medicine
VA Boston Health Care System
Boston, Massachusetts

Norman K. Hollenberg, MD, PhD
Professor, Department of Medicine
Harvard Medical School
Director of Physiologic Research Division
Department of Radiology
Brigham and Women's Hospital
Boston, Massachusetts

Willa A. Hsueh, MD
Chief
Division of Endocrinology, Diabetes, and Hypertension
University of California
Los Angeles School of Medicine
Los Angeles, California

David J. Hyman, MD
Professor
Medicine and Family & Community Medicine
Baylor College of Medicine
Chief, General Internal Medicine
Ben Taub General Hospital
Houston, Texas

Naveed Iqbal, MD
Clinical Pharmacology Fellow
Department of Medicine
Baylor College of Medicine
Houston, Texas

Joseph L. Izzo, Jr., MD
Professor of Medicine, Pharmacology and Toxicology
State University of New York at Buffalo
Clinical Director, Department of Medicine
Erie County Medical Center
Buffalo, New York

Edward J. Johns, BSc, PhD, DSc
Professor, Department of Physiology
University College Cork
Cork, Ireland

Daniel W. Jones, MD
Vice Chancellor for Health Affairs
Dean, School of Medicine
University of Mississippi Medical Center
Jackson, Mississippi

William B. Kannel, MD, MPH
Professor of Medicine
Department of Epidemiology
Boston University School of Medicine
Senior Investigator
Framingham Heart Study
Boston, Massachusetts

Norman M. Kaplan, MD
Clinical Professor of Medicine
Department of Internal Medicine
University of Texas Southwestern Medical School
Dallas, Texas

John B. Kostis, MD
Chairman, Department of Medicine
Robert Wood Johnson Medical School
New Brunswick, New Jersey

Jane Morley Kotchen, MD, MPH
Professor, Departments of Population Health and Medicine
Medical College of Wisconsin
Milwaukee, Wisconsin

Theodore A. Kotchen, MD
Professor of Medicine and Epidemiology
Associate Dean for Clinical Research
Medical College of Winsconsin
Milwaukee, Wisconsin

Lawrence R. Krakoff, MD
Professor, Department of Medicine
Mount Sinai School of Medicine
New York, New York
Chief, Department of Medicine
Englewood Hospital and Medical Center
Englewood, New Jersey

George Kunos, MD, PhD, FAHA
Scientific Director, NIAAA
National Institutes of Health
Bethesda, Maryland

Daniel T. Lackland, DrPH
Professor, Departments of Biometry and Epidemiology,
    and Medicine
Medical University of South Carolina
Charleston, South Carolina

Cheryl L. Laffer, MD, PhD
Associate Professor, Department of Medicine
Texas A&M Health Science Center, College of Medicine
Senior Staff, Medicine and Hypertension/Nephrology
Scott & White Memorial Hospital & Clinic
Temple, Texas

Edward G. Lakatta, MD
Chief, Laboratory of Cardiovascular Science
Intramural Research Program
National Institute on Aging, National Institutes of Health
Baltimore, Maryland

Guido Lastra, MD
Resident, Department of Internal Medicine
University of Missouri Columbia
Harry S. Truman VA Hospital
Columbia, Missouri

John J. Leddy, MD, FACSM
Associate Professor, Department of Orthopedics
Associate Director and Program Director
University Sports Medicine
State University of New York at Buffalo
Buffalo, New York

Romulo Leite, PhD
Research Scientist, Department of Physiology
Medical College of Georgia
Augusta Georgia

Thierry H. Le Jemtel, MD
Professor, Department of Medicine
Tulane University School of Medicine
Tulane University Hospital
New Orleans, Louisiana

Daniel Levy, MD
Director, Framingham Heart Study
Director, Center for Population Studies
National Heart, Lung, & Blood Institute
Bethesda, Maryland

Marshall D. Lindheimer, MD
Professor Emeritus
Departments of Medicine and Obstetrics and Gynecology
University of Chicago
Chicago, Illinois

Donald M. Lloyd-Jones, MD, ScM
Associate Professor, Department of Preventive Medicine
Northwestern University
Chicago, Illinois

Andrew J. Luisi, Jr., MD
Assistant Professor, Department of Medicine
Director of Nuclear Cardiology
State University of New York at buffalo
Buffalo, New York

Barry J. Materson, MD
Professor of Medicine
University of Miami Miller School of Medicine
Miami, Florida

Samy I. McFarlane, MD, MPH
Professor and Chief
Division of Endocrinology, Diabetes and Hypertension
Department of Medicine
State University of New York, Downstate Medical Center
Chief of Endocrinology, Kings County Hospital Center
Brooklyn, New York

John C. McGiff, MD
Professor and Chairman
Department of Pharmacology/Medicine
New York Medical College
Valhalla, New York

George A. Mensah, MD
Clinical Professor, Department of Medicine
Medical College of Georgia
Chief Medical Officer, National Center for Chronic Disease
 Prevention and Health Promotion
Centers for Disease Control and Prevention
Atlanta, Georgia

Franz H. Messerli, MD, FACC
Director, Hypertension Program
Division of Cardiology
St. Luke's Roosevelt Hospital
Columbia University
New York, New York

Mieczyslaw Michalkiewicz, DVM, PhD
Associate Professor, Department of Physiology
Medical College of Wisconsin
Milwaukee, Wisconsin

Nancy Houston Miller, RN
Associate Director, Stanford Cardiac Rehabilitation Program
Stanford University School of Medicine
Palo Alto, California

Gary F. Mitchell, MD
President
Cardiovascular Engineering, Inc.
Waltham, Massachusetts

Emile R. Mohler III, MD, MS
Associate Professor of Medicine
University of Pennsylvania School of Medicine
Philadelphia, Pennsylvania

Michael A. Moore, MD, FACP, FAHA
Clinical Professor
Department of Medicine/Nephrology
Hypertension and Vascular Disease Center
Wake Forest University School of Medicine
Winston-Salem, North Carolina

Barbara J. Morgan, PhD
Professor of Orthopedics and Rehabilitation
University of Wisconsin School of Medicine and Public Health
Madison, Wisconsin

Bruce Z. Morgenstern, MD
Professor of Clinical Pediatrics
University of Arizona College of Medicine
Phoenix, Arizona
Associate Professor of Pediatrics
Mayo Clinic, Scottsdale, Arizona
Chief, Division of Nephrology, Phoenix Children's Hospital
Phoenix, Arizona

Jerry L. Nadler, MD
Kenneth R. Crispell, Professor of Medicine
University of Virginia School of Medicine
Chief, Division of Endocrinology and Metabolism
University of Virginia Health System
Charlottesville, Virginia

Samer S. Najjar, MD
Staff Clinician, Laboratory of Cardiovascular Science
National Institute on Aging
National Institutes of Health
Baltimore, Maryland

Joseph V. Nally, Jr., MD
Clinical Professor of Medicine and Staff Nephrologist
Department of Nephrology and Hypertension
Cleveland Clinic Lerner College of Medicine
Cleveland, Ohio

Alberto Nasjletti, MD
Professor, Department of Pharmacology
New York Medical College
Valhalla, New York

Samar A. Nasser, PA-C, MPH
Physician Assistant, Department of Internal Medicine
Division of Translational Research and Clinical Epidemiology
Wayne State University
Detroit, Michigan

L. Gabriel Navar, PhD
Professor and Chair
Department of Physiology
Tulane University Health Sciences Center
New Orleans, Louisiana

Ana Navas-Acien, MD, PhD
Assistant Professor
Departments of Environmental Health Sciences and
 Epidemiology
Johns Hopkins University
Baltimore, Maryland

Carrie A. Northcott, PhD
Research Associate
Department of Pharmacology and Toxicology
Michigan State University
East Lansing, Michigan

Shannon M. O'Connor, BS
Research Assistant, Department of Internal Medicine
Division of Translational Research and Clinical Epidemiology
Wayne State University
Detroit, Michigan

Jeffrey W. Olin, DO
Professor of Medicine
Zena and Michael A. Wiener Cardiovascular Institute and
Marie-Josée and Henry R. Kravis Center for Cardiovascular
   Health
Director, Vascular Medicine
Mount Sinai School of Medicine
New York, New York

Suzanne Oparil, MD
Professor of Medicine, Physiology and Biophysics
Director, Vascular Biology and Hypertension Program of the
   Division of Cardiovascular Disease
University of Alabama at Birmingham
Birmingham, Alabama

Pál Pacher, MD, PhD, FAHA
Chief, Section of Oxidative Stress Tissue Injury
Laboratory of Physiological Studies
National Institutes of Health
Bethesda, Maryland

Gianfranco Parati, MD, FAHA, FESC
Professor, Department of Clinical Medicine and Prevention
University of Milano-Bicocca
Chief, Department of Cardiology
S. Luca Hospital, Instituto Auxologico Italiano
Milano, Italy

Jeanie Park, MD
Clinical Instructor
Department of Internal Medicine/Nephrology
University of Southern California Medical Center
Los Angeles, California

Valory N. Pavlik, PhD
Associate Professor
Department of Family and Community Medicine
Baylor College of Medicine
Houston, Texas

Stephen J. Phillips, MBBS, FRCPC
Professor, Department of Medicine
Dalhousie University
Director, Acute Stroke Program
Queen Elizabeth II Health Sciences Centre
Halifax, Nova Scotia

Xavier Pi-Sunyer, MD, MPH
Professor, Department of Medicine
Columbia University College of Physicians and Surgeons
Chief, Division of Endocrinology, Diabetes and Nutrition
St. Luke's-Roosevelt Hospital Center
New York, New York

Thomas G. Pickering, MD, DPhil
Professor, Department of Medicine
Director, Center for Behavioral Cardiovascular Health
Columbia University Medical College
New York, New York

Eduardo Pimenta, MD
Research Associate
Vascular Biology and Hypertension Program
University of Alabama at Birmingham
Birmingham, Alabama

David W. Ploth, MD
A.V. Williams, Jr., Professor of Medicine
Director, Division of Nephrology
Editor in Chief, The American Journal of The Medical Sciences
The Medical University of South Carolina
Charleston, South Carolina

Jorge Plutzky, MD
Associate Professor, Department of Medicine
Harvard Medical School
Director, Vascular Disease Prevention Program
Brigham and Women's Hospital
Boston, Massachusetts

James L. Pool, MD
Professor, Departments of Medicine and Pharmacology
Baylor College of Medicine
Houston, Texas

J. Howard Pratt, MD
Professor, Department of Medicine
Indiana University School of Medicine
Richard L. Roudebush VA Medical Center
Indianapolis, Indiana

Morton P. Printz, PhD
Professor, Department of Pharmacology
University of California, San Diego
La Jolla, California

L. Michael Prisant, MD, FAHA, FACC, FACP
Professor, Department of Medicine
Director of Hypertension and Clinical Pharmacology
Medical College of Georgia
Augusta, Georgia

Arshed A. Quyyumi, MD, FACC, FRCP
Professor of Medicine, Division of Cardiology
Emory University School of Medicine
Atlanta, Georgia

Mahboob Rahman, MD, MS
Associate Professor, Department of Medicine
Case Western Reserve University
Cleveland, Ohio

Leopoldo Raij, MD
Professor, Department of Medicine
Director of Hypertension, Renal and Hypertension Division
University of Miami Miller School of Medicine
Miami, Florida

C. Venkata S. Ram, MD, FACC, MACP
Clinical Professor, Department of Internal Medicine
University of Texas Southwestern Medical School
Director, Texas Blood Pressure Institute
Dallas, Texas

Efrain Reisin, MD
Victor Chaltiel Professor of Medicine and Chief
Section of Nephrology and Hypertension
Lousiana State University Health Science Center
New Orleans, Louisiana

Nour-Eddine Rhaleb, PhD
Associate Professor, Department of Physiology
Wayne State University
Senior Staff Scientist, Medicine/Hypertension and Vascular
    Research
Henry Ford Hospital
Detroit, Michigan

David Robertson, MD
Elton Yates Professor of Medicine, Pharmacology and Neurology
Director, Clinical Research Center
Vanderbilt University Medical Center
Nashville, Tennessee

Edward J. Roccella, PhD, MPH
Coordinator
National High Blood Pressure Education Program
National Institutes of Health
Bethesda, Maryland

Albert P. Rocchini, MD
Professor, Department of Pediatrics
Director, Peds Cardiology
University of Michigan
Ann Arbor, Michigan

Clive Rosendorff, MD, PhD, FRCP
Professor of Medicine
Mount Sinai School of Medicine
Detroit, Michigan
New York, New York
The James J. Peters VA Medical Center
Bronx, New York

Luis M. Ruilope, MD
Chief of Hypertension, Department of Nephrology
Hospital Universitario
Madrid, Spain

Frank M. Sacks, MD
Professor, Department of Nutrition
Harvard School of Public Health
Professor, Deparment of Medicine
Harvard Medical School and Brigham & Women's Hospital
Boston, Massachusetts

Michel E. Safar, MD
Professor, Department of Therapeutics
Paris Descartes University
Hôtel-Dieu Hospital
Paris, France

Willis K. Samson, PhD
Professor, Department of Pharmacology and Physiology
St. Louis University
St. Louis, Missouri

Ernesto L. Schiffrin, MD, PhD, FRSC, FRCPC, FACP
Professor and Chair for Research
Department of Medicine
McGill University
Montreal, Quebec

Carrie L. Schleis, MA
Principal Clinical Trial Leader
Medtronic Inc.
St. Paul, Minnesota

Ellen W. Seely, MD
Associate Professor, Department of Medicine
Harvard Medical School
Director, Clinical Research, Endocrinology,
    Diabetes & Hypertension, Department of Medicine
Brigham & Women's Hospital
Boston, Massachusetts

Yoram Shenker, MD
Professor, Department of Internal Medicine
University of Wisconsin School of Medicine and Public Health
Madison, Wisconsin

Alexander M. M. Shepherd, MD, PhD
Professor, Departments of Medicine and Pharmacology
University of Texas Health Sciences Center
San Antonio, Texas

Sheldon G. Sheps, MD
Emeritus Professor, Department of Medicine
Divisions of Cardiovascular Diseases, Nephrology and
    Hypertension
College of Medicine, Mayo Clinic
Rochester, Minnesota

Clarence Shub, MD
Consultant, Department of Cardiology
College of Medicine, Mayo Clinic
Rochester, Minnesota

Domenic A. Sica, MD
Professor of Medicine and Pharmacology
Chairman, Clinical Pharmacology and Hypertension
Department of Medicine
Virginia Commonwealth University Health System
Richmond, Virginia

Denise G. Simons-Morton, MD, PhD
Senior Scientific Advisor
Division of Prevention and Population Sciences
National Heart, Lung, and Blood Institute
Bethesda, Maryland

Alan R. Sinaiko, MD
Professor of Pediatrics and Adjunct Professor of Epidemiology
Medical School and School of Public Health
University of Minnesota
Minneapolis, Minnesota

Randal A. Skidgel, PhD
Professor, Department of Pharmacology
University of Illinois College of Medicine
Chicago, Illinois

Caren G. Solomon, MD
Associate Professor, Department of Medicine
Department of Medicine
Harvard Medical School
Brigham and Women's Hospital
Boston, Massachusetts

Virend K. Somers, MD, PhD
Professor of Medicine
Division of Cardiovascular Diseases
Mayo Clinic College of Medicine
Rochester, Minnesota

James R. Sowers, MD
Professor of Medicine, Physiology and Pharmacology
University of Missouri School of Medicine
University of Missouri Hospital and Truman VA Medical Center
Columbia, Missouri

J. David Spence, BA, MBA, MD, FRCPC, FAHA
Professor of Neurology and Clinical Pharmacology
University of Western Ontario
Director, Stroke Prevention & Atherosclerosis Research Centre
Robarts Research Institute
Stroke Team, Department of Neurology
University Hospital
London, Ontario

Jeremiah Stamler, MD
Professor Emeritus
Department of Preventive Medicine
Feinberg School of Medicine
Northwestern University
Chicago, Illinois

Stanko S. Stojilkovic, PhD
Head, Section on Cellular Signaling
Developmental Neuroscience Program
National Institute of Child Health and Human Development
Bethesda, Maryland

Scott Supowit, PhD
Associate Professor
Cell and Developmental Biology and Anatomy
University of South Carolina School of Medicine
Columbia, South Carolina

Sandra J. Taler, MD
Associate Professor, Department of Medicine
Division Of Nephrology
Mayo Clinic College of Medicine
Rochester, Minnesota

William T. Talman, MD
Professor, Department of Neurology
University of Iowa, Roy J. and Lucille A. Carver College
   of Medicine
Chief of Neurology-Veterans Affairs Medical Center
Iowa City, Iowa

Rajendra K. Tangirala, PhD
Assistant Professor of Medicine
Department of Medicine/Endocrinology, Diabetes and
   Hypertension
David Geffen School of Medicine at UCLA
Los Angeles, California

Addison A. Taylor, MD, PhD
Professor, Department of Medicine
Baylor College of Medicine
Houston, Texas

Bamidele Tayo, PhD
Assistant Professor
Department of Preventive Medicine and Epidemiology
Loyola University School of Medicine
Maywood, Illinois

Stephen C. Textor, MD
Professor of Medicine
Vice-Chair, Division of Nephrology and Hypertension
Mayo Clinic College of Medicine
Rochester, Minnesota

Thomas J. Thom, BA
Statistician
National Heart, Lung, and Blood Institute, NIH
US Department of Health and Human Services
Bethesda, Maryland

Rita C. Tostes, PhD
Associate Professor, Department of Pharmacology
University of Sao Paulo
Sao Paulo, Brazil

Peter P. Toth, MD, PhD
Clinical Associate Professor
Family and Community Medicine
University of Illinois College of Medicine
Peoria, Illinois
Director of Preventive Cardiology
Sterling Rock Falls Clinic
Sterling, Illinois

Rhian M. Touyz, MD, PhD
Professor of Medicine
University of Ottawa
Canada Research Chair in Hypertension
Senior Scientist, Kidney Research Center
Ottawa Health Research Institute
Ottawa, Ontario

Raymond R. Townsend, MD
Professor, Department of Medicine
Department of Medicine
University of Pennsylvania
Philadelphia, Pennsylvania

David J. Triggle, PhD, DSc (Hon.)
Professor
School of Pharmacy
State University of New York at Buffalo
Buffalo, New York

Douglas E. Vaughan, MD
Professor of Medicine and Pharmacology
Chief, Division of Cardiovascular Medicine
Vanderbilt University Medical Center
Nashville, Tennessee

Donald G. Vidt, MD
Consultant, Department of Nephrology and Hypertension
Cleveland Clinic
Cleveland, Ohio

Ralph E. Watson, MD, FACP
Associate Professor, Department of Medicine
Director, Hypertension Clinic
Michigan State University
East Lansing, Michigan

Stephanie W. Watts, PhD
Professor of Pharmacology and Toxicology
Michigan State University
East Lansing, Michigan

R. Clinton Webb, PhD
H.S. Kupperman Chair in Cardiovascular Disease
Professor and Chairperson of Physiology
Medical College of Georgia School of Medicine
Augusta, Georgia

Michael A. Weber, MD
Professor of Medicine
State University of New York, Downstate College
   of Medicine
Brooklyn, New York

Alan B. Weder, MD
Professor, Department of Internal Medicine
University of Michigan
Ann Arbor, Michigan

Myron H. Weinberger, MD
Professor, Department of Medicine
Indiana University School of Medicine
Indianapolis, Indiana

Matthew R. Weir, MD
Professor of Medicine
University of Maryland School of Medicine
Director, Division of Nephrology
University of Maryland Hospital
Baltimore, Maryland

Adam Whaley-Connell, DO, MSPH
Assistant Professor of Medicine
University of Missouri Columbia
Columbia, Missouri

Paul K. Whelton, MD, MS
Vice President for Health Sciences
Professor, Preventive Medicine and Epidemiology
Stritch School of Medicine, Loyola University
   of Chicago
President and Chief Executive Officer
Loyola University Health System
Maywood, Illinois

William B. White, MD
Professor of Medicine and Cardiology
University of Connecticut School of Medicine
Chief, Division of Hypertension & Clinical Pharmacology
Calhoun Cardiology Center
University of Connecticut Health Center
Farmington, Connecticut

Bryan Williams, MD
Professor of Medicine
Department of Cardiovascular Sciences
University of Leicester School of Medicine
Leicester, United Kingdom

Michael D. Williams, MD
Fellow, Department of Endocrinology and Metabolism
University of Virginia
Charlottesville, Virginia

Peter W.F. Wilson, MD
Professor, Department of Medicine
Cardiology Division
Emory University School of Medicine
Atlanta, Georgia

Nathaniel Winer, MD
Professor of Medicine
Division of Endocrinology, Diabetes and Hypertension
State University of New York Health Sciences Center
   at Brooklyn
Director of Diabetes, Thyroid Clinics
Kings County Hospital Center
Brooklyn, New York

Philip A. Wolf, MD
Professor, Department of Neurology
Framingham Heart Study
Boston University School of Medicine
Boston, Massachusetts

Nathan D. Wong, PhD, MPH
Professor and Director
Heart Disease Prevention Program
Division of Cardiology
University of California Irvine
Irvine, California

Jackson T. Wright, Jr., MD, PhD
Professor of Medicine
Director, Clinical Hypertension Program
Case Western Reserve University
Cleveland, Ohio

J. Michael Wyss, PhD
Professor of Cell Biology and Medicine
Director, Center for Community OutReach Development
University of Alabama at Birmingham
Birmingham, Alabama

William F. Young, Jr., MD, MSc
Professor of Medicine
Division of Endocrinology, Diabetes, Metabolism, and Nutrition
Mayo Clinic College of Medicine
Rochester, Minnesota

Jason X.-J. Yuan, MD, PhD
Professor and Associate Chair for Research
Department of Medicine
University of California, San Diego
La Jolla, California

SECTION I ■ ION TRANSPORT AND SIGNAL TRANSDUCTION

CHAPTER A1 ■ SIGNAL TRANSDUCTION: RECEPTORS

GRETI AGUILERA, MD

KEY POINTS

- Receptors are protein complexes that recognize specific hormones and translate extracellular hormone levels into intracellular events.
- The guanyl nucleotide protein (G protein)–coupled receptor superfamily is the largest group of plasma membrane receptors.
- Hormone ligand binding activates the receptors, usually downregulates receptor number or affinity, and reduces tissue sensitivity.
- Receptors modulate their biological activity by interacting at the protein–protein or signaling levels.

See also Chapters **A2, A3, A4,** and **A5**

Cell-to-cell communication, an essential component of integrated physiologic function in multicellular organisms, is mediated largely through informational molecules, such as hormones and neurotransmitters.

Major receptor types and functions

Extracellular signaling molecules, or first messengers, are recognized by specific receptor proteins in the target cell, which are of two types. Type 1 includes receptors located in the plasma membrane that recognize growth factors, catecholamines, insulin, cytokines, prostaglandins, and many other substances. Type 2 includes receptors for steroids and iodothyronines that are located in the cytoplasm or nucleus of the cell and control gene expression.

Receptors have two major functions: (a) recognition of a specific hormone ligand and (b) intracellular transmission of information leading to modification of cell function. Modified hormone analogs capable of binding the receptor without activating transduction mechanisms act as receptor antagonists.

Receptor binding properties

The use of radiolabeled ligands has made possible the identification and measurement of receptors for steroids, peptide hormones, and neurotransmitters in their various target tissues.

Receptor kinetics. In general, each ligand-receptor interaction is rapid and reversible, consistent with the time course of the biological effects of hormones. Binding kinetics depend on the rates of association and dissociation of the ligand-receptor complexes, which are affected by temperature and pH. The ratio between association and dissociation rates determines the association constant (K_a). The reciprocal of the association constant is the dissociation constant (K_d), which is usually expressed as the ligand concentration necessary to saturate the binding sites.

Receptor affinity. Ligand-receptor binding exhibits high affinity, which allows for significant binding despite low circulating levels of hormones. Receptor binding is always saturable, indicating a limited number of binding sites. Receptor affinity usually correlates well with tissue sensitivity to the biological effect of the hormone, but in a number of systems, full biological response is achieved with only partial receptor occupancy. The presence of excess or "spare" receptors may be important to maintain biological effects of hormones in physiologic or pathologic conditions involving alterations of receptor number.

Transduction mechanisms

In general, a requisite for a receptor molecule is the ability to communicate information to effector molecules (second messengers) inside the cell. The informational transduction can be carried out by the receptor itself or through activation of one or more intermediary signaling molecules or pathways.

Cell membrane (type 1) receptors. Interaction of hormones or neurotransmitters with cell-surface receptors leads to modification of cell function through a chain of events involving the generation of second-messenger molecules. Cell-surface receptors can be categorized into two major groups: (a) receptors with intrinsic enzymatic or ion channel activity and (b) receptors coupled to cellular effector molecules through a transduction protein. Molecular cloning and characterization of these receptors show that they are anchored to the cell membrane through one or several hydrophobic amino acid sequences. In general, the structure of these receptors consists of an extracellular domain, transmembrane regions, and one or more intracellular regions responsible for catalytic activity or coupling to intermediary proteins.

Intracellular (type 2) receptors. Intracellular receptors, such as steroid and thyroid hormone receptors, are dimeric proteins consisting of a hormone-binding subunit and a regulatory subunit. After ligand (first-messenger) binding, the regulatory subunit dissociates from the complex and the activated hormone-binding subunit interacts with DNA, influencing gene transcription. Activated receptors interact with DNA-responsive elements in the form of homodimers. Receptor-DNA binding activity can be modulated through formation of heterodimers with other transcription factors, and by recruitment of coactivators or corepressors on binding to responsive elements at the gene promoter level.

Type 1 receptors and intrinsic activity
Receptors with intrinsic activity

Tyrosine kinase dependent. Growth factor and insulin receptors include a tyrosine kinase domain and one or more tyrosine phosphorylation sites that are structural parts of the receptor molecule. Ligand interaction with these receptors results in receptor autophosphorylation, which leads to binding of phosphorylated receptor domains to signaling molecules. Examples include phosphatidylinositol kinase, guanosine triphosphatase (GTPase)-activating factor, phospholipase C, Src family kinases, or serine kinases.

Receptor-gated ion channels. Receptor-gated ion channels, in which the receptor is a structural component of the ion channel, also exhibit intrinsic activity. Examples are γ-aminobutyric acid $(GABA)_A$ receptors associated with Cl^- and HCO_3^- transport; nicotinic acetylcholine receptors associated with Na^+, K^+, and Ca^{2+} transport; N-methyl-D-aspartate (NMDA) and non-NMDA glutamate receptors associated with Na^+, K^+, and Ca^{2+} transport; 5- hydroxytryptamine $(HT)_3$ receptors associated with Na^+ and K^+ transport; and channel-opening adenosine triphosphate (ATP) receptors associated with Ca^{2+}, Na^+, and Mg^{2+} transport.

Receptors without intrinsic activity. A second group of cell-surface receptors lacks intrinsic activity and uses an intermediary protein such as adenylyl cyclase, phospholipase

C, ion channels, or tyrosine kinases for coupling to effectors. Two major types belong to this group: (a) the cytokine receptor superfamily, including growth hormone and prolactin receptors, which activate tyrosine kinases of the Janus kinase (JAK) family, and (b) the guanyl nucleotide–binding protein (G protein) receptor superfamily (GPCR).

G proteins are located on the intracellular side of the plasma membrane, where they can interact with the receptor and the effector signaling system. G proteins consist of three subunits, α, β, and γ, of which α has GTP binding and GTPase activity properties. Occupancy of the receptor by its ligand causes conformational changes in the associated G protein, allowing binding of the α subunit to GTP and dissociation from the βγ-complex. The activated α subunit activates an effector molecule, such as adenylyl cyclase or phospholipase C. This process is rapidly reversible on degradation of bound GTP by the intrinsic GTPase activity of the α subunit.

Although ligand binding is responsible for hormonal activation of receptors, there is evidence that unligated GPCRs exist in at least two states, an inactive conformation and a constitutively active conformation, which has affinity for the G protein in the absence of the agonist. Inverse agonists are ligand analogs, which preferentially stabilize the receptor in the inactive conformation, decreasing basal receptor activity in the absence of a ligand.

Receptor regulation

The effectiveness of a hormone depends on hormone concentration, the number and affinity of receptors in the target tissue, and postreceptor events. For a given set of conditions, changes in receptor number result in: (a) changes in sensitivity in tissues containing spare receptors, or (b) changes in magnitude of the response in tissues in which receptor number is limited. Although peptide hormone receptors undergo changes in number and affinity when exposed to their ligand (homologous regulation), the binding and activity of many receptors can be regulated by heterologous hormones.

Receptor downregulation. Increased hormone levels usually result in receptor loss and desensitization of the biological responses to the hormone. Mechanisms leading to receptor downregulation include negative cooperativity, in which partial receptor occupancy decreases the binding affinity of the remaining receptors (insulin receptor), internalization and lysosomal degradation of hormone-receptor complexes [epidermal growth factor, human chorionic gonadotropin, gonadotropin-releasing hormone (GnRH), insulin], and receptor phosphorylation, which can be heterologous (by second messenger–dependent kinases) or homologous (phosphorylation of agonist-occupied receptor by G protein receptor kinases). Guanyl nucleotides have been shown to reduce high-affinity binding in membrane preparations of a number of G protein–coupled receptors, probably through conformational changes in the receptor protein.

Receptor upregulation. Some peptide hormone receptors, such as adrenal angiotensin II, prolactin, V1b subtype vasopressin and GnRH receptors, have been shown to undergo upregulation after exposure to increased hormone levels.

Altered tissue sensitivity. In a number of conditions, receptor regulation can contribute to the sensitivity of the target tissue to a hormone. For example, downregulation of angiotensin II receptors could account for the low pressor responses to the peptide during Na^+ restriction and other clinical states of high renin secretion. Conversely, upregulation of angiotensin II receptors may contribute to the increase in sensitivity of the adrenal glomerulosa to AII during Na^+ restriction.

Receptor interactions

Receptors can physically interact with each other or at the signaling levels, resulting in changes in biological activity.

Dimerization. Receptor–receptor interaction through homo- or heterodimerization is a requirement for nuclear receptors, cytokine, and growth factor receptors. However, increasing evidence indicates that G protein–coupled receptors form homodimers (β-adrenergic, opioid, histamine H_2, M_1 and M_2 muscarinic, vasopressin V_1 and V_2, and somatostatin receptors), or heterodimers between receptors of the same or different families, as occurs between somatostatin 1 and 5 receptors, somatostatin and dopamine receptors, vasopressin V_{1b} and corticotropin releasing hormone, and GABA and dopamine receptors. For many of these receptors, dimerization plays an important role modulating binding affinity as well as receptor coupling to signaling systems and agonist mediated endocytosis.

Cross-phosphorylation. Simultaneous activation of multiple G protein–coupled receptors from different families in the same cell can modulate the binding and signaling properties of one of the receptors through cross-phosphorylation of the receptor itself of signaling proteins. For example, vasopressin V_{1b} receptor activation potentiates the stimulation of cyclic adenosine monophosphate (cAMP) by corticotrophin releasing hormone and also facilitates corticotrophin releasing hormone receptor downregulation (through phosphorylation), independent of dimerization. Also, G protein–coupled receptors can regulate cellular growth and differentiation by controlling the activity of mitogen-activated protein (MAP) kinases through cross-talk with receptor tyrosine kinases, such as the epidermal growth factor receptor.

Protein modulation. In addition to interaction among receptors themselves or with signaling coupling proteins, receptors can directly interact with other intracellular and extracellular proteins. The most dramatic example is the interaction of the calcitonin receptor-like receptor with novel proteins encoded by the same gene, called *receptor activity modifying proteins* (RAMPs). Interaction with different members of the RAMP family confers receptor specificity—the same receptor therefore functions as either an adrenomedullin or calcitonin-gene related peptide (CGRP) receptor.

Other proteins with specific receptor modulating properties are the AT_1 receptor-associated protein (ATRAP) shown to specifically downregulate AT_1 receptors, and a 24 kDa single transmembrane domain protein called *calcyon*, which induces calcium/phospholipid responses by the Gs-adenylyl cyclase coupled dopamine D_1 receptor. These protein–protein interactions allow a greater diversity of function for individual GPCRs within different cell backgrounds. The composition of protein complexes influences receptor properties such as subcellular localization, binding affinity and specificity, signaling and trafficking processes.

Suggested Readings

Bulenger S, Marullo M, Bouvier M. Emerging role of homo- and heterodimerization in G protein–coupled receptor biosynthesis and maturation. *Trends Pharmacol Sci* 2005;26:131–137.

Kahn RC, Smith RJ, Chin WW. Mechanism of action of hormones that act at the cell surface. In: Wilson JD, Foster DW, Kronenberg HM, et al. eds. *Williams textbook of endocrinology*. Philadelphia: WB Saunders, 1998.

Koshland DE. The structural basis of negative cooperativity: receptors and enzymes. *Curr Opin Struct Biol* 1996;6:757–761.

Milligan G, Kostenis E. Heterotrimeric G proteins: a short history. *Br J Pharmacol* 2006;147:S46–S55.

Rodbell M. The complex regulation of receptor-coupled G proteins. *Adv Enzyme Regul* 1997;37:427–435.

Smith NJ, Luttrell LM. Signal switching, crosstalk, and arrestin scaffolds: novel G protein–coupled receptor signaling in cardiovascular disease. *Hypertension* 2006;48:173–179.

Tsai MJ, Clark JH, Schrader WT, O'Malley BW. Mechanisms of action of hormones that act as transcription regulatory factors. In: Wilson JD, Foster DW, Kronenberg HM, Larsen PR, eds. *Williams textbook of endocrinology*. Philadelphia: WB Saunders; 1998.

Wess J. Molecular basis of receptor/G protein–coupling selectivity. *Pharmacol Ther* 1998;80:231–264.

CHAPTER A2 ■ GUANINE NUCLEOTIDE BINDING PROTEINS

JAMES C. GARRISON, PhD

KEY POINTS

■ Guanine nucleotide binding proteins (G proteins) transduce a wide variety of signals in differentiated target cells in response to ligands bound to receptors with seven transmembrane-spanning domains (G protein–coupled receptors).

■ G proteins communicate the signal of ligand binding by regulating the activity of intracellular effectors, such as adenylyl cyclase, phospholipase C-β, or ion channels, which in turn regulate the levels of second messengers such as cyclic adenosine monophosphate (cAMP), inositol phosphates, diacylglycerol (DAG), and potassium or calcium ions.

■ G proteins can be stimulatory or inhibitory; interactions of different G protein–coupled receptors can counterregulate physiologic effects within single cells such as those in the cardiac sinoatrial (SA) and atrioventricular (AV) nodes.

See also Chapters **A1, A3, A4,** and **A5**

G protein–coupled receptors

Many cell-surface receptors regulate intracellular effectors through a family of signal-transducing proteins termed *guanine nucleotide binding proteins*, or G proteins, that are common to virtually all cells. The specificity of response in a given tissue is achieved by several linked factors: differential cellular expression of the receptors that activate the signaling process, the nature of the intracellular signal [e.g., cyclic adenosine monophosphate (cAMP) or calcium (Ca^{2+})], the targets of these signals, and the downstream molecule(s) regulated by the signal. Because many of the targets of second messengers are protein kinases, the cellular response in certain tissues is further determined by the nature of the intracellular substrates expressed for the relevant kinases.

Ligand types.   G protein–coupled receptors are responsible for monitoring signals from neurotransmitters, hormones, endothelins, autacoids, lipids such as lysophosphatidic acid or sphingosine-1 phosphate, chemokines, light, odorants, and other sensory stimuli in the extracellular environment. Humans express approximately 800 types of G protein–coupled receptors; >60% of these receptors are involved in the sensory pathways of smell, vision, and taste. In the cardiovascular system, some of the major agonists for these receptors are acetylcholine (muscarinic receptors), serotonin, catecholamines, dopamine, angiotensin, vasopressin, endothelin, histamine, bradykinin, prostaglandins, thrombin, lysophosphatidic acid, sphingosine-1 phosphate, and adenosine.

Receptor structure.   G protein–coupled receptors share a characteristic structure composed of seven membrane-spanning domains and four intracellular loops responsible for direct interaction with the G proteins. The intracellular segments most responsible for recognition of G proteins include the third intracellular loop, between helices 5 and 6, and the carboxyl-terminal domain. G protein–coupled receptors are monomeric proteins with molecular weights ranging from 35,000 to 70,000 Kda and are members of the extended rhodopsin receptor family.

There are five major variations in the topological structure of receptors with seven transmembrane-spanning domains. Depending on the topology, the receptors are activated by the binding of ligands to sites within the seven transmembrane domains or to the extracellular loops of the molecule. Ligand binding causes conformational changes in the transmembrane-spanning domains of helices 3 and 6 in the receptor, which translate to activation of the G protein α subunit (see subsequent text).

Receptor isoforms.   It is common for multiple isoforms (or subtypes) of a receptor type to respond to a single ligand; for example, five isoforms of the muscarinic receptor all respond to acetylcholine and three isoforms of the β-adrenergic receptor respond to epinephrine. Usually, different receptor isoforms are expressed in different tissues and are coupled to different G proteins. For example, muscarinic M_2 receptors expressed in cardiac tissue activate G protein–dependent inwardly rectifying potassium (K^+) channels (GIRKs) by coupling to the G_i and G_o α subunits and releasing βγ subunits. Muscarinic M_3 receptors expressed in smooth muscle regulate contraction through the G_q α subunit, which activates phospholipase C-β and releases Ca^{2+}. Catecholamine receptors are also differentially expressed, with β_1-adrenergic receptors mainly expressed in cardiac and kidney tissue. α_1-Adrenergic receptors are especially important in vascular smooth muscle, where they mediate the effects of norepinephrine.

Receptor networks. G protein–coupled receptors can form complex regulatory networks in which a single receptor may couple to multiple G proteins and generate a variety of signals in a given cell. Conversely, multiple different types of receptors may interact with a single α subunit subtype of the G protein family and generate the same signal. The best-studied effectors regulated by G proteins are adenylyl cyclase (multiple tissues), cyclic guanosine monophosphate (cGMP) phosphodiesterase (retinal tissue), phospholipase C-β (multiple tissues), phosphatidylinositol 3-kinase (hematopoietic cells), and certain members of the Ca^{2+}, Na^+, or K^+ channel families (vascular, cardiac, and neural tissues).

G protein family

Basic structure and subunits. The heterotrimeric G proteins are themselves composed of three subunits: α subunits with molecular weights of 39 to 52 kDa, β subunits with molecular weights of 35 to 39 kDa, and γ subunits with molecular weights of 6 to 8 kDa. The α subunits can bind 1 mole of guanosine triphosphate (GTP) or guanosine diphosphate (GDP) per mole of α subunit. The β and γ subunits form a functional unit, called the $\beta\gamma$ *dimer,* which cannot be dissociated without loss of activity.

Structural diversity. There is significant diversity in the subunits making up the heterotrimer. Currently, 16 genes are known to encode α subunits, 5 encode β subunits, and 12 encode γ subunits. Alternative splicing of the genes for the α subunit yields 22 different α subunits; splicing of the 5 β subunit genes yields 7 different β subunits. The genes for the 12 γ subunits do not appear to be alternatively spliced. Although some sensory cells express only a limited subset of α and $\beta\gamma$ subunits (e.g., retinal tissue), most cells can express most of the known proteins that compose the heterotrimer (**Table A2.1**).

Both α and γ subunits are posttranslationally modified by lipid attachments, causing the heterotrimer to reside at the inner surface of the plasma membrane. The α subunit is modified by combination of palmitate or myristate; the γ subunits are modified by isoprenylation, farnesylation (in the case of $\gamma1$, $\gamma8$, and $\gamma11$) or geranylgeranyl in all other γ subunits.

Heterotrimer families. The G protein heterotrimers are grouped into four families according to the similarity in their amino acid sequences or the function of their α subunits (**Table A2.1**).

TABLE A2.1

PROPERTIES OF G PROTEIN α SUBUNITS

α Subunit	Tissue distribution	Effector (action)	Effect on message
G_s family			
$G_s{}^a$	Wide	Adenylyl cyclase ($\uparrow$)	Increase cAMP
G_{olf}	Brain	Adenylyl cyclase ($\uparrow$)	Increase cAMP
G_i family			
G_{i1}	Wide	Adenylyl cyclase ($\downarrow$)	Decrease cAMP
G_{i2}	Wide	Adenylyl cyclase ($\downarrow$)	Decrease cAMP
G_{i3}	Wide	Adenylyl cyclase ($\downarrow$)	Decrease cAMP
G_o	Neuronal	Ion channels ($\downarrow$)	Decrease Ca^{2+} current
		GRIN ($\uparrow$)	Increase neurite outgrowth
G_i and G_o through $\beta\gamma$		K^+ channels ($\uparrow$)	Increase K^+ current
		Phospholipase C-β ($\uparrow$)	Increase IP_3, DAG
		Ca^{2+} channels ($\downarrow$) (Both T and N type)	Decrease Ca^{2+} current
		PI 3-kinase (β and γ isoforms) ($\uparrow$)	Increase PIP 3
		Adenylyl cyclase ($\uparrow$) or ($\downarrow$)	Increase/Decrease cAMP
G_t	Rod and cone cells	cGMP phosphodiesterase ($\uparrow$)	Decrease cGMP
G_g	Tongue	cGMP phosphodiesterase ($\uparrow$)	Decrease cGMP
G_z	Brain	Adenylyl cyclase ($\downarrow$)	Decrease cAMP
G_q family			
G_q	Wide	Phospholipase C-β ($\uparrow$)	Increase IP_3, DAG
G_{11}	Wide	Phospholipase C-β ($\uparrow$)	Increase IP_3, DAG
G_{14}	Wide	Phospholipase C-β ($\uparrow$)	Increase IP_3, DAG
G_{15}	Hematopoietic cells	Phospholipase C-β ($\uparrow$)	Increase IP_3, DAG
G_{16}	Hematopoietic cells	Phospholipase C-β ($\uparrow$)	Increase IP_3, DAG
G_{12} family			
G_{12}	Wide	Rho GTP exchange factor ($\uparrow$)	Activate Rho targets
G_{13}	Wide	Rho GTP exchange factor ($\uparrow$) Na^+/H^+ antiporter	Activate Rho targets
		Na^+/H^+ Antiporter ($\uparrow$)	Change in cytoplasmic [ion]
		Radixin ($\uparrow$)	Increase transformation

cAMP, cyclic adenosine monophosphate; cGMP, cyclic guanosine monophosphate; IP, inositol triphosphate; DAG, diacylglycerol; GTP, guanosine triphosphate; PIP_3, phosphatidylinositol 3,4,5 triphosphate; GRIN, G protein regulated inducer of neurite outgrowth. ($\uparrow$) increased activity; ($\downarrow$) decreased activity.
^{a} The G_s and G_o α subunits have multiple splice variants.

Stimulatory. Members of the G_s (stimulatory) family include the G_s and G_{olf} proteins, which uniformly stimulate adenylyl cyclase to produce the second messenger cAMP.

Inhibitory. Members of the G_i (inhibitory) family are more diverse and include the G_t, G_{i1}, G_{i2}, G_{i3}, G_o, G_z, and G_g proteins. The α_i subunits inhibit adenylyl cyclase and regulate the gating of Ca^{2+} or K^+ ion channels by releasing the $\beta\gamma$ subunit. The α_t or α_g subunits stimulate cGMP phosphodiesterases, especially those involved in the senses of vision (α_t) and taste (α_g). The G_o α subunit may have a specific effector (G protein–regulated inducer of neurite outgrowth), which induces formation of fine processes in cultured neuronal cells.

G_q proteins. The G_q family includes G_q, G_{11}, G_{14}, G_{15}, and G_{16}. These α subunits stimulate phospholipase C-β to hydrolyze the membrane lipid phosphatidylinositol 4, 5-biphosphate, leading to formation of the second messengers inositol triphosphate (IP_3) and diacylglycerol (DAG). G_q and G_{11} are widely expressed and the G14, G15, and G16 α subunits are found in hematopoietic cells.

G_{12} proteins. The G_{12} family (including the G_{12} and G_{13} α subunits) can regulate the p115 Rho guanine nucleotide exchange factor (GEF), thereby providing a direct link between cell surface receptors coupled to large G proteins and pathways regulated by small G proteins such as *Rho*. The G_{12} and G_{13} α subunits may also interact with proteins such as radixin, which interacts with cytoskeletal elements to affect events such as cell migration and transformation. Receptors coupled to the G_{12} and G_{13} α subunits often couple to the Gq family of α subunits as well and thereby generate multiple signals in the cell.

Activity of G proteins

Receptor activation complexes and second messengers.

The basal state of the G protein signaling system consists of the receptor α-GDP-$\beta\gamma$ complex. When an agonist ligand binds to the receptor, the conformational change induced in the receptor causes the α subunit to release the bound GDP. The binding site becomes occupied with GTP from the cytoplasm, causing a conformational change in the α subunit and a reduction in its affinity for the $\beta\gamma$ subunit. This activation process generates two active signaling molecules, the α-GTP complex and the $\beta\gamma$ dimer. Both of these signals can activate effectors (**Figure A2.1**). The activated α-GTP complex regulates effectors such as adenylyl cyclase, the cGMP phosphodiesterase in the visual system or in the tongue or phospholipase C-β. Most of these interactions lead to an increase in the level of a second messenger in the cell, such as an increase in adenylyl cyclase activity causing a rise in cAMP levels, or an increase in phospholipase C activity causing a rise in IP_3, intracellular Ca^{2+}, and DAG. cAMP and Ca^{2+} activate the cAMP-dependent and Ca^{2+}/calmodulin-dependent protein kinases, respectively. These kinases then regulate the differentiated functions of the target cells.

Receptor occupancy and subunit interactions.

As receptor occupancy increases, a greater number of α subunits are activated, causing a larger cellular response. $\beta\gamma$ subunits also stimulate or inhibit adenylyl cyclase, phospholipase C-β, or muscarinic K^+ channels (GIRK channels) in cardiac tissue, and inhibit L- and N-type Ca^{2+} channels in neural tissue. Because of the high concentrations of G_i and G_o in neuronal plasma membranes, it is thought that $\beta\gamma$ dimers released from α subunits may play significant regulatory roles in signaling by receptors coupled to G_i and G_o. Therefore, receptors coupled to G_i or G_o may regulate

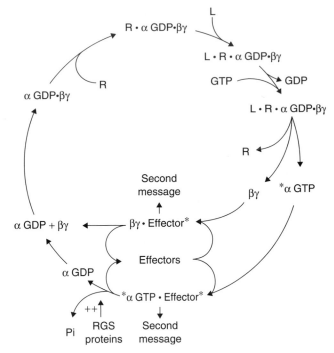

Figure A2.1 Sequence of activation and inactivation of G protein–coupled receptors and effectors. Binding of hormone or other ligand (L) to its receptor (R) causes dissociation of guanosine diphosphate (GDP) and binding of guanosine triphosphate (GTP) to the α subunit of the G protein heterotrimer. Ligand-receptor binding also causes dissociation of G protein subunits. Both the GTP-bound α subunit and $\beta\gamma$ subunit regulate the activity of various effectors. Hydrolysis of GTP to GDP and inorganic phosphate (Pi) terminates participation of G protein subunits and leads to their reassociation into the inactive heterotrimer. The regulators of G protein signaling (RGS) proteins markedly increase the rate of GTP hydrolysis by the α subunit and speed termination of the signal.

certain cell functions through the $\beta\gamma$ dimer and others through the α subunit. Important examples of regulation through the $\beta\gamma$ dimer in the cardiovascular system include modulation of the cardiac sinoatrial (SA) and atrioventricular (AV) nodes by GIRK channels, and activation of phospholipase C-β or phosphatidyl inositol 3-kinase in mast cells, leukocytes, neutrophils, and other white blood cells.

Signal termination and RGS proteins.

The G protein signal is terminated by the intrinsic guanosine triphosphatase (GTPase) activity of the α subunit, along with the actions of a family of proteins termed *regulators of G protein signaling* (RGS proteins). The GTPase activity of the α subunit hydrolyzes bound GTP to GDP, which remains bound to the α subunit, keeping the complex in the inactive conformation. The rate of hydrolysis of GTP to GDP by the α subunit is markedly stimulated (100- to 1,000-fold) by RGS proteins. In addition, when bound GTP is hydrolyzed by the α subunit, the affinity of the α subunit for the $\beta\gamma$ dimer increases and the GDP-bound form of the α subunit sequesters the $\beta\gamma$ subunit. These two events return the system to its basal state (**Figure A2.1**).

There are >30 members of the RGS family divided into six subfamilies that all share a 120-amino acid sequence that binds activated α subunits and catalyzes GTP hydrolysis. Many members of the family have other regulatory domains, implying that this family of proteins harbors multiple functions in the same molecule. An example is the p115 Rho GEF protein, which is

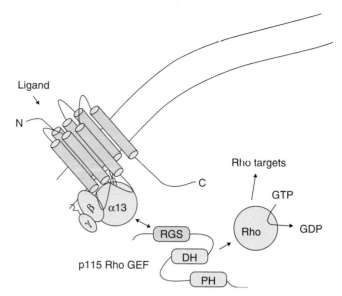

Figure A2.2 p115 Rho GEF; an example of a RGS protein with multiple functions. The RGS protein p115 Rho GEF has an RGS domain at its N-terminus and DH (Dbl homology) and PH (plextrin homology) domains near its C-terminus. The RGS domain can interact with Gα13 and the DH and PH domains can increase exchange of GTP for GDP on Rho (guanine nucleotide exchange activity or GEF activity). Binding of ligands to GPCRs coupled to Gα13 causes a conformational change in p115 Rho GEF and causes the DH and PH domains to interact with Rho. This event releases bound GDP from Rho and GTP exchanges onto the protein. Binding of GTP to Rho causes activation of Rho and promotes downstream events such as cytoskeletal rearrangements. RGS, regulators of G protein signaling; GPCRs, G protein–coupled receptors; GTP, guanosine triphosphate.

activated by the G13 α subunit and functions as a GEF for the small GTP binding protein Rho (**Figure A2.2**).

RGS proteins are emerging as very important determinants of the specificity of G protein signaling because specific members of the family form functional complexes with certain G protein–coupled receptors and effectors. Therefore, they act as scaffolds for signaling complexes in addition to their role in terminating the G protein signal. This mechanism allows for efficient organization of receptors, their cognate G proteins, effectors, and the mechanism for termination of the signal.

Effector regulation

Effector activation. The actions of the α-GTP complex and the βγ dimer initiate complex signaling patterns with certain common features. The activation of effectors by the α-GTP complex or the βγ dimer appears to occur by direct, high affinity protein–protein interactions, causing the effector to shift to a more active state. Activation of the effectors listed in **Table A2.1** causes these proteins to change the concentration of intracellular messengers such as cAMP, DAG, IP_3, Ca^{2+}, or K^+ ions. Adenylyl cyclase, ion channels, and phospholipase C-β are important effectors found in virtually all cells and regulate the response of organ systems to a large number of hormones, neurotransmitters, and autacoids. An important example of activation of adenylyl cyclase in the cardiovascular system is

β-adrenergic stimulation of cardiac rate and force of contraction. β-Adrenergic receptors activate adenylyl cyclase through G_s and increase the level of cAMP in all cardiac tissues. The rise in cAMP activates cAMP-dependent protein kinase, increases cardiac rate through the hyperpolarization and cyclic nucleotide (HCN)-activated channel in the SA and AV nodes and increases the force of contraction (through increasing the open time of N-type Ca^{2+} channels) in atrial and ventricular muscle. Phospholipase C-β plays a very important role in regulating contraction of smooth muscle by controlling the level of Ca^{2+} in the cytoplasm of these cells. The $α_1$-adrenergic receptor that regulates vascular tone is coupled to the G_q α subunit. Activation of this receptor by norepinephrine produces an active G_q–α-GTP complex that markedly stimulates phospholipase C-β, leading to increases in IP_3, DAG, intracellular Ca^{2+} levels (activating Ca^{2+}/calmodulin-dependent protein kinases) and ultimately to contraction of smooth muscle.

Effector inhibition. Adenylyl cyclase activity can be inhibited by receptors coupled to the G_i α subunit in most cells. Examples of cardiovascular receptors that inhibit adenylyl cyclase include the muscarinic M_2, $α_2$-adrenergic, adenosine A_1, and angiotensin AT_1 receptors. As noted in the preceding text, many second messengers generated by receptor activation lead to activation of protein kinases that produce a cellular response by increasing the phosphorylation state of important regulatory proteins in the target cells. This is the case for cAMP; activation of the inhibitory receptors mentioned earlier lowers the concentration of cAMP in the target cells, causing a smaller activation of the cAMP-dependent protein kinase, thereby reducing the responses stimulated by this messenger.

Counterregulatory effects of G proteins

In many tissues, it is common to find two or more receptors that regulate important functions by using opposing effects. In the SA node in the heart, the activity of the cardiac pacemaker cells is stimulated by norepinephrine acting on $β_1$-adrenergic receptors, which in turn stimulates adenylyl cyclase through the activated G_s α subunit and raises the level of cAMP, inducing pacemaker activity through the HCN channel. At the same time, the GIRK K^+ channel in the SA node can be activated by muscarinic M_2 receptors, opposing the actions of norepinephrine. M_2 receptors inhibit pacemaker activity by two mechanisms, inhibiting adenylyl cyclase and lowering cAMP and activating the GIRK K^+ channel via the βγ dimer. Both the decrease in cAMP and the increase in K^+ conductance slow the heart and oppose the rate-increasing effects of norepinephrine.

Suggested Readings

Abramow-Newerly M, Roy AA, Nunn C, et al. RGS proteins have a signalling complex. Interaction between RGS proteins and GPCRs, effectors and auxiliary proteins. *Cell Signal* 2006; **18**: 579–591.

Cabrera-Vera TM, Vanhauwe J, Thomas TO, et al. Insights into G protein structure, function, and regulation. *Endocr Rev* 2003; **24**: 765–781.

Downes GB, Gautam N. The G protein subunit gene families. *Genomics* 1999; **62**: 544–552.

Wettschureck N, Offermanns S. Mammalian G proteins and their cell type specific functions. *Physiol Rev* 2005; **85**: 1159–1204.

CHAPTER A3 ■ CYCLIC NUCLEOTIDES AND THEIR REGULATION

STANKO S. STOJILKOVIC, PhD

KEY POINTS

- Cyclic adenosine monophosphate (cAMP) is produced by plasma membrane–bound adenylyl cyclases (ACs); activity of these enzymes is regulated by numerous extracellular messengers through G_s and $G_{i/o/z}$ protein–coupled receptors.
- Cyclic guanosine monophosphate (cGMP) is produced by receptor-linked guanylyl cyclases (GCs) and nitric oxide–regulated soluble cytosolic GCs.
- cAMP and cGMP activate protein kinases (PKs) A and G, respectively, which (a) phosphorylate regulatory proteins in the plasma membrane, cytosol, and nucleus, (b) open cationic plasma membrane channels, and (c) regulate certain guanine nucleotide exchange proteins.
- Intracellular cyclic nucleotide concentration is controlled by phosphodiesterases (PDEs) and specific efflux pumps that transport cyclic nucleotides from the cytosol to the extracellular space.

See also Chapters **A1, A2, A4,** and **A5**

Cyclic 3′, 5′-adenosine monophosphate (cAMP) and cyclic 3′, 5′-guanosine monophosphate (cGMP) are intracellular (second) messengers produced from nucleotide triphosphates by a family of enzymes: adenylyl cyclases (ACs), particulate guanylyl cyclase (pGCs), and soluble guanylyl cyclase (sGC) (**Figure A3.1**). These enzymes are involved in a broad array of signal transduction pathways, including vision, cardiovascular regulation, and responses to numerous hormones and neurotransmitters.

Cyclic nucleotides

Cyclic adenosine monophosphate. cAMP, the first intracellular messenger identified (1957), is used in organisms from prokaryotes to mammals and is synthesized from adenosine triphosphate (ATP) by ACs. Most of its physiologic actions are mediated by cAMP-dependent protein kinase (PKA), which controls multiple aspects of cell function through phosphorylation of protein substrates. cAMP also directly regulates certain guanine nucleotide exchange factors (GEFs), hyperpolarization and cyclic nucleotide-activated (HCN) channels, and cyclic nucleotide-gated (CNG) channels.

Cyclic guanosine monophosphate. Two families of enzymes, pGCs and sGCs, hydrolyze guanosine triphosphate (GTP) to form cGMP using a mechanism stereochemically analogous to ACs. pGCs operate as part of the plasma membrane receptor complexes for several peptides. sGCs are activated by the cell-permeable messenger nitric oxide (NO). Many $G_{q/11}$ and G_s protein–coupled receptors also stimulate cGMP production in

a Ca^{2+}- and kinase-dependent manner. In contrast to cAMP, the intracellular messenger functions of cGMP are more restricted and are mediated indirectly through protein phosphorylation by cGMP-dependent protein kinase (PKG) and directly by activating CNG channels.

Adenylyl cyclases

Enzyme characteristics. The alignment of amino acid sequences of the catalytic domains of ACs, pGCs, and sGCs reveals a highly homologous region of approximately 220 residues long that was common to all three enzymes. These enzymes catalyze virtually identical reactions, indicating that the genes that code for the catalytic domains are derived from a common ancestor. Molecular cloning has confirmed that several structurally related plasma membrane–bound ACs are expressed in animal cells and are encoded by nine different genes. ACs contain two hydrophobic domains, each composed of six transmembrane helices and two cytoplasmic catalytic domains. An unusual soluble adenylyl cyclase activated by bicarbonate is present in the testis and kidney.

Activity and coupling. All isoforms of ACs produce cAMP in the absence of hormonal stimulation. This basal activity is markedly modulated by receptors coupled to heterotrimeric G proteins; enhanced on binding of G_s protein and reduced on binding of G_i, G_o, and G_z α subunits. The βγ dimers of G_i and G_o proteins also contribute to the control of AC2, AC4, and AC7 activity. In addition, the $G_{q/11}$-coupled calcium-mobilizing receptors indirectly modulate AC activity through Ca^{2+} and

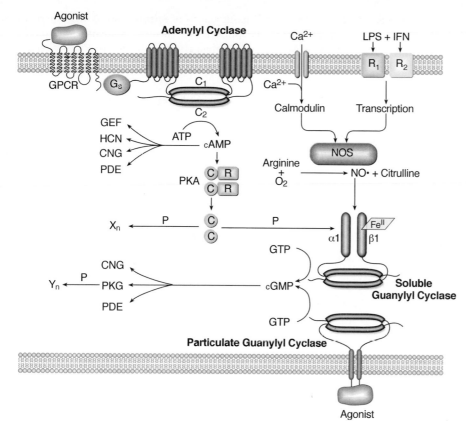

Figure A3.1 Schematic representation of cyclic nucleotide signaling pathway. GPCR, G protein–coupled receptors; GEF, guanine nucleotide exchange factor; HCN, hyperpolarization and cyclic nucleotide-activated channels; CNG, cyclic nucleotide-gated channels; PDE, phosphodiesterase; ATP, adenosine triphosphate; cAMP, cyclic adenosine monophosphate; LPS + IFN, lipopolysaccharide + interferon; NOS, nitric oxide synthase; NO, nitric oxide; GTP, guanosine triphosphate; cGMP, cyclic guanosine monophosphate; PKA, protein kinase A–C and R, catalytic and regulatory units; PKG, protein kinase G; X_n, PKA phosphorylated proteins, including L-type voltage-gated Ca^{2+} channels, ryanodine and $Ins(1,4,5)P_3$ receptors, troponin, and CREB, cAMP-responsive enhancer binding proteins; Y_n, PKG phosphorylated proteins, including $Ins(1,4,5)P_3$ receptors, Ca^{2+}-activated K^+ channels and CREB proteins.

protein kinase C (PKC) signaling pathways. Cytosolic Ca^{2+} directly inhibits AC5 and AC6 isoforms and indirectly inhibits AC9 (through the Ser/Thr protein phosphatase calcineurin) and AC3 (through Ca^{2+}-calmodulin kinase II). Ca^{2+} also stimulates AC1 and AC8 through calmodulin. AC2, AC4, AC5, and AC7 are activated by PKC; the AC2 subtype is most sensitive to such regulation. In contrast, PKA inhibits AC5 and AC6 isoforms, providing a form of negative feedback to cAMP formation. Forskolin activates all isoforms except AC9, whereas several 3′-adenosine nucleotide analogs bind to the activated pyrophosphate complexes of ACs and inhibit enzyme activity.

Guanylyl cyclases

Plasma membrane (particulate) guanylyl cyclases.
These enzymes contain an extracellular peptide receptor–operated domain and an intracellular catalytic domain connected by a single transmembrane domain. The active enzyme is believed to be a homodimer of approximately 120 kDa formed in the intracellular domain. Seven mammalian pGCs and a sea urchin enzyme have been identified and sequenced. Three of these have known peptide ligands (GC-A, atrial natriuretic peptide; GC-B, brain natriuretic peptide; GC-C, the heat-stable enterotoxin of *Escherichia coli* and endogenous intestinal peptide guanylin). The activated ligands for other enzymes (GC-D, olfactory epithelium; GC-E and GS-F, retina; and GC-G lung, intestine, skeletal muscle, testis) have not been determined. The activity of these enzymes is regulated by both Ca^{2+} and PKC. Disruption of the GC-A gene elevates blood pressure independent of dietary salt and induces marked cardiac hypertrophy.

Soluble (cytosolic) guanylyl cyclases.
sGCs are present in most mammalian tissues and are abundant in lung and smooth muscle, as well as in nonmammalian species, including *Drosophila* and *Caenorhabditis elegans*. On the basis of cDNA cloning, four sGC subunits have been identified: α1, α2, β1, and β2. The α1 and α2 subunits are interchangeable in terms of sGC activity when coexpressed with β1, but the α1β1 heterodimer is most common in mammalian tissues. In the absence of NO, sGC-derived cGMP production is negligible. The enzyme is also subjected to phosphorylation by PKA and PKC.

Cyclic adenosine monophosphate-dependent protein kinases

PKAs are present in all eukaryotic cells as the major mediators of the effects of cAMP. The existence of at least 12 forms of PKA provides for a considerable degree of diversity in the tissue-specific expression, intracellular localization, and activation properties of the individual enzymes. In the absence of cAMP, PKA is an inactive, asymmetric tetramer containing both two regulatory and two catalytic subunits that bind to each other with high affinity.

Regulatory subunits.
There are two categories of regulatory subunits and several isoforms of each regulatory subunit are expressed in most cells. The general structural features of the molecule are retained in all of the isoforms. Binding of cAMP to the regulatory subunit alters its affinity for the catalytic subunits by four orders of magnitude, leading to the formation of a dimeric regulatory subunit and two active monomeric catalytic subunits (**Figure A3.1**). The regulatory dimer can later reassociate with free catalytic subunits. Each regulatory monomeric subunit has two high-affinity binding sites for cAMP localized at the C-terminus. In some tissues, regulatory subunits are present in excess over catalytic subunits, allowing interaction with other cellular

proteins or structures. Selective increases in regulatory subunits occur in several tissues during cAMP-induced differentiation.

Catalytic subunits. Catalytic subunits are highly conserved between species. These subunits are encoded by multiple genes, giving rise to α, β and γ isoforms. The α-isoform appears to be expressed constitutively in most cells, whereas the expression of the β-isoform is tissue specific. Because each regulatory subunit can associate with any of the catalytic subunits, a wide variety of AC holoenzymes can exist. The conserved catalytic core shared by all PKAs extends approximately from residue 40 to residue 285 in the catalytic subunit and contains an ATP binding site and a cyclic nucleotide binding site. Catalytic subunits undergo at least two posttranslation covalent modifications, autophosphorylation (Thr^{197} and Ser^{338}), and myristoylation at the amino termini.

Anchoring proteins. In addition to the concentration of cyclic nucleotides in the cell, PKA spatial distribution and temporal profiles are important aspects of cAMP-dependent intracellular signaling. Earlier observations suggesting compartmentalization of cyclic nucleotides and more recent findings localizing PKAs to specific intracellular domains have lent support to this concept. A large and growing family of >50 PKA-kinase anchor proteins (AKAPs) is now known to determine the spatial distribution of PKA isoforms within the cell. All AKAPs contain a PKA-binding tethering domain and a unique targeting domain for the PKA-AKAP complex that is specific for individual downstream targets. This permits PKAs to remain near their target proteins, thereby increasing the efficiency and specificity of subcellular cAMP-dependent signaling in the cell membrane, nucleus, mitochondria, cytoskeletal elements, and vesicular systems.

Nuclear signaling by protein kinase. In contrast to cytosolic actions, enzyme activity in the nucleus is mediated by free catalytic subunits, which enter the nucleus by passive diffusion and phosphorylate transcriptional regulatory proteins, such as proteins that bind to cAMP-responsive enhancer elements (CREs) located in the promoter regions of numerous genes. In some CRE-binding (CREB) proteins, the phosphorylation of a specific serine residue (Ser133) by PKA promotes their transcriptional activation potential and stimulates gene expression. The same residue is also phosphorylated by Ca^{2+}-CaM-dependent PKAs and therefore serves to integrate signals from at least two distinct signaling pathways. An important subset of the CREB family is the CRE-modulator protein group, which is phosphorylated by PKA and Ca^{2+}–CaM-dependent kinases at the equivalent serine residue (Ser^{117}), as well as by PKC and mitogen-activated S6 kinase. Termination of PKA signaling in the nucleus is mediated by a heat-stable PKA inhibitor, which inactivates the catalytic subunit and activates a nuclear export signal, leading to export of this complex from the nucleus.

Role of protein kinase in cellular and organ function. The cAMP–PKA signaling pathway is involved in regulation of (a) cardiovascular function, (b) exocytotic events in normal and polarized secretory cells, (c) metabolism in adipose tissue, (d) steroidogenesis, (e) reproductive function, and (f) immune responses. Sympathetic stimulation of the heart through β-adrenergic receptors is associated with PKA-mediated phosphorylation of several proteins related to excitation–contraction coupling, including L-type Ca^{2+} channels, ryanodine receptors, troponin I, and myosin binding protein. The acute regulation of steroid biosynthesis in the adrenal glands and gonads involves PKA-mediated increase in cholesterol release from lipid droplets and cholesterol transport across the mitochondrial membrane.

The initiation and maintenance of sperm motility also involves PKA-dependent phosphorylation through unidentified proteins that includes AKAP82. Protein phosphorylation by PKA enhances insulin secretion, as well as secretion of pituitary hormones.

Cyclic guanosine monophosphate-dependent protein kinases

Structural properties. The marked amino acid sequence homologies between PKA and PKG and predicted similarities in their structures suggest that the two enzymes have evolved from an ancestral phosphotransferase. In contrast to PKAs, PKGs have a more limited distribution in mammalian tissues. In high concentrations they are present in cerebellar Purkinje cells, platelets, and intestinal epithelial cells. In other tissues, PKG is 10- to 100-fold lower than that of PKA. In mammals, there are two forms of this enzyme. Type I kinase is a soluble protein, consisting of two spliced forms that mediates effects of natriuretic peptides and NO in cardiovascular cells. On the other hand, type II kinase is a membrane-associated enzyme that transduces signals from the *E. coli* heat-stable enterotoxin STa, and from the endogenous intestinal peptide, guanylin. PKG operates as a dimer, although each monomer seems self-sufficient in its regulatory and catalytic properties.

Regulatory roles of cGMP-dependent protein kinases. In smooth muscle cells, there are several different phosphorylation events occurring in response to PKG activation that lead to inhibition of Ca^{2+} signaling and relaxation, including inhibition of Ca^{2+} release through phosphorylation of Ins(1,4,5)P3 receptors and inhibition of Ca^{2+} influx through blockade of voltage-gated Ca^{2+} channels and activation of Ca^{2+}-activated K^+ channels. PKG I also inhibits platelet activation, presumably through inhibition of Ca^{2+} signaling. In endothelial cells, cGMP inhibits a thrombin-stimulated increase in permeability. PKG I opposes the PKA-stimulated Ca^{2+} influx through voltage-gated Ca^{2+} channels in cardiac myocytes. It also appears that PKG I signals to the nucleus, including phosphorylation of CREB. On the other hand, PKG II plays a critical role in intestinal salt and water secretion, and in secretory diarrhea induced by microbial enterotoxins. The cystic fibrosis transmembrane conductance regulator, a chloride channel, is also activated by PKG II. New evidence has emerged supporting the role of this enzyme subtype in the kidney, brain, and bone functions. Mice lacking PKG show moderate hypertension.

Other cyclic nucleotide effectors

Cyclic nucleotide-gated channels. Molecular cloning has revealed >20 genes that encode different subtypes of CNG in invertebrates and vertebrates. They are nonselective voltage-dependent cation channels, formed by four α subunits, each containing a six-transmembrane-domain module similar to that of voltage-gated K^+ channels. β subunits do not form functional channels, but modulate the channel properties of α subunits. CNG channels open in response to direct binding of intracellular cyclic nucleotides and contribute to cellular control of the membrane potential and intracellular Ca^{2+} levels. Each α subunit has a cytosolic binding domain for cyclic nucleotides located in the last transmembrane segment of the channel. Maximal activation typically requires four bound ligands. cGMP-activated retinal rod receptor channels are abundant in the cone photoreceptors of the retina, and in ganglion, bipolar, and Muller glial cells, where they mediate light-induced neurotransmission. A similar cAMP/cGMP-sensitive channel participates in olfactory transduction and channels are also expressed in the central nervous system, pituitary, heart, kidney, and testis.

Hyperpolarization and cyclic nucleotide-activated channels. In a variety of spontaneously firing cells, including sinoatrial node cells, thalamic relay neurons, cochlear pyramidal cells, and inferior olive neurons in the brain stem, a pacemaking current termed the hyperpolarization-activated current (I_h) has been identified. Channels underlying I_h, termed *HCN channels*, are nonselective cation channels permeable to both K^+ and Na^+, with a reversal potential approximately −30 mV. On their activation, the plasma membrane depolarizes. Another unique property of I_h is its modulation by cyclic nucleotides, which bind directly to HCN channels, accelerating the kinetics of channel activation and shifting the voltage-dependence of activation toward more depolarized potentials. To date, four mammalian channel subunits, termed *HCN1-4*, have been cloned.

cAMP-regulated guanine nucleotide exchange factors. GEFs and guanosine triphosphatase(GTPase)-activating proteins regulate the activity of numerous Ras-related proteins, including Rap-1 and Rap-2, the small Ras-like GTPases. Two Rap-specific GEFs, called *Epac* (exchange protein activated by cAMP) provide an additional effector system for cAMP signaling. Epac1 has one and Epac2 has two cAMP binding moieties. The binding of cAMP to the C-terminal of Epac proteins induces a conformational change, leading to activation of the GEF domain.

Cyclic nucleotide phosphodiesterases

Phosphodiesterase actions. Cyclic nucleotide PDEs are enzymes responsible for the hydrolysis of cAMP and cGMP and represent the main pathway for elimination of cyclic nucleotides from most cells. PDEs contribute to local gradients of cyclic nucleotides in subcellular compartments and to the temporal and spatial specificity of cyclic nucleotide signaling. Inactivation of cyclic nucleotides by PDEs is important in retinal phototransduction, smooth muscle contraction, insulin secretion, and fertility. Another important function of PDEs is to coordinate the activities of cyclic nucleotide and Ca^{2+} signaling pathways, largely through the regulatory action of Ca^{2+}–CaM on PDE activity. PDEs are important drug targets in asthma and chronic obstructive pulmonary disease, cardiovascular diseases, neurologic disorders, and erectile dysfunction.

Phosphodiesterases subtypes. Mammalian cells contain >50 cyclic nucleotide PDEs that are classified into 11 families based on their amino acid sequences, substrate specificities, allosteric regulatory characteristics, and pharmacologic properties. They share a modular architecture, with a conserved central catalytic domain, N- and C-terminal regulatory domains, and N-terminal targeting domain. The substrate specificities of the PDEs families include cAMP-specific (PDE4, PDE7, and PDE8), cGMP-specific (PDE5, PDE6, and PDE9), and mixed specificity enzymes (PDE1, PDE2, PDE3, PDE10, and PDE11). The regulatory domains are binding domains for allosteric regulators, such as Ca^{2+}-calmodulin, and the N-terminus also contains sites that are targets for phosphorylation by PKAs.

Inhibitors. Common inhibitors of PDEs are xanthines such as caffeine and theophylline. Because xanthines are inhibitors of all PDEs, treatment with them produces a wide range of pharmacologic effects, including stimulation of the central nervous system, increased urine production, and relaxation of the bronchi and vascular smooth muscle. PDE5 inhibitors are indicated for erectile dysfunction and pulmonary hypertension. Their blood pressure (BP)-lowering effects are usually modest except in the presence of nitrate-donor drugs (especially organic nitrates) or α-blocking drugs.

Cyclic nucleotide efflux pumps

Lipid membranes are virtually impermeable to cyclic nucleotides and their extrusion against a concentration gradient is consistent with operation of an ATP-dependent and probenecid-sensitive transport mechanism in the plasma membrane, termed the *cyclic nucleotide efflux pump*. Despite extensive knowledge of their kinetic properties and inhibitor profiles, the molecular identity of these transporters is elusive. Recently, the multidrug resistance proteins 4, 5, and 8 have been identified as potential ATP-dependent cyclic nucleotide efflux pumps.

Suggested Readings

Bender AT, Beavo JA. Cyclic nucleotide phosphodiesterases: molecular regulation to clinical use. *Pharmacol Rev* 2006;58:488–520.

Kruh GD, Belinsky MG. The MRP family of drug efflux pumps. *Oncogene* 2003; 22:7537–7552.

Lohmann SM, Vaandrager AB, Smolenski A, et al. Distinct and specific functions of cGMP-dependent protein kinases. *Trends Biochem Sci* 1997; 22:307–312.

Lucas KA, Pitari GM, Kazerounian S, et al. Guanylyl cyclases and signaling by cyclic GMP. *Pharmacol Rev* 2000;52:375–413.

Tasken K, Aandahl EM. Localized effects of cAMP mediated by distinct routes of protein kinase A. *Physiol Rev* 2004;84:137–167.

CHAPTER A4 ■ SIGNAL TRANSDUCTION: INOSITOL PHOSPHOLIPIDS AND INOSITOL PHOSPHATES

TAMAS BALLA, MD, PhD

KEY POINTS

■ Phosphoinositides, a minor fraction of virtually all cell membrane phospholipids, are formed by inositol ring phosphorylation of phosphatidylinositol (PI) by specific inositol lipid kinases.

■ A major signaling mechanism by which cell-surface receptors regulate several cellular functions is phospholipase C (PLC)-mediated hydrolysis of membrane PI(4,5)P$_2$, which releases inositol 1,4,5-trisphosphate and diacylglycerol (DAG), the primary messengers that regulate calcium release and protein kinase C (PKC) activity.

■ Specific phosphoinositide isoforms serve as localization signals for protein modules on key regulatory proteins and contribute to protein signaling complexes in specific membrane compartments.

■ Some phosphoinositide isoforms (e.g., 3-phosphorylated forms) not hydrolyzed by PLC are controlled by inositol lipid phosphatases.

See also Chapters **A1, A2, A3,** and **A5**

Inositol phospholipids [phosphoinositides, (PIs)] are found in all cellular membranes. Although they represent only a small fraction of the total cellular phospholipids, they have remarkable importance in regulating a wide range of cellular functions. PIs are synthesized by phosphorylation of various hydroxyls of the inositol ring of phosphatidylinositol (PI). These lipids are precursors of soluble inositol polyphosphates that become diffusible intracellular messengers, which control calcium (Ca^{2+}) signaling but they also function as docking sites to promote formation of molecular signaling complexes on the surface of cellular membranes. PIs are involved in the control of many cellular processes related to membrane traffic, including endo- and exocytosis. They also modify the characteristics of ion channels and transporters and regulate actin polymerization. Using their multiple regulatory roles, they ultimately control cell proliferation, differentiation, and apoptosis.

Phosphoinositides and Ca^{2+} signaling

Phospholipase C products. The first recognized change of inositol phospholipid metabolism was related to the increased hydrolysis of phosphoinositides by phospholipase C (PLC) when Ca^{2+} mobilizing surface receptors are stimulated with their agonist ligands. The main substrate of PLC action is PI 4,5-bisphosphate [PI(4,5)P$_2$], a minor component of the membrane phospholipid pool that is synthesized from PI through PI 4-phosphate [PI4P]. In agonist-stimulated cells,

PI(4,5)P$_2$ is rapidly hydrolyzed by PLC to form two second messengers, inositol 1,4,5-trisphosphate [Ins(1,4,5)P$_3$] and DAG (**Figure A4.1**).

Inositol 1,4,5-trisphosphate and calcium flux.

Ins(1,4,5)P$_3$ binds to specific receptors found in the endoplasmic reticulum (ER) to rapidly release stored Ca^{2+} into the cytosol. The resulting "Ca^{2+} transient" initiates acute cellular responses such as exocytosis, contraction, and neurotransmission. However, prolonged signaling (e.g., continuous contraction of vascular smooth muscle) cannot be sustained by ER Ca^{2+} release alone, and therefore depends on supplementation by Ca^{2+} entering the cell from the extracellular space. This Ca^{2+} influx occurs through plasma membrane Ca^{2+} channels that are activated either by changes of membrane potential (L- or T-channels) or by a mechanism that senses the depletion of the ER Ca^{2+} pools. Ins(1,4,5)P$_3$, therefore, both initiates and maintains specific Ca^{2+}-regulated cellular responses.

Ins(1,4,5)P$_3$ metabolism.

Following its production, Ins(1,4,5)P$_3$ becomes part of a recycling pathway that begins with rapid degradation by dephosphorylation to Ins(1,4)P$_2$, Ins4P, and inositol. Inositol is then reincorporated into the biosynthetic pathway in the ER to form PI and subsequently PI4P and PI(4,5)P$_2$ in other membranes. Some of the dephosphorylation steps are inhibited by lithium (Li$^+$) ions, which may account for the therapeutic benefits of Li$^+$ treatment in manic-depressive disease. In addition to being degraded to inositol, Ins(1,4,5)P$_3$ is also phosphorylated to Ins(1,3,4,5)P$_4$, a

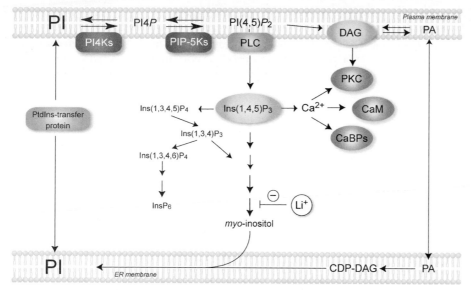

Figure A4.1 Signaling by phosphoinositides. The primary action of agonist stimulation is the activation of PLC enzymes that hydrolyze the lipid $PI(4,5)P_2$ to generate the messengers, $Ins(1,4,5)P_3$ and diacylglycerol (DAG). The Ca^{2+} mobilizing effect of $Ins(1,4,5)P_3$ together with the regulation by DAG of specific protein kinases (of the PKC family) leads to the activation of numerous Ca^{2+}-dependent kinases and ultimately to the phosphorylation of downstream regulatory proteins. $Ins(1,4,5)P_3$ can be metabolized either by dephosphorylation or can be converted to higher inositol phosphates. PI, phosphatidylinositol; PA, phosphatidic acid; PLC, phospholipase C; PKC, protein kinase ER, endoplasmic reticulum; CDP, cytidine diphosphate C; CaM, calmodulin; CaBPs, other calcium-binding proteins.

molecule that also may participate in Ca^{2+} regulation and as an intermediate in the formation of higher inositol phosphates ($InsP_5$ and $InsP_6$).

Diacylglycerol. DAG formed by activated PLC in the plasma membrane behaves as a comessenger with the $Ins(1,4,5)P_3$-induced rise of Ca^{2+}, causing activation of protein kinases, particularly certain isoforms of PKC. PKC is a member of an expanding family of serine threonine kinases with only some of its subclasses being regulated by DAG. PKCs phosphorylate numerous key regulatory proteins, receptors, ion channels, and enzymes in cell membranes, cytoplasm, and nucleus. DAG can also regulate other proteins such as ion channels either directly or by conversion to phosphatidic acid (PA).

Phospholipase C

Multiple forms of PLC identified have been designated as α, β, γ, δ, ε, and ζ. These subtypes contain several conserved regions interrupted by dissimilar amino acid sequences. Two such domains (X and Y) form the catalytic site of the enzyme, and others, termed SH2 and SH3 that have homology with the *src* oncogene bind to phosphotyrosine residues and proline-rich sequences. Some PLC enzymes also contain pleckstrin homology (PH) domains that recognize phosphoinositides and perhaps other regulatory proteins. Within the Ca^{2+}-phosphoinositide signaling system, phospholipases β and γ appear to be the major enzymes responsible for generating the second messengers that activate cell responses to hormones and growth factors.

Activation of phospholipase C-β enzymes. PLC-β enzymes are activated by subunits of heterotrimeric guanosine triphosphate (GTP) binding proteins following stimulation of receptors of the G protein–coupled variety. The β-isozyme of PLC exists in four forms ($β_1$–$β_4$), two of which ($β_1$ and $β_3$) are activated by G protein α subunits. The $β_2$ form is activated by βγ dimers derived from dissociation of the heterotrimeric proteins G_i/G_o, although βγ subunits can stimulate the other isoforms to a lesser degree. Cells of hematopoietic origin contain relatively high amounts of the $β_2$ enzyme; this explains why pertussis toxin treatment almost completely eliminates PLC activation (through their G protein–coupled receptors) in such cells. However, G protein–coupled receptors in most cells activate PLC

in a pertussis toxin–insensitive manner through the α subunits of $G_{q/11}$ proteins.

Activation of phospholipase Cγ enzymes. PLCγ enzymes are activated by tyrosine phosphorylation either by receptor- or nonreceptor tyrosine kinases that respond to growth factors (e.g., platelet-derived growth factor and epidermal growth factor). PLCγ enzymes have two forms: $γ_1$ is expressed ubiquitously, whereas $γ_2$ is restricted to hematopoietic and immune cells. These enzymes contain an extra stretch of regulatory sequence inserted between the two parts of their conserved catalytic domains (X and Y). This insertion contains two SH2 and one SH3 domains sandwiched between what appears to be two halves of a PH domain. PLCγ binds to the phosphorylated tyrosines of several growth factor receptors or adaptor molecules and is subsequently recruited to the plasma membrane, where it is phosphorylated on critical tyrosine residues. Membrane association and tyrosine phosphorylation increase the activity of the enzyme, probably through association with other regulatory proteins. An additional feature of PLCγ is its regulation by $PI(3,4,5)P_3$, especially during PLCγ2 activation of immune cells. This is believed to result from the increased recruitment of PLCγ to the plasma membrane through interaction of its N-terminal PH domain with $PI(3,4,5)P_3$ molecules.

Other phospholipase C forms. Although all PLC forms can be activated by Ca^{2+} ions, PLCδ (δ1–δ4) enzymes are regulated primarily by changes in cytosolic Ca^{2+} concentration. PLCζ is a small PLC isoform responsible for generation of $Ins(1,4,5)P_3$ in the egg after fertilization. PLCε, on the other hand, is a large enzyme that is activated by small GTP binding proteins of the Ras superfamily and heterotrimeric G protein βγ subunits.

$Ins(1,4,5)P_3$ receptors

Characteristics. $Ins(1,4,5)P_3$ formed during activation of PLC binds with high affinity to specific ER receptors. Ca^{2+} stored in the ER is then released through the $InsP_3$ receptor-channel during agonist stimulation. In some cells, $Ins(1,4,5)P_3$ receptors are also present in the plasma membrane. The receptor is a large protein of 260 to 300 kDa in size that forms a tetramer and functions as a Ca^{2+} channel. After $Ins(1,4,5)P_3$ binding, Ca^{2+} moves through the $Ins(1,4,5)P_3$ receptor channel along its concentration gradient from intracellular stores to the cytosol.

Molecular variants and architecture. The three major forms of Ins(1,4,5)P$_3$ receptors (type I, type II, and type III) have a great deal of sequence homology and similar domain structure. The type I Ins(1,4,5)P$_3$ receptor has several splice variants, some of which are only expressed in neurons, and others only in peripheral tissues. Most tissues contain more than one form of the receptor, and these can even form heterotetramers. Ins(1,4,5)P$_3$ receptors contain a N-terminal Ins(1,4,5)P$_3$-binding domain that binds ligand even if expressed separately from the rest of the receptor-channel. The C-terminal part of the molecule contains a six transmembrane domain unit that functions as the channel domain. The region between the Ins(1,4,5)P$_3$-binding and the channel domain is the regulatory domain, where there are numerous phosphorylation sites as well as binding sites for other regulators [e.g., adenosine triphosphate (ATP), Ca^{2+}, calmodulin, or immunophilins].

Functional features. In addition to Ins(1,4,5)P$_3$-induced Ca^{2+} release, the most unique feature of the Ins(1,4,5)P$_3$ receptor is its ability to mediate Ca^{2+}-induced Ca^{2+} release. In this respect the receptor behaves like its structural relative, the ryanodine receptor, which is very abundant in heart and striated muscle. Ca^{2+}-induced Ca^{2+} release through the Ins(1,4,5)P$_3$ receptor is caused by the positive effect of small (nanomolar) increases in Ca^{2+} (above resting cytosolic levels) on channel opening. In contrast, Ca^{2+} in the micromolar range causes channel inactivation. According to current models, Ins(1,4,5)P$_3$ determines the threshold level of Ca^{2+} at which Ins(1,4,5)P$_3$ channels open. Ca^{2+} increases in the absence of Ins(1,4,5)P$_3$ are not sufficient to open the channel. Once Ins(1,4,5)P$_3$ channels are activated, however, Ins(1,4,5)P$_3$ concentrations have little positive effect because subsequent Ca^{2+} release is governed primarily by the filling-state of the Ca^{2+} pools and also by inactivation of the Ins(1,4,5)P$_3$ channel by Ca^{2+} and Ins(1,4,5)P$_3$ itself. This biphasic regulation of the Ins(1,4,5)P$_3$ receptor channel by Ca^{2+} is the underlying mechanism for the oscillatory cytosolic Ca^{2+} signals observed in many cells during stimulation with low agonist concentrations.

Inositol polyphosphates

Metabolism. Large amounts of highly phosphorylated inositols (e.g., InsP$_4$, InsP$_5$, and InsP$_6$) are present in mammalian, avian, and plant cells. Their relationships to the second messenger Ins(1,4,5)P$_3$ and its metabolite Ins(1,3,4,5)P$_4$ vary between lower eukaryotes and vertebrates, but an enzymatic pathway leading from Ins(1,4,5)P$_3$ to InsP$_6$ has been identified by which Ins(1,3,4)P$_3$ [a metabolite of Ins(1,3,4,5)P$_4$] is converted to Ins(1,3,4,6)P$_4$ with subsequent production of InsP$_5$. Isotope labeling studies have showed that labeling of the highly phosphorylated inositols with myo-inositol is very slow, with changes visible only after prolonged agonist stimulation. The labeling of InsP$_5$ and Ins(3,4,5,6)P$_4$/Ins(1,4,5,6)P$_4$ has been found to correlate with the growth rate of cells. Some highly phosphorylated inositols also contain pyrophosphate groups attached to their rings. The more rapid turnover and regulation of these pyrophosphorylations may indicate that they could be involved in acutely regulated cellular responses.

Functions. The function(s) of these compounds in mammalian cells are largely unknown. In avian erythrocytes, Ins(1,3,4,5,6)P$_5$ regulates the binding of oxygen to hemoglobin, whereas higher inositides may function as neurotransmitters in the rat brain stem. Ins(3,4,5,6)P$_4$ has been shown to affect Ca^{2+}-dependent chloride currents and InsP$_5$/InsP$_6$ bind to the clathrin adaptor protein, AP-2.

Recent studies in yeast have identified two genes that play a critical role in mRNA export from the nucleus. One of the enzymes, Ipk2, synthesizes Ins(1,4,5,6)P$_4$ from Ins(1,4,5)P$_3$, and is a regulator of one of the known transcriptional complexes. The other enzyme, Ipk1, is an Ins(1,3,4,5,6)P$_5$ 2-kinase, that produces InsP$_6$ or phytic acid. It is not yet understood how these inositol phosphates function in yeast or mammalian cells, but experimental yeast studies indicate the potential importance of these compounds in transcriptional regulation.

Regulation of cell membrane signals. Phosphoinositides not only serve as precursors of the second messengers [Ins(1,4,5)P$_3$ and DAG] but also function as regulators of signaling proteins on the surface of various membranes. Numerous regulatory proteins are stimulated by different isomers of inositol phospholipids, and several protein motifs have been identified that interact with inositides and mediate their regulators. These include PH domains, phox-homology (PX) domains, epsin N-terminal homology (ENTH), and FERM domains and perhaps many others found in regulatory proteins. Because these domains can recruit proteins to sites where inositides are formed in the membranes, local production and degradation of these lipids is an effective way of controlling the dynamics of protein signaling complexes in localized membrane compartments.

Many molecules are regulated by the phosphoinositide composition of membranes, including ion channels and transporters, clathrin adaptor proteins (and hence endocytosis of receptors), enzymes such as PLC and phospholipase D (PLD), kinases such as Akt and Btk, and actin polymerization. Phosphoinositides usually act together with small GTP binding proteins to recruit and regulate proteins on the cytoplasmic leaflet of cell membranes. The tight control of their formation by multiple phosphoinositide kinases, along with their degradation by the inositide phosphatases, provides for the fine regulation of these multiple effectors. Overproduction or impaired degradation of the phosphoinositides has been identified in several human diseases, including cancer, and such abnormalities are being investigated on multiple levels.

Phosphoinositide kinases

Phosphatidylinositol 4-kinases. Several groups of enzymes that produce phosphoinositides have been isolated and identified. PI 4-kinases phosphorylate PI on the 4-position of the inositol ring to produce PI4P, some of which is converted to PI(4,5)P$_2$. PI4P is probably a regulator molecule because the different forms of PI 4-kinases (type II and type III forms) serve nonredundant functions. The existence of PI4P binding proteins and PI 4-kinases in the Golgi further suggests that this lipid has a regulatory role. Type II PI 4-kinases are also present in endosomes and the trans-Golgi network and have been shown to recruit heterotetrameric adaptor proteins to these compartments.

Phosphatidylinositol 3-kinases. This important group of PI kinases (type I PI kinase enzymes) phosphorylate inositol lipids on the 3-position of the inositol ring and are regulated by growth factor receptors and oncogenic tyrosine kinases. The 3-phosphorylated inositides are not hydrolyzed by any known PLC forms and they exert regulatory functions by binding to specific protein modules present in many signaling proteins. PI 3-kinases are classified into the following three groups.

Class I enzymes. The regulation of class I enzymes is best understood. The activity and cellular localization of the 110 kDa catalytic subunit of 3 of the 4 class I isoforms (α, β, and δ) is regulated by a closely associated p85 regulatory subunit, which has two SH2 and one SH3 domains that interact with tyrosine-phosphorylated and proline-rich sequences. Activation of growth factor receptors, or soluble tyrosine kinases, brings the p85/p110 complex to the cell membrane, where tyrosine phosphorylation of p85 leads to an increased catalytic activity of the complex. Little is known about smaller splice variants of p85 lacking the SH3 domain (p55 and p50). A fourth and somewhat different member of the class I PI 3-kinases is PI3Kγ, which is primarily regulated by $\beta\gamma$ subunits of heterotrimeric G proteins either directly or through another adaptor protein, p101.

Class II enzymes. Class II PI 3-kinases are larger (170–220 kDa) proteins that contain the characteristic lipid kinase catalytic and unique domains, but also possess a C-terminal C2 domain that may mediate Ca^{2+} and phospholipid regulation of the enzyme. Class II enzymes can phosphorylate PI and PI4P but the latter is the most likely physiologic substrate. Relatively little is known about the function and regulation of class II PI 3-kinases but they are important in receptor endocytosis and vesicular trafficking.

Class III enzyme. The single class III PI 3-kinase (also called *hVps34*) specifically phosphorylates PI and its function is crucial for vacuolar sorting in yeast. The mammalian enzyme is probably also involved at multiple steps of endocytic membrane trafficking, together with an associated 150 kDa protein, the mammalian homolog of the yeast vps15p. Little is known about the regulation of these proteins in mammalian cells.

Phosphatidylinositol phosphate kinases. These enzymes use monophosphorylated PI as substrate and are classified into the following three groups based on their substrate preference.

Type I phosphatidylinositol phosphate (PIP) kinases. These enzymes phosphorylate PI4P to form PI(4,5)P$_2$, mostly in the plasma membrane. Three isoforms of these enzymes (α, β, and γ) have been isolated. The gamma form has multiple splice variants each showing distinctive expression and association with unique proteins in the plasma membrane. PIP5KIγ plays an important role in synaptic vesicle exocytosis and recycling and one of its splice variant associates with focal adhesions. All PIP5K isoforms regulate actin polymerization by producing PI(4,5)P$_2$ and are presumed to control the activity of various PI(4,5)P$_2$-regulated ion channels and transporters.

Type II PIP kinases. These enzymes that phosphorylate PI5P to PI(4,5)P$_2$ are structural relatives of the type I enzymes. Three forms of this family (α, β, and γ) have been described; although their significance is largely unknown, the elimination of the type IIβ form causes insulin hypersensitivity in mice and is therefore of particular interest.

Type III PIP kinase. This enzyme (also called *PIKfyve*) that phosphorylates PI3P to PI(3,5)P$_2$ is a homolog of the yeast Fab1p protein known to regulate vacuolar sorting in yeast. The enzyme is activated by osmotic stress; because it also controls Glut4 translocation in mammalian cells, it may have importance in regulating the effects of insulin on its target cells.

Phosphoinositide phosphatases

Several enzymes dephosphorylate inositol lipids and inositol phosphates at specific positions on the inositol ring. Interestingly, the positional substrate specificity of these enzymes is often more strict within the cellular context than *in vitro*, making it difficult to assess their respective contributions to the control of any particular inositol lipid or phosphate.

Group I 5-phosphatase. This enzyme, which dephosphorylates only water-soluble inositol phosphates [Ins(1,4,5)P$_3$ and Ins(1,3,4,5)P$_4$], regulates the levels of these soluble messengers and hence Ca^{2+} signaling. It is localized to the plasma membrane where these messengers are formed.

Group II 5-phosphatases. These enzymes dephosphorylate lipid PIs [PI(4,5)P$_2$ and PI(3,4,5)P$_3$] in addition to the soluble inositol phosphates. One of these enzymes, the oculocerebrorenal syndrome of Lowe (OCRL) protein, is mutated in a rare X-linked human disease, OCRL, that is characterized by renal tubular acidosis, mental retardation, early development of cataracts, retinal degeneration, and renal failure. The OCRL protein is believed to be associated primarily with the trans-Golgi network and is also present in lysosomal membranes but it is not clear how the defect in OCRL protein function leads to development of Lowe disease. Additional members of the group II 5-phosphatases are the synaptojanins (Snj1 and Snj2) that are believed to hydrolyze inositol lipids rather than inositol phosphates. In addition to containing a 5-phosphatase domain, synaptojanins also contain a Sac1 domain that presumably hydrolyses monophosphorylated inositides such as PI4P and PI3P. Synaptojanins have been implicated in synaptic vesicle trafficking, in association with other proteins important for the retrieval of exocytosed synaptic vesicles.

Group III 5-phosphatases. The enzymes src-homology 2–containing inositide 5' phosphatase (SHIP) and SHIP2 dephosphorylate only at the 5-position of inositide substrates that also have a phosphate group at position 3 of the inositol ring, that is, PI(3,4,5)P$_3$ [and possibly Ins(1,3,4,5)P$_4$]. They serve as important negative regulators (terminators) of the activation of PI(3,4,5)P$_3$-dependent pathways.

Group IV 5-phosphatases. Less is known about these enzymes that very effectively hydrolyze both PI(4,5)P$_2$ and PI(3,4,5)P$_3$. Interestingly, they are largely localized to the Golgi, where these inositol lipids have not been found in abundance, perhaps due to the presence of the enzyme.

Other inositide phosphatases. One of the tumor suppressor gene products, phosphatase and tensin homolog (PTEN), has been recently shown to be an inositol lipid phosphatase that removes the 3-phosphate group with relatively broad substrate specificity. PTEN antagonizes the effect of class I PI 3-kinases and probably exerts its tumor suppressor action by hydrolyzing PI(3,4,5)P$_3$. It is not clear if PTEN is functionally distinct, as it acts similarly to the SHIP 5-phosphatases that also antagonize growth factors that increase the level of PI(3,4,5)P$_3$. Another group of enzymes, the myotubularins, remove the 3-phosphate from 3-phosphorylated inositides [most likely PI3P and PI(3,5)P$_2$]. These enzymes, therefore, are regulators of vesicular trafficking. Finally, the Sac1 phosphatase is believed to act on monophosphorylated phosphoinositides (PI4P and PI3P) but little is known about the importance of this enzyme in mammalian cell systems.

Phosphatidylcholine signaling

In addition to the lipid second messengers derived from phosphoinositides, agonist stimulation of cell membrane receptors is associated with hydrolysis of phosphatidylcholine by many phospholipases (including phospholipase A$_2$, PLC, and PLD) to form DAG, phosphatidic acid, and arachidonic acid.

Phospholipase D and diacylglycerol. G proteins and PKC have been implicated in the activation of PLD, which leads to the release of PA and its subsequent conversion (through PA phosphohydrolase) to DAG. In a given cell type, various agonists stimulate the activation of PLC or PLD. The proportion of DAG generated from phosphatidylcholine (versus phosphoinositide breakdown) leads to secondary activation of PLD through PKC, causing a further increase in DAG from the hydrolysis of phosphatidylcholine and metabolism of PA.

Phospholipase D isoforms. Two major forms of phosphatidylcholine-specific PLD, PLD_1 and PLD_2, have been isolated and identified by molecular cloning. Both of these enzymes are regulated by phosphoinositides, especially $PI(4,5)P_2$. PLD_1 activity is also stimulated by the Arf family of small GTP binding proteins, as well as by PKC. Activation of PLD by cell-surface receptors has been well documented but the enzyme's role in vesicular trafficking is also important. This suggests that these enzymes, like inositide kinases, control multiple processes at specific membrane compartments within the cells.

Suggested Readings

Balla A, Balla T. Phosphatidylinositol 4-kinases: old enzymes with emerging functions. *Trends Cell Biol* 2006;16:351–361.

Berridge MJ. Inositol trisphosphate and diacylglycerol: two interacting second messengers. *Annu Rev Biochem* 1987;56:159–193.

Doughman RL, Firestone AJ, Anderson RA. Phosphatidylinositol phosphate kinases put PI4,5P(2) in its place. *J Membr Biol* 2003;194:77–89.

Engelman JA, Luo J, Cantley LC. The evolution of phosphatidylinositol 3-kinases as regulators of growth and metabolism. *Nat Rev Genet* 2006;7:606–619.

Exton JH. Phospholipase D-structure, regulation and function. *Rev Physiol Biochem Pharmacol* 2002;144:1–94.

Irvine RF, Schell MJ. Back in the water: the return of the inositol phosphates. *Nat Rev Mol Cell Biol* 2001;2:327–338.

Lemmon MA, Ferguson KM. Signal-dependent membrane targeting by pleckstrin homology (PH) domains. *Biochem Biophys Res Commun* 2000;350(Pt 1):1–18.

Majerus PW, Kisseleva MV, Norris FA. The role of phosphatases in inositol signaling reactions. *J Biol Chem* 1999;274(16):10669–10672.

Martin TF. PI(4,5)P(2) regulation of surface membrane traffic. *Curr Opin Cell Biol* 2001;13:493–499.

Rebecchi MJ, Pentyala SN. Structure, function, and control of phosphoinositide-specific phospholipase C. *Physiol Rev* 2000;80:1291–1335.

Robinson FL, Dixon JE. Myotubularin phosphatases: policing 3-phosphoinositides. *Trends Cell Biol* 2006;16(8):403–412.

Simonsen A, Wurmser AE, Emr SD, et al. The role of phosphoinositides in membrane transport. *Curr Opin Cell Biol* 2001;13(4):485–492.

CHAPTER A5 ■ PROTEIN PHOSPHORYLATION

GEORGE W. BOOZ, PhD AND KENNETH M. BAKER, MD

KEY POINTS

■ Protein phosphorylation plays an important role in the control of many cellular processes, including metabolism, membrane transport, volume regulation, protein synthesis, and gene expression.

■ The sequential activation of protein kinases (PKs) in distinct phosphorylation cascades is the principal means by which cells respond to external stimuli.

■ The activity of transcription factors can be regulated by phosphorylation in several ways including control of the cellular location of a transcription factor, modulation of DNA-binding activity or transactivation potential, and/or by recruitment of a coactivator.

■ Protein phosphorylation is critically important in regulating protein synthesis, primarily at the level of translation initiation; the associated cell growth is dependent on mitogens that activate the mitogen activated protein kinase (MAPK) or phosphatidylinositol (PI)3K cascades.

See also Chapters **A1, A2, A3,** and **A4**

For many cellular proteins, kinase-dependent phosphorylation triggers a conformational change that modifies the activity or function of that protein. An important feature of this type of covalent modification is that it is reversible through the action of a corresponding phosphatase. Protein phosphorylation–dephosphorylation therefore serves as a molecular switch for turning on and off cellular systems and events, including metabolism, membrane transport, volume regulation, protein synthesis, and gene expression. In general, phosphorylation is the "on-switch" but there are many examples of phosphorylation inhibiting the function of a protein, as with glycogen synthase kinase-3 (GSK-3) (see **Table A5.1** for abbreviations).

TABLE A5.1

SELECTED ABBREVIATIONS AND ACRONYMS

AMPK = AMP-activated protein kinase
ASK = Activator of S phase kinase
CaMK = Ca^{2+}/calmodulin-regulated kinase
CBP = CREB-binding protein
CRE = cAMP response element
CREB = CRE-binding protein
EGF = epidermal growth factor
eIF = eukaryotic initiation factor
ERK = extracellular signal–regulated kinase
FGF = fibroblast growth factor
FH = forkhead (transcription factor)
GEF = guanine nucleotide exchange factor
GPCR = G protein–coupled receptor
GSK-3 = glycogen synthase kinase-3
IKK = IκB kinase
IRS-1 = insulin receptor substrate-1
Jak = Janus kinase
JNK = c-Jun NH$_2$ terminal kinase
MAPK = mitogen activated protein kinase
MAPKAP = MAPK activated protein
MEK = MAPK kinase
MEKK = MEK kinase
MIP1 = MEKK2 interacting protein 1
MKK = MAP kinase kinase
MLK = mixed lineage kinase
Mnk = MAPK interacting kinase
mTOR = mammalian target of rapamycin
NFAT = nuclear factor of activated T cells
NFκB = nuclear factor-κB
PDGF = platelet derived growth factor
PDK1 = 3-phosphoinositide–dependent protein kinase 1
PI3K = phosphoinositide 3 kinase
PKA = protein kinase A
PKB = protein kinase B
PKC = protein kinase C
PKG = protein kinase G
PTB = phosphotyrosine binding
PTK = protein tyrosine kinase
Rheb = ras-homolog enriched in brain
RSKs = ribosomal S6 kinases
RTK = receptor tyrosine kinase
S6K = (ribosomal) S6 kinase
SAPK = stress-activated protein kinase
SH2 = Src-homology 2
SIN1 = stress-activated protein kinase-interacting 1
Smad = blend of Sma and Mad (mothers against decapentaplegic)
STAT = signal transducers and activators of transcription
TAK = TGF-beta-activated kinase
TIF-I = transcription initiation factor I
TSC1/TSC2 = tuberous sclerosis complex ½

Protein kinases

Sequential activation of protein kinases (PKs) within distinct phosphorylation cascades is the principal means by which cells respond to external stimuli. These cascades amplify and prolong an initial signal, allow for the integration of different signals, and often result in a sustained or even permanent cellular response to a transient external stimulus. Protein phosphorylation cascades, in particular those involving MAPKs, are critically important in development, growth, cellular survival, and programmed cell death (apoptosis). The importance of protein phosphorylation to the physiology of the cell is underscored by the fact that PKs represent an estimated 1.7% of all human genes.

Structure and function. PKs are structurally related by having a common catalytic domain that (a) binds and orients a substrate peptide/protein, a purine nucleotide triphosphate donor [adenosine triphosphate (ATP)/guanosine triphosphate (GTP)], and a divalent cation (Mg^{2+} or Mn^{2+}) and (b) facilitates the transfer of the γ-phosphate of the donor to a hydroxyl residue (serine, threonine, or tyrosine) on the substrate.

Subtypes. On the basis of the amino acid sequence of the catalytic domain, eukaryotic PKs can be organized into the following four groups that have related functions and share substrate preference.

AGC group (for protein kinases A, G, and C). The AGC group phosphorylates serine/threonine residues near the basic residues arginine and lysine. This group includes the cyclic nucleotide–dependent kinases PKA and PKG, PKCs, ribosomal S6Ks, PKB/Akt, and β-adrenergic receptor kinases.

Ca^{2+}/calmodulin-regulated kinase (CaMK) group. The CaMK group, which includes Ca^{2+}/calmodulin-regulated and related kinases, phosphorylates serine, or threonine residues near basic amino acids.

CMGC group [for cyclin-dependent kinases (CDKs), mitogen-activated protein kinases (MAPKs), glycogen synthase kinases (GSKs), and CDK-like kinases (CLKs)]. The CMGC kinases phosphorylate serine/threonine residues in proline-rich domains and include cyclin dependent kinases, GSK-3, MAPKs, and Clk (Cdk-like) kinase.

Protein tyrosine kinase (PTK) group. The PTK group includes receptor kinases [e.g., receptors for epidermal growth factor (EGF), platelet derived growth factor (PDGF), insulin, and fibroblast growth factor (FGF)] and nonreceptor kinases (e.g., the Jak and Src families), both of which phosphorylate tyrosine residues.

Other groups. Several recently described kinases fall outside of these major subgroups, including MAPK kinases (MEKs), MEK kinases (MEKKs), the Raf family, and mixed lineage kinases (MLKs).

Phosphorylation and intracellular signaling

Signaling cascades. Cells respond to external stimuli by a multitude of intracellular signaling cascades involving phosphorylation or dephosphorylation events that are linked to cell membrane receptors, channels, or integrins. These cascades serve to distribute a ligand's signal throughout the cell, resulting in short- and long-term responses. Signaling cascades can be activated by classical second messengers [e.g., cyclic adenosine monophosphate (cAMP), cyclic guanosine monophosphate (cGMP), Ca^{2+}, diacylglycerol] or by tyrosine kinases (both receptor and nonreceptor-activated).

One stimulus generally activates multiple signaling cascades, both second messenger and tyrosine kinase dependent. A cascade may involve a simple second messenger–kinase pair (e.g., cAMP–PKA) or a series of sequentially activated kinases (e.g., MAPK cascades). Cascades can exhibit branching, and one cascade can initiate another through formation of a second messenger or through activation of a tyrosine or serine/threonine kinase. Cross-talk can occur between cascades at the level of the membrane transducers, signaling components, or effector proteins, resulting in synergistic or antagonistic effects.

Recruitment and spatial organization of kinases and effector proteins.

Two important regulatory mechanisms for the control of intracellular signaling are (a) the recruitment of kinases and effector proteins to a particular subcellular location such as a receptor and (b) the organization of kinases in a phosphorylation cascade into complexes or modules, before or after stimulation.

Ordering events.

Ordering events confine a signal to the appropriate subcellular location, optimize the response time, and reinforce the specificity with which kinases interact with targets. Protein–protein or protein–lipid interactions form the basis of these ordering events, which are mediated by defined domains of 35 to 150 amino acids. Several domains important in protein–protein interactions recognize specific phosphotyrosine or phosphoserine/threonine motifs. SH2 domains bind to specific phosphotyrosine containing motifs, such as those found on receptors for cytokines, growth factors, and antigens. Specificity is conferred by the preference of the domain for the amino acids immediately following the phosphorylated tyrosine. Numerous adaptor, scaffold, and docking proteins, enzymes, cytoskeletal proteins, inhibitory factors, and transcription factors contain 1 or more SH2 domains. Phosphotyrosine binding (PTB) domains bind Asn-Pro-X-Tyr motifs, with some requiring phosphorylation of the tyrosine residue. The PTB domains of the docking proteins, insulin receptor substrate-1 (IRS-1) and Shc, exhibit this requirement. The forkhead-associated domain, which is found primarily in eukaryotic nuclear proteins, binds specific motifs phosphorylated by serine/threonine kinases.

14-3-3 proteins.

A family of proteins known as *14-3-3 proteins* form homo- and heterodimeric cuplike structures that bind discrete phosphoserine containing motifs. These 14-3-3 proteins function like adaptor or scaffold proteins and are involved in the regulation of mitogenesis, cell cycle progression, and apoptosis, by either enhancing or inhibiting the activity of the proteins they bind. Bad, the Rafs, various PKCs, MEKK1, and forkhead (FH) transcription factors are some of the proteins the 14-3-3 proteins bind.

Multisite phosphorylation and signal strength.

Phosphorylation of more than one site is a common feature of many proteins involved in intracellular signaling. Multisite phosphorylation of receptors or docking proteins allows for the activation of multiple signaling cascades by a single agonist. Phosphorylation of a protein on multiple sites can also determine the strength and duration of a signal; allow for different agonists to have synergistic, antagonistic, or redundant effects; or raise the threshold required for the activation of a protein.

The regulation of phosphorylase kinase by cAMP and Ca^{2+} signals in mammalian skeletal muscle is an example of multisite phosphorylation that is important in glycogenolysis during increased muscle activity. By increasing cAMP, adrenaline activates PKA, which phosphorylates the α- and β-regulatory subunits of phosphorylase kinase, thereby enhancing sensitivity of the catalytic subunit to regulation by the Ca^{2+}-regulated δ calmodulin subunit and maximizing kinase activity.

Mitogen-activated protein kinase phosphorylation cascades.

MAPKs belong to a family of serine/threonine kinases that play a central role in many basic cellular processes, including proliferation, differentiation, and apoptosis (**Figure A5.1**). MAPKs affect cellular processes and gene expression by phosphorylating structural or functional proteins and transcription factors or by activating other kinases. There are six mammalian MAPK families linked to distinct signaling cascades that are organized hierarchically into three-tiered modules. Activation of MAPKs requires phosphorylation of threonine and tyrosine residues by the family of cytosolic dual-specificity kinases (MAPKK). MAPKK activation in turn results from phosphorylation by serine/threonine kinases (MAPKKK). MAPKKKs are activated by small G proteins or other PKs, thereby linking the MAPK module to a cell-surface receptor or external stimulus.

Three phosphorylation cascades linked to the activation of ERK1/2, p38, and stress-activated protein kinase (SAPK)/c-Jun

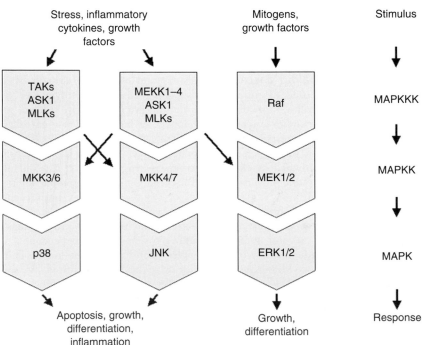

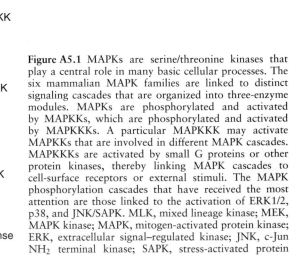

Figure A5.1 MAPKs are serine/threonine kinases that play a central role in many basic cellular processes. The six mammalian MAPK families are linked to distinct signaling cascades that are organized into three-enzyme modules. MAPKs are phosphorylated and activated by MAPKKs, which are phosphorylated and activated by MAPKKKs. A particular MAPKKK may activate MAPKKs that are involved in different MAPK cascades. MAPKKKs are activated by small G proteins or other protein kinases, thereby linking MAPK cascades to cell-surface receptors or external stimuli. The MAPK phosphorylation cascades that have received the most attention are those linked to the activation of ERK1/2, p38, and JNK/SAPK. MLK, mixed lineage kinase; MEK, MAPK kinase; MAPK, mitogen-activated protein kinase; ERK, extracellular signal–regulated kinase; JNK, c-Jun NH₂ terminal kinase; SAPK, stress-activated protein kinase.

NH2 terminal kinase (JNK) members of the MAPK family have received the most attention. The ERK1/2 MAPK cascade is activated by growth factors and mitogens and is involved in cellular growth and differentiation. The p38 and SAPK/JNK MAPK cascades are linked to a broad range of cellular responses such as growth, apoptosis, differentiation, or inflammation. They are activated by growth factors (generally weakly and dependent on cell type), inflammatory cytokines, and various stress stimuli (e.g., ultraviolet light, heat, reactive oxygen species, and protein synthesis inhibitors).

Extracellular signal–regulated kinase cascade

Tyrosine phosphorylation and docking. When activated by ligand binding, receptor tyrosine kinase (RTKs) undergo dimerization or conformational change, resulting in the autophosphorylation of multiple tyrosine residues in the cytoplasmic region of the receptor. These phosphorylated tyrosine residues serve as docking sites for various proteins with one or more SH2 or PTB domains. One such protein is the nonenzymic adaptor protein Shc, which has an SH3 domain that recognizes a left-hand polyproline type II helix domain in other proteins. Shc binds to a guanine nucleotide exchange factor (GEF) protein, mSOS, directly by the SH3 domain or through an adaptor protein, GRB2. mSOS binds to and activates the small G protein Ras by catalyzing the release of guanosine diphosphate (GDP). Activated Ras in turn recruits the MAPKKK Raf to the membrane, thereby triggering the cascade that results in ERK1/2 activation.

G protein–coupling and extracellular signal–regulated kinase activation. G protein–coupled receptors (GPCRs) promote ERK1/2 activation by multiple means. For example, G_q/G_o–coupled receptors may stimulate the ERK cascade through Ras by activating PKC, PI3K, or both. Such receptors may also activate the nonreceptor PTK, Pyk2, through increases in intracellular Ca^{2+}. Pyk2 in turn activates Src and/or leads to Shc phosphorylation. G_q/G_i–coupled receptors may also activate the ERK cascade independent of Ras through PKC-mediated activation of Raf. G_i–coupled receptors may be linked to the ERK cascade through activation of the Src family tyrosine kinases, resulting in Shc phosphorylation and formation of the Shc-GRB2-mSOS-Ras complex. Src family kinases are direct effectors of $G\alpha_i$ or may be turned on indirectly through $G\beta\gamma$-mediated activation of PI3K. Finally, GPCRs may activate the ERK cascade through transactivation of the PDGF or EGF receptors by either Ca^{2+}-dependent or -independent mechanisms.

Phosphoinositide 3 kinase phosphorylation

The phosphorylated lipid products of PI3K are involved in membrane ruffling and cytoskeletal changes, receptor endocytosis, activation of certain PKC isoforms, and translocation of PKB/Akt (henceforth called *Akt*) to the membrane.

Parallel activation of mitogen-activated protein kinase and phosphatidylinositol 3K. Agonists that stimulate MAPK activity commonly induce a parallel phosphorylation cascade that is linked to PI3K activation and has been implicated in enhanced protein synthesis, cell survival, and in mediating many of the cellular actions of insulin. PI3K represents a family of membrane proteins, composed of an 85-kd regulatory subunit and a 110-kd catalytic subunit, that phosphorylate the 3′-OH position of the inositol ring of inositol phospholipids or the serine or threonine residues on proteins such as IRS-1. Association of SH2 domains of the regulatory subunits with phosphorylated tyrosine residues leads to activation of PI3K. Ras and the $\beta\gamma$ subunit of heterotrimeric G proteins may also activate the catalytic subunit. A 101-kd regulatory protein, which is found in certain mammalian cell types, is directly activated by G proteins.

Phosphatidylinositol 3K intermediaries. After translocation to the membrane, Akt is activated through threonine and serine phosphorylation by PDK1 and "PDK2," respectively. PDK2 was recently identified as the kinase SIN1/MIP1, a subunit of the rictor-mTOR protein complex (mammalian target of rapamycin (mTOR) complex 2 or TORC2). There are numerous targets downstream of activated Akt, many of which impact on cell survival and protein synthesis. For example, activated Akt promotes cell survival by activating IκB kinase (IKK), and inhibiting Bad, caspase-9, and FH transcription factors. Akt activation promotes protein synthesis by inhibiting GSK-3 and activating mTOR. This activation of mTOR is achieved by Akt-mediated phosphorylation (AMP) and inactivation of the GTPase-activator protein TSC2 (in a dimer with TSC1), which allows the small G protein Rheb to accumulate in the GTP-bound form. Rheb-GTP in turn positively regulates mTOR. In this case, the serine/threonine kinase mTOR exists in a protein complex (mTOR complex 1 or TORC1) with raptor and mLST8. When activated, TORC1 positively regulates protein translation by phosphorylating p70 S6 kinase and 4E-BP. TORC1 may be activated independently of Akt and also appears to function as an intracellular sensor of amino acid levels (most often leucine). Conversely, TORC1 activity and protein synthesis is reduced by depletion of cellular ATP (and accumulation of AMP) through AMPK-mediated phosphorylation of TSC2.

Regulation of transcription factor activity

Transcription factors can be regulated by changes in their concentration or activity. Concentration changes result from the collective activities of multiple steps from transcription to translation, each of which may be regulated by protein phosphorylation. The activity of transcription factors can be regulated by phosphorylation in several ways.

Cellular localization of transcription factors. Four examples of transcription factors with this type of control are the Smads, NFκBs, signal transducers and activators of transcription (STATs), and cytoplasmic nuclear factor of activated T cells (NFATs).

Smads. The receptor-regulated Smads (R-Smads) are latent cytoplasmic transcription factors that become active at cognate receptors with serine kinase activity that bind the transforming growth factor β superfamily of ligands. Serine phosphorylation of Smads results in association with the common mediator Smad (coSmad), SMAD4 and translocation to the nucleus.

NFκB (nuclear factor-κB). The NFκB proteins are found in the cytoplasm bound to the anchor protein IκB in the nonstimulated state. Phosphorylation of IκB by IKK, PKC, or PKA, induces its proteolysis, thereby liberating the transcription factor and allowing it to move into the nucleus.

STATs. STATs are the only known transcription factors activated from a latent state by tyrosine phosphorylation. Cytoplasmic STATs are phosphorylated by the Jak or Src family of kinases, resulting in STAT dimerization (through intermolecular binding of their juxtaposed phosphorylated tyrosine residues and SH2 domains) and subsequent nuclear translocation.

NFATs. Cytoplasmic NFATs are activated by agonists that increase cell Ca^{2+}. Increased Ca^{2+} activates the phosphatase calcineurin, which dephosphorylates the NFATs and leads to nuclear translocation. NFATs are phosphorylated by several types of kinases, including GSK-3 and JNK.

DNA-binding activity. Phosphorylation can modulate the DNA-binding activity or transactivation potential of a transcription factor. For example, JNKs phosphorylate two sites in the N-terminal transactivation domain of c-Jun, thereby enhancing transactivation potential. ERKs phosphorylate an inhibitor domain in C/EBPβ, disrupting intramolecular binding with the transactivation domain and permitting DNA binding.

Coactivator recruitment. Phosphorylation (generally on serine) of a transcription factor may be required for recruitment of a coactivator. PKA-mediated CRE-binding protein (CREB) phosphorylation causes it to bind CREB-binding protein (CBP), which is required for CREB to function as a transcription factor. A conserved serine residue modulates STAT transcriptional activity in an isoform-specific manner: Phosphorylation may enhance transcriptional activity through recruitment of coactivators, prolong tyrosine phosphorylation and DNA binding, or interfere with tyrosine phosphorylation and activation.

Regulation of protein synthesis

Protein phosphorylation is critically important in regulating protein synthesis. Control occurs primarily at the level of translation initiation, which is correlated with cell growth and is influenced by mitogens that activate the MAPK or PI3K cascades.

Translation initiation. Translation initiation is a multistep process whereby the 40S ribosome subunit is positioned at the AUG initiation codon of the messenger RNA (mRNA) transcript. Attachment of the ribosome to the transcript is facilitated by a cap structure [7-methyl GTP] at the 5' terminus of all nuclear-encoded eukaryotic mRNAs.

eIF Proteins. Attachment requires the participation of eIFs and is initiated by eIF4F, which facilitates ribosomal binding of the 5' untranslated region of mRNA by unwinding its secondary structure. The protein eIF4F consists of three subunits: eIF4E, the cap-binding subunit present in rate-limiting amounts; eIF4A, an RNA helicase which acts in synergy with eIF4B and exhibits bidirectional RNA unwinding activity; and eIF4G, a scaffold protein that binds to ribosome-associated eIF3 and functions as a link between the ribosome and mRNA.

4E-BP Binding Proteins. The function of eIF4E is negatively regulated by 4E-BP binding proteins that compete with eIF4G for a common binding site on eIF4E. Phosphorylation of 4E-BPs decreases the affinity for eIF4E, thereby allowing cap-dependent translation initiation to occur and as a result protein synthesis is enhanced. 4E-BP hyperphosphorylation is induced by extracellular ligands including insulin and various growth factors that act through the sequential activation of PI3K, PDKs, and PKB/Akt. 4E-BP hyperphosphorylation may be dependent on its initial phosphorylation by mTOR. The phosphorylation states of eIF4G and eIF4B are also affected by this signaling cascade, but what significance this has on function has not been established. ERK activation may also result in 4E-BP hyperphosphorylation, after 4E-BP is initially phosphorylated by mTOR.

In addition to being under negative control through 4E-BP, eIF4E function appears to be positively regulated by phosphorylation on Ser209, after it is bound to eIF4G. In general, a strong correlation occurs between eIF4E phosphorylation and rates of protein synthesis and cell growth, but how Ser209 phosphorylation affects eIF4E function is not clear. Phosphorylation of eIF4E on Ser209 may play a key role in regulating *de novo* initiation of translation, as opposed to reinitiation. Recent evidence indicates that the kinases responsible for cellular phosphorylation of eIF4E are Mnk1 and 2, which are substrates for the ERK1/2 and p38 MAPKs.

Translation elongation. Protein elongation occurs with the movement of the ribosome one codon along the mRNA. In this process, the peptidyl-tRNA occupying the ribosomal A site migrates to the P site, the previous occupant of the P site is expelled along with the formation of a new peptide bond. In eukaryotes, the translocation step is promoted by eEF2. Phosphorylation of eEF2 by eEF2 kinase, a highly specific, calcium/calmodulin-dependent kinase, impairs its activity by inhibiting ribosomal binding. In turn, activity of eEF2 kinase, which does not belong to any of the four major groups of eukaryotic PKs, is inhibited by mTOR signaling at three separate serine residues, one of which has been shown to be a target for phosphorylation by S6K1 and other ribosomal S6 kinases (RSKs) downstream of ERK1/2. Therefore, enhanced mTOR activity also stimulates the elongation step of protein synthesis. In contrast, AMP-activated protein kinase (AMPK) phosphorylation of another serine residue activates eEF2 kinase, thereby slowing elongation when ATP levels are reduced.

Ribosomal biogenesis regulation. Hormones and mitogens also stimulate protein synthesis by inducing the upregulation of ribosome biogenesis, thereby increasing the translational capacity of the cell. The mRNAs that encode much of the translational machinery, including numerous ribosomal proteins, elongation factors, and the poly(A) binding protein, all contain a 5' terminal oligopyrimidine tract (5'TOP) adjacent to the cap that suppresses their translation under basal conditions. mTOR activation enhances 5'TOP mRNA translation, although the mechanism is unclear. Recent evidence has undermined the once-prevailing view that phosphorylation of the 40S ribosomal S6 protein by p70 S6K, a serine/threonine PK, is involved. Regulation of ribosome biogenesis occurs primarily at the level of transcription and involves all three nuclear RNA polymerases (Pol I - III). mTOR regulates Pol I transcription by controlling the activity of the regulatory factor TIF-IA. Recently, TORC1 was also shown to enhance Pol I-mediated 35S rRNA precursor transcription in yeast by binding directly to the rDNA promoter. mTOR may also enhance ribosome biogenesis by regulating phosphorylation of the ribosomal DNA transcription factor upstream binding factor (UBF).

Translation modulation by eIF2. Protein phosphorylation is important in the control of translation by eIF2, which functions to transfer the initiator methionyl–transfer RNA to the 40S subunit, thereby forming the 43S preinitiation complex. In its function, eIF2 binds and hydrolyzes GTP. For eIF2 to participate in another round of initiation, GDP must be exchanged for GTP in a process catalyzed by eIF2B. Amino acid deprivation, double-stranded RNA, and other stress stimuli activate kinases that phosphorylate eIF2, stabilize the eIF2-GDP-eIF2B complex, and inhibit global protein synthesis. At the same time, the translation of a select group of mRNAs involved in remediation or apoptosis is enhanced. GSK-3 also phosphorylates and inhibits eIF2B. Serine phosphorylation of GSK-3 by Akt, S6K, or MAPKAP-K1 relieves the inhibitory effect of GSK-3 on eIF2B. Therefore, eIF2B activity can be enhanced by growth factors through either the PI3K cascade (Akt, mTOR, and S6K activation) or ERK1/2 (MAPKAP-K1 and S6K activation) or by amino acids through mTOR.

RNA dynamics. Protein phosphorylation plays a role in the regulation of other aspects of protein synthesis, including the release of mRNA from the nucleus, RNA stability, and pre-RNA splicing. In part, this regulation involves phosphorylation or dephosphorylation of members of the SR (serine/arginine-residue) class of proteins that dynamically associate with mRNA molecules during their lifespan.

Suggested Readings

Brivanlou AH, Darnell JE. Signal transduction and the control of gene expression. *Science* 2002;295:813–818.

De Virgilio C, Loewith R. Cell growth control: little eukaryotes make big contributions. *Oncogene* 2006;25:6392–6415.

Hinnebusch AG. eIF3: a versatile scaffold for translation initiation complexes. *Trends Biochem Sci* 2006;31:553–562.

Huang Y, Steitz JA. SRprises along a messenger's journey. *Mol Cell* 2005;17:613–615.

Manning G, Whyte DB, Martinez R, et al. The protein kinase complement of the human genome. *Science* 2002;298:1912–1934.

Martin DE, Powers T, Hall MN. Regulation of ribosome biogenesis: where is TOR? *Cell Metab* 2006;4:259–260.

Wang X, Proud CG. The mTOR pathway in the control of protein synthesis. *Physiology* 2006;21:362–369.

Wek RC, Jiang HY, Anthony TG. Coping with stress: eIF2 kinases and translational control. *Biochem Soc Trans* 2006;34:7–11.

CHAPTER A6 ■ INTRACELLULAR pH AND CELL VOLUME

BRADFORD C. BERK, MD, PhD

KEY POINTS

■ Anion and cation transporters and exchangers regulate intracellular pH (pH_i) and cell volume.

■ Increased Na^+–H^+ exchange can cause cell swelling, sensitivity to pressors, and cell hypertrophy.

■ Na^+–H^+ exchange is increased in most hypertensive humans and some animal models; enzymes that regulate Na^+–H^+ exchange are expressed by candidate genes for essential hypertension.

See also Chapters A7, A8, and A10

Cells maintain a homeostatic balance by regulating critical variables around physiologic or pathologic "set points." Cell volume and intracellular pH (pH_i) are two such critical variables regulated by ion transport systems, including anion (HCO_3^-–Cl^-) and cation (Na^+–H^+) exchangers.

Regulation of intracellular pH

Vascular smooth muscle cells (VSMCs) maintain vessel tone by altering their contractile states and maintain vessel structure by altering their growth states. pH_i plays a critical role in both functions. Regulation of pH_i occurs through intracellular "buffering" and also as a result of transport of H^+ (or OH^-) across membranes through three ion transport mechanisms that participate in pH_i homeostasis: (a) Na^+–H^+ exchange, (b) Na^+-dependent HCO_3^-–Cl^- exchange, and (c) cation-independent HCO_3^-–Cl^- exchange (**Figure A6.1**).

Intracellular buffering. Intracellular buffering is complex and includes physicochemical buffering by the interaction of H^+ with cellular proteins and amino acids, subcellular compartmentalization, and metabolic consumption.

Na^+–H^+ exchange. Na^+–H^+ exchange is an electroneutral transport process that under physiologic conditions exchanges one intracellular H^+ for one extracellular Na^+. The Na^+–H^+ exchanger (NHE) participates in multiple cellular functions, including regulation of pH_i as well as the transport of salt and water.

It is now known that Na^+–H^+ exchange is mediated by a family of at least eight related Na^+–H^+ exchanger gene products (NHE-1 through NHE-8), each with unique tissue distribution and sensitivity to inhibition by pharmacologic agents. The NHE-1 isoform appears to be ubiquitous and is dominant in VSMCs. The primary function of NHE-1 is to regulate pH_i, as evidenced by the pH_i dependence of the rate of transport. Basal NHE-1 activity maintains normal VSMC pH_i at 0.3 to 0.5 pH units above the Donnan equilibrium for H^+. Rapid increases in Na^+–H^+ exchange activity occur on exposure to growth factors and vasoconstrictors. This stimulation is characterized

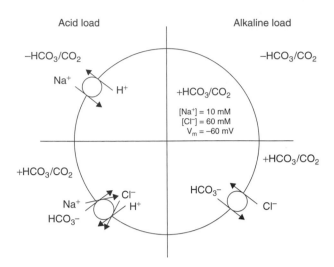

Figure A6.1 Regulation of intracellular pH. Shown are pH-regulatory ion transport mechanisms in response to an acid load (**left**) or an alkaline load (**right**). Nature of transport is also influenced by bicarbonate (**bottom**) or absence of bicarbonate (**top**). There is no regulatory ion transport process for alkaline loads in absence of bicarbonate, and cell relies on intracellular generation of protons.

by a change in affinity for intracellular H^+ and extracellular Na^+.

In the absence of CO_2–HCO_3^-, as might occur with decreased blood flow, the Na^+–H^+ exchanger is the dominant pH_i regulator. At normal pH_i (7.4), the Na^+–H^+ exchanger is inactive, indicating the existence of an intracellular H^+ sensor. The sensitivity of this intracellular site can be shifted to more acid pH_i by depletion of adenosine triphosphate (ATP) or to more alkaline pH_i by growth factor stimulation or cell shrinkage. The efficiency of Na^+–H^+ exchange in restoring pH_i of an acid-loaded cell is inversely proportional to the buffering power; only a few exchanges are required to induce a large pH recovery when buffering power is low.

Na-dependent HCO_3^-–Cl^- exchange.
In the presence of CO_2–HCO_3^-, the Na^+-dependent HCO_3^-–Cl^- exchanger is dominant. This transporter normally exchanges extracellular Na^+ and HCO_3^- for intracellular Cl^- (and probably H^+), with stoichiometry for Na^+/Cl^-/acid–base equivalents of 1:1:2. It can be distinguished from Na^+–H^+ exchange by its sensitivity to stilbene derivatives and resistance to amiloride.

Cation-dependent HCO_3–Cl^- exchange.
The cation-independent HCO_3^-–Cl^- exchanger transports anions across the cell membrane with a stoichiometry of 1:1 and is electroneutral. Like Na^+–H^+ exchange, HCO_3^-–Cl^- exchange has been shown to be mediated by a multigene family of transporters (AE1 through AE3).

At normal intracellular Cl^- and HCO_3^- concentrations, net transport of the exchanger would be one intracellular HCO_3^- for one extracellular Cl^-, producing intracellular acidification. Therefore, as shown in **Figure A6.1**, HCO_3^-–Cl^- exchange will lower pH_i in alkaline-loaded cells. There is no alkaline pH_i regulatory mechanism in the absence of HCO_3^-–CO_2 except for transporters that normally extrude H^+ by working in reverse.

Regulation of cell volume
Cells regulate their volumes by unloading excess water when swollen and by absorbing water when shrunken. Usually, cell

volume is corrected by altering the number of osmotically active particles in the cytoplasm, thereby causing obligate water movement.

Volume sensors. Several intracellular volume-sensing mechanisms have been discovered, including (a) cytoskeleton-membrane interactions that respond to cellular deformation, and (b) alterations in kinases that regulate shape (such as Rho kinase and myosin light chain kinase). Volume regulation is particularly important in VSMCs, which must undergo rapid transient volume changes during contraction and slower sustained volume changes during hypertrophy.

Transporters. Two mechanisms have been described that regulate volume in VSMCs: (a) Na^+–H^+ exchange and Cl^-–HCO_3^- exchange–coupled transport and (b) Na^+–K^+–$2Cl^-$ cotransport and Na^+, K^+–ATPase–coupled transport (**Figure A6.2**).

Na^+–H^+ and Cl^-–HCO_3^- are functionally coupled with pH_i regulation because H^+ adjusts Na^+–H^+ exchange and also determines the concentration of HCO_3^-. An example of the tight link between pH_i and volume regulation is the situation that occurs after sudden intracellular acidification. Because the buffering power is not infinitely large, some time is required for Na^+–H^+ exchange to restore pH_i to its basal level. The amount of time required depends on the buffering power and the rate of Na^+–H^+ exchange. During this time, cell volume changes due to the increased influx of Na^+ and water caused by activation of Na^+–H^+ exchange. H^+ ions are generated by intracellular metabolism, further "fueling" the exchange.

If Cl^-–HCO_3^- exchange is also stimulated, the initial rate of pH recovery will be faster because of exchange of intracellular Cl^- for extracellular HCO_3^-, which raises pH_i. Although the loss of intracellular Cl^- initially causes a decrease in cell volume, the ensuing coupled Na^+ per H^+ and Cl^-–HCO_3^- exchange exerts the opposite influence. The result of this coupling is the inward movement of Na^+ (by Na^+–H^+ exchange) and of Cl^- (by Cl^-–HCO_3^- exchange). The H^+ and HCO_3^- transported out of the cell in exchange for Na^+ and Cl^- are then converted through carbonic anhydrase into H_2O and CO_2, increasing cell volume (**Figure A6.2**). Key to this increase in cell volume are the facts that: (a) H^+ is generated from cell metabolism (and hence "created" *de novo*) and (b) the Na^+–K^+–$2Cl^-$ co-transporter can mediate a net influx of Cl^- accompanied by increases in intracellular Na^+ and K^+. The changes in intracellular Na^+ activate membrane Na^+, K^+–ATPase, which works to maintain cell homeostasis by extruding Na^+ in exchange for K^+. The net result is obligate inward movement of water and an increase in cell volume.

Na^+–H^+ exchange and vascular smooth muscle cell function
The Na^+ per H^+ exchanger may play a physiologic or pathogenic role (**Figure A6.3**) by modifying pH_i and altering signal transduction pathways.

Vascular smooth muscle tone. Increased activity of the Na^+ per H^+ exchanger could lead to increased vascular tone by two mechanisms. First, increased Na^+ entry may activate Na^+–Ca^{2+} exchange, leading to increased intracellular Ca^{2+}. This phenomenon is important in conditions of ischemia and reperfusion, such as occur with myocardial infarction, stroke, and microvascular occlusion. Second, increased pH_i enhances the Ca^{2+} sensitivity of the contractile apparatus, leading to an increase in contractility for a given intracellular Ca^{2+} concentration. Owing to the activation of NHE by both hyperplastic and

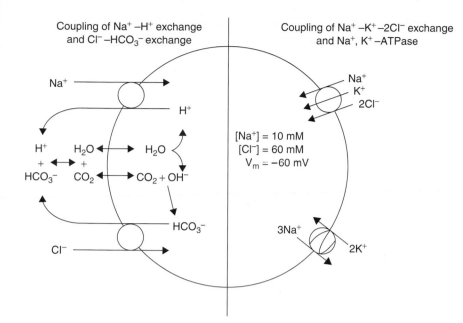

Figure A6.2 Coupling of several exchangers and sodium pump to regulate cell volume. Change in pH may regulate cell volume, and conversely, changes in cell volume may alter intracellular pH as discussed in text. Na^+, K^+–ATPase, sodium- and potassium-activated adenosine triphosphatase.

hypertrophic agents, it has been proposed that abnormal function of this protein may be involved in the pathophysiology of hypertension.

Growth effects. The effect of increased Na^+ per H^+ exchange on growth most likely relates to enhanced sensitivity to mitogens. Recent work has identified several NHE-1 kinases [p90RSK, ERK1/2, p160ROCK (a RhoA-activated kinase) and Nck-interacting kinase (NIK)] as well as several NHE-1 binding proteins [calcineurin B homologous protein (CHP), calmodulin, 14-3-3 heat shock protein 70, and ezrin] that may be altered in hypertension. In addition, upstream signaling mediators such as G proteins may exhibit enhanced activity that is transduced into increased NHE-1 activity

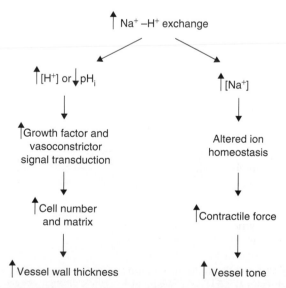

Figure A6.3 Effect of Na^+–H^+ exchange on vascular smooth muscle cell (VSMC) growth and tone. Increased activity leads to alterations in concentrations of H^+ and Na^+ that secondarily modulate signal transduction and contractile force. Chronic changes mediated by these alterations may lead to fixed structural abnormalities, such as medial hypertrophy and smooth muscle hyperplasia. pH_i, intracellular pH.

Na^+–H^+ exchange and hypertension

The abnormalities of vessel tone and growth seen in hypertension may be, in part, the result of changes in the regulation of cell volume and pH_i. Evidence for dysfunction of the Na^+ per H^+ exchanger in hypertension includes observations that its activity is increased in skeletal muscle, VSMCs, lymphocytes, platelets from spontaneously hypertensive rats, and platelets from hypertensive patients. Alterations in Na^+–H^+ exchange in hypertension can theoretically be divided into three categories: mutation in the gene, increased expression of the gene product, and altered posttranslational regulation of existing exchangers. However, restriction fragment length polymorphism analysis and single nucleotide polymorphism (SNP) studies have not demonstrated linkages between the human NHE-1 gene and essential hypertension.

There is clearly an increase in both NHE-1 phosphorylation and cell growth in cells derived from hypertensive rats and human hypertensive patients. However, there does not appear to be any alteration in NHE-1 mRNA or protein expression in the spontaneously hypertensive rat. These findings are consistent with the concept that increased activity of an NHE-1 kinase (or decreased activity of an NHE-1 phosphatase) is responsible for increased basal activity of the exchanger in tissues of hypertensive persons and animals. Alternatively, an NHE-1 regulatory protein whose activity is modulated by phosphorylation may be altered in hypertension. Studies with mutated or deleted NHE-1 proteins indicate that phosphorylation of NHE-1 shifts the pH range over which the "pH_i sensor" operates. Therefore, the primary alteration in Na^+–H^+ exchange in VSMCs in hypertension may involve a change in phosphorylation of an NHE-1 regulatory protein or in NHE-1 itself.

Suggested Readings

Berk BC. Regulation of the Na^+/H^+ exchanger in vascular smooth muscle. In: Fliegel L, Austin RG, eds. *The Na^+/H^+ exchanger*. Austin: Landes Co, 1996:47–67.

Berk BC, Vallega G, Muslin AJ, et al. Spontaneously hypertensive rat vascular smooth muscle cells in culture exhibit increased growth and Na^+/H^+ exchange. *J Clin Invest* 1989;83:822–829.

Chamberlin ME, Strange K. Anisosmotic cell volume regulation: a comparative view. *Am J Physiol* 1989;257:C159–C173.

Lifton RP, Hunt SC, Williams RR, et al. Exclusion of the Na$^+$–H$^+$ antiporter as a candidate gene in human essential hypertension. *Hypertension* 1991;17:8–14.

Orlov SN, Tremblay J, Hamet P. Cell volume in vascular smooth muscle is regulated by bumetanide-sensitive ion transport. *Am J Physiol* 1996;270:C1388–C1397.

Orlowski J, Grinstein S. Na$^+$/H$^+$ exchangers of mammalian cells. *J Biol Chem* 1997;272:22373–22376.

Rosskopf D, Dusing R, Siffert W. Membrane sodium-proton exchange and primary hypertension. *Hypertension* 1993;21:607–617.

Siczkowski M, Davies JE, Ng LL. Na$^+$–H$^+$ exchanger isoform 1 phosphorylation in normal Wistar-Kyoto and spontaneously hypertensive rats. *Circ Res* 1995;76:825–831.

Wakabayashi S, Fafournoux P, Sardet C, et al. The Na$^+$/H$^+$ antiporter cytoplasmic domain mediates growth factor signals and controls "H$^+$-sensing." *Proc Natl Acad Sci USA* 1992;89:2424–2428.

CHAPTER A7 ■ CELLULAR POTASSIUM TRANSPORT

JASON X.-J. YUAN, MD, PhD AND MORDECAI P. BLAUSTEIN, MD

KEY POINTS

■ High intracellular K$^+$ concentration in vascular smooth muscle cells is maintained by the Na$^+$, K$^+$ pump [Na$^+$,K–adenosine triphosphatase (ATPase)].

■ In vascular smooth muscle cells (VSMCs), activity of K$^+$ channels affects membrane potential, cytosolic free Ca^{2+} concentration, and tonic constriction.

■ Multiple types of K$^+$ channels are expressed in VSMC: voltage-gated, Ca^{2+}-activated, and adenosine triphosphate (ATP)-sensitive.

■ Endothelium-derived relaxing factors regulate vascular tone by affecting K$^+$ channel activity.

■ Dysfunction of K$^+$ channels in VSMC is associated with membrane depolarization, increased Ca^{2+} concentration, and arterial hypertension.

See also Chapters A6, **A8,** and A10

Na$^+$, K$^+$-adenosine triphosphatase and inward transport of K$^+$

Potassium ions are actively transported into virtually all mammalian cells against the electrochemical K$^+$-gradient caused by the ouabain-sensitive Na$^+$, K$^+$ pump [Na$^+$, K$^+$–adenosine triphosphatase (ATPase), which expels three Na$^+$ ions in exchange for two entering K$^+$ ions (**Figure A7.1**). Energy for this process is provided by hydrolysis of the terminal high-energy phosphate bond of adenosine triphosphate (ATP). The Na$^+$, K$^+$ pump can concentrate K$^+$ approximately 20-fold in cells and can therefore extrude Na$^+$ against approximately a 20-fold concentration gradient. This transport is electrogenic, with 1 net positive charge extruded during each cycle. The resulting current flow usually adds approximately 1 to 2 mV to the resting membrane potential (E_m) caused by ion gradients and permeabilities. The Na$^+$, K$^+$ pump can therefore compensate for the loss of K$^+$ through various types of K$^+$-permeable channels.

K$^+$ channels and depolarization

The E_m in vascular smooth muscle cells (VSMCs) depends on Na$^+$, K$^+$, and Cl$^-$ concentration gradients across the plasma membrane and the relative ion permeabilities (P) as given by:

$$E_m = 58\log\frac{(P_{Na}[Na^+]_{out} + P_K[K^+]_{out} + P_{Cl}[Cl^-]_{cyt})}{(P_{Na}[Na^+]_{cyt} + P_K[K^+]_{cyt} + P_{Cl}[Cl^-]_{out})}$$

where *out* and *cyt* refer to the extracellular (out) and cytosolic (cyt) ion concentrations. In resting VSMC, E_m is controlled primarily

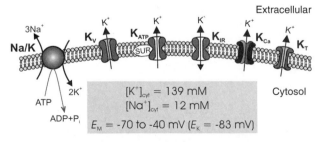

Figure A7.1 Schematic diagram showing inward transportation of K$^+$ through Na$^+$, K$^+$ ATPase (Na/K) and K$^+$ efflux through voltage-gated (K$_V$), ATP-sensitive (K$_{ATP}$), inward rectifier (K$_{IR}$), Ca^{2+}-activated (K$_{Ca}$), and two-pore domain (K$_T$) K$^+$ channels in the plasma membrane. The resting membrane potential (E_m), which is close to the K$^+$ equilibrium potential (E_K), is primarily determined by activities of the electrogenic Na$^+$, K$^+$ ATPase and various K$^+$ channels. ATPase, adenosine triphosphatase; ATP, adenosine triphosphate.

by K^+ permeability and gradient, because $P_K \gg P_{Cl} > P_{Na}$. K^+ permeability is directly related to the whole-cell K^+ current ($I_K = N \cdot i \cdot P_o$, where N is the number of membrane K^+ channels, i is the amplitude of the single-channel K^+ current, and P_o is the steady-state probability that the K^+ channel is open). When K^+ channels close, P_K and I_K decrease and the cell's E_m becomes less negative (i.e., the membrane depolarizes). When K^+ channel gene expression is inhibited, N and I_K decrease, also causing membrane depolarization.

K$^+$ currents and channels

At least five types of K^+ currents have been described in VSMC: background, voltage-gated, Ca^{2+}-activated, ATP-sensitive, and inward rectifier. These currents are carried by four corresponding K^+ channels: two-pore domain, voltage-gated, Ca^{2+}-activated, and inward rectifier. Voltage-gated and Ca^{2+}-activated channels are composed of two structurally distinct types of subunits: large pore-forming α subunits, and small cytoplasmic β subunits. The kinetics and gating of the K^+ channels encoded by certain α subunits can be dramatically affected by their associated β subunits. Different K^+ channel subunits (α and β) also coassociate *in vivo* to yield a larger number of functionally distinct K^+ channels.

Two-pore domain K$^+$ channels.

Two-pore domain K^+ (K_T) channels, which are voltage-insensitive and constitutively active, contribute to setting, maintaining, and regulating K^+ efflux and resting E_m in VSMC. K_T channels are not sensitive to classical K^+ channel blockers (e.g., 4-aminopyridine, or tetraethylammonia) but are sensitive to quinine, quinidine, and zinc. K_T channels are also regulated by changes in pH, arachidonic acid, general anesthetics, and mechanical stimulation. Acid-sensitive and mechanogated K_T currents play an important role in the regulation of vascular tone.

K_T channels have structures unlike any other K^+ channels. In contrast to other types of K^+ channels (see subsequent text), functional K_T channels are homo- or heterodimers (instead of tetramers) with four transmembrane domains and two ion-conducting pores. The known mammalian K_T channel subfamily consists of 14 members that can be functionally divided into five classes: weak inward rectifiers, acid-sensitive outward rectifiers, the lipid-sensitive mechanogated channels, the halothane-inhibited channels, and alkaline-activated background channels.

Voltage-gated K$^+$ channels.

Voltage-gated K^+ (K_V) channels of VSMC carry a rapidly inactivating A-type current, a slowly inactivating delayed rectifier current, and a noninactivating delayed rectifier current. All of these are activated within the range of resting E_m in VSMC, with unitary conductances of 5 to 65 picoSiemens (pS). Functionally, noninactivating or slowly inactivating delayed rectifier K_V currents are major determinants of resting E_m and therefore, intracellular Ca^{2+} concentration ($[Ca^{2+}]_{cyt}$) and tonic tension in VSMC. Inhibition of K_V channels by four aminopyridine (4-AP) or hypoxia depolarizes the pulmonary VSMC, induces Ca^{2+}-dependent action potentials, raises $[Ca^{2+}]_{cyt}$, and causes vasoconstriction. In contrast, activation of K_V channels by nitric oxide hyperpolarizes VSMC, closes voltage-gated Ca^{2+} channels, and causes vasodilation.

Native K_V channels are homo- or heterotetramers composed of four identical or similar α-subunits and probably four β-subunits. The α-subunit consists of six transmembrane domains (S1 through S6), a pore-forming region (H5, located in the

loop between the S5 and S6 domains), and cytoplasmic N- and C-termini. Segment S4 is the voltage sensor. There are at least 13 subfamilies of K_V channel α-subunits [$K_V 1$ through $K_V 11$, K_V long QT syndrome (LQT), and *eag*]. Four ($K_V 5$, $K_V 6$, $K_V 8$, and $K_V 9$) are electrically silent modulatory α-subunits, whereas the remainder are functional α-subunits. There are three subfamilies of β-subunits: $K_V \beta 1$ through $K_V \beta 3$.

Ca^{2+}-activated K$^+$ channels.

Ca^{2+}-activated K^+ (K_{Ca}) channels are the major Ca^{2+}-regulated channels. By opening when Ca^{2+} enters cells or $[Ca^{2+}]_{cyt}$ rises, K_{Ca} channels may contribute to negative feedback regulation of E_m and vascular tone. There are three types of K_{Ca} channels: small-conductance (4–14 pS; SK channels), intermediate-conductance (100–200 pS; IK channels), and large-conductance (200–285 pS; BK or maxi-K channels). Apamin blocks SK channels but negligibly affects BK and IK channels. BK channels are very sensitive to charybdotoxin (from scorpion venom) and tetraethylammonium. Voltage and Ca^{2+} gating for K_{Ca} channels are synergistic; therefore, K_{Ca} channels play a critical role in coupling changes in $[Ca^{2+}]_{cyt}$ to changes in E_m. K_{Ca} channels are half-maximally activated between +12 and +30 mV, and most are closed in VSMC under resting conditions [where $E_m = -60$ to -40 mV and $(Ca^{2+})_{cyt} = 50$–100 nmol/L]. Toxins that inhibit K_{Ca} channels enhance evoked membrane depolarization and elevation of $[Ca^{2+}]_{cyt}$ in stimulated VSMC. Normally, K_{Ca} channels control E_m and vascular tone by negative feedback regulation of the degree of membrane depolarization caused by myogenic factors and vasoactive substances.

The α subunit of the BK channel is encoded by the slowpoke gene (*Slo*), first identified in *Drosophila*. The channel protein shares extensive homology with the K_V channels of the Shaker ($K_V 1$) subfamily. In 1996, the small-conductance, apamin-sensitive K_{Ca} channel was also cloned; it has a membrane topology similar to those of K_V and BK channels; the β1 subunit of the BK channel tunes the Ca^{2+} sensitivity and voltage dependence of this channel. Deletion of the gene that encodes this subunit reduces the Ca^{2+} sensitivity of BK channels at any given E_m.

Inward rectifier K$^+$ channels.

Rectifiers conduct current in only one direction. K_{IR} channels conduct inward K^+ current (but little outward current) and can be blocked by intracellular Mg^{2+} or Cs^+ or external Ba^{2+}. K_{IR} channels in VSMC help set and regulate resting E_m, prevent membrane hyperpolarization by electrogenic Na^+, K^+–ATPase, mediate K^+-induced vasodilation, and minimize loss of cell K^+. In contrast to K_V, K_{Ca} or K_T channels, K_{IR} channels contain only two transmembrane domains (M1 and M2). Heteromultimeric combinations of different K_{IR} channel subunits form distinct K^+ additional channels; for example, the acetylcholine-sensitive, G protein–gated K^+ channel is a heteromultimer of two distinct types of K_{IR} subunits, $K_{IR} 3.1$ and $K_{IR} 3.4$.

Adenosine triphosphate-sensitive K$^+$ channels.

ATP-sensitive K^+ (K_{ATP}) channels are inhibited by intracellular ATP and activated by adenosine diphosphate (ADP). They fall into two categories: low-conductance (10–50 pS) and large-conductance (130 pS) channels that are voltage-independent. Sulfonylurea agents such as glibenclamide are selective blockers of K_{ATP} channels, whereas cromakalim and pinacidil are selective K_{ATP} channel openers. In coronary and cerebral arteries, metabolic regulation of basal tone and blood flow involves modulation of K_{ATP} channels. During hypoxia or ischemia, ATP falls and ADP rises. This activates K_{ATP} channels, hyperpolarizes VSMC, and contributes to vasodilation. K_{ATP} channels are heteromultimers: Four $K_{IR} 6.2$ (pore-forming) subunits and four sulfonylurea receptor (SUR1) subunits are required to form a K_{ATP} channel. $K_{IR}6.2$ also serves as the ATP sensor, whereas SUR1 confers sensitivity to sulfonylureas, channel openers like diazoxide, and ADP.

Role of K⁺ channels in regulating membrane potential, Ca²⁺ concentration, and vascular tone

Owing to the voltage dependence of sarcolemmal voltage-gated Ca^{2+} channels, E_m plays an important role in regulating intracellular Ca^{2+} in VSMC. Closure or inactivation of K^+ channels lowers E_m (depolarizes), which increases $[Ca^{2+}]_{cyt}$ by opening voltage-gated Ca^{2+} channels. This influx of Ca^{2+} causes vasoconstriction. In contrast, opening or activation of K^+ channels hyperpolarizes VSMC, closes voltage-gated Ca^{2+} channels, and causes vasodilation. Many vasodilators activate K^+ channels, including β-adrenergic agonists, muscarinic agonists, and nitroglycerin. Endothelium-derived relaxing factors (e.g., nitric oxide and prostacyclin) open K_V and K_{Ca} channels in pulmonary and systemic vessels. Antihypertensive drugs such as diazoxide and cromakalim also open K_{ATP} channels.

Ca^{2+} entry through voltage-gated Ca^{2+} channels raises $[Ca^{2+}]_{cyt}$. This activates Ca^{2+}- and ryanodine-sensitive sarcoplasmic reticulum (SR) Ca^{2+}-release channels. The coordinated opening of clusters of these SR channels produces "Ca^{2+} sparks," which contribute to the global elevation of $[Ca^{2+}]_{cyt}$ and VSMC contraction. Ca^{2+} sparks that occur in regions of SR adjacent to the plasma membrane may activate nearby BK channels or Ca^{2+}-activated Cl^- channels. Opening the latter depolarizes VSMC and thereby exerts positive feedback on the rise in $[Ca^{2+}]_{cyt}$. Opening of BK channels, however, hyperpolarizes VSMC and exerts a potent negative feedback effect on the $[Ca^{2+}]_{cyt}$ elevation and contraction. Therefore, SR Ca^{2+} release contributes to positive and negative feedback regulation of vascular smooth muscle contraction.

Dysfunctional K⁺ channels and hypertension

Defective K^+ channels and downregulated K^+ channel gene expression have been implicated in some types of hypertension and pulmonary hypertension. In systemic (renal and mesenteric) VSMC from spontaneously hypertensive rats, voltage-gated (K_V) and cromakalim-activated (K_{ATP}) K^+ channels are decreased compared with normotensive rats. In pulmonary VSMC from patients with idiopathic pulmonary arterial hypertension, K_V current is significantly attenuated compared with control cells. Hypoxia and the anorexic agent fenfluramine can cause pulmonary hypertension clinically and in pulmonary VSMC, both hypoxia and fenfluramine reduce the four AP-sensitive K_V current, depolarize E_m, and increase $[Ca^{2+}]_{cyt}$. These observations fit the view that dysfunctional K^+ channels in pulmonary and systemic VSMC may play an etiologic role in the development of pulmonary and systemic hypertension.

Suggested Readings

Blaustein MP. Physiological Effects of endogenous ouabain: control of intracellular Ca^{2+} stores and cell responsiveness. *Am J Physiol* 1993;264:C1367–C1387.

Blaustein MP, Zhang J, Chen J, et al. How does salt retention raise blood pressure? *Am J Physiol Regul Integr Comp Physiol* 2006;290:R514–R523.

Carl A, Lee HK, Sanders KM. Regulation of ion channels in smooth muscles by calcium. *Am J Physiol* 1996;271:C9–C34.

Cook NS. The pharmacology of potassium channels and their therapeutic potential. *Trends Pharmacol Sci* 1988;9:21–28.

Jaggar JH, Porter VA, Lederer WJ, et al. Calcium sparks in smooth muscle. *Am J Physiol Cell Physiol* 2000;278:C235–C256.

Lesage F, Lazdunski M. Molecular and functional properties of two-pore-domain potassium channels. *Am J Physiol Renal Physiol* 2000;279:F793–F801.

Nelson MT, Quayle JM. Physiological roles and properties of potassium channels in arterial smooth muscle. *Am J Physiol* 1995;268:C799–C822.

Yuan X-J. Voltage-gated K^+ currents regulate resting membrane potential and $[Ca^{2+}]_i$ in pulmonary arterial myocytes. *Circ Res* 1995;77:370–378.

Yuan X-J, Tod ML, Rubin LJ, et al. NO hyperpolarizes pulmonary artery smooth muscle cells and decreases the intracellular Ca^{2+} concentration by activating voltage-gated K^+ channels. *Proc Natl Acad Sci U S A* 1996;93:10489–10494.

CHAPTER A8 ◼ CALCIUM TRANSPORT AND CALMODULIN

DAVID J. TRIGGLE, PhD, DSc (Hon.)

KEY POINTS

- Intracellular calcium is a critical determinant of the stimulus–response paradigm, including excitation–contraction and stimulus–secretion coupling, gene activation, and cell death.
- Calcium is stored in intracellular pools, including mitochondria, sarcoplasmic reticulum (SR) of vascular smooth muscle cells (VSMC), and endoplasmic reticulum (ER) of neurons, from which it is transiently released through the action of the numerous receptors, pumps and channels that actively regulate intracellular calcium.
- Calmodulin, a Ca^{2+}-binding protein, is the most important transducer of intracellular Ca^{2+} signals; it can exist as Ca^{2+}-bound or unbound forms and functions in many different signal transduction pathways involving protein kinases, ion channels, protein phosphatases (e.g., calcineurin), and nitric oxide synthase.
- Calmodulin acts in a temporally and spatially heterogeneous manner that parallels the heterogeneous activation and distribution of Ca^{2+}; its expression is encoded by a family of nonallelic genes that are highly conserved across species.
- Movement of Ca^{2+} into cells occurs through ligand-gated (receptor-operated) channels and through six types of voltage-gated Ca^{2+} channels, two of which (T- and L-types) are of particular cardiovascular significance.

See also Chapters A6, A7, and **A10**

Intracellular calcium

Calcium is a cation of critical significance in many diverse cellular control mechanisms, serving as a ubiquitous second messenger and, in excitable cells, as a current-carrying species. Both roles serve to link events at the plasma membrane with cellular responses, including muscle contraction, hormone and neurotransmitter release, gene activation, cell cycling, fertilization, and cell death or destruction. Calcium is therefore both a physiologic and a pathologic cation—one that both brings us into and takes us out of this world.

Calcium gradients. During excitation, intracellular Ca^{2+} concentration rises by either (a) Ca^{2+} entry through the plasma membrane through voltage- or ligand-gated ion channels, or (b) release from intracellular stores. Ca^{2+} sensors that control the activities of pumps, enzymes, and other targets detect these increased Ca^{2+} levels and trigger events that restore intracellular Ca^{2+} to physiologically low pre-excitation levels.

In resting states, there is an extremely high Ca^{2+} gradient and intracellular free ionized Ca^{2+} is maintained at very low levels ($<5 \times 10^{-8}$ mol/L) despite high extracellular concentrations (in the millimolar range). Plasma Ca^{2+} levels are themselves tightly regulated through a triumvirate of hormones: vitamin D, parathyroid, and calcitonin. During stimulation, intracellular Ca^{2+} concentration can rise up to 200-fold (to approximately 10^{-5} mol/L); these elevated concentrations are coupled to cellular responses through a homologous group of Ca^{2+} binding proteins that serve as intracellular Ca^{2+} sensors, including the ubiquitous calmodulin.

Calcium sparks. Changes in intracellular Ca^{2+} are spatially and temporally heterogeneous, and localized "hot spots" or "sparks" are observed, together with waves of Ca^{2+} that are propagated through excited cells. These oscillations may represent a graded signal being converted into digital signals, the sequential activation of Ca^{2+}-demanding processes that require different timing of signals, or different concentrations of Ca^{2+}. Heterogeneity of Ca^{2+} mobilization likely serves as a mechanism that protects the cell against the deleterious consequences of persistently elevated Ca^{2+} levels.

Regulation of cellular calcium stores

Ca^{2+} movements are tightly regulated by the various Ca^{2+} regulatory processes depicted in **Figure A8.1**. These processes are not

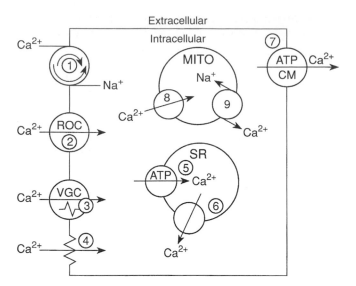

Figure A8.1 The regulation of cellular Ca^{2+} movements. (*1*) Na^+/Ca^{2+} exchanger; (*2*) Receptor-operated (ligand-gated) channels; (*3*) Voltage-gated channels; (*4*) Store-operated channels; (*5*) Adenosine triphosphate (ATP)–dependent Ca^{2+} uptake into sarcoplasmic reticulum; (*6*) Ca^{2+} release channel; (*7*) ATP-dependent pump across the plasma membrane; (*8,9*) Mitochondrial (MITO) transport processes. CM, calmodulin, ROC, receptor-operated channel; SR, sarcoplasmic reticulum; VGC, voltage-gated channel.

of equal importance in every cell type but all cells maintain mechanisms that permit Ca^{2+} influx, efflux, storage, and mobilization that are critical to the maintenance of overall cellular Ca^{2+} homeostasis. Adenosine triphosphate (ATP)-dependent pumps direct Ca^{2+} to two principal reservoirs: the [sarcoplasmic reticulum (SR) or endoplasmic reticulum (ER)] and the extracellular space.

Sources. Two principal sources of Ca^{2+} are used in cellular signaling: that which enters across the plasma membrane, or that released from intracellular stores (SR or ER or mitochondria). Ca^{2+} mobilization by either route can give rise to "elementary calcium events:" representing the opening of single channels. These elementary events can be visualized as the "sparks" and "puffs" seen in fluorescent dye-labeled cells.

Ligand-gated channels. Plasma membrane signals can increase intracellular Ca^{2+} through several processes. G protein–coupled receptors (e.g., the angiotensin AT1 receptor) and tyrosine kinases typically mobilize Ca^{2+} through inositol triphosphate (IP_3) receptors, with subsequent Ca^{2+} release from the ER stores. The IP_3 receptor of the plasma membrane is a large, relatively nonselective cation channel that mediates relatively slow Ca^{2+} entry, compared to the fast Ca^{2+} release mediated by IP_3 receptors in the ER. A second process involves intracellular Ca^{2+} release activated by Ca^{2+} entry. The channel involved here, the Ca^{2+} release-activated channel (CRAC), is associated with a transmembrane protein ORAI1 that is defective in patients with severe combined immune deficiency (SCID). Transient receptor potential channels (TRPs) may also be associated with store-operated Ca^{2+} release.

Voltage-gated channels. Of particular importance to the cardiovascular system is Ca^{2+} mobilization through voltage-gated channels (VGCs). Defects in Ca^{2+} regulation appear to contribute to a variety of pathologic states, including the abnormal vascular smooth muscle cells (VSMCs) tone or reactivity. Other "molecular diseases" associated with defects in Ca^{2+} channels include malignant hyperthermia (ryanodine receptor),

hypokalemic periodic paralysis, and hypertension (L-type voltage-gated Ca^{2+} channel).

Calmodulin

Expression of the intracellular Ca^{2+} signal requires the presence of intracellular sensors or receptors. Calmodulin and the other members (~200) of this protein family bind to calcium with micromolar affinity and undergo conformational changes linked to effector regulation. These proteins share a common Ca^{2+}-binding motif: the EF hand (a helix-loop-helix structure).

Structure. Calmodulin is a 148-residue protein with four EF hands, two each at the C- and N-terminal domains. Calcium binding to these hands is a cooperative process accompanied by significant conformational changes in protein structure. In these changes, the α-helical content of the protein increases. The C- and N-terminal domains become separated and then connected through the α-helix to form a dumbbell-shaped structure. The helix allows calmodulin to interact with many different effector proteins that typically contain calmodulin-binding domains constituted by 9 to 26 amino acid residue amphipathic helices. Because of this large number of interacting partners, calmodulin is a highly conserved species.

Function. Calmodulin is found in all neural, smooth muscle and nonmuscle cells, where it regulates large families of intracellular Ca^{2+}-dependent proteins, including cyclic nucleotide phosphodiesterase, adenylyl cyclase, Ca^{2+}-adenosine triphosphatase, phosphorylase kinase, phospholipase A_2, nitric oxide synthase, voltage-gated Ca^{2+} channels, IP_3 and ryanodine receptors, transcription factors (including the cyclic adenosine monophosphate response element binding protein), serum response factor and CAAT-enhancer binding protein, and the several proteins involved in vesicle-driven neurotransmitter release.

Interactions. Calmodulin interacts reversibly with many targets that have K_D values in the nanomolar range, but it also functions as an integral subunit of other targets including inducible nitric oxide synthase and the ryanodine receptor. The dynamic association of calmodulin with its target is determined by the limiting stoichiometric availability of the protein. Competition among targets facilitates cross-talk between multiple calmodulin-sensitive signaling pathways. Additional diversity and specificity of function are achieved through a variety of regulatory processes; these include use of fully, intermediate and non–Ca^{2+}-ligated forms of the protein, the use of at least eight different mRNAs, selective compartmentalization in the cell, posttranslational modification, and differential phosphorylation. Calmodulin exhibits exceptional conformational flexibility and in the presence of Ca^{2+} can adopt a number of conformations according to the target binding sequence.

Ca^{2+}/calmodulin-dependent protein kinases

Subtypes. Calmodulin activates members of the serine/tyrosine protein kinase family referred to as *Ca^{2+}/calmodulin-dependent protein kinases* (CaM kinases), including CaM kinases I, II, III, and IV, phosphorylase kinase, and myosin light-chain kinase. These kinases share a similar domain structure but differ functionally according to whether they can interact with several substrates (CaM kinase I, II, and IV) or have a single substrate (phosphorylase kinase, myosin light-chain kinase, and CaM kinase III). The general architecture of these kinases includes an N-terminal kinase domain followed by an autoinhibitory domain and a calmodulin-binding domain; for phosphorylase kinase and CaM kinase II, a C-terminal oligomerization domain is also present. The role of Ca^{2+}/CaM is to bind to the protein and remove the autoinhibitory domain that functions as a pseudosubstrate, allowing substrate access.

Localization and activation chacteristics. CaM kinases are also distinguished by their localization and activation characteristics. The multifunctional CaM kinases (I and II) are ubiquitously expressed in the cytoplasm, whereas CaM kinase IV is more limited in its nuclear and cytoplasmic localization. CaM kinase II, the best characterized of the CaM kinases, is encoded by four separate genes—α, β, γ, and δ—and their alternate splicing yields a total of 24 subtypes; every cell contains at least one subtype of this kinase. Activation of the CaM kinases depends on their primary interaction with calmodulin but may also be further achieved by phosphorylation. CaM kinases I and IV are phosphorylated in the activation loop embedded within the catalytic domain and CaM kinase IV also undergoes autophosphorylation to achieve further activation. This autoregulatory process confers significant activity on CaM kinase II even in the absence of Ca^{2+}/CaM ("autonomous activity") and provides an ability to translate Ca^{2+} transient frequencies into graded levels of effector activation. The CaM kinases are themselves part of a regulatory cascade being activated by other kinases—that is, CaM kinase kinases. CaM kinase I and IV are activated by CaM kinase kinases α and β, which may themselves be activated by other upstream kinases.

Calcium pumps

The two principal pumps involved in the control of poststimulus Ca^{2+} levels are located in the SR or ER and plasma membrane (**Figure A8.1**). Ca^{2+} activation of these pumps provides a critical link between Ca^{2+}-mobilizing processes and cellular recovery from elevated intracellular Ca^{2+} levels. The CaM-dependent adenosine triphosphatase of the plasma membrane is widely distributed across eukaryotic cells. In nonmuscle cells, the role of the plasma membrane pump appears to be minor. Both pumps are of the P-type and can be distinguished from the multimeric F- and V-types. The P-type pumps form an energized acylphosphate intermediate that is coupled to Ca^{2+} transport through the interconversion of E1 and E2 states. The cardiac isoform of the pump is regulated by phospholamban, an inhibitory protein which, when phosphorylated through adenosine monophosphate and CaM kinase, dissociates, removing the pump inhibition. Pump activity is also modulated by acidic phospholipids and polyunsaturated fatty acids, notably phosphatidylinositol and its phosphorylated derivatives. Additionally, inhibitors such as thapsigargin bind with subnanomolar affinity to the pump, trapping it in a "dead end" conformation.

Calcium channels

The two major types of calcium channels are widely distributed in excitable tissues. These are the voltage-sensitive (voltage-gated) channels and the (relatively) voltage-independent (ligand-gated) channels.

Voltage-gated Ca^+ channels. Voltage-gated Ca^{2+} channels are widely distributed in excitable tissues, including the cardiovascular system. They enjoy a heterogeneous tissue- and cell-specific expression that underlies in significant part their physiologic and pharmacologic specificities.

Subclasses. At least six major classes of voltage-gated Ca^{2+} channels exist in the cardiovascular and nervous systems: T, L, N, P, Q, and R (Ca_V1, Ca_V2, and Ca_V3) classes. These channels are distinguished by their electrophysiologic and pharmacologic characteristics, their functions, and their localizations. The T- ($Ca_V3.1$–3.3) and L-type ($Ca_V1.1$–1.4) channels are of particular importance to the functional pharmacology of the cardiovascular system. The L-type channel is the site of action of the therapeutically important Ca^{2+} channel blockers (including diltiazem, verapamil, nifedipine, and the second-generation 1,4-dihydropyridines such as amlodipine and isradipine).

Structure and function. Voltage-gated Ca^{2+} channels belong to an ion channel "superfamily" that includes Na^+ and K^+ channels. The channels have a heteromeric structure with the principal α subunit possessing the channel pore and gating mechanisms as well as the ligand binding sites. The properties of this channel subunit are substantially modified by the presence of other subunits, notably β subunits.

Regulation of activity. The activities of voltage-gated Ca^{2+} channels are regulated by their associations with calmodulin, parallel to the behavior of other ion channels, including Ca^{2+}-activated big conductance K^+ channels and cyclic nucleotide–gated channels. Calmodulin association with the L-type channels of the cardiovascular system is of particular importance mediating both channel closing during depolarization (Ca^{2+}-dependent inactivation or CDI) and prolonged opening during depolarization (Ca^{2+}-dependent facilitation or CDF). CDI of the CaV1.2 channel is mediated through the binding of a single calmodulin molecule.

Voltage-independent (ligand-gated) Ca^{2+} channels. Some evidence suggests that ligand-gated and store-operated channels may belong to the same protein family—the TRP channel type; α-adrenergic and angiotensin II receptors are examples of TRP channels. Two classes of ligand-gated Ca^{2+} channels control intracellular release of calcium: IP3- and ryanodine-sensitive channels that are linked to G protein–coupled receptors and to Ca^{2+} influx, respectively. Both types of channels show biphasic sensitivity to Ca^{2+} with low concentrations of Ca^{2+} serving to activate and mediate Ca^{2+} release and high Ca^{2+} serving to blunt or inhibit activation. The low-dose stimulatory effect of Ca^{2+} underlies the phenomenon of "Ca^{2+}-induced Ca^{2+} release", mediated through CRAC.

Suggested Readings

Carafoli E, Klee C, eds. *Calcium as a cellular regulator*. New York: Oxford University Press, 1999.

Haling DB, Aracena-Parks P, Hamilton SL. *Regulation of voltage-gated Ca^{2+} channels by calmodulin*. Science STKE 2005; re15., 2005.

Hook SS, Means AR. Ca^{2+}/CaM-Dependent kinases: from activation to function. *Annu Rev Pharmacol Toxicol* 2001; 41: 471–508.

Kortvely E, Gulya K. Calmodulin, and various ways to regulate its activity. *Life Sci* 2004;74:1065–1070.

Means AR. Regulatory cascades involving calmodulin-dependent protein kinases. *Mol Endocrinol* 2000;14:4–13.

Parekh AB. Cracking the calcium entry code. *Nature* 2006;441:163–165.

Soderling TR, Chang B, Brickey D. Cellular signaling through multifunctional Ca^{2+}/calmodulin-dependent protein kinase II. *J Biol Chem* 2001;276:3719–3722.

Toutenhoofd SL, Strehler EE. The calmodulin multigene family as a unique case of genetic redundancy: multiple levels of regulation to provide spatial and temporal control of calmodulin pools. *Cell Calcium* 2000;28:83–96.?

Triggle DJ. Calcium channel antagonists: clinical uses – past, present and future. *Biochem Pharmacol* 2007;74:1–9.

Sonkusare S, Fraer M, Marsch JD, et al. New strategies to circumvent hypertension. *Mol Interv* 2006;6:311–314.

CHAPTER A9 ■ REACTIVE OXYGEN SPECIES AND MEDIATORS OF OXIDATIVE STRESS

RHIAN M. TOUYZ, MD, PhD

KEY POINTS

■ The major reactive oxygen species (ROS) in cardiovascular biology are superoxide, hydroxyl (OH·) ion, hydrogen peroxide, nitric oxide (NO·), and peroxynitrite.
■ Many vascular enzyme systems generate superoxide but nonphagocytic nicotinamide adenine dinucleotide phosphate [NAD(P)H] oxidase is the most important; NAD(P)H oxidases are a group of related enzymes (the Nox family) of which seven members have been characterized (Nox1, Nox2, Nox3, Nox4, Nox5, Duox1, and Duox2).
■ NAD(P)H oxidase is regulated by growth factors, cytokines, physical forces, and vasoactive agents.
■ Superoxide and hydrogen peroxide are signal transduction intermediates that activate signaling cascades and reduction–oxidation-sensitive transcription factors that regulate cell growth, endothelial function, inflammatory responses, and extracellular matrix deposition.
■ Oxidative stress, a consequence of increased formation of ROS or decreased antioxidant reserve, can cause cardiovascular damage.

See also Chapters **A25,** A30, A31, **A63,** and A65

Metabolism of biologically important reactive oxygen species

Reactive oxygen species (ROS), also termed *oxygen-derived species* or *oxidants,* are produced as intermediates in reduction–oxidation (redox) reactions leading from O_2 to H_2O. ROS are reactive chemical entities comprising two major groups: free radicals [e.g., superoxide ($\cdot O_2^-$), hydroxyl (OH·), nitric oxide (NO·)], and nonradical derivatives of O_2 (e.g., H_2O_2, $ONOO^-$) (**Table A9.1**). A free radical is any species capable of independent existence (therefore the term *free*) that contains one or more unpaired electrons. The unpaired electron imparts high reactivity and renders the radical unstable. Nonradical derivatives are less reactive and more stable with a longer half-life than free radicals. When oxygen accepts electrons to its orbitals, it is "reduced" and functions as a strong oxidizing agent. The sequential univalent reduction of O_2 is

$$O_2 \xrightarrow{e-} \cdot O_2^- \xrightarrow{e-} H_2O_2 \xrightarrow{e-} OH \cdot \xrightarrow{e-} H_2O + O_2$$

Superoxide radical. Superoxide is produced by the 1-electron reduction of O_2 by enzymatic catalysis or by electron leaks from electron transfer reactions: $O_2 \rightarrow \cdot O_2^-$. In biologic fluids, $\cdot O_2^-$ is short-lived owing to its rapid reduction to H_2O_2 by superoxide dismutase (SOD). Superoxide can act as an oxidizing agent (and is reduced to H_2O_2) or as a reducing agent (donating its extra electron to NO· to form $ONOO^-$). NO· reacts with $\cdot O_2^-$ at rates near diffusion-limitation and is therefore one of the few biomolecules able to "out compete" SOD for $\cdot O_2^-$. Hence, in most biologic systems, unless NO· levels are very high, production of $\cdot O_2^-$ usually results in H_2O_2 formation.

Hydrogen peroxide. Of the many ROS generated in vascular cells, H_2O_2 seems to be particularly important because it is relatively stable and uncharged. Hydrogen peroxide is lipid

TABLE A9.1

BIOLOGICALLY IMPORTANT REACTIVE OXYGEN SPECIES

Free radicals (species with an unpaired electron)	
$\cdot O_2^-$	Superoxide anion radical
OH·	Hydroxyl radical
ROO·	Lipid peroxide
$RO_2\cdot$	Peroxyl
NO·	Nitric oxide
Nonradicals	
H_2O_2	Hydrogen peroxide
HOCl	Hypochlorous acid
$ONOO^-$	Peroxynitrite
O_3	Ozone
$^1O_2$	Singlet oxygen

soluble, easily diffusible within and between cells, and is stable under physiologic conditions. H_2O_2 is only a weak oxidizing and reducing agent and is generally poorly reactive. In the presence of myeloperoxidase and chloride ion, H_2O_2 forms hypochlorous acid, followed by the formation of other nonradical oxidants, including singlet oxygen ($^1O_2$). Hypochlorous acid is highly reactive and can damage biomolecules, both directly and by decomposing to form chlorine. H_2O_2 is also a precursor of OH·. The main source of H_2O_2 in vascular tissue is the dismutation of $\cdot O_2^-$: $2 \cdot O_2^- + 2H^+ \rightarrow H_2O_2 + O_2$. This reaction can be spontaneous or catalyzed by SOD. The SOD-catalyzed dismutation is favored when the concentration of $\cdot O_2^-$ is low and the concentration of SOD is high, which occurs normally. Three mammalian SOD isoforms are known: copper/zinc SOD (SOD1), mitochondrial SOD (Mn SOD, SOD2), and extracellular SOD (SOD3).

Hydroxyl radical. OH· radical is generated by two major reactions from H_2O_2: the Fenton reaction, in which H_2O_2 decomposes by accepting an electron from a reduced metal ($Fe^{2+} + H_2O_2 \rightarrow Fe^{3+} + OH\cdot + OH^-$), and the Haber-Weiss reaction, in which OH· is generated by the interaction of $\cdot O_2^-$ and H_2O_2 ($\cdot O_2^- + H_2O_2 \rightarrow O_2 + H_2O + OH\cdot$). OH· radicals are highly reactive (and unstable), and unlike $\cdot O_2^-$ and H_2O_2, which travel some distance from their sites of generation, OH· principally induces local damage.

Peroxynitrite. Peroxynitrite is a potent oxidant formed from the reaction between $\cdot O_2^-$ and NO· in a 1:1 stoichiometry: NO· $+ \cdot O_2^- \rightarrow ONOO^-$. A major regulator of $ONOO^-$ formation is the concentration of NO·. When the level of NO· increases and overcomes dismutation by SOD (e.g., during ischemia, reperfusion, or both), $ONOO^-$ is produced. This reaction is biologically significant because NO· and $\cdot O_2^-$ can antagonize each other's biologic actions and because $ONOO^-$ is a very powerful oxidizing species. The toxic effect of $ONOO^-$ and its protonated form, peroxynitrous acid, derive from oxidation of zinc fingers, protein thiols, and membrane lipids. Intermediates are formed from the heterolytic cleavage of $ONOO^-$ to OH· and nitronium ion (NO_2^+), catalyzed by the transition metal of SOD and myeloperoxidase. Nitration of protein tyrosine residues produces 3-nitrotyrosine, which is often used as an assay for $ONOO^-$ activity in tissue and blood.

Vascular ROS and nicotinamide adenine dinucleotide phosphate

General features. Superoxide anion, H_2O_2, OH·, and $ONOO^-$ are all produced to varying degrees in the cardiovascular system. Enzymes that generate (intra)cellular $\cdot O_2^-$ include mitochondrial oxidases, xanthine oxidase, cyclooxygenase, lipoxygenase, NO· synthase, heme oxygenases, hemoproteins (heme and hematin), peroxidases, and the nicotinamide adenine dinucleotide phosphate [NAD(P)H] oxidases (**Figure A9.1**). Oxygen derivatives, which are tightly regulated under physiologic conditions, act as second messengers to control cardiac, renal and vascular function, and structure. Biochemically, ROS act by oxidative modification of nucleic acids, sugars, lipids, and proteins. This leads to DNA damage and to regulated signaling through the inactivation of enzymes such as protein tyrosine phosphatases, which results in increased tyrosine kinase and mitogen-activated protein (MAP) kinase activity. To preserve the cellular redox balance, to control cell signaling and to prevent potentially damaging actions, ROS are scavenged by antioxidant systems, including

glutathione peroxidase (GTP), thioredoxin, catalase (CAT), SOD and antioxidant enzymes.

Perturbation of the balance between ROS production and scavenging results in oxidative stress (enhanced susceptibility of biological molecules to reaction with ROS) and presumably to pathophysiologic changes and cardiovascular disease. A central determinant of the specific biological consequences of cellular ROS production relates largely to the enzymatic source of ROS generation, especially with respect to redox signaling. In the cardiovascular system, the primary source of ROS is NAD(P)H oxidase.

NAD(P)H oxidase. This multisubunit enzyme catalyzes $\cdot O_2^-$ production by the 1-electron reduction of O_2 using NADPH or NADH [hence the parentheses in NAD(P)H] as the electron donor: $2O_2 + NADPH \rightarrow 2O_2^- + NADP^+ + H^+$. The prototypical NAD(P)H oxidase is found in neutrophils and has five subunits: p47phox ("phox" or *ph*agocyte *ox*idase), p67phox, p40phox, p22phox, and the catalytic subunit gp91phox (also termed *Nox2*) (**Figure A9.1**). In unstimulated cells p47phox, p67phox and p40phox, exist in the cytosol, whereas p22phox and gp91phox are in the membrane, where they occur as a heterodimeric flavoprotein, cytochrome b558. On stimulation, p47phox becomes phosphorylated and the cytosolic subunits form a complex that translocates to the membrane, where it associates with cytochrome b558 to assemble the active oxidase, which in turn transfers electrons from the substrate to O_2 to form $\cdot O_2^-$. Activation also requires participation of Rac 2 (or Rac 1) and Rap 1A. Although NAD(P)H oxidases were originally found in phagocytic cells involved in host defense and innate immunity, discovery of gp91phox homologs indicates that there is an entire family of NAD(P)H oxidases.

The new homologs, along with gp91phox, are now designated the Nox family of NAD(P)H oxidases. The family includes seven members, including Nox1, Nox2 (formerly termed *gp91phox*), Nox3, Nox4, Nox5, Duox1, and Duox2. They are expressed in many tissues and mediate diverse biological functions (**Tables A9.2, A9.3**). Nox1 is found in colon and vascular cells and plays a role in host defense and cell growth; Nox2 is the catalytic subunit of the respiratory burst oxidase in phagocytes, but is also expressed in vascular, cardiac, renal and neural cells; Nox3 is found in fetal tissue and the adult inner ear and is involved in vestibular function; Nox4, originally termed *Renox* (renal oxidase) because of its abundance in the kidney, is also found in vascular cells and osteoclasts; Nox5 is a Ca^{2+}-dependent homolog found in testis and lymphoid tissue but also in vascular cells. Duox1 and 2 are thyroid Nox enzymes involved in thyroid hormone biosynthesis. While all Nox proteins are present in rodents and man, mouse and rat genomes do not contain the *nox5* gene. The regulation and function of each Nox remains unclear but it is evident that Nox enzymes participate in normal biological responses. They are also believed to contribute to cardiovascular and renal disease, including hypertension and atherosclerosis. Nox1 has been implicated in the pathogenesis of Ang II-dependent hypertension because Nox1-deficient mice have reduced blood pressure (BP) and attenuated pressor responses to Ang II. As expected, mice that overexpress Nox1 exhibit enhanced pressor responses to Ang II and exaggerated vascular remodeling. Other NAD(P)H oxidase subunits, such as p22phox and p47 phox, have also been implicated in the pathogenesis of Ang II-dependent hypertension.

Regulation of NADPH activity. How NADPH components interact in cardiovascular cells to generate $\cdot O_2^-$ is not fully

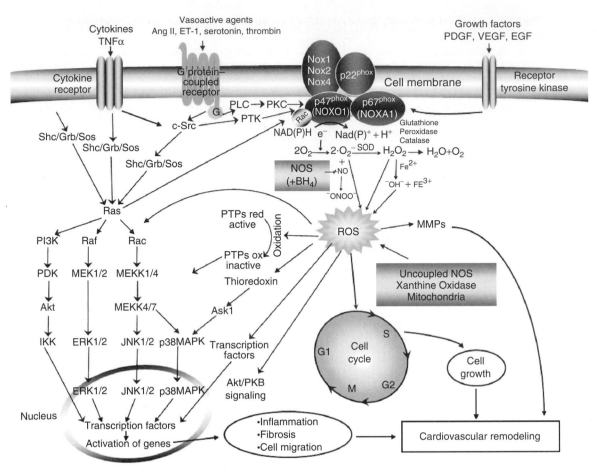

Figure A9.1 Generation of reactive oxygen species (ROS) in cardiovascular cells. The major source of $\cdot O_2^-$ in vascular cells is a multisubunit enzyme, [NAD(P)H] oxidase. Multiple Noxes, including Nox1, Nox2, Nox4, and Nox5 have been identified in cardiovascular cells. Other enzymes, including uncoupled nitric oxide synthase (NOS), xanthine oxidase, and mitochondrial enzymes, also contribute to $\cdot O_2^-$ formation in cardiovascular tissue, but their role is minor. $\cdot O_2^-$ is dismutated by superoxide dismutase (SOD) to form H_2O_2, which is converted by CAT or GTP to H_2O. ROS activate many signaling pathways, which regulate vascular function. Increased production of ROS leads to increased cell growth, altered vasomotor tone, inflammation and fibrosis, which contribute to cardiovascular remodeling and endothelial dysfunction, characteristic features of hypertensive vascular damage. $\downarrow$, decreased; $\uparrow$, increased; TNF, tumor necrosis factor; PDGF, platelet-derived growth factor; VEGF, vascular endothelial growth factor; EGF, epidermal growth factor; PTP, protein tyrosin phosphatase; PTPs red, reduced PTP (active form); PTP ox, oxidized PTP (inactive form); PDK, 3-phosphoinositide–dependent protein kinase; IKK, IκB kinase; MEK, mitogen-activated protein kinase kinase; MEKK, MEK kinase; ERK, extracellular signal-regulated kinase; JNK, c-Jun NH$_2$ terminal kinase; PKB, protein kinase B; MMP, matrix metalloproteinase; NOXO1, [NAD(P)H] oxidase organizer 1; NOXA1, NADPH oxidase activator 1.

known. All Noxes appear to have an obligatory need for p22phox, whereas Nox2 requires p47phox and p67phox for its activity. Nox1 may interact with the recently identified homologs of p47phox and p67phox, namely NAD(P)H oxidase organizer 1 (NOXO1) and NAD(P)H oxidase activator 1 (NOXA1). Oxidase activation involves Rac translocation, phosphorylation, and translocation of p47phox (possibly with p67phox and p47phox associated with cytochrome b558). Vascular NAD(P)H oxidase is responsive to several growth factors (platelet-derived growth factor, epidermal growth factor, and transforming growth factor β), cytokines (tumor necrosis factor-α, interleukin-1, and platelet aggregation factor), mechanical forces (cyclic stretch, laminar and oscillatory shear stress), metabolic factors (hyperglycemia, hyperinsulinemia, free fatty acids, advanced glycation end products (AGE) and G protein–coupled receptor agonists (serotonin, thrombin, bradykinin, endothelin, and angiotensin II (Ang II).

Ang II is an important and potent regulator of cardiovascular NAD(P)H oxidase through AT$_1$ receptor activation and stimulation of signaling pathways involving c-Src p21^{Ras}, PKC, PLD, and PLA$_2$. Ang II also influences NAD(P)H oxidase activation through transcriptional regulation of oxidase subunits.

Antioxidant defenses

Antioxidants are defined as substances present at low concentrations relative to an oxidizable substrate that significantly delay or prevent oxidation of that substrate. Living organisms have evolved a number of antioxidant defenses to survive chronic oxidative stress (**Table A9.4**). These mechanisms are different in their intracellular and extracellular compartments and include enzymatic and nonenzymatic types. The major intracellular enzymatic antioxidants are SOD, CAT, and GTP. SOD catalyzes

TABLE A9.2

TISSUE DISTRIBUTION, FUNCTION AND REGULATORS OF NOX ENZYMES

Enzyme	Site of expression	Function	Regulators
Nox1	Colon, vessels Muscle, prostate, uterus	Host defense? BP regulation	p22phox, NOXO1, NOXA1, Rac1
Nox2	Phagocytes Vessels, heart, Kidneys	Host defense Signaling?	p22phox, p47phox, p67phox, Rac1/2
Nox3	Fetal tissue, inner ear	Otoconia biosynthesis	p22phox, NOXO1, Rac1
Nox4	Kidney, vessels, bone	O_2 sensing? Vasoregulation? Erythropoietin synthesis? Signaling?	p22phox
Nox5	Lymph nodes, testes	Signaling?	?
Duox1/2	Thyroid, lung, salivary glands, GIT	Hormone synthesis Signaling? Host defense?	??

BP, blood pressure; GIT, gastrointestinal tract; NOXO1, NADPH oxidase organizer 1; NOXA1, NADPH oxidase activator 1; ?, possible function; ??, unknown regulator.

the dismutation of $\cdot O_2^-$ into H_2O_2 and O_2. H_2O_2 is then decomposed by CAT and GTP into H_2O and O_2. CAT is especially important when H_2O_2 concentrations are high. GTP uses reduced glutathione (GSH) to convert H_2O_2 to H_2O, and, in the process, oxidizes glutathione. This enzyme is important when H_2O_2 concentrations are low. GTP is the major enzyme protecting the cell membrane against lipid peroxidation, because GSH donates protons to the membrane lipids, maintaining them in a reduced state. Because of its extremely high reactivity, there are no specific scavengers of OH·. However, numerous nonspecific antioxidants, such as α-tocopherol (vitamin E) and ascorbic acid (vitamin C), scavenge OH· as well as other radicals. Low antioxidant bioavailability promotes cellular oxidative stress.

Pathophysiologic effects of cardiovascular NAD(P)H oxidases

ROS influence cell growth, migration, proliferation, and activation. Physiologically, NAD(P)H oxidase-derived ROS have been implicated in the regulation of vascular tone. H_2O_2 may

have direct or indirect vasodilator actions through decreased NO bioavailability by favoring quenching by $\cdot O_2^-$ to form $ONOO^-$. ROS, through the regulation of hypoxia-inducible factor-1 (HIF-1), are also important in O_2 sensing, which is essential for maintaining normal O_2 homeostasis. ROS appear to exert important effects on processes such as inflammation, endothelial dysfunction, cell proliferation, migration/activation, extracellular matrix deposition, fibrosis, angiogenesis, and cardiovascular remodeling. These processes may contribute directly or indirectly to hypertension, atherosclerosis, diabetes mellitus, cardiac failure, and myocardial ischemia-reperfusion injury.

Antioxidant therapy limitations. Treatment with antioxidants has been found to be effective in certain experimental animal disease models and in small clinical studies but data from large clinical trials have not demonstrated benefits. The poor response to antioxidant vitamins in man may be related to the need for much higher doses of scavengers needed to deliver sufficient quantities of active compound to injury sites at the appropriate moment. Newer research is focused on inhibiting specific Noxes rather than trying to scavenge existing ROS with biologically inefficient and nonspecific antioxidants such as vitamins C and E.

TABLE A9.3

MRNA EXPRESSION OF NOX ISOFORMS IN CARDIOVASCULAR CELLS

Enzyme	VSMC	Endothelial cells	Fibroblasts	Cardiomyocytes
Nox1	+	+	+	−
Nox2	+	+	+	+
Nox3	−	−	−	−
Nox4	+	+	+	+
Nox5	Human VSMCs	HUVEC	Human cardiac	−
Duox1	+	−	−	−

VSMC, vascular smooth muscle cells; HUVEC, human umbilical vein endothelial cells.
+, denotes presence of Nox isoform.
−, denotes absence of Nox isoform.

TABLE A9.4

ANTIOXIDANT DEFENSE MECHANISMS

Enzymatic defense enzymes	
Superoxide dismutase (SOD)	$2 \cdot O_2^- + 2H^+ \xrightarrow{SOD} H_2O_2 + O_2 \cdot$
Catalase (CAT)	$2H_2O_2 \xrightarrow{CAT} O_2 + H_2O$
Glutathione peroxidase	$2GSH + H_2O_2 \xrightarrow{GTP} GSSG + 2H_2O$
(GTP)	$2GSH + ROOH \xrightarrow{GTP} GSSG + ROH + H_2O$
Nonenzymatic scavengers	
Vitamins—A, β-carotene, C (ascorbic acid), E (α-tocopherol)	
Transferrin, lactoferrin	
Ceruloplasmin	
Urate	
Bilirubin	
Albumin	
Cysteine	
Flavonoids	
Sulfhydryl group	

GSH, reduced glutathione; GSSG, oxidized glutathione; R, lipid chain.

Suggested Readings

Babior BM. NADPH oxidase: an update. *Blood* 1999;93(5):1464–1476.

Berk BC. Redox signals that regulate the vascular response to injury. *Thromb Haemost* 1999;82(2):810–817.

Cave AC, Brewer AC, Panicker AN, et al. NADPH oxidases in cardiovascular health and disease. *Antioxid Redox Signal* 2006;8:691–727.

Dikalova A, Clempus R, Lassegue B, et al. Nox1 overexpression potentiates angiotensin II-induced hypertension and vascular smooth muscle hypertrophy in transgenic mice. *Circulation* 2005;112(17):2668–2676.

Droge W. Free radicals in the physiological control of cell function. *Physiol Rev* 2001;82:47–95.

Fridovich I. Superoxide anion radical, superoxide dismutases, and related matters. *J Biol Chem* 1997;272:18515–18517.

Geiszt M. NADPH oxidases: new kids on the block. *Cardiovasc Res* 2006;71:289–299.

Griendling KK, Sorescu D, Lassegue B, et al. Modulation of protein kinase activity and gene expression by reactive oxygen species and their role in vascular physiology and pathophysiology. *Arterioscler Thromb Vasc Biol* 2000;20:2175–2183.

Halliwell B, Gutteridge JMC. *Free Radicals in Biology and Medicine*, 3rd ed. New York: Oxford University Press, 2000.

Matsuno K, Yamada H, Iwata K, et al. Nox1 is involved in angiotensin II-mediated hypertension: a study in Nox1-deficient mice. *Circulation* 2005; 112(17):2677–2685.

McIntyre M, Bohr DF, Dominiczak AF. Endothelial function in hypertension. The role of superoxide anion. *Hypertension* 1999;34:539–545.

Thannickal VJ, Fanburg BL. Reactive oxygen species in cell signaling. *Am J Physiol* 2000;279:L1005–L1028.

Touyz RM, Schiffrin EL. Reactive oxygen species in vascular biology: implications in hypertension. *Histochem Cell Biol* 2004;122(4):339–352.

CHAPTER A10 ■ VASCULAR SMOOTH MUSCLE CONTRACTION AND RELAXATION

RITA C. TOSTES, PhD; ROMULO LEITE, PhD AND R. CLINTON WEBB, PhD

KEY POINTS

- The dynamic degree of phosphorylation of myosin light chain (MLC) regulates the interaction of myosin and actin and the contraction of vascular smooth muscle cells (VSMCs).
- Regardless of the external stimulus, intracellular events controlling VSMC contraction are ultimately dependent on: (a) the intracellular calcium ion (Ca^{2+}) concentration and (b) the degree of phosphorylation and cross-bridge cycling between the contractile proteins myosin and actin.
- Ca^{2+}-dependent activation of MLC kinase and Ca^{2+}-independent regulation of MLC phosphatase (MLCP) together dynamically determine the proportional degrees of MLC phosphorylation and tonic VSMC contraction.
- Following removal of a contractile stimulus, dilation occurs as a result of decreased intracellular Ca^{2+} and increased MLCP activity.

See also Chapters A1, A2, A3, A4, A5, and **A8**

In order for the organism to respond efficiently to a wide variety of external and internal stresses, local and systemic blood flow must be continuously adjusted. The tonic contractile state of vascular smooth muscle cells (VSMCs) is the primary determinant of arterial luminal diameter, which affects pressure and flow characteristics. Physiologic adjustments in arteriolar tone depend on the contractile state of VSMC, which responds to a wide variety of systemic and local physiologic influences, including the sympathetic nervous system, vasoactive hormones, autocrine and paracrine agents (such as endothelium-derived factors), and local chemical signals.

VSMC contraction can be initiated by changes in membrane potential, but mainly depends on changes in input signals from receptor-activated signaling cascades or from alterations in mechanical deformation (stretch/changes in load or length). Regardless of the external stimulus, intracellular events controlling VSMC contraction ultimately depend on (a) the intracellular calcium ion (Ca^{2+}) concentration and (b) the degree of phosphorylation and cross-bridge cycling between the contractile proteins myosin and actin.

Alterations in the regulatory processes maintaining intracellular Ca^{2+} and MLC phosphorylation, as well as their upstream regulatory products, are possible contributors to vasoconstriction and impaired vasodilation in chronic hypertension.

Calcium and vasoconstriction

Ca^{2+}–calmodulin-dependent activation of myosin light chain.

Phosphorylation of the 20-kDa light chain of myosin (MLC) enables the myosin–actin interaction to occur. The sequence is initiated by Ca^{2+}–calmodulin-dependent activation of MLC kinase (MLCK). As the intracellular Ca^{2+} concentration $[(Ca^{2+})_i]$ increases, Ca^{2+} combines with calmodulin, a member of the family of EF -hand Ca^{2+}-binding proteins, causing a conformational change in the calmodulin molecule.

The Ca^{2+}–calmodulin complex interacts with MLCK, exposing its catalytic site and leading to MLCK activation, which then phosphorylates Ser19 of MLC (**Figures A10.1**). In all muscle cells, energy released from adenosine triphosphate (ATP) by myosin adenosine triphosphatase (ATPase) activity results in the cycling of myosin–actin cross-bridges and VSMC contraction.

Cellular calcium flux.

Cytosolic Ca^{2+} increases on either Ca^{2+} entry from the extracellular space or its release from intracellular stores, mainly the sarcoplasmic reticulum (SR). Ca^{2+} entry is mainly mediated by Ca^{2+} channels in the plasma membrane. Voltage-gated Ca^{2+} channels, such as L-type Ca^{2+} channels, open in response to changes in the membrane potential of the cell, brought on by receptor activation or by increased intraluminal pressure/stretch of the smooth muscle cell.

Ligand-dependent vasoconstriction

Binding of a vasoconstrictor agonist (e.g., norepinephrine, angiotensin II, or endothelin) to heterotrimeric G protein–coupled receptors stimulates phospholipase C (PLC) activity, resulting in the production of inositol trisphosphate (IP₃) and diacylglycerol (DAG) from the membrane lipid phosphatidylinositol 4,5 bisphosphate (PIP₂). The binding of IP₃ to receptors on the SR results in the release of Ca^{2+} into the cytosol, whereas DAG, along with Ca^{2+}, activates protein kinase C (PKC), which phosphorylates specific target proteins, such as L-type Ca^{2+} channels.

Intracellular calcium waves and sparks.

Receptor activation also causes increased Ca^{2+} oscillations or "wave" activity in VSMCs. Within the vessel wall, individual cells may exhibit asynchronous Ca^{2+} oscillations (Ca^{2+} transients) during agonist stimulation. Therefore, in contrast to the "global" $[Ca^{2+}]_i$ measured by conventional imaging methods, the actual intracellular $[Ca^{2+}]_i$ signal varies both spatially and temporally, as has been

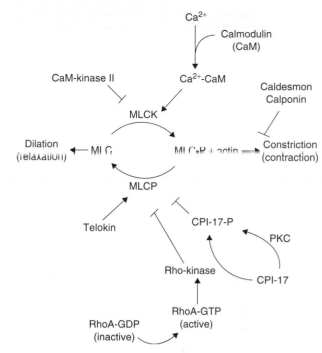

Figure A10.1 Contractile regulation of vascular smooth muscle. Activity of myosin light chain kinase (MLCK) and myosin light chain phosphatase (MLCP) dynamically regulate the phosphorylation state of the 20-kDa light chain of myosin (MLC), and therefore the interaction of myosin and actin for contraction. Various signaling molecules can affect MLCK and MLCP activation, and therefore modulate cellular contraction. CaM, calmodulin; CaM-kinase II, Ca^{2+}/CaM-dependent protein kinase; CPI-17, 17-kDa smooth muscle–specific myosin phosphatase inhibitor; PKC, protein kinase C; GDP, guanosine diphosphate; GTP, guanosine triphosphate. (Courtesy of: Tostes RC, Leite R, Webb RC. Department of Physiology, Medical College of Georgia, Augusta, Georgia 30912.)

demonstrated by high-resolution confocal microscopy. In addition to the plasma membrane and SR, mitochondria have recently been shown to contribute to the regulation of intracellular Ca^{2+} distribution (see Chapter A8). Ca^{2+} oscillations depend on the function of the SR and are primarily associated with IP₃-induced Ca^{2+} release. Highly localized increases in $[Ca^{2+}]_i$ termed Ca^{2+} *sparks* occur in close proximity to the cell membrane after activation of ryanodine receptors in the SR. Sparks can influence the activity of neighboring KCa channels, modulating membrane potential and therefore voltage-dependent Ca^{2+} inflow.

Vasodilation through intracellular Ca^{2+}-lowering

Vasodilation occurs when intracellular Ca^{2+} is decreased. Several mechanisms have been implicated in the lowering of cytosolic Ca^{2+}, including Ca^{2+}, Mg-ATPases in the SR and in the plasma membrane, Na^+-Ca^{2+}–exchangers and, in some cases, mitochondria.

Ca^{2+}, Mg-adenosine triphosphatases.

Ca^{2+} uptake into the SR, which is dependent on ATP and magnesium (Mg^{2+}), decreases intracellular Ca^{2+} and elicits ATP hydrolysis and VSMC relaxation in parallel. Phosphorylated SR Ca^{2+}, Mg-ATPase binds two Ca^{2+} ions, which are then translocated to the luminal side of the SR and released. Mg^{2+} binds to the catalytic site of Ca^{2+}, Mg-ATPase to mediate the reaction, which is inhibited by vanadate, thapsigargin, cyclopiazonic acid, and phospholamban. Phosphorylation of phospholamban removes its inhibitory effect and stimulates ATP-dependent Ca^{2+} uptake. SR Ca^{2+}-binding proteins, such as calsequestrin and calreticulin, also contribute to decreased intracellular Ca^{2+} levels. Plasma membranes also contain Ca^{2+}, Mg-ATPases that aid the removal of Ca^{2+} from the cell. This enzyme differs from the SR protein in that it has an autoinhibitory domain that can be bound by calmodulin causing stimulation of the plasma membrane Ca^{2+} pump. It has been reported that the membrane Ca^{2+}, Mg-ATPases are localized in caveolae/rafts (sphingolipids and cholesterol membrane-rich domains involved in the lateral sorting of certain proteins during signal transduction events), with concentrations 18- to 25-fold higher in the caveolae membrane compared with the noncaveolae portion.

Na^+/Ca^{2+} exchange.
Due to colocalization with Na^+, K^+-ATPase on the plasma membrane near superficial portions of the SR, Na^+/Ca^{2+} exchangers are capable of functioning cooperatively with SR Ca^{2+}, Mg-ATPases to decrease intracellular Ca^{2+}. Membrane potential as well as transmembrane gradients of Na^+ and Ca^{2+} control its bidirectional activity, with the ultimate driving force being the Na^+,K^+-ATPase. This low affinity antiporter is closely coupled to intracellular Ca^{2+} and Na^+ levels.

Blockade of voltage-gated Ca^{2+} channels.
Voltage-gated L-type Ca^{2+} channels located on plasma membranes are important in Ca^{2+} influx and VSMC contraction. L-channel antagonists (dihydropyridine, phenylalkylamines, and benzothiazepines) bind to distinct receptors on the channel protein, inhibit Ca^{2+} entry, and promote vasorelaxation. Ca^{2+}-entry blockade is clinically effective in controlling hypertension.

Myosin light chain phosphatase activity and vasorelaxation

Overall MLC phosphorylation (and therefore tonic VSMC contraction) also depends on the Ca^{2+}-independent activity of MLC phosphatase (MLCP), which removes high-energy phosphates from MLC, promoting vasorelaxation (**Figure A10.1**). Dephosphorylated MLC leads to VSMC relaxation through the detachment of actin–myosin cross-bridges (**Figure A10.1**).

Ca^{2+}-dependent phosphorylation.
Lowering intracellular Ca^{2+} decreases the rate of myosin phosphorylation and increases MLCP activity, which is potentiated by phosphorylation of cytosolic inhibitor proteins. These proteins release the bound MLCP catalytic subunits, which then bind with the targeting subunits and together increase the affinity for MLC.

Subunit regulation of myosin light chain phosphatase.
MLCP consists of three major subunits: a 37-kDa catalytic subunit (PP1c), a 20-kDa variable subunit and a 110- to 130-kDa myosin-binding subunit (MYPT1), the latter of which, when phosphorylated, causes feedback inhibition of the enzymatic activity of MLCP. At the same time, MLCP activity in phasic smooth muscle contraction is stimulated by the 16-kDa protein, telokin.

RhoA.
The small G protein RhoA and its downstream target, Rho-kinase, play a direct role in the regulation of MLCP activity. Similar to other small G proteins from the Rho family, RhoA is activated on the binding of guanosine triphosphate (GTP). In the inactive state, RhoA is primarily cytosolic, and is bound to guanosine diphosphate (GDP) and a guanine dissociation inhibitor (GDI), which functions to stabilize the bound GDP. Exchange of GDP for GTP, and subsequent activation of RhoA, is facilitated by Rho-specific guanine nucleotide exchange factors (RhoGEFs), which can be activated by heterotrimeric receptor G protein subunits after agonist-receptor binding. The hydrolysis of bound GTP that results in the activation of RhoA requires the catalytic presence of a GTPase activating protein (GAP). The posttranslational addition of a geranyl phosphate onto RhoA enables its membrane binding, and in addition to GTP binding, is necessary for its activation.

Rho-kinase.
In the active state, RhoA engages downstream effectors, such as Rho-kinase, a serine/threonine kinase that phosphorylates the myosin-binding subunit of MLCP (MYPT1 Thr853), inhibiting its activity, and therefore promoting the phosphorylated state of MLC (**Figure A10.1**). When the bound GTP is hydrolyzed to GDP, RhoA returns to the inactive basal state. Y-27632, a selective inhibitor of Rho-kinase, induces relaxation of isolated agonist-contracted vasculature, and lowers blood pressure (BP) in hypertensive, but not normotensive, rats. Increased vasodilator response to Rho-kinase inhibition in hypertensive as compared to normotensive humans has also been demonstrated, suggesting that Rho-kinase contributes to elevated peripheral resistance.

Other modulators.
MLCP is inhibited by a downstream mediator of DAG/PKC, the 17-kDa smooth muscle–specific myosin phosphatase inhibitor (CPI-17) as well as by the phosphatase holoenzyme inhibitor (PHI)-1, one of the newest members of the family of protein phosphatase inhibitor proteins. Several kinases, including PKC and Rho-kinase, have been shown to phosphorylate CPI-17 (CPI-17 Thr38) and PHI-1, leading to inhibition of MLCP, thereby facilitating VSMC contraction. Phosphorylated CPI-17 is able to bind to the catalytic subunit of MLCP (PP1c) to inhibit the enzyme's activity. Therefore, Ca^{2+}-sensitization may involve Rho-kinase–mediated and PKC-mediated phosphorylation of CPI-17 to increase MLC phosphorylation and prolong smooth muscle contraction. In some circumstances, VSMC contraction is independent of either Ca^{2+} or MLC phosphorylation, depending instead on a mechanism involving PKC, as occurs during VSMC contraction elicited by phorbol dibutyrate (PDBu) and phosphatidylinositol 3-kinase (PI3-K). Calmodulin-dependent PKA II decreases the sensitivity of MLCK for Ca^{2+}, promoting vasodilation.

Caldesmon and calponin

Independent of MLC, proteins such as caldesmon and calponin modulate actin or actomyosin ATPase activity and influence cross-bridge cycling. Caldesmon is an actin-binding protein capable of inhibiting actomyosin ATPase activity and stabilizing actin filaments against actin-severing proteins. Caldesmon is encoded by a single gene that is alternatively spliced to generate two major isoforms: the longer, smooth muscle–specific h-caldesmon, and a shorter, non–muscle l-caldesmon. Caldesmon is a substrate of PKC, cdc2 kinase and Erk1/2 mitogen activated protein kinase (MAPK), and phosphorylation by either of these kinases induces its dissociation from actin, leading to the exposure of the myosin-binding sites on the actin surface, allowing actomyosin interactions and reversal of the inhibitory effects of caldesmon on the thin filament-associated protein.

Calponin and SM22α are also actin-binding proteins thought to modulate blood vessel contractility through inhibition of actomyosin ATPase activity and actin filament organization, respectively. Although these factors affect myosin or actin, the physiologic importance of these regulatory events still needs further investigation (**Figure A10.1**).

Suggested Readings

Barany M, Barany K. Protein phosphorylation during contraction and relaxation. In: Barany M, ed. *Biochemistry of smooth muscle contraction*, San Diego: Academic Press, 1996:321–339.

Hai C, Murphy R. Ca^{2+}, crossbridge phosphorylation, and contraction. *Annu Rev Physiol* 1989;51:285–298.

Hilgers RH, Webb RC. Molecular aspects of arterial smooth muscle contraction: focus on Rho. *Exp Biol Med (Maywood)* 2005;230:829–835.

Hirano K, Hirano M, Kanaide H. Regulation of myosin phosphorylation and myofilament Ca^{2+} sensitivity in vascular smooth muscle. *J Smooth Muscle Res* 2004;40:219–236.

Ito M, Nakano T, Erdodi F, et al. Myosin phosphatase: structure, regulation and function. *Mol Cell Biochem* 2004;259:197–209.

Morgan K. The role of calcium in the control of vascular tone as assessed by the Ca^{2+} indicator aequorin. *Cardiovasc Drugs Ther* 1990;4:1355–1362.

Ogut O, Brozovich FV. Regulation of force in vascular smooth muscle. *J Mol Cell Cardiol* 2003;35:347–355.

Somlyo A, Wu X, Walker L, et al. Pharmacomechanical coupling: the role of calcium, G-proteins, kinases and phosphatases. *Rev Physiol Biochem Pharmacol* 1999;134:201–234.

Su X, Smolock EM, Marcel KN, et al. Phosphatidylinositol 3-kinase modulates vascular smooth muscle contraction by calcium and myosin light chain phosphorylation-independent and -dependent pathways. *Am J Physiol* 2004;286:H657–H666.

Uehata M, Ishizaki T, Satoh H, et al. Calcium sensitization of smooth muscle mediated by a Rho-associated protein kinase in hypertension. *Nature* 1997;389:990–994.

SECTION II ■ VASOACTIVE SUBSTANCES

CHAPTER A11 ■ CATECHOLAMINE SYNTHESIS, RELEASE, REUPTAKE, AND METABOLISM

DAVID S. GOLDSTEIN, MD, PhD AND GRAEME EISENHOFER, PhD

KEY POINTS

- Norepinephrine [(NE), noradrenaline], epinephrine (EPI) (adrenaline), and dopamine (DA), the endogenous catecholamines, are chemical effectors of the sympathetic nervous, adrenomedullary hormonal, and dihydroxyphenylalanine (DOPA)-dopamine autocrine/paracrine systems.
- The main determinants of delivery of NE to its receptors are sympathetic nerve traffic and reuptake through the cell membrane NE transporter (Uptake-1).
- Catecholamines are metabolized by multiple enzymes, and plasma levels and urinary excretion rates of those metabolites have different sources and meanings.

See also Chapters **A12** and **C169**

Three endogenous catecholamines in humans, norepinephrine (NE) (noradrenaline), EPI (adrenaline), and dopamine (DA), act as effector chemicals of the sympathetic nervous, adrenomedullary hormonal, and dihydroxyphenylalanine (DOPA) DA autocrine/paracrine systems. All three systems play important roles in tonic and phasic cardiovascular regulation and responses.

Catecholamine synthesis

The enzymatic rate-limiting step in catecholamine synthesis is conversion of tyrosine to the catechol amino acid, 3,4-DOPA, catalyzed by tyrosine hydroxylase (TH) in **Figure A11.1**. This step requires tetrahydrobiopterin as a cofactor. A variety of cell types outside the central nervous system, including sympathetic neurons, adrenomedullary cells, and gastrointestinal parenchymal cells, express TH. Many tissues express L-aromatic-amino-acid decarboxylase (LAAAD), which catalyzes conversion of DOPA to

DA, using pyridoxal phosphate as a cofactor. Carbidopa inhibits this enzyme. In the kidneys, the main source of DA production is uptake and decarboxylation of DOPA by tubular cells.

After translocation of DA into vesicles that contain dopamine-ß-hydroxylase (DBH), DA undergoes conversion to NE, with ascorbic acid a cofactor. Phenylethanolamine-N-methyltransferase (PNMT), a cytoplasmic enzyme, catalyzes donation of a methyl group from S-adenosyl-methionine to NE, producing EPI (**Figure A11.2**).

Catecholamine release

Release of NE from sympathetic nerve endings and of EPI from adrenomedullary cells is by exocytosis, where vesicles containing the catecholamines fuse with the cell membrane, porate, and the vesicular contents diffuse into the extracellular fluid. The exocytosis results from processes initiated by depolarization

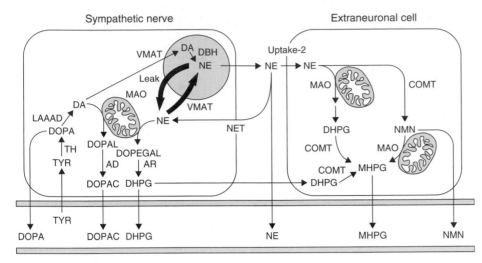

Figure A11.1 Diagram of steps in catecholamine biosynthesis, release, cellular uptake, and metabolism. VMAT, vesicular monoamine transporter; DA, dopamine; DBH, dopamine-ß-hydroxylase; NE, norepinephrine; NET, norepinephrine transporter; MAO, monoamine oxidase; LAAAD, L-aromatic-amino-acid decarboxylase; DOPA, dihydroxyphenylalanine; TH, tyrosine hydroxylase; TYR, tyramine; AD, alcohol dehydrogenase; AR, aldehyde reductase; DOPAC, dihydroxyphenylacetic acid; DHPG, dihydroxyphenylglycol; COMT, catechol-O-methyltransferase; NMN, normetanephrine.

of the cell membrane and entry of ionized calcium into the terminal. Nicotine potently stimulates ganglionic transmission and adrenomedullary secretion. Glucagon and angiotensin II also evoke adrenomedullary secretion, by binding to specific receptors on adrenomedullary cells.

Receptors on sympathetic nerves modulate release for a given amount of sympathetic nerve traffic. In humans, NE can feedback inhibit its own release, by occupying α-2 adrenoceptors on noradrenergic terminals. α-2 Adrenoceptor agonists such as clonidine therefore decrease release of NE from sympathetic nerves. Circulating EPI can augment NE release, by occupying β-2 adrenoceptors on the terminals. NE release can also occur nonexocytotically in response to drugs that displace vesicular NE (the most well known is tyramine) and in the setting of anoxic ischemia.

Catecholamine reuptake

Neuronal reuptake (Uptake-1) through the cell membrane norepinephrine transporter (NET) is the main means of inactivation of NE released from sympathetic nerves (**Figure A11.1**), especially in the heart. Tricyclic antidepressants and cocaine inhibit Uptake-1. Most of the NE taken up into the terminals is translocated into storage vesicles, through the vesicular monoamine transporter (VMAT). Reserpine inhibits the vesicular translocation. Nonneuronal uptake (Uptake-2), mediated by at least three different extraneuronal cell membrane transporters and followed by intracellular metabolism, is the main means of inactivation of circulating catecholamines.

Catecholamine metabolism

Catecholamines in cells undergo a complex metabolic fate, dependent on the actions of multiple enzymes, including monoamine oxidase (MAO), aldose reductase/aldehyde reductase (AR), aldehyde/alcohol dehydrogenase (AD), catechol-O-methyltransferase (COMT), and monoamine-preferring phenolsulfotransferase (PST).

Under resting conditions, the main determinant of NE turnover (irreversible loss of NE from a tissue) is net leakage from the vesicles into the axoplasm, an ongoing process independent of sympathetic nerve traffic (**Figure A11.1**). Some of the NE in the axoplasm is metabolized by MAO-A, which is present in the mitochondrial outer membrane. The resultant aldehyde, dihydroxyphenylglycolaldehyde (DOPEGAL) is mainly converted to dihydroxyphenylglycol (DHPG), catalyzed by AR. DHPG is the main neuronal metabolite of NE. During sympathetic stimulation, released NE is taken back up into the axoplasm through the Uptake-1 process, providing a second source of production of DHPG. Most of the DHPG produced in sympathetically innervated organs undergoes conversion to

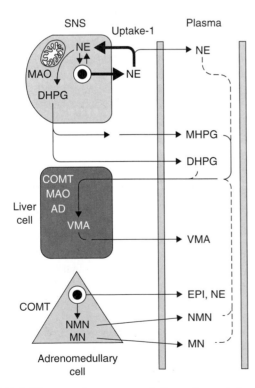

Figure A11.2 Diagram of sources and fate of catecholamines and their metabolites in plasma. SNS, Sympathetic Nervous System; NE, norepinephrine; MAO, monoamine oxidase; DHPG, dihydroxyphenylglycol; MHPG, methoxyhydroxyphenylglycol; COMT, catechol-O-methyltransferase; AD, alcohol dehydrogenase; VMA, vanillylmandelic acid; EPI, epinephrine; NE, norepinephrine; NMN, norepinephrine; MN, metanephrine.

methoxyhydroxyphenylglycol (MHPG) catalyzed by COMT, within the organ (**Figure A11.1**). In the liver, MHPG is converted to vanillylmandelic acid (VMA), catalyzed by AD (**Figure A11.2**), and in mesenteric organs MHPG is converted to MHPG-sulfate, catalyzed by PST. Therefore, the main end products of NE metabolism are VMA, MHPG, and MHPG-sulfate.

Adrenomedullary cells express COMT, which catalyzes conversion of NE to normetanephrine (NMN) and conversion of EPI to metanephrine (MN). Plasma levels of NMN arise partly from extraneuronal uptake of NE released from sympathetic nerves and partly from leakage of NE from storage vesicles into the cytoplasm of adrenomedullary cells (**Figure A11.2**). More than 90% of plasma MN is derived from EPI leaking from storage vesicles in adrenomedullary cells. Ongoing leakage and intracellular O-methylation help explain the extraordinary sensitivity of plasma unconjugated metanephrines (NMN and MN) for diagnosing pheochromocytoma.

DA in neuronal and extraneuronal cells is metabolized by MAO to form dihydroxyphenylacetaldehyde (DOPAL), which is rapidly metabolized further by AD to form dihydroxyphenylacetic acid (DOPAC, **Figure A11.1**). DOPAC in turn is O-methylated through COMT to form homovanillic acid, the main end product of DA metabolism. DA in nonneuronal cells is also extensively sulfoconjugated by monoamine-preferring PST to form DA sulfate. Another major end product of DA metabolism is 3-methoxytyramine sulfate, formed from the actions of COMT and monoamine-preferring PST on DA.

Human plasma normally contains six unconjugated catechols—DOPA, DA, NE, EPI, DHPG, and DOPAC—and two unconjugated metanephrines—NMN and MN (**Figure A11.2**). Because of the different sources of these compounds in sympathetic nerves, the adrenal medulla, and nonchromaffin cells, and the different enzymes and sites of enzymatic reactions leading to their formation, plasma levels of catechols and MNs have distinctly different meanings in terms of functions and dysfunctions of catecholamine systems.

Suggested Readings

Eisenhofer G, Kopin IJ, Goldstein DS. Catecholamine metabolism: a contemporary view with implications for physiology and medicine. *Pharmacol Rev* 2004;56:331–349.

Goldstein DS. *The autonomic nervous system in health and disease.* New York: Marcel Dekker Inc; 2001.

Goldstein DS. *Adrenaline and the inner world: an introduction to scientific integrative medicine.* Baltimore: The Johns Hopkins University Press; 2006.

Goldstein DS, Eisenhofer G, Kopin IJ. Sources and significance of plasma levels of catechols and their metabolites in humans. *J Pharmacol Exp Ther* 2003;305:800–811.

CHAPTER A12 ■ ADRENERGIC AND DOPAMINERGIC RECEPTORS AND ACTIONS

KATHLEEN H. BERECEK, PhD AND ROBERT M. CAREY, MD, MACP

KEY POINTS

- There are nine different adrenergic receptor (AR) subtypes in three main classes ($\alpha 1$, $\alpha 2$, and β) and five dopaminergic receptor (DR) subtypes in two main classes, D_1-like and D_2-like.
- ARs and DRs are coupled to G proteins and affect cells by altering intracellular calcium, cyclic nucleotides, inositol phosphates, and protein phosphorylation.
- Receptor desensitization and downregulation reduce responses of cells to continuous exposure to catecholamines.
- Alterations in ARs and DRs and their functions may play a role in hypertension, cardiac ischemia, congestive heart failure, nocturnal asthma, and obesity.

See also Chapters **A11,** C132, C133, and C140

ADRENERGIC RECEPTORS

Biologic actions

Adrenergic receptors (ARs) mediate cellular responses to the catecholamines norepinephrine (NE) and epinephrine (EPI). These hormones are secreted by the adrenal gland and are also released as neurotransmitters from adrenergic neurons within the central nervous system and postganglionic peripheral sympathetic neurons. Drugs targeting AR are among the most widely used therapeutic agents in clinical medicine.

TABLE A12.1

TISSUE DISTRIBUTION, RESPONSES, AND PHARMACOLOGY OF ADRENERGIC RECEPTOR SUBTYPES

Receptor	Physiology		Pharmacology	
	Tissue	Response	Agonists	Antagonists
$\alpha_{1A,B,C}$	Smooth muscle: vascular, iris, radial ureter, pilomotor, uterus, sphincters (gut, bladder)	Contraction	Methoxamine Phenylephrine	Prazosin Terazosin
	Smooth muscle (gut)	Relaxation		Doxazosin
	Heart	Positive inotropic ($\beta_1 \gg \alpha_1$), cell growth, hypertrophy		Corynanthine Phentolamine
	Salivary gland	Secretion		Phenoxybenzamine
	Adipose tissue	Glycogenolysis		
	Sweat glands	Secretion		
	Kidney (proximal tubule)	Gluconeogenesis, Na^+ reabsorption		
$\alpha_{2A,B,C,D}$	Presynaptic autoreceptor on sympathetic nerve endings	Inhibition of norepinephrine release	Guanfacine Clonidine	Yohimbine Piperoxan
	Platelets	Aggregation, granule release	α-Methyl-NE	Rauwolscine
	Endocrine pancreas	Inhibition of insulin release	Tramazoline	Phentolamine
	Adipose tissue	Inhibition of lipolysis	Xylazine	Phenoxybenzamine
	Vascular smooth tissue	Contraction	Guanadrel	
	Kidney	Inhibition of renin release (?)	Oxymetazoline	
β_1	Heart	Positive inotropic effect, positive chronotropic effect, cell growth, hypertrophy	Isoproterenol Prenaterol	Propranolol Betaxolol
	Adipose tissue	Lipolysis	Dobutamine	Atenolol
	Kidney	Renin release		Practolol Metoprolol
β_2	Liver	Glycogenolysis, gluconeogenesis	Isoproterenol	Propanolol
	Skeletal muscle	Glycogenolysis, lactate release	Terbutaline	Butoxamine
	Smooth muscle: bronchi, uterus, gut, vascular (skeletal muscle), detrusor	Relaxation	Salbutamol Rimiterol Albuterol	High concentration of β_1-antagonists
	Endocrine pancreas	Insulin secretion (?)		
	Salivary gland	Amylase secretion		
β_3	Adipose tissue	Lipolysis	BRL 37344	
	Striated muscle	Thermogenesis		

? = possible action.
NE, norepinephrine.

Catecholamines released during physical or emotional stress trigger coordinated AR-mediated cardiovascular and metabolic responses that affect the regulation of virtually every organ system (see Table A12.1). Activation of cardiac AR increases heart rate and contractile strength, whereas activation of these receptors in vascular smooth muscle increases blood pressure (BP) and directs blood flow to essential organs. AR activation on liver and adipose cells triggers the liberation of glucose and fatty acids. Stimulation of AR in the lungs leads to bronchodilation and in the central nervous system, sedation, and analgesia. Inhibition of AR results in vasodilation, decreased BP, and heart rate, and strengthening of contraction and relaxation of prostate smooth muscle. In addition to their physiologic functions, ARs have been linked to pathogenic processes in the heart such as myocyte apoptosis and hypertrophy which contribute to pathologic structural remodeling of the heart and ultimately to heart failure.

Characteristics of adrenergic receptors

ARs are G protein–coupled transmembrane receptors. On binding to ligands, the G proteins dissociate from the intracellular domain of the AR to propagate signals by modulating the activity of downstream effector molecules such as adenylyl cyclase, phosholipases, and ion channels. Each type of AR preferentially couples to a particular class of $G\alpha$ proteins.

Subtypes. AR subtypes, their tissue distributions, and the responses they mediate are shown in **Table A12.1**. Pharmacologic and molecular cloning studies have identified three families of AR receptors, each with three subtypes: α_1 receptors (α_{1A}, α_{1B}, α_{1D}); α_2 receptors (α_{2A}, α_{2B}, α_{2C}); and β receptors (β_1, β_2, β_3). All three α_1-AR subtypes couple to the $G_{q\alpha}$ pathway, resulting in stimulation of phospholipase C (PC) and generation of the second messengers inositol (1,4,5)-trisphosphate (IP_3) and diacylglycerol (DAG), the mobilization of intracellular Ca^{2+}, the activation of protein kinase C (PKC) and in some tissues, activation of Na^+–H^+ and Na^+–Ca^{2+} exchangers and activation or inhibition of K^+ channels. All three α_2-AR subtypes couple to G_i which inhibit cyclic adenosine 3′,5′-monophosphate (cAMP)-dependent protein kinase A (PKA). All three β-AR subtypes are Gs-coupled receptors, which activate the adenylyl cyclase–cAMP–PKA pathway.

Also included in **Table A12.1** are the pharmacologic agents that stimulate or inhibit various AR subtypes. As shown in this table, individual AR subtypes are not restricted to a single tissue location, with most tissues containing more than one AR subtype. The response of a cell will depend on the concentration of NE and EPI in the tissue, the AR subtypes and kinetics of the receptors on the cell, and the second messenger system(s) altered by occupancy of these receptors.

Signal transduction pathways. PKA and PKC phosphorylate a variety of proteins to modify their functions *in vivo*. Activated Gi and Gq can also couple to mitogen-activated protein kinase (MAPK) cascades to induce cell apoptosis or cell growth. Through varied interactions with ion channels and second messengers, different AR subtypes enable NE and EPI to have a broad range of physiologic actions.

Traditionally, a linear signaling cascade of ligand-AR subtype G protein–second messenger effector has been the accepted view of AR signal transduction; however, recent studies of AR have not only shown subtype-specific signaling but also promiscuous G protein coupling, time-dependent switching of intracellular signaling pathways, interactions within or between AR families, and G protein–independent signaling pathways. The linear signaling pathway has been replaced by a complex multidimensional "signalome" in which an individual AR can dynamically couple to multiple G proteins or other signaling or scaffold proteins in a temporally and spatially regulated manner and AR can form homodimers or heterodimers, resulting in pharmacologically and functionally distinct receptor populations. Evidence has been given for functional and intermolecular interactions between α_1-and β-AR subtypes in regulating cardiac cell growth and contractility. In addition, persistent stimulation of β-AR subtypes results in a time-dependent switch of signaling pathways eliciting different and, at times, opposite functional roles of these receptors in regulating cardiac structure and function. These new findings may have important pathogenic and therapeutic implications in heart disease.

Pharmacology and function of adrenergic receptors

ARs can be characterized physiologically or pharmacologically. It is important to note that the endogenous catecholamines, NE, and EPI, are agonists for all AR subtypes, although with varying affinities.

α_1-adrenergic receptors. α_1-AR located on postsynaptic cells in smooth muscle, heart, liver, vas deferens, and brain regulate smooth muscle contraction (i.e., vascular tone), myocardial inotropy, and hepatic glucose metabolism. α_1-AR subtypes are stimulated by the agonists, methoxamine and phenylephrine, and inhibited by antagonists such as prazosin, phentolamine, and doxazosin.

α_2-adrenergic receptors. α_2-ARs are located on both sides of the synaptic cleft, that is, presynaptically and postsynaptically. α_2-ARs function as autoreceptors on the presynaptic nerve terminals that synthesize and release NE; when activated by catecholamines, these α_2-ARs inhibit subsequent NE release, thereby dampening the output of the sympathetic nervous system (SNS). Conversely, blockade of α_2-AR facilitates release of NE from sympathetic nerve terminals. α_2-ARs are stimulated by clonidine, guanfacine, and α-methyl NE (formed from α-methyldopa) and are inhibited by yohimbine and rauwolscine.

β_1-adrenergic receptors. Activation of β_1-AR stimulates the rate and strength of cardiac contraction, lipolysis in fat cells, and renin release from the kidneys. This receptor is stimulated by isoproterenol, dobutamine, and prenaterol and inhibited by β blockers such as propranolol, betaxolol, etc. β_2-AR stimulation relaxes smooth muscle cells in bronchi, vasculature, uterus, gut, and bladder. This receptor is stimulated by isoproterenol, terbutaline, albuterol, salbutamol, and rimiterol and is inhibited by IPS 339 and ICI 118,551. The order of potency for stimulation of β_1-AR by catecholamines is isoproterenol > EPI = NE whereas for β_2-AR, the order of stimulatory potency is isoproterenol > EPI > NE.

Receptor regulation

Following stimulation, both α- and β-AR decrease their responses to further stimulation, that is, they are "desensitized" rapidly and downregulated following prolonged exposure to catecholamines.

α-adrenergic receptors. α-ARs are subject to dynamic regulation by a variety of mechanisms including phosphorylation, protein–protein interactions, protein trafficking and transcription, which produce homologous and heterologous desensitization. The mechanism of desensitization appears to involve both phosphorylation of agonist-occupied receptors and uncoupling of the phosphorylated receptor from G protein by β-arrestins.

β-adrenergic receptors. Regulation of β-AR involves modifications at several loci, including the gene itself.

Receptor phosphorylation. One cascade that decreases β-adrenergic responses includes phosphorylation of agonist-occupied receptors, uncoupling of the receptors from G proteins, and internalization of receptors from the membrane into the cytoplasm. Immediately following agonist presentation, β-AR kinase catalyzes phosphorylation of consensus sequences near the carboxy terminus (cytoplasmic domain) of the receptor. Subsequent events, including the actions of G proteins, cause internalization of the receptor, after which the receptor can either be degraded or reinserted into the plasma membrane.

Heterologous desensitization. In addition to desensitization and downregulation induced by the agonist itself (homologous desensitization), β-AR display heterologous desensitization. In this case, β-ARs become less responsive to agonists following stimulation of the same cell by a nonadrenergic adenylyl cyclase activator, such as another neurotransmitter. This phenomenon is associated with cyclic AMP activation of protein kinases and subsequent phosphorylation and desensitization of the β-AR at β-AR kinase or other phosphorylation sites.

Gene regulation. Long-term regulation of β-AR occurs principally at the gene level. Stimulation of β-AR modifies both the transcription rate and the steady-state level of β-AR messenger RNA. cAMP-responsive elements in the promoter region of the gene, as well as exposure of cells to several humoral agents (i.e., glucocorticoids and thyroid hormone), modify the expression of β-AR.

Implications for disease states. Alterations in AR structure and function may play a role in numerous disease states such as hypertension, cardiac ischemia, heart failure, cardiac and vascular hypertrophy, hypothyroidism, diabetes, morbid obesity, and asthma. Increased expression of AR in myocardial ischemia and hypertension and decreased expression of β-AR in heart failure have been reported as well as genetic polymorphisms in β_2-AR in patients with asthma and β_3-AR in patients with morbid obesity. Identification and further characterization of AR subtypes may lead to the development of new therapeutic agents which are highly selective, more effective, and have fewer side effects than currently available agents.

DOPAMINERGIC RECEPTORS

Dopamine (DA) is an endogenous catecholamine that is a precursor of NE and EPI and serves as a neurotransmitter in its own right. DA is released by postganglionic sympathetic neurons, dopaminergic neurons, and nonchromaffin tissues, especially renal proximal tubules and gastrointestinal epithelial cells. The vast majority of circulating DA derives from the kidney. DA modulates a variety of physiologic functions, including behavior, movement, nerve conduction, hormone synthesis and release, ion transport, vascular tone, and BP.

General characteristics

Subtypes. Peripheral dopaminergic receptors (DRs) have been divided into two major types: D_1-like and D_2-like (**Table A12.2**). Molecular studies have revealed five major subtypes (D_1 through D_5). D_1-like receptors include D_1 and D_5. D_2-like receptors include D_2, D_3, and D_4 receptors. DRs contain the seven transmembrane domains that characterize other G protein–coupled receptors. The D_1-like receptors have no introns

and are encoded by a single exon, whereas the D_2-like family is encoded by a mosaic of exons and contains introns within its protein-coding regions. Therefore, it is likely that the D_1- and D_2-like receptors derive from two different gene families.

Signal transduction mechanisms. D_1-like and D_2-like receptors induce two different types of signal transduction. One of these, the adenylyl cyclase pathway, is obligatory for all cell systems. D_1-like receptors are associated with stimulation and D_2-like receptors with inhibition of adenylyl cyclase. The other pathways include activation of calcium or potassium channels and stimulation of phosphoinositide hydrolysis and differ in different cells.

Distribution. In peripheral tissues, DRs are distributed in the SNS, the pituitary gland, the cardiovascular system, kidney, and adrenal cortex. Molecular studies suggest that peripheral D_1- and D_2-like receptors are identical to those in the central nervous system. D_1-like DRs are located postsynaptically in the heart (atrial and ventricular myocardium and coronary vessels), arterial blood vessels (vascular smooth muscle cells), adrenal cortex (zona glomerulosa), and kidney (proximal tubule, thick ascending loop of Henle, cortical collecting duct, and vascular smooth muscle).

Biologic effects

D_1-like receptor renal effects and natriuresis. Stimulation of D_1-like receptors by fenoldopam, a selective D_1-like DR agonist, leads to vasodilation (renal and systemic), diuresis, natriuresis, and a decrease in systemic BP without postural hypotension or increased plasma renin activity. DA-induced natriuresis is caused by an increase in renal blood flow and a decrease in tubular Na^+ reabsorption.

In proximal tubule cells, inhibition of Na^+ transport from the tubule lumen is mediated by stimulation of adenylyl cyclase, increased PKA activity, and inhibition of Na^+/H^+ exchanger-3 (NHE-3) activity at the apical (brush border) membrane.

TABLE A12.2

CLASSIFICATION OF DOPAMINE RECEPTORS

Group	Pharmacologic class				
	D_1-like group		D_2-like group		
G protein–coupling	Gs		Gi/Go		
Signal transduction	+AC	+AC	−AC		
	+PLC		+K^+ channel		
			−Ca^{2+} channel		
Group–selective agonists	Fenoldopam[a]		Bromocriptine[b]		
Group–selective antagonists	SCH 23390 and 39166[a]		YM-09151[b]		
	SKF 83566[a]				
Molecular biologic subclass	D_1	D_5	D_2	D_3	D_4
Subclass-selective agonists	None	None	091356A	PD128907	PD168077
				Pramipexole	(+)N-propyl-norapomorphine
				Quinelorane	
Subclass-selective antagonists	None	None	L-741,6626	Nafadotride	U-101958
				U-99, 194A21	L-745,870
			L-741,742		
			Raclopride	(+)AJ76	NGD-94
				(+)S14297	

+, stimulatory; −, inhibitory; AC, adenylyl cyclase; PLC, phospholipase C.
[a]Selective for D_1-like dopamine receptor but cannot distinguish D_1 from D_5.
[b]Selective for D_2-like dopamine receptor but cannot distinguish subtypes.

In the medullary thick ascending loop of Henle, DA acts through D_1-like receptors to increase cAMP-dependent protein kinase, which phosphorylates a protein, DARPP-32 (DA-related phosphoprotein), which phosphorylates basolateral membrane Na^+/K^+ adenosine triphosphatase, causing inactivation of this enzyme. D_1-like receptor-selective antagonists include SCH-23390, SCH-39166, LE-300, and SKF-83566.

DA synthesized in and released from renal proximal tubule cells is thought to act as a paracrine substance (cell-to-cell mediator) stimulating D_1-like DR on these cells to inhibit Na^+ reabsorption in tonic manner. Approximately 50% of basal Na^+ excretion can be attributed to tonic activation of renal proximal tubule D_1-like receptors. A defect in proximal tubule D_1 receptor–G protein complex recycling is present in spontaneously hypertensive rats and in human essential hypertension. It is now thought that activating mutations in G protein–coupled receptor kinase-4 (GRK-4) hyperphosphorylate, internalize and desensitize the D_1 receptor in the renal proximal tubule of humans with essential hypertension. This defect promotes renal Na^+ reabsorption and is thought to contribute to the development of hypertension.

D_2-like receptor effects.

D_2-like DRs in the periphery are distributed both presynaptically and postsynaptically in the SNS. Presynaptic D_2-like DRs inhibit NE release from sympathetic neurons. Postsynaptic and nonneuronal D_2-like DRs are present in the endothelial and adventitial layers of blood vessels, on pituitary lactotrophs (where they inhibit prolactin secretion in response to DA), and in the adrenal zona glomerulosa (where they inhibit aldosterone secretion).

D_3 receptors, one of the D_2-like DR group, have been identified in glomeruli, proximal tubules, and blood vessels of the kidney, and a novel D_2-like receptor (the D_{2K} receptor) has been described in inner medullary collecting duct cells. The functions of the D_3 and D_{2K} receptors are unknown. However, knockout of the D_3

receptor in mice leads to angiotensin-dependent hypertension associated with increased renin secretion.

Aside from inhibition of NE, prolactin, and aldosterone secretion, the physiologic role of peripheral D_2-like DRs is not established, and it is unclear whether these receptors have a role in the pathophysiology of cardiovascular disease. Bromocriptine and domperidone are selective agonists at D_2-like receptors. Relatively specific agonists for the D_3 receptor include PD 128907, quinelorane, and pramipexole.

Suggested Readings

Brodde O-E, Bruck H, Leineweber K. Cardiac adrenoreceptors: physiological and pathophysiological relevance. *J Pharmacol Sci* 2006; 100: 323–337.

Carey RM. Renal dopamine system: paracrine regulator of sodium homeostasis and blood pressure. *Hypertension* 2001; 38: 298–302.

Felder RA, Jose PA. Mechanisms of disease. The role of GRK 4 in the etiology of essential hypertension and salt sensitivity. *Nat Clin Pract Nephrol* 2006; 2: 637–650.

Felder RA, Sanada H, Xu J, et al. G-protein coupled receptor kinase-4 gene variants in human essential hypertension. *Proc Natl Acad Sci U S A* 2002; 99: 3872–3877.

Kirstein SL, Insel PA. Autonomic nervous system pharmacogenomics: a progress report. *Pharmacol Rev* 2004; 56: 31–52.

Lefkowitz RJ. Historical review: A brief history and personal retrospective of seven transmembrane receptors. *Trends Pharmacol Sci* 2004; 25: 413–422.

Molenaar P, Parsonage WA. Fundamental considerations of β-adrenoceptor subtypes in human heart failure. *Trends Pharmacol Sci* 2005; 26: 368–374.

Philipp M, Hein L. Adrenergic receptor knockout mice: distinct function of 9 adrenergic receptor subtypes. *Pharmacol Ther* 2004; 101: 65–74.

Shannon R, Chaudhry M. Effect of $α_1$ adrenergic receptors in cardiac pathophysiology. *Am Heart J* 2006; 152: 842–850.

Smith NJ, Luttrell LM. Signal switching, crosstalk and arrestin scaffolds: novel G protein-coupled receptor signaling in cardiovascular disease. *Hypertension* 2006; 48: 173–179.

Xiao R-P, Zhu W, Zheng M, et al. Subtype specific $α_1$ and β-adrenoceptor signaling in the heart. *Trends Pharmacol Sci* 2006; 27: 330–337.

Yasuda K, Matsunaga T, Adachi T, et al. Adrenergic receptor polymorphisms and autonomic nervous system function in human obesity. *Trends Endocrinol Metab* 2006; 17: 269–275.

CHAPTER A13 ■ PRORENIN AND RENIN

WILLIAM H. BEIERWALTES, PhD

KEY POINTS

■ The renal juxtaglomerular (JG) cells are the primary site of renin synthesis, storage and release.
■ Renin release is initiated by the synthesis of preprorenin, which is converted to inactive prorenin and stored in JG granules, where it is activated before its regulated release.
■ Active renin is secreted in response to four regulatory mechanisms: the renal baroreceptor, the macula densa, renal nerves, and humoral factors.
■ Renin is the rate-limiting step in the formation of the vasoconstrictor peptide angiotensin II.

See also Chapters A14, A15, A16, A17, A18, A25, and **C135**

Renin-angiotensin cascade

Renin catalyzes the rate-limiting step in a cascade that forms angiotensin II (Ang II) and its congeners (**Figure A13.1**). Renin is a monospecific aspartyl proteolytic enzyme whose only substrate is angiotensinogen; a 60,000-Da peptide formed within the liver and released into the general circulation. The target bond of renin action is located between leucine in position 10 and valine in position 11, between the body of the angiotensinogen molecule and its amino-terminal decapeptide. The decapeptide released from the substrate is Ang I, which in turn is changed by angiotensin-converting enzyme (ACE) into the potent vasoactive hormone Ang II. Because renin catalyzes the critical rate-limiting step in the formation of Ang II, renin activity is generally used as an index of the endogenous formation of Ang II and its concentration reflects the importance of the signals that control renin synthesis and release.

Renin synthesis in juxtaglomerular cells

The juxtaglomerular (JG) cells are the locus for renin synthesis, storage, and release. The human renin gene has ten exons and nine introns. The initial step in renin synthesis is translation of renin mRNA into a 404- amino acid inactive preprorenin protein. This is an intermediate form, which is transported into the rough endoplasmic reticulum. The 23-amino acid "pre" sequence is cleaved, leaving prorenin, an inactive form of the enzyme (47,000 Da), which is passed through the Golgi apparatus, glycosylated, and deposited in lysosomal granules. There, the carboxyl-terminal 43-amino acid "pro" sequence is cleaved to form the enzymatically active form of renin (40,000 Da). It is thought that cleavage and activation within the granules are initiated by the enzyme cathepsin B. Once the pro sequence is removed, unmasking the active aspartyl residues of the molecule, secretion or release of active renin occurs in response to various

regulatory stimuli (discussed in the subsequent text). Renin-storing granules migrate to the cellular surface, where they release active enzyme by exocytosis into the vascular lumen and possibly into the renal interstitium. There is basal (or constitutive) release of active renin into the circulation, accounting for both basal plasma renin activity and circulating levels of Ang II.

Prorenin

Prorenin release and its presence in the circulation, which under basal conditions is two-fold to 10-fold greater than circulating active renin, are not regulated by acute control mechanisms and may only reflect synthesis. Generally, circulating prorenin and active renin levels are well correlated, but the percent of active renin may increase in response to specific stimuli and also in some disease states. It is now proposed that various cells have prorenin receptors which bind the circulating inactive renin and may (a) reversibly activate it on the cell surface, (b) bind and internalize the prorenin to digest it, acting as a "clearance" receptor, or (c) internalize and activate the prorenin to serve as a critical enzymatic step in an intracellular renin-angiotensin system. The utility or the regulation of such diverse binding of circulating prorenin is an active area of investigation.

When active renin secretion is stimulated in most mammals, circulating inactive renin tends to be diminished, presumably as the result of more prorenin being channeled into granular storage and/or activated. The kidney is the primary source of synthesis and secretion of active renin; alternatively, prorenin has been found in a number of extrarenal sources, including the adrenal glands, the pituitary, and the submandibular glands. These extrarenal ("tissue") renin-angiotensin systems are discussed in Chapter A18. Renal renin is synthesized, stored, and released by the JG cells—a cell type commonly felt to be derived from vascular smooth muscle (although this origin is being questioned). The JG

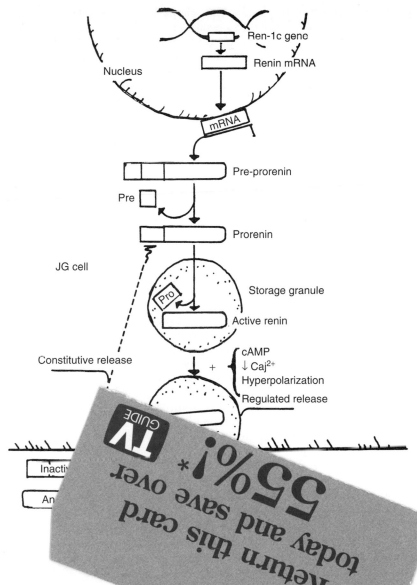

Figure A13.1 Cascade of renin synthesis, activation, and ...ease in the JG cell of the renal afferent arteriole, leading ... enzymatic formation of Ang II. JG, juxtaglomerular; cAMP; cyclic adenosine monophosphate, mRNA; messenger ribonucleic acid.

cells are located in the vasc... the afferent arteriole, where they a... densa. In response to chronic sodium de... other stimuli of renin), there is a unique "recruitme... afferent arteriolar cells upstream, which become renin-p... as renin secretion and plasma renin activity increase under these conditions.

Renin gene expression is mediated by hormones through hormone response elements for androgens and thyroxin. Sodium restriction also leads to renin expression in the JG cell, as does chronic increases in cyclic adenosine monophosphate (cAMP), whereas angiotensin II has been proposed as a negative (feedback) regulator of renin gene expression.

Signal transduction mechanisms

Cyclic adenosine monophosphate.
The primary second messenger in the pathway for stimulating renin secretion is cAMP. All known acute and chronic stimuli of renin operate through activation of adenylyl cyclase production of cAMP in the JG cell. Unlike most secretory responses, renin release is inhibited, not stimulated, by increased intracellular calcium, so there is an relation between intracellular calcium concentration and ... release. It is now known that this paradoxical relation ...een adenylyl cyclase and calcium is due to the colocalization ...ne renin-containing granules in the JG cell and adenylyl ...lase isoform type 5, which is inhibited by μM increases in ...tracellular calcium. Therefore, while any stimulus that activates JG cell adenylyl cyclase also stimulates renin release, the level of intracellular calcium inversely modifies the activity of the enzyme, and therefore cAMP production.

Calcium.
It is not completely clear how JG cell intracellular calcium is modulated, but release of intracellular calcium stores depends on ionic gradients, membrane calcium channels, electrical depolarization, and modulation of signal transduction mechanisms. Sequestration of intracellular calcium or JG cell hyperpolarization leads to decreased JG cell calcium and increased renin release. Depolarizing, (inhibitory) humoral factors include vasoconstrictors such as angiotensin, α-adrenergic agonists, thromboxane, endoperoxides [prostaglandin (PG)H$_2$], adenosine A$_1$ agonists, and endothelin-1.

Cyclic guanosine monophosphate.
The cyclic nucleotide cyclic guanosine monophosphate (cGMP), may act as another inhibitory second messenger. Factors that stimulate guanylyl

cyclase, such as atrial natriuretic factor and nitric oxide (NO), in the absence of stimulation of cAMP, inhibit renin release (*note: as discussedin the subsequent text, cGMP in the presence of cAMP may also facilitate renin release*). It is possible that some of these inhibitory factors stimulate phospholipase C, leading to release of intracellular calcium from sequestered stores that would also inhibit renin release.

Other factors. In contrast, autacoids such as prostacyclin, endothelium-derived hyperpolarizing factor, and NO may hyperpolarize both vascular smooth muscle cells and JG cells, decreasing influx of calcium across cell membranes. Integration of these humoral or regulatory mechanisms into the more classic pathways of renin stimulation remains the focus of considerable investigation.

Physiologic regulation of renin release

The classic pathways regulating active renin secretion include the renal baroreceptor, the macula densa, and renal nerves.

Renal baroreceptor. The renal baroreceptor is an intrarenal vascular receptor in the afferent arteriole that stimulates renin secretion in response to reduced renal perfusion pressure, and attenuates renin secretion as renal perfusion is elevated. The renal baroreceptor is perhaps the most powerful regulator of renin release. Chronic stimulation of the renal baroreceptor by reduced perfusion pressure contributes to the hyperreninemic phase of renovascular hypertension, and chronic activation can lead to both increased renin secretion and synthesis. Conversely, high renal perfusion pressure suppresses renin, possibly through adenosine production, shear-mediated nitric oxide synthase (NOS) type 3 cGMP production, and myogenic-induced cellular depolarization permitting calcium entry.

Macula densa. The macula densa is a modified plaque of cells in the distal tubule of the nephron, located at the end of the loop of Henle and adjacent to the afferent arteriole, the JG cells, and extraglomerular mesangium. All of these components make up the JG apparatus, which sends a feedback signal when the macula densa senses a chronic change in distal tubular salt delivery. Decreased NaCl delivery leads to induction of macula densa cyclooxygenase-2 (COX-2) and NOS-1. COX-2 produces PGE_2, which acts on the adjacent JG cells through prostaglandin type E (EP) -4 receptor to stimulate adenylyl cyclase, cAMP production and consequently renin release. NOS-1 produces NO and subsequently cGMP, which acts on phosphodiesterase-3 in the JG cells to block the degradation of cAMP, thereby exaggerating cAMP-mediated stimulation of renin secretion. Chronic sodium loading creates the reverse scenario, removing this pathway for stimulating adenylyl cyclase and therefore suppressing renin

release. The macula densa mechanism is most likely a chronic adaptive system for regulating renin rather than an acute mediator, although diuretics such as furosemide suppress macula densa sodium reabsorption and stimulate renin release through the macula densa pathway.

Sympathetic nerves. JG cells are directly innervated by sympathetic nerves and stimulation of the renal nerves causes an increase in renin from the JG cells through a β-adrenergic–mediated stimulation of JG cell adenylyl cyclase activity. The renal nerves are stimulated through a pathway that involves cardiac mechanoreceptors, aortocarotid pressoreceptors, chemoreceptors, and vagal afferent fibers. Several central neural reflex pathways mediate stimulation of efferent sympathetic renal nerve traffic and the subsequent stimulation of renin secretion. Renal nerve–mediated renin secretion provides an acute pathway by which rapid activation of the renin–angiotensin system can be provoked by such stimuli as stress and posture.

Humoral factors. Although the three pathways discussed in the preceding text are the "classic" regulators of renin release, a series of humoral factors has also been implicated. The primary stimulatory intracellular "second messenger" for renin release is cAMP, and activation or inhibition of adenylyl cyclase in the JG cell is the target of many factors, including arachidonic acid products, and numerous vasoactive factors including angiotensin, endothelin, atrial natriuretic peptide and more. Because angiotensin, the biologically active end product of this system is so integrally linked to renin synthesis and activity, the factors and pathways controlling renin represent a critical arena of integration in understanding renal and cardiovascular function and the control of blood pressure.

Suggested Readings

Bader M, Ganten D. Regulation of renin: new evidence from cultured cells and genetically modified mice. *J Mol Med* 2000;78:130–139.

Hsueh WA, Baxter JD. Human prorenin. *Hypertension* 1991;17:469–477.

Jan Danser AH, Deinum J. Renin, prorenin and the putative (Pro)renin receptor. *Hypertension* 2005;46:1069–1076.

Keeton TK, Campbell WB. The pharmacologic alteration of renin release. *Pharmacol Rev* 1980;32:81–227.

Kurtz A, Wagner C. Role of nitric oxide in the control of renin secretion. *Am J Physiol Renal Physiol* 1998;275:F849–F862.

Kurtz A, Wagner C. Cellular control of renin secretion. *J Exp Biol* 1999;202:219–225.

Navar LG, Inscho EW, Majid SA, et al. Paracrine regulation of the renal microcirculation. *Physiol Rev* 1996;76:425–536.

Ortiz-Capisano MC, Ortiz PA, Harding P, et al. Decreased intracellular calcium stimulates cAMP and renin release via calcium-inhibitable adenylyl cyclase. *Hypertension* 2007;49:162–169.

Sigmund CD, Gross KW. Structure, expression and regulation of the murine renin genes. *Hypertension* 1991;18:446–457.

CHAPTER A14 ■ ANGIOTENSINOGEN

MORTON P. PRINTZ, PhD

KEY POINTS

■ Angiotensinogen is the protein from which a family of angiotensins is formed by proteolytic cleavage reactions.

■ Systemic and tissue angiotensinogen synthesis is under complex multifactorial control by a variety of molecules.

■ Arterial pressure is dependent on both systemic and tissue angiotensinogen concentration.

See also Chapters A13, A15, A16, A17, and A18

Angiotensinogen is the only known precursor protein for the entire family of angiotensin peptides, angiotensin I, II, III (des-Asp^1-angiotensin II), IV (des-Asp^1-Arg^2-angiotensin II), and angiotensin (1–7) (des-Phe^8-angiotensin II) and therefore, the site(s) of biosynthesis of angiotensinogen and the locations of the protein define the existence of various angiotensin systems. On the basis of many years of research, it may also be concluded that there are two generic angiotensin systems in mammals defined by the source of angiotensinogen: the classical, or "systemic," where angiotensinogen, mainly of hepatocyte origin, is transported through the systemic circulation to accessible tissue targets thereby providing the source of the angiotensin peptides, and the "tissue" consisting of cells that synthesize angiotensinogen and release the prohormone locally. The ability of systemic (blood-borne) angiotensinogen to egress the vascular compartment into extravascular, extracellular space, confounds exclusive separation of these two angiotensin systems, except for the brain angiotensin system which is sheltered from systemic angiotensinogen by the blood–brain barrier.

Biochemistry and molecular genetics

Pre-proangiotensinogen is the product of a single gene, 11,800 bases in length, and is synthesized, processed, and glycosylated in a species- and tissue-dependent manner. The human angiotensinogen gene consists of five exons and four introns with exon 1 encoding the 5′-nontranslated portion of the mRNA for angiotensinogen, whereas the signal peptides and coding region for angiotensin I are encoded by exon 2. The other three exons contain the balance of information for the protein as well as the 3′-nontranslated region, a major site for mRNA stability and lifetime. Most of the reported physiologic and pathophysiologic factors that affect systemic angiotensinogen synthesis operate through transcriptional regulation. The 3′-nontranslated sequences of

angiotensinogen mRNA contain recognition sequences for cytosolic proteins that determine the lifetime of the mRNA.

Systemic and tissue angiotensinogens are distinguishable by their patterns of glycosylation and product profile. The angiotensin I decapeptide is located on the N-terminus of secreted angiotensinogen, immediately after the signal peptides. In the systemic angiotensin system, the decapeptide angiotensin I is released from the N-terminus of angiotensinogen by the action of renin. Although renin mRNA has been identified in some extrancural tissues, alternative modes of proteolytic release of angiotensin peptides have been documented. Tissue angiotensinogen may be a substrate for a variety of proteases including cathepsin G, tonin, chymase, and even an intracellular form of renin. The brain protease(s) responsible for the release of either angiotensin I, or directly angiotensin II, from brain angiotensinogen remain controversial.

Within the blood of healthy subjects, men and women, 95% of the circulating systemic angiotensinogen is monomeric with a molecular weight of approximately 62,000 Da. The balance, approximately 5% of the total, appears to circulate as a high-molecular-weight (or "heavy") form, 110,000 to 500,000 Da. During pregnancy when plasma angiotensinogen levels are elevated, the proportion of high-molecular-weight angiotensinogen increases, especially in the setting of pregnancy-induced hypertension. Differences in the kinetics of renin releasing angiotensin I from angiotensinogen have been reported for the high-molecular-weight form, but the significance of the heavy form of angiotensinogen remains unknown. Studies suggest that formation of heavy angiotensinogen may involve either disulfide bond formation between monomeric angiotensinogens, or complex formation with other circulating proteins. Angiotensinogen is classed as a member of the serpin family of protease inhibitors, although no serpin function for angiotensinogen has been identified. Yet this may explain the origin of the heavy angiotensinogen. At this time, any pathophysiologic significance of heavy angiotensinogen remains to be established.

In contrast to renin, the half-life of systemic plasma angiotensinogen is quite long, up to 16 hours. The steady-state plasma level of angiotensinogen is determined primarily by the rate of synthesis and secretion from hepatocytes, and by the rate of egress from the vascular compartment into extravascular space, including the peritoneal cavity. Cleavage by plasma renin accounts for only 5% to 10% of the total rate of elimination of angiotensinogen from the circulation. The kinetics of disappearance of tissue angiotensinogen is more difficult to define. In plasma, angiotensinogen constitutes an extremely small fraction of the total pool of plasma proteins; however, brain angiotensinogen comprises up to 2% of total cerebrospinal fluid protein.

Control of systemic and tissue angiotensinogen release

Hepatocyte angiotensinogen is constitutively secreted with little intracellular storage. Plasma levels of angiotensinogen vary with the respective degrees of transcriptional regulation (into mRNA), mRNA lifetime, and secreted protein lifetime in the circulation. A variety of signal molecules can exert transcriptional control of angiotensinogen, including glucocorticoids, estrogens, thyroid hormone, insulin, and selected cytokines. These and other regulators of transcription act through specific regulatory DNA sequences in the angiotensinogen promoter regions of the gene. A positive feedback pathway enhances transcription by angiotensin II acting through the AT_1 subtype angiotensin receptor on hepatocytes. In a similar manner, much evidence indicates that tissue angiotensinogen mRNA formation is also transcriptionally regulated, with upstream inhibitory sequences likely conveying tissue specificity. Currently much research focuses on defining transcriptional control mechanisms that dictate synthesis of brain and adipocyte angiotensinogens.

Angiotensinogen and hypertension

Experimental animals.   Several lines of evidence continue to suggest that angiotensinogen contributes to the hypertensive phenotype in genetic forms of hypertension in man and some animal models. A variety of studies show that plasma angiotensinogen levels or functionality of the angiotensinogen gene can influence arterial pressure. Genetic engineering and the use of antisense constructs have established that brain angiotensinogen concentrations determine levels of arterial pressure in both rat and mouse models. Varying the copy number in mice leads to proportional changes in arterial pressure. This suggests that control of the lifetimes of angiotensinogen (and probably renin) may be more important than the lifetime of the active peptides. However, it is still premature to infer that angiotensinogen levels have a direct causal association with genetic hypertension in animals or the human disorder of essential hypertension.

Population genetics.   It is now established that the angiotensinogen gene contains several single nucleotide polymorphisms (SNPs) that may define different populations of inherited haplotypes. Yet classic genetic efforts to demonstrate involvement of the angiotensinogen gene in genetic hypertension of humans or rodents have met with limited and mixed success. Population studies continue to explore the role of T174M and M235T diallelic polymorphisms within the coding sequence as potential contributors to human hypertension or associated cardiovascular disease. In addition, the M235T polymorphism exhibits linkage disequilibrium with an A (–6) G polymorphism in the 5′-promoter sequence. Additional SNPs have been reported and efforts increasingly focus on the role of various haplotype combinations in predicting the frequency of hypertension in selected ethnic populations. Several of the haplotypes vary considerably in frequency of occurrence, further obfuscating any simple relation between variants of angiotensinogen and chronic hypertension.

Suggested Readings

Dickson ME, Sigmund CD. Genetic basis of hypertension. Revisiting angiotensinogen. *Hypertension* 2006;48:14–20.

Kumar A, Yanna L, Patil S, et al. A haplotype of the angiotensinogen gene is associated with hypertension in African Americans. *Clin Exp Pharmacol Physiol* 2005;32:495–502.

Lavoie JL, Liu X, Bianco RA, et al. Evidence supporting a functional role for intracellular renin in the brain. *Hypertension* 2006;47:461–466.

Nakajima T, Jorde LB, Ishigami T, et al. Nucleotide diversity and haplotype structure of the human angiotensinogen gene in two populations. *Am J Hum Genet* 2002;70:108–123.

Ramaha A, Celerier J, Patston PA. Characterization of different high molecular weight angiotensinogen forms. *Am J Hypertens* 2003;16:478–483.

CHAPTER A15 ■ ANGIOTENSIN I–CONVERTING ENZYME AND NEPRILYSIN (NEUTRAL ENDOPEPTIDASE)

RANDAL A. SKIDGEL, PhD AND ERVIN G. ERDÖS, MD

KEY POINTS

- Angiotensin-converting enzyme (ACE) hydrolyzes inactive angiotensin I to generate the active pressor angiotensin II and also inactivates the vasodilator bradykinin.
- ACE is found on endothelial cells, especially in the lung, retina, and brain. It is also present in testes and in high concentration on microvillar structures in the choroid plexus, proximal tubules of the kidney, placenta, and intestine.
- Neprilysin cleaves a variety of peptides, including angiotensin I, bradykinin, enkephalins, substance P, atrial natriuretic peptide (ANP) and amyloid ß peptide.
- Neprilysin is widely distributed in the body in kidney, brain, and male genital tract, but its expression is low in endothelial cells. Neprilysin is a marker (CD10) of the malignant cells in acute lymphoblastic leukemia.

See also Chapters A13, A14, A16, A17, A18, A26, and **C136**

ANGIOTENSIN I–CONVERTING ENZYME

Activity

Angiotensin-converting enzyme (ΛCE) converts the inactive decapeptide angiotensin (Ang) I to the active octapeptide Ang II by cleaving the C-terminal histidyl-leucine dipeptide. The enzyme is not specific for Ang I because it cleaves a variety of other peptides, including bradykinin, luteinizing hormone–releasing hormone, enkephalins, substance P and acetyl-Ser-Asp-Lys-Pro. On the basis of enzyme kinetics, ACE is a better "kininase" than "converting enzyme" or "enkephalinase" because of the very low K_m of bradykinin. Therefore, ACE generates the vasoconstrictor Ang II, whereas it inactivates the vasodilator bradykinin (**Figure A15.1**). ACE inhibitors interfere with both reactions, prolonging the half-life of bradykinin while inhibiting the formation of Ang II. ACE is a metalloenzyme that utilizes zinc as a cofactor and also needs chloride ions to cleave most substrates; Ang I conversion is entirely chloride dependent, whereas bradykinin hydrolysis is less affected. Some of the beneficial cardiovascular actions of ACE inhibitor therapy are attributed to prolonging and potentiating the effect of bradykinin on its receptors.

Molecular aspects

General properties. Human ACE has a molecular weight of 150,000 to 180,000 Da, of which 146,000 Da is protein and the balance carbohydrate. Most ACE is membrane bound on the plasma membrane of various cell types. ACE is inserted into the membrane by a short hydrophobic region near its C-terminus that is connected by a juxtamembrane stalk to the C-domain. Proteolytic cleavage of the stalk by a zinc-dependent metalloprotease releases ACE from the plasma membrane. The secretase may be a member of the ADAM (*a disintegrin and metalloprotease*) family. Released ACE can be detected in many fluid compartments including blood, urine, pulmonary and amniotic fluid, cerebrospinal fluid, lymph, and semen.

Structure. ACE has two active centers located within the highly homologous N- and C-domains that likely evolved through gene duplication. A unique ACE isoform containing only the C-domain is expressed in testis because this tissue-specific transcription is dependent on a promoter within intron 12 of the ACE gene. Endothelial (or somatic) ACE contains two zinc ions and two inhibitor-binding sites per molecule, consistent with the finding that both active sites are functional. The K_m values for the classic substrates (Ang I or bradykinin) do not differ much between the active centers on the N- and C-domains, but the turnover number of the C-domain is higher *in vitro*. Some other physiologic peptides are preferentially cleaved by the N-domain active site including the hemoregulatory tetrapeptide acetyl-Ser-Asp-Lys-Pro, Ang 1–7, enkephalin-Arg[6]-Phe[7], and luteinizing hormone–releasing hormone. The rates of dissociation of inhibitors from the active centers of the two domains differ as does the duration of their inhibition.

The crystal structures of the separate N- and C-domains have been determined but the complete somatic ACE structure has not. Testicular (C-domain) ACE is essentially an all-helical

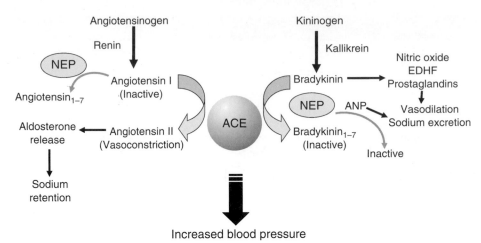

Figure A15.1 By cleaving peptide hormones, angiotensin I–converting enzyme (ACE) and neprilysin (NEP) can participate in the regulation of blood pressure. ACE converts the inactive angiotensin I to the active angiotensin II, which causes vasoconstriction, aldosterone release, and sodium retention. ACE also inactivates bradykinin, a peptide that stimulates production of nitric oxide, endothelial-derived hyperpolarizing factor (EDHF) and prostaglandins and causes vasodilation and natriuresis. NEP converts angiotensin I to angiotensin 1–7, which generally opposes the actions of angiotensin II. However, NEP may also contribute to hypertension because it inactivates the atrial natriuretic peptide (ANP) and bradykinin.

ellipsoid with a deep central groove dividing the molecule into two subdomains with two bound chloride ions and one zinc. An N-terminal "lid" likely restricts access of large substrates, consistent with the preference of ACE to cleave peptides of <13 residues. The structure of the N-domain is very similar to that of the C-domain, but contains only one bound chloride ion. Very likely, subtle variations in the structure and conformation of the two active sites is why the two domains differ in substrate specificity and inhibitor binding.

Distribution

In vascular beds, ACE is bound to the plasma membrane of endothelial cells, where it cleaves circulating peptides such as Ang I or bradykinin. Small vessels of the lung, retina, and brain are especially rich in ACE. Some epithelial cells in humans have more ACE than endothelial cells. The human kidney contains five to six times more ACE per unit of wet weight than the lung; the proximal tubular brush border is a major site of kidney ACE. Other microvillar structures of epithelial linings in the small intestine, choroid plexus, and placenta are also very rich in ACE. ACE is concentrated in some regions of the brain, especially the choroid plexus, but also the subfornical organ, area postrema, substantia nigra, and locus caeruleus.

Genetic aspects

Genetic strains. The effects of overall ACE levels and targeted expression on blood pressure (BP) and renal development have been studied in genetically altered mice. Knockout of the ACE gene impairs renal development and decreases systolic BP by approximately 35 mm, but varying the ACE concentration (from 62% to 213% of normal) by altering ACE gene copy number from one to four does not affect BP. However, streptozotocin-induced diabetes caused higher BP and albumin excretion in mice with three ACE genes. Deletion of ACE expression in the endothelium and targeted expression in liver cells using an albumin promoter yielded mice with approximately 80% the normal value of plasma ACE and 15% of normal renal ACE. In such animals, BP and renal development are normal.

Insertion/deletion polymorphism. Studies of the human ACE gene reveal an insertion/deletion (I/D) polymorphism in a noncoding region, corresponding to the presence or the absence of a 287-base pair sequence in intron 16. Individuals homozygous for the insertion polymorphism (I/I) have lower levels of ACE activity in plasma than do those with the D/D genotype. The correlation of this polymorphism with cardiovascular and renal diseases is the subject of many studies, with varying results. Some investigations associate the D allele with an increased risk for hypertension, atherosclerosis, myocardial infarction, or diabetic nephropathy, whereas the I allele interestingly has been suggested to confer enhanced endurance performance in athletes.

NEPRILYSIN (NEUTRAL ENDOPEPTIDASE)

Neprilysin (NEP) was originally identified in renal proximal tubules as neutral endopeptidase 24.11. It was also called *enkephalinase* in the brain and common acute lymphoblastic leukemia antigen (CALLA) or CD10 because it is found on lymphocytes in acute lymphoblastic leukemia.

Actions

NEP belongs to a family of related proteins (*M13* peptidase family) that notably includes the endothelin converting enzyme. NEP cleaves bradykinin, enkephalin, and the chemotactic peptide fMet-Leu-Phe at the same sites as ACE, but other vaso- and neuropeptides at different sites. In general, NEP hydrolyzes peptide substrates at the amino ends of hydrophobic amino acids such as phenylalanine. Whereas ACE action releases a dipeptide and an active octapeptide (Ang II) from Ang I, NEP forms a tripeptide and an active heptapeptide (Ang 1–7, see Chapter A16). NEP also cleaves bradykinin, endothelin, substance P, chemotactic peptide fMet-Leu-Phe, amyloid ß peptide and the atrial natriuretic peptides (ANPs) which are substrates of particular interest.

Structure

Human NEP is a type II integral membrane glycoprotein of 742 residues. In contrast to ACE, the large extracellular domain is inserted into the cell membrane by an uncleaved signal peptide near its N-terminus with a short N-terminal cytosolic domain. A single active center is present in the extracellular domain that contains the canonic HEXXH motif; glutamic acid is an important catalytic residue and the two histidines (and a glutamic acid 60 residues downstream) act as the zinc coordinating ligands. The crystal structure of the extracellular domain of NEP is marked by the presence of two separate α-helical lobes. The larger

N-terminal region contains the active site residues and resembles the structure of the related bacterial protease thermolysin. The smaller C-terminal region (absent in thermolysin) likely restricts access of substrate to the active site and explains why NEP preferentially cleaves relatively shorter oligopeptides. The structure of NEP is stabilized by six disulfide bonds. Although not related in overall sequence, the active site residues and catalytic mechanisms of ACE and NEP are quite similar, which has simplified the development of combined ACE/NEP inhibitors.

Distribution

ACE and NEP are both highly concentrated in some of the same tissues, including the microvilli of brush borders (e.g., proximal tubules) and in the male genital tract, but their distribution differs in other organs and cell types. In general, vascular endothelial cells express more ACE, whereas epithelial cells and fibroblasts are richer in NEP. Owing to its presence in neutrophil cell membranes, NEP is involved in chemotactic peptide metabolism, and in the brain and the lungs, in enkephalin, amyloid ß peptide and substance P hydrolysis; the latter peptide released from sensory nerves can cause pain and contract pulmonary smooth muscle.

Clinical implications

Theoretically, inhibiting NEP (and the breakdown of ANP and bradykinin, **Figure A15.1**) could be beneficial in patients with hypertension or congestive heart failure. Molecules that inhibit both ACE and NEP ("vasopeptidase" inhibitors) are highly effective in lowering BP but have not been found sufficiently safe relative to angioedema risk to be released for routine clinical use.

Suggested Readings

Bernstein KE, Xiao HD, Frenzel K, et al. Six truisms concerning ACE and the renin-angiotensin system educed from the genetic analysis of mice. *Circ Res* 2005;96:1135–1144.

Corradi HR, Schwager SLU, Nchinda AT, et al. Crystal structure of the N domain of human somatic angiotensin I-converting enzyme provides a structural basis for domain-specific inhibitor design. *J Mol Biol* 2006;357:964–974.

Corvol P, Williams TA. Peptidyl-dipeptidase A/angiotensin I-converting enzyme. In: Barrett AJ, Rawlings ND, Woessner JF, eds. *Handbook of proteolytic enzymes*, 2nd ed. Amsterdam: Elsevier Science, 2004:332–346.

Erdös EG, Skidgel RA. Neutral endopeptidase 24.11 (enkephalinase) and related regulators of peptide hormones. *FASEB J* 1989;3:145–151.

Erdös EG, Skidgel RA. Metabolism of bradykinin by peptidases in health and disease. In: Farmer SG, ed. *The kinin system. Handbook of immunopharmacology.* London, UK: Academic Press;1997:112–141.

Gafford JT, Skidgel RA, Erdös EG, et al. Human kidney "enkephalinase," a neutral metalloendopeptidase that cleaves active peptides. *Biochemistry* 1983; 22:3265–3271.

Jones A, Montgomery HE, Woods DR. Human performance: a role for the ACE genotype? *Exerc Sport Sci Rev* 2002;30:184–190.

Skidgel RA, Erdös EG. Angiotensin converting enzyme (ACE) and neprilysin hydrolyze neuropeptides: a brief history, the beginning and follow-ups to early studies. *Peptides* 2004;25:521–525.

Turner AJ. Neprilysin. In: Barrett AJ, Rawlings ND, Woessner IF, eds. *Handbook of proteolytic enzymes.* 2nd ed. Amsterdam: Elsevier Science, 2004:419–426.

Wohlfart P, Wiemer G. Interactions between the renin-angiotensin and the kallikrein-kinin system. In: Unger T, Schölkens BA, eds. *Handbook of experimental pharmacology,* Vol. 163, Angiotensin, part 2. Springer-Verlag New York, 2004:359–373.

CHAPTER A16 ■ ANGIOTENSIN FORMATION AND DEGRADATION

CARLOS M. FERRARIO, MD AND MARK C. CHAPPELL, PhD

KEY POINTS

- A family of angiotensins is derived from angiotensin (Ang) I through the action of converting enzymes, chymase (CHYM), aminopeptidases, and tissue endopeptidases (EPs).
- CHYMs (angiotensin convertases) and angiotensin-converting enzyme (ACE) 2 degrade Ang I and Ang II to other effectors of the renin-angiotensin system, such as Ang (1–9) Ang II and Ang (1–7); these enzymes are resistant to ACE inhibitors.
- Blockade of ACE initially reduces Ang II levels, which may increase during chronic therapy, possibly due to the actions of tissue CHYMs and upregulation of ACE gene expression.
- The vasodepressor and antigrowth functions of Ang (1–7), acting as a competitive endogenous inhibitor of Ang II, contribute to the antihypertensive effects of ACE inhibition and Ang II receptor blockade.
- ACE 2 may play a role in regulating the pathologic actions of Ang II in the heart, the vasculature, and the kidneys by degrading this peptide to Ang (1–7).

See also Chapters A13, A14, A15, A17, and A18

In mammalian systems, the concentration of a peptide hormone such as angiotensin (Ang) II at its receptor is controlled by numerous factors, including those that influence its synthesis, secretion, and biologic removal. Major mechanisms by which peptides are removed include enzymatic degradation by peptidases, hemodynamic factors, and endocytosis of the ligand-receptor complex.

Metabolic pathways

Figure A16.1 illustrates the enzymatic pathways responsible for the production and metabolism of the active angiotensins.

Angiotensin-converting enzyme and tissue endopeptidases. Ang I, the prohormone decapeptide, is cleaved to the octapeptide Ang II primarily by angiotensin-converting enzyme (ACE) and to the heptapeptide Ang (1–7) by tissue EPs. One form of chymase (CHYM, angiotensin convertase) has been implicated in an alternative pathway for the production of Ang II. Multiple EPs can form Ang (1–7) from Ang I, including prolyl EP (EC 3.4.21.26), neprilysin (NEP) (EC 3.4.24.11), thimet oligopeptidase (EC 3.4.24.15), and endothelin-converting enzyme (EC 3.4.24.71). NEP can also cleave Ang II and Ang (1–7) forming the inactive peptide fragment Ang (1–4).

Angiotensin-converting enzyme 2. A homolog of ACE, termed *ACE2*, has been identified in several cardiovascular organs including the heart, blood vessels, and the kidney. In contrast to ACE, ACE2 exhibits a very high specificity for Ang II and directly generates Ang (1–7) (**Table A16.1**). This enzyme constitutes an important regulatory step for reducing Ang II and increasing Ang (1–7). Localization of ACE2 to cardiac myocytes and renal tubules in the rat and the presence of ACE2 polymorphisms correlate with diabetic nephropathy and primary essential hypertension suggesting a critical role for this enzyme in regulating Ang II disposition and function.

Aminopeptidases. Aminopeptidases constitute another route for Ang II metabolism. Glutamyl aminopeptidase (EC 3.4.11.7) cleaves Ang II to Ang III [Ang (2–8)], and arginyl aminopeptidase (EC 3.4.11.6) converts Ang III to Ang IV [Ang (3–8)].

Endocytosis. Another determinant of the duration of action of angiotensin peptides is endocytosis. AT_1 receptors are the primary mediators of intracellular transport of Ang II, but the internalization of the ligand–receptor complex may also be influenced by the AT_2-receptor subtype.

Function of alternative pathways

The possibility of forming two different active angiotensin peptides [Ang II and Ang (1–7)] from a common substrate, Ang I, could allow cells to selectively regulate production of one or the other product. Further processing of these two active peptides into smaller fragments may add another level of specificity specialization to the signaling process. The role of ACE, ACE2, and NEP in regulating the balance between constriction (Ang II) and dilation [Ang (1–7) and bradykinin] in peripheral tissues may be important in the regulation of blood pressure (BP) and the

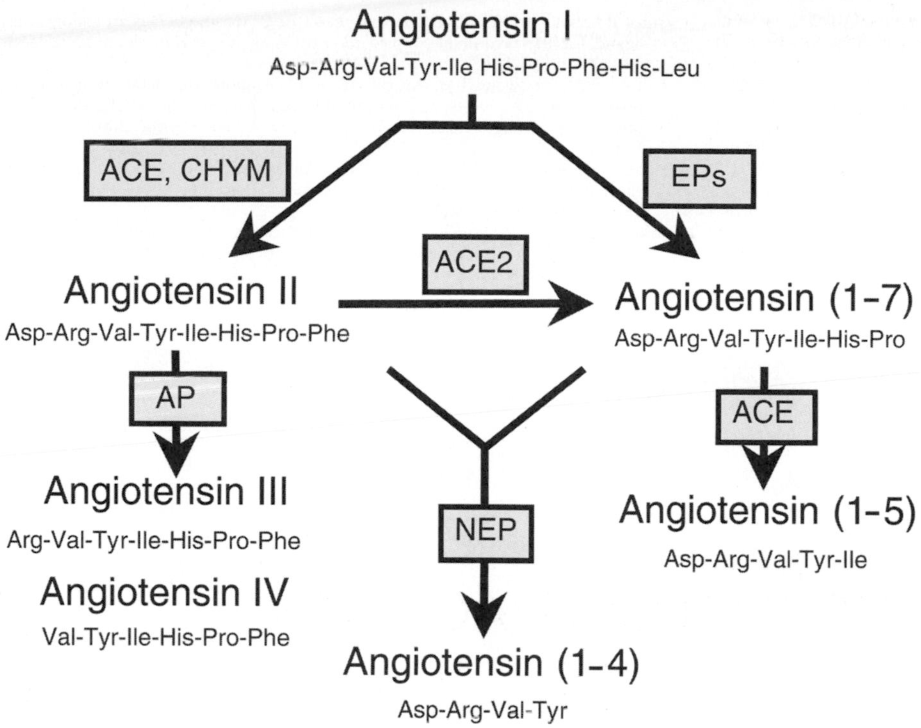

Angiotensin I
Asp-Arg-Val-Tyr-Ile His-Pro-Phe-His-Leu

| ACE, CHYM | | EPs |

Angiotensin II
Asp-Arg-Val-Tyr-Ile-His-Pro-Phe

ACE2

Angiotensin (1–7)
Asp-Arg-Val-Tyr-Ile-His-Pro

AP

Angiotensin III
Arg-Val-Tyr-Ile-His-Pro-Phe

Angiotensin IV
Val-Tyr-Ile-His-Pro-Phe

NEP

ACE

Angiotensin (1-5)
Asp-Arg-Val-Tyr-Ile

Angiotensin (1-4)
Asp-Arg-Val-Tyr

Figure A16.1 Proteolytic pathways that contribute to the formation and metabolism of products derived from angiotensin I. ACE, angiotensin-converting enzyme; AP, aminopeptidases; CHYM, chymase; EPs, endopeptidases; NEP, neprilysin.

structural changes associated with hypertension. The occurrence of angiotensinogen-derived peptides of amino acid sequences longer than Ang I has been recently reported. Ang I–Leu-Tyr [Ang (1–12)], a precursor of Ang II and, possibly, Ang (1–7) exists in high concentrations in small intestine, the heart, and the kidneys. Ang (1–12) is cleaved from angiotensinogen through a non–renin dependent pathway.

Angiotensin metabolic changes during angiotensin-converting enzyme inhibition
Incomplete angiotensin-converting enzyme inhibition.
Inhibition of ACE initially increases the concentration of Ang I and decreases Ang II and aldosterone. However, whether plasma levels of Ang II remain fully suppressed during chronic ACE inhibition is debated. In some studies in hypertension, trough Ang II levels may increase with time ("ACE escape"). In heart failure, chronic ACE inhibition is associated with reduced plasma Ang II levels. ACE inhibition uniformly increases renin and circulating

Ang I, which may, by mass action, exceed the inhibitory capacity of an ACE inhibitor in plasma or tissues. Dissociation of the therapeutic effects of ACE inhibitors and the levels of plasma Ang II may indicate incomplete blockade of ACE.

Angiotensin (1–7). Chronic inhibition of ACE also raises the plasma and tissue concentration of Ang (1–7) in both humans and animals. Ang (1–7) is an endogenous competitive inhibitor of native Ang II; blockade of Ang (1–7) activity or synthesis reduces the antihypertensive effects of ACE inhibition and Ang II receptor blockers. Ang (1–7) can be degraded to the inactive product Ang (1–5) by ACE and the reaction's kinetics are comparable to that of bradykinin; therefore, ACE inhibitors have two actions that can increase levels of Ang (1–7). New findings using the mixed or combined ACE-NEP inhibitor omapatrilat reveal augmented renal excretion of Ang (1–7) in humans and animals. Elevated levels of Ang (1–7) may contribute to the diuretic and BP-lowering actions of both ACE and NEP inhibitors as well as Ang II receptor blockers by direct coupling of the peptide to the *mas* receptor. Since ACE2 gene expression in heart, kidney, and brain is modulated by Ang II acting through the AT_1 receptor, a regulatory mechanism has been found for modulating the pathologic actions of Ang II.

Chymases. One form of mast cell CHYM expressed in hypertension and injury provides another route for the formation of Ang II during chronic ACE-inhibitor therapy. The relative importance of alternative Ang II generating pathways in counteracting the antihypertensive effects of ACE inhibitors is the subject of continuing debate.

TABLE A16.1

SUBSTRATE PROPERTIES OF HUMAN
ANGIOTENSIN-CONVERTING ENZYME 2

Substrate	K_m (μmol/L)	K_{cat}/K_m (mmol/L/s)	Bond
Angiotensin II	2.0	1,800	Pro-Phe
Angiotensin I	6.9	4.9	His-Leu
Apelin-13	6.8	2,000	Pro-Phe
Casomorphin	31	220	Pro-Ile
Dynorphin A	5.5	2,900	Leu-Lys
[des-Arg⁹]-Bradykinin	290	220	Pro-Phe
Neurotensin	300	190	Pro-Arg

Suggested Readings

Albiston AL, McDowall SG, Matsacos D, et al. Evidence that the angiotensin IV (AT(4)) receptor is the enzyme insulin-regulated aminopeptidase. *J Biol Chem* 2001;276:48623–48626.

Crackower MA, Sarao R, Oudit GY, et al. Angiotensin-converting enzyme 2 is an essential regulator of heart function. *Nature* 2002;417:822–828.

Ferrario CM, Jessup J, Chappell MC, et al. Effect of angiotensin-converting enzyme inhibition and angiotensin II receptor blockers on cardiac angiotensin-converting enzyme 2. *Circulation* 2005;111:2605–2610.

Ferrario CM, Smith RD, Brosnihan KB, et al. Effects of omapatrilat on the renin angiotensin system in salt sensitive hypertension. *Am J Hypertens* 2002;15: 557–564.

Ferrario CM, Trask AJ, Jessup JA. Advances in biochemical and functional roles of angiotensin-converting enzyme 2 and angiotensin-(1–7) in regulation of cardio-vascular function. *Am J Physiol Heart Circ Physiol* 2005;289(6):H2281–H2290.

Guo C, Ju H, Leung D, et al. A novel vascular smooth muscle chymase is upregulated in hypertensive rats. *J Clin Invest* 2001;107:703–715.

Luque M, Martin P, Martell N, et al. Effects of captopril related to increased levels of prostacyclin and angiotensin-(1–7) in essential hypertension. *J Hypertens* 1996;14:799–805.

Santos RA, Simoes E Silva AC, Maric C, et al. Angiotensin-(1–7) is an endogenous ligand for the G protein-coupled receptor *mas. Proc Natl Acad Sci U S A* 2003;100:8258–8263.

Shaltout HA, Westwood BM, Averill DB, et al. Angiotensin metabolism in renal proximal tubules, urine and serum of sheep: evidence for ACE2-dependent processing of angiotensin II. *Am J Physiol Renal Physiol* 2007;292:F82–F91.

Tallant EA, Ferrario CM, Gallagher PE. Angiotensin-(1–7) inhibits growth of cardiac myocytes through activation of the *mas* receptor. *Am J Physiol Heart Circ Physiol* 2005;289:H1560–H1566.

Vickers C, Hales P, Kaushik V, et al. Hydrolysis of biological peptides by human angiotensin-converting enzyme-related carboxypeptidase. *J Biol Chem* 2002;277:14838–14843.

CHAPTER A17 ■ ANGIOTENSINS: ACTIONS AND RECEPTORS

THEODORE L. GOODFRIEND, MD

KEY POINTS

■ Angiotensin II (Ang II), by activating receptors of the AT$_1$ subtype, stimulates aldosterone secretion, constricts blood vessels, amplifies sympathetic nervous outflow, increases renal sodium retention, and promotes cell growth in the cardiovascular system.

■ Ang II effects are amplified or attenuated by other autacoids, such as nitric oxide, eicosanoids, steroids, and growth factors, many of which are released in response to Ang II.

■ A second subtype of Ang II receptor, AT$_2$, predominant in the fetus, injured tissue, and a few adult organs including brain and adrenal medulla, affects growth and vascular tone in ways that oppose actions mediated by AT$_1$.

■ Two shorter peptides, formed from Ang II (Ang 1–7 and Ang 3–8), bind to specific macromolecules and have actions distinct from those of Ang II in the brain and other organs.

See also Chapters A15, A16, **A18,** and **C137**

Angiotensins comprise a family of four biologically active peptides derived from renin substrate (angiotensinogen). They exert a wide array of acute functional, and chronic structural effects on the cardiovascular system and other tissues, mediated by four receptors.

General characteristics

Angiotensins. Angiotensins are peptides ranging in length from 6 to 10 amino acids. They can be classified by Roman numerals [e.g., angiotensin II (Ang II)] or by Arabic numbers referring to amino acid sequence, starting with the *N*-terminal aspartic acid of Ang I (e.g., Ang 1–7). Ang I (Ang 1–10), a peptide with no known biologic role, serves as a precursor of smaller Ang peptides. Ang I is cleaved by converting enzyme to yield Ang II

(Ang 1–8), the peptide with the greatest cardiovascular potency. Ang III (Ang 2–8) is more lipid-soluble than Ang II and is found in relatively high concentrations in the brain and cerebrospinal fluid. Ang IV (Ang 3–8) and Ang 1–7 are both found in human blood and have effects in the vasculature and brain with potential relevance to human physiology and disease.

Receptor activation patterns. There are two well-charac-terized receptors for Ang II, denoted AT$_1$ and AT$_2$ (the subscript numbers of which should not be confused with the Roman numerals or amino acid numerals that define the peptides.) Both receptor subtypes have strong affinity for Ang II and virtually none for Ang I. The gene for AT$_1$ is located on human chromosome 3; the gene for AT$_2$ is located on the X chromosome. Both subtypes are typical of receptors that have seven membrane-spanning sequences, but they share only 34% of their amino acid sequences. AT_1 receptors, the subtype that mediates most of the classic effects of Ang II, are blocked by the angiotensin receptor blockers (ARBs) drug class.

There is no specific receptor for Ang III (Ang 2–8) but the AT_2 subtype has a relatively high affinity for that peptide. A protein with specificity for Ang IV has been described and identified as insulin-regulated aminopeptidase (IRAP), a proteolytic enzyme that is not a classical signal-transducing receptor. Ang 1–7 is tightly bound by a G protein–coupled membrane-spanning receptor previously identified as "Mas." Ang 1–7 also binds weakly to the two classical AT receptors. Ang II biologic actions at its receptors can be mimicked by certain antibodies, including those found in some women with preeclampsia. In vascular smooth muscle cells (VSMC), mechanical stretch can activate AT_1 receptors without the participation of Ang II.

Cellular actions of Ang II
AT_1 receptor mechanisms
Rapid signal transduction. Ang II binding to AT_1 receptors on the cell membrane causes dissociation of G proteins, (especially Gq/11) associated with the intracellular loops of the receptor, activation of phospholipase C, and cleavage of phosphoinositides to form inositol trisphosphate (IP_3) and diacylglycerol (DAG). IP_3 releases calcium (Ca^{2+}) from intracellular stores whereas activated AT_1 receptors also open Ca^{2+} channels in the cell membrane. Calcium and DAG stimulate protein kinase C, which phosphorylates and activates various cell-specific signaling proteins that are responsible for the rapid changes in function initiated by Ang II, most notably VSMC contraction and aldosterone synthesis. Ang II stimulates two other phospholipases: phospholipase A2, which provides arachidonic acid as a substrate for enzymes that form eicosanoids, and phospholipase D, which cleaves phosphatidyl choline. Because phosphatidyl choline is so prevalent, phospholipase D creates enough DAG to prolong Ang II-dependent stimulation of targets after phosphatidyl inositol is depleted.

In some target cells, Ang II stimulates the membrane Na^+/H^+ exchanger, leading to slight intracellular alkalinization. Ang II also affects levels of cyclic adenosine monophosphate (cAMP) and cyclic guanosine monophosphate (cGMP) in several cell types with the magnitude and direction of changes varying from cell to cell.

Ang II stimulates formation of reactive oxygen species, such as superoxide, that mediate and amplify some of the actions of Ang II. Superoxide inactivates nitric oxide, and reactive oxygen species inactivate some protein phosphatases. These actions promote vasoconstriction and growth stimulated by Ang II. Although they are short lived, oxygen-free radicals play an important role in the relatively prolonged growth responses to Ang II.

Gene transcription and protein synthesis. Binding of Ang II to membrane AT_1 receptors initiates a series of events that involve gene transcription and protein synthesis. These gene-expression responses engage several cascades of protein phosphorylation, each of which includes several protein kinases. Among the kinases close to the AT_1 receptor are Src and Jak2. At the other end of the cascades are proteins such as signal transduction and activation of transcription (STAT), MEK, and extracellular signal-regulated protein kinase (ERK) that directly or indirectly regulate gene transcription. Some of the phosphorylation reactions accelerated by Ang II binding to AT_1 receptors are mediated by G proteins

released from the receptor, whereas others are independent of G proteins.

In many cells, Ang II binding to AT_1 receptors enlists peptide growth factors (and their respective receptors), including epidermal growth factor (EGF) and vascular endothelial growth factor (VEGF). To involve these factors, Ang II either releases them from sites where they are inactive, increases their synthesis, and/or increases expression of their respective receptors. When the phosphorylation cascades initiated by these local growth factors are added to those directly initiated by the AT_1 receptor, it appears that almost every known protein kinase is activated by Ang II. The direct actions of Ang II and local growth factors in vessels, heart, and kidney are abetted by blood-borne aldosterone, whose release from the adrenal is stimulated by circulating Ang II.

Receptor regulation. The AT_1 receptor is associated with a protein called *angiotensin receptor–associated protein* (ATRAP) that restrains signal transduction. Direct control of the receptor is exerted by two other proteins, arrestin and dynamin, that usher the Ang II–AT_1 receptor complex to clathrin-coated pits and thence to degradative sites inside the cell. This is a mechanism for rapid downregulation or desensitization that is common to most G protein–linked receptor systems. Internalization does not occur when antagonists (ARBs) bind to the AT_1 receptor. The AT_1 receptor can dimerize and can also form heterodimers with the principal bradykinin receptor (BK2); both doublets have more signal-transducing power than the AT_1 monomer acting alone. Heterodimers of AT_1 and AT_2 are weaker signal transducers than AT_1 monomers or homodimers. The AT_2 receptor subtype is not internalized or acutely downregulated by either Ang II or any known drugs.

AT_2 receptor mechanisms.
Binding of Ang II to AT_2 receptors activates cellular phosphatases, and the resulting protein dephosphorylation counteracts the activating effects of protein kinases on cell growth and other processes. The G protein associated with AT_2 receptors is a member of the Gi class, a classical inhibitory intracellular mediator. AT_2 antagonizes AT_1 in other ways. In the kidney, AT_2 receptors stimulate formation of the vasodilators bradykinin and nitric oxide. Another inhibitory mechanism mediated by AT_2 is hyperpolarization of cell membranes by opening potassium channels. AT_2 activation affects levels of cAMP and cGMP, but the specific magnitude and direction of these changes varies from cell to cell. AT_2 receptors can form heterodimers with the AT_1 receptor, creating a complex that weakens AT_1 signal transduction. Almost every mechanism engaged by the AT_2 receptor antagonizes those engaged by AT_1.

AT_4 and mas (angiotensin 1–7) receptor mechanisms.
Although Ang IV and Ang 1–7 can bind weakly to AT_1 and AT_2, they are more avidly bound by other macromolecules. The IRAP that binds Ang IV is actually a proteolytic enzyme whose activity is inhibited by Ang IV but it is often called the AT_4 receptor. The presumption is that at least some of the cerebral effects of the hexapeptide Ang IV are mediated by prolonging the lifespan of other substrates of the aminopeptidase, including enkephalin and oxytocin.

Ang 1–7 is avidly bound by a protein ("Mas") that was first discovered as a protooncogene, then found to display hallmarks of a transmembrane receptor with no known cognate ligand (aka an "orphan receptor"). It is now recognized that the effects of Ang 1–7 that cannot be explained by weak interactions with AT_1 or AT_2 are mediated by strong activation of Mas.

Mas is a G protein–coupled receptor whose signal transduction involves protein phosphorylation and subsequent release of nitric oxide and eicosanoids. When it binds to AT_2, Ang 1–7 activates mechanisms that oppose classical Ang II actions, resulting in vasodilation of some vascular beds.

Regulation of receptor density and responsiveness

The number of angiotensin receptors available for activation by Ang II depends on synthesis of the receptors themselves as well as internalization and degradation of the peptide–receptor complex. Synthesis of AT_1 receptors is increased by insulin, glucocorticoids, aldosterone, EGF, and some eicosanoid products of lipoxygenase, and decreased by nitric oxide, dopamine, and adrenomedullin. Synthesis of AT_2 receptors is increased by estrogen, tissue injury, and in the myocardium of failing hearts. Density of both receptor subtypes in the myometrium varies during pregnancy and after parturition.

In essential hypertension of animals and humans, virtually all of the pressor and growth-stimulating aspects of Ang II action are increased, from elevation of intracellular Ca^{2+} to production of amplifying autacoids. So far, it has not been possible to identify a single element of the signaling cascade that is solely responsible for this hyperreactivity. Many polymorphisms have been described in the genes coding for AT_1 and AT_2, and at least two have been linked statistically with elevations of blood pressure (BP) in humans or its treatment with ARBs. Considering the many factors that can modulate hormone action, and the many other mechanisms involved in pressure regulation, it is unlikely that more than a small fraction of human hypertension can be explained by abnormal angiotensin receptors.

Physiologic effects of angiotensin II

Short-term actions mediated by AT_1 receptors

Cardiovascular homeostasis. The best-established biologic effects of Ang II are listed in **Table A17.1**, and some are depicted in **Figure A17.1**. Most of the rapid actions comprise a concerted response that supports the circulation when hemorrhage or dehydration depletes plasma volume. These actions include stimulation of vasoconstriction, which reduces the capacitance of the vascular tree, and aldosterone secretion, direct tubular sodium reabsorption, and release of antidiuretic hormone, which conserve intravascular fluid volume. Most other rapid homeostatic actions of Ang II can be viewed as adjuncts to circulatory rescue: increased sympathetic nervous system activity, increased cardiac contractility, increased thirst, intestinal fluid absorption, promotion of blood coagulation by facilitating platelet aggregation, and inhibiting clot lysis by formation of an inhibitor of plasminogen activation (PAI-1). In the absence of volume contraction, the rapid actions of Ang II can elevate BP above baseline. This is particularly evident in renovascular hypertension wherein angiotensin formation is increased despite a normal plasma volume.

Central nervous system. Angiotensin receptors of all subtypes are found in many regions of the brain. Some sites are in circumventricular organs, which lack the usual blood–brain barrier and can be activated by angiotensins present in the circulation. Other sites are behind the blood–brain barrier and are probably activated by angiotensins formed from substrate and enzymes resident in the brain itself. Ang II and III in the brain increase release of antidiuretic hormone, stimulate thirst, and

TABLE A17.1

ANGIOTENSIN TARGETS AND ACTIONS

Target organ or cell	Action (stimulatory unless indicated)
Vascular smooth muscle	Vasoconstriction, hypertrophy, hyperplasia, migration
Vascular endothelium	Prostaglandin, nitric oxide, endothelin and PAI-1 production, cell growth, angiogenesis
Vascular connective tissue	Extracellular matrix synthesis
Myocardium	Inotropy, hypertrophy
Platelets	Aggregation by catecholamines
Monocytes and leukocytes	Chemotaxis, adhesion, oxidative burst
Bone marrow	Erythropoiesis
Adrenal glomerulosa	Aldosterone secretion
Adrenal medulla	Catecholamine release
Adrenal fasciculata	Cortisol secretion
Posterior pituitary	Antidiuretic hormone release
Kidney	Embryogenesis, efferent arteriolar vasoconstriction
Juxtaglomerular cells	Inhibit renin release
Mesangial cells	Contraction, proliferation, fibrogenesis
Proximal tubule	Sodium reabsorption
Sympathetic neurons	Norepinephrine release
Brain	Pressor center activation, baroreceptor blunting, antidiuretic hormone synthesis, thirst, prostaglandin release, memory enhancement
Intestine	Salt and water absorption (AT_2)
Liver	Glycogenolysis, angiotensinogen synthesis

PAI-1, plasminogen activator inhibitor-1.

increase BP by effects on hypothalamic and brain stem neurons that increase sympathetic nerve traffic.

Feedback interactions. Some actions of Ang serve as afferent limbs of negative and positive feedback loops. Ang II directly inhibits release of renin by the juxtaglomerular cells (a negative feedback effect), and stimulates release of angiotensinogen by the liver (a positive feedback effect).

Long-term actions mediated by AT_1 receptors

Cell growth and organ hypertrophy. Administration of subpressor doses of Ang II to animals for days or weeks causes AT_1 receptor–mediated trophic changes in the heart and blood vessels, including hypertrophy of myocardial and vascular contractile cells, with deposition of collagen and other macromolecules of the extracellular matrix. The histologic changes induced by prolonged elevations of Ang II, sometimes called *arterial remodeling*, make arterial smooth muscle cells more numerous, bigger and more sensitive to all vasoconstrictors. Drugs that block the formation of Ang II (ACE inhibitors) or block AT_1 receptors (ARBs) can retard or reverse left ventricular hypertrophy and other structural cardiovascular manifestations of human hypertension.

Inflammation. Ang II stimulates migration and activity of monocytes and other peripheral leukocytes by generation of

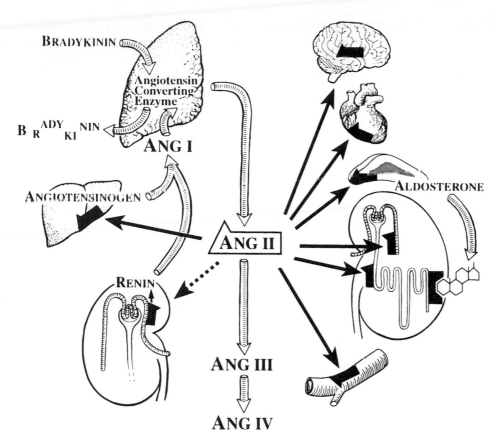

Figure A17.1 Schematic of classical, circulating (blood-borne) renin-angiotensin-aldosterone system. *Tubular arrows* on left show pathway of formation of angiotensin (Ang) II and degradation of bradykinin by enzymes in blood and lung. *Arrows in center* show cascade of proteolytic cleavages that form smaller congeners of Ang II. *Solid arrows* to organs indicate stimulatory actions of Ang II through AT_1 receptors, and dashed arrow shows its inhibition of renin release. *Solid symbols* at end of *arrows* indicate angiotensin receptors. Not shown are the formation and actions of Ang (1–7) and Ang IV (Ang 3–8), the different actions mediated by other receptors, and the synthesis of angiotensin within tissues independent of the blood-borne system.

chemoattractant proteins and by direct binding to AT_1 receptors on circulating mononuclear cells. It is not clear exactly how Ang II alters the activities of circulating cells, but it is known that cytokine release is stimulated. Ang II, through the AT_1 receptor, activates the transcription factor nuclear factor kappa B (NF-B), which triggers transcription of genes whose products cause many features of inflammation.

Embryogenesis. One of the most important slow effects of Ang II is on the developing fetus. Experiments with ACE inhibitors, ARBs, and gene deletions in animals, along with experience with ACE inhibitors and ARBs in humans, clearly show that Ang II is essential for normal embryogenesis. The organ whose development suffers most from loss of Ang II action is the kidney, which becomes hypoplastic. A variety of other abnormalities have been observed in animals and humans when the renin-angiotensin axis is perturbed during fetal life. It is not clear whether the AT_1 or AT_2 receptor subtype is most critical for embryogenesis, although the AT_2 isoform predominates in the fetus.

Erythropoietic and hematologic effects. Ang II, through the AT_1 receptor, synergizes with erythropoietin to increase red cell production. This is most evident in patients whose hematocrit drops a few percent on treatment with drugs that block angiotensin formation or action. Ang II and Ang IV stimulate synthesis of PAI-1 by cells of the vessel wall. The resulting decrease in plasmin activity prolongs clot survival and may also promote deposition of other macromolecules in the vessel wall.

Other actions. There are receptors for Ang II in locations where the function of the peptide is obscure. For example, the rat bladder contracts when exposed to Ang II *in vitro*, but there is no known parallel effect in humans. Tissues of the male and female reproductive tract display angiotensin receptors, but the roles of the peptide in the function of the ovary, uterus, placenta, testis and

spermatozoa are unknown. Similar mystery shrouds the function of Ang II receptors in adipocytes, synovium, skin, peripheral nerves, anterior pituitary, pancreas, retina, and immune system. Effects of Ang II on a variety of epithelial cells are suggested by the presence of receptors there. Although a specific effect may be unclear for a given target, Ang II can affect vascular tone, stimulate angiogenesis, induce production of reactive oxygen species, and promote inflammation rather ubiquitously. A good example of this is the recent attention on the possible role of Ang II in tumors of the breast and prostate where the peptide appears to stimulate growth and angiogenesis.

Actions mediated by AT_2 receptors

Fetal development. AT_2 is the predominant subtype in fetal mammals. It is important in the development of the kidney. Because they mediate vasodilation, AT_2 receptors may protect the fetus from ischemia that might result from any maternal angiotensin that crosses the placenta. In normal adult mammals, the AT_2 subtype is found almost exclusively in some regions of the brain, the uterus, the adrenal medulla, and the kidneys, but in much smaller amounts than in the fetus. Wherever it is found, the AT_2 receptor appears to mediate actions that antagonize those of the AT_1 isoform.

Vasodilation. Activation of AT_2 receptors by Ang II initiates a vasodilatory cascade that begins with release of bradykinin, followed by production of nitric oxide and generation of intracellular cGMP. In addition, AT_2 receptors mediate release of prostaglandins, notably in the kidneys, and inhibition of cell growth. Because ARBs interfere with feedback inhibition of renin release, they cause increased plasma levels of Ang II, but they leave the AT_2 receptor open to the peptide. This has led to speculation that activation of AT_2 subtypes mediate some of the antihypertensive properties of these drugs.

Apoptosis, natriuresis, and other effects. There is evidence that Ang II, when it binds to AT_2, induces apoptosis. This is most evident during embryogenesis where proper organ structure depends on programmed cell death as well as appropriate growth. In the adult kidney, AT_2 receptors promote natriuresis, a process mediated by bradykinin and nitric oxide. Levels of AT_2 receptors in the adult heart are lower than those of AT_1, but they rise dramatically after myocardial infarction, as they do after injury in other tissues. The function of these receptors in injured tissue is unknown, but they may facilitate healing by preventing vasoconstriction that might otherwise occur by Ang II acting through AT_1.

Modulation of angiotensin II actions

Hormones and autacoids. Several classic peptide and non-peptide hormones and autacoids are affected by Ang II, and, in turn, modify the direct actions of Ang II. Aldosterone, catecholamine, and antidiuretic hormone release are increased by Ang II, and they work with Ang II to protect or expand circulating blood volume and maintain BP. Aldosterone also amplifies the actions of Ang II to release PAI-1 from endothelium and to stimulate fibrosis in the heart and blood vessels. Ang II stimulates release of endothelin and thromboxane from endothelium, and both of those autacoids contribute to vasoconstriction.

The slower actions of Ang II to stimulate growth, fibrosis, and inflammation in the cardiovascular system are amplified by growth factors such as platelet-derived growth factor, EGF, insulin-like growth factor, basic fibroblast growth factor, and transforming growth factor β. By contrast, the vasodilators nitric oxide and prostacyclin released from blood vessels under the influence of Ang II protect the kidney and other vital organs from excessive vasoconstriction.

Oxidative stress. Along with aldosterone, thromboxane, catecholamines, growth factors, and endothelin, Ang II exerts some of its effects on the cardiovascular system by stimulating the production of reactive oxygen species. Those derivatives of oxygen, such as peroxide and superoxide, can damage cell membrane lipids, intracellular structural proteins, and nucleic acids, and can combine with nitric oxide. When the net effect is deleterious, the phenomenon is called *oxidative stress*, but some of these highly reactive molecules participate in adaptive Ang II actions.

Biologic effects of other angiotensins

Ang 1–7 binds with low affinity to the AT_1 receptor, and is a weak agonist there, so the net effect of large amounts of that peptide is to partially inhibit classical Ang II actions. In addition, Ang 1–7 induces formation of nitric oxide and vasodilator prostaglandins and retards vascular smooth muscle growth by a mechanism that probably involves AT_2 and Mas receptors. Ang IV (Ang 3–8) has effects on the brain that favorably affect memory in rodents. This may be achieved by inhibiting degradation of other peptides cleaved by IRAP (aka AT_4). Ang IV also stimulates the release of PAI-1 from endothelial cells.

Suggested Readings

Carey RM, Siragy HM. Newly recognized components of the renin-angiotensin system: potential roles in cardiovascular and renal regulation. *Endocr Rev* 2003; 24: 261–271.

Goodfriend TL. Angiotensin receptors: history and mysteries. *Am J Hypertens* 2000; 13: 442–449.

Hunyady L, Catt KJ. Pleiotropic AT1 receptor signaling pathways mediating physiological and pathogenic actions of angiotensin II. *Mol Endocrinol* 2006; 20: 953–970.

Johren O, Dendorfer A, Dominiak P. Cardiovascular and renal function of angiotensin II type-2 receptors. *Cardiovasc Res* 2004; 62: 460–467.

Struthers AD, MacDonald TM. Review of aldosterone- and angiotensin II-induced target organ damage and prevention. *Cardiovasc Res* 2004; 61: 663–670.

CHAPTER A18 ■ TISSUE RENIN-ANGIOTENSIN SYSTEMS

NANCY J. BROWN, MD

KEY POINTS

■ Many tissues can synthesize angiotensin (Ang) II independent of the classic circulating renin-angiotensin system (RAS).

■ Local uptake and activation of prorenin and renin through the renin receptor may amplify the effects of low local expression.

■ Locally formed angiotensins play an important role in the regulation of blood pressure and promote inflammation, fibrosis, and remodeling.

■ Tissue Ang II is a target for antihypertensive and vasoprotective effects of drugs.

See also Chapters A13, A14, A15, A16, A17, C135, and C137

Classically, the renin-angiotensin system (RAS) has been viewed as a circulating endocrine system in which renin, produced by the juxtaglomerular cells, cleaved angiotensinogen (AGT) produced in the liver, to form angiotensin (Ang) I. Ang I was further degraded to the potent vasoconstrictor Ang II through angiotensin-converting enzyme (ACE), particularly at the pulmonary endothelium. It is now appreciated that the tissue RAS has important paracrine, autocrine, and even intracrine effects.

Renin

Tissue Ang I and Ang II may be produced by the effects of circulating, kidney-derived renin or through locally produced renin. Renin expression has been demonstrated in the adrenal cortex, the brain, the pituitary gland, the ovary, the vasculature, and the heart. Renin 1A, a transcript that lacks the coding region for the secretory signal peptide, is expressed in adrenal, brain, and heart tissue. Renin and renin 1A expression are increased in the heart following myocardial infarction. However, for the most part, studies in nephrectomized rats suggest that the production of cardiac angiotensins depends on the uptake of circulating renin, rather than *in situ* production. In contrast, local renin expression contributes to the vascular synthesis of Ang II in nephrectomized animals.

Angiotensinogen

Tissue Ang II concentrations exceed plasma concentrations and vary considerably among different tissues, suggesting Ang II can be synthesized *in situ*. The liver is the largest source of AGT but AGT is also expressed in glial cells, neurons, pituitary cells, fibroblasts, and adipocytes. Vascular AGT is expressed primarily in the adventitia and surrounding fatty tissue. The local production of AGT is increased in the heart during pressure overload and following myocardial infarction. Thyroid hormone, glucocorticoids, estrogen, and high salt intake also increase cardiac AGT expression.

Angiotensin-converting enzyme and other angiotensin-generating enzymes

Although a small amount of ACE circulates in the serum, ACE functions primarily as an ectoenzyme on the cell surface where it hydrolyzes peptides such as Ang I. ACE is expressed in endothelial cells, monocytes, T lymphocytes, and adipocytes, and, in a smaller germinal form in the testes. ACE expression is upregulated in atherosclerotic plaques and in the heart after injury. In addition to producing Ang II, ACE may contribute to the effects of the tissue renin-angiotensin system (RAS) by functioning as a signaling molecule on the cell surface. Enzymes other than ACE may also contribute to the local generation of Ang II. Chymase, a serine protease belonging to the chymotrypsin family, is found in mast cells and contributes to the generation of Ang II in the heart and vasculature. Other enzymes may function to counteract the effects of locally produced Ang II. ACE2, expressed in endothelial cells, hydrolyzes Ang I to Ang 1–9 and Ang II to Ang 1–7.

Aldosterone

In addition to being synthesized by the adrenal gland, aldosterone can be synthesized in the brain and vasculature. The heart expresses steroidogenic acute regulatory protein and aldosterone synthase; however, the weight of evidence suggests that cardiac aldosterone, like renin, is derived from circulating aldosterone. Mineralocorticoid receptors (MR) are expressed in nonepithelial tissues such as the brain, cardiomyocytes of the heart, and endothelial and smooth muscle cells of the vasculature. In the heart, which lacks 11β-hydroxysteroid dehydrogenase (HSD2), the enzyme that converts cortisol and corticosterone to the non-MR binding cortisone and 11-dehydrocorticosterone, the MR is occupied by glucocorticoids, which circulate at 1,000-fold excess in the plasma compared to aldosterone. Furthermore, in the heart, glucocorticoids may act as antagonists, rather than agonists, at the MR.

Increased efficiency of the tissue renin-angiotensin system

Given the low levels of expression of renin in tissues such as the heart, the efficiency of the local RAS requires either the uptake of circulating prorenin or renin or the amplification of the effects of locally produced renin. Internalization of prorenin or renin by the mannose 6-phosphate/insulin-like growth factor II (MP/IGFII) receptor results in the intracellular activation of prorenin; however, this receptor is felt to function primarily as a clearance receptor. On the other hand, binding of prorenin or renin to the newly described "renin receptor" induces a conformational change and increased activity of prorenin and renin, thereby intensifying the effect of low levels of expression. In addition to activating the cell-surface receptors AT_1 and AT_2, Ang II can be internalized to act at intracellular sites. Ang II produced from Ang I, restricted to the extracellular compartment, appears to be internalized through AT_1 receptor–dependent endocytosis. Because extracellular Ang II is degraded by angiotensinases more rapidly than receptor-bound Ang II, AT_1 receptor antagonists may increase the degradation of tissue Ang II by displacing it from the receptor.

Function of the tissue renin-angiotensin system

The tissue RAS plays an important role in the regulation of reproduction through effects in the pituitary, the testes, and the ovaries. However, this chapter focuses on the roles of the tissue RAS relevant to hypertension and its adverse effects.

Cardiovascular remodeling. All the components of the RAS are expressed in the heart and vasculature (See **Figure A18.1**). Uptake of circulating renin by cardiomyocytes contributes to Ang I formation in the heart. Cardiac ACE expression is increased following myocardial infarction and in the hearts of patients with atrial fibrillation. Chymase derived from mast cells also converts Ang I to Ang II. In contrast to the circulating RAS, the cardiac RAS is upregulated by high salt intake. Locally produced Ang II induces hypertrophy through activation of tyrosine kinase and RhoA cascades, including activation of mitogen-activating protein (MAP) kinase and Janus kinase/signal transducers and activators of transcription (JAK/STAT) pathways. Ang II induces inflammation and fibrosis, in part through increased synthesis of growth factors such as endothelin and transforming growth factor-β. Aldosterone also stimulates the generation of reactive oxygen species, cardiac inflammation, and fibrosis. Locally produced Ang II may act in part by transactivating cardiac MR.

Vascular inflammation. Atherosclerosis is a low-grade inflammatory process marked initially by the recruitment of inflammatory cells and the accumulation of lipids. Monocytes and

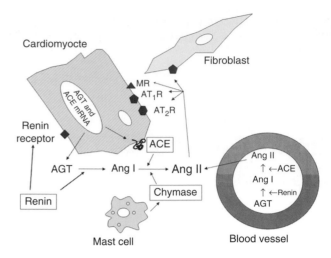

Figure A18.1 Schematic representation of the renin-angiotensin system (RAS) in the heart. Renin may be taken up from the plasma or formed locally particularly in the vasculature. Angiotensinogen (AGT) and angiotensin-converting enzyme (ACE) expression is upregulated during pressure overload or following myocardial infarction. Chymase, produced by mast cells, can also convert angiotensin (Ang) I to Ang II. Locally produced Ang II can act through the AT_1 or AT_1 receptor (R) or may transactivate the mineralocorticoid receptor (MR).

macrophages express AGT, renin, ACE, and the AT_1 receptor. Upregulation of the RAS during monocyte differentiation to macrophages may play a role in monocyte migration into the vascular wall. Ang II generates reactive oxygen species and uptake of oxidized low-density lipoprotein by macrophages leads to the formation of foam cells. ACE is upregulated in atherosclerotic plaques and locally produced Ang II can induce oxidative stress and stimulate the release of metalloproteases contributing to the pathogenesis of plaque rupture.

Kidney disease. In addition to producing renin, the kidney contains all of the components of a local RAS. AGT and ACE expression are greatest in the proximal tubules. Mesangial cells also express renin and ACE. Ang II affects glomerular blood flow and filtration through constriction of the afferent and efferent arterioles and promotes growth and fibrosis. In addition, renin stimulates mesangial expression of profibrotic molecules through direct Ang II-independent, renin receptor-dependent mechanisms. Interruption of the RAS has become the mainstay in preventing the development of renal injury in predisposed patients.

Central regulation of blood pressure. Ang II, acting at specific nuclei within the brain, increases blood pressure, sympathetic outflow, vasopressin release and drinking behavior, and attenuates the baroreflex response. The separation of the brain from the systemic circulation by the blood–brain barrier and the local expression of many components of the RAS provide evidence for a brain RAS. For example, glial cells throughout the brain express AGT. Regions of the brain responsible for blood pressure regulation express both ACE and the AT_1 receptor. The role of local renin production in the generation of Ang II in the brain is controversial. Renin is expressed in low levels, in the pineal gland, pituitary, choroid plexus, hypothalamus, cerebellum, and amygdala. The renin receptor is expressed in the brain and may magnify the effect of locally expressed renin. Renin 1A expression has been identified in the brain, raising the possibility of intracellular Ang II generation. Alternatively, Ang II may be formed by renin-independent pathways, such as through tonin expressed by astrocytes. In addition, Ang II degrading enzymes are expressed in the brain and may produce peptide fragments such as Ang III [Ang (2–8)], and Ang IV [Ang (3–8)], which also act centrally to increase blood pressure.

Obesity. Adipose tissue expresses AGT, ACE, renin, and the AT_1 receptor. Studies in adipose-specific AGT transgenic mice as well as in obese humans suggest that components derived from adipose tissue may contribute to circulating concentrations of the RAS in obesity. Ang II inhibits the differentiation of preadipocytes and induces insulin-resistance through interactions between the AT_1 and insulin receptors. Ang II also induces adipocytes expression of inflammatory cytokines and the prothrombotic plasminogen activator inhibitor-1.

Overview

Ang II is produced locally in many tissues vital to the regulation of blood pressure and end organ damage. Local production of Ang II may rely on tissue uptake of circulating renin or on the local expression of renin. The renin receptor may function to amplify the effects of small amounts of locally produced prorenin or renin. Tissue Ang II may also be produced by nonrenin proteases such as chymase and tonin. Locally produced Ang II may act through its extracellular receptors, may act intracellularly or may transactivate the MR. Locally generated Ang II contributes significantly to inflammation and remodeling.

Suggested Readings

Chai W, Danser AH. Is angiotensin II made inside or outside of the cell? *Curr Hypertens Rep* 2005;7:124–127.

Fleming I, Kohlstedt K, Busse R. The tissue renin-angiotensin system and intracellular signaling. *Curr Opin Nephrol Hypertens* 2006;15:8–13.

Funder JW. Mineralocorticoid receptors and cardiovascular damage: it's not just aldosterone. *Hypertension* 2006;47:634–635.

Miyazaki M, Takai S. Tissue angiotensin II generating system by angiotensin-converting enzyme and chymase. *J Pharmacol Sci* 2006;100:391–397.

Nguyen G. Renin/prorenin receptors. *Kidney Int* 2006;69:1503–1506.

Paul M, Poyan MA, Kreutz R. Physiology of local renin-angiotensin systems. *Physiol Rev* 2006;86:747–803.

Sakai K, Sigmund CD. Molecular evidence of tissue renin-angiotensin systems: a focus on the brain. *Curr Hypertens Rep* 2005;7:135–140.

CHAPTER A19 ■ ADRENAL STEROID SYNTHESIS AND REGULATION

CELSO E. GOMEZ-SANCHEZ, MD

KEY POINTS

- The adrenal cortex synthesizes aldosterone in the zona glomerulosa and cortisol in the zona fasciculata.
- Aldosterone synthesis and secretion is regulated primarily by angiotensin II (Ang II) and potassium.
- The adrenal cortex also synthesizes less potent sodium-retaining steroids, including deoxycorticosterone (DOC), 18-oxocortisol, 18-hydroxydeoxycorticosterone, and 19-nordeoxycorticosterone, which can be clinically significant in patients with adrenal adenomas or other syndromes of mineralocorticoid excess.
- Metabolism of cortisol in mineralocorticoid target organs determines whether the mineralocorticoid receptor responds selectively to aldosterone.
- Small amounts of aldosterone can be synthesized in extra-adrenal organs where they may have a paracrine or autocrine function.

See also Chapters **A20** and **C167**

Adrenal cortex

The adrenal cortex contains three distinct areas that are involved in adrenal steroid biosynthesis. Each of these areas plays different physiologic and therefore pathophysiologic roles. Cells of the outer portion of the adrenal, the zona glomerulosa, synthesize aldosterone, the most important mineralocorticoid hormone. The next layer, or zona fasciculata (fasciculata-reticularis in some species), is the site of synthesis of the most important glucocorticoids, cortisol in species (including the human) that express the cytochrome P-450 17α-hydroxylase or corticosterone in those that do not have cytochrome P-450 17α-hydroxylase. The innermost layer of the cortex, the zona reticularis, is the site of synthesis of adrenal androgens. There is a relatively narrow progenitor zone of cells that do not appear to produce steroids that is located between the zona glomerulosa and fasciculata.

Regulation of steroid biosynthesis

Adrenocorticotropic hormone (ACTH) is responsible for the trophic regulation and the maintenance of steroidogenic capacity of the zona fasciculata. Acute increases in ACTH or its administration results in the rapid release of both cortisol and aldosterone. The acute effects of ACTH are mediated by a cyclic adenosine monophosphate–mediated process resulting in the rapid mobilization of cholesterol for steroidogenesis through a labile protein (i.e., StAR or steroidogenic acute regulatory protein). Continued ACTH stimulation does not result in sustained aldosterone synthesis. Chronic aldosterone regulation is primarily under the control of angiotensin II (Ang II) and extracellular potassium (K^+). Changes in vascular volume or sodium (Na^+) ingestion affect aldosterone secretion by variably altering levels of Ang II.

Synthetic pathways

Most of the enzymes required for the synthesis of cortisol and aldosterone from cholesterol are the same (**Figure A19.1**), except for those involved in terminal synthetic reactions.

Initial steps. Cholesterol is the fundamental building block for steroid synthesis; high-density lipoprotein (HDL) and low-density lipoprotein (LDL) in plasma transport most of the cholesterol used by the adrenal gland for steroid synthesis. After deposition in intracellular lipid droplets, cholesterol is transported into the mitochondria by an incompletely understood mechanism that involves StAR and a peripheral benzodiazepine receptor. In the inner mitochondrial membrane, the cytochrome P-450 side-chain cleavage enzyme performs successive hydroxylations of cholesterol, eliminating a portion of the side chain, to generate pregnenolone.

17-hydroxylation. In the zona fasciculata, pregnenolone is hydroxylated to 17α-hydroxy pregnenolone by microsomal cytochrome P-450 17α-hydroxylase.

Isomeration. Pregnenolone in the zona glomerulosa and 17α-hydroxypregnenolone in the zona fasciculata are then oxidized and isomerized by the microsomal enzyme 3β-ol dehydrogenase 4-5 isomerase to generate progesterone and

17α-hydroxyprogesterone, which are then hydroxylated by microsomal cytochrome P-450 21-hydroxylase to DOC and 11-deoxycortisol.

11-hydroxylation. DOC and 11-deoxycortisol then diffuse into the mitochondria of the zona glomerulosa and zona fasciculata, respectively, where two similar enzymes transform them to aldosterone and cortisol. In humans, two cytochrome P-450-11β-hydroxylases have been described: the 11β-hydroxylase in the fasciculata and aldosterone synthase in the glomerulosa. Genes for these enzymes are located on chromosome 8q24.3, separated by approximately 40 kilobases (kb), with nine exons spread over 7 kb of DNA and a sequence homology of 95% in the coding region and 90% in the introns.

Aldosterone synthase. Aldosterone synthase, a cytochrome P-450 on the inner mitochondrial membrane of the zona glomerulosa, binds DOC and catalyzes three successive hydroxylations, converting DOC into corticosterone (11-hydroxylation), corticosterone to 18-hydroxycorticosterone (18-OH-B), and 18-OH-B to a germinal diol that spontaneously dehydrates to form aldosterone. Aldosterone synthase is a relatively inefficient, partial-processing enzyme from which a significant portion of the products of each enzymatic hydroxylation escapes from the enzyme only to be secreted. As a consequence, the zona glomerulosa secretes significantly greater quantities of corticosterone and 18-OH-B than it does aldosterone. These free metabolites are less efficient substrates for aldosterone synthase, especially 18-OH-B, which adopts a stable hemiacetal form that is a very poor substrate for the enzyme.

Cortisol synthesis. In the zona fasciculata, 11-deoxycortisol also passively enters the mitochondria where it is hydroxylated by the cytochrome P-450 11β-hydroxylase to cortisol. Not all of the pregnenolone is hydroxylated to 17α-hydroxy pregnenolone in the human zona fasciculata; as in the zona glomerulosa, the remaining pregnenolone is successively hydroxylated to form DOC and corticosterone. Because the mass of fasciculata tissue is far larger than that of the glomerulosa, most of the DOC and corticosterone in plasma originates in the zona fasciculata.

Other mineralocorticoids

Aldosterone is the most important mineralocorticoid, but other adrenal corticosteroids also have variable mineralocorticoid activity, including DOC, 18-oxocortisol, 19-nordeoxycorticosterone (19-norDOC), and 18-hydroxydeoxycorticosterone (18-OH-DOC). 11β-hydroxylase has the ability, but to a lesser degree, to hydroxylate DOC or 11-deoxycortisol in other positions of the steroid molecule, including the 18 position (to generate 18-OH-DOC) and the 19 position (to generate 19-OH-DOC). The degree of alternative hydroxylations for this enzyme is species dependent.

Deoxycorticosterone. Increased production of DOC occurs in individuals with 11β-hydroxylase deficiency or in adrenal tumors having incomplete expression of this enzyme.

18-hydroxydeoxycorticosterone. In the rat, approximately 25% of DOC is transformed into 18-OH-DOC. Although it has weak mineralocorticoid properties, 18-OH-DOC is produced in large enough amounts to participate in the development of hypertension in the Dahl salt-sensitive rat. In this animal, a high-salt diet suppresses aldosterone, but not corticosterone or 18-OH-DOC (a side product of 11β-hydroxylase) production. The human 11β-hydroxylase synthesizes a much smaller proportion of 18-OH-DOC, but there are cases of mineralocorticoid

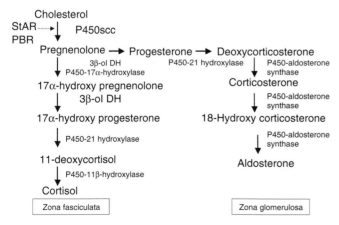

Figure A19.1 Biosynthesis of adrenal steroids in the human zona fasciculata and glomerulosa. StAR, steroidogenic acute regulatory protein; PBR, peripheral benzodiazepine receptor; DH, dehydrogenase.

hypertension in which increased secretion of 18-OH-DOC has been demonstrated.

19-nordeoxycorticosterone and 19-noraldosterone.

The steroid 19-norDOC, a potent mineralocorticoid, was initially identified in the urine of rats undergoing adrenal regeneration. 19-Hydroxylation of DOC by the 11β-hydroxylase occurs in small quantities and the product is further processed, probably by successive hydroxylations, to form 19-oxoDOC and 19-oicDOC. 19-NorDOC is formed extraadrenally, probably in the kidney, by the decarboxylation of the adrenal precursor 19-oicDOC. 19-NorDOC has been found to be elevated in the urine of some rat models of genetic hypertension and in very rare cases of hypertension associated with adrenal adenomas. Another 19-nor steroid, 19-noraldosterone, a mineralocorticoid with similar potency to that of aldosterone, is also excreted in excessive amounts (but less so than aldosterone) in patients with primary aldosteronism. The biosynthetic pathway for the formation of this steroid is unknown.

Extraadrenal synthesis

Steroid transformations occur outside steroid-producing glands. Testosterone action is mediated to a significant degree by its peripheral conversion to estradiol, a reaction catalyzed by the aromatase enzyme, and also by conversion to 5α-dihydrotestosterone by 5α-reductases. In addition, *de novo* synthesis of pregnenolone, progesterone, DOC, and their reduced derivatives occurs in the brain to form neurosteroids. Corticosterone and aldosterone can be formed in vascular tissue and brain by the same steroidogenic enzymes present in the adrenal, which are also expressed in small amounts in these tissues. It is likely that corticosterone and aldosterone formed in vascular and brain tissue have a paracrine rather than an autocrine role, because their contribution to circulating steroid levels is negligible in that aldosterone and corticosterone levels become unmeasurable in plasma after adrenalectomy.

Target cell metabolism and receptor specificity

The mineralocorticoid receptor exhibits similar affinity for aldosterone, corticosterone, and cortisol. Under normal conditions, corticosterone and cortisol are secreted and circulate in 100- to 1,000-fold greater quantities than aldosterone. Aldosterone is able to successfully compete for its receptor in mineralocorticoid target cells such as those of the kidney tubule because specificity of the mineralocorticoid receptor for aldosterone is conferred by the coexpression of enzymes that metabolize cortisol or corticosterone into inactive compounds such as cortisone or 11-dehydrocorticosterone in these cells. The 11β-hydroxysteroid dehydrogenase-2 is a NAD+-dependent, high affinity, unidirectional enzyme which, when expressed in the same cell as the mineralocorticoid receptor, protects the receptor from binding by more abundant glucocorticoids. Congenital or acquired (by ingestion of licorice or derivatives) deficiency of the 11β-hydroxysteroid dehydrogenase-2 enzyme results in the syndrome of apparent mineralocorticoid excess. In these cases, cortisol is able to reach the receptor and produce transactivation. An isoform of 11β-hydroxysteroid dehydrogenase-2 (**Figure A19.2**), 11β-hydroxysteroid dehydrogenase-1 is an NADP+-dependent, low-affinity, bidirectional enzyme that preferentially reduces cortisone to cortisol. In circumstances in which NADP+ is not available, as in hexose-6-phosphate dehydrogenase deficiency, the 11β-hydroxysteroid dehydrogenase-1 acts as a dehydrogenase converting cortisol to cortisone.

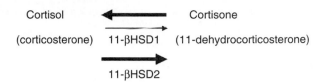

Figure A19.2 Regulation of the formation of cortisol and cortisone in peripheral tissues by the 11β-hydroxysteroid dehydrogenase (11-βHSD) enzymes.

Hepatic and renal metabolism of adrenal steroids

In the human, aldosterone is metabolized in the liver and kidney. In the liver, the principal metabolite (~30%–40%) is 3α,5β-tetrahydroaldosterone, which is excreted in the urine as a 3-glucuronide, and, in the kidney, aldosterone is conjugated at the 18-position to form aldosterone-18-oxo-glucuronide (~5%–10%). This renal metabolite is acid sensitive and generates aldosterone when incubated at pH 1. It is the most commonly measured urinary metabolite used in the diagnosis of alterations of aldosterone secretion.

Further metabolism of the glucocorticoids occurs primarily in the liver, where cortisol is reduced at the third and the fifth position of the steroid molecule to form tetrahydrocortisol (5β reduction) and allotetrahydrocortisol (5α reduction). Cortisone is similarly reduced at the third and fifth positions of the steroid molecule to form tetrahydrocortisone. These metabolites are excreted in the urine as glucuronide conjugates. The measurement of the ratio of tetrahydrocortisol plus allotetrahydrocortisol over tetrahydrocortisone is used for estimation of *in vivo* 11β-hydroxysteroid dehydrogenase-2 activity.

Syndromes with abnormal steroid synthesis

In aldosterone-producing adenomas and in glucocorticoid-suppressible aldosteronism (also known as *glucocorticoid-remediable aldosteronism, or GRA*), 11-deoxycortisol can be metabolized by aldosterone synthase to generate the aldosterone analogs 18-hydroxycortisol and 18-oxocortisol. Some aldosterone-producing adenomas express the 17α-hydroxylase and aldosterone synthase. In GRA, there is a gene duplication resulting from the crossover of the genes CYP11B1-11β-hydroxylase) and CYP11B2 (aldosterone synthase) with the formation of an additional gene that has sequences for the promoter region and first exons of the 11β-hydroxylase, followed by most of the coding region from the aldosterone synthase gene. This results in an enzyme expressed in the zona fasciculata and regulated by ACTH that can synthesize aldosterone from DOC or 18-hydroxycortisol and form 18-oxocortisol from 11-deoxycortisol. 18-Oxocortisol has approximately 2% of the mineralocorticoid activity of aldosterone and produces a hypertensive state when infused in rats or sheep. The large amounts of 18-oxocortisol produced in GRA play a role in the pathogenesis of hypertension in this syndrome.

Suggested Readings

Auchus RJ, Miller WL. The principles, pathways and enzymes of human steroidogenesis. In: DeGroot LJ, Jameson JL, eds. *Endocrinology.* 5th ed, Chapter 116. Philadelphia: Elsevier Science, 2006.

Compagnone NA, Mellon SH. Neurosteroids: biosynthesis and function of these novel neuromodulators. *Front Neuroendocrinol* 2000;21:1–56.

Connell JM, Davies E. The new biology of aldosterone. *J Endocrinol* 2005;186:1–20.

Hewitt KN, Walker EA, Stewart PM. Mini-review: hexose-6-phosphate dehydrogenase and redox control of 11{beta}-hydroxysteroid dehydrogenase type 1 activity. *Endocrinology* 2005;146:2539–2543.

Melby JC, Griffing GT, Gomez-Sanchez CE. 19-Nor-deoxycorticosterone (19-nor-DOC) in genetic and experimental hypertension in rats and in human

hypertension. In: Biglieri EG, Melby JC, eds. *Endocrine Hypertension*. New York: Raven Press, 1990:183–194.

Stocco DM. Star protein and the regulation of steroid hormone biosynthesis. *Annu Rev Physiol* 2001;63:193–213.

White PC. Inherited forms of mineralocorticoid hypertension. *Hypertension* 1996; 28:927–936.

White PC, Mune T, Agarwal AK. 11-Beta-hydroxysteroid dehydrogenase and the syndrome of apparent mineralocorticoid excess. *Endocr Rev* 1997;18:135–156.

CHAPTER A20 ■ MINERALOCORTICOID RECEPTORS

TAE-YON CHUN, PhD AND J. HOWARD PRATT, MD

KEY POINTS

■ Aldosterone binding to mineralocorticoid receptors (MRs) increases expression of Sgk1, which leads to phosphorylation of certain proteins and increased numbers of epithelial sodium channels.

■ The enzyme 11β-hydroxysteroid dehydrogenase type 2 prevents cortisol from serving as a ligand for MR, thereby conferring selectivity for aldosterone.

■ MR-mediated responses to aldosterone in cardiovascular and renal tissues result in necrosis and fibrosis if salt intake is high.

See also Chapters **A19, C131, and C167**

Aldosterone's principal functions, increased sodium (Na^+) reabsorption and potassium (K^+) secretion in the distal nephron, are initiated by binding of aldosterone to the mineralocorticoid receptor (MR). The phylogenetic emergence of the MR, and therefore its biologic role, predates that of aldosterone synthase. MRs are expressed in the kidney, colon, sweat glands, brain, vasculature, and heart. MRs belong to the family of nuclear receptors [a large family that includes receptors for other steroid hormones, thyroid hormone, vitamin D, retinoic acid, and peroxisome proliferator-activated receptors (PPARs)] that, when coupled to a selective ligand, function as transcription factors. MRs have taken on new relevance with the growing interest in aldosterone as an important mediator of hypertension and cardiovascular disease.

Mineralocorticoid receptor selectivity: 11β-hydroxysteroid dehydrogenase type 2

Cortisol is a ligand for MR, with an affinity equal to that of aldosterone. Despite much higher circulating levels of cortisol than aldosterone, the specificity of MR for aldosterone is maintained by the enzyme 11β-hydroxysteroid dehydrogenase type 2 (11βHSD2), which is expressed in close proximity to the MR. Oxidation of cortisol by 11βHSD2 forms cortisone, which has no affinity for MR, leaving aldosterone as the singular ligand activating this receptor.

There are nonepithelial sites where MRs do not coexist with 11βHSD2, such as in brain and possibly the heart, where cortisol may be the principal MR ligand. When 11βHSD2 is deficient, as occurs with licorice ingestion or with mutation in the 11βHSD2 gene (the syndrome of apparent mineralocorticoid excess), increased retention of Na^+ contributes to what is not uncommonly severe hypertension. Some studies have suggested that lesser degrees of 11βHSD2 deficiency may contribute to common forms of salt-sensitive hypertension.

Mineralocorticoid receptor–induced NA reabsorption

Aldosterone increases Na^+ reabsorption in the renal cortical collecting duct through at least two mechanisms that are temporally distinct.

Rapid effects. A common denominator is increased expression of serum- and glucocorticoid-induced kinase 1 (Sgk1) (**Figure A20.1**). An increase in Sgk1 leads to phosphorylation and inactivation of Nedd4-2, a ubiquitin ligase that functions in its unphosphorylated state to internalize and inactivate Na^+ channels [epithelial Na channel (ENaC)] and to limit Na^+ reabsorption in the distal nephron. MR activation results in an accumulation of ENaC units at the cell surface because their usual rates of inactivation by Nedd4-2 are reduced. It is therefore believed that Sgk1 is an immediate early gene with rapid effects on the

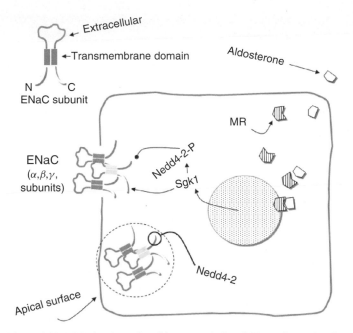

Figure A20.1 Mechanisms for aldosterone-induced Na reabsorption by the epithelial Na channel (ENaC). Aldosterone coupled to mineralocorticoid receptor (MR) increases transcription of Sgk1. Sgk1 phosphorylates the ubiquitin ligase, Nedd4-2, thereby disabling its ability to internalize ENaC. In addition, Sgk1 increases *expression of αENaC*. ENaC is composed of 4 subunits: 2αs, 1β, and 1γ. Na$^+$ exits the cell at the basolateral side by way of the Na$^+$ pump (not shown).

residency time of ENaC at the cell surface (through inhibition of Nedd4-2), an influence that parallels the fluctuations in aldosterone levels.

Longer-term effects. A slower effect of MR activation of Na$^+$ reabsorption occurs through increases in transcription of the gene for the α subunit of ENaC. In this case, Sgk1-mediated phosphorylation results in chromosomal derepression of α *ENaC* transcription. The more delayed increase in expression of α-*ENaC* probably receives input from other factors in addition to aldosterone to allow a more sustained level of ENaC activity.

Syndromes of mineralocorticoid receptor variation

Loss-of-function mutations in MR result in pseudohypoaldosteronism type 1, a salt-losing disorder that can be life threatening in the neonatal period. A mutation in MR (S810L) that permitted recognition of progesterone as an activating ligand was identified in individuals with hypokalemia and hypertension during pregnancy. Similar mutations have not been identified in other families or individuals with hypertension but the occasional appearance of similar phenotypes suggests that other molecular variations or differences in the untranslated region of the gene may exist.

Effects of mineralocorticoid receptor blockade

Nonepithelial mineralocorticoid receptor effects. Nonclassical aldosterone targets include cardiomyocytes, renal interstitium, and endothelium. Many of the well-known adverse effects of angiotensin II may be a consequence of elevated aldosterone levels as demonstrated in models where adrenalectomy or MR blockade ameliorates disease or injury. In almost all cases, concomitant increases in Na$^+$ ingestion are required for the deleterious effects of excess aldosterone to be fully recognized.

Hypertension. Some patients with hypertension, particularly older individuals, demonstrate a pattern of elevated plasma aldosterone level with suppressed plasma renin activity that is consistent with primary aldosteronism. Most of these individuals have bilateral adrenal hyperplasia and often the blood pressure (BP) is highly responsive to MR blockade (spironolactone or eplerenone) or inhibition of ENaC (amiloride). Some hypertensive patients with normal plasma or urinary aldosterone levels but suppressed renin secretion may also demonstrate remarkable improvement in BP control with the addition of a small dose of MR antagonist.

Heart failure. Two clinical trials have shown that the MR antagonists spironolactone and eplerenone can improve the natural history of heart failure: the Randomized Aldactone Evaluation Study (RALES) and the Eplerenone Post-Acute Myocardial Infarction Heart Failure Efficacy and Survival Study (EPHESUS). In both trials, the MR antagonist was added to angiotensin-converting enzyme (ACE) inhibition, suggesting a specific benefit of MR blockade beyond the effects of decreasing angiotensin II generation. The doses of antagonists in both studies were small and with minimal, if any, effect on BP. Some investigators have postulated that MR activation induces the formation of inflammatory cytokines but the precise mechanism for the favorable outcomes in both the RALES and EPHESUS remain a topic of active debate.

Suggested Readings

Bridgham JT, Carroll SM, Thornton JW. Evolution of hormone-receptor complexity by molecular exploitation. *Science* 2006;312(5770):97–101.

Mune T, Rogerson FM, Nikkila H, et al. Human hypertension caused by mutations in the kidney isozyme of 11 beta-hydroxysteroid dehydrogenase. *Nat Genet* 1995;10(4):394–399.

Pearce D, Kleyman TR. Salt, sodium channels, and SGK1. *J Clin Invest.* 2007;117(3):592–595.

Pearce D, Verrey F, Chen SY, et al. Role of SGK in mineralocorticoid-regulated sodium transport. *Kidney Int* 2000;57(4):1283–1289.

Pitt B, Remme W, Zannad F, et al. Eplerenone, a selective aldosterone blocker, in patients with left ventricular dysfunction after myocardial infarction. *N Engl J Med* 2003;348(14):1309–1321.

Pitt B, Zannad F, Remme WJ, et al. The effect of spironolactone on morbidity and mortality in patients with severe heart failure. *N Engl J Med* 1999;341:709–717.

Saha C, Eckert GJ, Ambrosius WT, et al. Improvement in BP with inhibition of the epithelial sodium channel in blacks with hypertension. *Hypertension* 2005;46(3):481–487.

Staub O, Abriel H, Plant P, et al. Regulation of the epithelial Na$^+$ channel by Nedd4 and ubiquitination. *Kidney Int* 2000;57(3):809–815.

Zhang W, Xia X, Reisenauer MR, et al. Aldosterone-induced Sgk1 relieves Dot1a-Af9-mediated transcriptional repression of epithelial Na channel alpha. *J Clin Invest* 2007;117(3):773–783.

CHAPTER A21 ■ ENDOTHELIN

ERNESTO L. SCHIFFRIN, MD, PhD, FRSC, FRCPC, FACP

KEY POINTS

■ Endothelin (ET)-1 is a potent 21-amino acid vasoconstrictor peptide produced by the endothelium.
■ ET-1 may be overexpressed in blood vessels, kidney, and heart in salt-sensitive and severe forms of hypertension in experimental animals, and in blood vessels of humans with atherosclerosis or stage 2 hypertension.
■ Orally active ET receptor antagonists have been effective in some forms of experimental hypertension, heart failure, and primary pulmonary hypertension.
■ Preliminary reports suggest that orally active ET antagonists may be effective in lowering blood pressure in resistant hypertension.

See also Chapters A10, **C140,** and **C142**

Three endothelins (ETs) have been recognized in mammals (ET-1, ET-2, and ET-3) (**Figure A21.1**). These 21-amino acid peptides were originally identified as products of vascular endothelial cells but are now known to be produced in different organs. They are important regulators of cardiovascular function, including smooth muscle tone, but also affect digestive tract function, endocrine glands, the renal and genitourinary system, and the nervous system.

Synthesis and release

Endothelial cells cleave proendothelin (183 residues) from the 203-residue preproendothelin and subsequently convert it to big ET (39 amino acids) by the action of ET-converting enzyme (ECE), a neutral metalloendopeptidase that is inhibited by phosphoramidon but not thiorphan. Different ECE isoforms may cleave big ET to form active 21-residue ET inside or outside endothelial cells.

The main ET secreted by endothelium is ET-1, which is released in response to stimulation by high pressure and low shear stress; low pressure or high shear inhibits ET-1 production. ET release is also promoted by angiotensin II (Ang II), vasopressin, catecholamines, and transforming growth factor β among other factors. ET-1 produced by endothelial cells is mainly secreted abluminally and plasma ET results from spillover from the vascular wall or from pituitary secretion. Plasma concentrations of immunoreactive ET probably do not reliably reflect tissue ET-1 production, particularly by the endothelium of blood vessels.

Endothelin receptors

ET receptors (ET_A and ET_B) are 7-transmembrane domain receptors with <70% sequence homology. ET_A and ET_B, which are encoded by genes located in different chromosomes, are G protein–coupled receptors that activate phospholipase C, causing intracellular calcium (Ca^{2+}) mobilization, and activation of protein kinase C, mitogen-activated protein (MAP) kinases, certain protooncogenes, and the Na^+/H^+ antiporter (causing intracellular alkalinization). Extracellular Ca^{2+} influx into smooth muscle cells (SMCs) of some vascular beds, activation of phospholipases (A_2 and D), and stimulation of nonreceptor tyrosine kinases are other pathways that participate in the intracellular signaling mediated by ET receptors. ET_A receptor stimulation increases oxidative stress in an NAD(P)H oxidase–dependent manner in some but not all species.

Endothelial ET-1 acts on ET_A and ET_B receptors to induce contraction, proliferation, and cell hypertrophy (**Figure A21.2**). ET-1 may also act on endothelial ET_B receptors, inducing release of nitric oxide and prostacyclin, which explains ET-1's bifunctional constrictor and relaxant properties. It is unknown which effect is more important, although this probably varies according to the vascular bed. Mitogen-activated protein kinase stimulation of protooncogenes such as c-*jun*, c-*myc*, and c-*fos* may participate in the mitogenic and hypertrophic effects of ETs, whereas promotion of apoptosis may counterbalance ET-induced cellular growth.

Pathophysiology

Vascular effects. ET activation causes constriction and hypertrophy of blood vessels (**Figure A21.2**) and promotes vascular fibrosis. In several rat models, including stroke-prone spontaneously hypertensive rats (SPSHRs), rats infused with Ang II (a known stimulant of ET-1 production), or those administered aldosterone, vascular ET-1 expression is increased. In these models, ET antagonists lower blood pressure (BP) and reduce small

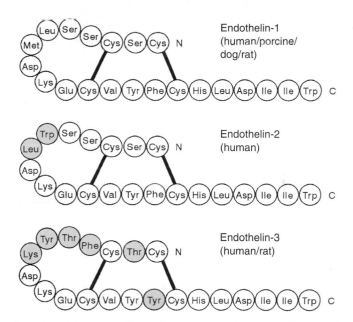

Figure A21.1 Structure of endothelin-1, -2, and -3. N and C are the N-terminal and C-terminal ends, respectively.

artery hypertrophic remodeling. Such effects on blood vessels and the heart are probably exerted by the paracrine or autocrine effects of locally released ET, acting through ET receptors in the immediate vicinity.

SMC growth and migration stimulated by ET-1 may contribute to foam cell formation through stimulation of inflammatory mediators (e.g., NFκB), adhesion molecules (e.g., intercellular adhesion module-1 or ICAM-1, and vascular cell adhesion molecule-1 or VCAM-1), or chemokines (e.g., monocyte chemoattractant protein-1 or MCP-1). In the aorta and conduit arteries, ET-1 production is enhanced in part as a result of endothelial damage, hypertension, oxidized low-density lipoprotein cholesterol,

and increased oxidative stress. All these processes contribute to progression of both vascular disease and atherosclerosis (Figure A21.3).

Cardiac effects. ET_A receptors are present in cardiomyocytes and fibroblasts, and ET-1 mediates the extensive cardiac fibrosis and microvascular remodeling that is found in deoxycorticosterone acetate (DOCA)-salt and aldosterone-infused rats. ETs have positive chronotropic and inotropic effects on cardiac muscle and may induce cell hypertrophy. In the coronary circulation, the small number of endothelial ET_B receptors suggests that ET acts mainly as a coronary vasoconstrictor.

Renal effects. In the kidney, ET receptors are mainly present in blood vessels and mesangial cells. Although ET_A receptors predominate in the kidney those ET_B receptors present may have pathophysiologic significance, particularly in the distal tubules, where their stimulation promotes sodium excretion.

Developmental effects. The role of the ET system in development has been emphasized by gene disruption experiments: Inactivation of the ET-1 or the ET_A receptor genes in mice results in brachial cleft abnormalities, inducing malformations of the mandibula, upper airway, and aortic arch (resembling the Pierre Robin syndrome), with hypoxia and hypercapnia. Surprisingly for a vasoconstrictor system, this is associated with elevation of BP, a paradoxical result that may be explained in part by the balance of its opposing effects on vasoconstriction (by ET_A or ET_B smooth muscle receptors) and vasorelaxation (by ET_B endothelial receptors, which stimulate the release of endothelial-derived nitric oxide, and prostacyclin) as shown in **Figure A21.2**. The slight BP elevation found in this syndrome may also result from hypoxia and hypercapnia, acting through sympathetic activation.

Inactivation of ET-3 or ET_B-receptor genes results in pigmentary abnormalities and in aganglionic megacolon, underscoring the role of ET-3 and the ET_B receptor in migration of neural crest cells (in this case, melanocytes and neurons of the myenteric plexus). In humans, mutations in the ET_B-receptor gene have been discovered in some of the familial and sporadic forms of Hirschsprung's disease. These results show that ET-1 is the main

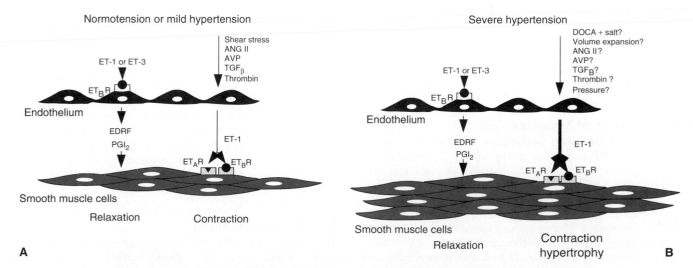

Figure A21.2 Endothelin-1 (ET-1) may play either a vasorelaxant role or a vasoconstrictor role in different vascular beds in normotension and in stage 1 hypertension (**A**). In stage 2 hypertension (**B**), enhanced expression of ET-1 produces a predominant vasoconstrictor effect associated with enhanced growth, resulting in a contribution to elevated blood pressure. Growth of the vascular wall is accentuated and contributes to further elevate blood pressure and to complications of hypertension. ET_BR, ET_B receptor; EDRF, endothelium-derived relaxing factor; PGI_2, prostacyclin; ANG, angiotensin; AVP, arginine vasopressin; TGFβ, transforming growth factor β; ET_AR, ET_A receptor; DOCA, deoxycorticosterone acetate.

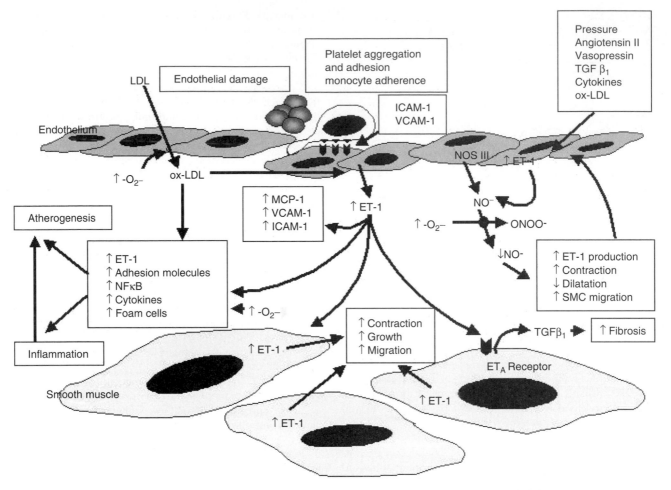

Figure A21.3 Endothelin-1 (ET-1) production is enhanced in part as a result of endothelial damage, hypertension, and oxidized low-density lipoprotein (LDL) cholesterol. The latter is enhanced by increased oxidative stress. Smooth muscle cell (SMC) growth and migration are stimulated. Foam cells are formed, and inflammatory mediators (NFκB), adhesion molecules such as ICAM-1 and VCAM-1, and chemokines such as monocyte chemoattractant protein (MCP-1), are upregulated. Macrophages produce cytokines, and an inflammatory reaction is triggered, in large measure resulting from endothelial dysfunction. All these processes contribute to progression of vascular disease and atherosclerosis. NO, nitric oxide; NOS III, nitric oxide synthase III; oxLDL, oxidized low-density lipoprotein; NFκB, nuclear factor kappa B; TGFβ$_1$, transforming growth factor β$_1$.

ligand of the ET$_A$ receptor, whereas ET-3 is the main endogenous ligand of the ET$_B$ receptor.

Animal models of hypertension

Variation in endothelin activation. In many hypertensive models, plasma ET is normal but in severe hypertension, the ET system seems to be activated, especially in low-renin, salt-sensitive models. Other hypertensive models, including 1-kidney Goldblatt hypertensive rats, cyclosporine-induced hypertensive rats, and fructose-fed hypertensive rats, may also exhibit an ET-dependent component. Mice that overexpress the human prepro-ET-1 gene (targeted to the endothelium by the Tie-2 promoter) exhibit hypertrophic remodeling of small arteries associated with endothelial dysfunction and enhanced expression of inflammatory mediators.

Salt-sensitive hypertension in rats. The ET system is activated in salt-dependent rat models of hypertension, including the DOCA-salt hypertension, DOCA-salt–treated SHR, aldosterone infusion, and Dahl salt-sensitive rats. In all of these models, ET-1

is overexpressed in the endothelium. BP also responds to ET receptor antagonists and severe hypertrophic remodeling of small arteries regresses with ET antagonist treatment.

Renovascular and spontaneous hypertension in rats. Two-kidney one-clip (Goldblatt) renovascular hypertensive rats (generally considered to be at least partly Ang II-dependent) and SHRs without deoxycorticosterone or salt do not have an activated ET system. In these models, there is eutrophic rather than hypertrophic remodeling of small arteries.

Human hypertension

The role of ETs in the pathophysiology of hypertension is still unclear. **Figure A21.2** summarizes the current view of the potential implication of ET-1 in BP elevation and vascular hypertrophy, and **Figure A21.3** the mechanisms whereby ET-1 contributes to vascular injury and the progression of atherosclerosis in stage 2 hypertension.

Endothelin activation. Severity of BP elevation and salt sensitivity may be common denominators for activation of the vascular

ET system in humans and experimental animals. In humans, ET plasma levels are usually normal but certain subpopulations of hypertensive subjects may exhibit chronic activation of the ET system. In blacks, especially in stage 2 hypertension, salt sensitivity is a common finding. Other forms of hypertension in which ETs may be involved in humans include rare cases of hemangioendotheliomas that produce ET, chronic renal failure, erythropoietin- and cyclosporine-induced hypertension, pheochromocytoma, and pregnancy-induced hypertension. Using *in situ* hybridization radioautography, the expression of the ET-1 gene has been shown to be enhanced in small arteries from gluteal subcutaneous biopsies in hypertensive patients. ET expression is also enhanced in large vessels in association with extensive atherosclerosis.

Endothelin blockade. In healthy subjects, the acute intravenous administration of a mixed ET receptor antagonist results in minimal lowering of BP. In hypertensive patients, endothelial dysfunction improves acutely with nonselective ET blockade (by combined infusion of BQ-123, an ET_A blocker, and BQ-788, an ET_B blocker). In stage 1 essential hypertension, one study showed a moderate BP-lowering effect after 4 weeks of oral administration of the combined ET_A receptor antagonist/ET_B receptor antagonist bosentan. ET_A-selective ET antagonists are currently being evaluated for the treatment of resistant hypertension.

Genomics

Some polymorphisms have been identified in components of the ET system, including EDN1 K198N in the coding region of the prepro-ET-1 gene, which has been related to increased vascular reactivity in obese individuals with hypertension. A polymorphism of ECE-1b (ECE1 C-388A) in the 5'-regulatory region of the ECE-1b gene has been associated with increased promoter activity in two cohorts of hypertensive patients. In untreated hypertensive German women, the A allele of this polymorphism has a codominant effect on daytime and night time systolic and diastolic BP. In a French cohort, women homozygous for the A allele had significantly higher systolic, diastolic, and mean BP levels. The A allele may raise expression of ECE-1b, resulting in increased production of ET-1. The EDN1 K198N polymorphism of the prepro-ET-1 gene is not correlated with BP in either men or women, but interacted with the ECE1 C-338A variant to influence systolic and mean BP levels in women. The ECE-1b effect could be related to interactions between sex hormones and the ET system.

Primary pulmonary hypertension

ET antagonism has been shown to improve outcomes in primary pulmonary hypertension, and the combined ET_A receptor antagonist/ET_B receptor antagonist bosentan has been approved by the U.S. Food and Drug Administration (FDA) for this indication. Other compounds such as ambrisentan and sitaxsentan, which are both selective ET_A receptor antagonists, are in the late stages of development for use in primary pulmonary hypertension.

Suggested Readings

Amiri F, Virdis A, Neves MF, et al. Endothelium-restricted overexpression of human endothelin-1 causes vascular remodeling and endothelial dysfunction. *Circulation* 2004;110:2233–2240.

Campia U, Cardillo C, Panza JA. Ethnic differences in the vasoconstrictor activity of endogenous endothelin-1 in hypertensive patients. *Circulation* 2004;109:3191–3195.

Cardillo C, Kilcoyne CM, Waclawiw M, et al. Role of endothelin in the increased vascular tone of patients with essential hypertension. *Hypertension* 1999;33:753–758.

Funalot B, Courbon D, Brousseau T, et al. Genes encoding endothelin-converting enzyme-1 and endothelin-1 interact to influence blood pressure in women: the EVA study. *J Hypertens* 2004;22:739–743.

Goddard J, Johnston NR, Hand MF, et al. Endothelin-a receptor antagonism reduces blood pressure and increases renal blood flow in hypertensive patients with chronic renal failure: a comparison of selective and combined endothelin receptor blockade. *Circulation* 2004;109:1186–1193.

Krum H, Viskoper RJ, Lacourciere Y, et al. Bosentan Hypertension Investigators. The effect of an endothelin-receptor antagonist, bosentan, on blood pressure in patients with essential hypertension. *N Engl J Med* 1998;338:784–790.

Li JS, Larivière R, Schiffrin EL. Effect of a nonselective endothelin antagonist on vascular remodeling in deoxycorticosterone acetate-salt hypertensive rats. Evidence for a role of endothelin in vascular hypertrophy. *Hypertension* 1994;24:183–188.

Pu Q, Fritsch Neves M, Virdis A, et al. Endothelin antagonism on aldosterone-induced oxidative stress and vascular remodeling. *Hypertension* 2003;42:49–55.

Rubin LJ, Badesch DB, Barst RJ, et al. The Bosentan Randomized Trial of Endothelin Antagonist Therapy Study Group. Bosentan therapy for pulmonary arterial hypertension. *N Engl J Med* 2002;46:896–903.

Schiffrin EL. Vascular endothelin in hypertension. *Vasc Pharmacol* 2005;43:19–29.

CHAPTER A22 ■ VASOPRESSIN AND NEUROPEPTIDE Y

ALLEN W. COWLEY, Jr., PhD AND MIECZYSLAW MICHALKIEWICZ, DVM, PhD

KEY POINTS

■ Vasopressin is a potent vasoconstrictor as well as a stimulus to water retention; it plays a significant role in normalizing blood pressure (BP) during conditions of acute hypotension.

■ The long-term effect of vasopressin on BP depends on water intake and counterregulatory mechanisms, but elevated levels of vasopressin may contribute to hypertension in a subset of human subjects.

■ Neuropeptide Y (NPY) acts centrally as an inhibitory neurotransmitter reducing sympathetic outflow and BP.

■ At the neurovascular synapse, NPY accentuates the vasoconstrictor effects of sympathetic nerves and pressor hormones; its role in short- and long-term regulation of BP remains to be established.

See also Chapters A10, A23, C108, and **C141**

VASOPRESSIN

Physiologic regulation

Arginine vasopressin (AVP), also known as *antidiuretic hormone*, is a nonapeptide released from the posterior pituitary gland in response to (a) reduced cardiopulmonary blood volume, (b) decreased arterial blood pressure (BP), or (c) increased plasma osmolality.

Plasma osmolality. AVP release is mediated directly by receptors in the hypothalamus, which can sense osmotic changes of <1%. An increase from normal concentrations of 3 pg/mL plasma AVP to only 9 pg/mL reduces renal medullary blood flow and exerts powerful antidiuretic effects by increasing water permeability of the renal collecting ducts. These effects make AVP the major determinant of the rate of renal water excretion. Under normal physiologic conditions, osmolality is the principal signal modulating AVP release.

Pressure and volume signals. Stimulation of AVP release is elicited by sudden decreases in central blood volume and cardiac stretch during "unloading" (stimulation) of cardiac mechanoreceptors (cardiopulmonary baroreflex) or during acute decreases in arterial pressure with unloading of aortocarotid baroreceptors. During hypovolemia or other conditions that reduce cardiac "preload," however, the hypovolemic stimulus can easily override the effect of the osmotic feedback loop so that AVP can be released despite significant hyponatremia. Very high concentrations of plasma AVP (20–400 pg/mL) can be attained during volume depletion and/or hypotension.

Vasopressin receptors

There are currently three firmly established vasopressin receptors known to play a relevant role in physiologic functions.

V_1 receptors. The V_1 receptor gene is expressed in blood vessels from a wide variety of organs, including the kidneys. V_1 receptors are linked to membrane phosphatidylinositol turnover, phospholipase C stimulation, and increased cytosolic free calcium (Ca^{2+}) V_1 receptors participate in the regulation of vascular tone and AVP stimulation of these receptors mediates vasoconstrictor responses of blood vessels. V_1 receptors are linked directly to stimulation of myocardial hypertrophic growth factors and also mediate glycogenolytic responses of hepatocytes. V_1 receptors are also found in distal segments of the mammalian nephron and promote prostaglandin E_2 generation. Pharmacologic studies have found that V_1 receptors at pre- or postsynaptic sites predominately mediate the interactions between AVP and sympathetic neurons.

V_2 receptors. V_2 receptors are known to mediate the antidiuretic activity of vasopressin through stimulation of adenylyl cyclase and thereby alter the expression of aquaporin channels in the renal collecting ducts, leading to water retention. V_2 receptors in cells of the ascending limb of the loop of Henle also stimulate Na^+–K^+–Cl^- cotransport at this site.

V₃ receptors. V_3 receptors are less well understood but appear to be involved in the release of adrenocorticotropic hormone.

Vasodilatory responses. Vasodilation is observed in some parts of the systemic circulation (such as skeletal muscle) in response to selective vasopressin V_2 agonists, but V_2 receptor messenger RNA and proteins have not been found in blood vessels. Vasodilation after V_2 stimulation may be mediated through the release of paracrine hormones from the interstitial or parenchymal cells surrounding the vessels.

Vasopressin antagonists

Selective nonpeptidergic receptor blockers have been developed for the V_1 and V_2 receptors, as well as agents that have affinity for both receptor subtypes. The vaptans (such as relcovaptan) represent currently used V_1 receptor antagonists and tolvaptan and lixivaptan represent V_2 receptor antagonists. Used largely as pharmacologic tools, they have also been explored as therapeutic agents in cardiovascular and/or renal diseases.

Physiologic effects

AVP circulates normally at very low concentrations, ranging from 1 to 3 pg/mL. AVP is one of the most potent vasoactive peptides circulating in the blood; concentrations that are well within the physiologic range (10–20 pg/mL) can produce significant renal vasoconstriction and greatly blunt the pressure-diuresis-natriuresis relationship.

Hemodynamic effects. Constrictive effects of AVP on skin, kidneys, and splanchnic and coronary beds are offset by vasodilation in skeletal muscle, resulting in a variable effect on systemic BP. AVP enhances the sympathoinhibitory influence of the arterial baroreflex and the central nervous system, which further buffers the hemodynamic effect of this powerful vasoconstrictor substance. As a result of these forces, only slight elevations of arterial pressure are normally observed with physiologic elevations of plasma AVP, and therefore the antidiuretic action of AVP occurs without limitation by pressure-induced diuresis.

Autonomic nervous system interactions. In the absence of autonomic reflex mechanisms, the pressor activity of vasopressin is increased 9,000-fold. AVP has been found to participate in BP maintenance, especially when other pressor systems are endogenously or pharmacologically impaired such as in diabetic patients with autonomic neuropathy and quadriplegic patients with reduced baroreceptor-mediated sympathetic nervous system responses. The latter exhibit marked reductions of mean arterial pressure (from 75 → 58 mm Hg) in response to selective V_1 receptor blockade. Greater pressor effects and a greater contribution of AVP to orthostatic BP maintenance in the elderly have been observed, perhaps due to a degree of autonomic nervous system impairment. Interestingly, race has also been found to be an important element in that blacks exhibit greater fall in mean arterial pressure in response to V_1 receptor blockade than do non-blacks.

Hypertension

Animal models. AVP is elevated in many forms of experimental hypertension, but its contribution to the elevated pressure in these models is not entirely clear. AVP is a potent vasoconstrictor and can play an important role in BP normalization after rapid hemorrhage. As shown in dogs, AVP release can bring about a rapid compensation of arterial pressure (70%↑) in the absence of the autonomic reflexes and renin release. Despite the vasoconstrictor and fluid-retaining effects of AVP, chronic administration of the endogenous peptide does not result in sustained hypertension in rats, dogs, or humans. Yet, chronic administration of a selective V_1 agonist intravenously or into the medullary interstitial space of the rat lowers blood flow to the renal medulla and produces sustained hypertension. The difference between the pressor action of the selective agonist and that of AVP itself is probably accounted for by the lack of a depressor V_2 effect.

Several studies have now demonstrated that AVP-stimulated nitric oxide (NO) release from the renal medulla is mediated by V_2 receptor activation of the phosphoinositide pathway and the mobilization of Ca^{2+} from both intracellular and extracellular pools. Sustained increases of medullary interstitial NO have been found by microdialysis in response to chronic elevations of plasma AVP. However, it has also been shown that V_2 receptors are downregulated after dehydration when plasma AVP is elevated. This downregulation of V_2 receptors with sustained elevations of AVP could contribute to the so-called *vasopressin escape* mechanism and is consistent with the failure of AVP to cause a sustained elevation of blood volume and arterial pressure. Recently, it was found that Dahl salt-sensitive rats exhibit lower medullary levels of NO synthase activity, messenger RNA, and protein and that in this strain of rats, chronic intravenous administration of very small amounts of AVP does result in sustained hypertension. It has been demonstrated that stimulation of NO release with AVP is necessary to prevent sustained hypertension with AVP infusion.

Human hypertension. The contribution of AVP to the maintenance of arterial hypertension in humans remains unclear and it is unknown whether changes in AVP concentrations in essential hypertension are primary or secondary. Plasma AVP levels are significantly elevated (5–20 pg/mL) in approximately 30% of male hypertensive patients and are directly correlated with systolic and diastolic BP in men. By contrast, as few as 7% of female hypertensive subjects exhibit elevated plasma AVP. Plasma AVP levels can be higher (>20 pg/mL) in the malignant phase of hypertension or in congestive heart failure. AVP elevations of this magnitude could contribute to chronic redistribution of cardiac output and influence regional blood flow, body fluid volume status, and autonomic reflex mechanisms. Plasma AVP levels are higher in blacks than in whites, and selective vasopressin V_1 receptor inhibition was shown to lower mean arterial pressure in blacks (28 mm Hg) but not in whites.

The plasma AVP levels usually found in hypertensive humans are lower than those needed to produce pressor responses in healthy subjects. However, sustained plasma levels of 10 to 20 pg/mL could result in fluid retention, volume expansion, and a rise of arterial pressure. The extent to which this occurs depends on the level of daily water intake. If hypertension does occur, as observed with chronic intravenous infusion of AVP with a fixed water intake, significant elevations of pressure are sustained for only 1 to 2 weeks because of *vasopressin escape*. Escape from the fluid-retaining effects of AVP results from pressure-induced diuresis similar to that observed in patients with the syndrome of inappropriate antidiuretic hormone. It is possible that some human subjects resemble the genetically inbred Dahl S rat and fail to produce sufficient renal NO in response to AVP, thereby enabling small elevations of this peptide to contribute to the chronic hypertensive state.

NEUROPEPTIDE Y

Neuropeptide Y (NPY) is one of the most abundant peptides of the mammalian nervous systems. It has been implicated in controling numerous physiologic processes, including thirst, appetite, BP, and energy metabolism.

Localization

Central nervous system. In the central nervous system, NPY is expressed in regions involved in cardiovascular and metabolic regulation, including the hypothalamus, the ventrolateral medulla, the nucleus tractus solitari, the locus coeruleus, and preganglionic sympathetic neurons of the lateral column of the spinal cord. It acts as a potent inhibitory neurotransmitter, reduces sympathetic outflow, mediates central leptin signaling and stimulates appetite. NPY receptors are expressed on the vasopressinergic neurons of the paraventricular nucleus and their stimulation potentiates vasopressin release from the neuronal lobe of the pituitary gland.

Peripheral nerves. In the peripheral nervous system, NPY is expressed in sympathetic ganglia and fibers innervating blood vessels, as well as the heart, and the kidney. A striking feature of this peptide is its close coexistence with norepinephrine in peripheral adrenergic neurons and the potent vasoconstrictor effect in many vascular beds.

Neuropeptide receptors

Of the six proposed NPY receptor subtypes, Y_1, Y_2, and Y_5 are believed to be the most relevant for control of cardiovascular functions.

Y_1 receptors. Y_1 receptors are postsynaptic, coupled to the inhibition of adenylate cyclase, and act to increase intracellular calcium. Central Y_1 receptor signaling mediates the hypotensive effect of NPY, whereas stimulation of peripheral Y_1 receptors results in direct vasoconstriction or potentiation of the vasoconstrictor effects of norepinephrine, angiotensin, or serotonin in some vessels. Small resistance arteries of the coronary, splanchnic, or cerebral vascular beds are particularly sensitive to NPY.

Y_2 receptors. Y_2 receptors are predominantly presynaptic, and they decrease intracellular calcium by inhibiting N-type calcium channels in nerve terminals. At presynaptic membranes in the central nervous system, vasculature, heart, and kidney, this receptor inhibits the release of neurotransmitters, including norepinephrine and glutamate.

Y_5 receptors. NPY stimulates diuresis and natriuresis through Y_5 receptor activation. The peptide hypertrophic effects on cardiomyocytes and blood vessels also appear to be mediated by this receptor.

Actions

Sympathetic and hemodynamic effects. Exogenous NPY elicits either a hypertensive or hypotensive effect, depending on the site of its administration. Injection of NPY into discrete areas of the central nervous system (such as the third ventricle, the paraventricular nucleus, the nucleus tractus solitarius, or ventrolateral medulla) causes a potent decrease in BP and heart rate in a pattern similar to α_2 agonists and norepinephrine itself. The hypotensive effects of centrally admnistered NPY are associated with reduced renal sympathetic nerve traffic and reduced norepinephrine release. Quite the opposite, acute administration of NPY into the systemic circulation effectively increases BP. Systemic or central administration of NPY increases the sensitivity of the aortic baroreceptor reflex. Recently, a cardiomyocyte hypertrophic effect and an angiogenic effect in skeletal muscle has been demonstrated with NPY. Elevated plasma NPY levels have been found in conditions of intense and prolonged sympathetic activation, including stress, exercise, hemorrhage, or myocardial infarction.

Renal effects. In contrast to the antidiuretic effects of most vasoconstrictor neurotransmitters and hormones, NPY enhances diuresis and natriuresis *in vivo* in anesthetized animals. NPY has been reported to reduce renin release, elevate plasma atrial natriuretic peptide, and directly modify Na, K-ATPase activity on renal proximal tubules. The antihypertensive and natriuretic effects of NPY indicate that this signaling molecule can enhance pressure-diuresis-natriuresis and reduce pressure sensitivity to salt.

Hypertension

NPY release is enhanced in some animal models of hypertension and in a subset of patients with essential hypertension, including hypertensive children. NPY content is reduced in the brain of the spontaneously hypertensive rat (SHR). In addition, the sympatholytic and BP-reducing effects of centrally administered NPY are diminished in the SHR.

Central NPY Y_1 receptor blockade prevents the antihypertensive effect of endogenous NPY while blockade of this receptor in the periphery blocks stress-induced vasoconstriction. NPY or NPY Y_1 receptor gene deletion in mice does not significantly affect baseline BP. However, transgenic NPY overexpression under a natural promoter in rats is associated with lower sympathetic nervous activity and BP in L-NAME, DOCA, and Goldblatt models of hypertension. The NPY locus cosegregates with high BP in the SHR and NPY gene polymorphism is associated with increased BP, accelerated development of left ventricle hypertrophy, and atherosclerotic progression in humans.

Suggested Readings

Bakris G, Bursztzen M, Gavras I, et al. Role of vasopressin in essential hypertension: racial differences. *J Hypertens* 1997;15:545–550.

Bischoff A, Rascher W, Michel MC. Bradykinin may be involved in neuropeptide Y-induced diuresis, natriuresis, and calciuresis. *Am J Physiol* 1998;275:F502–F509.

Cowley AW Jr, Liard JF. Cardiovascular actions of vasopressin. In: Gash DM, Boer GJ, eds. *Vasopressin: principles and properties.* New York: Plenum Publishing, 1987:389–433.

Lee EW, Michalkiewicz M, Kitlinska J, et al. Neuropeptide Y induces ischemic angiogenesis and restores function of ischemic skeletal muscles. *J Clin Invest* 2003;111:1853–1862.

Michalkiewicz M, Knestaut KM, Bytchkova EY, et al. Hypotension and reduced catecholamines in neuropeptide Y transgenic rats. *Hypertension* 2003;41:1056–1062.

Michalkiewicz M, Zhao G, Jia Z, et al. Central neuropeptide Y signaling ameliorates L-NAME hypertension in the rat through a Y1 receptor mechanism. *Hypertension* 2005;45:780–785.

de Paula RB, Plavnik FL, Rodrigues CI, et al. Contribution of vasopressin to orthostatic blood pressure maintenance in essential hypertension. *Am J Hypertens* 1993;6:794–798.

Streefkerk JO, van Zwieten PA. Vasopressin receptor antagonists: pharmacological tools and potential therapeutic agents. *Auton Autacoid Pharmacol* 2006;26:141–148.

Westfall TC. Neuropeptide Y and sympathetic control of vascular tone in hypertension. *EXS* 2006;95:89–103.

Yuan B, Cowley AW Jr. Evidence that reduced renal medullary nitric oxide synthase activity of Dahl S rats enables small elevations of arginine vasopressin to produce sustained hypertension. *Hypertension* 2001;37:524–528.

CHAPTER A23 ■ CALCITONIN GENE-RELATED PEPTIDES AND ADRENOMEDULLIN-DERIVED PEPTIDES

DONALD J. DIPETTE, MD AND SCOTT SUPOWIT, PhD

KEY POINTS

- Calcitonin gene–related peptide (CGRP) and adrenomedullin (ADM) belong to a superfamily of closely related substances that include calcitonin and amylin.
- CGRP and ADM affect both normal cardiovascular function and cardiovascular disease states because of their effects on peripheral vasodilation, with CGRP being the most potent vasodilator known to date.
- CGRP is primarily released from perivascular sensory nerves, whereas ADM is produced by vascular cells and the adrenal gland.
- CGRP and ADM effects are mediated by stimulation of a shared G protein–coupled receptor, CLR (calcitonin-like receptor), whose ligand specificity is determined by coexpression of either of two chaperone proteins called *receptor activity modifying proteins*: RAMP1 for CGRP and RAMP2 for ADM. A functional CGRP (or ADM) receptor must also contain a third peptide, the receptor component protein (RCP), which couples the receptor to the cellular signal transduction pathway(s).

See also Chapters A8 and **A34**

The potent vasodilator activity of calcitonin gene-related peptide [CGRP (a neuropeptide)] and adrenomedullin (ADM) (acting as a circulating endocrine/paracrine factor) and their widespread distributions in peripheral tissues suggest a role in normal and diseased organ function.

CALCITONIN GENE–RELATED PEPTIDE

Synthesis and localization of calcitonin gene–related peptide

There are two forms of CGRP, α and β, which differ in only two amino acids in rats and three in humans. α-CGRP is derived from tissue-specific splicing of the calcitonin/CGRP gene. Whereas calcitonin is produced mainly in the C cells of the thyroid, α-CGRP synthesis occurs almost exclusively in specific regions of the central and peripheral nervous systems. The β-CGRP gene does not produce calcitonin but β-CGRP peptide is synthesized in the central nervous system (CNS) and in intestinal neurons. The biological activities of both peptides are similar in most vascular beds.

CGRP and its receptors are widely distributed in the nervous and cardiovascular systems. In the periphery, prominent sites of CGRP synthesis are the dorsal root ganglion (DRG) neurons of sensory nerves that terminate peripherally on blood vessels. These neurons project to the laminae I/II of the dorsal horn of the spinal cord and to the CNS. A dense perivascular CGRP neural network is seen around the blood vessels in all vascular beds. In these vessels, CGRP-containing nerves are found at the junctions of the adventitia and the media and in the tunica media. It is thought that circulating CGRP is largely derived from these perivascular nerve terminals and represents a spillover phenomenon related to the release of these peptides to promote vasodilation or other tissue functions. Receptors for CGRP have been identified in the media and intima of resistance vessels as well as in the endothelial layer.

Release of calcitonin gene–related peptide from sensory nerve terminals

CGRP-rich nerve fibers are components of the primary afferent nervous system, comprising principally capsaicin-sensitive C- and Aδ-fiber nerves that respond to chemical, thermal, and mechanical stimuli. These afferent nerves are believed to "sense" metabolic and humorally mediated events in the periphery and to transmit this information to the CNS. They may also have an efferent function because DRG neuron-derived peptides are released at peripheral sensory nerve terminals in the absence of afferent nerve stimulation. The continuous release of peptides from DRG neurons may reflect a paracrine function, implying that these neurons participate in the continuous regulation of local blood flow and other tissue activities. Sensory nerve terminals can either increase or decrease release CGRP in response to numerous factors, including hydrogen ions, nerve growth factor, vascular wall tension, bradykinin, prostaglandins, endothelin, sympathetic nervous system activation, and various renin-angiotensin-aldosterone system components.

Role of calcitonin gene–related peptide in hypertension

A direct role for CGRP in experimental hypertension has now been established. CGRP attenuates chronic hypoxic pulmonary hypertension and also acts as a compensatory depressor mechanism to partially attenuate the blood pressure (BP) increase in four models of experimental hypertension: (a) deoxycorticosterone-salt, (b) subtotal nephrectomy-salt, (c) N^{ω}-nitro-L-arginine methyl ester (L-NAME)-induced hypertension during pregnancy, and (d) the two-kidney one-clip model. In contrast, in the spontaneously hypertensive rat (SHR), there is an age-dependent reduction in sensory nerve CGRP synthesis and release suggesting that the absence of CGRP may contribute to the development and maintenance of high BP.

The important question regarding the long-term participation of CGRP is being studied using α-CGRP knockout (KO) mice in which long-term radiotelemetric monitoring is established. Basal BP is significantly elevated in these animals compared to their wild type (WT) counterparts. More importantly, when BP is further elevated in these mice by deoxycorticosterone (DOC)-salt administration, hypertension-induced damage of the heart and kidney is significantly enhanced occurring by way of both BP-dependent and BP-independent mechanisms that may involve increased oxidative stress.

Although CGRP administration can acutely decrease high BP in humans, it is not clear what role CGRP plays in chronic human hypertension. Data concerning circulating levels of immunoreactive calcitonin gene-related peptide (iCGRP) in hypertensive humans are conflicting, perhaps due to a variety of factors including the assay systems, heterogeneity of the condition, severity, and duration of the hypertension, degree of end-organ damage, and the type of treatment regimen in use.

ADRENOMEDULLIN

Synthesis and tissue distribution of adrenomedullin

ADM was discovered in 1993 in peptide extracts from pheochromocytoma cells, hence the name. It is a 52-amino acid peptide with a unique 6-amino acid ring structure formed by an intramolecular disulfide bond between residues 16 and 21. This feature is similar to the structure found in CGRP and is required for agonist activity. Pre-proadrenomedullin consists of 185 amino acids; cleavage at the signal peptide between Thr21 and Ala22 yields a truncated propeptide with 164 residues that contains ADM. Three proteolytic processing sites are found in proadrenomedullin. The first paired basic amino acids, Lys43-Arg44, is a representative proteolytic cleavage site. It is preceded by Arg41-Gly42 residues that can be amidated at the C-terminus to yield proadrenomedullin N-terminal 20 peptide (PAMP). Although PAMP and ADM are derived from the same precursor, PAMP does not dilate the vasculature despite inhibiting sympathetic nerve transmission. Because the ADM gene is more highly expressed in endothelial cells than in the adrenal medulla, PAMP is now regarded as a secretory product similar to nitric oxide and endothelin. The binding sites for ADM are abundant and include a variety of tissues such as kidney, brain, spleen, heart, and adrenal glands.

Adrenomedullin and proadrenomedullin N-terminal 20 peptide in hypertension

CNS administration of ADM in rats dilates the peripheral vasculature, reduces thirst, and attenuates salt appetite. It also attenuates aldosterone secretion, increases renal blood flow, and stimulates sodium excretion. These physiologic effects contribute significantly to the role of ADM in regulating BP. In Dahl salt-sensitive rats, plasma ADM, cardiac ventricle ADM concentrations, and ADM mRNA levels are higher during high than with low-salt intake. Also plasma ADM correlates well with the weight of the left ventricle suggesting that ADM participates in the pathophysiology of salt-dependent hypertension and plays a role in cardiac hypertrophy. Human ADM gene delivery delays the BP rise and protects against cardiovascular remodeling and renal injury in several rat models of hypertension. As with CGRP, the ADM protective activity against hypertension-induced end-organ damage is mediated, at least in part through the inhibition of oxidative stress. In deoxycorticosterone acetate (DOCA) treated SHRs with malignant hypertension, plasma ADM and renal tissue ADM are significantly elevated. Chronic ADM infusion in Dahl salt-sensitive rats improves reduced glomerular filtration and renal histopathology and prolongs life without having lowered mean arterial pressure, suggesting that ADM has both renal and vascular protective effects.

In the conscious, unrestrained rat, the hypotension evoked by PAMP is accompanied by less reflex tachycardia than that evoked by amplitude modulation (AM). This finding suggests a modulatory interaction between PAMP and sympathetic nervous outflow. Using a mesenteric artery perfusion model, PAMP decreased norepinephrine overflow in a dose-dependent manner, indicating that it possesses presynaptic sympathoinhibitory actions that may depend on inhibiting calcium influx from N-type calcium channels.

Plasma ADM levels are increased in hypertensive patients and there is a progressive rise in ADM in proportion to the level to which BP is chronically elevated as well as the degree of end-organ damage. Plasma ADM levels are directly proportional to serum creatinine levels and inversely related to glomerular filtration rates in hypertensive patients. These associations suggest that ADM may be released to compensate for these hypertension-associated abnormalities. Neither acute nor chronic salt loading affects plasma ADM levels in normotensives or essential hypertensives.

Suggested Readings

Brain SD, Grant AD. Vascular actions of calcitonin gene-related peptide and adrenomedullin. *Physiol Rev* 2004;84:903–934.
Hinson JP, Kapas S, Smith DM. Adrenomedullin, a multifunctional regulatory peptide. *Endocr Rev* 2000;21:138–167.
Poyner DR, Sexton PM, Marshall I, et al. The mammalian calcitonin gene-related peptides, adrenomedullin, amylin, and calcitonin receptors. *Pharmacol Rev* 2002;54:233–246.

Supowit, SC, Rao A. Bowers MC, et al. Calcitonin gene-related peptide protects against hypertension-induced heart and kidney damage. *Hypertension* 2005;45:109–114.
Wimalawansa SJ. Calcitonin gene-related peptide and its receptors:molecular genetics, physiology, pathophysiology, and therapeutic potentials. *Endocr Rev* 1996;17:533–585.

CHAPTER A24 ■ ACETYLCHOLINE, γ-AMINOBUTYRIC ACID, SEROTONIN, ADENOSINE, AND ENDOGENOUS OUABAIN

JOHN M. HAMLYN, PhD

KEY POINTS

- Acetylcholine dilates blood vessels through muscarinic receptors in vascular smooth muscle and the central nervous system (CNS); acetylcholine slows the heart and constricts blood vessels through nicotinic receptors in autonomic ganglia.
- Serotonin vasodilates through central and peripheral 5-hydroxytryptamine$_1$ (HT) receptors, and vasoconstricts through 5-HT$_2$ receptors.
- Adenosine is a direct vasodilator, whereas γ-aminobutyric acid (GABA) has tonic central depressor effects.
- Ouabain, an endogenous steroidal glycoside produced in the adrenal cortex, inhibits sodium- and potassium-activated adenosine triphosphatase (ATPase), leading to vascular smooth muscle constriction, increased sympathetic outflow, elevated blood pressure (BP); plasma ouabain is often increased in human hypertension.

See also Chapters A6, A7, and **C140**

ACETYLCHOLINE

Synthesis and actions

Acetylcholine (ACh) is a neurotransmitter with widespread cardiovascular and noncardiovascular actions that is synthesized in nerve terminals. Active uptake of choline is followed by acetylation, with subsequent storage in secretory vesicles. In response to electrical stimulation and fusion of secretory vesicles with presynaptic membranes, ACh is released into the synapse, where it is rapidly degraded by neuronal acetylcholinesterase. ACh serves as the primary neurotransmitter for (a) ganglionic and postganglionic parasympathetic neurons, (b) preganglionic sympathetic neurons and the adrenal medulla, (c) motor end plates in skeletal muscle; and (d) some neurons within the central nervous system (CNS).

Muscarinic effects. Postganglionic parasympathetic effects of ACh are mediated by muscarinic receptors. Cardiovascular muscarinic effects include vasodilation and negative chronotropic and inotropic effects. Five functional subtypes of muscarinic receptors have been identified: M$_2$ receptors mediate the cardiac and coronary artery effects of ACh and M$_3$ receptors mediate endothelium-dependent vascular responses. M$_1$ and M$_3$ receptors directly mediate vascular smooth muscle constriction that can be blocked by atropine. Vasodilatory effects of ACh are mediated through endothelial M$_3$ receptors that cause nitric oxide release. ACh also stimulates release of prostacyclin and endothelium-derived hyperpolarizing factor, which further contribute to vasodilation. To date, there is no evidence that either neurally derived or circulating ACh is a significant regulator of vascular tone *in vivo*, and accordingly, atropine has minimal effects on systemic vascular resistance. Tonic vagal release of ACh is a predominant regulator of heart rate, particularly in young, healthy individuals in whom atropine administration often increases heart rate by 30 to 40 beats per minute.

Nicotinic effects. Autonomic ganglionic neurotransmission is mediated by $\alpha2\beta4$ nicotinic receptors that inhibit sympathetic and parasympathetic postganglionic neurons, and lead to arterial and venous dilation, increased blood flow, and decreased venous return. Postural hypotension is a particularly prominent response to nicotinic stimulation. Ganglionic blockers such as trimethaphan and mecamylamine were among the first compounds found to lower blood pressure (BP) in humans. Because the vagal effects of nicotinic blockers tend to predominate, ganglionic blockers commonly cause tachycardia.

Central effects

Cholinergic neurotransmission within the CNS is involved in the regulation of BP. The most important sites of action appear to be the rostral ventrolateral medulla (RVLM) (**see Chapter A37**) and several areas within the hypothalamus. Administration of muscarinic antagonists into the cerebrospinal fluid or directly into the hypothalamus or RVLM decreases BP in most experimental forms of hypertension. However, normal animals are relatively unresponsive to muscarinic antagonists. Therefore, although central cholinergic neurons appear to play no important role in normal BP regulation, they may be of some importance once hypertension has developed.

SEROTONIN

Synthesis and metabolism

Serotonin, or 5-hydroxytryptamine (5-HT) (**Figure A24.1**), is synthesized in a two-step process involving hydroxylation of tryptophan to 5-hydroxytryptophan followed by decarboxylation. Serotonin is present in the enterochromaffin cells of the gastrointestinal tract, in the central and peripheral nervous systems, and in platelets. Within neural cells, serotonin is stored in granular vesicles similar to those of catecholamines. *De novo*

synthesis occurs only in the enterochromaffin cells and the nervous system. Serotonin released from enterochromaffin cells is metabolized almost entirely in the liver. The remainder of intestinal and neurally derived serotonin is captured by high-affinity uptake systems in platelets and nerves. As a result, circulating concentrations of serotonin are extremely low.

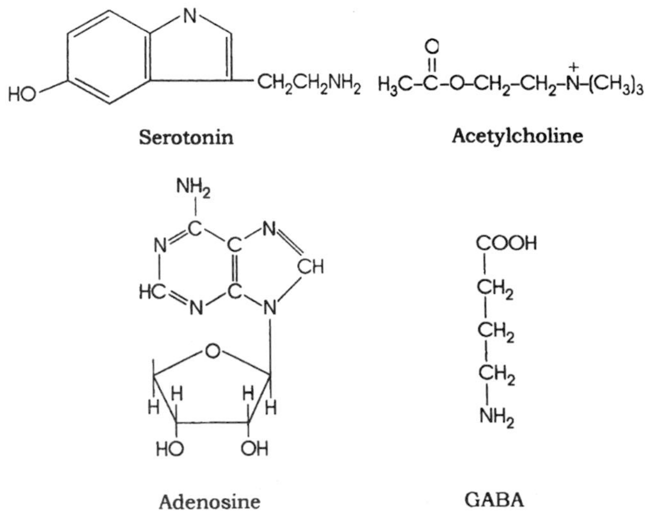

Cardiovascular effects

Serotonin may have either vasoconstricting or vasodilating effects, depending on the state of the endothelium and the specific vessel type it is being exposed to. Different receptor subtypes mediate the different vasoactive actions of serotonin. Vasodilation is mediated through endothelial 5-HT$_{1A}$ receptors, which cause release of nitric oxide, prostacyclin, and endothelium-derived hyperpolarizing factors. Vasoconstrictive effects are mediated through smooth muscle 5-HT$_2$ receptors. Serotonin-induced vasoconstriction is enhanced in chronic hypertension, perhaps partly owing to endothelial damage and loss of vasodilating effects. In animal models where hypertension is caused by administration of deoxycorticosterone (DOC) and high salt diet, there is a switch from 5-HT$_{2A}$ to 5-HT$_{2B}$ receptors in vascular smooth muscle along with enhanced vasoconstrictor effects of serotonin. Treatment of DOC-salt hypertensive rats with a 5-HT$_{2B}$ receptor antagonist decreases BP dramatically.

Central effects

Serotonin effects within the CNS are also dimorphic and central administration of serotonin may either increase or decrease BP. Activation of 5HT$_{1A}$ receptors in the RVLM results in a decrease in BP through reduced sympathetic outflow, particularly in renal sympathetic nerves. At the same time, activation of 5HT$_2$ receptors in the RVLM increases renal and splanchnic sympathetic activity, with accompanying vasoconstriction, and increased BP. Therefore, the effects of serotonin antagonists on BP can be neutral. Nevertheless, in models with increased hypothalamic serotonin levels, as occurs during the development of hypertension in the spontaneously hypertensive rats (SHRs), central administration of 5,6-dihydroxytryptamine lowers BP.

ADENOSINE

Synthesis and metabolism

Adenosine is a nucleoside composed of adenine and d-ribose. When combined with phosphate, energy-storing mono-, di-, and triphosphate forms (AMP, ADP, and ATP) are synthesized. Adenosine itself is ubiquitous in body tissues and is formed by breakdown of adenine nucleoside polyphosphates or hydrolysis of S-adenosylmethionine and S-adenosylhomocysteine. Adenosine production is increased during periods of tissue ischemia, and through its powerful local vasodilatory actions, may ameliorate the effects of ischemia. Adenosine is rapidly metabolized with a half-life of 1 to 7 seconds. Plasma levels are in the range of 1.5 $\times10^{-7}$ mol/L in healthy individuals.

Receptors and actions

Four types of adenosine receptors have been characterized. Cardiac effects are mediated mainly by A$_1$ receptors, which inhibit adenylyl cyclase and activate K$^+$ channels. Adenosine suppresses sinus node automaticity and atrioventricular nodal

Figure A24.1 Structures of serotonin, acetylcholine, adenosine, and γ-aminobutyric acid (GABA).

conduction and decreases inotropy. A_{2A} and A_{2B} receptors stimulate adenylyl cyclase and cause vasodilation. Adenosine has direct vasodilatory effects in coronary and systemic vascular beds and causes hypotension in anesthetized individuals. Adenosine administration has minor effects on BP in conscious individuals but results in decreased vagal tone and reflex activation of the sympathetic nervous system. Adenosine is commonly used in the treatment of supraventricular tachycardias and as a test agent for coronary artery disease, where its vasodilatory activity in relatively normal regions of the coronary circulation produces a "steal" effect, revealing perfusion defects in regions of ischemia.

γ-AMINOBUTYRIC ACID

γ-Aminobutyric acid (GABA) is an inhibitory amino acid neurotransmitter distributed throughout the CNS. Tonic release of GABA by neurons in the posterior hypothalamus and ventral medulla plays a modulatory role in BP homeostasis. Administration of $GABA_A$ agonists into these brain regions decreases BP, whereas $GABA_A$ antagonists increase BP. $GABA_B$ receptors in the anterior hypothalamus also mediate increases in BP. In the SHR model, GABA content and $GABA_A$ receptors are decreased in the posterior hypothalamus. As a result, these animals are unresponsive to hypothalamic injection of GABA antagonists and have been described as lacking tonic GABA-nergic input.

ENDOGENOUS OUABAIN

Endogenous "ouabain" (EO) is a mammalian steroidal counterpart of the plant glycoside ouabain (**Figure A24.2**). The vast majority of analytical work indicates that the EO isolated from human plasma and bovine adrenal glands is identical with ouabain but the (co)existence of one or more isomers of EO remains under investigation. Human EO, like its plant counterpart, is a high-affinity, reversible, and specific inhibitor of the mammalian sodium pump (Na/K–ATPase), which confers cardiac inotropic and vasopressor activity.

Biosynthesis

Circulating EO levels are primarily dependent upon adrenocortical function. EO biosynthesis is secondary to cholesterol side chain cleavage. The early events in EO biosynthesis occur through an aldosterone-like pathway and appear to be mediated by cells primarily located in the adrenal zona glomerulosa. The later events in EO biosynthesis and the mechanism of EO secretion are not known. The adrenocortical source and the active regulated secretion of EO by adrenal stimulants are some of the classical hallmarks of a mammalian hormone system. Like aldosterone, EO secretion in rats and humans is stimulated by angiotensin II, and volume depletion. Adrenocorticotropic hormone is a stimulus to EO secretion in rats and humans. Approximately 50% of patients with primary hyperaldosteronism have elevated plasma EO.

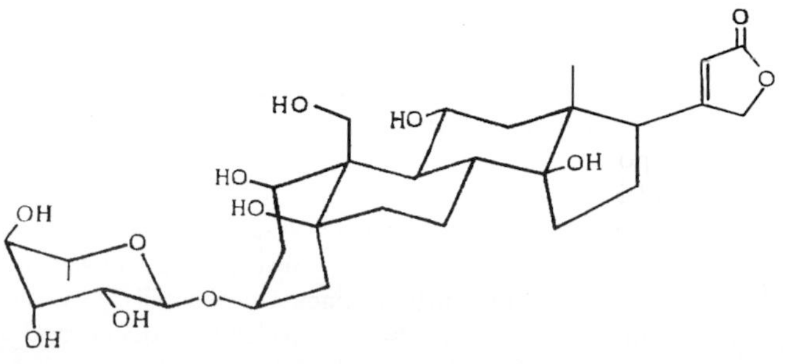

Actions

Most mammals express four catalytically active α subunit isoforms of the sodium (Na^+) pump. Each α subunit is encoded by its own gene and has a single conserved high-affinity binding site for the cardiac glycosides. All known actions of EO and ouabain follow from their ability to bind and occupy this receptor site. In addition to Na^+ pumps, a new class of high-affinity ouabain binding sites has been described in the adrenal cortex, brain, and kidney. The prevalence of these novel binding sites is typically <1% of total Na^+ pump density and their identity and function are not known. Recent experiments with transgenic mice show that the pathologic significance of EO in the cardiovascular system is due primarily to EO occupation of the α1 and α2 isoforms of the Na^+ pump and that the downstream effects are mediated by the vascular Na^+–Ca^{2+} exchanger.

Ouabain binding to Na^+ pump isoforms tends to increase intracellular Na^+ concentrations, thereby lowering the Na^+ gradient. This leads to augmented influx of calcium (Ca^{2+}) through the Na^+–Ca^{2+} exchanger and increased intracellular Ca^{2+}. Augmentation of many Ca^{2+}-dependent cellular responses follows, including increased arterial myogenic tone and neurogenic activity. In addition to this mechanism, ouabain stimulates an src-kinase activated signaling cascade by binding to Na^+ pumps in membrane caveolae. Although the signaling cascade triggers cell growth, its significance in hypertension is currently not known.

Hypertension and cardiac disease

Several lines of evidence link EO with cardiovascular dysfunction: (a) many white patients with essential hypertension (~45%) have elevated circulating levels of EO and (b) plasma EO levels correlate with BP. High dietary salt intake raises plasma EO in humans and in the rat, and sustained plasma levels of ouabain that mimic the elevated levels of EO in essential hypertension exert a slow pressor effect with sustained hypertension. The BP elevation is dose dependent, highly correlated with circulating ouabain, resembles human essential hypertension hemodynamically, and is influenced by gender and renal function. Elevated plasma EO has also been linked with cardiac cell growth *in vitro* and *in vivo* and predicts worsening heart failure in humans. A novel class of pharmacologic agents is under development that antagonizes receptor binding of EO. One of these agents (rostafuroxin) reduces BP in some forms of experimental hypertension and is in early phase III trials in essential hypertension.

Figure A24.2 Structure of ouabain. The A/B and C/D rings are both *cis*-fused. A 5-member lactone ring is attached at C_{17} in the β-orientation. The deoxy-L-sugar rhamnose is linked to C_3. The steroid nucleus of ouabain is heavily oxygenated (positions 1, 3, 5, 14, and 19). Endogenous ouabain (EO) may have one or more steroidal isomers.

Suggested Readings

Blaustein MP. The physiological effects of endogenous ouabain: control of cell responsiveness. *Am J Optom Physiol Opt* 1993;264:C1367–C1387.

Chalmers J, Arnolda L, Llewellyn-Smith I, et al. Central neurons and neurotransmitters in the control of blood pressure. *Clin Exp Pharmacol Physiol* 1994;21:819–829.

Ckuba T. Cholinergic mechanism and blood pressure regulation in the central nervous system. *Brain Res Bull* 1998;46:475–481.

DeWardener HE. The hypothalamus and hypertension. *Physiol Meas* 2001;71:1599–1658.

Hindle AT. Recent developments in the physiology and pharmacology of 5-hydroxytryptamine. *Br J Anaesth* 1994;73:395–407.

Huang BS, Leenen FH. Brain renin-angiotensin system and ouabain-induced sympathetic hyperactivity and hypertension in Wistar rats. *Hypertension* 1999;34(1):107–112.

Manunta P, Hamilton BP, Hamlyn JM. Salt intake and depletion increase circulating levels of endogenous ouabain in normal men. *Am J Physiol Regul Integr Comp Physiol* 2006;290(3):R553–R559.

Manunta P, Stella P, Rivera R, et al. Left ventricular mass, stroke volume, and ouabain-like factor in essential hypertension. *Hypertension* 1999;34(3):450–456.

Pelleg A, Porter RS. The pharmacology of adenosine. *Pharmacotherapy* 1990;10:157–174.

Ramage AG. Central cardiovascular regulation and 5-hydroxytryptamine receptors. *Brain Res Bull* 2001;56:425–439.

Schoner W, Scheiner-Bobis G. Endogenous cardiac glycosides: hormones using the sodium pump as signal transducer. *Semin Nephrol* 2005;25(5):343–351.

Walch L, Brink C, Norel X. The muscarinic receptor subtypes in human blood vessels. *Therapie* 2001;56:223–226.

Xie Z, Askari A. Na(+)/K(+)-ATPase as a signal transducer. *Eur J Biochem* 2002;269(10):2434–2439.

Zhang J, Lee MY, Cavalli M, et al. Sodium pump α2 subunits control myogenic tone and blood pressure in mice. *J Physiol* 2005;569(Pt 1):243–256.

CHAPTER A25 ■ VASCULAR AND RENAL NITRIC OXIDE

LEOPOLDO RAIJ, MD

KEY POINTS

■ Endothelial cells contain the constitutive form of nitric oxide (NO) synthase, which produces NO through L-arginine metabolism.

■ Release of NO can be augmented acutely by (a) increases in blood flow velocity or shear stress and (b) a variety of hormones, autacoids, and by-products associated with vasoconstriction or blood coagulation.

■ Endothelium-derived NO inhibits contraction and proliferation of the underlying vascular smooth muscle, adhesion of leukocytes and platelets, and platelet aggregation; endothelial NO bioavailability is decreased in many vascular diseases, including hypertension and atherosclerosis.

■ NO regulates renal function and blood pressure (BP) through its effects on tubular sodium reabsorption, tubuloglomerular feedback (TGF), renal hemodynamics, and pressure-natriuresis.

See also Chapters A2, A3, **A9, A10, A26,** A62, **A63, A64,** and **C140**

Nitric oxide (NO) is an endogenously produced, freely diffusible gas with a half-life of several seconds. NO functions as an endogenous intracellular and intercellular messenger that is involved in many pathophysiologic responses, especially regional blood flow regulation and sodium (Na^+) per water excretion. Cardiovascular and renal health also depends on the pleiotropic effects of NO.

Nitric oxide synthases

NO is produced from the guanidine-nitrogen terminal of L-arginine by nitric oxide synthases (NOS).

Nitric oxide synthase isoforms. Three NOS isoforms have been characterized, purified, and cloned: neuronal (nNOS or NOS1), inducible (iNOS or NOS2), and endothelial (eNOS or NOS3). These NOS isoforms are encoded by three different genes on different chromosomes and have approximately 50% to 60% homology with each other and the cytochrome P-450 enzymes. They share a common basic structure, organization, and requirement for substrate cofactors, including oxygen, reduced nicotinamide adenine dinucleotide phosphate, and tetrahydrobiopterin.

Distribution.

Nitric oxide synthase 1. Neuronal NOS (nNOS or NOS1) is expressed in neural tissue, skeletal muscle, and myocardium. NOS1 is expressed abundantly in macula densa cells, Bowman's capsule, and the inner medullary collecting ducts and in lesser quantities in efferent arterioles, and the thick ascending limb.

Nitric oxide synthase 2. Expression of NOS2 is induced in nearly all tissues in response to cytokines, endotoxin, and other proinflammatory stimuli. In the kidney, NOS2 is expressed in

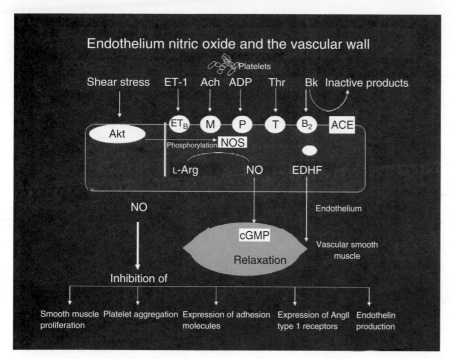

Figure A25.1 Selected humoral factors that cause the release of nitric oxide (NO) from nitric oxide synthase (NOS) in the endothelium: ET-1, Endothelin1; Ach, acetylcholine; ADP, adenosine diphosphate; Thr, thrombin; Bk, bradykinin. Receptors in circles: ET_B, endothelin type B; M, muscarinic; P, purinergic; T, thrombin; B_2, bradykinin type 2; ACE, angiotensin-converting enzyme. NOS, nitric oxide synthase; L-Arg, L-Arginine; EDHF, endothelium-dependent hyperpolarizing factor; cGMP, cyclic guanosine monophosphate.

vascular smooth muscle, mesangial, medullary interstitial, and tubular epithelial cells.

Nitric oxide synthase 3. NOS3 is expressed in the endothelium (**Figure A25.1**) and myocardium. Endothelial cells of the renal vasculature and tubular epithelial cells of the collecting duct and thick ascending limb of Henle's loop express NOS3.

Nitric oxide synthase regulation

General characteristics. NOS1 and NOS3 are constitutively expressed, calmodulin-dependent enzymes that were originally described as being primarily regulated by intracellular calcium (Ca^{2+}). Regulation of NOS2 had been thought to occur primarily through changes in expression of the enzyme. The overall activity of NOS enzymes can be modulated by numerous physical and hormonal factors, including cofactor availability, protein–protein interactions, and phosphorylation state.

Vascular nitric oxide synthase 3 regulation

Acylation. NOS3 in peripheral cell membrane protein undergoes specific acylation reactions that alter its activity and location within the cell. N-myristoylation of NOS3 targets the enzyme to the Golgi apparatus, where it undergoes cysteine palmitoylation. The myristoylated and palmitoylated NOS3 is then targeted to the caveolae, which are cholesterol and sphingolipid-enriched cell membrane vesicle structures in the endothelium and other cell types. Caveolin-1, a major coat protein responsible for assembly of caveolae, directly interacts with and inhibits NOS3 in endothelial cells.

Intracellular calcium and calmodulin. Agonists that raise intracellular Ca^{2+} levels (e.g., bradykinin, acetylcholine, and thrombin) promote calmodulin binding to NOS3 and caveolin-1 dissociation from the enzyme, resulting in an activated NOS3–calmodulin complex. Heat shock protein 90 (Hsp90) also facilitates calmodulin-induced displacement of caveolin-1 from NOS3. Once intracellular Ca^{2+} levels return to the resting state, calmodulin dissociates and caveolin-1 reassociates with NOS3. G protein–coupled receptors resident in caveolae, including the

B2 kinin, angiotensin (Ang) II type 1 (AT_1), and endothelin type B (ET_B) receptors, have also been reported to contribute to the NOS3-membrane complex and regulate NOS3 activity.

Shear stress. Changes in shear stress and blood flow are important in the control of endothelium-derived NO release. During increased shear stress, there is enhanced NOS3 activation through dissociation from caveolin-1 and increased association with calmodulin. The tyrosine kinase c-Src modulates NOS3 expression in response to shear stress through a short-term increase in NOS3 transcription and a longer-term stabilization of NOS3 mRNA.

Humoral factors. Ang II, glucose, hydrogen peroxide, and transforming growth factor-β also increase NOS3 expression. Mediators that decrease NOS3 expression include RhoA/Rho-kinase, oxidized low-density lipoprotein, lipopolysaccharide, and tumor necrosis factor-α. Moreover, the NOS3 promoter gene possesses consensus sequences that are potential binding sites for transcription factors, such as AP-1 complex, nuclear factor-κB, and interleukin-6.

Direct phosphorylation of NOS3 by the serine/threonine protein kinase Akt results in its activation. Shear stress, vascular endothelial growth factor, insulin, and estrogen also trigger Akt-mediated phosphorylation of NOS3, leading to NOS3 activation. Hsp90 may function as a scaffold for eNOS and Akt. In response to endothelial cell stimulation, eNOS and Akt appear to be recruited to an adjacent region on the same domain of Hsp90, which facilitates eNOS phosphorylation and enzyme activation.

Substrates and cofactors. NOS3 is a tightly coupled enzyme system that is also affected by perturbations in availability of substrates (e.g., L-arginine), cofactors (e.g., BH4), and by competitive endogenous NOS inhibitors such as asymmetric dimethylarginine (ADMA). Experimental and clinical studies have demonstrated that BH4 deficiency is associated with impaired endothelium-dependent relaxation. Because NO effects on the vascular cells are dependent on the concomitant production of O_2^- in the microenvironment where NO is synthesized and released, changes in the endothelial redox state may have a profound impact on endothelial NO bioavailability.

Nitric oxide signal transduction

Guanylyl cyclase. The receptor for NO is soluble (cytosolic) guanylyl cyclase (GC), a heterodimer with α and β subunits. Activation of this enzyme is mediated by the binding of NO to the heme moiety of GC, which forms a nitrosyl-heme adduct. As a result, the heme iron is shifted out of the plane of the porphyrine ring configuration, initiating the binding and hydrolysis of guanosine triphosphate (GTP) to form cyclic guanosine monophosphate (cGMP). The increased level of cGMP activates the cGMP-dependent protein kinase I, which in turn phosphorylates a number of proteins involved in the relaxation of vascular smooth muscle, cell proliferation, expression of adhesion molecules, and aggregation of platelets. Recent elegant studies have demonstrated that most GC receptors function as spare receptors that increase NO sensitivity, suggesting that the bioavailability of NO is the critical parameter for NO/cGMP signaling.

Phosphodiesterases. The cGMP signal is terminated by the action of the cyclic nucleotide-hydrolyzing phosphodiesterases (PDEs), with PDE1, PDE3, and PDE5 being of importance in the vascular system.

Nitric oxide and endothelial function

Vasodilation. Endothelial NO is also a key mediator of tonic vasodilation. The signaling pathway for insulin stimulation of NO production is through activation of phosphatidylinositol 3-kinase, which subsequently results in Akt phosphorylation. Interestingly, this signaling pathway is also required for insulin-mediated glucose metabolism. Some factors, including increase in oxidative stress, free fatty acids, and advanced glycation end products, contribute to endothelial dysfunction as well as insulin resistance. Clinically, impairment in insulin-mediated NO production in the endothelium is associated with hypertension and cardiovascular and metabolic diseases.

Antithrombotic effects. One of the central functions of the endothelium is to maintain blood fluidity through the production of factors that inhibit blood coagulation and platelet aggregation and promote fibrinolysis. NO release from endothelium as well as from platelets plays a crucial role in the maintenance of fluidity by preventing coagulation. Local platelet aggregation, resulting in the release of serotonin and adenosine diphosphate (ADP), local activation of the coagulation cascade, and the production of thrombin cause a massive local NO response. NO-induced vasodilation helps to eliminate "microaggregates," whereas the release of NO toward the lumen, in synergy with prostacyclin, inhibits platelet adhesion and aggregation and prevents vascular occlusion. Indeed, it has been reported that NOS3 is present in platelets and patients with acute coronary syndrome manifested impairment of NO production in the vasculature as well as in platelets.

Endothelial dysfunction and disease

Loss of endothelial NO bioactivity, as manifested by reduced endothelium-dependent relaxation, has been shown to be an independent risk factor for major adverse cardiovascular events.
Vasoconstriction. The underlying mechanisms of NO-induced endothelium-dependent relaxation are multifactorial. In addition

to its direct vasodilatory effect, NO counteracts agonist–induced vasoconstriction and downregulates Ang II type 1 (AT1) receptor expression. NO also inhibits the production and action of endothelin-1.

Impaired endothelium-dependent relaxation is often associated with an increase in vascular oxidative stress from the production of endogenous reactive oxygen species (ROS), especially O_2^-, in excess of antioxidant capacity. Both O_2 and $ONOO^-$ have been demonstrated to oxidize tetrahydrobiopterin (BH4), which lead to eNOS uncoupling and a subsequent shift to the production of O_2^- instead of NO.

Hypertension and vascular function. Inhibition of NO production upregulates endothelial angiotensin-converting enzyme (ACE) activity, increases production of Ang II and superoxide anion (O_2^-), induces vasoconstriction, and causes pronounced and sustained hypertension.

The contribution of NO to endothelium-dependent vasorelaxation may differ in large (conduit) and resistance arteries. In the conduit artery, NO is a primary mediator of endothelium-dependent relaxation, whereas in resistance arteries, endothelium-derived hyperpolarizing factor (EDHF) appears to be a more important mediator than NO. Mice lacking the NOS3 gene have a slightly higher arterial blood pressure (BP) than wild type animals, whereas frank hypotension occurs in mice that overexpress the NOS3 gene.

Vascular remodeling. NO plays a central role in the pathophysiology of vascular remodeling of resistance and conduit arteries through modulation of vascular smooth muscle cell (VSMC) proliferation, extracellular matrix deposition, and macrophage adhesion and migration. NO inhibits total protein and collagen synthesis in VSMC and activates certain matrix metalloproteinases in the vessel wall. The inhibitory effects of NO on vascular wall growth has also been verified in *in vivo* models of vascular injury: (a) NOS inhibitor–treated animals, (b) mice genetically deficient in eNOS, (c) transgenic mice that overexpress NOS3 in the endothelium, and (d) animals that overexpress eNOS in VSMC or adventitia through NOS3 gene transfer. Clinically, endothelial dysfunction is associated with impaired NO bioavailability and structural changes in the coronary arteries and is a risk factor for coronary heart disease.

Atherosclerosis. Endothelial dysfunction associated with reduced NO bioavailability is a harbinger of atherosclerosis. Endothelial NO inhibits VSMC migration and proliferation, platelet aggregation, leukocyte–endothelial adhesion, and plasminogen activator inhibitor-1 activation, suggesting that NO has antiinflammatory and antiatherogenic properties. Physical or biochemical injury to the endothelium impairs NO production, resulting in enhanced thrombus formation, aberrant vessel tone, and dysregulated VSMC growth. Interaction of NO with ROS reduces NO bioavailability and yields reactive nitrogen/oxygen species that induce protein nitration.

In apo-E–deficient mice, inhibition of NOS results in a significant inhibition of NO-mediated vascular responses and increases aortic atherosclerotic plaque surface area. High-density lipoprotein (HDL) cholesterol exerts antiatherogenic effects, at least in part, by promoting endothelial NO production. HDL regulates the subcellular distribution of NOS3 by maintaining the lipid environment in caveolae, where NOS3 is colocalized with other signaling molecules. Furthermore, HDL directly upregulates NOS3 mRNA expression and stimulates NOS3 activity through activation of the phosphatidylinositol 3-kinase/Akt pathway.

Cardiomyocytes

In the cardiac myocyte, NO activity is predominantly determined by its site of production, which in turn is controlled by spatial localization of the NOS enzymes. NOS3 is localized primarily to caveolae of the sarcolemma and t tubules, where its function is regulated by interaction with caveolin-3 and is linked to multiple cell-surface receptors, including muscarinic, β-adrenergic, and bradykinin receptors. Activation of NOS3 results in negative inotropy and chronotropy. NOS1 has been localized to the sarcoplasmic reticulum, where it influences Ca^{2+} cycling and thereby exerts positive inotropic effects in the heart. NOS enzyme activity and subcellular localization are altered after myocardial infarction and in heart failure.

Kidney

NO plays an important role in the control of renal function and regulation of BP through its effects on tubular Na^+ reabsorption, tubuloglomerular feedback (TGF), renal hemodynamics, and pressure-natriuresis. The diuretic and natriuretic effects of NO are mediated by direct inhibition of epithelial transport mechanisms in the proximal tubule, thick ascending limb, and cortical collecting duct cells. NO effects also depend on associated changes in peritubular hemodynamics and interstitial pressure, although NO-induced natriuresis and diuresis is not accompanied by proportional renal hemodynamic changes. NOS inhibitors administered intrarenally elicit substantial reductions in urine flow and in Na^+ and potassium (K^+) excretion.

Renal tubular effects

Nitric oxide synthase regulation.
In isolated, perfused thick ascending limbs, increasing luminal flow stimulates NOS3 activity and NO production through phosphorylation of serine 1179 by PI3-kinase. However, unlike endothelial cells, activation of NOS3 in the thick ascending limb leads to Hsp90-dependent translocation from intracellular compartments to the luminal membrane.

Transporters.
NO inhibits the absorption of sodium chloride in the proximal tubule and thick ascending limb by stimulating soluble guanylyl cyclase. Subsequent generation of cGMP leads to the inactivation of the Na^+/H^+ exchangers on the luminal membranes of the proximal tubule and thick ascending limb as well as the $Na^+-K^+-2CL^-$ cotransporter on the luminal membrane of the thick ascending limb.

Na channels and water permeability.
The mechanism by which NO inhibits Na^+ absorption appears to involve a direct effect on apical Na^+ channels. Activation of both soluble guanylyl cyclase and cGMP-dependent protein kinase is involved in the effect of NO on water permeability. NO signaling may also be a mediator that links the activity of basolateral $Na^+-K^+-ATPase$ activity to the basolateral K^+ channels and K^+ conductance in the collecting duct. In the collecting duct, NO inhibits Na^+ absorption and vasopressin-stimulated osmotic water permeability.

Renal hemodynamics

Renal blood flow.
Intrarenal NO helps to maintain the normally low renal vascular resistance. In response to inhibition of NO synthesis with L-arginine analogs, there is an increase of 30% to 50% in renal vascular resistance and a decrease of 25% to 40% in renal blood flow. Responses to NOS inhibition are reversed by the administration of the NO substrate L-arginine, substantiating that the responses to NOS inhibition are due to inhibition of endogenous NO generation.

In vivo studies have suggested that NO plays an important role in maintaining renal hemodynamics near the normal range in kidneys in response to elevated Ang II levels. In Ang II-infused hypertensive rats, inhibition of NOS decreases afferent and efferent arteriolar diameters, more so in afferent than efferent arterioles. Adding a NO donor blunts Ang II-induced vasoconstriction in afferent but not efferent arterioles.

Autoregulation.
Although NOS inhibition consistently reduces renal blood flow, corresponding glomerular filtration rate (GFR) responses are less consistent, with no change or only slight reductions in GFR depending on the dose and duration. NOS inhibition does not interfere with the ability of the kidney to autoregulate renal blood flow in response to alterations in renal arterial pressure but NOS inhibition decreases the autoregulatory plateau in proportion to the decrease in basal renal blood flow.

Pressure-natriuresis.
Pressure-natriuresis, the increase in Na^+ excretion caused by increased renal perfusion pressure, is NO dependent. On the basis of *in vivo* and *in vitro* data, intrarenal NO generation in response to acute elevations in renal arterial pressure directly inhibits distal tubular Na^+ reabsorption and increases Na^+ excretion. In experiments conducted in rats treated for 8 weeks with an NOS inhibitor, renin-angiotensin system blockade normalized BP but had no effect on the pressure-natriuresis, implying that BP reduction is not enough to overcome chronic renal NO deficiency. Alterations in shear stress that accompany increased renal arterial pressure may alter tubular natriuretic mechanisms, vascular tone, and renal interstitial hydrostatic pressure.

Tubuloglomerular feedback.
TGF is the homeostatic mechanism whereby increases or decrease in sodium chloride delivery to the macula densa signal the afferent arterioles to constrict or dilate to maintain stability of the filtered load. An increase in sodium chloride delivery to the macula densa stimulates apical Na^+/H^+ exchange, raises intracellular pH, activates NOS1, and increases NO generation. NO blunts the TGF response by stimulating generation of cGMP and activating cGMP-dependent protein kinase within the macula cells. Blocking luminal Na^+/H^+ exchange prevents the rise in pH of the macula densa cells and augments TGF, similar to selective NOS1 inhibition. Raising intracellular pH without increasing luminal sodium chloride also induces NO production. NO modulates TGF responsiveness, at least partially, by counteracting vasoconstriction. NOS1 is responsible for the resetting of TGF and glomerular hemodynamics after sustained changes in salt intake or proximal tubular reabsorption.

Suggested Readings

Félétou M, Vanhoutte PM. Endothelium-derived hyperpolarizing factor: where are we now? *Arterioscler Thromb Vasc Biol* 2006;26:1215–1225.

Fleming I, Busse R. Molecular mechanisms involved in the regulation of the endothelial nitric oxide synthase. *Am J Physiol Regul Integr Comp Physiol* 2003;284:R1–R12.

Herrera M, Ortiz PA, Garvin JL. Regulation of thick ascending limb transport: role of nitric oxide. *Am J Physiol Renal Physiol* 2006;290:1279–1284.

Kone BC, Kuncewicz T, Zhang W, et al. Protein interactions with nitric oxide synthases: controlling the right time, the right place, and the right amount of nitric oxide. *Am J Physiol Renal Physiol* 2003;285(2):F178–F190.

Majid DS, Navar LG. Nitric oxide in the control of renal hemodynamics and excretory function. *Am J Hypertens* 2001;14(6 Pt 2):74S–82S.

Mergia E, Friebe A, Dangel O, et al. Spare guanylyl cyclase NO receptors ensure high NO sensitivity in the vascular system. *J Clin Invest* 2006;116:1731–1737.

Schulman IH, Zhou MS, Raij L. Interaction between nitric oxide and angiotensin II in the endothelium: role in atherosclerosis and hypertension. *J Hypertens* 2006;24(Suppl 1):S45–S50.

Yu J, Bergaya S, Murata T, et al. Direct evidence for the role of caveolin-1 and caveolae in mechanotransduction and remodeling of blood vessels. *J Clin Invest* 2006;116:1284–1291.

Zhou MS, Adam AG, Jaimes EA, et al. In salt-sensitive hypertension, increased superoxide production is linked to functional upregulation of angiotensin II. *Hypertension* 2003;42(5):945–951.

Zimmet JM, Hare JM. Nitroso-redox interactions in the cardiovascular system. *Circulation* 2006;114:1531–1544.

CHAPTER A26 ■ KININS

OSCAR A. CARRETERO, MD AND NOUR-EDDINE RHALEB, PhD

KEY POINTS

- Kinins are potent vasodilators cleaved from kininogens by kallikreins.
- Kinins stimulate release of nitric oxide, prostaglandins, and other mediators.
- Kinin formation increases with stimulation of secretory activity in some glands and with inflammation in some cases.
- Kinins are natriuretic and diuretic, and they mediate part of the cardioprotective effect of angiotensin-converting enzyme (ACE) inhibitors.

See also Chapters **A10, A15,** and **A25**

Kinins are vasodepressor autacoids that play an important role in the regulation of cardiovascular and renal function. In mammals, the main kinins are bradykinin and lysyl-bradykinin (kallidin). They are released from substrates known as *kininogens* by enzymes called *kininogenases* (**Figure A26.1**). The main kininogenases, plasma and tissue (glandular) kallikrein, are separate enzymes with different functions and are encoded by different genes.

Kallikrein–kinin bioregulation

The two main kininogens, *high-molecular-weight kininogen* and *low-molecular-weight kininogen*, are synthesized in the liver and found in very high concentrations in plasma. They are encoded by a single gene, but their separate messenger RNAs are generated by different splicing of the gene transcript. Kinins, the active peptide products of the system, are released by the action of plasma kallikrein on high-molecular-weight kininogen. All kininogens also inhibit thiol proteases, such as cathepsin M and H, and calpains.

Kinins are destroyed by enzymes known as *kininases*, which are located mainly in the endothelial cells of the capillaries of the lungs and other tissues. The best-known kininases are angiotensin-converting enzyme (ACE, also known as *kininase II*), neutral endopeptidases (NEPs) 24.11 and 24.15, aminopeptidases, and carboxypeptidase N (known as *kininase I*) (**Figure A26.1**).

However, even after inhibition of most of these enzymes, the half-life of kinins *in vivo* is <15 seconds, suggesting that other peptidases are also important in the metabolism of these peptides. The kallikrein–kinin system is especially important in the venous circulation because kinins are generated principally in the systemic microcirculation and kininases are very prominent in the lung.

Receptors

Kinins act mainly as local autocrine and paracrine hormones *through* their actions on two different receptors: B_1 and B_2. B_1 receptors are selectively activated by des-Arg^9-bradykinin or des-Ar^{10}-kallidin, whereas B_2 receptors are activated by bradykinin or kallidin. In wild-type animals and humans, most of the known physiologic effects of kinins are mediated by B_2 receptors, which belong to the family of peptide hormone receptors with seven membrane-spanning regions linked to G proteins.

B_1 receptor expression is constitutively present in vascular and visceral tissues in humans, dogs, and pigs but B_1 receptor expression is increased in inflammatory states and in the presence of lipopolysaccharides such as endotoxin. Certain pleiotropic effects of B_1 receptors have also been observed. When no B_2 receptors are present, as in B_2 receptor knockout mice, B_1 receptor expression can be upregulated and the B_1 receptor itself can transduce some of the cellular and hemodynamic properties usually ascribed to B_2 receptors.

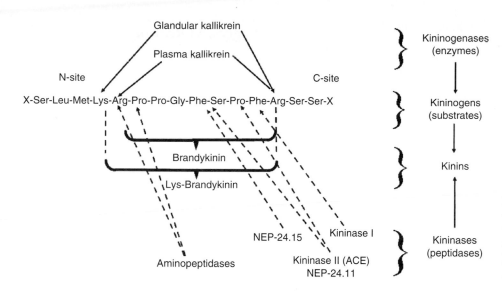

Figure A26.1 *Solid arrows* indicate kininogen cleavage by the main kininogenases, glandular, and plasma kallikrein. *Broken arrows* indicate sites of kinin cleavage by kininases [kininase I, kininase II (ACE [angiotensin-converting enzyme]), neutral endopeptidases (NEP) 24.11 and 24.15, and aminopeptidases].

Pathophysiology

In some organs, kinins appear to play an important role in the regulation of blood flow to meet metabolic or functional demands. ***Kidney.*** Kinins play an important role in the regulation of the renal microcirculation as well as water and sodium (Na$^+$) excretion. Renal kallikrein is located in the connecting cells of the tubules and kinin receptors are present in the collecting duct. The natriuretic and diuretic effects of kinins are mediated in part by the stimulation of prostaglandin E$_2$ by B$_2$ receptor-mediated stimulation of cyclooxygenases. Kinins stimulate nitric oxide release from endothelial cells, thereby generating cyclic guanosine monophosphate (cGMP), which inhibits Na$^+$ transport in cortical collecting duct cells. *In vivo*, bradykinin causes natriuresis and diuresis without affecting glomerular filtration rate. Kinins also relax the ureters and bladder.

The diuretic and natriuretic effects of NEP 24.11 inhibitors are due in part to the simultaneous blockade of NEP-dependent degradation of kinins and endogenous natriuretic peptides. These two peptides normally act in synergy to inhibit water and Na$^+$ transport in the nephron and blocking either peptide suppresses the natriuretic and diuretic effects of NEP inhibitors. ***Salivary and sweat glands.*** In the submandibular salivary glands, kallikrein secretion and vasoconstriction are increased by sympathetic nerve stimulation along with kinin-mediated vasodilation. The vasodilation is greatly magnified by ACE inhibitors, which block kininase II. Other glands of the gastrointestinal tract also contain kallikrein, and it is likely that the kallikrein–kinin system mediates postprandial vasodilation. Similarly, exocrine (sweat) glands contain a kallikrein-like enzyme, and it is possible that kinins also participate in the regulation of sweat formation as well as the skin vasodilatation observed during sweating. ***Inflammation.*** Kininogenase, low- and high-molecular-weight kininogens, and NEP 24.11 are all present in leukocytes. Kinins can also stimulate release of cytokines such as interleukin-1 from monocytes. Prostaglandins, nitric oxide, endothelium-derived hyperpolarizing factor, and tissue plasminogen activator mediate some of the effects of kinins. Kinins mediate part of the local vasodilation and edema observed during inflammation. ***Thrombosis.*** The bradykinin cascade interacts with the hemostatic system in several ways. Plasma kallikrein, high-molecular-weight kininogen, and Hageman factor are involved in the intrinsic pathway of blood clotting and in fibrinolysis. Kinins induce formation of nitric oxide and prostaglandin I$_2$, which inhibit platelet aggregation. Kinins are also potent stimulators of the release of tissue plasminogen activator and may promote fibrinolysis. These effects may help explain some of the beneficial properties of ACE inhibitors in patients with heart disease.

Hypertension

Decreased activity of the kallikrein–kinin system may play a role in some forms of experimental and human hypertension but the relationship between kinins and hypertension is complex. ***Animal models.*** Urinary and arterial tissue kallikrein are decreased in experimental renovascular hypertension, whereas in mineralocorticoid hypertension, circulating kinins and urinary kallikrein excretion are increased. A restriction fragment-length polymorphism for the kallikrein gene family in spontaneously hypertensive rats has been linked to high blood pressure (BP). On the other hand, hypertension is not a feature of mice lacking B$_2$ receptors or rats that are kininogen-deficient. The potentially important role of the kallikrein–kinin system in salt-sensitivity is demonstrated by bradykinin B$_2$ receptor knockout mice, which develop hypertension when fed a high-Na$^+$ diet. ***Human hypertension.*** Low urinary kallikrein excretion in children is one of the major genetic markers associated with a family history of essential hypertension and children with high urinary kallikrein excretion are less likely to have a genetic background of hypertension.

Therapeutic implications

Blood pressure responses to angiotensin-converting enzyme inhibition. Increased tissue kinin concentrations and potentiation of kinin effects may be involved in the therapeutic effect of ACE inhibitors. This hypothesis is supported by the following facts: (a) ACE is one of the main peptidases that hydrolyze kinins; (b) tissue and urinary kinins increase after treatment with ACE inhibitors, possibly promoting vasodilatation and increased Na$^+$ and water excretion; (c) inhibition of the kallikrein–kinin system with a kinin antagonist partially blocks the acute, but not the chronic, hypotensive effects of ACE inhibitors; and (d) in kininogen- or kinin-deficient Brown Norway rats with experimental renovascular hypertension, the acute antihypertensive effect of ACE inhibitors is significantly reduced in both magnitude and duration.

Ischemia and preconditioning.

Kallikrein and other system components are present in the heart, arteries, and veins. The release of kinins into the coronary sinus of isolated perfused hearts is markedly enhanced during acute ischemia. In chronic ischemia, repeated brief periods of oxygen deficit render the myocardium more resistant to subsequent ischemic injury, a phenomenon called *ischemic preconditioning*. Kinins appear to be involved because the preconditioning effect (similar to the BP response to ACE inhibition) is greatly attenuated in B_2 receptor knockout mice and in kinin-deficient rats with experimental myocardial infarction.

Cardiac and vascular remodeling.

ACE inhibitors reverse cardiac remodeling and improve function in heart failure due to myocardial infarction. In rats with heart failure, the benefit of ACE inhibitors can be blunted or eliminated by simultaneous administration of a bradykinin blocker, strongly suggesting that kinins have a favorable influence on remodeling. Similarly, kinins may play an important role in the beneficial effects of ACE inhibitors or angiotensin receptor blockers (ARBs) on atherosclerosis.

Angiotensin-converting enzyme inhibitor-induced angioedema.

Uncommonly (0.1%–0.7% of patients), ACE inhibitors cause oropharyngeal angioedema with potential airway compromise. This idiosyncratic response is not well understood but bradykinin may be involved because tissue levels of bradykinin are increased by ACE inhibitors and the profile of effects of the peptide—(local vasodilation, increased vascular permeability, and systemic hypotension) are consistent with findings in this abnormality.

Suggested Readings

Bhoola KD, Figueroa CD, Worthy K. Bioregulation of kinins: kallikreins, kininogens, and kininases. *Pharmacol Rev* 1992;44:1–80.

Carretero OA, Scicli AG. The kallikrein-kinin system. In: Fozzard HA, et al. eds. *The Heart and cardiovascular system. Scientific foundations*, Vol. 2. New York: Raven Press, 1991;1851–1874.

Liu Y-H, Yang X-P, Mehta D, et al. Role of kinins in chronic heart failure and in the therapeutic effect of ACE inhibitors in kininogen-deficient rats. *Am J Physiol Heart Circ Physiol* 2000;278:HSO7–H514.

Liu Y-H, Yang X-P, Sharov VG, et al. Effects of angiotensin-converting enzyme inhibitors and angiotensin II type 1 receptor antagonists in rats with heart failure. Role of kinins and angiotensin II type 2 receptors. *J Clin Invest* 1997;99:1926–1935.

Margolius HS. Tissue kallikreins and kinins: regulation and roles in hypertensive and diabetic diseases. *Annu Rev Pharmacol Toxicol* 1989;29:343364.

Milia AF, Gross V, Plehm R, et al. Normal blood pressure and renal function in mice lacking the bradykinin B_2 receptor. *Hypertension* 2001;37:1473–1479.

Nasjletti A, Malik KU. The renal kallikrein-kinin and prostaglandin systems interaction. *Annu Rev Physiol* 1981;43:597–609.

Nussberger J, Cugno M, Amstutz C, et al. Plasma bradykinin in angio-oedema. *Lancet* 1998;351:1693–1697.

Rhaleb N-E, Peng H, Alfie M, et al. Effect of ACE inhibitor on DOCA-salt- and aortic coarctation-induced hypertension in mice. Do kinin B_2 receptors play a role? *Hypertension* 1999;33:329–334.

Rhaleb N-E, Yang X-P, Nanba M, et al. Effect of chronic blockade of the kallikrein-kinin system on the development of hypertension in rats. *Hypertension* 2001;37:121–128.

Tschope C, Heringer-Walther S, Koch M, et al. Upregulation of bradykinin B_1-receptor expression after myocardial infarction. *Br J Pharmacol* 2000;129:1537–1538.

Xu J, Carretero OA, Sun Y, et al. Role of the B_1 kinin receptor in the regulation of cardiac function and remodeling after myocardial infarction. *Hypertension* 2005;45:747–753.

Yang X-P, Liu Y-H, Scicli GM, et al. Role of kinins in the cardioprotective effect of preconditioning. Study of myocardial ischemia/reperfusion injury in B_2 kinin receptor knockout mice and kininogen-deficient rats. *Hypertension* 1997;30:737–740.

CHAPTER A27 ■ ENDOGENOUS NATRIURETIC PEPTIDES

WILLIS K. SAMSON, PhD AND DOMENIC A. SICA, MD

KEY POINTS

- Endogenous natriuretic peptides (NPs) are produced in many tissues, including cardiac myocytes and vascular endothelial cells, generally in response to increased mechanical stretch and volume overload.
- Renal effects include generalized vasodilation, inhibition of renin release, and inhibition of sodium reabsorption in the thick ascending limb of Henle's loop.
- Systemic effects include vasodilation, central inhibition of sympathetic outflow, blunting of adrenal catecholamine release, blunting of the actions of angiotensin-II and aldosterone, lipolysis, and modulation of bone growth.
- NPs are elevated in dilated cardiomyopathies; determination of plasma levels of pro–brain natriuretic peptide (BNP) or BNP provides supplementary diagnostic and prognostic information in heart failure (HF).
- Parenteral BNP (nesiritide) can be used for treatment of pulmonary edema; however, recent data suggest that the risks of such therapy may outweigh the benefits demonstrated to date.

See also Chapters **A10, A25,** and C151

Three homologous peptides, products of unique genes, have been identified as members of the natriuretic peptide (NP) family. These peptides include atrial natriuretic peptide (ANP), BNP, and C-type natriuretic peptide (CNP). They are produced primarily in the heart and blood vessels and together exert potent adrenal, vascular, and renal actions all seemingly coordinated to unload the vascular tree (e.g., inhibition of aldosterone release, increased glomerular filtration, natriuresis, diuresis, and inhibition of sympathetic tone).

Natriuretic peptide subclasses

Atrial natriuretic peptide. The first to be identified, ANP, was found to be the factor present in granules in atrial myocytes, which when purified exerted significant hypotensive and natriuretic actions in experimental animals. In addition, urodilatin is an NP (isolated in human urine), derived from the same common precursor as ANP.

Brain natriuretic peptide. A second peptide was identified in cardiac extracts that originally had been thought to be uniquely produced in the brain (therefore the name brain natriuretic peptide). However, it is now clear that BNP is primarily a product of the myocardium and not abundantly produced in the brain. Circulating BNP concentrations are typically lower than those of ANP except in the instance of HF where it can be found in much higher concentrations.

C-type natriuretic peptide. The third member of the family, CNP is produced in the brain, but even more widely in the vascular endothelium and is felt to act in a paracrine fashion on vascular smooth muscle cells. CNP is a potent vasoactive agent with a prominent venodilator effect. Its release from the vascular endothelium is stimulated by shear stress as well as local factors, which include transforming growth factor (TGF)-β, tumor necrosis factor (TNF)-α, and some interleukins (e.g., IL-1).

Natriuretic peptide receptors

It is not surprising that all three NPs share common biologic receptors. The peptides and their respective receptors [natriuretic peptide receptor (NPR)] are identified in **Figure A27.1.** A hierarchy of ligand binding exists for these three receptors, as follows: (NPR)-A (guanylyl cyclase [GC]-A) ANP ≥ BNP > CNP; NPR-B (GC-B) CNP > ANP ≥ BNP; NPR-C ("clearance" receptor) ANP ≥ CNP ≥ BNP.

Natriuretic peptide receptor-A and B. Two of the NPRs, NPR-A and NPR-B, are membrane-bound GCs that signal through the formation of cyclic guanosine monophosphate (cGMP), and are therefore also referred to as *GC-A* and *GC-B* respectively.

Natriuretic peptide receptor-C. A third receptor, NPR-C, is devoid of guanylyl cyclase activity but shares structural homology with NPR-A and NPR-B in the extracellular domains.

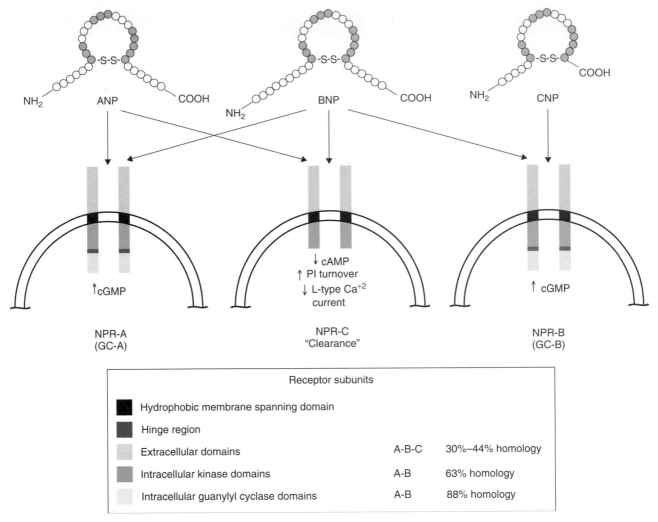

Figure A27.1 Structures of the members of the natriuretic peptide family and their receptors demonstrating shared homology domains among the receptors. ANP, atrial natriuretic peptide; BNP, brain natriuretic peptide; CNP, C-type natriuretic peptide; cAMP, cyclic adenosine monophosphate; cGMP, cyclic guanosine monophosphate; NPR, natriuretic peptide receptor; GC, guanylyl cyclase.

NPR-C was originally thought to be a biologically inactive clearance receptor but it is now recognized that ligand binding to this receptor results in inhibition of cyclic adenosine monophosphate (cAMP) formation, probably through a G_i protein. In some cells, this results in inhibition of L-type calcium channels. Mutations of the NPR-C result in increased NP levels and enhanced biologic effects of those peptides, including bone overgrowth and hypotension.

Biologic actions

As predicted by the hypotensive and natriuretic actions of NPs, receptors are present throughout the vascular tree, and in the heart, adrenal gland, lung, brain and kidney.

Blood vessels. In blood vessels, ANP increases microvascular permeability and favors transvascular fluid exchange and its administration results in hemoconcentration. NPR-B is responsible for the vasodilatory effects of CNP in response to vascular injury and also works through a conserved series of cytoprotective signal transduction pathways and antimitogenic actions. These effects may prove therapeutically advantageous in the clinical setting of ischemia/reperfusion.

Heart. ANP may also play an important protective role during tissue ischemia since the peptide exerts antiinflammatory actions through suppression of inflammatory cytokine production. In the lung, ANP exerts vasodilatory and bronchodilatory actions. In fact overexpression of ANP in mice protects against hypoxia-induced hypertension. Activation of the NPR-A inhibits pressure-induced cardiac remodeling, and both ANP and BNP inhibit cardiac hypertrophy and fibroblast remodeling. In this regard, deletion of the BNP gene in mouse models results in cardiac fibrosis, a process that is BP independent.

Renal effects. Direct renal effects of the NPs were the initial hallmark of their biologic action.

Atrial natriuretic peptide. Acting through the NPR-A, ANP produces natriuresis and diuresis due to renal hemodynamic and direct tubular actions. The increase in renal blood flow and glomerular filtration produced by ANP does not persist as long as the natriuretic response, suggesting separate and distinct pathways. In addition to direct tubular effects to inhibit sodium (Na^+) and water reabsorption, ANP acts in the juxtaglomerular apparatus to also reduce renin release. The natriuresis induced by ANP is not accompanied by a concomitant kaliuresis.

Brain natriuretic peptide. BNP has pharmacologic actions that are qualitatively similar to those of ANP. The spectrum of renal actions ascribed to ANP have also been demonstrated in experimental animals and humans with BNP, but BNP kinetics and effects are quantitatively different (usually more powerful) than those of ANP, particularly in pathophysiologic settings.

C-type natriuretic peptide. Diuresis and natriuresis appear not to occur with CNP.

Neurohumoral systems. The natriuretic and diuretic actions of ANP are complemented by actions of the peptide in the central nervous system (CNS) to inhibit Na$^+$ appetite and thirst. The zona glomerulosa cells contain specific NP binding sites and ANP (or BNP) inhibits aldosterone synthesis and blocks the release of aldosterone that occurs following angiotensin-II infusions. In addition, many of the actions of angiotensin-II are antagonized by ANP. Although plasma ANP and BNP do not cross the blood–brain barrier, they can access hormonally sensitive sites outside this barrier (such as the subfornical organ or area postrema) and thereby potentially affect cardiovascular control mechanisms. As in the periphery, ANP opposes many of the central actions of angiotensin-II. Pharmacologic levels of ANP and BNP also inhibit antidiuretic hormone (ADH) production and release from the posterior pituitary.

Adipose tissue. Lipolytic actions of ANP and BNP in humans have been ascribed to the expression of the NPR-A by adipocytes.

Bone. The unexpected finding of the presence of NPR-B on chondrocytes led to the discovery that CNP stimulates long bone growth and mutations of the NPR-B or CNP itself result in dwarfism. The importance of signaling through the NPR-B was further demonstrated in transgenic overexpression studies where increased CNP levels, or reduced clearance of the peptide, resulted in skeletal overgrowth.

Control of natriuretic peptide release and secretion

Natriuretic peptide synthesis. Cleavage of human pro–atrial natriuretic peptide (126 amino acids) releases mature ANP, a 28-amino-acid carboxy-terminal fragment.

BNP originates from a 134-amino acid prepropeptide that is cleaved into a precursor molecule, proBNP108. Upon release from cardiac myocyte secretory granules, proBNP108 is cleaved to NT-proBNP and BNP by the protease corin. NT-proBNP is a biologically inert molecule (76 amino acids); BNP is the biologically active counterpart.

Two CNP molecules, 22 and 53 amino acids in length, are derived from a single pro-CNP precursor. The 22-amino acid form predominates in the CNS, anterior pituitary, kidney, vascular endothelial cells, and plasma. It is more potent than the 53-amino acid form.

Natriuretic peptide release. The major stimuli for the release of ANP and BNP are (i) increased tension across the myocardium caused by increased blood volume or pressure, (ii) increased mechanical effort (heart rate), (iii) neurohumoral factors such as endothelin, angiotensin-II, adrenal steroids, inflammatory cytokines, growth factors, prostaglandins, thyroid hormones, and α-adrenergic agents. Although constitutive release of the peptides occurs under normal conditions, production and secretion can be upregulated in volume overload states such as HF or after ischemic events (e.g., acute myocardial infarction).

Natriuretic peptide clearance. All three NPs are cleared from tissue and the circulation by a combination of sequestration through the NPR-C and enzymatic degradation by neutral endopeptidase 24.11 (neprilysin). Neutral endopeptidase inhibitors reduce degradation and therefore increase plasma levels of the NPs. The clinical effectiveness of neutral endopeptidase inhibitors as antihypertensive agents is limited because of accompanying neurohumoral counterregulatory responses. Single molecules have been developed that contain angiotensin-converting enzyme (ACE) inhibitor and neutral endopeptidase inhibitor moieties. These agents are potent antihypertensive medications but a high rate of angioedema is a major barrier to their clinical development.

Natriuretic peptides and cardiovascular disease

Plasma levels of ANP and BNP are elevated in a variety of disease states including dilated cardiomyopathy, myocardial infarction, pulmonary arterial hypertension, chronic renal failure, and cirrhosis. These elevations may reflect the activation of compensatory mechanisms designed to correct imbalances in fluid and electrolyte homeostasis. In contrast to ANP and BNP, circulating CNP levels are not consistently elevated in patients with HF, although atrial and ventricular CNP content is increased.

Hypertension. The importance of the NPs in cardiovascular function is demonstrated by the hypertensive state displayed by mice engineered to lack either ANP or a functional NPR-A. Gene titration studies have demonstrated further the importance of NP signaling through NPR-A in the maintenance of resting blood pressure (BP). In humans, ANP infusion reduces BP more so in hypertensive than normotensive subjects; however, the clinical development of synthetic ANP as a potential antihypertensive agent has been limited by its lack of oral bioavailability. The clinical use of BNP as a potential antihypertensive agent still requires further clarification although the technology now exists to permit its oral administration without enzymatic degradation, therefore allowing adequate bioavailability.

Heart failure

Diagnosis. In dilated cardiomyopathies, the increase in synthesis and release of BNP (which is greater than the corresponding ANP response) provides a rationale for the diagnostic use of plasma BNP or NT-proBNP levels to help differentiate HF from other causes of dyspnea. The half-life of BNP is 18 minutes compared with 90 to 120 minutes for NT-proBNP, which is likely the basis for the prevailing differences in the circulating concentrations of these two substances. Commercial assays for BNP and NT-proBNP, to some extent, both measure, proBNP but the proportion of either indicator that is proBNP is highly variable.

Although BNP has provided ancillary diagnostic and prognostic information in dilated cardiomyopathies, the value of BNP and NT-proBNP in HF with preserved systolic function (diastolic dysfunction) is unclear. Moreover, there often appears to be a limited correlation between BNP or NT-proBNP levels and a patient's clinical response once therapy is under way. BNP is elevated by concurrent kidney or lung diseases, so the actual clinical value of BNP determinations is less than what was expected.

Treatment. A recombinant form of BNP (nesiritide) decreases pulmonary capillary wedge pressure, systemic vascular resistance, right atrial pressure and a range of neurohormone concentrations in patients with symptomatic left ventricular dysfunction. Renal function may occasionally worsen in nesiritide-treated patients, possibly related to the degree and duration of the BP reduction. The clinical significance of this change in renal function is not well documented and it is unknown whether mortality is increased. Accordingly, the initial enthusiasm for the use of nesiritide in pulmonary edema has been tempered.

Suggested Readings

Clerico A, Recchia FA, Passino C, et al. Cardiac endocrine function is an essential component of the homeostatic regulation network: physiological and clinical implications. *Am J Physiol* 2005;290:H17–H29.

Colucci, WS, Elkayam U, Horton DP, et al. The Nesiritide Study Group. Intravenous nesiritide, a natriuretic peptide, in the treatment of decompensated congestive heart failure. *N Engl J Med* 2000;343:246–253.

John SW, Veress AT, Honrath U, et al. BP and fluid-electrolyte balance in mice with reduced or absent ANP. *Am J Physiol* 1996;271:R109–R114.

Kostis JB, Packer M, Black HR, et al. Omapatrilat and enalapril in patients with hypertension: the omapatrilat cardiovascular treatment *vs.* enalapril (OCTAVE) trial. *Am J Hypertens* 2004;17:103–111.

Lafontan M, Moro C, Sengenes C, et al. An unsuspected metabolic role for atrial natriuretic peptides: the control of lipolysis, lipid mobilization, and systemic nonesterified fatty acids levels in humans. *Arterioscler Thromb Vasc Biol* 2005;25:2032–2042.

Levin ER, Gardner DG, Samson WK. Natriuretic peptides. *N Engl J Med* 1998;339:321–328.

Melo LG, Steinhelper ME, Pang SC, et al. ANP in regulation of arterial pressure and fluid-electrolyte balance: lessons from genetic mouse models. *Physiol Genomics* 2000;3:45–58.

Potter LR, Abbey-Hosch S, Dicket DM. Natriuretic peptides, their receptors, and cyclic guanosine monophosphate-dependent signaling functions. *Endocr Rev* 2006;27:47–72.

Rademaker MT, Richards AM. Cardiac natriuretic peptides for cardiac health. *Clin Sci* 2005;108:23–36.

Samson WK, White MM. Fluid/mineral balance: atrial natriuretic peptide. In: Squire LR, ed. *New encyclopedia of neuroscience.* Oxford:Elsevier Science, 2006.

CHAPTER A28 ■ VASOACTIVE GROWTH FACTORS

CARRIE A. NORTHCOTT, PhD AND STEPHANIE W. WATTS, PhD

KEY POINTS

■ Classic peptide growth factors can elicit contraction or relaxation of vascular smooth muscle.
■ Agonists of heptahelical receptors that alter arterial tone also modify smooth muscle cell growth.
■ Activation of tyrosine kinase mediates both contraction and growth in vascular smooth muscle.
■ Signaling paradigms of vascular contraction are more complicated than originally thought; this interaction underscores the interrelation of growth and contractility in arterial smooth muscle.

See also Chapters A25 and A61

Definitions

Growth factor: an extracellular polypeptide signaling molecule that stimulates a cell to grow or proliferate

Heptahelical receptor: a protein, the transmembrane portions of which traverse the plasma membrane seven times

Growth: an increase in cell number or cell size

Introduction

Decades of research have established the effect of hormones on arterial contraction and smooth muscle cell growth. Both arterial function and structure are significantly abnormal in conditions of human and experimental hypertension. The central point of this chapter is that substances that stimulate heptahelical receptors or substances that stimulate receptor tyrosine kinase(s) alter both smooth muscle contractility *and* cellular growth potential.

Growth factors and growth factor receptors

Growth factors are peptides that stimulate in various ways a group of receptors that traverse the plasma membrane typically but one time. For example, epidermal growth factor (EGF) interacts with one of its monomeric receptors (ErbB1, ErbB3, ErbB4) to cause dimerization of the monomer or alternatively it combines with ErbB2, an epidermal growth factor receptor (EGFR) for which no known agonist has been identified. Dimerization of stimulated monomers results in activation of a tyrosine kinase intrinsic to the receptor, located on the cytoplasmic C-terminal end of the receptor. The activated tyrosine kinase phosphorylates tyrosine residues within src homology 2 (SH2) domains of its activated partner. Tyrosine-phosphorylated SH2 domains are sites of protein–protein interactions, and scaffolding of proteins (Grb 2, Sos) that enable signal transduction pathways to proceed. The extracellular signal-regulated kinase (Erk) known as *mitogen-activated protein kinase* (MAPK) is one pathway that depends on such a sequence of events. The end result of activation of the Erk-MAPK pathway is translocation of MAPK to the nucleus, where the MAPK phosphorylates and alters activation of transcription factors involved in the processes of growth. The Erk-MAPK pathway is a "growth pathway" just as a substance that activates this pathway is a "growth factor."

In 1986 it was demonstrated that platelet-derived growth factor (PDGF) caused a potent and concentration-dependent contraction of isolated rat aorta. Since that time, numerous substances considered to be classical growth factors have been shown to modify arterial tone acutely (**Table A28.1**). One mechanism by which growth factors modulate smooth muscle tone is through modulation of caldesmon activity. Caldesmon, a substrate of Erk MAPK, in its unphosphorylated state inhibits the actinomysin ATPase necessary for contraction to occur; when phosphorylated by Erk MAPK, this inhibition is lifted and contraction is allowed to proceed. Growth factors also activate L-type calcium channels; the mechanism by which this occurs is not well understood.

Growth factors are not typically thought of as substances that can modify arterial tone. One reason for this belief is that plasma levels of growth factors are low (e.g., plasma EGF in humans is estimated at approximately 30 picomolar). However, plasma levels of growth factors are not necessarily indicative of local receptor activation because plasma membrane and extracellular matrix proteins are reservoirs for growth factors. The action of matrix metalloproteases, which are necessary for growth factor release, contribute to acute and locally high concentrations of growth factors in the arterial wall and promote both growth and contractile effects. **Table A28.1** lists some of the *acute* contractile and growth-promoting effects of growth factors and cytokines.

Heptahelical receptors

Heptahelical or G protein–coupled receptors are the single largest family of plasma membrane molecules involved in signal transduction. Heptahelical receptors interact with heterotrimeric G proteins (α, $\beta\gamma$) to transduce the external signal of receptor activation to an internal signal. Once activated, both the α and $\beta\gamma$ subunit of the G protein stimulate effector molecules, which include phospholipase C-β1, adenylyl cyclase, ion channels, that lead to a biological response. For example, activation of the angiotensin AT_1 or endothelin ET_A receptor in arterial smooth muscle results in activation of phospholipase C-β1 through the G protein Gq. Phospholipase C hydrolyses phosphatidylinositol in the plasma membrane to release diacylglycerol and inositol (1,4,5) trisphosphate (IP3). Diacylglycerol activates classical

TABLE A28.1

NONTRADITIONAL VASOACTIVE PEPTIDES

Substance	Vessel	Contractile effect	Growth effect on arterial smooth muscle
Basic fibroblast growth factor	Coronary arterioles	Relaxation	+
		Endothelium-dependent	
Ceramide C2	Rat aorta	Relaxation	−
Epidermal growth factor	Rabbit and rat aorta	Contraction	+
Insulin	Coronary artery	Relaxation (complex)	+ (complex)
Insulin-like growth factor-I	Coronary artery	Relaxation	+
Interleukin-1β	Rat aorta	Relaxation, decrease of agonist contraction	+ (complex—acts synergistically with growth factors)
Interleukin-6	Rat aorta	Decreased PE contraction	+ (through stimulating PDGF)
	Rat aorta	Decreased heptahelical receptor–mediated contractions	
	Human artery	Contraction	
Parathyroid hormone–related protein	Rat mesenteric artery	Relaxation	
	Uterine artery		
Platelet-activating factor	Mesenteric veins	Contraction	+
Platelet-derived growth factor	Rat aorta	Contraction	+
	Rat mesangial cells	Contraction	+
Tumor necrosis factor α	Rat aorta	Decreased Ach relaxation/increase PE contraction	+ (complex)
	Mouse carotid artery	Relaxation	
	Human artery	Contraction	
Vascular endothelial growth factor	Coronary postcapillary venular endothelial cells	Relaxation	
	Rat aorta	Relaxation	
	Cavernous smooth muscle cells		+

+, increase; −, decrease; PE, α adrenergic agonist phenylephrine; Ach, muscarinic receptor agonist acetylcholine; PDGF, platelet-derived growth factor.

TABLE A28.2

HEPTAHELICAL RECEPTOR AGONISTS, CONTRACTILITY AND GROWTH

Substance	Artery/cell	Contractile effect	Growth effect on arterial smooth muscle
Adrenomedullin	Rat mesangial cells	Relaxation	−
Angiotensin II (*through* AT$_1$ receptor)	Multiple	Contraction	+
Atrial natriuretic peptide	Multiple	Relaxation	−
Bradykinin	Multiple	Relaxation/contraction	−
Endothelin-1 (through ET$_A$ receptor)	Multiple	Contraction	+
Norepinephrine	Multiple	Contraction	+
Serotonin	Multiple	Contraction	+
Thrombin	Multiple	Contraction/relaxation	+
Vasoactive intestinal polypeptide	Smooth muscle cells	Relaxation	−

forms of protein kinase C, whereas IP3 releases calcium (Ca^{2+}) from intracellular stores located in the sarcoplasmic reticulum. Both events—activation of protein kinase C and release of Ca^{2+}—promote smooth muscle contraction.

The literature is replete with reports of heptahelical receptor agonists affecting smooth muscle contraction. Associated effects of heptahelical receptor agonists on growth of smooth muscle was attributed in past decades to stimulation of phospholipase C through G proteins, but it is now clear that heptahelical receptors are directly linked to growth pathways triggered by growth factor receptors. In **Table A28.2**, a small number of these studies are reported and a general trend has emerged. First, agonists of heptahelical receptors that contract arterial smooth muscle typically stimulate smooth muscle cell growth. Conversely, agonists that relax smooth muscle inhibit growth of smooth muscle cells (**Table A28.2**). There are exceptions to this trend; a prime example is insulin, which causes an endothelium-dependent relaxation but can act as a smooth muscle cell mitogen.

Recent research suggests that activation of heptahelical receptors may lead to biological events that are not G protein-dependent, hence the use of the describer heptahelical. For example, a diverse group of heptahelical receptor agonists can activate the Erk-MAPK pathway. This occurs by a mechanism both dependent and independent of G protein stimulation. Agonists of heptahelical receptors can also activate the EGFR tyrosine kinase.

Mechanism of interaction with growth pathways

In the later half of the 1990s, it was demonstrated that several heptahelical receptor agonists activate the tyrosine kinase intrinsic to the EGFR ErbB1. This process, called *transactivation*, defines the complicated and no longer separate signal transduction of heptahelical and growth factor receptors. In vascular smooth muscle, angiotensin II, endothelin-1, thrombin, arachidonic acid activate the EGFR-mediated signaling and growth. EGFR transactivation can occur independently of EGF release but may also occur in a manner that depends upon local release of an EGF-like growth factor. Transactivation by heptahelical receptors has been described for the PDGF receptor as well. The role of transactivation in smooth muscle contraction is unclear. **Figure A28.1** depicts the cellular interaction of the two described signal transduction pathways—growth factor and heptahelical

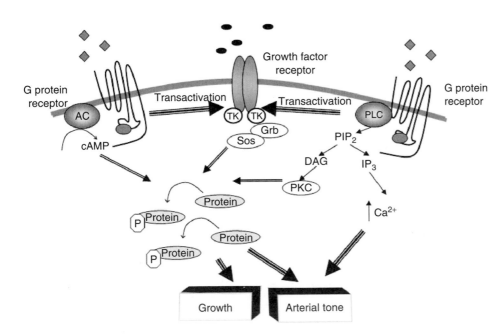

Figure A28.1 Depiction of interaction of the heptahelical G protein coupled and growth factor receptors in control of vascular tone and growth. TK, tyrosine kinase; AC, adenylyl cyclase; cAMP, cyclic adenosine monophosphate; Sos and Grb, scaffolding proteins; DAG, diacyl glycerol; PKC, protein kinase C; PLC, phospholipase C; P, phosphorylation.

receptors—as a demonstration of the significant overlap in these two systems.

Suggested Readings

Berk BC. Vascular smooth muscle growth: autocrine growth mechanisms. *Physiol Rev* 2001;81:999–1030.
Gerthoffer WT, Singer CA. Secretory functions of smooth muscle: cytokines and growth factors. *Mol Interv* 2002;2:447–456.
Hollenberg MD. Tyrosine kinase pathways and the regulation of smooth muscle contractility. *Trends Pharmacol Sci* 1994;15:108–114.

Marinissen MJ, Gutkind JS. G-protein coupled receptors and signaling networks: emerging paradigms. *Trends Pharmacol Sci* 2001;22:368–376.

Web Sites

G Proteins. http://www.gpcr.org functions in 2007.
Signal Transduction. http://stke.sciencemag.org 2007.
Signal Transduction. http://vlib.org/Science/Cell_Biology/signal_transduction.html 2007.
Signal Transduction. http://www.biocarta.com 2007.

CHAPTER A29 ■ PLASMINOGEN ACTIVATION AND THE RENIN-ANGIOTENSIN SYSTEM

DOUGLAS E. VAUGHAN, MD

KEY POINTS

■ The plasminogen activator (PA) (i.e., fibrinolytic) system is one of the endogenous defenses against intravascular thrombosis.
■ Activity of the fibrinolytic system is highly dependent on the balance between tissue-type plasminogen activation and plasminogen-activator inhibitor 1 (PAI-1).
■ Angiotensin and aldosterone play important roles in regulating vascular PAI-1 production, whereas bradykinin is an extremely potent stimulus of vascular tissue-type plasminogen activation release.
■ Angiotensin-converting enzyme (ACE) plays a critical role in regulating vascular fibrinolytic balance.

See also Chapters A15, A34, and A65

The renin-angiotensin-aldosterone system (RAAS) plays an integral role in cardiovascular homeostasis through its effects on vascular tone and volume; pharmacologic interruption of this system has found widespread clinical application. Independent of its effects on blood pressure (BP), RAAS activation may also be a risk factor for the development of ischemic heart disease, perhaps involving deleterious effects of the RAAS on the plasminogen activator (PA) system.

Fibrinolytic balance

The PA/plasmin (i.e., fibrinolytic) system serves as one of the endogenous defense mechanisms for the prevention of intravascular thrombosis. As such, it complements the effects of the protein anticoagulants (proteins C and S, antithrombin III, heparin cofactor II, etc.) and the short-acting, endothelial-derived platelet inhibitors [nitric oxide (NO) and prostacyclin].

The activity of the fibrinolytic system is ultimately dependent on generation of the protease plasmin, which is produced from its inactive precursor (plasminogen) by the action of PAs. In mammals, two PAs have been identified: tissue-type plasminogen activator (t-PA) and urokinase-type plasminogen activator (u-PA). Although both of these activators are synthesized in the endothelium, t-PA is felt to be the primary PA in plasma. Normally, there is an abundant supply of plasminogen in plasma that is available for activation and conversion to plasmin. However, little, if any, plasmin is produced because: (a) t-PA circulates in trace concentrations in plasma; (b) t-PA is a relatively inefficient PA in solution in the absence of fibrin; and (c) t-PA is inhibited by the presence of very specific and rapid acting, plasminogen-activator inhibitors (PAIs) that are also present in plasma. The most important inhibitor of t-PA in the blood is PAI-1.

Genetic expression of plasminogen-activator inhibitor 1

The gene for PAI-1 is located on human chromosome number 7, spans approximately 12 kilobases, and is composed of nine

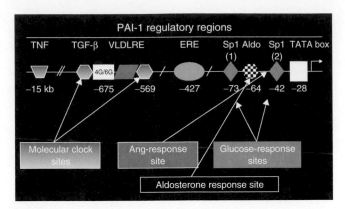

Figure A29.1 Schematic representation of the promoter region of PAI-1. RE, response element; TNF, tumor necrosis factor; TGF-β, transforming growth factor β; VLDL, very low-density lipoprotein; E, estrogen; Aldo, aldosterone.

introns and eight exons. Regulatory elements in the PAI-1 gene include AP-1 sites, a glucocorticoid response element (GRE, which also mediates the aldosterone response), a very low-density lipoprotein (VLDL) response site, and two Sp1 sites that appear to mediate glucose responsiveness. Recent studies have localized an angiotensin-responsive region that conforms with a methyl ethyl ketone (MEK) response element located between −89 and −50 in the promoter and requires Sp1 and AP-1 coactivation (**Figure A29.1**).

Physiology and regulation of plasminogen-activator inhibitor 1

PAI-1 is readily detectable in plasma samples, and mean PAI-1 antigen levels in healthy adults vary between 15 and 30 ng/mL. Plasma PAI-1 levels correlate with systolic BP in healthy middle-aged men and women. Older populations tend to have higher PAI-1 levels and mean PAI-1 antigen levels of 50 to 60 ng/mL are not uncommon in middle-aged male subjects.

Sources and interactions. Plasma PAI-1 is derived from several sources, including the vascular endothelium, adipose tissue, and liver. Platelets store large quantities of PAI-1 that are secreted following platelet aggregation. Endothelial cells in culture synthesize PAI-1 at relatively high rates, although it is not clear that this is true *in vivo.* Several different fates are possible for PAI-1 after it is synthesized and secreted. Because PAI-1 concentrations exceed t-PA by a 4:1 ratio on a molar basis, most PAI-1 likely circulates briefly in plasma before it is removed through hepatic clearance. Because the circulating half-life of PAI-1 is approximately 5 minutes, only a fraction of the secreted active PAI-1 has the opportunity to react with plasma t-PA to form inert covalent complexes. This suggests that PAI-1 may serve other functions as well. There appears to be no endogenous mechanism for recycling PA–PAI-1 complexes, which are cleared through the low-density lipoprotein-related (LRP) receptor and the VLDL receptor.

Vitronectin. PAI-1 is present in the extracellular matrix of blood vessels, where it associates with vitronectin. Tissue PAI-1 is derived from adjacent endothelium, vascular smooth muscle cells (VSMC), and monocytes, and is frequently found to accumulate in areas of inflammation. The relative abundance of vitronectin in the subendothelial matrix provides a mechanism for preserving PAI-1 activity. It is likely that vitronectin-bound PAI-1 represents the

physiologically relevant form of the inhibitor in the extracellular matrix that blocks engagement of specific integrin receptors and thereby impairs cellular migration.

Plasminogen-activator inhibitor 1 stimulants. Several diverse agents stimulate endothelial PAI-1 production. PAI-1 is an acute phase reactant and inflammatory cytokines such as interleukin 1 (IL-1) and tumor necrosis factor α (TNF-α) induce PAI-1 production and promote vascular inflammation and atherosclerosis. Growth factors and hormones that regulate PAI-1 production include transforming growth factor β (TGF-β), epidermal growth factor (EGF), thrombin, insulin, angiotensin II (Ang II), Ang IV, and aldosterone.

Diurnal variation. There is a well-recognized circadian variation in plasma PAI-1; this fluctuation in PAI-1 activity is responsible for the diurnal variation in net fibrinolytic activity. PAI-1 levels peak in the early morning and correspond with a nadir in net fibrinolytic activity, whereas the afternoon fall in plasma PAI-1 facilitates a peak in endogenous fibrinolysis. These diurnal fluctuations may have important clinical consequences, as the morning peak in PAI-1 corresponds with the circadian peak in sympathetic and RAAS activity and with a higher incidence of acute myocardial infarction (MI) and stroke.

Renin-angiotensin-aldosterone system activation. Studies from this laboratory indicate that activation of the RAAS prolongs and exaggerates the morning peak in PAI-1. In salt-depleted, healthy human subjects and in hypertensive subjects treated with hydrochlorothiazide, there is a correlation between serum aldosterone and plasma PAI-1 levels; treatment with spironolactone abolishes this correlation. Furthermore, it may be more than coincidence that the efficiency of t-PA in therapeutic thrombolysis appears to be reduced during early morning hours, when PAI-1 levels are at their highest. The basic mechanisms that are responsible for this diurnal regulation of PAI-1 are poorly understood, although recently it has been reported that transcription factors involved in peripheral circadian gene expression regulate PAI-1 promoter activity *in vitro.*

Renin-angiotensin-aldosterone system—plasminogen-activator inhibitor 1 interactions

As illustrated in **Figure A29.2**, angiotensin-converting enzyme (ACE) is strategically located to play a crucial role in regulating the interaction between the RAAS and fibrinolysis. In addition to catalyzing the activation of Ang II, ACE is also responsible for

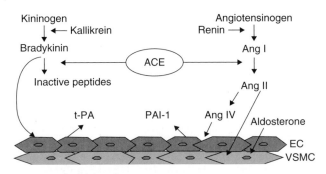

Figure A29.2 The dual functional roles of ACE and the strategic location of ACE in regulating vascular fibrinolytic balance. ACE, angiotensin-converting enzyme; t-PA, tissue-type plasminogen activator; PAI, plasminogen-activator inhibitors; Ang, angiotensin; VSMC, vascular smooth muscle cells; EC, endothelial cell.

the rapid degradation of bradykinin. ACE inhibitors potentiate the hemodynamic effects of exogenous bradykinin, whereas endogenous bradykinin contributes to the acute hypotensive effects of ACE inhibition. Importantly, bradykinin is one of the most potent stimuli for the release of t-PA in animals. Whereas systemic infusion of bradykinin induces a moderate (fourfold) increase in plasma t-PA levels, local infusions of bradykinin into humans stimulate the acute release of t-PA, yielding a >50-fold increase across the vascular bed through a B_2 receptor dependent, prostacyclin- and NO-independent mechanism. Arterial t-PA is augmented by the administration of ACE inhibitors but not angiotensin-receptor blockers.

Plasminogen-activator inhibitor 1 and human disease

Ischemic cardiovascular disease.
There is substantial experimental and epidemiologic evidence that PAI-1 may contribute to the development of ischemic cardiovascular disease. PAI-1 excess has been identified in youthful survivors of acute MI and plasma PAI-1 activity is increased in MI survivors who have recurrent MI. A large prospective, nested, case–control study identified a strong association between elevated plasma levels of PAI-1 (antigen and activity) and increased risk of MI in middle-aged men and women, independent of other conventional risk factors. Low plasma fibrinolytic activity, which likely reflects increased PAI-1 activity, appears to be a leading determinant of risk for ischemic heart disease in younger men.

Epidemiologic links are probably more than just casual associations because transgenic mice, that overexpress a stable form of human PAI-1 in response to murine pre-proendothelin promoter, and develop spontaneous macrovascular coronary thrombosis and MI. This mouse model is unique because it develops occlusive coronary disease following a single gene manipulation. Plasminogen-deficient and combined t-PA/u-PA-deficient mice express a phenotype that is characterized by impaired wound healing and reduced thrombolytic capacity but not occlusive coronary disease.

There is a growing body of evidence that therapeutic interruption of the RAAS impacts on vascular fibrinolytic balance in clinical populations. In the Healing and Early Afterload Reducing Therapy (HEART) study, the effects of ramipril (10 mg) on plasma t-PA and PAI-1 were studied in 120 subjects in a randomized, double-blind, placebo-controlled trial of survivors of an anterior MI; ramipril reduced plasma PAI-1 levels by >40% during the post-MI phase.

Hypertension and arteriosclerosis.
PAI-1 also appears to play a role in hypertension and arteriosclerosis. Long-term inhibition of nitric oxide synthase (NOS) induces hypertension and perivascular fibrosis in experimental animals and has also been found to induce expression of PAI-1 in vascular tissues and that ACE inhibition prevents vascular PAI-1 accumulation in this model. In response to long-term NOS inhibition by N^{ω}-nitro-L-arginine methyl ester (L-NAME) in PAI-1—deficient (PAI-1$^{-/-}$) and wild-type (WT) male mice, systolic BP increased (to 141 $\pm$ 3 mm Hg) in WT animals (vs. 112 $\pm$ 4 mm Hg in PAI-1$^{-/-}$ mice,

p <0.0001). The extent of coronary perivascular fibrosis also increased significantly in L-NAME–treated WT mice (p <0.01 vs. PAI-1$^{-/-}$ mice). These findings suggest that PAI-1 deficiency is sufficient to protect against the structural vascular changes that accompany hypertension in the setting of long-term NOS inhibition and that direct inhibition of vascular PAI-1 activity may provide a new therapeutic strategy for the prevention of arteriosclerotic cardiovascular disease.

Diabetes.
Plasma PAI-1 levels are increased in individuals with obesity, insulin resistance and type 2 diabetes mellitus. Recently, two large epidemiologic studies identified PAI-1 as one of the most robust nonmetabolic predictors of the development of type 2 diabetes. Numerous factors may contribute to the increases in PAI-1 associated with insulin resistance, including hyperglycemia and inflammation, and RAAS activation. ACE inhibition reduces PAI-1 levels in patients with obesity and insulin resistance.

Atherosclerosis.
RAAS activation is believed by some investigators to promote the development of atherosclerosis and ischemic cardiovascular disease independent of its effects on BP. Some of the most striking data comes from recent experimental studies demonstrating a remarkable acceleration in the development of atherosclerosis in ApoE$^{-/-}$ mice that receive chronic infusions of Ang II. ACE inhibitor therapy has not been definitively shown to reduce the progression of atherosclerotic lesions in humans but does reduce the incidence of cardiovascular death and MI by >20% in high-risk subjects.

Suggested Readings

Brown NJ, Kim KS, Chen YQ, et al. Synergistic effect of adrenal steroids and angiotensin II on plasminogen activator inhibitor-1 production. *J Clin Endocrinol Metab* 2000;85(1):336–344.

Brown NJ, Kumar S, Painter CA, et al. ACE inhibition versus angiotensin type 1 receptor antagonism: differential effects on PAI-1 over time. *Hypertension* 2002;40(6):859–865.

Festa A, D'Agostino R Jr, Tracy RP, et al. Elevated levels of acute-phase proteins and plasminogen activator inhibitor-1 predict the development of type 2 diabetes: the insulin resistance atherosclerosis study. *Diabetes* 2002;51(4):1131–1137.

Hou B, Eren M, Painter CA, et al. Tumor necrosis factor alpha activates the human plasminogen activator inhibitor-1 gene through a distal nuclear factor kappaB site. *J Biol Chem* 2004;279(18):18127–18136.

Kaikita K, Fogo A.B, Ma L, et al. Plasminogen activator inhibitor-1 deficiency prevents hypertension and vascular fibrosis in response to long-term nitric oxide synthase inhibition. *Circulation* 2001;104(7):839–844.

Kerins DM, Hao Q, Vaughan DE. Angiotensin induction of PAI-1 expression in endothelial cells is mediated by the hexapeptide angiotensin IV. *J Clin Invest* 1995;96(5):2515–2520.

Rosenberg RD, Aird WC. Vascular-bed--specific hemostasis and hypercoagulable states. *N Engl J Med* 1999;340(20):1555–1564.

Sawathiparnich P, Kumar S, Vaughan DE, et al. Spironolactone abolishes the relationship between aldosterone and plasminogen activator inhibitor-1 in humans. *J Clin Endocrinol Metab* 2002;87(2):448–452.

Stefansson S, Lawrence DA. The serpin PAI-1 inhibits cell migration by blocking integrin alpha V beta3 binding to vitronectin. *Nature* 1996;383(6599):441–443.

Thogersen AM, Jansson JH, Boman K, et al. High plasminogen activator inhibitor and tissue plasminogen activator levels in plasma precede a first acute myocardial infarction in both men and women: evidence for the fibrinolytic system as an independent primary risk factor. *Circulation* 1998;98(21):2241–2247.

Vaughan DE, Rouleau J-L, Ridker PM, et al. Effects of ramipril on plasma fibrinolytic balance in patients with acute anterior myocardial infarction. *Circulation* 1997;96:442–447.

Van Guilder GP, Hoetzler GL, Smith DT, et al. Endothelial t-PA release is impaired in overweight and obese adults but can be improved with regular aerobic exercise. *Am J Physiol Endocrinol Metab* 2005;289(5):E807–E813.

CHAPTER A30 ■ PROSTAGLANDINS AND P450 METABOLITES

ALBERTO NASJLETTI, MD AND JOHN C. MCGIFF, MD

KEY POINTS

■ Prostaglandins and other eicosanoids are produced from arachidonic acid (AA) by the action of tissue cyclooxygenases (COXs), cytochromes, and lipoxygenases.

■ Prostacyclin (prostaglandin I_2) and prostaglandin E_2 are vasodilators that counteract the pressor effects of norepinephrine and angiotensin II and stimulate diuresis and natriuresis.

■ Thromboxane A_2, prostaglandin H_2, and prostaglandin F_2 are vasoconstrictors that blunt renal salt excretion.

■ 20-Hydroxyeicosatetraenoic produced by cytochrome P450 (CYP) 4A enzymes has vasoconstrictor activity and exhibits complex effects on salt and water excretion.

See also Chapters A9, **A31, A49,** and **C144**

Arachidonic acid (AA) is liberated from tissue phospholipids by hormone-regulated phospholipases (**Figure A30.1**). Once free, AA is processed by cyclooxygenases (COXs), cytochrome (CYP450) P450 oxygenases, or lipoxygenases to form an abundance of eicosanoids capable of affecting a variety of vascular and renal functions.

CYCLOOXYGENASE-DERIVED EICOSANOIDS

Synthesis

The constitutive form of COX-1, is expressed in most tissues, including blood vessels, kidney, and platelets. The inducible form, COX-2, is usually undetectable but can be expressed in response to cytokines and growth factors. COXs catalyze the metabolism of AA to the endoperoxide prostaglandin H_2 (PGH_2), which is subsequently converted to thromboxane A_2 (TxA_2) by thromboxane synthase, to prostaglandin I_2 (PGI_2, or prostacyclin) by prostacyclin synthase, or to prostaglandins E_2 (PGE_2), D_2, or $F_2\alpha$ by specific isomerases (**Figure A30.1**).

Vasodilator prostaglandins

The prostaglandins PGE_2 and PGI_2 dilate resistance vessels, reduce release of norepinephrine from sympathetic nerves, attenuate the vasoconstrictor responses to angiotensin II and other constrictor hormones, and facilitate renal excretion of salt and water.

The vasodilatory action of PGE_2 is linked to activation of EP_2 and EP_4, which are distinct G protein–coupled receptors. Mice lacking EP_2 receptors develop hypertension when placed on a high salt diet, implying that the actions of PGE_2 on this receptor serve an antihypertensive function. Inhibition of COX augments vascular resistance, increases vascular responsiveness to angiotensin II and other constrictor hormones, increases antidiuretic responsiveness to vasopressin, and blunts the pressure–natriuresis response.

Collectively, these observations support the concept that PGE_2 and PGI_2 serve as counterregulatory influences to pressor mechanisms mediated by the renin-angiotensin system, the sympathetic nervous system, and vasopressin. Conversely, PGE_2 and PGI_2 stimulate renin secretion, and COX inhibitors reduce plasma renin activity.

Vasoconstrictor eicosanoids

TxA_2 and its immediate precursor, PGH_2, stimulate contraction of vascular smooth muscle directly through activation of shared receptors and indirectly by enhancing sympathetic nervous activity. In the kidney, activation of TxA_2/PGH_2 receptors results in renal vasoconstriction as well as salt and water retention. PGH_2 may mediate endothelium-dependent vasoconstriction.

Long-term systemic infusion of a synthetic agonist for TxA_2/PGH_2 receptors produces sustained elevation of blood pressure (BP), part of which is attributable to activation of central pressor mechanisms. Treatment with inhibitors of thromboxane synthase lowers BP in high renin models of experimental hypertension in rats.

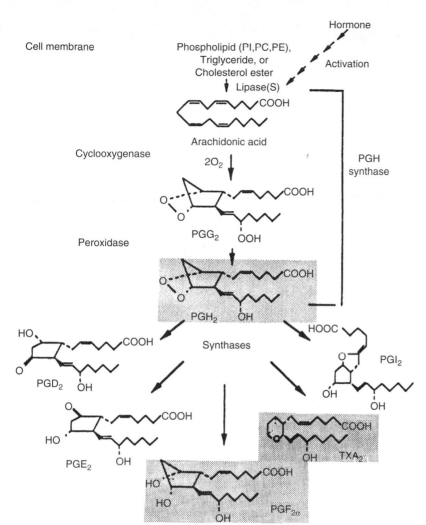

Figure A30.1 Formation of prostaglandins by the cyclooxygenase pathway. Shading indicates prostanoids that are prohypertensive. PGD_2, prostaglandin D_2; PGE_2, prostaglandin E; $PGF_{2\alpha}$, prostaglandin $F_{2\alpha}$; PGG_2, prostaglandin G_2; PGH_2, prostaglandin H_2; PGI_2, prostaglandin I_2; TXA_2, thromboxane A_2. (Reproduced from Smith WL. Prostanoid biosynthesis and mechanisms of action. *Am J Physiol* 1992;263:F181–F191, with permission.)

Blood pressure responses to cyclooxygenase inhibition

BP can increase, decrease, or remain unaffected during treatment with COX inhibitors. This variability in BP response is not unexpected, because COX-derived eicosanoids subserve vasodilatory and vasoconstrictive functions. In general, COX inhibitors have little effect on BP in healthy subjects but are likely to increase BP in patients with salt-sensitive hypertension, such as in the case of the elderly or diabetic patient with hypertension. On the other hand, COX inhibitors can decrease BP in normotensive and hypertensive conditions in which the renin-angiotensin system is stimulated, presumably by disrupting prostanoid-mediated renin secretion and vasoconstrictor mechanisms. The net BP response to inhibition of COX thereby seems to reflect the sum of alterations in BP regulatory mechanisms involving a prostaglandin component.

CYTOCHROME P450—DERIVED EICOSANOIDS

The wide distribution of the CYP monooxygenases in the vasculature and transporting epithelia and the diverse circulatory and renal effects of CYP-derived AA products suggest their possible participation in BP regulation.

Synthesis

CYP catalyzes transformation of AA by three types of oxidative reactions.

Epoxidation. Epoxidation of AA forms four epoxyeicosatrienoic acids (EETs) (**Figure A30.2**), characterized by the position of the epoxide oxygen (5,6-, 8,9-, 11,12-, or 14,15-EET), which are readily degraded by epoxide hydrolases (**Figure A30.2**). The 5,6- and 11,12-EETs are the most important, having the greatest vascular smooth muscle relaxing activity. The 5,6-EET can be further metabolized by COX to a bioactive product (**Figure A30.2**). Endothelial cells manufacture EETs, which stimulate calcium-activated potassium channels in vascular smooth muscle, producing hyperpolarization and vasodilation. Endothelium-derived EETs mediate the nitric oxide–independent action of bradykinin and other vasodilators and attenuate the vasoconstrictor action of angiotensin II.

Dietary salt loading upregulates EET production in the kidney. EETs subserve antihypertensive functions, because inhibitors of EET synthesis increase BP in tandem with heightening vasoconstrictor responsiveness to pressor hormones. Interference with the degradation of EETs lowers BP and vasoconstrictor responsiveness.

Allylic oxidation. Allylic oxidation of AA forms hydroxyeicosatetraenoic acids (HETEs), one of which, 12(R)-HETE, is a potent inhibitor of sodium- and potassium-activated adenosine

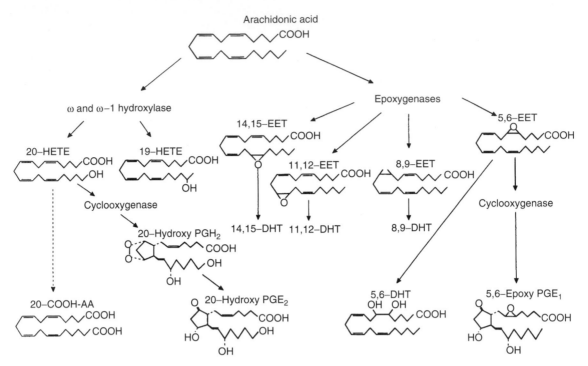

Figure A30.2 Pathways of arachidonic acid (AA) metabolism catalyzed by cytochrome P450 enzymes. 20-Hydroxyeicosatetraenoic acid (HETE) and 5,6-epoxyeicosatrienoic acid (EET) can be metabolized through cyclooxygenase to 5,6-EET and 20-COOH-AA prostaglandin analogs as shown. DHT, dihydroxyeicosatrienoic acid; PGH_2, prostaglandin H_2; PGE_1, prostaglandin E_1; PGE_2, prostaglandin E_2.

triphosphatase and exists in high levels in the vasculature in response to ischemic insults.

Hydroxylation. ω-Hydroxylation of AA by CYP oxygenases of the 4A family yields 20-HETE (**Figure A30.2**), which exhibits several properties that may affect BP. For example, 20-HETE inhibits the activity of calcium (Ca^{2+})-activated potassium channels in vascular smooth muscle, which promotes accumulation of Ca^{2+} in the cytosol, and leads to vasoconstriction. This action of 20-HETE is central to its ability to sensitize the vasculature to vasoconstrictor hormones and other constrictor stimuli. 20-HETE has been shown to have a role in the pathogenesis of salt-sensitive forms of essential hypertension.

20-hydroxyeicosatetraenoic acid

Regulation and effects. 20-HETE contributes to the mechanisms underlying preglomerular renal vasoconstriction in response to elevation of renal perfusion pressure and activation of the tubuloglomerular feedback mechanism. 20-HETE also inhibits sodium reabsorption in the proximal tubule and in the medullary thick ascending limb of the loop (mTAL) of Henle, which are actions attributable to inhibition of sodium- and potassium-activated adenosine triphosphatase and of the Na^+–K^+–$2Cl^-$ cotransporter, respectively. Accordingly, 20-HETE produced by arterial vessels may mediate prohypertensive functions by fostering vasoconstriction at renal and extrarenal sites. Conversely, 20-HETE produced by renal tubular structures may mediate antihypertensive functions by promoting sodium excretion as well as in playing a role in the pressure–natriuresis response. Another product of AA metabolism by CYP, 19-HETE, may also contribute to BP regulation, as it was shown to antagonize the vascular actions of 20-HETE.

Cytochrome P450 isoform regulation. The multiplicity of CYPs metabolizing AA is complicated further by the diversity of mechanisms by which the isoforms are regulated. The rat renal CYP 4A isoforms (4A1, 2, 3, and 8), which generate 20-HETE, may exhibit antihypertensive or prohypertensive properties, based on differential distribution of the 4A isoforms among tubular segments and vasculature of the kidney. 20-HETE constricts preglomerular arterioles and also modulates ion movement in the mTAL, each site presumably served by a different cohydroxylase isoform that is subject to different regulatory factors.

Renal effects. Increased Cl^- transport in the mTAL is critical to BP elevation in the Dahl salt-sensitive rat and is attributable to deficient production of 20-HETE, which reduces the activity of the Na^+–K^+–$2Cl^-$ cotransporter responsible for Cl^- reabsorption. In agreement with this concept, induction of CYP4A ω-hydroxylase with clofibrate normalizes BP in the Dahl salt-sensitive rat. Conversely, in the spontaneously hypertensive rat, 20-HETE production at renal and vascular sites is increased and may contribute to the hypertension. For example, 20-HETE produced in preglomerular vessels may elevate BP by promoting renal vasoconstriction, which reduces the glomerular filtration rate and facilitates salt and water reabsorption by decreasing renal interstitial pressure. Supporting this idea, BP in spontaneously hypertensive rats was decreased by interventions that decrease 20-HETE synthesis. 20-HETE also acts as a second messenger for the renal tubular and vascular actions of endothelins. The dependence of the renal functional effects of endothelins on generation of 20-HETE was shown in the deoxycorticosterone acetate/salt-induced hypertension model in rats. The appearance of severe renal injury and rapid elevation of BP coincided with increased production of endothelins and 20-HETE. The pressor response and proteinuria were markedly attenuated by inhibition of CYP450 metabolism of AA.

Suggested Readings

Breyer MD, Jacobson HR, Breyer RM. Functional and molecular aspects of renal prostaglandin receptors. *J Am Soc Nephrol* 1996;7:8–17.

Keen HL, Brands MW, Smith MJ Jr, et al. Thromboxane is required for full expression of angiotensin hypertension in rats. *Hypertension* 1997;29:310–314.

Makita K, Takahashi K, Karara A, et al. Experimental and/or genetically controlled alterations of the renal microsomal cytochrome P450 epoxygenase induce hypertension in rats fed a high salt diet. *J Clin Invest* 1994;94:2414–2420.

Nasjletti A, Arthur C. Corcoran memorial lecture: the role of eicosanoids in angiotensin-dependent hypertension. *Hypertension* 1997;31:194–200.

Omata K, Abraham NG, Schwartzman ML. Renal cytochrome P450-arachidonic acid metabolism: localization and hormonal regulation in SHR. *Am J Physiol* 1992;262:F591–F599.

Oyekan AO, McGiff JC. Cytochrome P450-derived eicosanoids participate in the renal functional effects of ET-1 in the anesthetized rat. *Am J Physiol* 1998;274:R52–R61.

Quilley J, Bell-Quilley CP, McGiff JC. *Hypertension: pathophysiology, diagnosis, and management*. New York:Raven Press, 1995.

Roman RJ. P450 metabolites of arachidonic acid in the control of cardiovascular function. *Physiol Rev* 2002;82:131–186.

Sacerdoti D, Escalante B, Abraham NG, et al. Treatment with tin prevents the development of hypertension in spontaneously hypertensive rats. *Science* 1989;243:388–390.

CHAPTER A31 ■ LIPOXYGENASE PRODUCTS

MICHAEL D. WILLIAMS, MD AND JERRY L. NADLER, MD

KEY POINTS

■ Arachidonic acid is oxidized by lipoxygenase (LO) enzymes to form eicosanoid molecules such as leukotrienes and hydroxyeicosatetraenoic acids (HETEs).

■ LO-derived eicosanoids may affect endothelial function, vascular smooth muscle contraction and growth, aldosterone secretion, cytokine release and inflammation, and oxidation of low-density lipoproteins.

■ Current evidence supports a role for 5-, 12-, and 15-LO pathway activation in the pathogenesis of inflammation that may lead to atherosclerosis.

■ Antagonists of 5-LO and leukotriene action are in clinical use but no inhibitors of 12- or 15-LO are currently available.

See also Chapters A9, **A30,** and C144

Eicosanoid synthesis

The term *eicosanoids* refers to a group of biologically active lipids formed by the oxidation of 20-carbon fatty acids. Arachidonic acid is the primary fatty acid involved in eicosanoid synthesis and is a precursor for several classes of eicosanoid molecules that play important roles in inflammation and vascular function. Free arachidonic acid is released from cell membrane phospholipids by phospholipases, which can be activated by the binding to cell-surface receptors of inflammatory cytokines, vasoactive peptides, and growth factors.

The metabolism of arachidonic acid into eicosanoids is mediated by three major oxidative pathways, as depicted in **Figure A31.1.** The cyclooxygenase (COX) pathway, which is inhibited by aspirin and other nonsteroidal antiinflammatory drugs (NSAIDs), converts arachidonic acid to prostaglandins. The cytochrome P-450 pathway forms epoxides, which have potent vasoconstrictive or vasodilatory properties, particularly in the renal vasculature. Other chapters will discuss the COX and cytochrome P-450 pathways in further detail. This chapter will focus on the lipoxygenase (LO) pathway, which involves a group of nonheme iron-containing oxidase enzymes known as *lipoxygenases*. LO enzymes metabolize arachidonic acid into hydroxyeicosatetraenoic acids (HETEs) and leukotrienes. LOs are classified as 5-, 12-, or 15-LO based on their ability to insert molecular oxygen at the corresponding carbon position of arachidonic acid.

Mechanisms of action

Possible mechanisms through which LO products produce their inflammatory effects include increased intracellular free calcium levels and activation of protein kinase C. Products of 12- and 15-LO, particularly 12(S)-HETE and 15(S)-HETE, activate mitogen-activated protein (MAP) kinase, stress-activated kinases, and proinflammatory transcription factors, which suggests a role for these molecules in cell proliferation and inflammation. It has recently been proposed that 12- and 15-LO may be important for generating the inflammatory cytokine interleukin 12 (IL-12). IL-12 and its downstream transcription factor STAT-4 (signal transducer and activator of transcription) promote development of T_H1 cells and induction of genes involved in inflammation and

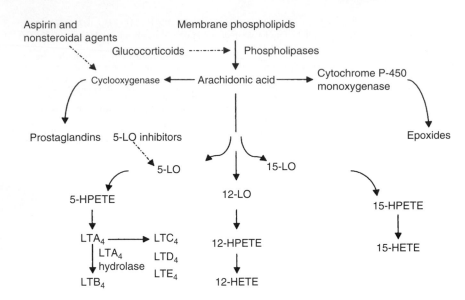

Figure A31.1 Pathways of arachidonic acid metabolism. Broken line illustrates possible areas for inhibition. LO, lipoxygenase; HPETE, hydroperoxyeicosatetraenoic acid; LTA_4, leukotriene A_4; LTB_4, leukotriene B_4; LTC_4, leukotriene C_4; LTD_4, leukotriene D4; LTE_4, leukotriene E_4; HETE, hydroxyeicosatetraenoic acid.

endothelial dysfunction. Some of the potential biologic effects of 12- and 15-LO products are outlined in **Table A31.1**.

Inhibition of arachidonic acid metabolism

Antiinflammatory agents are used clinically to block various pathways of arachidonic acid metabolism. For example, glucocorticoids inhibit phospholipase activity and prevent the release of arachidonic acid from cell membrane phospholipids. Aspirin and other NSAIDs inhibit COX and the production of prostaglandins. COX-2 selective antiinflammatory agents specifically block the action of the COX-2 cyclooxygenase enzyme primarily in inflammatory cells, which mediates response to tissue injury.

There are several antagonists of LO enzyme activity available for clinical use, primarily used in the treatment of asthma. Zileuton, for example, inhibits the 5-LO pathway and blocks the synthesis of leukotrienes. Zafirlukast and montelukast do not affect 5-LO directly, but block the activity of leukotriene D_4 at its receptor. No inhibitors of the 12- or 15-LO enzyme pathways are currently available for clinical use.

Leukotrienes

The generation of leukotrienes from arachidonic acid through the 5-LO pathway contributes to a variety of inflammatory processes

and is also thought to play a role in vascular pathology. 5-LO is present in inflammatory cells including neutrophils, eosinophils, macrophages, and mast cells. Activation of these cells leads to translocation of 5-LO to cell membranes, where arachidonic acid is presented by 5-lipoxygenase activating protein (FLAP). 5-LO then catalyzes the conversion of arachidonic acid first into 5-hydroperoxyeicosatetraenoic acid (5-HPETE) and then into leukotriene A_4 (LTA_4). LTA_4 can then be converted by LTA_4 hydrolase into leukotriene B_4 (LTB_4), which has potent chemoattractant properties and increases binding of inflammatory cells to vessel walls. Alternatively, LTA_4 can be converted to leukotriene C_4 (LTC_4) by LTC_4 synthase and subsequently cleaved into leukotriene D_4 (LTD_4) or leukotriene E_4 (LTE_4). These three leukotrienes, formerly known as the *slow-reacting substance of anaphylaxis*, have potent vasoconstrictive properties and also cause increased microvascular permeability.

5-LO is also present in the endothelium, and in that setting converts arachidonic acid primarily into 5-HETE. Vascular endothelial and smooth muscle cells have very limited capacity to produce leukotrienes, but they may mediate the conversion of intermediate products into leukotrienes under certain conditions.

New research has shown a positive association between genetic variants of FLAP, 5-LO, and LTA_4 hydrolase and risk for cardiovascular disease. Further ongoing studies will address the potential to prevent myocardial infarction (MI) or stroke with inhibitors of one or more of these pathways.

Hydroperoxides and hydroxyeicosatetraenoic acids

Activity of 12- and 15-LO has been demonstrated in several vascular tissues and cells including endothelial cells, monocytes, vascular smooth muscle cells, aorta, and coronary arteries. New studies in insulin-resistant animal models suggest that 12-LO expression is markedly increased in visceral fat cells. These LO pathways first convert arachidonic acid into unstable hydroperoxides or hydroperoxyeicosatetraenoic acids (HPETEs). HPETE molecules are subsequently metabolized into a variety of products, including the more stable 12(S)- and 15(S)-HETE as shown in **Figure A31.1**. In addition to its recognized presence in vasculature, 12-HETE can be produced by platelets, adrenal glomerulosa cells, pancreatic β

TABLE A31.1

POTENTIAL ROLES OF THE 12- AND 15-LIPOXYGENASE PATHWAYS IN CARDIOVASCULAR DISORDERS

Induction of proinflammatory cytokine expression in macrophages
Mediation of angiotensin II action on blood vessels and adrenal glomerulosa (particularly 12-lipoxygenase pathway)
Inhibition of prostacyclin synthesis
Direct vasoconstriction of certain vascular beds
Growth-promoting effect on vascular smooth muscle cells
Oxidative modification of low-density lipoprotein
Promotion of monocyte binding to human endothelium
Progression of atherosclerosis

cells, and mesangial and glomerular cells within the renal cortex. 15-HETE can also be formed by monocytes under the influence of IL-4 and IL-13. 12-LO expression and activity in various tissues is stimulated by the presence of growth factors such as angiotensin II and platelet-derived growth factor, and inflammatory cytokines such as IL-1β.

Lipoxins

Lipoxins are a group of antiinflammatory eicosanoids produced by the transcellular metabolism of arachidonic acid. These molecules can be formed from 15(S)-HPETE or 15(S)-HETE by the action of 5-LO, or from leukotriene A$_4$ through 12- or 15-LO. Aspirin-triggered lipoxins can also be formed by the reaction of aspirin with COX-2 followed by 5-LO.

Lipoxins appear to counteract the inflammatory effects of leukotrienes, thereby providing a negative feedback mechanism through which inflammatory cascade activation may be stopped. These molecules have several beneficial effects. For example, lipoxin A$_4$ inhibits the leukotriene-induced chemotaxis, attachment, and transendothelial migration of neutrophils. It also limits changes in vascular permeability and suppresses leukotriene-related smooth muscle contraction. Some lipoxins also have the capacity to reduce endothelial cell migration and angiogenesis. Very exciting recent studies have shown that omega-3 fatty acids can form new families of antiinflammatory lipids termed *resolvins* and *protectins*.

Lipoxygenase activity and atherosclerosis

In addition to the role of the 5-LO pathway, emerging evidence suggests that the activity of 12- and 15 LO and their products are important in the pathogenesis of atherosclerotic cardiovascular disease. The 15-LO enzyme is found in macrophage-rich atherosclerotic areas of blood vessel walls, suggesting a function in atherogenesis. A very recent study found markedly increased 12- and 15-LO expression in the carotid arteries of obese, insulin-resistant Zucker rats compared to lean controls. Low-density lipoprotein receptor (LDL-R)–deficient and apolipoprotein E (apo-E)–deficient mice that also underexpress 12- and 15-LO show considerably fewer and smaller atherosclerotic lesions than do LDL-R or apo-E–deficient mice with normal LO expression after several weeks of feeding with a high-fat diet. In addition, mice bred to overexpress 12- and 15-LO demonstrate increased monocyte binding to endothelial cells and early development of atherosclerotic lesions compared to wild-type mice. Treatment of porcine vascular smooth muscle cells with 12(S)-HETE leads to smooth muscle cell hypertrophy and increased production of matrix proteins, two factors that are important in the pathogenesis of vascular disease. New studies also indicate that products of the 12-LO pathway induce the expression of highly proinflammatory cytokines and chemokines such as tumor necrosis factor, IL-1 and IL-12, and monocyte chemoattractant protein. These findings suggest potential for specific targeted therapy against certain LO enzymes in the prevention and treatment of atherosclerosis.

Suggested Readings

Dwyer JH, Allayee H, Dwyer KM, et al. Arachidonate 5-lipoxygenase promoter genotype, dietary arachidonic acid, and atherosclerosis. *N Engl J Med* 2004;350(1):29–37.Jan 1;

George J, Afek A, Shaish A, et al. 12/15-lipoxygenase gene disruption attenuates atherogenesis in ldl receptor-deficient mice. *Circulation* 2001;104:1646–1650.

Helgadottir A, Mandescu A, Helgason A, et al. A variant of the gene encoding leukotriene A4 hydrolase confers ethnicity-specific risk of myocardial infarction. *Nat Genet* 2006;38(1):68–74.Jan;

Huo Y, Zhao L, Hyman MC, et al. Critical role of macrophage 12/15-lipoxygenase for atherosclerosis in apolipoprotein E-deficient mice. *Circulation* 2004;110:2024–2031.

Lewis RA, Austen KF, Soberman RJ. Leukotrienes and other products of the 5-lipoxygenase pathway. Biochemistry and relation to pathobiology in human diseases. *N Engl J Med* 1990;323(10):645–655.Sep 6;

Lotzer K, Funk CD, Habenicht AJ. The 5-lipoxygenase pathway in arterial wall biology and atherosclerosis. *Biochim Biophys Acta* 2005;1736(1):30–37.

Natarajan R, Nadler JL. Lipid inflammatory mediators in diabetic vascular disease. *Arterioscler Thromb Vasc Biol* 2004;24:1542–1548.

Pei H, Gu J, Thimmalapura PR, et al. Activation of the 12-lipoxygenase and signal transducer and activator of transcription pathway during neointima formation in a model of the metabolic syndrome. *Am J Physiol Endocrinol Metab* 2006;290:E92–102.

Reilly KB, Srinivasan S, Hatley ME, et al. 12/15-lipoxygenase activity mediates inflammatory monocyte/endothelial interactions and atherosclerosis *in vivo*. *J Biol Chem* 2004;279:9440–9450.

Serhan CN. Resolution phases of inflammation: novel endogenous anti-inflammatory and proresolving lipid mediators and pathways. *Annu Rev Immunol* 2007;25:101–137.

Zhao L, Funk CD. Lipoxygenase pathways in atherogenesis. *Trends Cardiovasc Med* 2004;14:191–195.

CHAPTER A32 ■ PEROXISOME PROLIFERATOR–ACTIVATED RECEPTORS

SANJEEV A. FRANCIS, MD AND JORGE PLUTZKY, MD

KEY POINTS

- Peroxisome proliferator–activated receptors (PPARs) are ligand-activated nuclear transcription factors of three known isotypes (α, γ, and δ) that regulate genes for lipid metabolism, adipogenesis, insulin sensitivity, and inflammation.
- Very low-density lipoprotein (VLDL) hydrolysis by lipoprotein lipase and high-density lipoprotein (HDL) hydrolysis by endothelial lipase are pathways for PPAR activation.
- Fibrates lower triglycerides and raise HDL through PPARα activation, whereas thiazolidinediones (TZDs), improve insulin sensitivity by activating PPARγ.

See also Chapters A34 and A47

The term *peroxisome proliferator–activated receptor* (PPAR) arose from the observation that some compounds increase the size and number of peroxisomes in animal models. It is now known that PPARs represent a class of nuclear receptors in humans. PPARs have been the subject of intense study for their role in metabolism and more recently in vascular biology and atherosclerosis. PPAR ligands in widespread therapeutic use include fibrates for dyslipidemia and thiazolidinediones (TZDs) as insulin-sensitizing agents used in the treatment of diabetes.

Peroxisome proliferator–activated receptor subtypes and gene expression

PPARs are ligand-activated transcription factors that include PPARα, PPARγ, and PPARβ/δ subtypes. Like other nuclear receptors (e.g., estrogen receptor and thyroid hormone receptor), PPARs contain both ligand-binding domains and DNA binding domains (**Figure A32.1**). Amino acid sequences diverge most around the ligand-binding domains, thereby accounting for receptor specificity among ligands. Through ligand-binding, PPARs form a heterodimeric complex with another nuclear receptor, retinoic X receptor, which is activated by its own ligand (9-*cis* retinoic acid). Together, this complex promotes release of corepressors and recruitment of coactivators, allowing specific expression of target genes with defined PPAR response elements in their promoters. PPARs can also repress gene expression through newly discovered effects, for example, SUMOylation.

Biologic actions of peroxisome proliferator–activated receptors

Peroxisome proliferator–activated receptor α.

Fatty acid metabolism. Many lines of evidence establish PPARα as a central regulator of fatty acid and lipid metabolism (**Table A32.1**), including fatty acid transport and oxidation, as well as apolipoprotein expression (A-I, A-II, and C-III). PPARα-deficient mice have increased free fatty acid levels and develop fatty liver arising from an inability to metabolize fatty acids. Synthetic fibrates (gemfibrozil and fenofibrate), used clinically to lower triglycerides and raise high-density lipoprotein (HDL), are PPARα agonists.

Vascular and antiinflammatory effects. PPARα is expressed in vascular as well as inflammatory cells including monocytes, macrophages, and lymphocytes. In vascular smooth muscle cells (VSMCs), PPARα activators inhibit interleukin (IL)-1, thereby inhibiting production of IL-6 and prostaglandin production by cyclooxygenase-2. Aortic explants of PPARα-deficient mice demonstrate prolonged inflammatory responses and increased IL-6 production. PPARα agonists also inhibit expression of tissue factor, a major procoagulant that contributes to plaque formation. In endothelial cells (EC), PPARα activators limit expression of cytokine-induced vascular cell adhesion molecule-1 (VCAM-1) and monocyte adhesion, probably through changes in nuclear factor kappa B (NFκB) activity. Consistent with these findings, synthetic PPARα agonists decrease circulating levels of the inflammatory markers, IL-6 and C-reactive protein. Some studies

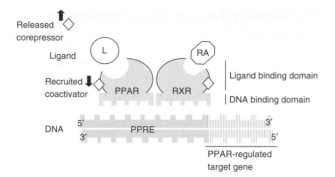

Figure A32.1 Schematic drawing of the peroxisome proliferator–activated receptor (PPAR)–RXR transcriptional complex. The interaction between a cognate ligand and the ligand-binding domain of a given PPAR isotype activates a PPAR–RXR transcriptional complex. The activated PPAR binds to specific PPAR response elements (PPRE) present on target genes through the PPAR DNA binding domain. In order for PPAR to function as a ligand-activated transcription factor, it must associate with another nuclear receptor RXR and form a heterodimeric complex. RXR, which is an obligate heterodimeric partner for many receptors as well as capable of homodimeric binding, has its own purported ligand (9-*cis* retinoic acid). Accessory molecule release (corepressors) and recruitment (coactivators) also help determine PPAR activity and responses. Distinct PPAR ligands, even for the same PPAR isotype, can interact with the PPAR ligand-binding domain in unique ways and hence induce specific responses. RXR, retinoid X receptor.

implicate PPARα in blood pressure changes in corticosteroid-dependent hypertension.

Peroxisome proliferator–activated receptor γ. PPARγ,
a key mediator in metabolic syndromes such as diabetes and obesity, was first identified as a part of a transcriptional complex necessary for adipocyte differentiation (**Table A32.1**). PPARγ is highly expressed in adipose tissue whereas PPARγ overexpression in fibroblasts results in differentiation toward an adipocyte-like phenotype. Homozygous PPARγ–deficient mice that are not viable die *in utero* and lack white fat. PPARγ also influences lipid metabolism, with target genes such as hydroxymethylglutaryl coenzyme A synthetase and apolipoprotein A-I. Consistent with this finding, TZDs can raise HDL although their lipid effects, including those on triglycerides, can be variable among specific agents.

Peroxisome proliferator–activated receptor δ. Although
PPARα and PPARγ have been more extensively studied, PPARδ is an intriguing molecule with potential relevance to metabolic and vascular issues. PPARδ is widely expressed in essentially all tissues, suggesting a fundamental role in homeostasis and cellular function. Like other PPARs, PPARδ is reportedly activated by certain fatty acids and by prostacyclin. Early studies with PPARδ agents have revealed significant increases in HDL, although such agents may find their use limited by side effects. PPARδ may limit inflammation, promote fatty acid oxidation, and increase exercise endurance.

Natural peroxisome proliferator–activated receptor ligands

Naturally occurring PPAR ligands include fatty acids, especially oxidized linoleic acid (in the form of 9- or 13- hydroxy octadecadienoic acid), which activates PPARγ and -α. PPAR activation and ligand generation has been shown to occur through specific pathways of lipoprotein metabolism such as very low-density lipoprotein (VLDL) hydrolysis by lipoprotein lipase. This key enzyme in triglyceride metabolism can generate PPARα ligands and activate a PPARα transcriptional cassette. HDL hydrolysis by endothelial lipase can also activate PPARs through a distinct mechanism.

Peroxisome proliferator–activated receptors in disease

Experimental atherosclerosis. PPARα and PPARγ activa-
tion suppress inflammation and atherosclerosis in mice and have actions on lymphocytes, macrophages, VSMCs, and EC. PPARγ ligands suppress cytokine-induced chemokine expression in vascular endothelium and colonic epithelium, the latter suggesting a potential role for PPAR agonists in inflammatory bowel disease. PPARγ activation also inhibits expression of cytokines and matrix metalloproteinases (enzymes known to be important in regulation of vascular wall composition and atherosclerotic plaque stability), as well as decreases VSMC cell cycle progression. Although PPARγ can induce expression of a fatty acid transported and oxidized by low-density lipoprotein (LDL) receptor CD36, it does not

---

TABLE A32.1

SYNTHETIC PEROXISOME PROLIFERATOR–ACTIVATED RECEPTOR (PPAR) LIGANDS IN CLINICAL USE AND SELECTED EXAMPLES OF CLINICALLY RELEVANT METABOLIC AND VASCULAR PPAR-REGULATED TARGET GENES

Nuclear receptor	Synthetic ligands	Metabolic targets	Vascular targets
PPARγ	Thiazolidinediones:	GLUT 4 (+)	Matrix metalloproteinase-9 (−)
	Pioglitazone (Actos)	AP2 (+)	Specific cytokines (−)
	Rosiglitazone (Avandia)	Adiponectin (+)	Specific chemokines (−)
PPARα	Fibrates:	Fatty acid β-oxidation (+)	Vascular cell adhesion molecule 1 (−)
	Gemfibrozil (Lopid)	Apolipoprotein A-I (+)	Tissue factor (−)
	Fenofibrate (Tricor)	Lipoprotein lipase (+)	Interleukin 6 (−)

+, gene induced; −, gene repressed.

appear to promote foam cell formation. It also increases expression of the cholesterol efflux transporter adenosine triphosphate binding cassette protein-1 (ABCA-1).

Genetic studies. In humans, dominant negative mutation in PPARγ is associated with severe insulin resistance, diabetes, hypertension, and a specific form of lipodystrophy. A PPARγ mutation has been found in association with severe obesity in a subset of German patients, and a single nucleotide polymorphism of PPARγ has been linked to decreased risk of diabetes and myocardial infarction (MI). PPARα variants in humans have also been reported.

Clinical trials with PPAR agonists

Fibrates and cardiovascular disease. Clinical trials of fibrates have yielded mixed results for cardiovascular (CV) endpoints. The Veteran's Administration-HDL Intervention Trial (VA-HIT) showed a decrease in CV events in patients with diabetes treated with gemfibrozil. Of note, none of these patients were taking statins. The Fenofibrate Intervention and Event Lowering in Diabetes (FIELD) trial used fenofibrate in a larger cohort with diabetes but did not show any significant benefit on the primary endpoint (CV death or nonfatal MI), although it has been postulated that concomitant statin use in the placebo group minimized between-group differences. Notably, important secondary endpoints, such as nonfatal MI and microvascular disease, were improved by fenofibrate. The ongoing Action to Control Cardiometabolic Risk in Diabetes (ACCORD) trial is testing the effect of combination therapy with a fibrate and a statin on CV events.

Thiazolidinediones.

Hyperglycemia. TZDs were serendipitously discovered to bind to PPARγ and to exert insulin-sensitizing effects. TZDs can delay the onset of diabetes in individuals at risk for diabetes [Diabetes REduction Approaches with ramipril and rosiglitazone Medications (DREAM) study] and also have strong durability of effects over time, as reported in A Diabetes Outcome Progression Trial (ADOPT).

Atherosclerosis. PPARγ effects on inflammatory and vascular targets *in vitro* and atherosclerotic mouse models *in vivo* raised the prospect that TZDs might also decrease CV events. Surrogate marker studies support this hypothesis; PPARγ agonists lower C-reactive protein as well as other CV risk markers. In the Carotid Intima-Media Thickness in Atherosclerosis Using Pioglitazone (CHICAGO) study, pioglitazone slowed the progression in carotid artery intima-media thickness, a surrogate marker for CV risk, over an 18-month period compared with glimepride despite similar glycemic control. In the Prospective Pioglitazone Clinical Trial in Macrovascular Events (PROactive) trial, pioglitazone treatment of patients with diabetes and significant macrovascular disease did not show a difference in a broad aggregate (and perhaps poorly chosen) primary cardiovascular disease (CVD) endpoint that included peripheral vascular disease and revascularization. Yet the more focused, objective secondary endpoint of all-cause mortality, nonfatal MI, and stroke was significantly lowered by pioglitazone compared to placebo. A known side effect of TZDs is fluid retention. In both PROactive and DREAM, increased "heart failure/edema" was observed without increased heart failure mortality. The lack of standard endpoint adjudication in PROactive makes interpretation difficult but it is likely that the aggregated "heart failure" endpoint was simply peripheral edema.

Other clinical effects of thiazolidinediones

Blood pressure. A consistent observation in the TZD trials has been a modest but statistically significant reduction in systolic blood pressure. In addition to the clear improvement in metabolic parameters with TZDs, animal models have shown that treatment with TZDs may blunt expression of angiotensin-II receptors in the vasculature. Recent work has also suggested that certain angiotensin receptor blockers, for example, telmisartan, losartan metabolites, may activate PPARγ. These findings, along with PPARγ effects on VSMCs and the clinical significance of these responses, remain under active investigation.

Edema and tubular sodium transport. Recent work identifying the epithelial Na^+ channel (ENaC) in the collecting duct of the distal nephron as a PPARγ target gene mediating sodium and volume retention may help explain TZD-induced edema. In a murine model, pioglitazone-induced volume retention was prevented by concomitant treatment with amiloride, a known inhibitor of EnaC-mediated salt absorption.

Weight gain. TZDs tend to increase appetite and body weight, potentially limiting clinical acceptability, but this weight change appears to include a potentially beneficial shift from visceral to subcutaneous fat.

Fatty liver disease. Currently available TZDs (pioglitazone and rosiglitazone) are not hepatotoxic and may have utility in treating some steatohepatoses.

Unresolved issues and future prospects

The evidence for PPARs as regulators of key transcriptional pathways relevant to diabetes, dyslipidemia, and atherosclerotic complications continues to focus attention on these nuclear receptors as drug targets. Large clinical trials have provided some data supporting the extensive preclinical evidence of beneficial effects of PPAR modulation, but have also left open many unanswered questions that have limited widespread use of these agents for reducing CV risk. The complex and overlapping antidiabetic, hypolipidemic, and antiinflammatory effects of these agents, as well as their potential for nontranscriptional and PPAR-independent effects, makes dissection of primary mechanisms accounting for their effects difficult to separate. The complexity of this system, including distinct effects that are specific to a given synthetic ligand, may well explain the adverse effects seen with dual PPARα/δ agonists whose development has largely been abandoned. At the same time, this biologic complexity, various metabolic, vascular and inflammatory targets under PPAR control, and the prospect that PPARs may integrate diverse cardiometabolic responses suggests that development of more sophisticated PPAR modulators is still an attractive option.

Suggested Readings

Ahmed W, Orasanu G, Nehra V, et al. High-density lipoprotein hydrolysis by endothelial lipase activates PPARα: a candidate mechanism for high-density lipoprotein-mediated repression of leukocyte adhesion. *Circ Res* 2006;98:490–498.

Barish GD, Narkar VA, Evans RM. PPARδ: a dagger in the heart of the metabolic syndrome. *J Clin Invest* 2006;116(3):590–597.

Barroso I, Gurnell M, Crowley VE, et al. Dominant negative mutations in human PPARγ associated with severe insulin resistance, diabetes mellitus and hypertension [See Comments]. *Nature* 1999;402:880–883.

Brown JD, Plutzky J. Peroxisome proliferator-activated receptors as transcriptional nodal points and therapeutic targets. *Circulation* 2007;115:518–533.

Lefebvre P, Chinetti G, Fruchart J, et al. Sorting out the roles of PPARα in energy metabolism and vascular homeostasis. *J Clin Invest* 2006;116:571–580.

Lehrke M, Lazar M. The many faces of PPARγ. *Cell* 2005;123:993–999.

Li AC, Brown KK, Silvestre MJ, et al. Peroxisome proliferator-activated receptor gamma ligands inhibit development of atherosclerosis in LDL receptor-deficient mice. *J Clin Invest* 2000;106:523–531.

Parulkar AA, Pendergrass ML, Granda-Ayala R, et al. Nonhypoglycemic effects of thiazolidinediones. *Ann Intern Med* 2001;134:61–71.

Plutzky J. PPARs are therapeutic targets: reverse cardiology? *Science* 2003;302:406–407.

Wilson TM, Brown PJ, Sternbach DD, et al. The PPARs: from orphan receptors to drug discovery. *J Med Chem* 2000;43:527–550.

Ziouzenkova O, Perrey S, Asatryan L, et al. Lipolysis of triglyceride-rich lipoproteins generates PPAR ligands: evidence for an anti-inflammatory role for lipoprotein lipase. *Proc Natl Acad Sci U S A* 2003;100:2730–2735.

CHAPTER A33 ■ ENDOCANNABINOIDS

GEORGE KUNOS, MD, PhD, FAHA AND PÁL PACHER, MD, PhD, FAHA

KEY POINTS

- Endocannabinoids are endogenous lipid ligands that bind to the receptors that mediate the biological effects of marijuana.
- The two best-characterized endocannabinoids, arachidonoyl ethanolamide (anandamide) and 2-arachidonoylglycerol (AG), interact with two G protein–coupled endocannabinoid receptors, CB_1 and CB_2.
- Cannabinoids and their endogenous counterparts, acting through CB_1 receptors, cause hypotension through negative chronotropic, inotropic vasodilator, and presynaptic sympathoinhibitory effects; antiinflammatory actions are mediated through CB_2 receptors on immune cells.
- Endocannabinoids have been implicated in the hypotension associated with shock and advanced liver cirrhosis and may contribute to obesity/metabolic syndrome.

See also Chapters A46 and **C157**

Endocannabinoids, endogenous lipid ligands with a broad range of biological actions similar to those of cannabis (CB), interact with the same set of CB receptors as marijuana. Circulating levels of endocannabinoids are too low to generate hormone-like effects, but endocannabinoids generated by many different cell types are thought to be autocrine or paracrine mediators acting in close proximity to their sites of release. In the central nervous system, endocannabinoids act as retrograde messengers. They are synthesized in and released from postsynaptic neurons in response to a rise in intracellular calcium or stimulation of metabotropic receptors. Depolarization-induced suppression of inhibitory or excitatory neurotransmission is mediated by presynaptic inhibition of GABA or glutamate release, respectively, factors that regulate synaptic strength or "plasticity." Similar to prostanoids, endocannabinoids are not stored in neurons, but are synthesized and released "on demand." Once released, retrograde diffusion in the synapse allows the molecules to reach and activate cannabinoid receptors on presynaptic axon terminals that inhibit transmitter release from presynaptic neurons.

Regulation of endocannabinoids

Synthesis. Arachidonoyl ethanolamide (anandamide) is generated by the transacylation of membrane phophatidylethanolamine (PE) to yield *N*-arachidonoyl PE, which is then hydrolyzed into arachidonoyl ethanolamide and phosphatidic acid. 2-Arachidonoyl glycerol (2-AG) is formed from glycerophospholipids by the sequential actions of phospholipase C, generating diacylglycerol (DAG), which is then hydrolyzed by DAG lipase to generate 2-AG.

Clearance. Endocannabinoids are cleared from the extracellular space by cellular uptake through a putative membrane transporter, followed by enzymatic degradation. Anandamide is selectively degraded by the membrane-associated enzyme, fatty acid amidohydrolase (FAAH) into arachidonic acid and ethanolamine, whereas 2-AG is selectively degraded by a monoglyceride lipase (MGL). There are reasonably selective inhibitors of anandamide transport, FAAH, and MGL, which potentiate certain endocannabinoid-mediated biological responses.

Cannabinoid receptors

Subtypes. The biological effects of endogenous, plant-derived and synthetic cannabinoids are mediated by cannabinoid receptors. To date, two G protein–coupled cannabinoid receptors have been identified by molecular cloning: CB_1 receptors, expressed at very high levels in the brain and at much lower levels in many peripheral tissues, and CB_2 receptors, expressed predominantly

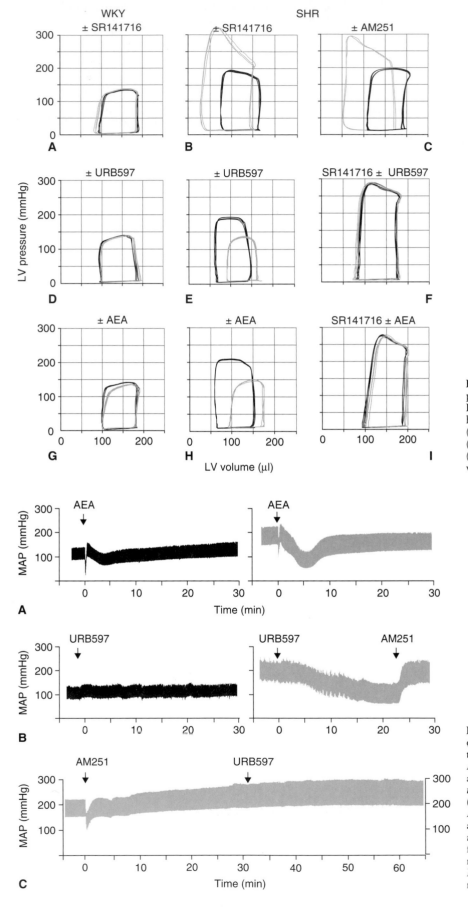

Figure A33.1 Representative left ventricular (LV) pressure–volume loops from normotensive Wistar Kyoto (WKY, panels *A, D, G*) and spontaneously hypertensive rats (SHR, *B, C, E, F, H, I*) before (*black*) and after (*gray*) treatment with CB$_1$ antagonist (SR141716), FAAH inhibitor (URB597), anandamide (AEA) or their combinations. (Reproduced from (6) with permission of Lippincott Williams & Wilkins.)

Figure A33.2 Representative recordings of the effects of anandamide (10 mg/kg i.v., AEA), the FAAH antagonist URB597 (10 mg/kg i.v.), the CB$_1$ antagonist AM251 (1 mg/kg i.v.) or their combinations on mean arterial pressure in anesthetized normotensive (*black tracings*) or angiotensin II-induced hypertensive rats (*gray tracings*). Note that the hypotensive effect of AEA and URB597 is potentiated in hypertensive rats and is prevented or reversed by AM251. The *arrows* indicate the injection of the drugs. (Reproduced from Pacher P, Bátkai S, Kunos G. Blood pressure regulation by endocannabinoids and their receptors. *Neuropharmacology* 2005;48:1130–1138, with permission of Elsevier.)

in cells of the immune and hematopoietic systems. Anandamide can also activate TRPV$_1$ vanilloid receptors, although at concentrations higher than required for CB$_1$ receptor activation.

Coupling. Both CB$_1$ and CB$_2$ receptors couple to adenylyl cyclase through Gi/Go proteins, resulting in cyclase inhibition. Cannabinoids also inhibit L-type and N-type calcium channels, activate certain potassium channels, activate all three types of multifunctional mitogen-activated protein kinases (including p44/42, p38, and JUN terminal kinase), and activate the PI3 kinase pathway.

Physiologic effects of cannabinoids

The mechanisms underlying the *in vivo* cardiovascular effects of cannabinoids are complex and may involve neuronal, cardiac, and vascular effects or their combinations.

Nervous system effects. Cannabinoids can influence cardiovascular function by modulating autonomic outflow through sites of action in the central and peripheral nervous systems. Both sympathetic and parasympathetic nerve terminals have presynaptic CB$_1$ receptors, stimulation of which suppresses norepinephrine and acetylcholine release, respectively. Sympathoinhibition may account for the bradycardia of chronic marijuana use and may contribute to hypotension. Parasympathetic inhibition has been implicated in the isolated tachycardia accompanying acute marijuana use.

Cardiac effects. Acute exposure to smoked marijuana usually causes isolated tachycardia, whereas chronic use can lead to hypotension and bradycardia. CB$_1$ receptors are present in the human myocardium and their activation results in negative inotropy. In anesthetized rodents, THC or anandamide elicit hypotension, bradycardia, decreased cardiac contractility, and decreased cardiac output but these hemodynamic responses are blunted or absent in conscious normotensive animals. The cardiovascular depressor effects of anandamide are devoid of a centrally mediated component, but certain potent synthetic cannabinoids may cause sympathoexcitation through sites of action in the brain.

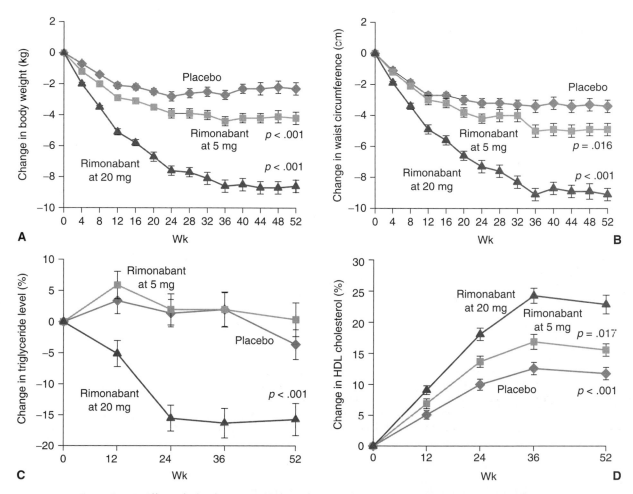

Figure A33.3 Effect of placebo or rimonabant for 52 weeks on body weight, waist circumference, plasma triglyceride levels, and high-density lipoprotein (HDL) cholesterol levels. Body weight and waist circumference were measured at randomization (week 0) and every 4 weeks thereafter until week 52, and plasma HDL cholesterol and triglyceride levels were measured at randomization (week 0) and every 3 months thereafter until week 52. Values are shown as means ±SE for all patients for whom measurements were taken at each visit (*lines*); *p* values were obtained after the repeated-measures analysis. The *p* values correspond to the mean difference between the rimonabant groups and the placebo group. SE, standard error. (Reproduced from Despres JP, Golay A, Sjostrom L, et al. Effects of rimonabant on metabolic risk factors in overweight patients with dyslipidemia. *N Eng J Med* 2005;353:2121–2134, with permission of the Massachusetts Medical Society.)

All cannabinoid effects in rodents are mediated by CB_1 receptors, as indicated by their absence in CB_1 receptor knockout mice.

Vascular effects. In isolated vascular preparations, anandamide elicits vasodilation that has both endothelium-dependent and -independent components. The endothelium-independent effect has been attributed to $TRPV_1$ receptors on sensory nerve endings that mediate the release of the vasodilator peptide CGRP. The endothelium-dependent, pertussis toxin–sensitive mesenteric vasodilator effect of anandamide may be mediated by a G protein–coupled receptor distinct from CB_1 or CB_2, because it remains unchanged in mice lacking both CB_1 and CB_2 receptors. In the cerebral and coronary circulations, CB_1 receptors and CB_1-mediated vasodilation have been documented.

Antiinflammatory effects. Cannabinoids have immunomodulatory and antiinflammatory effects, mediated predominantly by CB_2 receptors situated on immune cells. These could be therapeutically exploited in conditions associated with increased inflammatory cell infiltration, such as atherosclerosis and myocardial infarction, or cardiac transplantation.

Implications for human disease

Hypertension. The CB_1 receptor–mediated hypotensive effect of cannabinoids is potentiated in hypertensive rodents compared to normotensive animals, and the effect is due to a decrease in cardiac output and contractility. Inhibition of FAAH, which results in elevated tissue levels of anandamide without causing behavioral effects, also reduces BP and cardiac contractility in hypertensive but not normotensive animals. Conversely, CB_1 receptor antagonists, which do not affect BP in normotensive animals, cause a pressor effect due to increased cardiac contractility in various experimental models of hypertension (**Figures A33.1 and A33.2**). These findings suggest that the endocannabinoid system becomes tonically active in some forms of hyperdynamic hypertension, where elevated BP is dependent on inappropriately high heart rate or contractility. In clinical studies of the metabolic syndrome using the CB_1 antagonist rimonabant, BP reductions have been small and inconsistent.

Hypotension. The profound hypotension that can be elicited by stimulation of CB_1 receptors suggests a role for endocannabinoids in hypotensive states. This is supported by findings that CB_1 antagonists can prevent or reverse the hypotension associated with hemorrhagic, endotoxic or cardiogenic shock, or with advanced liver cirrhosis. Possible mediators of hypotension in these states may be macrophage- or platelet-derived endocannabinoids, whose levels are significantly elevated in these conditions.

Metabolic syndrome. Animal studies indicate that endocannabinoids acting at CB_1 receptors in the central nervous system (CNS) increase appetite, whereas cannabinoid-dependent lipogenesis in adipose tissue and liver occurs at least in part through peripheral CB_1 receptor stimulation. In obese rodents chronically treated with the CB_1 antagonist rimonabant, food intake was reduced only transiently, whereas the reduction in body weight was maintained throughout the treatment. Accordingly, in recent phase III clinical trials involving obese individuals with the metabolic syndrome, chronic treatment with rimonabant resulted not only in weight loss and reduced waist circumference, but also improved glucose tolerance, reduced plasma triglycerides, and increased HDL cholesterol. Decreased plasma insulin and leptin and increased plasma adiponectin levels were also observed (**Figure A33.3**).

Atherosclerosis and myocardial infarction. CB_2 receptor-expressing immune cells are present both in human and mouse atherosclerotic plaques. Accordingly, orally administered THC inhibits atherosclerosis progression in a mouse model through activation of CB_2 receptors. THC treatment also diminished the proliferative capacity of lymphoid cells, production of interferon-γ, and macrophage chemotaxis. Furthermore, CB_2 receptor activation protects the heart from ischemia/reperfusion injury by reducing the extent of leukocyte-dependent myocardial damage *in vivo*. Although the bulk of the evidence suggests that these effects are mediated by CB_2 receptors, studies to date have not convincingly documented the presence of CB_2 receptors in primary cardiomyocytes, only in endothelial cells.

Suggested Readings

Bátkai S, Járai Z, Wagner JA, et al. Endocannabinoids acting at vascular CB_1 receptors mediate the vasodilated state in advanced liver cirrhosis. *Nat Med* 2001;7:827–832.

Bátkai S, Pacher P, Osei-Hyiaman D, et al. Endocannabinoids acting at CB_1 receptors regulate cardiovascular function in hypertension. *Circulation* 2004;110:1996–2002.

Despres JP, Golay A, Sjostrom L, et al. Effects of rimonabant on metabolic risk factors in overweight patients with dyslipidemia. *N Engl J Med* 2005;353:2121–2134.

Howlett AC, Breivogel CS, Childers SR, et al. Cannabinoid physiology and pharmacology: 30 years of progress. *Neuropharmacology* 2004;47(Suppl 1):345–358.

Járai Z, Wagner JA, Varga K, et al. Cannabinoid-induced mesenteric vasodilation through an endothelial site distinct from CB_1 or CB_2 receptors. *Proc Natl Acad Sci U S A* 1999;96:14136–14141.

Mackie K. Cannabinoid receptors as therapeutic targets [Review]. *Annu Rev Pharmacol Toxicol* 2006;46:101–122.

Pacher P, Batkai S, Kunos G. The endocannabinoid system as an emerging target of pharmacotherapy. *Pharmacol Rev* 2006;58:389–462.

Piomelli D. The molecular logic of endocannabinoid signaling. *Nat Rev Neurosci* 2003;4:873–884.

Pi-Sunyer FX, Aronne LJ, Heshmati HM, et al. Effect of rimonabant, a cannabinoid-1 receptor blocker, on weight and cardiometabolic risk factors in overweight and obese patients. *J Am Med Assoc* 2006;295:761–775.

Wagner JA, Varga K, Ellis EF, et al. Activation of peripheral CB_1 cannabinoid receptors in haemorrhagic shock. *Nature* 1997;390:518–521.

CHAPTER A34 ■ ACTIVE PRODUCTS OF ADIPOCYTES

NATHANIEL WINER, MD

KEY POINTS

- Intraabdominal (visceral) fat cells are metabolically active, sense energy stores, and affect appetite.
- Adipocytes secrete one substance that promotes insulin sensitivity (adiponectin) and a myriad of substances that promote insulin resistance [tumor necrosis factor α (TNF-α), interleukin (IL)-6, adipsin, adrenomedullin (AM), angiotensin (Ang) II, apelin, 11β-hydroxysteroid dehydrogenase (11βHSD), resistin, retinol-binding protein-4 (RBP-4), visfatin, and others].
- Adipocytes produce substances with direct and indirect effects on blood vessel function and disease, including renin-angiotensin components, apelin, plasminogen-activator inhibitor-1 (PAI-1), and monocyte chemoattractant protein-1 (MCP-1).

See also Chapters A23, A29, **A35, A36, A47,** A65, B90, and C157

Adipose tissue as an endocrine organ

Recent research in obesity has revealed that adipose tissue functions not as a passive storage depot, but rather as an endocrine organ, producing a variety of secreted factors that can affect appetite, energy storage, insulin signaling and sensitivity, inflammation, and vascular function. With increasing intraabdominal (visceral) fat, adipocytes secrete disproportionately greater amounts of free fatty acids (FFA) and proinflammatory adipokines [e.g., tumor necrosis factor α, (TNF-α)] and less antiinflammatory adipokines (e.g., adiponectin, Acr30). Unbalanced production of pro- and antiinflammatory adipokines may play a role in the development of insulin resistance, which may contribute to the development of metabolic syndrome, hypertension, and atherosclerosis.

Leptin and energy balance

Leptin (see Chapter A35), one of the first identified adipocyte hormones, is a metabolic signal of energy sufficiency. Caloric restriction and weight loss cause a rapid decline in leptin, which stimulates hypothalamically mediated increases in appetite and decreases in energy expenditure. Elevated levels of leptin characterize most forms of human obesity but leptin treatment fails to cause weight reduction, indicating a degree of leptin resistance. Leptin resistance may result from defective leptin signal transduction or blood–brain transport. Other endocrine actions of leptin include stimulation of the proliferation and differentiation of hematopoietic cells, modulation of immune cell cytokine production, enhancement of endothelial cell growth and angiogenesis, acceleration of wound healing, and an antiosteogenic effect on bone mass.

Adiponectin and insulin sensitivity

Adiponectin (see Chapter A36) is expressed in differentiated adipocytes and circulates at high levels in the blood. Plasma adiponectin concentrations correlate inversely with levels of glucose, insulin, triglyceride, and body mass index (BMI), and positively with high-density lipoprotein–cholesterol levels and insulin-stimulated glucose disposal. The decrease in adiponectin before the onset of obesity and insulin resistance and its rise with weight reduction in nonhuman primates or after treatment with thiazolidinediones (TZDs) in mice suggests a pathogenic role of these conditions. Moreover, polymorphisms in the adiponectin gene are associated with obesity and insulin resistance. Adiponectin increases insulin sensitivity by enhancing tissue fat oxidation, reducing plasma FFA, and lowering liver and muscle intracellular triglyceride content. Adiponectin increases nitric oxide production in endothelial cells, stimulates angiogenesis, and suppresses the expression of adhesion molecules in vascular endothelial cells and cytokines in macrophages. Therefore, adiponectin, unlike other adipocyte-derived hormones, has unique antidiabetic, antiinflammatory, and antiatherogenic actions. It is also possible that hypoadiponectinemia facilitates atherosclerosis.

Products that promote insulin resistance

Adipocytes produce a myriad of products (some not included here) that strongly affect insulin signaling and insulin sensitivity. Many of these substances also have multiple actions in a variety of tissues, including proinflammatory and vasoactive properties. *Tumor necrosis factor α.* TNF-α is a 26-kDa transmembrane protein that is cleaved into a 17-kDa biologically active protein expressed by adipocytes and stromovascular cells. In most human studies, plasma TNF-α levels correlate with adiposity and insulin resistance. In adipose tissue, TNF-α represses genes involved in uptake and storage of nonesterified fatty acids (NEFA) and glucose, suppresses transcription factor genes regulating adipogenesis and lipogenesis, and changes expression of adiponectin and interleukin 6 (IL-6). In the liver, TNF-α alters expression of genes involved in glucose uptake and metabolism, fatty acid oxidation and synthesis of cholesterol and fatty acids. TNF-α also impairs insulin signaling.

Interleukin 6. IL-6 is a cytokine that circulates in multiple glycosylated forms ranging from 22 to 27 kDa in size. Weight loss reduces expression and circulating levels of IL-6, and increased plasma IL-6 is a risk factor for cardiovascular disease (CVD). Administration of IL-6 induces hyperlipidemia, hyperglycemia, and insulin resistance. Like TNF-α, IL-6 decreases insulin signaling in peripheral tissues, inhibits adipogenesis and decreases adiponectin secretion. Mice with a targeted deletion of IL-6 develop maturity-onset obesity and associated metabolic abnormalities, which are reversed by IL-6 replacement, suggesting that IL-6 is involved in causing these conditions.

Adrenomedullin. Adrenomedullin (AM) (see Chapter A23), a peptide originally isolated from human pheochromocytoma, is a multifunctional regulatory peptide that is produced and secreted by various types of cells, including cultured adipocytes and adipose tissue. Inflammatory cytokines such as TNF-α stimulate AM expression in adipocytes; AM expression in adipose tissue and plasma AM are increased in obese subjects. Unlike subcutaneous adipose tissue, AM expression in visceral adipose tissue is associated with the metabolic syndrome [BMI, waist circumference, systolic blood pressure (SBP), high-density lipoprotein (HDL) cholesterol, homeostatic model assessment (HOMA) index, TNF-α messenger RNA (mRNA) level, plasminogen-activator inhibitor-1 (PAI-1) levels, and triglycerides]. AM may also have natriuretic, antiapoptotic, and antiinflammatory properties, as well as inhibitory effects on migration of vascular smooth muscle cells, oxidative stress production, and insulin secretion. Taken together, it appears that AM in visceral and omental adipose tissue may initiate the complications of the metabolic syndrome, while simultaneously blunting its consequences through simultaneous antioxidant and vasodilator effects.

Adipsin and acylation stimulating protein. Adipsin is a complement component that catalyzes production of ASP, both of which correlate with obesity, insulin resistance, dyslipidemia, and CVD. ASP, a cleavage product of complement C3, is an adipocyte-derived protein that has potent anabolic effects on human adipose tissue to increase glucose uptake and NEFA storage through translocation of glucose transporters (GLUT1, GLUT3, and GLUT4) from intracellular sites to the cell surface and activation of diacylglycerol acyltransferase (DGAT) to stimulate triglyceride synthesis. In addition, ASP inhibits hormone-sensitive lipase in adipocytes, independently and additively to insulin. ASP is an important factor in regulating metabolic balance. The absence of ASP production in male and female ASP knockout mice results in increased energy expenditure. Although male and female mice deal differently with impaired triglyceride synthesis, animals of both genders exhibit a lean, insulin sensitive phenotype despite significant hyperphagia.

Retinol-binding protein 4. In insulin-resistant states the expression of the GLUT4 is downregulated in adipocytes and not in skeletal muscle, leading to impaired insulin-stimulated glucose transport, a defect that precedes glucose intolerance.

Retinol-binding protein 4 (RBP4), the only specific transport protein for retinol (vitamin A) in the circulation, increases in mice with a selective knockout of GLUT4 in adipocytes. Injection of purified RBP4 or transgenic overexpression of RBP4 in mice impairs insulin signaling in muscle and induces the hepatic expression of the gluconeogenic enzyme, phosphoenolpyruvate carboxykinase. Conversely, genetic deletion of RBP4 enhances insulin sensitivity. Similarly, fenretinide, a synthetic retinoid that increases urinary excretion of RBP4, normalizes serum RBP4 levels and improves insulin resistance and glucose intolerance in mice with obesity induced by a high-fat diet. Serum RBP4 levels correlate with the magnitude of insulin resistance in subjects with obesity, impaired glucose tolerance, components of the metabolic syndrome, or type 2 diabetes and in nonobese, nondiabetic subjects with a strong family history of type 2 diabetes. Elevated serum RBP4 levels are normalized by rosiglitazone, an insulin-sensitizing drug. Therefore, RBP4 is an adipocyte-derived molecule that may contribute to the pathogenesis of type 2 diabetes. Pharmacologic targeting of RBP4 could provide a new approach to treatment of type 2 diabetes.

Visfatin. The amino acid sequence of visfatin corresponds to a protein previously identified as pre–B cell colony-enhancing factor (PBEF), a 52-kDa cytokine expressed in lymphocytes. Visfatin, normally concentrated in the visceral fat of both humans and mice, increases in plasma during the development of obesity. Visfatin, like insulin, induces tyrosine phosphorylation of the insulin receptor and insulin receptor substrates-1 and -2 in the liver, binding of phosphatidylinositol 3 kinase (PI3K) to IRS-1 and IRS-2; and phosphorylation of Akt and mitogen-activated protein kinase (MAPK); it also reduces plasma glucose in mice. However, in contradistinction to insulin, plasma visfatin levels do not change significantly on fasting or feeding in mice, although heterozygous visfatin-deficient mice show modestly higher plasma glucose levels during fasting, feeding, and glucose tolerance testing compared to wild-type mice. The findings that plasma visfatin levels increase in proportion to visceral fat accumulation and that the adipocytokine has an insulin-mimetic action may be relevant to the metabolic syndrome. However, the absence of a correlation between plasma visfatin levels and insulin sensitivity in humans indicates the need for further studies.

Resistin. Resistin (named from its ability to induce resistance to insulin) is a 12-kDa polypeptide whose expression in rodents is 15-fold greater in visceral than in subcutaneous fat. Resistin impairs glucose tolerance and insulin action in mice and has been proposed as a link between obesity and type 2 diabetes, since higher levels of expression of the gene and protein are seen in visceral adipose tissue in both central obesity and diabetes. Incubation of cultured adipocytes with resistin decreases insulin-stimulated glucose uptake, an effect that is blocked by antiresistin antibodies. TZDs downregulate both resistin mRNA and protein *in vitro*. In subjects with metabolic syndrome, resistin levels predict coronary artery calcification, unlike C-reactive protein (CRP) levels. Plasma resistin levels correlate with markers of inflammation and are predictive of coronary atherosclerosis in humans, independent of CRP. In human type 2 diabetes, resistin is produced mainly in macrophages and elevated serum resistin levels may reflect subclinical inflammation. Resistin reduces glucose uptake, and the insulin-sensitizing and glucose-lowering actions of the TZDs may be partly due to suppression of resistin expression.

11β-hydroxysteroid dehydrogenase type 1. The enzyme 11β-hydroxysteroid dehydrogenase type 1 (11β-HSD1), which converts hormonally-inactive cortisone in humans and

11-dehydrocorticosterone in mice to hormonally active cortisol and corticosterone, respectively, is highly expressed in visceral adipose tissue. Obesity, diabetes, hypertension, dyslipidemia, hypertension, CVD, and polycystic ovarian syndrome have been linked to inappropriate regulation of glucocorticoid metabolism by 11β-HSD1 and pharmacologic inhibition of 11β-HSD1 in humans increases insulin sensitivity. Transgenic overexpression of 11β-HSD1 in mouse adipocytes increases adipose tissue glucocorticoid concentrations and development of features of the metabolic syndrome without affecting serum glucocorticoids, whereas targeted deletion of 11β-HSD1 in all tissues results in a reduction of high-fat diet-induced weight gain, preferential subcutaneous fat distribution, improved glucose tolerance and insulin sensitivity, and atheroprotective lipid profiles.

Products causing insulin resistance with major vascular effects

Renin-angiotensin system. Peptides of the renin-angiotensin system (RAS) found in adipose tissue include renin, angiotensinogen, angiotensin (Ang) I, Ang II, angiotensin receptors type 1 (AT$_1$) and type 2 (AT$_2$), and ACE-1. Ang II, acting through the AT$_1$ receptor, mediates vasoconstriction, cardiomyocyte and vascular smooth muscle growth, aldosterone secretion, and salt and water retention, all of which play a key role in blood pressure (BP) regulation. Additionally, Ang II stimulates superoxide radical formation, expression of adhesion molecules in vascular cells, and reduces nitric oxide bioavailability (see Chapter A47).

Apelin. Apelin was first isolated from bovine stomach extracts as an endogenous ligand of APJ transmembrane receptors; apelin and its receptor are expressed in the brain, heart, stomach, skeletal muscle, vascular cells, and adipose tissue. Isoforms of varying length have biologic activity and like Ang I and Ang II, apelin is cleaved and inactivated by the carboxypeptidase angiotensin-converting enzyme (ACE) type 2. In streptozotocin-treated mice, deficiency of insulin is associated with decreased expression of apelin in adipocytes. Apelin expression in fat cells is inhibited by fasting and normalized by refeeding and plasma levels of apelin are higher in obese men than in their lean counterparts. Treatment of human adipocyte explants with insulin increases apelin expression sixfold, suggesting that insulin exerts a direct control on apelin gene expression in adipocytes. Overall, apelin appears to be an adipose tissue–derived signaling hormone possibly related to obesity-associated variations in insulin sensitivity.

Apelin has several other cardiovascular actions, including a potent positive inotropic effect in a rat heart model and a modulating effect on Ang II pressor activity. The systolic BP rise following Ang II administration in APJ knockout mice is absent in wild-type mice. SBP is reduced in Ang II-treated AT$_1$/APJ double-knockout mice compared to that of Ang II-treated AT$_1$ knockout mice, suggesting that, like AT$_2$ receptors, APJ receptors may mediate effects opposite those of AT$_1$ receptors. In the Dahl salt-sensitive rat heart failure model, reduced APJ and apelin are increased by the AT$_1$ receptor blocker telmisartan, suggesting that restoration of apelin signaling may mediate the beneficial effect of RAS modulation.

Plasminogen-activator inhibitor. PAI-1 (see Chapter A29), a member of the serine protease inhibitor family, is the primary inhibitor of fibrinolysis. Plasma PAI-1 levels are elevated in obesity and insulin resistance, correlate with all components of the metabolic syndrome, and are a risk factor for type 2 diabetes and CVD. Circulating PAI-1 levels fall with weight loss and insulin sensitivity increases with metformin or TZD treatment. Similar changes occur in mice with targeted deletion of PAI-1, suggesting a link with obesity and insulin resistance.

Monocyte chemoattractant protein 1. Monocyte chemoattractant protein 1 (MCP-1), a chemokine that recruits monocytes to sites of inflammation, is expressed and secreted by adipose tissue. Monocyte migration is the primary step in the development of atherosclerosis (see Chapter A65). Circulating monocytes adhere to the endothelial layer of the vessel wall, migrate into the vascular interstitium, and phagocytize oxidized low-density lipoprotein cholesterol, resulting in the formation of lipid-laden foam cells, which accumulate within the arterial wall to form fatty streaks. These early lesions later evolve into advanced atherosclerotic plaques containing necrotic lipid cores covered by a fibrous cap, which can rupture to produce a clot and lead to myocardial infarction. In obesity adipose tissue is infiltrated by macrophages which, when activated, secrete TNF-α and IL-6, contributing to insulin resistance. Insulin resistance and obesity in rodents is associated with macrophage-mediated infiltration of adipose tissue and an increase in adipocyte expression and blood levels of MCP-1. Cultured adipocytes incubated with MCP-1 show reduced insulin-stimulated glucose uptake and insulin receptor tyrosine phosphorylation, decreased adipocyte growth and differentiation, and accumulation of monocytes in blood vessel walls.

Suggested Readings

Eckel RH, Grundy SM, Zimmet PZ. The metabolic syndrome. *Lancet* 2005;365: 1415–1428.

Haffner SM, Miettinen H, Gaskill SP, et al. Metabolic precursors of hypertension. The San Antonio Heart Study. *Arch Intern Med* 1996;156:1994–2001.

Hall JE. The kidney, hypertension and obesity. *Hypertension* 2003;41(3 Part 2): 625–633.

Kershaw EE, Flier JS. Adipose tissue as an endocrine organ. *J Clin Endocrinol Metab* 2004;89:2548–2556.

Lia Y, Jianga C, Wanga X, et al. Adrenomedullin is a novel adipokine: adrenomedullin in adipocytes and adipose tissues. *Peptides* 2007;28:1129–1143.

Lyon CJ, Law RE, Hsueh WA. Minireview: adiposity, inflammation, and atherogenesis. *Endocrinology* 2003;144:2195–2200.

Wassink AMJ, Olijhoek JK, Visserin FLJ. The metabolic syndrome: metabolic changes with vascular consequences. *Eur J Clin Invest* 2007;37:8–17.

CHAPTER A35 ■ LEPTIN

WILLIAM G. HAYNES, MD

KEY POINTS

■ Leptin is an adipocyte-derived hormone that acts in the central nervous system to decrease appetite and increase thermogenesis.

■ Leptin increases sympathetic nerve activity (SNA) to thermogenic and cardiovascular tissues, including brown adipose tissue (BAT) in animals, skeletal muscle, adrenal gland, and kidney, resulting in increased energy expenditure and elevated arterial pressure.

■ Leptin expression and plasma leptin concentrations are elevated in obesity; selective resistance to the actions of leptin may contribute to the sympathetic, cardiovascular, and renal changes associated with obesity.

See also Chapters **A34** and **A47**

Adipose tissue was formerly considered almost exclusively as a passive storage depot for energy-dense triglycerides but it is now clear that adipocyte-derived hormones (including leptin, tumor necrosis factor α, angiotensinogen, adiponectin, resistin, visfatin, and vaspin) profoundly affect food intake, thermogenesis, and lipid and glucose metabolism. Leptin causes sympathetic, renal, and metabolic effects that may contribute to altered blood flow and pressure regulation in obesity. Adiponectin has a variety of potential cardiovascular roles (see Chapter A36) other adipocyte-derived hormones are also of potential interest.

LEPTIN

Regulation of fat cell mass

Body fat stores are regulated to maintain energy reserves and to prevent excessive changes in body weight. A central tenet of the "lipostat hypothesis" is that a negative feedback signal from adipose tissue to the central nervous system exists. Parabiosis experiments demonstrated that obesity in *ob* mice is due to lack of a circulating factor that acts to decrease body weight, whereas obesity in *db* mice is due to insensitivity to this same substance. Positional cloning identified leptin as the mutated gene responsible for obesity in the *ob* mouse strain (named *leptin* from the Greek *leptos* for "thin" (**Figure A35.1**). Leptin is a 167-amino acid protein expressed and secreted exclusively from adipocytes that circulates in blood at low levels (5–15 ng/mL) in lean subjects, with approximately 50% as the free form.

Leptin regulation

Leptin expression and plasma leptin concentrations are proportional to adipose tissue mass in animals and humans with obesity,

other than those with leptin deficiency. Decreased adipose tissue mass in obesity leads to low leptin concentrations. Food intake, insulin, and corticosteroids increase leptin expression, whereas cold temperature and catecholamines also decrease leptin expression. Sympathetic blockade increases leptin expression and plasma leptin levels, suggesting that endogenous sympathetic activity physiologically suppresses leptin expression and secretion.

Leptin is too large to readily penetrate the blood–brain barrier by passive diffusion. Entry of leptin into cerebrospinal fluid (CSF) appears to occur through a saturable specific transport mechanism that mediates binding and endocytosis of leptin by brain capillaries. Although high plasma leptin concentrations may saturate the blood–brain transport mechanism, CSF leptin concentrations are still high in obese subjects.

Receptors and signal transduction

Ob-Rb Receptors. The full leptin receptor (Ob-Rb) is a protein containing a single transmembrane domain with similarities to the class I cytokine receptors. It possesses two peptide motifs in a long intracellular C-terminal tail that activates the janus kinase/signal transducer and activator of transcription (JAK/STAT) pathway. The gene for the leptin receptor appears to encode for at least six alternatively spliced variants of the receptor. The Ob-Rb form encodes for the full receptor, including a long intracellular tail. Full-length leptin receptors are abundantly expressed in the hypothalamus, especially in the arcuate nucleus, which has a more porous blood–brain barrier.

Other receptors. Ob-Ra, Rc, and Rd leptin receptors have premature terminations with short intracellular tails, and may act to transport leptin across the blood–brain barrier. The Ob-Re form lacks the transmembrane domain and may therefore be

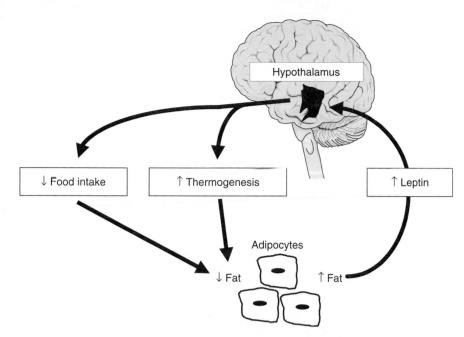

Figure A35.1 Leptin is a protein produced exclusively by adipocytes. Increases in adipose cell mass and insulin stimulate leptin expression and secretion. Leptin then circulates to cross the blood–brain barrier by a receptor-mediated saturable process. Leptin binds to leptin receptors in the hypothalamus, where it suppresses appetite and increases thermogenesis. Together, these actions decrease adipose cell mass. Therefore, leptin forms the afferent signaling component (adipostat) of a negative feedback loop that should maintain stable body fat stores. ↑, increased; ↓, decreased.

secreted as a soluble receptor, perhaps contributing to binding and inactivation of circulating leptin. Leptin receptor messenger RNA (mRNA) is expressed in adipose tissue, heart, kidney, liver, spleen, pancreatic islets, and testis, although the presence of the full-length receptor splice variant (Ob-Rb) has not been demonstrated in all these tissues. Full-length leptin receptor mRNA and protein has been demonstrated in vascular endothelial cells.

Signal transduction pathways. Leptin receptor signaling occurs through a number of intracellular mediators. The JAK/STAT pathway is essential for regulation of energy homeostasis by leptin, but not for its control of reproductive function, growth or glucose homeostasis. Other signaling mechanisms involved in the regulation of food intake by leptin include activation of phosphoinositol-3 kinase and mitogen-activated protein (MAP) kinase, and inhibition of AMP-activated protein kinase (AMPK). Therefore, the intracellular signaling mechanisms triggered by leptin appear more complicated than originally thought, with several downstream cascades involved in the actions of leptin.

Leptin actions
Sympathetic nervous system. Systemic and intracerebroventricular administration of leptin increases directly measured sympathetic nerve activity (SNA) to thermogenic brown adipose tissue (BAT) in rodents. Quite low doses of leptin increase SNA to kidney, hind limb, and adrenal gland, and chronic leptin administration also increases blood pressure in animals. In humans, high circulating levels of leptin correlate closely with markers of sympathetic activation, although this association weakens somewhat after adjusting for adiposity.

Neuropeptide modulation. Several hypothalamic neuropeptides mediate the effects of leptin on SNA, including α-melanocyte stimulating hormone (α-MSH), corticotrophin-releasing factor (CRF), and neuropeptide Y (NPY). In the neural melanocortin system, (α-MSH is derived from pro-opiomelanocortin and acts on melanocortin-4 receptors to decrease appetite and weight. Leptin is known to stimulate pro-opiomelanocortin expression in the arcuate nucleus. Leptin appears to increase renal and hind limb SNA through activation of a hypothalamic melanocortin system

acting on melanocortin-4 receptors (**Figure A35.2**). Hypothalamic expression of CRF-mRNA is upregulated by leptin, which appears to facilitate sympathetic activation of a hypothalamic CRF system. Leptin also downregulates hypothalamic NPY expression.

Vascular effects. Leptin has a number of nonsympathetic actions relevant to the cardiovascular system, although the physiologic relevance of some of these have not been demonstrated. First, high doses of leptin increase endothelial generation of nitric oxide (NO) in isolated blood vessels, although this has not been shown at more physiologic doses. With opposing increases in sympathetic activity and endothelial NO, leptin effects appear similar in nature to the cardiovascular actions of insulin. Second, leptin may also promote angiogenesis, although the mechanism and physiologic significance are unknown. Third, high local renal concentrations of leptin can cause natriuresis and diuresis. Fourth, leptin appears to increase insulin-mediated glucose uptake (insulin sensitivity), even in the absence of changes in food intake and adiposity. Fifth, leptin receptors have been demonstrated on platelets, and physiologic concentrations of leptin appear to promote platelet aggregation with obese leptin-deficient mice being protected from thrombosis. Finally, leptin also appears to have direct mitogenic effects on vascular smooth muscle and possibly cardiomyocytes, so could contribute to vascular and ventricular hypertrophy, as well as atherosclerosis. Strikingly, very obese mice with genetic leptin deficiency or resistance are actually *protected* from neointima formation after injury, and experimental atherosclerosis. The diverse and fundamental actions of leptin on neurobiology, metabolism, and cardiovascular function and structure suggest that animal models with complete genetic leptin deficiency (ob/ob) or resistance (db/db) should only be used as tools for exploring leptin biology, and should not be used as models of diabetes or insulin resistance.

Leptin resistance
Most obese humans have high circulating leptin concentrations. Obese subjects with normal leptin concentrations may be more likely to gain weight subsequently. However, for most obese humans, inadequate leptin production does not appear to underlie

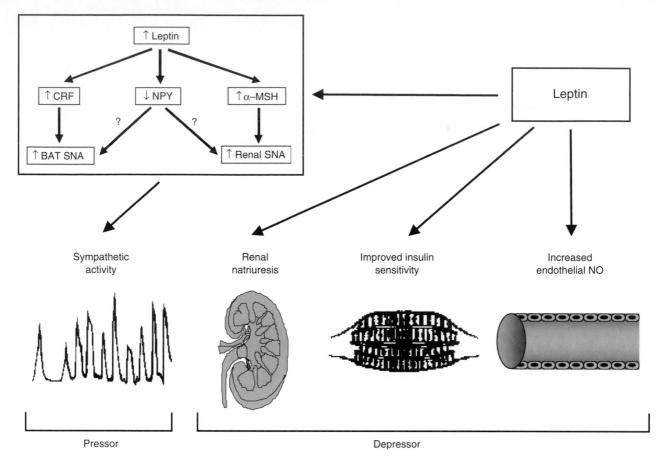

Figure A35.2 Leptin has multiple actions that may increase (sympathoactivation) or decrease arterial pressure (natriuresis, insulin sensitization, and vasodilatation), although physiologically the overall effect of leptin is pressor. The inset panel shows proposed mechanisms for sympathoactivation. Increases in renal sympathetic nerve activity (SNA) caused by leptin appear to be mediated by increased (α-melanocyte stimulating hormone (α-MSH), whereas increases in brown adipose tissue (BAT) SNA appear to be mediated by corticotropin-releasing factor (CRF). The role of neuropeptide Y (NPY) remains unclear. ↑, increased; ↓, decreased; NO, nitric oxide.

obesity. Indeed, circulating hyperleptinemia suggests a state of leptin resistance in human obesity.

Heterogeneity. There is emerging evidence that leptin resistance may differ across species, animal models, and races and spare some actions of leptin. In genetic and diet-induced murine obesity, there is resistance to the metabolic effects of leptin (anorexia and weight loss) with preservation of its sympathoexcitatory and pressor effects. Plasma leptin concentration correlates significantly with muscle SNA in obese subjects, supporting animal data suggesting selective leptin resistance. Relative preservation of leptin-induced sympathoactivation might then contribute to obesity-related sodium chloride retention, hypertension, vascular and myocardial hypertrophy, and cardiac arrhythmias.

Mechanisms. Several mechanisms have been suggested to explain the phenomenon of leptin resistance: (a) decreased transport of leptin across the blood–brain barrier, (b) a defect in the leptin receptor, or (c) impaired downstream signaling in the hypothalamus. The last possibility appears most important. Potential signaling mechanisms include leptin stimulation of hypothalamic suppressor of cytokine signaling (SOCS) proteins, which is preserved in obesity. Obesity is associated with preserved

ability of leptin to activate hypothalamic SOCS-3, which may then inhibit JAK tyrosine kinase activation by leptin. Another potential mechanism is activation of protein tyrosine phosphatase 1b (PTP1b), which also inhibits leptin signaling. Mice lacking either SOCS-3 or PTP1b exhibit enhanced leptin sensitivity and are protected from diet-induced obesity. However, the mechanisms underlying selective leptin resistance are likely more complicated than upregulation of these pathways. In obese mice, there is evidence that only the arcuate nucleus of the hypothalamus exhibits leptin resistance in terms of STAT3 activation. This may reflect relatively easy access of circulating leptin to the arcuate nucleus, with consequent activation of SOCS-3 and PTP1b. If leptin could directly activate other nuclei responsible for sympathetic activation (i.e., in the ventromedial and dorsomedial hypothalamus), this might explain selectivity in resistance. An additional mechanism for selective leptin resistance could be divergent signaling pathways for leptin (JAK, PI3K, MAP kinases), which appear to mediate different actions of leptin on thermogenic versus cardiovascular sympathetic nerve traffic. Further investigation of pathways and inhibitors of leptin signaling should yield novel therapeutic approaches.

Leptin and hypertension

Given the multiple cardiovascular actions of leptin (**Figure A35.2**), its overall impact on arterial pressure depends crucially on the balance achieved by its various effects. Several studies have suggested that chronic hyperleptinemia can increase arterial pressure, renal vascular resistance, and heart rate, consistent with sympathetic activation; sympathetic blockade prevents this pressor effect. Systemic pressor doses of leptin do not produce natriuresis despite an increase in arterial pressure. Intriguingly, arterial pressure is significantly lower in obese leptin-deficient mice than in lean controls. The rare human cases of complete leptin deficiency also tend to have normal or low arterial pressure despite severe obesity, with attenuated pressor responses to sympathetic stimuli. These data support the concept that leptin contributes to the physiologic maintenance of arterial pressure. In addition, the overall pressor effect of leptin suggests that many of the postulated nonsympathetic depressor actions of leptin are perhaps not physiologically relevant at concentrations achieved *in vivo* in humans or animals.

Suggested Readings

Bates SH, Stearns WH, Dundon TA, et al. STAT3 signalling is required for leptin regulation of energy balance but not reproduction. *Nature* 2003;421:856–859.

Fukuhara A, Matsuda M, Nishizawa M, et al. Visfatin: a protein secreted by visceral fat that mimics the effects of insulin. *Science* 2005;307:426–430.

Haynes WG, Morgan DA, Walsh SA, et al. Receptor-mediated regional sympathetic nerve activation by leptin. *J Clin Invest* 1997;100:270–278.

Howard JK, Cave BJ, Oksanen LJ, et al. Enhanced leptin sensitivity and attenuation of diet-induced obesity in mice with haploinsufficiency of Socs3. *Nat Med* 2004;10:734–738.

Minokoshi Y, Alquier T, Furukawa N, et al. AMP-kinase regulates food intake by responding to hormonal and nutrient signals in the hypothalamus. *Nature* 2004;428:569–574.

Munzberg H, Flier JS, Bjorbaek C. Region-specific leptin resistance within the hypothalamus of diet-induced-obese mice. *Endocrinology* 2004;145:4880–4889.

Niswender KD, Schwartz MW. Insulin and leptin revisited: adiposity signals with overlapping physiological and intracellular signaling capabilities. *Front Neuroendocrinol* 2003;24:1–10.

Zhang Y, Proenca R, Maffei M, et al. Positional cloning of the mouse *obese* gene and its human homologue. *Nature* 1994;372:425–432.

Zabolotny JM, Bence-Hanulec KK, Stricker-Krongrad A, et al. PTP1B regulates leptin signal transduction *in vivo*. *Dev Cell* 2002;2:489–495.

CHAPTER A36 ■ ADIPONECTIN

WILLA A. HSUEH, MD AND RAJENDRA K. TANGIRALA, PhD

KEY POINTS

- Adiponectin secreted by adipocytes circulates at levels in inverse proportion to the degree of visceral adiposity and insulin resistance.
- Adiponectin enhances skeletal muscle glucose uptake and suppresses hepatic glucose production.
- Adiponectin production is stimulated by thiazolidinediones [ligands to peroxisome proliferator–activated receptor γ (PPAR γ)] and may be a therapeutic target in type 2 diabetes.
- Adiponectin correlates with high-density lipoprotein cholesterol and has antiinflammatory actions that improve endothelial dysfunction and attenuate atherosclerosis in mouse models, perhaps related to attenuation of the effects of tumor necrosis factor α (TNF-α).

See also Chapters **A34** and **A47**

Adiponectin (Acrp 30, Adipo Q, apMI, GBP28), the most abundant protein secreted by the adipocyte, has emerged as a potential therapeutic target for diabetes and cardiovascular disease. Distinct from other adipokines, adiponectin enhances insulin-mediated skeletal muscle glucose uptake, suppresses hepatic glucose production, inhibits inflammation, improves endothelial dysfunction, and attenuates atherosclerosis in mouse models prone to diabetes and vascular injury.

Physiology

Structure. Adiponectin belongs to the soluble defense collagen superfamily and demonstrates homology with collagens VIII and X, complement factor C1q and the TNF family, which play crucial roles in inflammation, immunity, and atherosclerosis. Adiponectin encodes a 244 amino acid/30 kDa protein that contains two structurally distinct domains, an *N*-terminal collagenous domain and a *C*-terminal complement C1q-like globular domain which has a striking structural similarity to tumor necrosis factor α (TNF-α).

Adiponectin is abundantly expressed in the plasma, ranging in concentration from 2 to 30 mg per dL. It circulates as trimers and higher-order complexes; the state of these oligomers influences their biological activity, such that the higher molecular weight forms are biologically more active.

Receptors. Adiponectin activates two receptors: AdipoR1 in a variety of tissues and AdipoR2 found primarily in the liver. Activation of either receptor enhances the 5′ adenosine monophosphate–activated protein kinase (AMPK) cell signaling pathway, which mediates glucose metabolism and transport, and improves endothelial function.

Insulin resistance and diabetes

Genetic aspects. Adiponectin is encoded by apM1 (adipose most abundant gene transcript 1), a 3-exon gene that maps to human chromosome 3q27. This region of chromosome 3 was recently shown to link with obesity and diabetes. Studies in different ethnic populations have identified genetic variations in adiponectin that associate with disease phenotypes. An intronic variant, SNP276, is associated with type 2 diabetes and insulin resistance, and missense mutations in exon 3 are associated with lower plasma adiponectin levels and type 2 diabetes. A strong genetic contribution to the expression of circulating levels of adiponectin has also been established from several family studies.

Role in insulin resistance. Evidence that adiponectin is required for normal insulin action is provided by studies in adiponectin knockout mice. Both homozygous and heterozygous adiponectin knockout mice develop insulin resistance (especially diet-induced), suggesting that hypoadiponectinemia is directly related to insulin resistance. Lipoatrophic mice are also hypoadiponectinemic and develop insulin resistance, which reverses with adiponectin administration. Intraperitoneal injection of recombinant full-length adiponectin into wild-type mice and models of type 1 and type 2 diabetes significantly reduces plasma glucose levels without stimulating insulin secretion. In these diverse models, adiponectin appears to reduce plasma glucose levels through inhibition of hepatic glucose production, an effect that appears to be mediated by inhibition of gluconeogenesis through suppression of phosphoenolpyruvate carboxykinase (PEPCK) and glucose-6-phosphatase expression. Adiponectin also suppresses fatty acid influx into the liver, which is accelerated in the metabolic syndrome contributing to hepatic insulin resistance and liver damage.

Visceral obesity and metabolic syndrome. Plasma adiponectin levels are negatively associated with all components of the metabolic syndrome: fasting insulin/glucose ratio; free fatty acids, triglycerides, total cholesterol, and small, dense low-density lipoprotein cholesterol (LDLC); systolic and mean arterial blood pressure (BP); body mass index (BMI), waist-to-hip ratio, and visceral fat. In contrast to other adipokines, adiponectin expression and plasma levels are reduced in the metabolic syndrome, diabetes and cardiovascular disease, and there is a strong negative correlation with adiponectin and visceral fat and insulin resistance.

Since adiponectin is an insulin-sensitizing hormone, reduced plasma adiponectin levels in obese subjects helps to explain the well-known relationship between visceral fat deposition and insulin resistance. Adiponectin levels positively correlate with high-density lipoprotein (HDL) cholesterol, independent of age, gender, BMI, and insulin sensitivity. Normalization of these components through diet, exercise, or drug therapy is associated with a corresponding increase in adiponectin levels. Adiponectin expression is suppressed by the same cytokines, catecholamines, and glucocorticoids that induce insulin resistance. In ob/ob mice, adrenalectomy elevates adiponectin gene expression and plasma levels and improves or normalizes insulin sensitivity. Taken together, these observations implicate adiponectin as an important antidiabetogenic hormone.

Human studies. Plasma adiponectin levels are higher in women than in men, and increase with weight loss. Recent studies have shown that plasma adiponectin levels are only modestly affected by infusion of fatty acids, insulin and glucose administration, and acute energy restriction. Thiazolidinediones (PPAR-γ agonists) increase adiponectin RNA expression and plasma protein levels by two- to threefold in either nondiabetic or type 2 diabetic patients, a response that is much more consistent and potent than any other pharmacologic intervention observed to date. Conversely, plasma adiponectin levels are significantly reduced in human subjects who have insulin-resistant diabetes due to a dominant-negative PPAR-γ genotype. Inhibition of the renin-angiotensin-aldosterone system or endocannabinoid receptor-1 blockade in humans modestly increases circulating adiponectin levels.

Vascular function and atherosclerosis

Endothelial function. Adiponectin improves endothelium-dependent vasodilation in a mouse model of obesity, diabetes, and cardiovascular disease. The correlation of brachial artery endothelial dysfunction with low plasma adiponectin has been reported in subjects with diabetes and coronary artery disease (CAD). Plasma adiponectin (high-molecular weight form) also correlates with endothelium-dependent coronary blood flow in insulin-resistant, nondiabetic subjects with no known coronary disease (Hsueh and Lyon, unpublished observations).

Both globular and full-length adiponectin stimulate endothelial nitric oxide synthase (eNOS) activity and globular adiponectin suppress basal and stimulated low-density lipoprotein (LDL)–induced endothelial cell superoxide formation, as well as angiotensin II-mediated apoptosis, TNFα-induced NFB signaling, TNFα-induced monocyte cell adhesion, and expression of vascular cell adhesion molecule-1 (VCAM-1), intracellular adhesion molecule-1 (ICAM-1), and E-selectin.

Vascular smooth muscle function. Vascular smooth muscle cell (VSMC) proliferation and migration are integral processes in the development of fibroatheromatous plaques, as a response to sequester and repair the site of injury on the vessel wall. VSMC proliferation or migration responses to several growth factors [platelet derived growth factor (PDGF)-BB, epidermal growth factor (EGF), and heparin-binding epidermal growth factor (HB-EGF)] in cell culture are attenuated by prior exposure to adiponectin. Adiponectin-deficient mice demonstrate severe increases in neointimal formation and VSMC proliferation in response to vascular injury, and neointimal thickening in response to injury is normalized to wild-type levels in adiponectin-deficient mice after adenoviral transfection with adiponectin vector.

Atherosclerotic plaques. Adiponectin regulates acyl-coA: cholesterol acyltransferase (ACAT) expression and reduces macrophage cholesteryl ester formation. Vascular inflammation not only contributes to the initiation and progression of atherosclerotic plaque formation, but also plays an important role in plaque destabilization by promoting matrix degradation by matrix metalloproteases (MMPs), which initiates a cascade leading to thrombosis and acute cardiovascular events. Human monocyte–derived macrophages incubated with adiponectin demonstrate no change in the expression of MMP-9 (implicated in plaque destabilization), but demonstrated dose-dependent increases in the expression of interleukin (IL)-10 (an antiinflammatory cytokine) and tissue-inhibitor of metalloprotease-1 (TIMP-1).

Cardiovascular diseases

Hypertension. Adiponectin may influence BP regulation in obesity-related hypertension through its ability to enhance endothelial nitric oxide (NO) production. Administration of adiponectin to the obese hypertensive KKAy mouse is associated with a lowering of BP. High salt diet in adiponectin knockout mice increases BP, which can be lowered by adenoviral delivery of adiponectin. In humans, hypoadiponectinemia has been identified as a risk factor for the development of hypertension.

Myocardial infarction. Recent cross-sectional studies have shown an inverse relationship between low circulating adiponectin levels and cardiovascular disease. Studies in ethnic populations indicate that groups with lower circulating adiponectin levels have increased risk of type 2 diabetes and atherosclerotic cardiovascular disease. Furthermore, a recent large case–control study has shown the association of high adiponectin levels with a decreased risk of myocardial infarction in men.

Suggested Readings

Berg AH, Combs TP, Du X, et al. The adipocyte-secreted protein Acrp30 enhances hepatic insulin action. *Nat Med* 2001;7:947–953.

Combs TP, Berg AH, Obici S. Endogenous glucose production is inhibited by the adipose-derived protein Acrp30. *J Clin Invest* 2001;108:1875–1881.

Iwashima Y, Katsuya T, Ishikawa K, et al. Hypoadiponectinemia is an independent risk factor for hypertension. *Hypertension* 2004;43:1318–1323.

Kubota N, Terauchi Y, Yamauchi T, et al. Disruption of adiponectin causes insulin resistance and neointimal formation. *J Biol Chem* 2002;277:25863–25866.

Matsuda M, Shimomura I, Sata M, et al. Role of adiponectin in preventing vascular stenosis. The missing link of adipo-vascular axis. *J Biol Chem* 2002;277:37487–37491.

Menzaghi C, Ercolino T, Di PR, et al. A haplotype at the adiponectin locus is associated with obesity and other features of the insulin resistance syndrome. *Diabetes* 2002;51:2306–2312.

Ohashi K, Kihara S, Ouchi N, et al. adiponectin replenishment ameliorates obesity-related hypertension. *Hypertension* 2006;47:1108–1116.

Pischon T, Girman CJ, Hotamisligil GS, et al. Plasma adiponectin levels and risk of myocardial infarction in men. *JAMA* 2004;291:1730–1737.

Trujillo ME, Scherer PE. Adiponectin—Journey from an adipocyte secretory protein to biomarker of the metabolic syndrome. *J Intern Med* 2005;257:167–175.

Yamauchi T, Kamon J, Ito Y, et al. Cloning of adiponectin receptors that mediate antidiabetic metabolic effects. *Nature* 2003;423:762–769.

Yamauchi T, Kamon J, Minokoshi Y, et al. Adiponectin stimulates glucose utilization and fatty-acid oxidation by activating AMP-activated protein kinase. *Nat Med* 2002;8:1288–1295.

Yamauchi T, Kamon J, Waki H, et al. Globular adiponectin protected ob/ob mice from diabetes and ApoE-deficient mice from atherosclerosis. *J Biol Chem* 2003;278:2461–2468.

SECTION III ■ VASOREGULATORY SYSTEMS

CHAPTER A37 ■ CENTRAL NERVOUS SYSTEM IN ARTERIAL PRESSURE REGULATION

J. MICHAEL WYSS, PhD

KEY POINTS

- Tonic activity of the central and peripheral sympathetic nervous system (SNS) continuously and differentially regulates the constriction of peripheral veins and arterioles and contributes to control of heart rate, blood flow, and blood pressure (BP).
- Nuclei in the medulla oblongata maintain tonic SNS activity based on sensory input from baroreceptors and chemoreceptors, with additional modulation by other brain centers, including the hypothalamus.
- The hypothalamus coordinates BP through alterations in neurohormonal release and by regulation of brainstem cardiovascular nuclei.
- Cerebral cortical and subcortical areas alter cardiovascular function to meet the demands of cortically driven behaviors.

See also Chapters **A38, A39, A40,** A41, A43, and **C154**

Although the cardiovascular system is capable of maintaining blood flow and cardiac function in the absence of any nervous system input, addition of neural control mechanisms allows very precise, short-term (second-to-second and minute-to-minute) cardiovascular regulation. Studies over the last 30 years demonstrate that the nervous system can also contribute to long-term cardiovascular and blood pressure (BP) regulation. In several animal models and in subsets of human hypertensive patients, chronic activation of the nervous system appears to contribute to persistent hypertension and the resulting target organ damage.

The final common pathway for the contribution of the nervous system to chronic arterial pressure control involves the sympathetic and parasympathetic divisions of the autonomic nervous and the associated neurohormonal systems primarily regulated by the hypothalamus. Most experimental evidence suggests the parasympathetic nervous system is much less involved in BP regulation and hypertension than the sympathetic nervous and neurohormonal systems.

Peripheral autonomic nervous system

Efferent nerves. The autonomic nervous system includes sympathetic and parasympathetic divisions and the associated afferent (sensory) feedback nerves that affect each division. Sympathetic and parasympathetic motor neuron cell bodies are found in peripheral ganglia.

In the sympathetic nervous system (SNS), neuron cell bodies lie in ganglia that are immediately lateral to the spinal cord (paravertebral) or anterior to the vertebral column (prevertebral).

The prevertebral neurons primarily innervate visceral organs, including the heart and kidney, whereas the paravertebral neurons project more prominently to blood vessels throughout the body. Irrespective of their location, all sympathetic ganglia neurons synapse with preganglionic neurons that lie in the thoracic portion of the spinal cord.

Parasympathetic motor neuronal cell bodies are located in ganglia that are very close to the organ that is innervated. These ganglion cells are innervated by neuronal cell bodies that are in the medulla (for organs above the transverse colon) or the sacral spinal cord (for organs below the transverse colon).

Afferent nerves. Sensory afferent feedback from the innervated tissue is projected back through the ganglia to the central nervous system (CNS). Most sympathetic afferents terminate in the spinal cord at the level that correlates with the position of the preganglionic cell bodies (e.g., the lower thoracic spinal cord is the usual location of renal sympathetic preganglionic neurons and provides most of the renal "sympathetic" sensory feedback to the CNS). Parasympathetic sensory innervation follows the projection pattern of the motor fibers, and most of it terminates in the dorsal brain stem.

Cardiovascular monitoring systems

An intricate and interactive set of feedback mechanisms continuously regulates flow and pressure.

Baroreceptors. The brain continuously monitors arterial pressure through stretch receptors (mechanoreceptors) attached to vagal and glossopharyngeal axons innervating the aortic arch and carotid bifurcation (aortocarotid or "high-pressure" barore-ceptors). In parallel, blood volume is monitored by branches of the vagus nerve innervating the cardiac atria and ventricles (cardiopulmonary or "low-pressure" baroreceptors). Baroreceptors located elsewhere in the body (e.g., the kidney) serve a similar function. Although baroreflex abnormalities do not appear to lead directly to hypertension, the loss of these reflexes greatly increases BP lability and thereby accelerates end-organ damage.

Chemoreceptors. Chemoreceptors sensitive to vascular O_2 deficiency, CO_2 excess, and H^+ excess are found in the carotid bodies and adjacent to the aorta. These receptors are not as important to arterial pressure regulation as are the mechanoreceptors under usual conditions but appear to play a role in arterial pressure regulation during extreme conditions such as hypoxia.

Osmoreceptors. Osmoreceptors found in several areas of the brain and in the periphery can also modify arterial pressure; recent studies have highlighted the importance of hepatic osmoreceptors in cardiovascular regulation.

Local modulation of neurotransmission. Less conventional forms of synaptic transmission may be important to the role of the SNS in arterial pressure regulation. Kopp et al., have demonstrated that neurotransmitters released from efferent (motor) nerve terminals in the kidney can alter the ability of afferent (sensory) axons to send information to the CNS. Similarly, Kruelen et al., have shown that some peripheral afferent nerves directly innervate neurons in the sympathetic ganglia and give rise to sensory feedback control that does not go through the CNS.

Neurohormones. Other neurotransmitters and neuromodulators released by sensory neurons can have profound effects on the target organs. Perhaps the best example is calcitonin gene–related peptide (CGRP); release of CGRP from peripheral afferent neurons onto the blood vessels, is a potent cause of vasodilation. Recent studies in the rat suggest that the release of CGRP is inhibited by α_2-adrenoreceptor activation. Therefore, the overabundance of norepinephrine in a target tissue could engender vasoconstriction not only directly by stimulation of α_1-adrenoceptors, but also indirectly through inhibition of CGRP release.

Peripheral sympathetic abnormalities in hypertension

Several aspects of peripheral sympathetic function may contribute to certain forms of hypertension with available evidence pointing to two main peripheral abnormalities in hypertensive animal models.

Increased neurons and varicosities. Some genetic models of hypertension in the rat have more than normal numbers of sympathetic postganglionic neurons or sympathetic release sites (varicosities) for norepinephrine. This is suggestive of an increased sympathetic activation of organs and appears to be related to a failure of the nervous system to appropriately prune down the number of postganglionic neurons or varicosities during development. Abnormalities in peripheral norepinephrine transporters have also been described.

Altered sensory feedback. Increased sensory feedback from vital organs or diminished baroreflex control appears to contribute to some forms of hypertension. Irrespective of cause, in several animal models of hypertension, an overactive SNS appears to promote greater vasoconstriction in the periphery. In these models, increased sympathetic activity appears to be

most important during the early phases of the condition and less important during its maintenance phase.

Regulation of arterial pressure by the spinal cord and medulla

Preganglionic neurons in the intermediolateral cell column of the thoracic spinal cord mediate CNS regulation of the peripheral SNS. Preganglionic neurons are directly regulated by descending inputs from the cervical spinal cord, brain stem, and diencephalon, and from peripheral sensory inputs. Under usual physiologic conditions, the SNS is not regulated *en masse* but rather in regional or organ-specific manner and in patterns that facilitate differential responses of the organism to complex stimuli. For instance, during defense behaviors, blood flow shifts to skeletal muscle and brain and decreases to the gut and kidney. In contrast, cooling of the hand leads to blood flow restriction in the upper extremity. Although the spinal cord components of the SNS may contribute to certain aspects of hypertension, most research points to abnormalities at higher centers of the CNS as the primary neuronal contributors to hypertension. The medulla, the most caudal portion of the brain, contains four major neuronal complexes that are importantly involved in cardiovascular control (Table A37.1).

Nucleus tractus solitarius. The nucleus tractus solitarius (NTS) is the primary site of the brain for the receipt of cardiovascular information from the periphery. The NTS is responsible for integrating signals from baroreceptors, chemoreceptors and other "parasympathetic feedback" mechanisms and initiating appropriate responses. Additionally, the NTS receives input from forebrain and brain stem neurons involved in cardiovascular regulation. NTS projections modify preganglionic sympathetic and parasympathetic activity and modulate the release of vasopressin from the hypothalamus. Cardiovascular neurons in the NTS are organized in functionally distinct regions. Stimulation of the middle third of the NTS causes depressor and bradycardic responses, whereas stimulation of the midline region of the more posterior commissural NTS increases BP and heart rate.

Reis et al. demonstrated that NTS lesions result in acute fulminating hypertension in rats and less severe hypertension in other species. Lesions of the NTS in cats and dogs increase BP lability but have relatively little effect on mean BP. However, in rats and, perhaps, in humans, primary abnormalities in the NTS may contribute to hypertension by increasing SNS activity. Lesions of the commissural NTS prevent hypertension in several animal models. Other studies demonstrate that γ-aminobutyric acid A ($GABA_A$) and $GABA_B$ receptors are in separate locations in the NTS, and stimulation of pre- versus postsynaptic receptors may differentially suppress baroreflex responses, contributing to hypertension in some animal models.

In the early stage of hypertension in hypertensive rats and in humans, BP tends to rapidly rise during the waking hours and then fall to approximately normal levels during the sleeping hours. If the baroreflex resets to the higher and lower arterial pressures during each phase, then it may fail to appropriately buffer the rise and fall of arterial pressure during the 24-hour period. Such an effect could increase stress on the vessels during the early wake period, when SNS activity is high, ultimately worsening the hypertension.

Area postrema. The area postrema, which lies dorsal to the NTS and lacks a blood–brain barrier, monitors blood levels of hormones and neurotransmitters. Stimulation of area

TABLE A37.1

MAJOR AREAS OF THE CENTRAL NERVOUS SYSTEM THAT MODIFY ARTERIAL PRESSURE AND MAY PLAY A ROLE IN HYPERTENSION

Level of the central nervous system	Area of the brain	Primary effect on arterial pressure
Cerebral cortex	Neocortex and amygdala	Alterations in arterial pressure related to behavior and emotion
Forebrain circumventricular areas	Organum vasculosum lamina terminalis, subfornical organ	Modifies arterial pressure relative to plasma concentration of sodium and angiotensin II, respectively
Hypothalamus	Anterior and preoptic nuclei	Primarily decrease arterial pressure
	Lateral and posterior nuclei	Primarily increase arterial pressure
	Paraventricular and supraoptic nuclei	Primarily increase arterial pressure and vasopressin release
Brain stem	Nucleus of the solitary tract	Receives baroreflex and related sensory input to the brain
	Rostroventrolateral medulla	Tonic sympathetic nervous system activation; tonic arterial pressure drive
	Caudal ventrolateral medulla	Modulates activity of the rostroventrolateral medulla
	Area postrema	Changes in arterial pressure related especially to circulating substances (e.g., angiotensin II)
Spinal cord	Intermediolateral cell column	Final central nervous system formatting for sympathetic nervous system control of BP

BP, blood pressure.

postrema neurons by circulating or local angiotensin II (Ang II) decreases baroreflex sensitivity and increases sympathetic activity. Conversely, arginine vasopressin binds to V_1 receptors in the area postrema, inhibits sympathetic nervous activity, and increases baroreflex sensitivity.

The area postrema is critical for the development of hypertension in high renin models such as the mRen rat, and area postrema lesions normalize arterial pressure in several hypertensive animal models. The area postrema does not appear to modulate salt-sensitive hypertension in rats. Two forebrain areas, that is, organum vasculosum of the lamina terminalis and subfornical organ, also lack a blood–brain barrier and are able to monitor plasma concentrations of sodium and Ang II.

Rostroventrolateral medulla. The rostroventrolateral medulla (RVLM) contains the motor neurons that provide tonic drive to the preganglionic spinal cord motor neurons that directly regulate peripheral sympathetic nervous activity. Therefore, the RVLM is the nodal point for the regulation of sympathetic nervous outflow. Descending projections to the RVLM originate in the lateral parabrachial nuclei and periaqueductal gray, paraventricular hypothalamic nuclei, and other parts of the forebrain. Activation of most of these RVLM inputs increases sympathetic nervous activity and thereby constricts peripheral vessels and raises BP. Glutamate and American Medical Publishers Association (AMPA) receptors are the primary mode of activation of RVLM neurons, but acetylcholine (ACh) is used by excitatory inputs from the lateral parabrachial nucleus, posterior hypothalamus, and lateral septal area to RVLM.

RVLM drive to the preganglionic sympathetic neurons provides the background of vasoconstriction, cardiac contractility, and catecholamine release that set the basal state of arterial pressure. Increased RVLM firing increases arterial pressure, whereas inhibition of the RVLM or its output decreases arterial pressure. The RVLM (like the preganglionic neurons) is known to play a permissive role in almost any form of CNS-driven hypertension and studies suggest that its contribution is pivotal. Inhibitory

input to RVLM neurons is blunted in spontaneously hypertensive rats (SHRs), and Ang II microinjections into this region elicit greater responses in SHRs than in normotensive control rats. Further, ACh content is elevated in RVLM in two models of hypertension [SHRs and deoxycorticosterone acetate (DOCA)-salt rats]; inhibition of ACh-esterase in the RVLM increases arterial pressure in these models.

Caudal ventrolateral medulla. The caudal ventrolateral medulla (CVLM) is composed of neurons that are scattered in the ventral medulla from the RVLM to the spinomedullary junction. These neurons provide tonic and baroreflex-mediated inhibition to the RVLM neurons, likely through GABA-ergic projections. Although the role of CVLM in hypertension is unclear, the activity of CVLM neurons in young SHR is depressed, raising the possibility that loss of sympathoinhibition from this nucleus may contribute to some forms of hypertension.

Regulation of arterial pressure by the hypothalamus

Medullary neurons are responsible for the sensory reception and final motor output by which the brain regulates arterial pressure but higher brain areas provide the descending integration that coordinates arterial pressure and behavioral responses (**Table A37.1**). A role for the hypothalamus in chronic hypertension has been inferred from experimentation with regional ablation, electric stimulation, and neuronal transplantation studies.

Lateral posterior hypothalamus. Transplantation of the hypothalamus from a genetically hypertensive rat induces hypertension in a genetically normotensive recipient. The lateral and posterior hypothalamus contains predominantly sympathoexcitatory neurons, whereas the anterior and preoptic regions tend to be sympathoinhibitory. In rats made hypertensive by administration of the steroid DOCA in conjunction with a high salt diet, stimulation of the posterior or lateral hypothalamus increases arterial pressure and heart rate, whereas lesions of the posterior hypothalamus reduce arterial pressure. In the posterior hypothalamus of SHRs, imbalances in norepinephrine, ACh, and GABA may contribute to hypertension.

Paraventricular nucleus. Many of the magnocellular neurons of the paraventricular nucleus (PVN) and the associated supraoptic nucleus synthesize and release vasopressin into the circulation. The parvocellular neurons in PVN project nerve fibers to several CNS cardiovascular control nuclei, including the RVLM, area postrema, NTS, and the intermediolateral nucleus of the spinal cord; parvocellular neurons appear to alter cardiovascular function through these connections. Activity of parvocellular neurons in the PVN is influenced by glutamate and Ang II, both of which directly increase sympathetic activity. SHRs display abnormal regulation of parvocellular neurons in the PVN and the interaction between PVN neurons and Ang II appears to be altered in various forms of hypertension. Leptin has been found to modify PVN neuronal activity, potentially contributing to arterial pressure elevations in obesity.

Anteroventral third ventricle. The anterior hypothalamus contains several areas that are important in cardiovascular control, including the anteroventral third ventricle. Lesions of the anteroventral third ventricle prevent the development of hypertension and attenuate established hypertension in several animal models. The median preoptic nucleus appears to be able to affect BP control and is in turn modulated by inputs from circumventricular organs and brainstem nuclei. Other preoptic nuclei regulate vasopressin release and water balance and contribute at least indirectly to arterial pressure control.

Anterior hypothalamus. The anterior hypothalamic nucleus and the preoptic area provide important sympathoinhibitory influences, most of which are mediated by projections to sympathoexcitatory nuclei in the diencephalon and brain stem. Stimulation of these nuclei elicits a decrease in arterial pressure and heart rate, whereas lesions in the anterior hypothalamic area increase arterial pressure. In SHRs, diets high in salt exacerbate hypertension, at least in part by reducing sympathoinhibitory drive from the anterior hypothalamic nucleus.

Regulation of arterial pressure by the basal ganglia and cerebral cortex

Subcortical nuclei that may play a role in arterial pressure changes include the basal ganglia, the septal nuclei, and the amygdala (Table A37.1).

Amygdala. The amygdala regulates defense ("fight-or-flight") responses and has the closest potential linkage to hypertension. Stimulation of the amygdala results in elevated sympathetic activity and a corresponding increase in arterial pressure. Lesions of the amygdala attenuate the development of hypertension in SHRs, whereas stress-induced glutamate release in the amygdala is enhanced in SHRs compared to controls.

Hippocampus. Experimental and clinical observations indicate that the cortex affects cardiovascular function and that several cortical regions are asymmetrically involved. The hippocampus contributes to arterial pressure regulation, in part, through opioid-mediated hypotensive effects. In the rat, 70% of insular cortex neurons display significant responses to baroreceptor manipulations, whereas <35% of neurons in the surrounding cortex show similar activity.

Insular cortex. Most of the insular cortex neurons that respond to baroreceptor changes reside in the right (vs. the left) posterior insular cortex. In the monkey, cardiovascular information also converges on insular cortex neurons, and approximately twice as many of the baroreceptor-sensitive neurons are in the right (compared to left) cerebral hemisphere. In humans, the left (compared to the right) insular cortex appears to dominate parasympathetic control of the cardiovascular system. Strokes that significantly involve the left insular cortex are associated with an increase in sympathetic tone and a decrease in the phase relationship between heart rate and BP. These observations point to the potential importance of the insular cortex in both chronic and acute regulation of cardiovascular function and suggest that right–left asymmetries in the brain may be important in optimal cardiovascular control.

Infralimbic cortex. In addition to the insular cortex, other areas of the cerebral cortex contribute to cardiovascular control. Stimulation of infralimbic cortex (and to a lesser extent the prefrontal cortex) alters arterial pressure and many of its neurons project fibers to the lateral hypothalamus, the periaqueductal gray, and the medulla. These forebrain areas can also therefore influence arterial pressure, heart rate, and baroreflex gain.

Suggested Readings

Colombari E, Sato MA, Cravo SL, et al. Role of the medulla oblongata in hypertension. *Hypertension* 2001;38:549–554.

Coruzzi P, Parati G, Brambilla L, et al. Effects of salt sensitivity on neural cardiovascular regulation in essential hypertension. *Hypertension* 2005;46:1321–1326.

Esler M, Straznicky N, Eikelis N, et al. Mechanisms of sympathetic activation in obesity-related hypertension. *Hypertension* 2006;48:787–796.

Loewy AD. Anatomy of the autonomic nervous system. In: Loewy AD, Speyer KM, eds. *Central regulation of autonomic functions.* New York:Oxford University Press, 1990:3–16.

Lopes HF, Silva HB, Consolim-Colombo FM, et al. Autonomic abnormalities demonstrable in young normotensive subjects who are children of hypertensive parents. *Braz J Med Biol Res* 2000;33:51–54.

Mifflin SW. What does the brain know about blood pressure? *News Physiol Sci* 2001;16:266–271.

Oparil S, Chen YF, Berecek KH, et al. The role of the central nervous system in hypertension. In: Laragh JH, Brenner BM, eds. *Hypertension: pathophysiology, diagnosis and management,* 2nd ed. New York:Raven Press, 1995:713–740.

Oppenheimer SM, Kedem G, Martin WM. Left-insular cortex lesions perturb cardiac autonomic tone in humans. *Clin Auton Res* 1996;6(3):131–140.

Osborn JW, Collister JP, Carlson SH. Angiotensin and osmoreceptor inputs to the area postrema: role in long-term control of fluid homeostasis and arterial pressure. *Clin Exp Pharmacol Physiol* 2000;27:443–449.

Peng N, Wei CC, Oparil S, et al. The organum vasculosum of the lamina terminalis regulates noradrenaline release in the anterior hypothalamic nucleus. *Neuroscience* 2000;99(1):149–156.

CHAPTER A38 ■ ARTERIAL BAROREFLEXES

MARK W. CHAPLEAU, PhD

KEY POINTS

- Baroreceptor nerve endings in the carotid sinuses and aortic arch detect momentary changes in arterial pressure and initiate reflex circulatory adjustments to reduce blood pressure (BP) variability and its adverse consequences.
- Baroreflex sensitivity is determined by arterial compliance (carotid sinuses, aortic arch), ion channels that mediate mechanosensory transduction in baroreceptor terminals, central nervous system mechanisms, and efferent neurocardiac and neurovascular responsiveness.
- The baroreflex resets to higher pressure levels during hypertension, a phenomenon that helps preserve baroreflex buffering at the ambient pressure level.
- Endothelial dysfunction, oxidative stress, platelet activation, angiotensin II, and aldosterone may contribute to decreased baroreflex sensitivity in patients with cardiovascular disease.

See also Chapters **A37, A39, A40, A43, C117,** and **C154**

Arterial baroreceptors are stretch-sensitive sensory nerve endings located in the carotid sinuses and aortic arch that function as arterial pressure sensors (**Figure A38.1**). Afferent (sensory) baroreceptor activity is transmitted to the nucleus tractus solitarii in the medulla oblongata, where the signals are integrated and relayed through a network of central neurons that determine efferent autonomic outflow.

Baroreflex function

Cellular mechanisms of baroreceptor activation. Baroreceptors are activated as a result of deformation during vascular distension. The mechanism of activation is thought to involve opening of mechanosensitive ion channels in the sensory nerve endings (**Figure A38.2**). Emerging evidence points to members of three evolutionarily conserved ion channel families as mechanotransducers in baroreceptor terminals: epithelial sodium channels (ENaCs), acid sensing ion channels (ASICs), and transient receptor potential (TRP) channels. Mechanically induced depolarization opens voltage-dependent sodium (Na^+) and potassium (K^+) channels and generates action potentials at the "spike initiating zone" near the peripheral endings at frequencies proportional to the depolarization (**Figure A38.2**).

Buffering of arterial pressure fluctuations. The arterial baroreflex is the primary mechanism for buffering of acute fluctuations in arterial pressure that occur during physiologic adaptations such as postural change, behavioral and physiologic stress, or changes in blood volume. Increases in blood pressure (BP) and baroreceptor activity evoke reflex parasympathetic activation, sympathetic inhibition, and decreases in heart rate

(HR) and vascular resistance; all of these act in concert to oppose the rise in BP. Conversely, decreased baroreceptor activity during a fall in BP produces reflex-mediated increases in HR and vascular resistance. The baroreflex also influences secretion of vasopressin and renin, which further contributes to BP regulation.

The baroreflex provides moment-to-moment negative feedback regulation that minimizes potentially damaging BP variability. The extreme BP lability observed in baroreceptor-denervated animals and patients with "baroreflex failure," who often manifest significant target organ damage, underscores the importance of the reflex in buffering changes in BP.

Tonic sympathoinhibitory function. In addition to responding to changes in pressure, ongoing baroreceptor activity tonically inhibits basal sympathetic nerve activity under resting conditions and limits release of vasopressin and renin. The powerful tonic inhibitory influence of baroreceptor activity is easily appreciated by observing the profound autonomic changes and increase in BP that occur acutely after baroreceptor denervation.

Baroreflex resetting during acute and chronic hypertension

Rapid baroreflex resetting. After the initial increase in baroreceptor activity associated with an acute rise in arterial pressure, baroreceptor activity declines over a period of seconds to minutes despite the elevated BP. The mechanism of this "adaptation" involves mechanical viscoelastic relaxation and activation of 4-aminopyridine−sensitive K^+ channels. Similarly, on return of BP to lower levels after periods of acute hypertension, baroreceptor activity is suppressed, with a net resetting of the

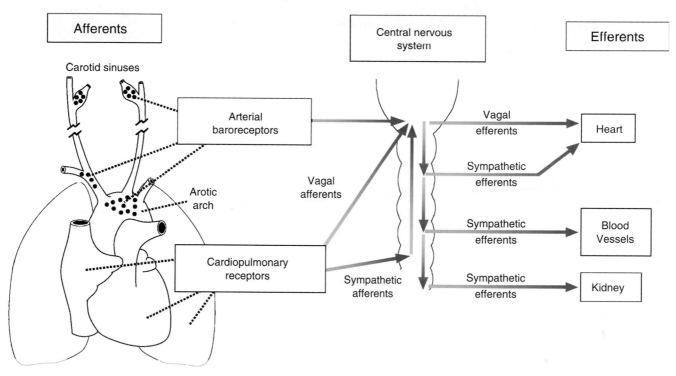

Figure A38.1 Cardiopulmonary and arterial baroreflex neural pathways involved in cardiovascular homeostasis and blood pressure (BP) regulation. Locations of arterial baroreceptors are indicated by filled circles. For discussion of cardiopulmonary baroreflexes, see Chapter A39.

baroreceptor pressure-activity curve to a higher BP level (**Figure A38.3**). This "postexcitatory depression" and baroreceptor resetting is caused in part by activation of an electrogenic Na^+ pump, which hyperpolarizes baroreceptor nerve endings. Rapid resetting does not alter the slope of the BP-baroreceptor activity curve nor does it attenuate maximum baroreceptor activity. Rapid baroreceptor resetting is usually accompanied by resetting of the arterial pressure-HR and pressure-sympathetic nerve activity relations that enable effective buffering of BP fluctuations at the new higher level of pressure (**Figure A38.3**).
Chronic baroreflex resetting. In chronic hypertension, baroreceptors are reset to still higher pressures (**Figure A38.3**).

The resting level of baroreceptor activity returns to near "normal" levels despite the high pressure, whereas baroreflex sensitivity to changes in pressure, that is, the slope of pressure-activity curve, is decreased. Structural consequences of hypertension including decreased arterial compliance and cardiac hypertrophy contribute to the decrease in baroreflex sensitivity.

Neurohumoral and paracrine modulation of baroreflex in disease

Hormonal modulation. In addition to vascular and cardiac structural changes, neurohumoral activation contributes to

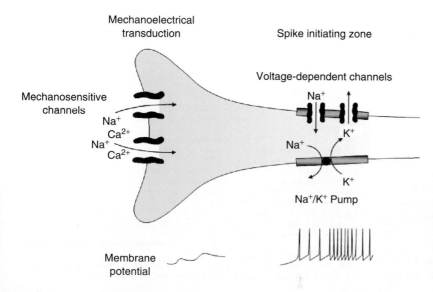

Figure A38.2 Model of baroreceptor nerve terminal. Mechanosensitive ion channels are thought to mediate mechanoelectrical transduction. Opening of mechanosensitive channels allows Na^+ and Ca^{2+} influx and depolarization of the endings. Sufficient depolarization opens voltage-dependent Na^+ and K^+ channels at the "spike initiating zone," triggering action potentials at frequencies related to the magnitude of depolarization. An electrogenic Na^+ pump maintains Na^+ and K^+ gradients and influences membrane potential.

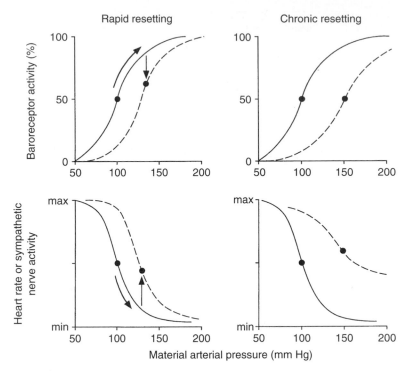

Figure A38.3 Shown are effects of acute and chronic hypertension on baroreceptor pressure–afferent activity (*top*) and pressure–heart rate (HR) or sympathetic activity (*bottom*) relations. **Left:** Initial responses to increased pressure are increased baroreceptor activity and reflex decreases in HR and sympathetic activity. Sustained acute hypertension results in baroreceptor adaptation, a return of HR and sympathetic activity toward control, and a shift in the baroreceptor function curves to the right. **Right:** In chronic hypertension, resting baroreceptor activity is relatively normal, function curves are shifted further to the right, and the slope and range of the curves may be decreased.

baroreflex impairment in hypertension and heart failure. Angiotensin (Ang II) resets the baroreflex function curve to higher pressures *independently* of its effect on BP. This action is mediated in part through effects of circulating Ang II on the area postrema, a circumventricular region that lacks a blood–brain barrier and contains neurons that project to the vasomotor control centers. Central actions of Ang II also decrease baroreflex sensitivity. Aldosterone inhibits baroreceptor afferent activity and exerts central actions that decrease baroreflex sensitivity.

Paracrine modulation. Paracrine factors produced near baroreceptor endings modulate baroreceptor activity through effects on vascular tone or ion channels in sensory terminals. For example, in atherosclerosis and hypertension, factors released from activated platelets and reactive oxygen species may contribute to decreased baroreceptor sensitivity. Furthermore, excessive sympathetic drive in Ang II-dependent hypertension and heart failure has been attributed to excess oxidative stress in the central nervous system.

Clinical aspects

Family history studies. Baroreflex sensitivity is decreased in normotensive subjects with a family history of hypertension. These and other data suggest that genetic factors may influence baroreflex sensitivity independently of BP.

Pharmacologic therapies. Baroreflex sensitivity can be restored, at least in part, by effective treatment of hypertension. Rapid baroreflex resetting occurs during decreases as well as increases in BP in normotensive and hypertensive subjects. The shift of the baroreflex function curve to lower pressures soon after therapy helps to stabilize BP at the lower level. Reversal of vascular and cardiac structural changes with longer periods of treatment further improves baroreflex sensitivity. Antioxidants, angiotensin-converting enzyme (ACE) inhibitors, and angiotensin AT_1 receptor antagonists increase baroreflex sensitivity in animals and patients with hypertension and heart failure, and in aging.

Baroreceptor stimulation therapy for hypertension. Recent studies have resurrected the concept that the baroreflex may contribute to long-term control of arterial pressure and have renewed interest in the use of chronic baroreceptor stimulation for treatment of hypertension. Clinical trials testing such device therapy in patients with drug-resistant hypertension are ongoing.

Baroreflexes and sudden death. The baroreceptor reflex influences electrical properties of the heart through modulation of parasympathetic and sympathetic nerve activity. Myocardial infarction, heart failure, and diabetes are associated with ventricular arrhythmias. Animal and clinical studies have demonstrated that decreased baroreflex sensitivity for control of HR predicts susceptibility to arrhythmias and sudden death in these pathologic states, suggesting the baroreflex may protect the heart from arrhythmias. Therefore, measurement of baroreflex sensitivity may be beneficial in screening high-risk patients; computer-based assessment of baroreflex sensitivity from recordings of spontaneous fluctuations in BP and HR may make this more feasible.

Suggested Readings

Brooks VL. Chronic infusion of angiotensin II resets baroreflex control of heart rate by an arterial pressure-independent mechanism. *Hypertension* 1995;26:420–424.

Brooks VL, Sved AF. Pressure to change? Re-evaluating the role of baroreceptors in the long-term control of arterial pressure. *Am J Physiol Regul Integr Comp Physiol* 2005;288:R815–R818.

Chapleau MW, Li Z, Meyrelles SS, et al. Mechanisms determining sensitivity of baroreceptor afferents in health and disease. In: Chapleau MW, Abboud FM, eds. *Neuro-cardiovascular regulation: from molecules to man*, Vol. 940. The New York Academy of Sciences. 2001:1–19.

Chapleau MW, Lu Y, Abboud FM. Mechanosensitive ion channels in blood pressure-sensing baroreceptor neurons. In: Hamill OP, ed. *Current topics in membranes*, Vol. 59. Elsevier Science, 2007;541–567.

Drummond HA, Price MP, Welsh MJ, et al. A molecular component of the arterial baroreceptor mechanotransducer. *Neuron* 1998;21:1435–1441.

Felder RB, Francis J, Zhang Z-H, et al. Heart failure and the brain: new perspectives. *Am J Physiol Regul Integr Comp Physiol* 2003;284:R259–R276.

Filippone JD, Sloand JA, Illig KA, et al. Electrical stimulation of the carotid sinus for the treatment of resistant hypertension. *Curr Hypertens Rep* 2006;8(5):420–424.

Korner P. Baroreceptor resetting and other determinants of baroreflex properties in hypertension. *Clin Exp Pharmacol Physiol Suppl* 1989;15:45–64.

Korner PI. Cardiac baroreflex in hypertension: role of the heart and angiotensin II. *Clin Exp Hypertens* 1995;17:425–439.

La Rovere MT, Bigger JT Jr, Marcus FI, et al. Baroreflex sensitivity and heart-rate variability in prediction of total cardiac mortality after myocardial infarction. *Lancet* 1998;351:478–484.

Monahan KD, Eskurza I, Seals DR. Ascorbic acid increases cardiovagal baroreflex sensitivity in healthy older men. *Am J Physiol Heart Circ Physiol* 2004;286:H2113–H2117.

Parati G, Di Rienzo M, Mancia G. How to measure baroreflex sensitivity: from the cardiovascular laboratory to daily life. *J Hypertens* 2000;18:7–19.

Persson PB, Kirchheim HR. *Baroreceptor reflexes: integrative functions and clinical aspects.* Berlin: Springer-Verlag New York, 1991.

Piccirillo G, Nocco M, Noise A, et al. Influence of vitamin C on baroreflex sensitivity in chronic heart failure. *Hypertension* 2003;41:1240–1245.

CHAPTER A39 ■ CARDIOPULMONARY BAROREFLEXES

MARK E. DUNLAP, MD

KEY POINTS

- The cardiopulmonary baroreflex (CPBR) arc includes stretch fibers in the heart and lungs that act as volume sensors, relaying information about central blood volume to the brain stem, where signals are integrated with those from the arterial baroreflexes and other systems to modulate sympathetic nervous outflow.
- CPBRs exert potent tonic inhibitory influences over sympathetic outflow and play an important role in systemic blood pressure (BP) and volume homeostasis.
- Important interactions exist between CPBRs and other neurohormonal systems.
- Abnormalities of cardiopulmonary reflexes may be important in disease states such as hypertension, heart failure (HF), myocardial ischemia, and in how the effects of smoking and the aging process evolve.

See also Chapters **A37, A38, A40,** A41, and A43

Cardiopulmonary baroreflex system

The cardiopulmonary baroreflex (CPBR) system is comprised of a set of sensory afferent fibers that respond to central (intrathoracic) volume signals to modulate the outflow of sympathetic efferent nerve fibers, thereby contributing importantly to blood pressure (BP) and volume regulation (see Chapter A40).

Reflex arcs controlling blood volume. CPBRs exert minimal effects on parasympathetic outflow. Myelinated and unmyelinated vagal afferent (sensory) fibers arise from the left ventricle, left atrium, and pulmonary veins, although the unmyelinated fibers mediate most of the baroreflex responses. The afferent cell bodies lie in the nodose ganglia, from which they send projections to the nucleus tractus solitarius (NTS) in the brain stem. NTS activity modulates the outflow of sympathetic nerve traffic from the brain stem nuclei that control efferent sympathetic outflow to the heart, kidneys, and blood vessels. Blood volume, cardiac preload, cardiac output, and peripheral vasoconstriction are therefore under direct control of the CPBR. Nitric oxide is an important modulator of these central projections, because inhibition of nitric oxide synthase within the NTS attenuates cardiopulmonary reflexes.

Afferent fibers. Cardiopulmonary receptors are activated by mechanical and chemosensitive stimuli acting through different sets of receptors. As left ventricular filling pressure rises, nerve traffic in the afferent fibers increases, leading to sympathoinhibitory responses. Therefore, there are similarities of these responses to arterial baroreceptors, both of which are activated by stretch and each results in decreased sympathetic outflow from the central nervous system (CNS).

Sensory receptors

Chemoreceptors. Chemosensitive receptors exert their primary effects during pathologic states, especially during ischemia, hypoxia, and heart failure (HF). Activation of these receptors in the setting of an inferior myocardial infarction leads to bradycardia and hypotension owing to powerful inhibition of sympathetic outflow and concurrent stimulation of parasympathetic outflow, an effect known as the *von Bezold-Jarisch reflex.*

Polymodal (excitatory) receptors. A parallel set of afferent fibers also course in the sympathetic nerves. As opposed to the cardiopulmonary receptors that lead to sympathoinhibitory responses, these sympathetic afferent fibers bring to bear excitatory influences that increase sympathetic outflow. Evidence from animal experiments suggests that these endings are polymodal and respond to chemical and mechanosensitive stimuli. Although these pathways play an important role during pathologic conditions (e.g., they mediate the sensation of angina during myocardial ischemia), the contribution of these fibers to tonic circulatory control is less clear.

Volume (preload) and sympathetic activity
Sympathetic response to acute preload reduction. During either assumption of upright posture or application of lower body negative pressure in humans, blood volume decreases in the central (intrathoracic) compartment, thereby decreasing central venous pressure and reducing right and left ventricular filling pressures or "preload." These reductions in filling pressure reduce the degree of distension of the left ventricle, thereby "unloading" or deactivating the cardiopulmonary baroreceptors and their afferent nerves and causing reflex increases in brain stem sympathetic outflow and vascular resistance (**Figure A39.1**) . At low levels of filling pressure reduction (e.g., lower body negative pressure changes of 5–10 mm Hg), changes in sympathetic activity and vascular resistance occur before changes in BP or heart rate, indicating that the arterial baroreflex system, which controls parasympathetic and sympathetic outflow, is not engaged. The

CPBR is therefore much more selective for sympathetic responses and acts as a "feed-forward" mechanism in anticipation of an impending reduction in cardiac output and arterial pressure.

Integrated compensatory responses. With progressively greater decrements in filling pressure (as with severe dehydration or subacute hemorrhage), the CPBR becomes more fully engaged, but other compensatory responses also occur. Cardiac output is diminished owing to decreased preload through the Frank-Starling mechanism, leading to engagement of arterial baroreflexes and to reflex increases in heart rate. The net increases in sympathetic outflow and vascular resistance protect against systemic hypotension, especially orthostatic hypotension. CPBR inactivation during zero gravity helps explain the transient orthostatic intolerance that is a common occurrence after space flight.

Interactions with other systems
Hormonal modulation. The CPBR is involved in controlling the release of several peptides involved in hemodynamic and volume homeostasis, including renin, vasopressin, and endothelin. The CPBR also is modulated by several other neurohormones. For example, vasopressin has been shown to sensitize the CPBR, thereby augmenting their overall sympathoinhibitory influence. Natriuretic peptides, released by distension of the atria and ventricle, also exert a net inhibitory effect on sympathetic outflow. Atrial natriuretic peptide has other complex effects, including sensitization of vagal afferent fibers and probable neuromodulatory activity at other central or ganglionic sites.

Carotid baroreflex interactions. Cardiopulmonary and arterial baroreceptors send projections to the NTS and other medullary sites and appear to converge on the same synapses, thereby having some impact on one another. For example, unloading of the CPBR improves carotid baroreflex control of BP, with the greatest effects occurring after a certain threshold filling pressure is achieved. The significance of this finding is that arterial baroreflex sensitivity is heightened when humans are in the upright position, thereby achieving the tightest beat-to-beat control over BP.

Pain and other responses. There also appears to be an interaction between CPBR and central analgesia centers, because loading CPBR by leg elevation leads to lower pain scores in response to painful stimulation. This suggests that there is a central convergence of neurons from several different systems. Such interplay among different neurohormonal systems underscores the redundant yet sensitive mechanisms by which these reflexes are involved in controlling systemic pressure and volume homeostasis.

Baroreflex blunting
Smoking. Smoking appears to directly impair the function of the CPBR response itself such that vasodilator responses to CPBR loading are converted to vasoconstrictor responses. This effect on CPBR function could explain some of the deleterious effects of smoking on the vasculature.

Aging and sympathetic activity. Resting sympathetic activity increases with advancing age in humans. This has led investigators to question whether age-associated alterations in CPBR might contribute to the age-related sympathoexcitation present in normotensive and hypertensive individuals. Indeed, vasodilatory responses to volume loading are attenuated in older

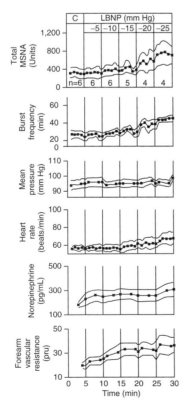

Figure A39.1 Sympathetic response to acute preload reduction. LBNP, lower body negative pressure; MSNA, muscle sympathetic nerve activity. (From Rowell LB. *Human cardiovascular control.* New York: Oxford University Press, 1993:95, with permission.)

people. However, when sympathetic nerve responses have been measured directly in older humans, sympathoinhibitory responses provoked by CPBR unloading are usually preserved. Therefore, the reduced vascular responses to volume loading observed in the elderly are more likely the result of attenuated responses of the vasculature or alterations in ventricular mechanics rather than alterations of the reflex itself.

Aging and ventricular stiffness. Age-related alterations in CPBR function would not be expected to cause increased sympathetic activity unless the sensitivity of the CPBR is abnormally low at both extremes of the relationship between preload and BP. This is theoretically possible given the types of age-related changes in cardiac structure and function that have been observed, especially increased myocardial stiffness. Mechanoreceptors are transducers that "measure" degree and rate of stretch as well as heart rate. A stiff ventricle would be expected to cause a smaller difference between end-diastolic and end-systolic cardiac stretch and would also tend to decrease the rate of mechanoreceptor unloading with each cardiac cycle. Another factor that could contribute to reduced variation in stroke volume is the decrease in heart rate variability (and thereby the variability of cardiac filling time) that occurs with age. In all of these cases, a stiffer myocardium is associated with reduced unloading of cardiac mechanoreceptors and blunting the ability of the CPBR to limit sympathetic outflow. Of note, CPBR blunting during chronic cardiac underfilling and overfilling also would be predicted, as in dilated cardiomyopathies, where increased wall tension and myocardial stiffness result from increased chamber diameter and further reduce stroke distance. The diminished sensory input in all of these situations is in some ways similar to cardiac deafferentation which leads to increased sympathetic outflow.

Hypertension and ventricular hypertrophy

Early changes. CPBR function actually appears to be augmented in the early stages of hypertension in normotensive subjects with a family history of hypertension compared to subjects without a family history of hypertension. CPBR reflexes are similarly enhanced in borderline hypertensive rats given a high salt diet. Saline loading itself augments CPBR sensitivity in normotensive subjects without a family history of hypertension.

Established hypertension and left ventricular hypertrophy. CPBRs become progressively more blunted as left ventricular hypertrophy (LVH) progresses and the cardiac walls become less distensible. Because some studies in humans have failed to demonstrate abnormal CPBR in fully developed hypertension, it is likely that the net response depends on the relative contributions of augmented responses and the degree of LVH present. LVH appears to attenuate the CPBR, possibly owing to altered ventricular compliance, and there is increased CPBR sensitivity with regression of LVH, suggesting that hypertension is associated with functional (not irreversible) alterations in CPBR function. This lends support to the importance of treating hypertension with agents that promote regression of cardiac hypertrophy because normalization of ventricular mass leads to improved sympathoinhibitory responses to CPBR stimulation.

Suggested Readings

Arosio E, De Marchi S, Rigoni A, et al. Effects of smoking on cardiopulmonary baroreceptor activation and peripheral vascular resistance. *Eur J Clin Invest* 2006;36(5):320–325.

Dias AC, Vitela M, Colombari E, et al. Nitric oxide modulation of glutamatergic, baroreflex, and cardiopulmonary transmission in the nucleus of the solitary tract. *Am J Physiol Heart Circ Physiol* 2005;288(1):H256–H262.

Floras JS. Sympathoinhibitory effects of atrial natriuretic factor in normal humans. *Circulation* 1990;81:1860–1873.

Grassi G, Giannattasio C, Cleroux J, et al. Cardiopulmonary reflex before and after regression of left ventricular hypertrophy in essential hypertension. *Hypertension* 1988;12(3):227–237.

Hasser EM, DiCarlo SE, Applegate RJ, et al. Osmotically released vasopressin augments cardiopulmonary reflex inhibition of the circulation. *Am J Physiol* 1988;254(5 Pt 2):R815–R820.

Iwase N, Takata S, Ogawa J, et al. The effects of sodium loading on cardiopulmonary baroreflexes. *Clin Exp Pharmacol Physiol* 1989;15:109–111.

Pawelczyk JA, Raven PB. Reductions in central venous pressure improve carotid baroreflex responses in conscious men. *Am J Physiol* 1989;257(5 Pt 2): H1389–H1395.

Rowell LB. *Human cardiovascular control.* New York:Oxford University Press, 1993.

Tanaka H, Davy KP, Seals DR. Cardiopulmonary baroreflex inhibition of sympathetic nerve activity is preserved with age in healthy humans. *J Physiol* 1999;515(Pt 1):249–254.

Ueda M, Nomura G, Shibata H, et al. Assessment of cardiopulmonary baroreflex function in hypertensive and normotensive subjects with or without hypertensive relatives. *Clin Exp Pharmacol Physiol* 1989;15:89–92.

CHAPTER A40 ■ RENAL SYMPATHETIC NERVES AND EXTRACELLULAR FLUID VOLUME REGULATION

EDWARD J. JOHNS, BSc, PhD, DSc

KEY POINTS

■ Renal sympathetic nerves directly control renin release, tubular sodium reabsorption and arteriolar tone; normal physiologic levels of renal nerve activity primarily modulate renin secretion and sodium and water excretion.
■ Cardiopulmonary receptors respond to changes in circulating volume in the venous circulation and inversely control renal sympathetic nerve activity.
■ The periodic intake of salt and water during everyday activity causes reflex suppression of renal nerve activity, ensuring that extracellular fluid volume (ECFV) homeostasis is maintained.
■ Renal sympathetic nerve activity is maladaptively increased in hypertension, heart failure and cirrhosis, thereby supporting the cardiovascular system at the expense of excessive volume retention.

See also Chapters **A37, A38, A39, A41,** and **A42**

Renal sympathetic innervation

The kidney is innervated only by the sympathetic nervous system with postganglionic fibers arising from spinal segments T_{10-11} to L_{2-3}, with great variability among individuals. Sympathetic nerves are characterized by strings of varicosities along their axons that contain the neurotransmitter, norepinephrine. Renal sympathetic nerve fibers track mainly through the cortex of the kidney, passing in close proximity to renal resistance vessels (afferent and efferent arterioles), and nephrons, especially proximal convoluted tubules and thick ascending limbs of the loops of Henle.

Functions of renal sympathetic nerves

Low-level activation of the renal nerves has little influence on renal hemodynamics, acting instead to increase renin secretion and tubular sodium and water reabsorption. High rates of renal nerve activity cause short-term reductions in both renal blood flow and glomerular filtration but have little influence on fluid balance. In contrast, a small rise in renal nerve activity for extended periods can have a major impact on extracellular fluid volume (ECFV). The actions of the renal sympathetic nerves on these various functions are summarized in **Figure A40.1**.

Tubular sodium reabsorption. Tubular epithelial cells are stimulated by norepinephrine released at neuroeffector junctions, with an ensuing activation of α-adrenoceptors on basolateral membranes. This causes an increase in sodium (Na^+)–hydrogen (H^+) exchanger activity at the apical membrane, allowing sodium to enter the cell, whereupon it is pumped out of the cell through Na–K–adenosine triphosphatase (ATPase) located in

basolateral membranes. Water of hydration follows Na^+ ions through (transcellular route) and between (paracellular route) these high-permeability epithelial cells.

Renin-angiotensin-aldosterone system stimulation. Neurally-mediated release of renin occurs when norepinephrine stimulates $β_1$-adrenoceptors on the juxtaglomerular (granular) cells of the afferent arterioles located at the entrance to the

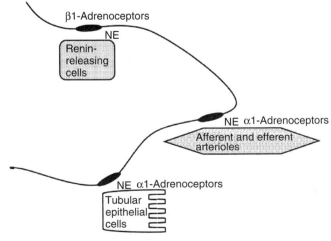

Figure A40.1 The innervation of the afferent and efferent resistance arterioles, renin-containing (juxtaglomerular) cells, epithelial cells of the kidney, and the norepinephrine (NE) stimulated adrenoceptors involved.

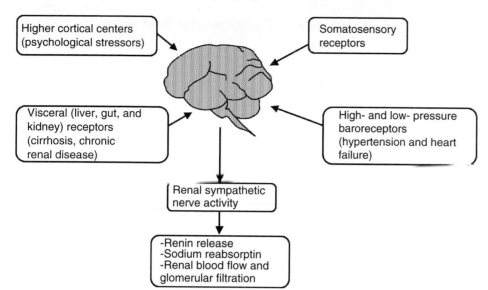

Figure A40.2 Sensory systems providing input to the central nervous system and the pathways of sympathetic nerve-mediated renal functional responses.

glomerulus. The subsequent generation of angiotensin II (Ang II) has both intra- and extra- renal actions that affect renal Na^+ and fluid handling as mediated by AT_1 receptor stimulation. Within the kidney, Ang II constricts afferent and efferent arterioles; constriction of the efferent arterioles is especially important in maintaining glomerular filtration pressure in low flow and/or hypotensive states. Ang II also acts rapidly and directly on proximal epithelial cells to increase fluid reabsorption. Aldosterone release prompted by Ang II, in addition, results in distal nephron and collecting duct Na^+ reabsorption. Together, these neural effects regulate fluid volume homeostasis in such a way that both rapid and/or chronic adaptive responses are possible.

Reflex regulation of renal sympathetic activity. Sensory information from many body systems is integrated in the hypothalamus and brainstem guiding autonomic regulation of sympathetic and parasympathetic nerves (**Figure A40.2**). Afferent fibers stimulated by mechanoreceptors and chemoreceptors in the somatic (muscle and skin) and visceral (gut, liver, and kidneys) systems provide input to the central nervous system and generally disinhibit (stimulate) efferent sympathetic nerves. Higher cortical neurons also provide input to cardiovascular control centers by way of psychological stressors and environmental conditions. The most important regulators of efferent renal sympathetic nerve activity are the high pressure (aortocarotid) and low-pressure (cardiopulmonary) baroreceptors.

Aortocarotid baroreceptors. Stretch receptors (mechanoreceptors) embedded in the walls of the carotid sinus and aortic arch are stimulated by distension (e.g., pulsatile flow), causing reflex sympathoinhibition. Therefore, the frequency of sympathetic nerve bursts approximates heart rate. The magnitude of sympathetic bursts is also influenced by respiration, being larger in inspiration than expiration. When blood pressure (BP) is increased or decreased by pharmacologic agents in experimental studies, the inverse changes in sympathetic nerve activity and heart rate can be used to generate "gain curves" that represent the sensitivity of baroreflex control. As BP rises or falls during normal activity and in response to stressful situations or exercise, the magnitude of change in sympathetic outflow is determined by the sensitivity of the baroreflex as can be seen in the construct of gain curves.

Cardiopulmonary baroreceptors. Stretch receptors within the large central veins, cardiac atria, and ventricles are sensitive to cardiothoracic (central) blood volume. If central volume is increased, central venous pressure and atrial filling pressure rise, stretching the cardiopulmonary mechanoreceptors. Increased nerve activity is then sensed by the vagus nerve with an ensuing reflex inhibition of renal sympathetic nerve activity and a subsequent reduction in tubular fluid reabsorption, resulting in a natriuresis and diuresis. The impact of this reflex arc has been most elegantly demonstrated in unilateral renal denervation studies, where acute saline infusion finds increases excretion of Na^+ from the innervated kidney more so than from the denervated kidney. Moreover, studies in man using lower-body negative pressure to reduce central volume demonstrate a rise in plasma norepinephrine and plasma renin activity and an antinatriuresis.

When there are periodic increases and decreases in fluid balance (e.g., food and drink or fluid loss during exercise), the cardiopulmonary–renal baroreflex arc adjusts vascular tone and alters renal function to the needs of the organism at the time. If there is a rapid rise or fall in fluid volume, the initial dynamic adjustment of fluid balance is through the renal nerves. In chronic situations of volume overload, some of the retained Na^+ and water migrates into the interstitial space, causing total extracellular fluid and Na^+ to increase. In this instance, return to a more normal homeostatic state occurs through humoral mechanisms (aldosterone and antidiuretic hormone) that are to a degree less immediate in their effect. These interactions are illustrated in **Figure A40.3**.

Hepatoreceptors. Receptors in the liver can be activated by pressure and tonicity increases within the portal vein circulation, causing renal sympathoexcitation. This reflex arc assumes added importance in the postprandial state, when there are large fluid shifts within the small intestine.

Somatosensory receptors. Within skeletal muscle, mechanoreceptors are activated by the degree of tension in the tissue and chemoreceptors are depolarized by metabolic and acid–base changes, including lactic acid production. Nociceptors residing within the skin also have an important input. Activation of each of these classes of receptors leads to short-term sympathoexcitation from which follows Na^+ retention. These additional input signals

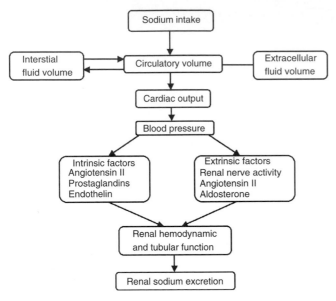

Figure A40.3 The factors involved in the physiologic balancing of sodium intake and excretion. Various degrees of activation of each of these steps contribute to the final state of sodium balance.

interact with those of the cardiovascular baroreflexes; their impact on fluid balance depends heavily on the ongoing input level of the aortocarotid and cardiopulmonary baroreceptors.

Reno renal reflexes. Sensory receptors within the renal collecting system can be activated by increased pressure within the pelvis (mechanoreceptors) or by changes in ionic concentration or composition of the urine passing through the pelvis. These nerves appear to provide neural cross talk between the two kidneys. For example, activation of pelvic sensory receptors in one kidney leads to contralateral renal sympathoinhibition, diuresis, and natriuresis. In this way, should urine flow from one kidney be obstructed, at least initially, the other kidney can compensate by increasing fluid excretion. Inappropriate activation of these receptors in chronic kidney disease (CKD) can contribute to the raised sympathetic nerve activity and hypertension that is a characteristic of this disease state.

Phasic regulation of extracellular fluid volume

Regulation of ECFV occurs in phases, with rapid and slow responses. Acute intake of fluid will result, within a few minutes, in a decreased renal sympathetic nerve activity and raised renal excretion of Na^+ and water. Thereafter, other intrinsic renal mechanisms aid in the mobilization of fluid, including a reduction in intrarenal Ang II concentrations, altered prostaglandin production, and changes in oncotic pressure of the plasma. At a later stage, a fine-tuning of the ECFV takes place through aldosterone and vasopressin-induced mobilization of Na^+ and water, respectively, which may take several hours.

Disorders of extracellular fluid volume regulation

Several pathophysiologic states are associated with disordered ECFV regulation and raised systemic and renal sympathetic outflow, including hypertension, heart failure, and cirrhosis. In hypertension, the increased sympathetic drive may originate from the central nervous system itself, either through higher cortical input pathways and/or from other sources of dysregulated sensory input. Heart failure is a state of systemic underperfusion, where decreasing cardiac output progressively fails to meet the metabolic needs of the body. A major systemic response to this hypoperfusion state is reflex sympathoexcitation, presumably intended to drive the heart and restore output. In cirrhosis, raised venous pressure and reduction in functioning liver mass activates hepatic receptors and in so doing engenders reflex sympathoexcitation.

An important renal consequence in all these states is neurally-dependent Na^+ retention leading to an increased ECFV. In hypertension, this contributes to the persistence of the hypertensive state. In heart failure, any rise in ECFV generally increases preload, which both compromises the function of the failing heart and contributes to congestive symptomatology. As cirrhosis evolves and volume expansion occurs there is also a concomitant decrease in plasma proteins and oncotic pressure, factors which together exacerbate the edema state.

There are two primary therapeutic strategies in these pathophysiologic conditions: (1) reducing sympathetic drive to the kidney and hence any neurally-induced Na^+ retention and (2) use of diuretics and vasoactive drugs that affect renal tubular reabsorptive processes in such a manner that excess Na^+ and water is mobilized.

Suggested Readings

Bie P, Wamberg S, Kjolby M. Volume natriuresis *vs.* pressure natriuresis. *Acta Physiol Scand* 2004;181(4):495–503.

DiBona GF. Sympathetic nervous system and the kidney in hypertension. *Curr Opin Nephrol Hypertens* 2002;11(2):197–200.

DiBona GF. Physiology in perspective: the wisdom of the body. Neural control of the kidney. *Am J Physiol Regul Integr Comp Physiol* 2005;289(3):R633–R641.

Esler M, Kaye D. Sympathetic nervous system activation in essential hypertension, cardiac failure and psychosomatic heart disease. *J Cardiovasc Pharmacol* 2000;35(7 SUPPLEMENT-REFSuppl 4):S1–S7.

Grisk O, Rettig R. Interactions between the sympathetic nervous system and the kidneys in arterial hypertension. *Cardiovasc Res* 2004;61(2):238–246.

Johns EJ. Angiotensin II in the brain and the autonomic control of the kidney. *Exp Physiol* 2005;90(2):163–168.

Lohmeier TE, Hildebrandt DA, Warren S, et al. Recent insights into the interactions between the baroreflex and the kidneys in hypertension. *Am J Physiol Regul Integr Comp Physiol* 2005;288(4):R828–R836.

Miki K, Hayashida Y, Shiraki K. Role of cardiac-renal neural reflex in regulating sodium excretion during water immersion in conscious dogs. *J Physiol* 2002;545(Pt 1):305–312.

Seeliger E, Wronski T, Ladwig M, et al. The 'body fluid pressure control system' relies on the Renin-Angiotensin-aldosterone system: balance studies in freely moving dogs. *Clin Exp Pharmacol Physiol* 2005;32(5–6):394–399.

Wurzner G, Chiolero A, Maillard M, et al. Renal and neurohormonal responses to increasing levels of lower body negative pressure in men. *Kidney Int* 2001;60(4):1469–1476.

CHAPTER A41 ■ SYSTEMIC HEMODYNAMICS AND REGIONAL BLOOD FLOW REGULATION

THOMAS G. COLEMAN, PhD AND JOHN E. HALL, PhD

KEY POINTS

■ Regional and organ blood flows are precisely regulated to satisfy the metabolic needs of the individual tissues, ranging from relatively constant flow to the brain or highly variable flow to skeletal muscle (for different activity levels) or skin (for temperature regulation).

■ Regional blood flow regulation is relatively normal in essential hypertension, with most organs showing a normal flow and an elevated vascular resistance proportional to the increase in systemic blood pressure (BP).

■ Exercise-induced vasodilation is impaired in essential hypertension.

■ The kidney sometimes shows decreased blood flow in long-standing hypertension; a potential sign of a renal defect contributing to hypertension.

See also Chapters **A37,** A38, A39, **A40,** A42, and A43

This whole body pattern of flow and resistance in mammals is determined by regional blood flow characteristics. Cardiac output is therefore the mathematical sum of all regional blood flows and total peripheral resistance is the parallel sum of all regional vascular resistances (**Figure A41.1**). The whole body hemodynamic pattern seen most often in established essential hypertension, at least in nonobese supine humans, is one of increased total peripheral resistance and normal cardiac output. Early in hypertension, however, inappropriately high cardiac output is common.

Principles of blood flow regulation

The metabolic state of a tissue is dependent on the relationship between metabolism and blood flow (**Figure A41.2**). The following discussion travels counterclockwise around **Figure A41.2**, beginning at top center. Blood flow through a tissue is equal to the pressure gradient across the tissue divided by the vascular resistance of the tissue. The pressure gradient is arterial pressure minus venous pressure; because this latter pressure is relatively small, it is often omitted. Therefore,

Blood flow = arterial pressure/vascular resistance

EQUATION (A41.1)

According to the theory of Poiseuille, vascular resistance is proportional to the viscosity of the blood and the length of the vessel and inversely proportional to the radius of the vessel raised to the power of 4. Under normal conditions, the radius is the most important of these 3 factors.

Resistance ∝ (viscosity × length)/radius^4 EQUATION (A41.2)

The radius of small, high-resistance vessels (arterioles) is determined by the tension generated by the smooth muscle in the vessel wall. Tension is influenced by local metabolic factors that are determined by the balance between metabolic need and nutrient transport. Nutrient transport is a function of blood flow, completing the circular and stable relationship. In addition to local metabolic factors, smooth muscle tension can be modified by overriding neural and humoral factors. This is particularly important in the control of skin blood flow and in preserving blood flow to vital organs in cardiovascular crises, such as severe hemorrhage.

Normal regional blood flow regulation

Regional blood flows differ widely and in some cases are highly variable. Many tissues have a blood flow of 3 to

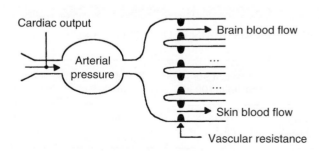

Figure A41.1 Flow and resistance.

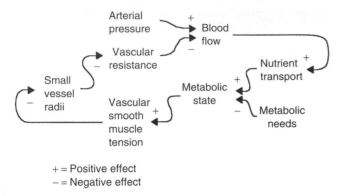

+ = Positive effect
– = Negative effect

Figure A41.2 Interrelationships between pressure, resistance, blood flow, and metabolic state.

5 mL/minute/100 g, a value that just meets basal metabolic demands. In contrast, the brain and heart have flows of 50 to 100 mL/minute/100 g because of their relatively high rates of metabolism. The kidney has a blood flow of 360 mL/minute/100 g, a value that greatly exceeds its metabolic needs (**Table A41.1**).

Cerebral blood flow. Cerebral blood flow is relatively constant because of autoregulation, yet it is very sensitive to CO_2 tension in the brain. CO_2 tension, in turn, is a function of blood flow; increased flow washes out excess cerebral CO_2. This interrelationship tends to keep brain pH constant and, in general, provides a stable environment for cerebral neural function. The stimulatory effect of cerebral CO_2 on ventilation and the ability of ventilation to remove excess CO_2 provide an additional stabilizing factor for the cerebral environment as well as other tissues.

Myocardial blood flow. Myocardial blood flow is proportional to myocardial oxygen use, which, in turn, is proportional to myocardial workload. Under normal conditions, the heart extracts approximately 50% of the oxygen delivered to it. This percentage is close to the practical maximum and is approximately twice the whole body oxygen extraction. Therefore, it is not increases in extraction but rather increases in coronary blood flow that satisfy myocardial oxygen demands during increased myocardial workload.

Skeletal muscle blood flow. Muscular flow is proportional to skeletal muscle workload and generally to cardiac output, ranging from a low of 4 mL/minute/100 g at rest to approximately 100 mL/minute/100 g during strenuous exercise. Because a trained athlete's body typically contains >20 kg of skeletal muscle, total muscle blood flow can approach 20 L per minute in trained individuals during strenuous exercise. Adequate flow delivers enough oxygen, fatty acids, and glucose to maintain muscle phosphocreatine stores.

Skin blood flow. Cutaneous and subcutaneous flow regulates heat loss from the body by metering the flow of heat from the core to the surface of the body, where heat is lost to the environment. Skin blood flow is controlled by the central nervous system through sympathetic nerves. Normal skin blood flow is <250 mL/minute/m^2 of surface area, but marked increases and decreases from that value occur as needed. Even with severe vasoconstriction, skin blood flow is usually great enough to meet the basic metabolic demands of the skin.

Renal blood flow. Renal blood flow is relatively constant and very large, averaging approximately 20% of cardiac output. On a unit weight basis, the kidney has twice the oxygen consumption of the brain but seven times the blood flow (**Table A41.1**). A high renal blood flow makes possible a high rate of glomerular filtration, usually 100 to 125 mL per minute, from a total renal plasma flow of 660 mL per minute. The total plasma volume is thereby processed by the kidney (i.e., filtered and reabsorbed) >60 times each day.

Control of salt and water excretion (natriuresis)

Renal sodium (Na^+) excretion rises or falls in a very precise way to match dietary Na^+ intake; with a half-time of response of <2 days. Renal blood flow, in partnership with renal nerve activity and the renin-angiotensin system, helps to maintain control of Na^+ excretion while keeping the glomerular filtration rate relatively steady. When dietary Na^+ intake is decreased, renal blood flow decreases, associated with decreased Na^+ filtration and excretion and increased fractional Na^+ reabsorption, renin secretion, angiotensin formation, and renal vascular resistance (**Figure A41.3**). The very high and relatively fixed kidney blood flow supports the basic functions of the kidney: filtering unwanted metabolites and controlling Na^+ balance. High, fixed flow may also be related in some way to erythropoiesis, by which the kidney is able to detect with great precision not only hypoxemia but also anemia. High renal blood flow is also characteristic of the early phases of diabetes and in some cases, essential hypertension.

Importance of systemic pressure in regional blood flow regulation

Determinants of arterial pressure. Arterial pressure is determined by the balance between the filling effect of cardiac output and the draining ("runoff") effect of the regional circulations (**Figure A41.1**). Tissue expansion drains additional blood from the arterial tree. If arterial pressure is to be held constant, the blood diverted to the periphery must be replaced by an increase in rate of blood flow (i.e., cardiac output). Several mechanisms make important contributions to this response. Vasodilation itself increases venous return and,

---

TABLE A41.1

KIDNEY VERSUS BRAIN BLOOD FLOW AND OXYGEN USE

	Oxygen use (mL/min/100 g)	Blood flow (mL/min/100 g)	Organ weight (g)
Kidney	7.6	360	330
Brain	3.3	50	1,400

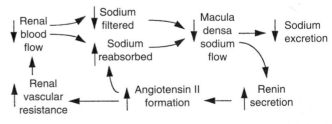

Figure A41.3 Events occurring when dietary sodium intake, and thereby renal blood flow, is decreased.

therefore, cardiac output. Repetitive contractions of skeletal muscle pump blood back to the heart, and venous valves prevent backflow. Sympathetic nervous activation causes peripheral venoconstriction, increased central venous pressure and increased heart rate and myocardial contractility. These factors combine to provide sufficient cardiac output and arterial pressure for adequate regional flow regulation.

When cardiac outflow is inadequate, as in heart failure or chronic hypovolemia, neural and humoral signals lead to enhanced systemic vasoconstriction that overrides normal flow control in many organs. This response initially sustains arterial pressure and blood flow to the brain and heart but eventually, chronic hypoperfusion leads to the syndrome of heart failure.

Responses to exercise. Regional blood flow regulation requires an adequate systemic arterial pressure, as illustrated by the response to physical exercise in patients with autonomic dysfunction. As a normal person begins to exercise, skeletal muscle resistance decreases, whereas cardiac output and skeletal muscle flow increase markedly; mean arterial pressure remains relatively constant whereas pulse pressure increases. As persons with autonomic dysfunction begin to exercise, skeletal muscle resistance decreases but cardiac output and skeletal muscle blood flow increase only modestly. Consequently, arterial pressure plummets, exercise is not well tolerated, and syncope is common.

Essential hypertension

Systemic hemodynamics. Early hemodynamic changes in hypertension often include increased or inappropriately high resting cardiac output, especially in obesity, as has been shown in the Tecumseh and Strong Heart studies; vascular resistance tends to be normal or inappropriately high in proportion to the chronic level of blood pressure (BP). The hemodynamic pattern seen at rest most often in nonobese subjects with established essential hypertension is normal blood flow with elevated vascular resistance.

Regional hemodynamics. In chronic hypertension, regional blood flows are generally not impaired; although blood flow "reserve" may be reduced in circumstances requiring increased blood flow (e.g., exercise). Oxygen consumption is also normal. Cerebral blood flow shows a normal value of approximately 50 mL/minute/100 g tissue in essential hypertension (**Table A41.2**) but coronary blood flow is elevated in proportion to the degree of ventricular hypertrophy. Blood flow per unit weight of heart muscle is normal, with a value of

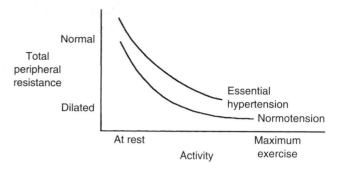

Figure A41.4 Relationship between total peripheral resistance and physical activity in normotensive and hypertensive individuals.

approximately 80 mL/minute/100 g. Splanchnic blood flow is slightly reduced in essential hypertension, having a typical value of 750 mL/minute/m^2 of surface area compared with 800 mL/minute/m^2 in normotensive subjects. Skin blood flow is normal.

Control of skeletal muscle blood flow is for the most part normal in essential hypertension, but several peculiarities have been identified. Skeletal muscle dilates subnormally in response to exercise in essential hypertension, as characterized by the minimum attainable vascular resistance. This impairment is probably due to structural limitations imposed by vessel wall hypertrophy. In addition, skeletal muscle blood flow per gram of tissue at rest is somewhat elevated.

Renal hemodynamics. Renal blood flow has been observed to be increased, normal, or decreased in essential hypertension. These flow data must be interpreted with regard to the special functional needs of the kidney. For instance, dietary protein, dietary Na$^+$, and weight gain all require increases in renal blood flow, whereas nephron damage and nephron loss lead to decreases. Renal blood flow tends to be normal or increased early in hypertension, particularly in obese subjects, whereas flow is generally reduced in longer-standing hypertension and nonobese subjects. It has been repeatedly postulated that inadequate renal blood flow is a pathophysiologic factor in essential hypertension.

Exercise responses. The hemodynamic response to exercise is altered in hypertension. The maximum level of exercise, quantified by oxygen uptake, is depressed in proportion to the severity of hypertension. Arterial pressure is high before exercise and can increase further during exercise. In the presence of the vasodilation defect noted in the preceding text, elevated BP boosts blood flow through the skeletal muscle (**Equation A41.1**), but it also creates a detrimental increase in cardiac afterload that limits cardiac output and exercise performance. At each level of exercise below maximum, cardiac output and skeletal muscle blood flow are maintained normally, but at the expense of a higher vascular resistance (**Figure A41.4**) and higher arterial pressure; the resistance and pressure influences cancel each other (**Equation A41.1**) to yield a normal flow.

Renovascular hypertension

In experimental renal artery stenosis, increased renal preglomerular resistance produces a predictable rise in arterial pressure that is proportional to the severity of the constriction. The immediate response to preglomerular vasoconstriction is a decrease in renal blood flow (**Equation A41.1**). A secondary increase in arterial pressure then follows, which is due to a combination of increased

---

TABLE A41.2

CEREBRAL HEMODYNAMICS IN ESSENTIAL HYPERTENSION

	Cerebral blood flow (mL/min/100 g)	Vascular resistance (mm Hg/mL/ min/100 g)	Mean arterial pressure (mm Hg)
Healthy subjects	54	1.6	86
Essential hypertension	54	3.0	159

renin secretion and renal Na^+ retention, with hyperreninemia having an important early role and Na^+ retention having an important chronic role. The eventual hemodynamic picture is elevated total peripheral resistance, normal cardiac output and plasma renin activity, and decreased renal blood flow.

Suggested Readings

Amery A, Julius S, Whitlock LS, et al. Influence of hypertension on the hemodynamic response to exercise. *Circulation* 1967;36:231–237.

Bevegard S, Jonsson B, Karlof I. Circulatory responses to recumbent exercise and head-up tilting in patients with disturbed sympathetic cardiovascular control (postural hypotension). *Acta Med Scand* 1962;172:623–636.

Coleman TG, Guyton AC, Young DB, et al. The role of the kidney in essential hypertension. *Clin Exp Pharmacol Physiol* 1975;2:571–581.

Goldblatt H, Lynch J, Hanzal RF, et al. Studies on experimental hypertension, I: the production of persistent elevation of systolic blood pressure by means of renal ischemia. *J Exp Med* 1934;59:347–379.

Hollenberg NK, Merrill JP. Intrarenal perfusion in the young "essential" hypertensive: a subpopulation resistant to sodium restriction. *Trans Assoc Am Physicians* 1970;83:93–101.

Kety SS, Hafkenschiel JH, Jeffers WA, et al. The blood flow, vascular resistance, and oxygen consumption of the brain in essential hypertension. *J Clin Invest* 1948;27:511–514.

Ljungman S, Aurell M, Hartford M, et al. Blood pressure and renal function. *Acta Med Scand* 1980;208:17–25.

Rowe GG, Castillo CA, Maxwell GM, et al. A hemodynamic study of hypertension including observations on coronary blood flow. *Ann Intern Med* 1961;54:405–412.

Wilkins RW, Culbertson JW, Rymut AA. The hepatic blood flow in resting hypertensive patients before and after splanchnicectomy. *J Clin Invest* 1952;31:529–531.

CHAPTER A42 ■ LOCAL AUTOREGULATION OF TISSUE BLOOD FLOW

ROBERT L. HESTER, PhD AND JOHN E. HALL, PhD

KEY POINTS

- In many tissues, local regulatory mechanisms match blood flow with local metabolic needs over a wide range of arterial pressures; in some tissues local blood flow regulation serves other functions such as maintenance of an adequate glomerular filtration rate (GFR) in the kidneys.
- Several mechanisms contribute to local tissue blood flow regulation: (i) metabolic factors, including formation of metabolites (e.g., CO_2) or delivery of O_2 and nutrients; (ii) myogenic activation of vascular smooth muscle due to increased circumferential stress; (iii) vascular conducted responses that propagate electric potentials upstream; (iv) release of endothelial-derived relaxing or hyperpolarizing factors; and (v) tubuloglomerular feedback (TGF) in the kidney.
- In most forms of hypertension, vascular resistance is elevated through acute and chronic mechanisms that maintain normal tissue blood flows despite increased perfusion pressure.

See also Chapters **A40, A41,** A61, and A62

A fundamental principle of circulatory function is the ability of each tissue to regulate its own blood flow according to local metabolic and functional needs.

General types of regulation

Local control of blood flow involves short-term and long-term mechanisms.

Short-term mechanisms. Some local regulatory mechanisms can be activated within seconds or minutes to cause constriction or dilation of the vasculature. For example, when tissue perfusion pressure is reduced, there is a transient decrease in the supply of nutrients and oxygen to the tissues and an accumulation of metabolic waste products. This, in turn, causes relaxation of constricted blood vessels and a return of tissue blood flow toward normal. Other short-term controls, such as the myogenic response, also alter vascular resistance in response to changes in blood pressure (BP) and help to maintain tissue blood flow at the appropriate level.

Long-term mechanisms. Long-term blood flow regulation takes place over days or weeks and involves structural changes in the blood vessels, such as thickening of vessel walls and decreased numbers of capillaries (rarefaction) in some tissues when BP is chronically elevated. Together, the short-term and long-term mechanisms maintain the required levels of blood flow to ensure normal tissue function. For example, a high renal blood flow (RBF) is needed to maintain a high glomerular filtration rate (GFR) and special feedback systems are present in the kidneys to ensure optimal GFR regulation. For nonrenal tissues such as brain, heart and skeletal muscle, a balance between oxygen and nutrient delivery and metabolic demand is essential for proper tissue function.

Cellular mechanisms

Several mechanisms contribute to the physiologic control of blood flow in nonrenal organs, including formation of metabolites (e.g., CO_2) or delivery of O_2 and nutrients, myogenic responses, vascular conducted responses that propagate electric potentials upstream, and the release of endothelium-derived relaxing factors such as nitric oxide (NO) and prostaglandins (PGs), or hyperpolarizing factors. Each of these mechanisms plays a role in basal blood flow control as well as during changes in tissue metabolism.

Metabolic control. Adequate supply of oxygen and nutrients and removal of the waste products of metabolism are necessary for the tissue to function normally. Tissue oxygen delivery can be regulated through either changes in blood flow or changes in oxygen loss from hemoglobin (i.e., oxygen extraction). When tissue metabolic rate is raised, a combination of increases in blood flow and oxygen extraction may contribute to greater oxygen delivery. However, in tissues with a high resting metabolic rate (e.g., the heart) the ability to further increase oxygen extraction is limited. Therefore, decreased vascular resistance and increased blood flow are needed to meet the oxygen delivery and metabolic demands of the muscle when it is subjected to increased work load, as occurs at the time of heavy exercise.

When there is a mismatch between O_2 and nutrient delivery and tissue metabolism, various metabolic factors contribute to the changes in blood flow that then match it to the metabolism of the tissue. For example, during decreased tissue perfusion pressure, reductions in blood flow cause accumulation of tissue metabolites, which then dilate the vasculature and return blood flow toward normal. Conversely, increased arterial pressure tends to raise blood flow and decreases tissue levels of vasodilator metabolites which, in turn, causes vasoconstriction and normalization of blood flow. During increases in tissue metabolic rate, such as occurs with skeletal muscle exercise, metabolites released from tissue cause vasodilation and increases in blood flow as well as oxygen and nutrient delivery.

Several factors have been proposed as metabolic controllers of blood flow, including oxygen, carbon dioxide, adenosine, and potassium. Hypoxia vasodilates arterioles, and this may depend, in part, on NO and/or arachidonic acid (AA) metabolites released from the vascular endothelium (see the following text). Carbon dioxide is a potent vasodilator of cerebral blood vessels and appears to play a major role in regulation of cerebral blood flow. Potassium ions are thought to activate inward-rectifying potassium channels (K_{IR}) causing hyperpolarization of smooth muscle and vasodilation. However, no single metabolite can fully account for local blood flow autoregulation during changes in perfusion pressure or during physiologic conditions associated with changes in tissue metabolism.

Myogenic control. Myogenic control of blood flow refers to the inherent ability of blood vessels to constrict in response to increased intravascular pressure, independent of neural or hormonal influences. This response is especially pronounced in high

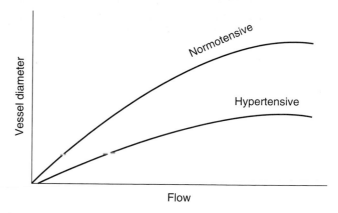

Figure A42.1 Hypertension results in an increased myogenic response. (Adapted from: Falcone JC, Granger HJ, Meininger GA, et al. Enhanced myogenic activation in skeletal muscle arterioles from spontaneously hypertensive rats. *Am J Physiol* 1993;265:H1847–H1855.)

resistance arterioles and involves stretch-induced depolarization of vascular smooth muscle cells (VSMC), a rise in intracellular calcium due to opening of voltage-sensitive calcium channels, and an increase in vessel tone and vascular resistance. With a decrease in intravascular pressure, there is hyperpolarization of vascular smooth muscle and a decrease in vascular resistance. It is unlikely that the myogenic response can completely account for tissue blood flow autoregulation because it does not directly involve changes in blood flow. The myogenic response does prevent excessive stretch of blood vessels when BP is increased and therefore also contributes to stabilization of tissue blood flow. In small (~100 μm) arterioles, chronic hypertension may lead to augmented myogenic responses as a result of structural changes in blood vessels and a change in the intrinsic activation state of the arterioles (**Figure A42.1**).

Vascular conducted responses. There are alterations in vascular constriction or dilation that ascend (i.e., are propagated upstream) from small arterioles to larger arterioles through electrical potential changes in gap junctions between endothelial cells or VSMCs. These "conducted responses" have been shown to occur *in vivo*, independent of other control mechanisms, and allow coordinated changes in resistance in the vasculature. In hypertension, vascular conducted responses are attenuated *in vivo* but their pathophysiologic significance is still unclear.

Endothelium-dependent mechanisms. A major mechanism of blood flow control is the release of endothelium-derived factors that can dilate arterioles to increase blood flow, or constrict arterioles to decrease blood flow. Vasoactive factors released by endothelial cells include NO, PGs, and cytochrome P-450 products. These factors can be released in response to agonists, increases in shear rate, or metabolic changes. Flow-mediated vasodilation is an endothelium-dependent mechanism whereby increases in vascular wall shear stress initiate the release of endothelium-derived relaxing factors, which then increase arteriolar diameter and thereby the blood flow. Chronic hypertension results in impaired flow-mediated vasodilation, which may be due to decreased NO or PG release (**Figure A42.2**).

Nitric oxide. NO, formed from arginine, is a key vasodilator released from the endothelium and plays a significant role in normal cardiovascular function and in pathophysiologic states. Tonic release of NO is important in vascular control as inhibition of NO release by nonmetabolized arginine analogs causes vasoconstriction in most tissues. NO release is impaired

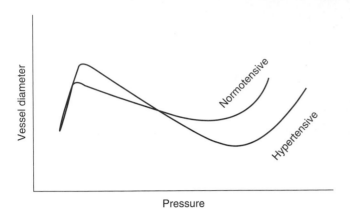

Figure A42.2 There is impaired flow-dependent vasodilation during hypertension. (Adapted from: Koller A, Huang A. Shear stress-induced dilation is attenuated in skeletal muscle arterioles of hypertensive rats. *Hypertension* 1995;25:758–763.)

in hypertension and dyslipidemia due to endothelial dysfunction, possibly through increased oxidative stress.

Prostanoids. AA metabolites are endothelial factors involved in local vascular control. AA is metabolized by three enzyme systems: cyclooxygenase (COX), cytochrome P-450, and lipoxygenase. Metabolism by COX leads to the formation of the vasodilator prostanoids and the vasoconstrictor thromboxane (TXA$_2$). Cytochrome P-450 enzymes produce vasodilatory epoxyeicosatrienoic acids (EETs), and vasoconstrictor hydroxyepoxyeicosatrienoic acids (HETEs). The lipoxygenase pathway yields leukotrienes, which are primarily involved in the inflammatory response. Prostacyclin (PGI$_2$) is considered to be the principal vasodilator released by vascular endothelial cells. In hypertension the elevated oxidative stress may result in a shift in production of the vasodilator PGI$_2$ to synthesis of the vasoconstrictors PGH$_2$ and TXA$_2$. The increase in vasoconstrictor AA metabolites, coupled with a decrease in vasodilator PGI$_2$ levels, may contribute to altered vascular regulation in hypertension.

Eicosanoids. Cytochrome P-450 metabolites play an important role in blood flow control, and may be more important in the vascular responses to hypertension. The formation of 20-HETE in vascular smooth muscle is stimulated by angiotensin (Ang) II, endothelin and norepinephrine, which are elevated in some forms of hypertension, and is inhibited by NO, which may be decreased during hypertension. 20-HETE also plays an important role as an oxygen sensor in the microcirculation, with an increase in 20-HETE release during hyperoxia, which would be observed during an increase in blood flow.

Chronic blood flow responses to vasoactive substances

The powerful role of local regulatory mechanisms in matching metabolic needs of the tissues with blood flow is illustrated by the chronic blood flow responses to vasoconstrictors and vasodilators. For example, Ang II administration may cause a transient decrease in blood flow and cardiac output (the sum of blood flows in all tissues) but usually has little long-term effect on cardiac output or blood flow to most tissues, except the kidneys; the converse occurs with vasodilators.

Renal autoregulation of blood flow and glomerular filtration rate

Renal blood flow. RBF is regulated through a combination of mechanisms including: (i) tubuloglomerular feedback (TGF) and (ii) myogenic control. The TGF system is designed to maintain a relatively constant sodium chloride delivery to the distal tubule. The myogenic mechanism in the kidneys acts to buffer the effects of transient changes in BP just as it does in other tissues. Oxygen and nutrients normally delivered to the kidneys far exceed their metabolic needs; on weight basis, the kidneys consume approximately twice as much oxygen as the brain, but the blood flow to the kidneys is normally almost seven times that of brain tissue. The major function of such high RBF is to permit a high GFR. Therefore, autoregulation of RBF maintains a relatively constant GFR and precise control of renal excretion of water and electrolytes.

Tubuloglomerular feedback and renal autoregulation.

RBF and GFR autoregulation are accomplished, at least in part, by a special feedback mechanism that links changes in sodium chloride concentration at the macula densa cells in the early distal tubule with the control of renal arteriolar resistance. This *tubuloglomerular feedback* (TGF) ensures a relatively constant delivery of sodium chloride to the distal tubule and is therefore directed toward preventing excessive fluctuations in renal sodium excretion (**Figure A42.3**). Under most circumstances, this mechanism autoregulates RBF and GFR in parallel through changes in afferent arteriolar resistance, although there are circumstances where GFR may be independently increased or decreased in order to stabilize sodium chloride delivery to the macula densa.

The macula densa cells sense changes in sodium chloride concentration in the tubular fluid and, through mechanisms that are still not entirely clear, cause changes in the diameter

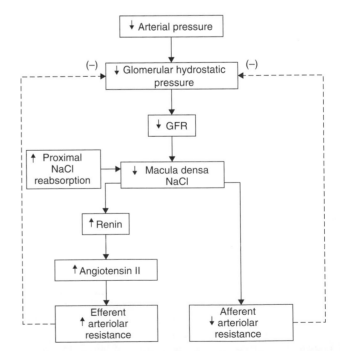

Figure A42.3 Tubuloglomerular feedback mechanism for autoregulation of glomerular filtration rate (GFR) during changes in renal perfusion pressure. (Adapted from: Guyton AC, Hall JE. *Textbook of medical physiology*, 12th ed. Elsevier Science, 2006.)

of the adjacent afferent arterioles. When GFR is reduced (e.g., renal artery stenosis), there is decreased tubular flow rate and a diminished delivery of sodium chloride to the macula densa, which has two effects: (i) to reduce afferent arteriolar resistance and increase glomerular hydrostatic pressure, which then facilitates the return of GFR toward normal, and (ii) stimulation of renin release from the juxtaglomerular cells, resulting in increased Ang II formation and constriction of efferent arterioles, which further increases glomerular hydrostatic pressure and returns GFR toward normal even in the face of a reduction in RBF. Conversely, an increased GFR raises tubular flow rate and sodium chloride concentration at the macula densa, causing constriction of the afferent arterioles, decreased renin secretion, reduced glomerular hydrostatic pressure, and once again a return of GFR toward normal. The precise mechanisms that link changes in macula densa sodium chloride concentration with changes in afferent arteriolar tone and renin release have not been fully elucidated but may include adenosine, AA, metabolites, and NO.

Renal TGF and myogenic mechanisms provide the kidneys with a highly developed process of autoregulation that permits a relatively constant GFR and RBF during large changes in renal perfusion pressure. This, in turn, ensures a steady rate for renal clearance of metabolic waste products despite variations in arterial pressure. There are circumstances, however, in which TGF may increase or decrease GFR and RBF. For example, disturbances that impair the sodium chloride reabsorption in tubular segments before the macula densa increase sodium chloride concentration at the macula densa cells which, in turn, causes constriction of afferent arterioles and reduces GFR and RBF below normal levels. Conversely, excessive reabsorption of sodium chloride in the proximal tubules or loop of Henle reduces sodium chloride concentration at the macula densa, initiating feedback-mediated dilation of afferent arterioles and increased RBF and GFR. Therefore, TGF serves the special needs of the kidneys to maintain a relatively constant delivery of electrolytes and waste products to the distal nephron.

Blood flow regulation in hypertension

In most patients with sustained hypertension, there is an increase in vascular resistance, but cardiac output and blood flow in most tissues often remain relatively normal. In the kidneys, RBF and GFR are often normal despite the elevated BP, most likely due to autoregulation through the TGF and myogenic mechanisms. For nonrenal tissues, each of the previously described mechanisms may play a role in the normalization of blood flow in the face of increased BP. Following an increase in BP and blood flow, the acute autoregulatory vasoconstrictor response occurs as a result of: (i) washout of vasoactive metabolites and increased oxygen delivery to the tissues, (ii) increased myogenic constriction, (iii) decreased release of endothelial vasodilatory factors, and (iv) increased release of endothelial vasoconstrictor factors. These autoregulatory mechanisms work to normalize

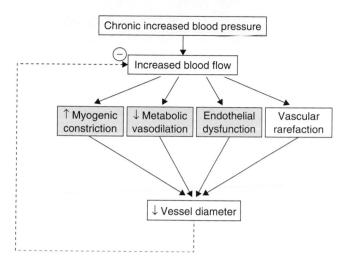

Figure A42.4 Control mechanisms responsible for autoregulation in nonrenal tissues during the development of hypertension. When pressure is elevated myogenic activity decreases vascular diameter. An overperfusion of the tissue also results in metabolic autoregulation to decrease flow. Hypertension results in endothelial dysfunction, resulting in decreased release of vasodilators and an increased release of vasoconstrictors. Long-term vessel structure and density are responsible for the chronic elevation in peripheral resistance.

blood flow over the short term, with structural changes in the vasculature contributing to chronic increase in vascular resistance. Long-term changes in the anatomy of the vasculature include vascular remodeling and VSMC hypertrophy, which reduce vessel diameter. In tissues such as skeletal muscle, there are also decreases in the number of vessels (rarefaction) (**Figure A42.4**). Changes in vascular structure serve to normalize blood flow, tissue delivery of oxygen and nutrients, and removal of metabolic waste products, in spite of elevated BP. A consequence of the structural alterations in individual microvessels and microvascular networks is that blood flow "reserve" may be reduced, which may limit increases in blood flow at higher levels of metabolic demand (e.g., during exercise), resulting in impairment of tissue function.

Suggested Readings

Barton CH, Ni Z, Vaziri ND. Enhanced nitric oxide inactivation in aortic coarctation-induced hypertension. *Kidney Int* 2001;60:1083–1087.

Bell PD, Lapointe JY, Peti-Peterdi J. Macula densa cell signaling. *Annu Rev Physiol* 2003;65:481–500.

Falcone JC, Granger HJ, Meininger GA. Enhanced myogenic activation in skeletal muscle arterioles from spontaneously hypertensive rats. *Am J Physiol* 1993;265:H1847–H1845.

Koller A, Huang A. Shear stress-induced dilation is attenuated in skeletal muscle arterioles of hypertensive rats. *Hypertension* 1995;25:758–763.

Lombard JH. Special issue on microcirculatory adaptations to hypertension. *Microcirculation* 2002;9:221–223.

Roman RJ. P-450 metabolites of arachidonic acid in the control of cardiovascular function. *Physiol Rev* 2002;82:131–185.

CHAPTER A43 ■ RESPIRATION AND BLOOD PRESSURE

GIANFRANCO PARATI, MD, FAHA, FESC; JOSEPH L. IZZO, Jr., MD AND BENJAMIN GAVISH, PhD

KEY POINTS

- Cyclic respiratory movements cause variation in heart rate and blood pressure (BP) at the respiratory frequency.
- The mechanisms of respiratory-induced cardiovascular (CV) variability are mechanical, neural, and metabolic, involving volume alterations, cardiopulmonary and arterial baroreceptors, and chemoreceptors.
- A number of pathologic conditions, [heart failure (HF), chronic obstructive pulmonary disease, obstructive sleep apnea (OSA), and cardiac tamponade] are characterized by marked respiration-induced changes in BP and heart rate.
- Regular use of slow-breathing exercises reduces sympathetic activity, improves baroreflex sensitivity, and is accompanied by vasodilation, BP lowering, and improved blood oxygenation.

See also Chapters A37, A39, and A55

In 1733, Hales first noticed that blood pressure (BP) decreases during inspiration and increases during expiration (*Traube-Hering waves*). Heart rate follows the opposite pattern, increasing during inspiration and decreasing during expiration. In humans, BP varies with each phase of the respiratory cycle in proportion to the rate and depth of breathing, the abdominal or thoracic pattern of respiration, the subject's posture, and the presence or absence of respiratory sinus arrhythmia (RSA).

Hemodynamic responses to variations in intrathoracic pressure

Venous return to the right heart is increased during inspiration and reduced during expiration. In addition to changes in intrathoracic pressure, inspiration compresses the abdominal venous compartment, enhancing venous return from the lower body. Respiration-related changes in venous return lead to opposite changes in venous inflow to the right and left heart chambers, with falls in stroke volume and BP during inspiration and increases during expiration. The BP reduction during inspiration may be particularly pronounced in specific pathologic conditions, especially those in which intrathoracic pressure varies widely, leading to "pulsus paradoxus". Respiratory oscillations of BP are enhanced in the upright posture, where venous return is limited by gravity. At moderate breathing rates, BP falls during most of inspiration, whereas at slow breathing rates, BP tends to rise during inspiration. At respiratory frequencies higher than

six breaths per minute, the amplitude of the respiration-induced BP oscillations is inversely proportional to the respiratory rate (**Figure A43.1**).

Neural control mechanisms

Optimal maintenance of tissue perfusion and adequate transport of O_2 and CO_2 into cells under variable metabolic conditions demands a continuous interplay between respiratory, cardiac, and vascular systems. Respiratory movements and ventilation stimulate sensory inputs that are integrated in the brain stem to modulate sympathetic nervous outflow and physiologic variability in the cardiovascular (CV) system.

Baroreflexes. In animal models, the effects of respiration on heart rate and BP are dependent on neural control mechanisms. In healthy humans, RSA originates from a direct effect of respiratory oscillations on medullary neuron firing rates, which determine sympathetic outflow to the heart. BP changes secondary to respiratory movements influence heart rate through the arterial baroreflex as suggested by the observation that the arterial baroreflex input–output relationship, which is not constant during the respiratory cycle, is affected by inputs from the cardiopulmonary stretch receptors. This implies that baroreflex sensitivity varies as a function of the respiratory phase and is enhanced during expiration, at least at lower breathing rates. In humans with cardiac or pulmonary disease, neural control is often altered or absent.

The heart and peripheral vessels are importantly modulated by central respiratory influences and by reflexes originating from

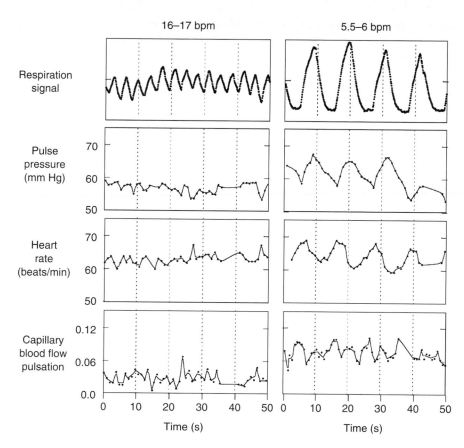

Figure A43.1 Acute effects of different breathing rates. Fluctuations in pulse pressure, heart rate, and capillary blood flow were monitored non-invasively in a normotensive subject. Synchronization of changes in pulse pressure and heart rate with the respiration signal occurs along with increased amplitude of changes at slow breathing. The trend toward opposite changes in pulse pressure and heart rate is probably owing to baroreflex influences. The capillary blood flow pulsations (derived from analysis of skin laser Doppler signal) increase considerably during slow breathing. Chronic effects differ in that BP falls as the result of reduction in sympathetic outflow that has been entrained by the slow breathing exercise. bpm, breaths per minute; beats/min, beats per minute; BP, blood pressure.

cardiopulmonary stretch receptors and arterial baroreceptors, leading to respiratory-related changes in heart rate, sympathetic activity, and total peripheral resistance (**Figure A43.2**). It has also been shown that the neural effects of cyclic variations in respiratory activity may influence the afferent signals arising from other peripheral vascular receptors and directed to the central nervous system (CNS).

Chemoreceptors. Blood gas changes have both a direct action on peripheral vascular resistance and a reflex effect on the heart and peripheral circulation through changes in peripheral

arterial chemoreceptor activity. The cardiopulmonary reflex and local stretch of the sinus node (responsible for a change in the spontaneous depolarization rate of cardiac pacemaker cells) interact with respiratory-related oscillations in $PaCO_2$ (and arterial pH) characterized by a time constant longer than normal breathing.

Syndromes of disordered breathing

Changes in respiration characterize a number of pathologic conditions in humans, ranging from chronic obstructive pulmonary

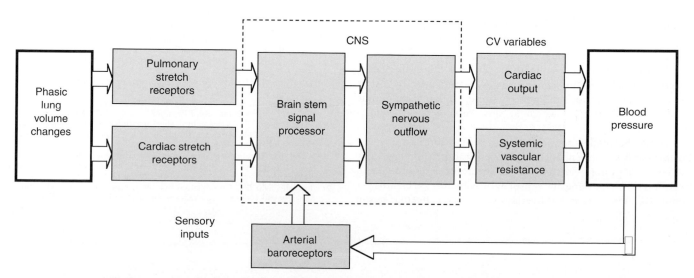

Figure A43.2 Schematic illustrating the modulating effects of phase lung volume changes on BP, with focus on reflex mechanisms. CNS, central nervous system; CV, cardiovascular; BP, blood pressure.

disease to chronic heart failure (HF) and obstructive sleep apnea (OSA). Under these conditions, changes in the features of phasic breathing may affect cardiac and vascular function, and thereby contribute to CV risk.

Cheyne-stokes respiration. In patients with severe HF, there is considerable variation in respiratory rate, including periods of apnea. There are also marked periodic swings in BP synchronous with the periodic breathing pattern of Cheyne-Stokes respiration. This syndrome has been shown to carry an adverse prognosis.

Obstructive sleep apnea syndrome. Recurrent episodes of upper airway obstruction during sleep lead to sleep fragmentation, arterial blood oxygen desaturation, chemoreflex stimulation, reduction in arterial baroreflex sensitivity, increase in sympathetic neural activity, and increased BP. All these changes may contribute to the increased rate of CV complications in OSA patients. In severe OSA, assessing the transfer function between changes in arterial oxygen saturation and the associated BP swings may help in quantifying the increase in CV risk.

Pulsus paradoxus. An exaggerated reduction in the amplitude of the arterial pulse during inspiration (a systolic BP decrease exceeding 12 mm Hg) is observed in cases of severely impaired cardiac filling or exaggerated swings in intrathoracic pressure. This condition, known as *pulsus paradoxus,* is an important physical finding of cardiac tamponade and results from the marked inspiratory decline of left ventricular stroke volume owing to a markedly decreased end-diastolic volume. Owing to the increased intrapericardial pressure, the intraventricular septum shifts toward the left ventricle during inspiration, further decreasing left ventricular preload in addition to the expected reduction in pulmonary venous return that occurs during this phase of breathing. Other clinical conditions associated with pulsus paradoxus are severe asthma, chronic obstructive pulmonary disease, and more rarely, constrictive pericarditis, pulmonary embolism, pregnancy, marked obesity, and partial obstruction of the superior vena cava.

Slow breathing and cardiovascular control mechanisms

Respiratory-induced reflex modulation of sympathetic activity and peripheral resistance can be affected by breathing rate. Reducing the breathing rate (from 15–20 to 6–10 breaths/minute) increases tidal volume while maintaining minute ventilation. There is increased cardiopulmonary stretch–receptor stimulation, which in turn reduces sympathetic efferent fiber discharge, resulting in vasodilation. This process is accompanied by a shift from smaller-amplitude "thoracic breathing" to larger-amplitude "abdominal breathing;" which at slow rates is more energy-efficient.

Arterial baroreflex sensitivity at breathing rates of 3 to 12 breaths per minute is enhanced during expiration; this expiratory enhancement is not evident at higher breathing rates. Of special interest is slow breathing at a rate of approximately six breaths per minute (0.1 Hz), a rate that overlays spontaneous fluctuations in sympathetic neural traffic and peripheral vascular tone. Breathing at 0.1 Hz (i.e., once every 10 seconds) appears to enhance and further synchronize spontaneous BP oscillations at this frequency, known as *Mayer waves.* Breathing at very low frequencies (slower than four breaths/minute) is usually inconvenient and is associated with a drop in Po_2 and an increase in Pco_2, which activate chemoreceptors to accelerate the breathing rate.

Therapeutic effects of slow breathing

Syndromes characterized by systemic vasoconstriction can in theory be improved by using slow breathing techniques to reduce sympathetic outflow and allow systemic vasodilation.

Blood pressure lowering. Slow breathing exercises can be performed without assistance ("yoga breathing") or can be performed with assistance from a device that guides breathing. Device-guided slow breathing (RESPeRATE used for 15 minutes daily) has been demonstrated in small studies to reduce systolic BP by 5 to 10 mm Hg and has been approved for use as an adjunct to lifestyle modifications and drug therapy in hypertensive patients. The clinical impact of different breathing patterns (inspiration/expiration ratio, amount of respiratory effort) and the effects of differences in patient's compliance are under investigation.

Other benefits. Slow breathing treatment also has potential applications in other areas of CV medicine, especially as a non-pharmacologic approach to aid patients with HF. In these patients, slow (and deep) breathing may optimize respiratory effort and increase blood O_2 saturation. A slow breathing–induced improvement in blood oxygenation, accompanied by a BP reduction, has also been shown to occur in healthy subjects acutely exposed to hypobaric hypoxia at high altitude.

Suggested Readings

Bernardi L, Spadaccini G, Bellowon J, et al. Effect of breathing rate on oxygen saturation and exercise performance in chronic heart failure. *Lancet* 1998; 351:1308–1311.

Castiglioni P, Bonsignore MR, Insalaco G, et al. Signal processing procedures for the evaluation of the cardiovascular effects in the obstructive sleep apnea syndrome. *Comput Cardiol* 2001;28:221–224.

Daly M de B. Interactions between respiration and circulation. In: Cheniack NS, Widdicombe JG, eds. *Handbook of physiology.* Bethesda: American Physiological Society, 1986:529–594.

Eckberg DL, Nerhed C, Wallyn G. Respiratory modulation of muscle sympathetic and vagal cardiac outflow in man. *J Physiol* 1985;365:181–196.

Eckberg DL, Orshan CR. Respiratory and baroreceptor reflex interactions in man. *J Clin Invest* 1977;59:780–785.

Gottlieb Tirala L. *The cure of high blood pressure by respiratory exercises.* New York: Westerman Inc., 1936.

Hirsch JA, Bishop B. Respiratory sinus arrhythmia in humans: how breathing pattern modulates heart rate. *Am J Physiol* 1981;241:H620–H629.

Parati G, Carretta R. Device-guided slow breathing as a non-pharmacological approach to antihypertensive treatment: efficacy, problems and perspectives. *J Hypertens* 2007;25:57–61.

Pinski MR. Cardiopulmonary interactions associated with airflow obstruction. In: Hall JB, Corbridge TC, Rodrigo C, et al. eds. *Acute asthma—assessment and management.* New York: McGraw-Hill, 2000:105–123.

Triedman JK, Saul JP. BP modulation by central venous pressure and respiration. Buffering effects of heart rate reflexes. *Circulation* 1994;89:169–179.

CHAPTER A44 ■ PULSATILE BLOOD FLOW AND SHEAR STRESS

MICHEL E. SAFAR, MD AND GARY F. MITCHELL, MD

KEY POINTS

- In contrast to diastolic or mean blood pressure (BP), systolic and pulse pressures are not constant along the arterial tree.
- In the central compartment, cyclic (pulsatile) blood flow is the most prominent feature. In the downstream microcirculation, pulsation is "damped" and blood flow is more constant.
- Arterial pressure gradients are affected by cyclic changes in flow along an artery and should be expressed as values that oscillate around a mean.
- Physical forces transduced by deformation of endothelial cell cytoskeletons ("mechanotransduction") change endothelial cell structure and function.

See also Chapters **A45, A58,** A59, **C112,** and **C146**

The arterial system includes two different functional compartments: (i) large central arteries and (ii) small peripheral arterioles and capillaries. In the central compartment, cyclic (pulsatile) blood flow is the most prominent feature. In the downstream microcirculation, pulsation is "damped" and blood flow is more constant. Pressure and flow in the second compartment is very difficult to measure because of the small size of vessels. In contrast, in the first compartment, although blood flow is higher and easier to determine, the pulsatile nature of the flow requires a series of assumptions in order to obtain a clinically relevant variable to be used in clinical investigations. These assumptions have distinct limitations that have in turn limited the study of pulsatile hemodynamics. For example, cardiac output (or mean blood flow) is commonly reported whereas cardiac stroke volume (an index of pulsatile flow) is not. Using mean flow data ignores critical associations of blood flow in conduit vessels together with their associations with endothelial function and shear stress.

Poiseuille's law and the circulation

Theory. In almost all studies of the interaction between blood flow and the vessel wall, either *in vitro* or *in vivo*, the tangential force (τ) on a vessel is calculated on the basis of Poiseuille's law. This force is usually derived from the measured steady flow q, the lumen radius r and the medium viscosity η according to the equation: $\tau = 4\eta q/\pi r^3$. In clinical studies, shear stress calculated from whole blood viscosity and shear rate (γ) is estimated from the measured blood flow velocity and the internal diameter of the artery, according to the equation: $\gamma = 8v_m/d$, where v_m is the

mean center-line flow velocity of the blood and d the end-diastolic internal arterial diameter.

Limitations. Although shear stress calculated as described in the preceding text might hold *in vitro* (provided that the conditions met Poiseuille's law), this ideal cannot be achieved in arteries *in vivo*. Instead, the presence of non-Newtonian fluids, distensible vessels, varying flow rates and velocities, and nonlaminar flow due to short entrance lengths are significant considerations. Acceleration and deceleration of pulsatile blood flow, for example, adds inertial forces to the constant kinetic energy of steady motion. Pressure and flow waves also change in size and shape as they travel through the circulatory system, and the diameter of vessels varies with time throughout the cardiac cycle. Therefore, meaningful analysis of pulsatile flow must take into consideration a wide variety of factors that are absent in variables derived from steady flow parameters.

Pulsatility and variations in pressure gradients

When blood flow velocity is measured continuously in the femoral artery or the ascending aorta, peak flow velocity precedes the peak pressure, although the increase in flow starts more or less synchronously with the pressure rise (**Figure A44.1**). At first approximation, this aspect would appear to violate the laws of inertia but the paradox was resolved by McDonald, who realized that the pressure gradient along the artery determines pulsatile flow just as it determines steady-state flow in the Poiseuille equation. The pressure gradient is usually measured by recording the pressure at two sites a short distance apart along an artery and subtracting the pressure at the downstream site from the

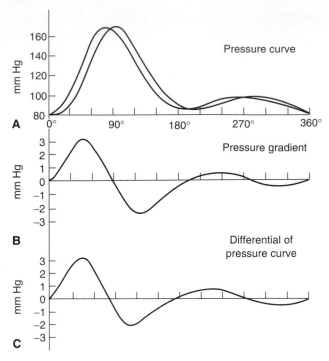

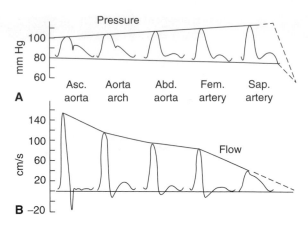

Figure A44.1 A diagram that shows how a traveling pressure wave creates an oscillatory pressure gradient. **A:** Two pressure waves recorded a short distance apart in the femoral artery of a dog. The downstream wave is identical to the upstream one. **B:** The pressure gradient (mm Hg/cm) derived by subtracting the pressure at the downstream site from that at the upstream one at 15-degree intervals and dividing by the distance between recording sites. (It should be noted that this gives a gradient opposite in sign to the usual mathematical convention for slopes). **C:** The derivative with respect to time of the upstream pressure wave (dp/dt). The form of this curve and that of the pressure gradient [which in the limiting case of a very small interval is the derivative with respect of distance (dp/dz)] is very similar. In this case, the only difference is due to the transmission time over the interval necessary to determine the gradient. The vertical lines demonstrate the small phase differences that this creates. In the presence of the usual distortion of the wave as it travels, this similarity between time derivative no longer holds with any precision.

Figure A44.2 Diagrammatic representation of change in pressure (**A**) and flow waves (**B**) between the ascending aorta and peripheral arteries. There is a progressive rise in amplitude of the pressure pulse and decrease in amplitude of the flow pulse. asc, ascending; abd, abdominal; fem, femoral; sap, saphenous.

upstream pressure at each moment (**Figure A44.1A**). The crest of the pressure wave reaches the upstream recording site a short time before it reaches the downstream site, so the upstream pressure peak is momentarily higher than the corresponding downstream site; this yields a pressure gradient sloping downstream. A short time later, however, when the pressure wave crest reaches the downstream site, the pressure gradient now slopes in the opposite direction. Any secondary 'bumps' in the waveform cause similar oscillations.

The resultant pressure gradient, therefore, is one that oscillates about a mean, as shown in **Figure A44.1B**. As there are traveling waves in all arteries, all arterial pressure gradients are of this form. This pressure gradient is directly related to changes in momentary flow, whereas the gradient and flow always occur synchronously in Poiseuille flow. Such observations have led to reexploration of the relationship between central and peripheral pressure and flow in humans.

Pulse wave transmission in humans

In contrast to diastolic or mean blood pressure (BP), systolic and pulse pressures are not constant along the arterial tree. The development of Doppler ultrasound allows flow pulses to be

recorded noninvasively from the great vessels of the chest and abdomen and peripheral arteries in humans. A diagrammatic comparison of the differences in arterial pressure and flow waves as the pulsations travel away from the heart is presented in **Figure A44.2**. In general, mean pressure falls slightly and pulse pressure increases (due to increased systolic pressure). By the time it reaches the iliac (saphenous) artery, pulse pressure is often double that at the root of the aorta. Flow oscillation, in contrast, diminishes markedly. Such behavior can only be explained by the presence of closed-end type reflections from the small peripheral vessels; in the absence of any reflections, damping would cause parallel decreases in pressure and flow oscillations. Ultimately, most of the damping of pressure oscillations is dependent the smallest arteries and largest arterioles, as indicated by the broken lines (**Figure A44.2**). The increase in the ratio of the pulsatile amplitude to the corresponding flow amplitude is the result of increased impedance of the vessel.

Pulse wave analysis

Fourier analysis. The oscillatory nature of large arterial pressure and flow and the information contained in the wave shapes can be reduced by Fourier analysis; after the mean value of the wave is determined, its shape can be described by a series of sine waves (harmonics). Further mathematical analyses are also possible. The technique to derive a series of sine waves from a given pressure or flow signal is mathematically simple and unique and the cumbersome calculation has been considerably improved by digital computers. An example of a Fourier analysis of an aortic pressure wave is given briefly in **Figure A44.3**. Similar calculations can be made with flow. The harmonic zero reflects the mean value, which represents a sine wave with an infinite period. The frequency of the first harmonic (f) is heavily dependent on heart rate, and higher harmonics have a frequency of $2f$, $3f$, and so forth. When all the sine waves are resolved, their addition leads to the mathematical reconstruction of the pulse wave signal.

Arterial impedance (pressure–flow) characteristics. Evaluations of pulsatile pressure–flow relations in the central aorta provide a comprehensive assessment of the steady flow and pulsatile loading characteristics of the arterial system. In recent

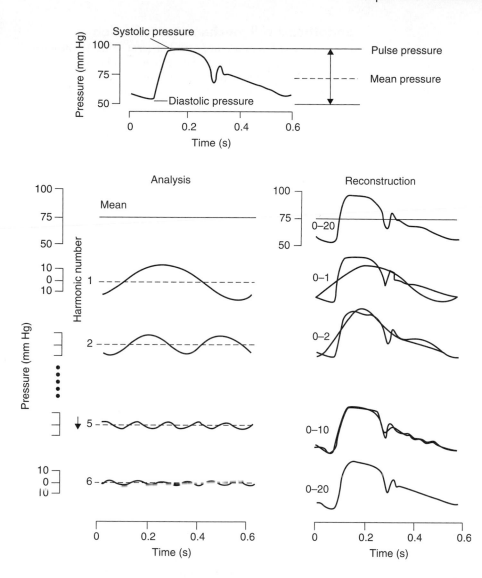

Figure A44.3 Blood pressure curve: pulsatile versus steady component; definition from Fourier analysis (see **text**).

years, techniques to accurately assess velocity profiles in arterioles have used fluorescently labeled particles as flow tracers. In large arteries, ultrasonography or magnetic resonance imaging (MRI) can be used.

Technical aspects. Pressure waveforms obtained by tonometry waveforms are signal-averaged using the electrocardiogram (ECG) as a fiducial point. The averaged systolic and diastolic cuff pressures are used to calibrate the peak and trough, respectively, of the signal-averaged brachial pressure waveform. Mean arterial pressure is calculated digitally by integrating the calibrated brachial pressure waveform. Diastolic and mean brachial pressures are then used to calibrate the carotid, radial, and femoral pressure tracings. Pulse wave velocity to each peripheral site (brachial, radial, and femoral) is then calculated from the delay between the appearance of the pressure waveform foot in the carotid and peripheral sites. The inflection point, t_i (**Figure A44.4**), between the peak of the forward pressure wave and the foot of the reflected wave is identified from the calibrated carotid pressure waveform (**Figure A44.4**). The time delay from the foot of the carotid waveform (t_{foot}) to the inflection point is calculated as a measure of the round-trip time between the central aorta and the dominant reflecting site. Left ventricular flow velocity is calculated by spectral analysis of the digitized broadband Doppler audio signal. Spectra are signal-averaged using the ECG as a fiducial point. The leading edge of the averaged spectral envelope is traced to provide a signal-averaged flow velocity waveform. The diameter of the left ventricular outflow tract from trailing edge to leading edge is measured, and the orifice area calculated assuming a circular orifice. Each point on the flow velocity waveform is multiplied by orifice area to generate a volume flow waveform.

Derived variables. Impedance is a term that relates changes in pressure to corresponding changes in arterial flow. Characteristic impedance (Z_c) can be estimated in the time domain as shown in **Figure A44.4**. When pressure waveforms are decomposed into forward (P_f) and backward (P_b or reflected) waves in the time domain, their ratio (P_b/P_f) is an index of global wave reflection.

Arterial shear stress

The pressure pulse induces distension of the artery wall, resulting in mainly radial and circumferential wall strain, (the increase in diameter and cross-sectional area in peak systole relative to end-diastole, **Figure A44.2**). The tangential stress (or wall shear stress) is the product of wall shear rate and blood viscosity, with wall shear rate being defined as the radial derivative of blood flow velocity at the wall.

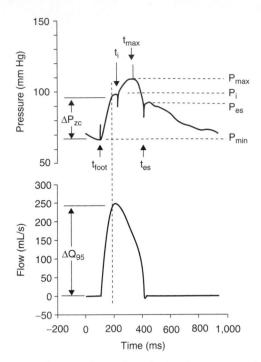

Figure A44.4 Definition of waveform landmarks, augmentation index (AI), and characteristic impedance. The timing of the waveform foot (t_{foot}), inflection point (t_i) signaling the return of the reflected wave, peak pressure (t_{max}), and end-systole (t_{es}) are identified on the calibrated carotid pressure waveform, relative to $t = 0$ at the peak of the QRS. The point at which flow reaches 95% of its peak value is located on the flow tracing (Q_{95}). The change in pressure from the foot to the time of Q_{95} is determined (P_{Zc}). Characteristic impedance is computed from the ratio of these two values: $Z_c = P_{Zc}/Q_{95}$. AI is the ratio $(P_{max}-P_i)/(P_{max}-P_{min})$. If P_i precedes P_{max}, AI is positive. If P_i follows P_{max}, AI is negative. The systolic ejection period is $t_{es}-t_{foot}$. (Reproduced with permission from: Mitchell, GF, Tradif J-C, Arnold JM, et al. Pulsatile hemodynamics in congestive heart failure. *Hypertension* 2001;38:1433–1439.)

Nonparabolic flow profiles. Characteristics of pulsatile blood flow in a branching arterial system deserve special attention. Arterial flow velocity is not fully parabolic (laminar) because of the short duration, amplitude variation, and short entrance lengths of the arterial pulsations (**Figure A44.5**). Observed flow velocity profiles are flattened parabolas, so the shear rate (i.e., the velocity gradient relative to the arterial radius, dv/dr), is lower in the center of the vessel and higher near the artery wall. At the same time, blood viscosity is higher in the center of the vessel due to the pattern of red blood cell streaming. The artery wall is exposed to the thin layer of plasma and blood platelets, which are dispersed from the center of the vessel due to collision with the larger red blood cells. Cross-sectional velocity profiles are not only flattened, but often also skewed due to vessel curvature effects. Therefore, mean wall shear stress is usually far from constant along the arterial tree, consistent with the theory of minimal energy expenditure.

Human arteries. Only in the human elastic common carotid artery is mean wall shear stress within the limits of the value predicted by theory, that is, 1.5 Pa ± 50%. In healthy human muscular arteries, mean wall shear stress is substantially lower (0.3 to 0.5 Pa in the femoral artery and 0.4 to 0.5 Pa in the brachial artery). The lower mean wall shear stress in the peripheral arteries can be explained by the high peripheral resistance in the former two arteries and the corresponding high reflection coefficients, which increase wave reflection but reduce mean wall shear stress.

Endothelial cell mechano-transduction

Biomechanical forces are important determinants of endothelial cell function and therefore of endothelial influences in health and disease. The interaction between biomechanical forces and endothelial cell function, often called *mechanotransduction* of physical signals acting on the luminal side of an endothelial cell, deforms and alters the endothelial cell's cytoskeleton, thereby sending the deformation signal to other sites in the cell. Deformation signals are especially sensed at critical cell junctions, including: (i) basal adhesion points where the endothelial cell is attached to the extracellular matrix, (ii) cell junctions, and (iii) nuclear membranes.

Cell structure. Endothelial cells tend to align with the axis of wall shear stress: the higher the wall shear stress, the more elongated the cells. Changes in endothelial cell phenotype are associated with alterations in intracellular stress fiber distribution, arrangement and number. Changes in endothelial cell shape and alignment probably directly affect flow patterns, especially in smaller arteries or arterioles.

Vasoactive substance production. Wall shear stress regulates arterial diameter by modifying the local production of vasoactive mediators, whereas changes in wall shear stress and circumferential strain influence endothelial gene expression. *In vitro*, endothelial genes that can be upregulated by alterations in shear stress include transcription factors, growth factors, adhesion molecules and enzymes; these effects can be transient or more permanent. Of interest, intercellular adhesion molecule-1 (ICAM-1) is upregulated by increased shear stress but vascular cell adhesion molecule-1 (VCAM-1) responses depend on the type of shear stress applied.

Implications for human disease

Endothelial dysfunction. Flow, and, hence, shear stress, is increased by (i) the administration of vasodilators or (ii) reactive hyperemia. The induced increase in arterial diameter (usually brachial artery) is recorded by ultrasonography or MRI. The arterial dilatory response during acutely increased in shear stress is used in clinical research studies to test the integrity of the endothelium. In patients with hypertension and atherosclerosis, increased volume flow is accompanied by reduced arterial dilation, which is interpreted as disturbed endothelial cell function. In community-based studies, impaired flow-mediated arterial dilation is proportional to the aggregated presence of risk factors such as smoking, hypercholesterolemia, advancing age, higher systolic BP or increased body mass index.

It is important to note that, although apparently straightforward, the test currently in use is subject to substantial criticism. Atherosclerosis is rarely present in the brachial artery. Further, flow-mediated dilation is enhanced if evaluated following a brief exercise test and varies substantially with acute changes in food intake. Furthermore, variability in the vasodilatory responses are largely determined by downstream (microvascular) responses to ischemia rather than local factors. Additional confounding occurs because abnormalities in resting or reactive arterial flow are themselves risk factor-dependent. Therefore, diameter responses must be normalized by flow change in order to allow for proper interpretation.

Atherosclerosis. Atherosclerotic lesions preferentially originate in areas of disturbed flow and low shear stress. Genes are differentially expressed in areas of laminar, turbulent or diminished flow; *in vitro*, shear stress levels of 1.0 to 1.5 Pa induce

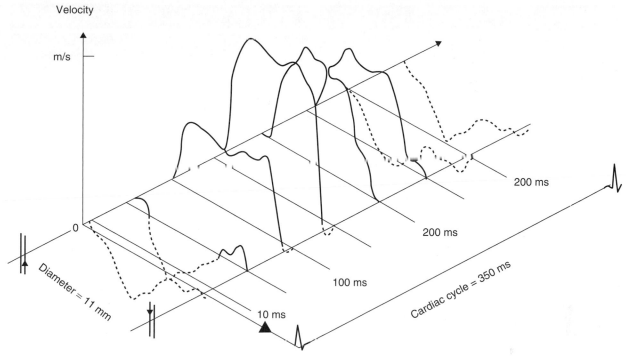

Velocity

m/s

0

Diameter = 11 mm

10 ms

100 ms

200 ms

200 ms

Cardiac cycle = 350 ms

Figure A44.5 A set of velocity profiles in the descending thoracic aorta of a dog recorded with a pulsed Doppler flowmeter. Profiles are recorded at 50 m per second intervals and are drawn obliquely to represent the time sequence; reserve flow is shown by a *dashed line*.

atheroprotective endothelial gene expression profiles, whereas reduced shear stress (approximately 0.4 Pa) stimulates the expression of an atherogenic phenotype.

Suggested Readings

Benjamin EJ, Larson MG, Keyes MJ, et al. Clinical correlates and heritability of flow-mediated dilation in the community: the Framingham Heart Study. *Circulation* 2004;109:613–619.

Davies PF, Shi C, Depaola N, et al. Hemodynamics and the focal origin of atherosclerosis: a spatial approach to endothelial structure, gene expression, and function. *Ann N Y Acad Sci* 2001;947:7–16. Discussion 16–17.

McDonald DA. *Blood flow in arteries.* London: Edward Arnold, 1960:101–145.

Mitchell GF, Parise H, Vita JA, et al. Local shear stress and brachial artery flow-mediated dilation. the Framingham Heart Study. *Hypertension* 2004;44:134–139.

Mitchell GF, Tardif J-C, Arnold JM, et al. Pulsatile hemodynamics in congestive heart failure. *Hypertension* 2001;38:1433–1439.

Nichols WW, O'Rourke M. *McDonald's blood-flow in arteries. Theoretical, experimental and clinical principles*, 5th ed. London: Edward Arnold, 2005:95–402.

Pannier BM, Lacolley PJ, Gharib C, et al. Twenty-four hours of bed rest with head-down tilt: venous and arteriolar changes of limbs. *Am J Physiol* 1991;260:H1043–H1050.

Peronneau PA, Hinglais JR, Pellet MM. Doppler ultrasonic pulsed flowmeter: velocity profiles studied in blood vessels. *Proceedings of the 23rd Annual Conference on Engineering in Medicine and Biology.* Washington, DC; 1970.

Reneman RS, Arts T, Hoeks APG. Wall shear stress—an important determinant of endothelial cell function and structure—in the arterial system *in vivo.* Discrepancies with theory. *J Vasc Res* 2006;43:251–269.

Safar ME, O'Rourke MF. In: Birkenhäger H, Reid JL, eds. *Handbook of hypertension, arterial stiffness in hypertension*, Vol. 23. Edinburgh: Elsevier Science, 2006:3–398.

SECTION IV ■ PATHOPHYSIOLOGY OF PRIMARY AND SECONDARY HYPERTENSION

CHAPTER A45 ■ AGING, ARTERIAL FUNCTION, AND SYSTOLIC HYPERTENSION

STANLEY S. FRANKLIN, MD, FACP, FACC AND GARY F. MITCHELL, MD

KEY POINTS

■ In adolescents and young adults, isolated systolic hypertension (ISH) is the predominant subtype and is associated with increased cardiac stroke volume, or in women, increased aortic impedance due to smaller aortic diameter.

■ Between 20 to 50 years of age, diastolic hypertension predominates, associated with increases in vascular resistance, mean arterial pressure (MAP) and wave reflection, with decreased pulse pressure (PP) amplification between the aorta and brachial artery.

■ After the age of 50 to 60 years, ISH again predominates, associated with increased central arterial stiffness, pulse wave velocity (PWV), and PP.

■ With aging there is a gradual shift in the BP-risk relationships from diastolic to systolic and eventually to PP.

See also Chapters A44, A56, **A58,** A59, A61, B76, **C112,** and **C146**

Physiology

Steady-state versus pulsatile flow. The arterial system has dual interrelated functions: (a) to provide a sufficient quantity of blood to various tissues of the body (the conduit function) and (b) to convert highly pulsatile flow into more continuous flow at the level of the small arteries (the cushioning, compliance, or capacitance function). The low intrinsic resistance to mean flow in large arteries allows for relatively efficient transfer of mean arterial blood pressure (MAP) between the ascending aorta and the peripheral arteries. MAP is the integrated mean of the pulsatile arterial pressure waveform, and as such, represents the interaction of mean cardiac output and systemic vascular resistance (SVR) across the cardiac cycle. In the presence of a relatively constrained range for resting cardiac output, MAP represents the static or steady state component of the circulation and is closely related to SVR.

In a youthful arterial system, flow pulsatility is dampened primarily by elastin-containing central arteries—the thoracic aorta and its most proximal branches, which provide the bulk of the cushioning function by expanding during systole to store some but not all of each stroke volume. Elastic recoil during diastole, which allows peripheral run-off of the stored blood, is dependent on the degree of cushioning function having been provided by the central circulation. Therefore, diastolic blood flow to peripheral tissues is highly dependent on the stiffness of the central arteries.

Determinants of blood pressure components

The two major physiologic components of blood pressure (BP) are MAP and pulse pressure (PP). MAP is simply the interaction of cardiac output (CO) and SVR, that is, $MAP = CO \times SVR$. PP depends on two major factors: (a) left ventricular ejection characteristics and (b) aortic impedance. The familiar peak or systolic blood pressure (SBP) and minimum or diastolic blood pressure (DBP) represent a weighted sum and difference of MAP and PP, respectively. The key point is that DBP rises with increased SVR but falls with increased arterial stiffness. PP represents a surrogate measurement of central elastic artery stiffness in the presence of a constant CO and heart rate. Therefore, central arterial stiffening is manifested by three factors: (a) a rise in PP leading to (b) a rise in SBP and (c) a fall in DBP.

Structural relations in the arterial wall. The elastic behavior of the arterial wall depends primarily on the composition and arrangement of the materials that make up the tunica media or middle layer of the arterial wall. In the media of the thoracic aorta and its immediate branches, concentric fenestrated sheets or lamellae of elastin are interspersed with spiraling, concentric rows of attached smooth muscle cells that together form contractile-elastic units. The alternating oblique pattern of these units exerts maximum force in a generally circumferential direction, an arrangement that is important for the balance of normal changes in intraluminal pressure and tension that occur during systole and diastole. In a young healthy person, the media of the

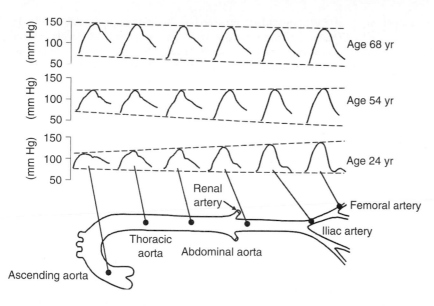

Figure A45.1 Pressure wave recorded along the arterial tree from the proximal ascending aorta to the femoral artery in three subjects aged 24, 54, and 68 years. (From: Nichols WW, Avolio AP, Kelly RP, et al. Effect of age and of hypertension on wave travel and reflections. In: O'Rourke MF, Safar ME, Dzau V, eds. *Arterial vasodilation: mechanisms and therapy.* London: Edward Arnold, 1993, with permission.)

thoracic aorta contains a predominance of elastin over collagen, but as one proceeds distally in the vascular tree, there is a rapid reversal of this proportioning, with more collagen than elastin in the peripheral muscular arteries, leading to progressively stiffer distal vessels.

Wave summation and pulse wave morphology. The morphology of any pulse wave results from the summation of incident (forward-traveling) and reflected (backward-traveling) pressure waves. Variable overlap between the forward and reflected wave contributes to variable augmentation of the central pressure waveform. The amount of augmentation depends on timing and amplitude of the reflected wave. Timing depends on both pulse wave velocity (PWV) and distance to the predominant or "effective" reflecting site. Amplitude depends on the amount of impedance mismatch at this effective reflecting site. A marked increase in stiffness or impedance at the reflecting site generates a larger reflected wave.

Pulse pressure amplification. PP amplification causes central aortic PP to be lower than peripheral vascular PP in a healthy young adult (**Figure A45.1**). PP amplification is induced by the central-to-peripheral stiffness gradient that occurs in the normal vascular tree acting together with progressive diminution in arterial diameter within the aorta and the large muscular arteries. This phenomenon is clinically important because alterations in brachial BP may not accurately reflect changes in central BP and pulsatile load in various conditions.

Aging, hypertension, and arterial function

Blood pressure and arterial stiffness. Elevated BP can increase arterial stiffness (and elastic modulus) by functional and structural mechanisms. With an increase in luminal pressure, the load-bearing elastic lamellae stretch and become stiffer and the loosely woven collagen web is progressively engaged. Since collagen is several orders of magnitude stiffer than elastin, transfer of load from elastin to collagen is associated with a marked nonlinear increase in functional stiffness (and elastic modulus) of the arterial wall. Contraction of vascular smooth muscle also tends to favor increased stiffness.

Wall composition. Central arterial elasticity is critically dependent on normal content and function of the matrix protein elastin, whose half-life of 40 years is one of the longest in the body. Despite this stability, fatigue of elastin fibers and lamellae from the accumulated cyclic stress of more than 2 billion aortic expansions often has occurred by the sixth decade of life. Eventual fracturing and disarray of elastin is accompanied by structural changes of the extracellular matrix that include proliferation of collagen and deposition of calcium. Humoral factors, cytokines, and oxidative metabolites may also play a pathogenic role. This pathologic process, classically termed *arteriosclerosis*, results in increased stiffness of the aortic wall at any ambient pressure.

Arterial diameter. Diameter is the most important determinant of a vessel's input impedance (impedance varies inversely with the 2.5 power radius). In hypertension, aortic and brachial diameters are increased. An important subgroup of those with isolated systolic hypertension (ISH) are shorter people, including women, with intrinsically smaller aortic diameters. In this case, aortic impedance can be increased even if wall elastic properties are normal because of the inverse geometric relationship between arterial diameter and impedance. Aortic radius increases by approximately 15 mm from age 30 to 80, likely as a result of a lifetime of pulsatile stretch. This mechanism offloads the age-related increase in systolic BP, PP, and forward pressure wave amplitude.

Arterial stiffness indicators.

Pulse wave velocity. Because pulse waves travel faster in stiffer arteries, PWV is a useful clinical surrogate for large artery stiffness. However, given that peripheral arteries are usually stiffer than central arteries, an intrinsic limitation of PWV is its dependence on both central and peripheral arterial characteristics, which are inherently different. Nevertheless, increased PWV has been shown to be a predictor of cardiovascular morbidity and mortality.

Limitations of pulse wave velocity. Importantly, not all arteries become stiff with age. Whereas long-term structural changes with aging cause increased stiffness of the thoracic aorta and its branches, the more peripheral muscular arteries (such as the brachial artery) retain their normal properties or may even become less stiff in people with hypertension. At least one explanation for this paradoxical relationship is that hypertension itself increases arterial diameter.

Age-related hemodynamic changes and blood pressure subtypes

Both cross-sectional and longitudinal population studies show that SBP rises progressively beginning in adolescence. In contrast, DBP initially increases with age, levels off at approximately age 50, and decreases after age 60. Interestingly, most of those who develop ISH do not have antecedent diastolic hypertension, strongly suggesting different etiologic and hemodynamic mechanisms for these two entities. Age-related patterns are now becoming clear. Not surprisingly, hypertension left untreated, regardless of the subtype, accelerates the development of aortic stiffness. This, in turn, can accentuate age-related arterial stiffening. Pulse wave propagation and reflection also vary considerably according to age (**Figure A45.2**).

Age less than 30 years. In adolescents and very young adults (mean age of 20), ISH and diastolic hypertension arise from different hemodynamic mechanisms. ISH, the predominant form of hypertension in this age-group, is usually associated with increased cardiac output/stroke volume. In contrast, diastolic hypertension is associated with increased vascular resistance and MAP. In young adults (late teens, early 20s) with full height and maximum elasticity of their central arteries, PWV is low but impedance mismatch is high. Therefore, there is a relatively large reflected wave but it returns to the aorta in mid-late diastole, leading to little or no augmentation of the central pressure.

Age 30 to 50 years. The proportional rise in SBP and DBP up to age 50 can best be explained by the dominance of SVR and MAP in systemic hemodynamics (**Table A45.1**). The transition at an age of 50 to 60, when DBP levels off and central pressure augmentation peaks, constitutes a near-balancing of increased resistance (and increased MAP and augmentation) with increased thoracic aortic impedance (and increased forward wave amplitude). Therefore, PP begins to increase after age 50 to 60. As a result of these changes, ISH, wide PP hypertension by definition (SBP $\geq$140 and DBP <90 mm Hg), becomes the main subtype of hypertension after the sixth decade of life.

Between 20 and 50 years of age, aortic PWV increases, but remains lower than peripheral PWV. The reflected wave returns slightly earlier in systole and the systolic ejection period lengthens, leading to increased overlap between the forward and reflected waves and a rapid increase in central pressure augmentation. As a result, central and peripheral systolic pressure peaks converge and PP amplification appears to abate.

Age more than 50 years. After age 50 to 60, the fall in DBP and the rapid widening of PP become surrogate indicators of central arterial stiffening. Indeed, after age 60, increased central arterial stiffness and forward wave amplitude (rather than increased SVR, MAP and augmentation) become the dominant hemodynamic factors in both normotensive and hypertensive individuals.

At approximately 50 to 60 years of age, however, aortic stiffness (measured by carotid-femoral PWV) reaches and then exceeds peripheral arterial stiffness (measured by carotid-brachial PWV). As a result, reflection at this interface is reduced with reflecting sites shifting distally. This "impedance matching" at the proximal reflecting sites leads to reduced reflection and therefore increased transmission of pulsatility distally, with a resultant increase in brachial artery PP. Increased pulsatility at the arteriolar level may have pathogenic implications for the microcirculation.

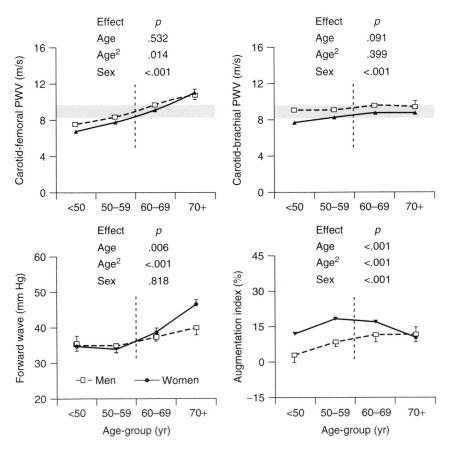

Figure A45.2 Changes in arterial properties in a health subset of the Framingham Offspring cohort. Means of regional pulse wave velocities and reflected wave variables are shown by sex and decade of age. Carotid-femoral PWV increased substantially with advancing age (age^2 term), whereas an insignificant increase in carotid-brachial PWV was found in these unadjusted analyses. As a result, carotid-femoral PWV exceeded carotid-brachial PWV in older participants. Aortic stiffening was accompanied by a proportional decrease in reflected wave transit time in younger but not older groups; therefore, distance to the effective reflecting site increased in older individuals. PWV, pulse wave velocity. (From: Mitchell GF, Parise H, Benjamin EJ, et al. Changes in arterial stiffness and wave reflection with advancing age in healthy men and women: The Framingham Heart Study. *Hypertension* 2004;43:1239–1245, with permission.)

TABLE A45.1

HEMODYNAMIC PATTERNS OF AGE-RELATED CHANGES IN BLOOD PRESSURE

Age (yr)	Diastolic BP (mm Hg)	Systolic BP (mm Hg)	Mean arterial pressure (mm Hg)	Pulse pressure (mm Hg)	Hemodynamics
30–49	↑	↑	↑	→↑	R > S
50–59	→	↑	→	↑↑	R = S
≥60	↓	↑	→↓	↑↑↑↑	S > R

↓, decrease; ↑, increase; →, no change; R, small-vessel resistance; S, large-vessel stiffness.

The combination of reduced proximal wave reflection and a distal shift of reflecting sites results in stabilization of central pressure augmentation after age 60.

Age, blood pressure, and coronary heart disease risk

Blood pressure components as risk predictors. SBP is superior to DBP as a predictor of coronary heart disease (CHD) risk after the age of 50. However, many recent studies, generally in older individuals, have shown PP to be slightly better than SBP in predicting risk. When both SBP and DBP were included together in a Cox model in individuals 50 to 79 years of age from the original Framingham cohort, CHD risk was inversely related to DBP at any given level of SBP, suggesting that PP predicted risk better than either SBP or DBP alone. From the age of 20 to 79 (**Figure A45.3**), there was a continuous, graded shift from DBP to SBP and eventually to PP as predictors of CHD risk. In individuals younger than 50 years of age, DBP was a stronger predictor than SBP. Age 50 to 59 was a transition period when all three BP indices were comparable predictors, and from 60 years of age onward, DBP was negatively related to CHD risk so that PP became superior to SBP. Overall, the power of DBP to predict risk disappears by middle age and is supplanted by SBP in individuals beyond 50 years of age. CHD events, which predominate beyond age 50, are therefore related more to the pulsatile stress of central elastic arterial stiffness during systole than to the steady state stress of peripheral arteriolar resistance during diastole.

Limitations of pulse pressure as a risk marker. Cuff PP cannot be used as a single measure of cardiovascular risk across the full adult age range, because PP may be normal in younger individuals with increased SVR and elevated MAP. Therefore, one must consider both physiologic components of BP—MAP and PP. SBP is useful in this regard because SBP goes up with an increase in either component (MAP or PP) and as such rises monotonically with age and level of cardiovascular risk. Furthermore, on average, elevated PP is a relatively late manifestation of age-related hemodynamic change and, as such, becomes markedly abnormal at a time (beyond age 60) when interventions to prevent cardiovascular events may prove less effective. PP *per se* is also not a useful marker of responsiveness to antihypertensive therapy. Central SBP can fall disproportionately in individuals with ISH when vasodilators are used. As a result, changes in peripheral SBP and PP may underestimate changes in central SBP and PP. Importantly, to date, no clinical trials have been conducted to establish the outcomes value of pharmacologic manipulation of PP or other measures of aortic stiffness.

Arterial stiffness and other cardiovascular disease risks

Increased PP may be a surrogate marker for several possible pathologic mechanisms, all originating from an underlying increase in central arterial stiffness and contributing to disorders of the myocardium.

Heart. Concentric left ventricular hypertrophy (LVH) is commonly associated with increased arterial stiffness. Increased aortic pulsatile load elevates left ventricular systolic wall stress and increases myocardial oxygen consumption while decreasing coronary flow reserve. Increased aortic pulsatile load is the major factor in the development of LVH and its concomitantly increased

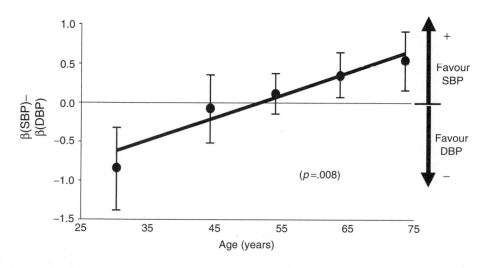

Figure A45.3 Difference in coronary heart disease prediction between systolic blood pressure (SBP) and diastolic blood pressure (DBP) as function of age. Difference in β coefficients (from Cox proportional-hazards regression) between SBP and DBP is plotted as function of age, obtaining this regression line: $\beta(SBP) - \beta(DBP) = -1.49848 + 0.0290 \times age$ ($p = .008$). (From Franklin SS, Larson MG, Khan SA, et al. Does the relation of blood pressure to coronary heart disease risk change with aging? The Framingham Heart Study. *Circulation.* 2001;103:1245–1249, with permission.)

coronary blood flow requirements. Simultaneously, the decrease in DBP (in the setting of a widened PP) further compromises the oxygen supply-to-demand ratio by reducing diastolic coronary flow.

Increased left ventricular afterload by itself may not explain all of the increased cardiac risks in the elderly with ISH. With age, the left ventricle becomes stiff, a maladaptive change that supports ventricular ejection and maintains matched coupling of the heart to the stiffer arteries, causing "coupling disease." Therefore, diastolic dysfunction and heart failure can result from the combination of an elevated cardiac afterload presented to a left ventricle unable to handle the pressure load.

Vasculature. Increased pulsatile stress leads to endothelial dysfunction with a greater propensity for developing coronary atherosclerosis and for rupture of unstable atherosclerotic plaques. Conversely, regardless of the direction of causality, wide PP may represent a marker for diffuse atherosclerosis.

High-risk conditions. Arterial stiffness and wide PP becomes an even stronger predictor of risk in middle-aged and older populations with risk factors such as diabetes, dyslipidemia, albuminuria, and in persons with prior cardiovascular events such as myocardial infarction or chronic kidney disease. Even after adjusting for the usual cardiovascular risk factors, there is evidence that increased arterial stiffness may increase pulsatile flow to the microcirculation and thereby predispose to cerebral white matter lesions, cognitive impairment, dementia, and chronic kidney disease.

Clinical assessment of arterial stiffness

The best current strategy for assessing risk in the elderly begins with determining the level of SBP elevation and is followed by the adjustment of risk upward when PP is wide (i.e., DBP is discordantly low). Because of the limitations of PP, alternative methods for estimating stiffness have been developed (see Chapter C112). Large artery stiffness (estimated by measurement of PWV), and increased pressure reflection (augmentation index) are independent risk factors for the development of cardiovascular disease (CVD). Measurement of central systolic BP may also allow better assessment of cardiovascular risk before the age of 50, possibly before hypertension develops and long before the onset of CVD.

Suggested Readings

Franklin SS, Gustin WG, Wong ND, et al. Hemodynamic patterns of age-related changes in blood pressure. The Framingham Heart Study. *Circulation* 1997;96:308–315.

Franklin SS, Larson MG, Khan SA, et al. Does the relation of blood pressure to coronary heart disease risk change with aging? The Framingham Heart Study. *Circulation* 2001;103:1245–1249.

Franklin SS, Pio JR, Wong ND, et al. Predictors of new-onset diastolic and systolic hypertension. The Framingham Heart Study. *Circulation* 2005;111:1121–1127.

Kass DA. Ventricular arterial stiffening: integrating the pathophysiology of hypertension. *Hypertension* 2005;46:185–193.

McEniery CM, Yasmin, Hall IR, et al. Normal vascular aging: differential effects on wave reflection and aortic pulse wave velocity. The Anglo-Cardiff Collaborative Trial (ACCT). *J Am Coll Cardiol* 2005;46:1753–1760.

McEniery CM, Yasmin, Wallace S, et al. Increased stroke volume and aortic stiffness contribute to isolated systolic hypertension in young adults. *Hypertension* 2005;46:221–226.

Mitchell GF, Lacourciere Y, Ouellet J-P, et al. Determinants of elevated pulse pressure in middle-aged and older subjects with uncomplicated systolic hypertension. *Circulation* 2003;108:1592–1598.

Mitchell GF, Parise H, Benjamin EJ, et al. Changes in arterial stiffness and wave reflection with advancing age in healthy men and women. The Framingham Heart Study. *Hypertension* 2004;43:1239–1245.

Nichols WW, O'Rourke ME. *McDonald's blood flow in arteries*, 5th ed. London, UK: Edward Arnold, 2005.

CHAPTER A46 ■ OBESITY-RELATED HYPERTENSION

EFRAIN REISIN, MD

KEY POINTS

- Obesity, specifically central adiposity, is strongly associated with chronic hypertension.
- The cause of hypertension in obesity is complex and multifactorial, including hemodynamic, metabolic, and endocrine mechanisms such as expanded blood volume, increased sympathetic nervous and renin-angiotensin activity, and altered leptin and adipokine release.
- The structural heart changes that occur in obesity-hypertension are characterized by eccentric and concentric left ventricular hypertrophy and mononuclear cell infiltration of the conduction system; these changes may increase the incidence of heart failure, arrhythmias, and sudden death.
- In the kidneys, obesity-hypertension results in glomerular hyperperfusion, hyperfiltration, and proteinuria, conditions that lead to glomerulomegaly, focal segmental glomerulosclerosis, tubulointerstitial fibrosis, and renal failure.

See also Chapters **A34,** A35, A36, **A48, A55, B90,** and **C157**

Epidemiologic studies have shown that the prevalence of obesity in children, adolescents, and adults is increasing worldwide. In the Framingham Heart Study, excess weight was associated with hypertension in 78% of men and 65% of women. Other investigators have found that central (truncal or visceral) obesity, rather than peripheral adiposity, is closely associated with hypertension. The cause of hypertension in obesity is complex and multifactorial, including hemodynamic, metabolic, and endocrine mechanisms (**Figure. A46.1**).

Mechanisms of obesity-related hypertension

Central obesity is the most common condition associated with insulin resistance and the consequent hyperinsulinemia. The resistance to insulin, however, is selective and not uniform in all tissues. In animal experiments insulin increases absorption of sodium in the diluting segment of the distal nephron, with a manifest effect of salt and water retention; it also increases adrenergic activity and causes vascular smooth-muscle hypertrophy. Insulin resistance and hyperinsulinemia may also impair the insulin-mediated vascular signaling pathways associated with vasorelaxation, mechanisms that may link hyperinsulinemia and insulin resistance to the development of hypertension.

Most of the insulin-resistance hypertension connection has been demonstrated in animal experiments. Acute and chronic studies that induce hyperinsulinemia in humans have failed to achieve consistent effects on blood pressure (BP) or other BP-raising mechanisms such as sodium reabsorption or sympathetic activity (SA). Consequently, the association between hyperinsulinemia and hypertension remains somewhat controversial. Some

investigators believe that insulin resistance and hyperinsulinemia may only minimally contribute to the relationship between obesity and hypertension.

Fluid volume distribution and systemic hemodynamic changes. Compared with lean hypertensives, individuals with obesity-hypertension have a higher total blood volume, which is largely redistributed centrally to the cardiopulmonary area, leading to augmented venous return, greater ventricular filling, and higher cardiac output. Total peripheral resistance in obese hypertensives remains less elevated than would be expected for the degree of hypertension but still may be considered "inappropriately" normal.

Sympathetic nervous system. Peripheral catecholamine levels or SA are not always elevated in obese compared to nonobese subjects; however, regional organ-specific SA in muscle and kidneys is elevated. The regionally elevated SA in obese subjects may, in part, explain the increased incidence of hypertension, arrhythmias, and angina pectoris that characterize obesity-hypertension.

Dogs made obese by overfeeding demonstrate activated renal sympathetic nerve traffic and increased BP. Renal denervation in these animals attenuates sodium retention and prevents the development of hypertension. Increased SA in the kidneys of obese patients has been found in several studies, and hyperleptinemia appears to be the most important mechanism that triggers the increase in SA in these subjects.

Leptin resistance and hyperleptinemia. Leptin is an amino-acid hormone produced almost exclusively by white adipose tissue. Leptin has an important activity in the regulation of food intake and may also increase BP through the enhancement

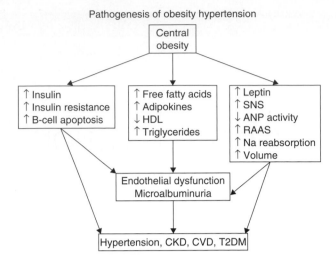

Figure A46.1 Pathogenesis of obesity-related hypertension. HDL, high-density lipoprotein; SNS, sympathetic nervous system; ANP, atrial natriuretic peptide; RAAS, renin-angiotensin-aldosterone system; CKD, chronic kidney disease; CVD, cardiovascular disease; T2DM, type 2 diabetes. (Adapted from Morse SA, Zhang R, Thakur V, et al. Hypertension and the metabolic syndrome. *Am J Med Sci* 2005;330:303–310.)

of SA. In animals, the acute infusion of leptin affects BP in an opposing way by the promotion of natriuresis and nitric oxide (NO) production. Conversely, chronic leptin administration decreases natriuresis and urinary excretion of NO metabolites but increases renal SA and BP.

In humans, a number of studies have found leptin to be positively correlated with systolic and diastolic BP in both obese and nonobese individuals. The strong correlation between serum leptin levels and adipose tissue mass suggests the existence of a selective leptin-resistant mechanism in human obesity. In summary, animal and human evidence demonstrated that hyperleptinemia that occurs in obesity due to a selective leptin resistance may be one of the most important mechanisms to explain the increased SA and the consequent obesity-induced hypertension.

Renin-angiotensin-aldosterone system. The role of the renin-angiotensin-aldosterone system (RAAS) in obesity-hypertension remains controversial. Some studies show RAAS activation in obese subjects despite the hypervolemia and sodium retention. Body mass index is positively correlated with plasma–angiotensinogen levels, plasma renin activity, plasma–angiotensin-converting enzyme concentrations, and plasma aldosterone levels. There may be higher expression of RAAS components in human adipose tissue, which appears to contain all components of the RAAS, and there may be a direct link between adipose tissue mass and hypertension. Increased aldosterone release may also occur in obesity-related hypertension.

Dyslipidemia, inflammatory cytokines. Elevated titers of autoantibodies to oxidized low-density lipoproteins (LDL) in patients with hypertension and increased peripheral-intimal media arteriolar thickness have been observed in hypertension. Increased oxidized LDL deposition may be related to hypertension through activation of local vascular RAAS components and decreased endothelial NO synthesis. Adipose tissue adipokines, which include inflammatory cytokines such as tumor necrosis factor α, interleukin-6, C-reactive protein, and plasminogen-activator inhibitor, may initiate and sustain the low-grade inflammatory state that appears to characterize the progression of hypertension

and arteriosclerosis. Obesity also increases various markers of oxidative stress in experimental animals and humans. A direct cause and effect relationship between markers of oxidative stress and hypertension has not been clearly established but superoxide radicals may elevate BP by decreasing the production of endogenous NO and interfering with endothelial-dependent vascular relaxation.

Impact of obesity-hypertension on the heart and kidneys

Cardiac changes. In obese individuals, ventricular dilation induces myocardial remodeling by adding contractile elements in series (eccentric hypertrophy). Hypertension in these patients restores wall stress to a normal level by thickening the myocardium, a process that adds contractile elements in parallel (concentric hypertrophy). The trends toward eccentric and concentric left ventricular hypertrophy may increase the risk for heart failure. Other studies in obese subjects show mononuclear infiltration in and around the sinoatrial node, with an increase of fat tissue throughout the conduction system and the interatrial septum. These changes and the regionally elevated SA may explain the increased rate of cardiac arrhythmias and sudden death in morbidly obese subjects.

Functional and structural renal changes. In obese animals, elevated interstitial hydrostatic pressure reduces medullary blood flow and induces tubular compression. These changes slow tubular flow and increase fractional tubular sodium reabsorption, which reduces the delivery of sodium chloride to the macula densa, causes feedback-mediated renal–vascular dilatation, increased glomerular filtration rate, and stimulation of the intrarenal RAAS. In most clinical studies, obesity in humans is associated with elevated effective renal plasma flow and glomerular filtration rate, increased glomerular pressure and fractional filtration, persistent glomerular hyperfiltration, and proteinuria. Hyperinsulinemia may also contribute to the functional and structural changes that occur in the kidneys as a consequence of obesity through preglomerular vasodilation, glomerular hypertension, glomerular hypertrophy, and mesangial cell expansion.

Other factors promoting renal degeneration may include leptin and cytokines secreted by the adipose tissue. Lipotoxicity caused by accumulation of albumin-bond fatty acid in proximal tubules may contribute to tubulointerstitial inflammation and fibrosis. Framingham data have shown that baseline body mass index predicts subsequent kidney disease, and biopsy studies in obese populations have shown a high incidence of glomerulomegaly and focal segmental glomerulosclerosis.

Suggested Readings

Aneja A, El-Atat F, McFarlane SI, et al. Hypertension and obesity. *Endocrinol Metab Clin North Am* 2003;32:823–854.

Engeli S, Negrel R, Sharma AM. Physiology and pathophysiology of the adipose tissue renin-angiotensin system. *Hypertension* 2000;35:1270–1277.

Esler M, Straznicky N, Eikelis N, et al. Mechanisms of sympathetic activation in obesity hypertension. *Hypertension* 2006;48:787–796.

Haynes WG. Role of leptin in obesity hypertension. *Exp Physiol* 2005;905:683–688.

Hall JE. The kidney, hypertension and obesity. *Hypertension* 2005;41:625–633.

Morse SA, Zhang R, Thakur V, et al. Hypertension and the metabolic syndrome. *Am J Med Sci* 2005;330:303–310.

Reisin E, Hutchinson HG. Obesity-hypertension: effects on the cardiovascular and renal systems: the therapeutic approach. In: Oparil S, Weber M, eds. *Hypertension*, 1st ed. Philadelphia: WB Saunders, 2000:206–211.

Sowers JR, Frohlich ED. Insulin and insulin resistance: impact on blood pressure and cardiovascular disease. *Med Clin North Am* 2004;88:63–82.

CHAPTER A47 ■ INSULIN ACTIONS AND INSULIN RESISTANCE

ADAM WHALEY-CONNELL, DO, MSPH; SAMY I. McFARLANE, MD, MPH AND JAMES R. SOWERS, MD, ASCI

KEY POINTS

■ Insulin resistance and hypertension (HTN) are part of a cluster of risk factors that also includes obesity and dyslipidemia; this constellation of risk factors has been termed the *cardiometabolic syndrome*.

■ Insulin resistance is associated with other subclinical markers of cardiovascular disease (CVD), including increased oxidative stress, chronic inflammation, activation of tissue renin-angiotensin-aldosterone systems (RAASs), impaired endothelial function, increased vascular reactivity, salt-sensitivity, and proteinuria.

■ Insulin resistance is a risk factor for the development of type 2 diabetes and HTN, along with target organ damage [chronic kidney disease (CKD), stroke, and coronary artery disease].

See also Chapters **A34,** A35, A36, **A48,** A49, **B90, C157,** and **C158**

In some populations, especially obese people, up to 50% have hypertension (HTN), insulin resistance or impaired glucose tolerance. This has led to the theory that HTN and insulin resistance share a common pathogenetic mechanism. In concert with this notion, human and animal studies demonstrate that pharmacologic or nonpharmacologic improvement in insulin resistance sometimes improves blood pressure (BP) control.

Cellular mechanisms of insulin action

Insulin receptors are found in many tissues, including pancreas, liver, vascular smooth muscle cells (VSMCs), neurons, mononuclear cells, and cardiomyocytes. Their wide distribution suggests an important role of insulin in all of these tissues.

Receptor activation and modulation. Insulin binds to classic G protein–coupled receptors. In the insulin-sensitive state, autophosphorylation of the β subunit of the receptor mediates noncovalent but stable balance between insulin receptor inactivation and insulin-dependent cellular activation through downstream kinases. Particularly important are tyrosine kinases that phosphorylate tyrosine residues after ligand binding at insulin receptors. Insulin receptor substrate-1 (IRS-1) is a pivotal substrate that regulates insulin signaling in skeletal muscle, adipose tissue, and the vasculature.

Glucose transport. IRS docking proteins bind to the enzyme PI3-kinase, a heterodimer consisting of a p85 regulatory subunit and a p110 catalytic subunit, through SH-2 domain interaction with the p85 subunit. Insulin stimulation increases PI3-kinase association with IRS, which then leads to activation of downstream enzymes. Subsequent translocation of the glucose transporter (GLUT 4) from the cytosol to the plasma membrane facilitates glucose transport.

Nuclear signaling. Several genes modulate insulin action at its target tissues, including those regulating insulin receptors and postreceptor insulin signaling (insulin receptor substrates and nuclear receptors such as PPAR-γ).

PC-1 proteins. PC-1 is a class II transmembrane glycoprotein that inhibits tyrosine kinase activity. The K121Q polymorphism of the PC-1 gene has been correlated with insulin resistance independent of the degree of obesity. Furthermore, IRS-1–associated PI-3 kinase activity may be impaired by Gly972Arg substitution in the IRS-1 gene.

Nuclear receptors. The nuclear receptor peroxisome proliferator-activated receptor γ (PPAR-γ) is expressed in adipose tissue. PPAR-γ regulates adipocyte differentiation, body weight, and glucose homeostasis. Although infrequent, mutations in the gene for this receptor have yielded significant information. Loss-of-function mutations lead to lipodystrophy, and gain-of-function mutations result in increased body fat mass. Therapeutic modulation of the PPAR-γ receptor with thiazolidinediones has been shown to reverse the insulin resistance that accompanies mutations of this gene. In humans, a Pro12Ala (substitution of Proline by Alanine) substitution has been detected in the PPAR-γ gene; thereby reducing the activity of PPAR-γ by 20% to 30%.

Systemic effects of insulin

In addition to its metabolic roles, insulin has several important effects on the brain, cardiovascular system, and kidney.

Vasodilation. Insulin is a powerful vasodilator that acts through two major mechanisms in VSMC: increased production of cyclic guanine nucleotide monophosphate (cGMP) and reduction of intracellular calcium (Ca^{2+}). Insulin receptor activation leads to vasorelaxation in part through increased endothelial nitric oxide (NO) production, which diffuses into adjacent myocytes and stimulates production of cGMP. This leads to attenuated phosphorylation of myosin-bound regulatory subunits and activation of myosin-bound protein phosphatase. Reduced phosphorylation of myosin light chain allows VSMC relaxation. In addition, insulin stimulates the activity of the Na^+–K^+ ATPase pump, which lowers intracellular sodium (Na^+). The enhanced transmembrane Na^+ gradient promotes increased Na^+–Ca^{2+} exchange across the cell membrane, reduces intracellular Ca^{2+}, and thereby causes vasorelaxation.

Sympathetic nervous activation. Acute insulin infusion activates the sympathetic nervous system (SNS) in animals and humans. This may be a necessary consequence of its vasodilator functions because if SNS activation did not occur, insulin would cause hypotension. From a metabolic standpoint, increased cardiac output increases the rate of delivery of insulin and substrate to peripheral tissues, thereby combating energy deficiency. Because insulin does not cross the blood–brain barrier, central sympathoexcitatory effects must be mediated through paraventricular nuclei outside the blood–brain barrier, either directly or through the actions of angiotensin II. In normotensive Sprague-Dawley (SD) rats with chronic hyperinsulinemia and HTN, renal denervation lowers BP, a finding that underscores the importance of renal sympathetic nerves in the maintenance of HTN.

Kidney. Insulin signaling also plays a complex balanced role in modulating salt and water excretion. While insulin-mediated renal vasodilation acts to reduce filtration fraction and Na^+ reabsorption, direct tubular effects enhance Na^+ reabsorption. This balanced effect ensures relative neutrality with respect to long-term salt balance. Insulin favors lower glomerular capillary pressures, which have two theoretically favorable effects on kidney function: diminished albumin leakage rates across the glomerulus and a reduced rate of development of glomerulosclerosis. This may explain why albuminuria and CKD are more prevalent in insulin resistant states.

Coagulation. NO-induced endothelial vasodilation has vascular protective actions that favor fibrinolysis, including decreases in plasminogen-activator inhibitor-1 (PAI-1) production. Increased NO production also diminishes platelet adhesion.

Obesity and insulin resistance

Insulin resistance denotes an impaired response to insulin in skeletal muscle, adipose, liver, and cardiovascular tissue. The actions of insulin and the appearance of insulin resistance have different implications in different organs. Insulin resistance is not absolute; some tissues may retain insulin sensitivity whereas others may not. However, mounting evidence supports that vascular tissue is influenced by the balance of insulin and its homologous peptide IGF-1. Several mechanisms for insulin resistance have been proposed; sometimes classified as prereceptor, receptor, or postreceptor defects. Altered signaling at the receptor level results in a cascade of events within target tissues that eventually results in impaired glucose transport. The increasing prevalence of the insulin resistance parallels the rise in prevalence of obesity, especially an increase in visceral fat.

Fatty acid metabolism. Visceral adipocytes have less ability to assimilate free fatty acids (FFA) than peripheral adipocytes and other tissues. Reduced adipocyte FFA uptake may contribute to increased circulating FFA and to insulin resistance as the excess FFA accumulate in nonadipose tissues, especially liver, skeletal muscle, and heart. When these excess FFA are metabolized, such as lineolic acid, in turn induce tumor necrosis factor α (TNF-α) and IL-1 as well as other inflammatory cytokines which then impairs insulin signaling.

Endocrine functions of adipocytes. Visceral fat is now widely recognized as an endocrine tissue capable of secreting metabolically active factors (adipokines) that are important in maintaining metabolic homeostasis (see Chapters A34–A36). Adipokines may contribute through complex mechanisms to the development of insulin resistance when food is plentiful, including alterations in skeletal muscle and cardiovascular cell function.

Adiponectin. Adiponectin is an adipocyte-derived plasma protein with insulin sensitizing, antiinflammatory, and antiatherogenic properties. Adiponectin levels are reduced in adipose tissue from obese humans and restored to normal with nonpharmacologic (weight loss and exercise) and pharmacologic treatments (blockers of the RAAS and PPAR-γ agonists).

Leptin. Another adipokine, leptin, acts primarily on the hypothalamus, where it regulates appetite and energy expenditure. In ob/ob mice deficient in leptin, replacement of leptin abrogates hyperglycemia and hyperinsulinemia without decreasing body weight. In humans, leptin levels correlate with the percentage of body fat, suggesting that obese humans become resistant to the central effects of leptin.

Inflammatory mediators. Visceral adipose tissue may contribute to insulin resistance and inflammation through increased production of TNF-α, IL-6, and resistin.

Visceral versus peripheral fat: cardiovascular impact

In contrast to visceral fat, peripheral adipose tissue tends to mediate against insulin resistance through secretion of leptin and adiponectin and assimilation of FFA. The implications of these findings are that adipocytes are related in complex ways to insulin resistance, HTN, and cardiovascular disease (CVD) (Figure A47.1). It is therefore important to differentiate visceral obesity from peripheral obesity in the assessment of potential cardiovascular impact. It is also implied that simple clinical indicators such as weight or body fat content will be confounded as CVD risk indicators.

Hypertension and insulin resistance

Complex interactions of both genetic and environmental factors are required for impaired insulin signaling, HTN, and the cardiometabolic syndrome (CMS).

Animal models. A genetic basis for the relationship between HTN and insulin resistance has been documented in several types of rat models: transgenic TG (mRen2)27 Ren2, Dahl hypertensive, spontaneously hypertensive (SHR), Zucker obese, and Goto-Kakizaki rats. In the last two models, regions of chromosomes 2, 3, and 19 are associated with insulin resistance and HTN.

Inflammation and oxidative stress. In experimental models with insulin resistance and HTN, caloric loads containing glucose and lipid (or mixed fast food with large amounts of saturated fats and carbohydrates) trigger transient increases in

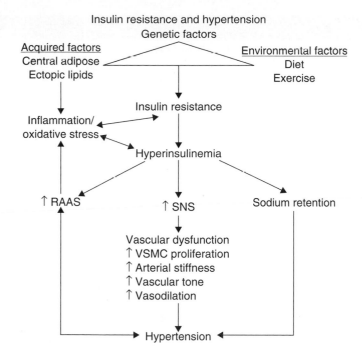

Insulin resistance and hypertension

Figure A47.1 This figure depicts the relationship between genetic, environmental, and acquired factors leading to insulin resistance and the compensatory hyperinsulinemia. This interaction then results in activation of the renin-angiotensin-aldosterone system (RAAS), increased sympathetic nervous system (SNS) activity, and sodium retention leading to vascular dysfunction and subsequent hypertension and cardiovascular risk. VSMC, vascular smooth muscle cell. (Adapted from Govindarajan G, Whaley-Connell A, Mugo M, et al. The metabolic syndrome as a cardiovascular risk factor. *Am J Med Sci.* 2005;330(6):311–318.)

inflammatory mediators. Activation of the nuclear factor-κβ (NF-κβ) and enhancement of the expression of nicotinamide adenine dinucleotide phosphate (NADPH) oxidase constituents leads to generation of superoxide anion (O_2^-) and other reactive oxygen species (ROS). In humans, glucose infusion can induce activation of the regulator of the transcription of matrix metalloproteinases [MMP, modulators of the transcription of tissue factor, (TF)], and PAI-1. The ensuing higher levels of MMPs (2 and 9), TF, and PAI-1 are believed to exacerbate endothelial dysfunction, microalbuminuria, and cardiovascular and renal injury.

Renin-angiotensin-aldosterone system. Insulin resistance is associated with RAAS activation that are mediated through angiotensin type 1 receptor (AT_1R), which partially inhibits the actions of insulin in vascular and skeletal muscle tissue. Angiotensin II (Ang II) alters insulin signaling through phosphatidylinositol-3-kinase (PI3-K) and protein kinase B (Akt) signaling pathways. RAAS activation also promotes increased generation of ROS through increased NADH and NADPH oxidase activity.

In concert, the collective inflammatory response, dysregulation of intracellular signaling pathways, and the actions of hyperinsulinemia independently on the vasculature support a contributory role of insulin resistance to HTN.

Inflammatory mediators. Insulin actions are also antiinflammatory in that they favor the accumulation of IkB, which blocks the proinflammatory and progrowth effects of NF-κβ.

TABLE A47.1

CARDIOVASCULAR DISEASE RISK FACTORS ASSOCIATED WITH VISCERAL ADIPOSITY

Insulin resistance/hyperinsulinemia
Hypertension
Dyslipidemia
↑ Plasminogen-activator inhibitor-1 (PAI-1)
↑ C-reactive Protein (CRP)
↑ Tumor necrosis factor α (TNF-α)
↑ Interleukin 6 (IL-6)
↑ Fibrinogen levels
Hyperviscosity
Premature atherosclerosis
Microalbuminuria

Adapted from Gill H, Whaley-Connell A, Muga M, et al. The central role of insulin resistance in the metabolic syndrome. *Am J Med Sci* 2005; 330(6):290–294.

Clinical studies. Human studies demonstrate that fasting insulin levels are directly correlated with BP. Yet HTN does not occur as a result of hyperinsulinemia alone because insulin infused into nonobese, normotensive individuals causes vasodilatation and BP lowering. In obesity, the beneficial effects of insulin are blunted, suggesting that obesity and insulin resistance contribute to a maladaptive vascular response.

Integrated view. The relationship between HTN and insulin resistance is complex and encompasses many confounding factors that all contribute to increased CVD risk. It involves not only vascular and hemodynamic changes induced by hyperinsulinemia as well as HTN, but also include a myriad of complex metabolic abnormalities (**Table A47.1**).

The role of insulin resistance/hyperinsulinemia and obesity appears to be part of the chronic low-grade inflammatory state characterized by dysfunctional adipose tissue, activation of the RAAS and SNS, oxidative stress, endothelial dysfunctional, and collectively increased risk of CVD. Appropriate cardiac glucose utilization fosters the beneficial effects of preconditioning on ischemic reperfusion injury. From a clinical standpoint, development of uniform criteria to easily diagnose CMS may help quantify and identify at-risk populations in whom intensive intervention could prevent CVD. Pharmacologic treatment strategies, most importantly RAAS inhibition, as well as nonpharmacologic approaches, specifically diet and physical activity, should be included in the treatment of insulin resistance/hyperinsulinemia to reduce BP subsequent CVD risk.

Suggested Readings

Marrero MB, Fulton D, Stepp D, et al. Angiotensin II-induced insulin resistance and protein tyrosine phosphatases. *Arterioscler Thromb Vasc Biol* 2004;24(11):2009–2013.

Sowers JR. Insulin resistance and hypertension. *Am J Physiol Heart Circ Physiol* 2004;286:H1597–H1602.

Wei Y, Sowers JR, Nistala R, et al. Angiotensin II-induced NADPH oxidase activation impairs insulin signaling in skeletal muscle cells. *J Biol Chem* 2006;281(46):35137–35146.

Whaley-Connell A, Palmer J, Sowers JR. Risk stratification and treatment options for hypertensive patients with metabolic syndrome and prediabetes. *Johns Hopkins Adv Stud Med* 2005;5(10C):S1011–S1018.

CHAPTER A48 ■ POLYCYSTIC OVARY SYNDROME

CAREN G. SOLOMON, MD AND ELLEN W. SEELY, MD

KEY POINTS

■ Polycystic ovary syndrome (PCOS) is associated with obesity and insulin resistance, known risk factors for hypertension.

■ Women with PCOS have higher blood pressures (BPs) and a higher prevalence of hypertension than do women with regular menstrual cycles.

■ It remains uncertain whether the increased risk for hypertension in PCOS is explained by the greater tendency to obesity in affected women.

See also Chapters A19, A46, C157, and C158

Polycystic ovary syndrome (PCOS, formerly called *Stein-Leventhal syndrome*) affects approximately 5% of women of reproductive age and is commonly associated with hypertension.

Clinical presentation

Signs and symptoms. Characteristic clinical features of PCOS include irregular menstrual cycles, hirsutism, and infertility. Androgen excess with clinical signs (e.g., hirsutism) or biochemical markers (e.g., elevated testosterone) is characteristic. Pathologically, the ovaries typically have multiple follicles that may be visualized on ultrasonographic examination but this finding may also be present in normally cycling women and is not sufficient in itself for the diagnosis of PCOS.

Diagnostic criteria. Although there is controversy regarding the diagnostic criteria, a commonly used definition for PCOS based on the Rotterdam 2003 consensus workshop is shown in **Table A48.1**.

TABLE A48.1

REVISED CRITERIA FOR THE DIAGNOSIS
OF POLYCYSTIC OVARY SYNDROME ACCORDING
TO THE ROTTERDAM 2003 CONSENSUS WORKSHOP

The definition requires the presence of two of three of the following: 1. Oligo and/or anovulation   2. Clinical and/or biochemical signs of hyperandrogenism   3. Polycystic ovaries   Other etiologies for these manifestations (such as congenital adrenal hyperplasia, androgen secreting neoplasm, and Cushing's syndrome) should be excluded.

Pathogenesis

Obesity, in particular, central obesity, is extremely common in women with PCOS, although up to 20% of women with PCOS are not obese. A closely related hallmark finding of this syndrome is insulin resistance that is out of proportion to the degree of obesity; even lean women with PCOS have been documented as being insulin resistant.

Insulin resistance may be a central cause of PCOS and may contribute to associated hypertension. Improvement in insulin resistance through weight loss in overweight PCOS women or therapy with insulin sensitizers can correct or improve many of the clinical abnormalities. Several studies support a relationship between PCOS and elevated blood pressure (BP), and have suggested a two- to three-fold increased prevalence of hypertension among women with this syndrome. However, many such reports have not adjusted for body mass index or have not specifically assessed the subgroup of lean women with PCOS for hypertension prevalence.

It is less clear whether BP is increased in PCOS independent of obesity. Some data support an association between PCOS and higher BP, measured either in the office or using ambulatory monitoring, even after adjustment for body mass index. However, other investigators have been unable to identify an independent association using either of these techniques. Available data have not convincingly demonstrated higher BPs among lean women with PCOS, suggesting that obesity may explain the overall higher risks for hypertension linked to this syndrome.

Associated disease risks

Pregnancy-associated hypertension. PCOS may also be associated with a higher risk of new-onset hypertension in pregnancy. However, as with essential hypertension, it remains controversial as to whether this risk is wholly explained by a

TABLE A48.2

CARDIOVASCULAR RISK FACTORS THAT HAVE BEEN REPORTED TO BE INCREASED IN FREQUENCY IN WOMEN WITH POLYCYSTIC OVARIAN SYNDROME (PCOS)

- Type 2 diabetes mellitus
- Insulin resistance/hyperinsulinemia
- Dyslipidemia
- Obesity (central)
- Hypertension
- Metabolic syndrome
- Elevated levels of C-reactive protein

greater body mass index, a recognized risk factor for hypertension development in pregnancy.

Coronary risk factors.   Several coronary risk factors in addition to hypertension are also more common in women with PCOS (**Table A48.2**). Type 2 diabetes mellitus is two to three times more frequent in women with PCOS than in weight-matched controls. Women with PCOS also have increased levels of triglycerides and lower levels of high-density lipoprotein (HDL) cholesterol relative to normally cycling women. Consistent with these observations, metabolic syndrome has been reported to be more frequent in women with PCOS. Endothelial dysfunction has also been described in these women. The relative contribution of obesity to these observations still remains unclear.

Coronary artery disease.   The presence of cardiometabolic risk factors in many women with PCOS would be expected to increase cardiovascular risk in this population and several observational reports have suggested increased atherosclerosis in PCOS. Prospective data are currently lacking to confirm an association between PCOS and an increased risk of cardiovascular events.

Suggested Readings

Boomsma CM, Eijkemans MJ, Hughes EG, et al. A meta-analysis of pregnancy outcomes in women with polycystic ovary syndrome. *Hum Reprod Update* 2006;12(6):673–683.

Conway GS, Agrawal R, Betteridge DJ, et al. Risk factors for coronary artery disease in lean and obese women with polycystic ovarian syndrome. *Clin Endocrinol (Oxf)* 1992;37:119–125.

Dahlgren E, Janson PO, Johannson S, et al. Women with polycystic ovary syndrome wedge resected in 1956 to 1965: a long term follow up focusing on natural history and circulating hormones. *Fertil Steril* 1992;57:505–513.

Meyer C, McGrath BP, Teede HJ. Overweight women with polycystic ovary syndrome and evidence of subclinical cardiovascular disease. *J Clin Endocrinol Metab* 2005;90:5711–5716.

Rotterdam ESHRE/ASRM. Revised 2003 consensus on diagnostic criteria and long-term health risks related to polycystic ovary syndrome (PCOS). *Hum Reprod* 2004;19:41–47.

Sampson M, Kong C, Patel A, et al. Ambulatory blood pressure profiles and plasminogen activator inhibitor (PAI-1) activity in lean women with and without the polycystic ovarian syndrome. *Clin Endocrinol (Oxf)* 1996;45:623–629.

Solomon CG. The epidemiology of polycystic ovary syndrome: prevalence and associated disease risks. *Endocrinol Metab Clin North Am* 1999;28:247–263.

Talbott E, Guzick D, Clerici A, et al. Coronary heart disease risk factors in women with polcystic ovary syndrome. *Arterioscler Thromb Vasc Biol* 1995;15:821–826.

CHAPTER A49 ■ SALT SENSITIVITY

FERNANDO ELIJOVICH, MD AND CHERYL L. LAFFER, MD, PhD

KEY POINTS

■ Salt-sensitivity of blood pressure (SSBP) is defined as blood pressure (BP) fluctuations in parallel with changes in salt balance; this phenomenon is found in some animal models and in more than half of human hypertensives.

■ Multiple genetic and physiologic abnormalities in vasoactive and natriuretic regulatory systems have been described in salt-sensitive (SS) animals and humans, but a single discrete etiology has yet to be established.

■ SS subjects have a worse cardiovascular prognosis than salt-resistant (SR) individuals, regardless of BP level.

■ Development of diagnostic markers and new therapies may lead to specific treatment for SS hypertensive and prehypertensive subjects.

See also Chapters A40, **A42**, A47, A50, **B93, B98,** and **C120**

Salt-sensitivity of blood pressure (SSBP) is the characteristic exhibited by some individuals and experimental animal models in which blood pressure (BP) increases or decreases significantly in response to a positive or negative salt balance. SSBP is an abnormality because: (a) it occurs less frequently (30%) than salt resistance in normotensive humans, (b) it associates with human and experimental hypertension, and (c) it is inconsistent with the classical physiologic concept that the normal balance between natriuretic and antinatriuretic systems makes the excretion of a salt load independent of renal perfusion pressure.

Furthermore, Weinberger et al., who studied a cohort of normotensive and hypertensive individuals for almost 3 decades, found that SSBP is a risk factor for cardiovascular morbidity and mortality, independent of BP.

Genetics

The BP response to salt loading or deprivation is genetically determined in animals and humans. The best evidence for this comes from inbreeding rodents for salt-sensitive (SS) and salt-resistant (SR) phenotypes, resulting in pure substrains after several generations (e.g., Dahl-SS and Dahl-SR, Milan-SS and Milan-SR, and Sabra-SS and Sabra-SR rats).

As opposed to clear dichotomization of the SS and SR phenotypes in inbred strains, the BP response to salt in humans is a continuous variable (suggesting multigenic etiology). Therefore, arbitrary cutoffs in the BP response to salt loading or deprivation have been used to classify subjects into SS and SR. Experimental paradigms have included long-term (weeks) dietary manipulation of salt balance or short-term (hours to days) intravenous salt loading followed by pharmacologically induced natriuresis.

Both experimental paradigms have yielded strong evidence for genetic factors determining the BP response to salt loading in humans. For example, SSBP is reproducible within an individual when different methods of measurement are used, is concordant in twins and non–twin siblings, and is sustained over time. It is remarkable that despite the different methodologies employed to classify subjects into SS and SR groups, a series of common clinical characteristics and biochemical markers have been found in SS subjects (**Table A49.1**). Association or linkage studies of gene polymorphisms with hypertension or with the response of BP to salt or to salt-deprivation also support genetic determination of SSBP, including studies about haptoglobin, adducin, $\alpha 2$ and β-adrenergic receptors, β subunit of the epithelial sodium channel (ENaC), angiotensinogen, and CYP4a11. However, the mechanisms by which the different products of these genes affect the BP response to salt have not been fully elucidated.

Gene–environment interactions

Notwithstanding the genetic influence on SSBP in humans, the SSBP phenotype is also influenced by acquired and environmental factors. Four observations demonstrate the influence of environmental factors on SSBP: (a) its apparent prevalence correlates with the magnitude of the salt load in healthy subjects, (b) its incidence is higher in older subjects, (c) it occurs more frequently in populations with low calcium and low potassium intake, and (d) it is highly prevalent in chronic renal disease. All these observations suggest a link between SSBP and renal sodium (Na^+) handling.

TABLE A49.1

CLINICAL AND BIOCHEMICAL CHARACTERISTICS OF SS HYPERTENSIVE SUBJECTS

Demographic
Increased prevalence in
  African Americans
  Elderly
  Obese
  Diabetes
  Chronic renal failure
Clinical
Exaggerated rates of
  Nocturnal nondipper status
  Microalbuminuria
  Left ventricular diastolic
    dysfunction
Delayed
  Half-life for urine sodium
    excretion
Biochemical
  Low plasma renin activity
  Blunted responses of renin,
    aldosterone, and norepinephrine
    to salt loading
  Increased plasma endothelin
  Commonly but not always insulin
    resistance
  Suppressed kallikrein-kinin system
  Excess activation of the arginine-
    vasopressin pressor system

Dietary
Increased prevalence in
  Nutritional potassium
    deficiency
  Nutritional calcium
    deficiency
Improves with
  Dietary potassium
    replacement
  Dietary calcium
    replacement
Target organ damage
Disproportionate rates of
  Left ventricular
    hypertrophy
  Heart failure and stroke
  Hypertensive
    nephrosclerosis
Compared to
  Ischemic heart disease

Renal mechanisms of salt-sensitivity of blood pressure

Guyton et al. suggested that salt balance in an intact animal is maintained by a counterregulatory balance between natriuretic and antinatriuretic systems. In an isolated kidney deprived of such regulatory mechanisms, an increase in perfusion pressure is required for restoration of salt balance after a salt load ("pressure-natriuresis"). Animals with SSBP must therefore have a defect in natriuresis (or chloruresis, because chloride excretion is probably the most important determinant of renal salt handling). SSBP will be expressed when salt does not normally stimulate a natriuretic system that remains "clamped" at a low-activity level. Alternatively SSBP animals may fail to suppress an antinatriuretic system (one that is "clamped" at a level inappropriate for the salt-replete state) (**Figure A49.1**).

Experiments with renal transplantation between SS and SR rodents strongly support the concept that the principal defect leading to SSBP is renal in origin because the SSBP trait "follows the transplanted kidney". An SR animal develops SSBP if given the kidney of an SS animal, whereas an SS animal becomes resistant to the pressor effect of salt on receipt of an SR kidney.

Influence of vasoregulatory and natriuretic systems

Innumerable lines of research in many laboratories have detected physiologic abnormalities in different vasoactive and renal regulatory mechanisms in SS animals and humans. However, the ultimate cause of SSBP remains elusive because these regulatory systems interact, making it very difficult to pinpoint a causal or primary pathway.

Renin-angiotensin-aldosterone system (RAAS). Salt loading inhibits and salt depletion stimulates the renin-angiotensin-aldosterone system (RAAS), thereby allowing large changes in salt intake to have minimal to no impact on BP. The regulation of salt balance through aldosterone effects on distal tubular Na^+ reabsorption is an important factor in this homeostatic pathway. "Clamping" the system at either very low or very high levels of angiotensin II produces SSBP in dogs. Hall et al. showed BP reduction during salt depletion in the presence of chronic angiotensin-converting enzyme (ACE) inhibition and BP increase by salt loading during chronic angiotensin II infusion. Variation in aldosterone responses to salt has been characterized by Williams and Hollenberg. Individuals who fail to increase plasma aldosterone in response to salt deprivation or angiotensin infusion and do not normally increase renal blood flow in response to salt loading ("nonmodulators") generally exhibit SSBP.

Endothelin. Endothelins are mainly known as potent vasoconstrictors and stimulators of cell growth but have important renal actions as well. Renal ETb receptors promote natriuresis through inhibition of Na–K–ATPase. Mice with specific knockout of the ET-1 gene in the collecting ducts and rats deficient in ETb receptor develop SS hypertension. Four clinical observations concerning endothelin are of particular interest: (a) urinary endothelin and Na^+ excretion exhibit parallel circadian rhythms, (b) they show a positive correlation during a salt load, (c) there is a negative correlation between urinary endothelin and mean arterial pressure in normotensive and hypertensive subjects, and (d) in human SS hypertension, urinary endothelin is diminished. Therefore, reduced basal urinary endothelin and blunted renal endothelin responsiveness during salt loading may contribute to the pathogenesis of impaired natriuresis in human SS hypertension. Whether pure

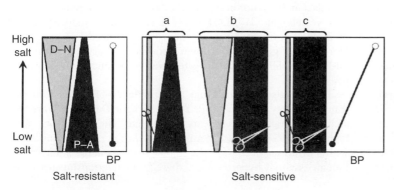

Figure A49.1 Schematic representation of the mechanisms that lead to salt-sensitivity of blood pressure (BP). In the left panel, when the salt-resistant animal is given a salt load (*bottom to top*), depressor and natriuretic mechanisms (*D-N*) are activated while pressor and antinatriuretic ones (*P-A*) are simultaneously inhibited. As a result, BP does not change (*vertical line*). In the right panel, possible abnormalities are depicted by (a) "clamping" of *D-N*, which remain unstimulated despite the salt load; (b) "clamping" of *P-A*, which remain active despite the salt-load; or (c) or a combination of both abnormalities. In any of these three situations, the animal becomes salt-sensitive, that is, BP increases in response to salt (*tilted line*).

ETa blockade (with ETb preservation) is useful in patients with SS hypertension remains to be tested.

Nitric oxide and oxidative stress.
Salt-stimulated production of neuronal nitric oxide synthase (nNOS)-derived nitric oxide (NO) is important for the regulation of renal blood flow and natriuresis in the rat. Also, nNOS inhibition leads to SS hypertension in rodents. Wilcox et al. showed that the antioxidant tempol abolishes the pressor response to salt and attenuates the hypertension in the spontaneously hypertensive rats (SHR), suggesting an imbalance between the generation of NO and oxygen radicals in these models. In humans with SS hypertension, a salt load paradoxically decreases excretion of NO metabolites. We have shown acute salt-induced increases in free isoprostanes in SS hypertensive subjects, suggesting perhaps that NO is diverted to the scavenging of salt-induced oxygen-free radicals. Alternatively, others have suggested that salt-stimulated production of an endogenous inhibitor of NO (asymmetric dimethylarginine) may play a role in SS hypertension.

Sympathetic nervous system.
DiBona et al. have characterized cardiorenal interactions in which the cardiac atria (and ventricles) act as volume sensors. Information about cardiac distension is transmitted by cardiopulmonary afferent nerves to brain stem integrator centers and then by renal sympathetic nerves to the kidney. This neurogenic renal vasodilator mechanism regulates renal blood flow and natriuresis. Disruption of this reflex by sinoaortic deafferentation in animals, or by cardiac transplantation in humans, leads to impaired natriuresis and SS hypertension. However, these models differ substantially from SS hypertension because they exhibit impaired natriuresis and subsequent volume expansion after salt administration. In contrast, in human SS hypertension, the increase in BP leads to restoration of salt balance, such that these patients do not differ from their SR counterparts in terms of renal Na^+ handling, but only in the level of BP required to modulate natriuresis. Blunting of the normal decrease in plasma or urinary norepinephrine and the concomitant increase in dopamine during salt loading occur in SS hypertension. The inability to suppress the sympathetic nervous system during salt loading could have substantial impact on renal and systemic hemodynamics, volume homeostasis, and BP levels in SSBP. In addition, alterations in dopaminergically mediated natriuresis could participate in the origin of SSBP. Furthermore, decreased activation of the dopamine D5 receptor may contribute to SSBP because it relates to increased oxidative stress, as demonstrated in D5 receptor knockout mice.

Behavior, gas exchange and natriuresis.
Although direct neural connections between the central nervous system (CNS) and the kidney are important, avoidance-conditioning stress induces SS hypertension in dogs, even after renal denervation. This nonsympathetic effect of stress has been attributed to a hypoventilatory response that increases Pco_2. The ensuing decrease in plasma pH blunts natriuresis, possibly by exaggerated renal Na^+–H^+ exchange. Human end tidal volume CO_2 (a good reflection of plasma Pco_2) is variable. Subjects with higher Pco_2 values have higher scores for worry, experiences of negative effects, and feelings of vulnerability on personality-trait scales, suggesting that slow breathing with high Pco_2 reflects a specific emotional pattern. This mechanism may participate in the exaggerated BP responses to some stressors, that is, mental arithmetic tests, in SS-hypertensive subjects.

Relationships between Pco_2 and digitalis-like compounds (ouabain immunoreactivity or marinobufagenin) have been demonstrated in both animals and humans suggesting a role for volume expansion in Pco_2-related SSBP. Anderson et al. showed that Pco_2 correlates with BP in normotensive women and predicts the salt-induced increase in BP and digitalis-like compounds in normotensive subjects of both genders. Moreover, end tidal volume CO_2 is higher in African Americans of both genders compared to whites, particularly in older subjects. This is consistent with slower urinary Na^+ excretion and greater SSBP in African Americans. It is not known whether different breathing patterns between races reflect genetic or cultural influences.

Arachidonic acid metabolites.
There is mounting evidence that products of cyclooxygenation, epoxygenation, and ω-hydroxylation of arachidonic acid play a major role in SSBP. For example, the cyclooxygenase 1 (COX-1) knockout mouse fails to increase the levels of the vasodilatory and natriuretic prostaglandin PGE_2 in response to a salt load. In this model and in experiments with COX-1 blockers, BP becomes sensitive to salt. One explanation for this effect is the role of PGE_2 in removing Na^+ channels (ENaC) from the cell membrane for proteasome recycling. It is noteworthy that the COX-1 knockout mouse shares with SSBP in humans a common feature, that is, a blunting of the sleep-related fall in BP. Aside from the salt-dependent form of hypertension that may occur during therapeutic administration of COX inhibitors, there is no clear evidence for direct participation of a deficit of PGE_2 in SS essential hypertension.

Epoxyeicosatrienoic acids (EETs), the products of epoxygenation of arachidonic acid, inhibit distal Na^+ reabsorption by altering the gating properties of ENaC. Increased synthesis of these compounds during salt loading is consistent with their participation in normal renal salt handling. In Dahl-SS rats, renal epoxygenase activity and urine EET excretion are diminished. Reduced expression of the CYP2c44 epoxygenase in CYP4a10 knockout mice and pharmacologic inhibition of the epoxygenase diminish synthesis of 11–12 EET and produce SS hypertension. In the knockout mouse, amiloride corrects the hypertension, supporting a role for ENaC hyperactivity.

20-hydroxyeicosatetraenoic acid (20-HETE), the major product of ω-hydroxylation of arachidonic acid has pro-(vasoconstriction) and antihypertensive (natriuresis) actions. The latter are exerted through blockade of potassium channels, thereby impairing the action of the $Na^+K^+2Cl^-$ cotransporter of the medullary thick ascending limb (mTAL) and also through inhibition of Na–K–ATPase. There is very strong evidence in three species that diminished renal 20-HETE content is linked to SSBP. There is a deficit in 20-HETE and the expression of CYP4A2 in the renal medulla of Dahl-SS rats with diminished chloride transport and blunted pressure-natriuresis. Moreover, congenic Dahl-SS strains harboring the region of chromosome 5 that contains the normal CYP4A genes, exhibit attenuated SSBP. In addition, stimulation by fenofibrate of CYP4a protein in renal tubules (not vessels) of C57BL/6J mice, a strain with reduced levels of 20-HETE, antagonizes angiotensin II–induced hypertension. Finally, our group has shown reduced urinary excretion of 20-HETE in SS essential hypertensives with concomitant insulin resistance.

There is also evidence that a defect in 20-HETE actions on transport plays a role in SSBP. Young Sprague Dawley rats are SS, a characteristic that disappears as they age. The young rats have high levels of 20-HETE but a poor correlation of this compound with natriuresis, both opposite to observations in the adult. In SS human essential hypertensives, there is no relationship between

20-HETE and Na^+ excretion, which is distinct from the tight correlation observed in SR subjects. Finally, population studies have linked risk of hypertension to a polymorphism of CYP4a11 that produces an enzyme with half the catalytic activity of the wild type protein.

Clinical significance

Research on the genetics and pathophysiology of SSBP has been stimulated by demonstration of the prognostic significance of the phenotype. Development of a specific biochemical or genetic marker to diagnose SSBP would replace the cumbersome methodology currently required to differentiate SS from SR subjects. Such a marker could be employed in risk profiling of hypertensive or prehypertensive subjects to determine the intensity of therapy. More importantly, unraveling of the causal mechanisms of SSBP may lead to development of pharmacologic therapy for the SS phenotype, regardless of the magnitude of BP elevation. This should contribute to decreased cardiovascular risk in prehypertensive and hypertensive SS subjects.

Suggested Readings

Anderson DE, Scuteri A, Agalakova N, et al. Racial differences in resting end-tidal CO_2 and circulating sodium pump inhibitor. *Am J Hypertens* 2001;14:761–767.

Campese VM, Romoff MS, Levitan D, et al. Abnormal relationship between sodium intake and sympathetic nervous system activity in salt-sensitive patients with essential hypertension. *Kidney Int* 1982;21:371–378.

DiBona GF, Sawin LL. Effect of arterial baroreceptor denervation on sodium balance. *Hypertension* 2002;40:547–551.

Elijovich F, Laffer CL. Participation of renal and circulating endothelin in salt-sensitive essential hypertension. *J Hum Hypertens* 2002;16:459–467.

Hall JE, Granger JP, Hester RL, et al. Mechanisms of sodium balance in hypertension: role of pressure natriuresis. *J Hypertens* 1986;4:657–665.

Laffer CL, Laniado-Schwartzman M, Wang MH, et al. Differential regulation of natriuresis by 20-hydroxyeicosatetraenoic acid in human salt-sensitive versus salt-resistant hypertension. *Circulation* 2003;107:574–578.

Nakagawa K, Holla VR, Wei Y, et al. Salt-sensitive hypertension is associated with dysfunctional Cyp4a10 gene and kidney epithelial sodium channel. *J Clin Invest* 2006;116:1696–1702.

Roman RJ, Hoagland KM, Lopez B, et al. Characterization of blood pressure and renal function in chromosome 5 congenic strains of Dahl S rats. *Am J Physiol* 2006;290:F1463–F1471.

Weinberger MH, Fineberg NS, Fineberg SE, et al. Salt sensitivity, pulse pressure, and death in normal and hypertensive humans. *Hypertension* 2001;37:429–432.

Wilcox CS. Oxidative stress and nitric oxide deficiency in the kidney: a critical link to hypertension? *Am J Physiol* 2005;289:R913–R935.

CHAPTER A50 ■ PATHOPHYSIOLOGY OF RENAL PARENCHYMAL HYPERTENSION

VITO M. CAMPESE, MD AND JEANIE PARK, MD

KEY POINTS

- Intravascular volume expansion is a major pathogenic factor in renal parenchymal hypertension, and dietary sodium restriction, diuretic therapy, and/or removal of excess volume with dialysis are important mainstays in the management of these patients.
- Excessive renin secretion relative to volume status has long been recognized as an important factor in the pathogenesis of hypertension among patients with renal parenchymal diseases.
- Sympathetic nervous system overactivity contributes to hypertension in patients with renal disease, and potential mechanisms include afferent stimuli from the injured kidneys to the brain, reduced central dopaminergic tone, reduced baroreceptor sensitivity, abnormal vagal function, increased $[Ca^{2+}]_1$ concentration, and increased plasma β-endorphin and β-lipotropin levels.
- Endothelial dysfunction, perhaps due to inhibition of nitric oxide (NO) synthesis, may contribute to hypertension in renal failure.

See also Chapters A51, **A69, B80, C115,** and **C156**

The association between hypertension and chronic renal disease has been recognized since the pioneering work of Richard Bright at Guy's Hospital in 1836. Renal disease is by far the commonest cause of secondary hypertension, which occurs in approximately 80% of patients with chronic renal failure, and it contributes to the progression of renal disease.

Cardiovascular disease is the leading cause of death in patients with end-stage renal disease (ESRD) and chronic kidney

FACTORS IMPLICATED IN THE PATHOGENESIS OF
HYPERTENSION ASSOCIATED WITH KIDNEY DISEASE

Sodium and volume excess
Activation of the renin-angiotensin-aldosterone system
Increase sympathetic nervous system activity
Baroreceptor dysfunction
Reduced endothelium-derived vasodepressor substances
Increased endothelium-derived vasoconstrictor substances
Oxidative stress
Divalent ions and parathyroid hormone
Structural changes in the arteries
Preexistent essential hypertension
Phospholipid antibodies syndrome
Drugs (steroids, cyclosporin, NSAIDs, sympathomimetics)
Erythropoietin
Vasopressin
Serotonin
Calcitonin-gene related peptide

NSAIDs, nonsteroidal antiinflammatory drugs.

disease (CKD). Hypertension is the single most important predictor of coronary artery disease in uremic patients, even more predictive than cigarette smoking or hypertriglyceridemia. The pathophysiology of hypertension in renal patients is multifactorial (**Table A50.1**), and oftentimes difficult to control. In addition, patients with renal failure exhibit an abnormal circadian pattern of blood pressure characterized by blunted nocturnal dipping, probably due to autonomic dysfunction or obstructive sleep apnea, contributing to increased cardiovascular morbidity. Because blood pressure is usually measured during the day, this may lead to the erroneous impression that blood pressure is adequately controlled.

Pathogenesis

Role of sodium and volume status.
Excessive intravascular volume is a major pathogenic factor in renal parenchymal hypertension. The mechanisms by which sodium excess leads to arterial hypertension in the uremic patient are complex. In early phases, sodium excess leads to volume expansion and to increased cardiac output. Later, hypertension is sustained by an increase in peripheral vascular resistance. Restriction of dietary sodium intake to <2 g per day helps to control volume status in these patients. Administration of diuretics, and/or removal of excess volume with dialysis are important adjuncts in the management of hypertension in these patients.

Role of the renin-angiotensin system.
The role of excessive renin secretion relative to the state of sodium/volume balance has long been recognized as an important factor in the pathogenesis of hypertension in patients with renal parenchymal diseases. Several factors support this notion. First, these patients do not have the normal suppression of plasma renin activity in relation to exchangeable sodium or blood volume. "Normal" plasma concentrations of renin are inappropriately high in relation to the state of sodium and volume balance. Secondly, a direct relationship between plasma renin activity and blood pressure frequently can be found. Thirdly, blood pressure can be effectively reduced in most of these patients by the administration of

angiotensin-converting enzyme inhibitors or angiotensin II blockers. Finally, bilateral nephrectomy results in normalization of blood pressure in most of these patients.

Role of the autonomic nervous system.
Both ESRD and CKD are characterized by a state of sympathetic overactivity, contributing to hypertension and cardiovascular risk. In patients with chronic renal failure, plasma norepinephrine levels are frequently but not always increased. This variability is probably related to the complex effects of uremia on prejunctional modulation of norepinephrine release and on plasma catecholamine clearance. However, muscle sympathetic nerve activity, when measured in real-time from the peroneal nerve of living human subjects, is not subject to such variation, and has been consistently higher in patients with ESRD as well as CKD when compared to controls. Converse and others found that muscle sympathetic nerve activity, which correlates with central sympathetic output, was significantly higher in dialysis patients than in healthy controls. However, interestingly, dialysis patients who had undergone bilateral nephrectomy had significantly lower muscle sympathetic nerve activity compared to dialysis patients who still had their native diseased kidneys. Muscle sympathetic nerve activity in bilaterally nephrectomized patients was as low as that of healthy controls, and this decrease in sympathetic nerve activity was associated with lower regional vascular resistance and mean arterial pressure. These findings support the notion that the diseased kidneys themselves play a role in sympathetic overactivity and play a role in the pathogenesis of hypertension in renal failure.

The pathogenesis by which the diseased kidneys themselves increase central sympathetic output has been further elucidated in animal studies. The kidney is not only an elaborate filtering device but also a sensory organ richly innervated with afferent nerves. There are two main functional types of renal sensory receptors and afferent nerves: renal baroreceptors, which increase their firing in response to changes in renal perfusion and intrarenal pressure, and renal chemoreceptors, which are stimulated by ischemic metabolites or uremic toxins. Activation of renal chemoreceptors or baroreceptors and renal afferent nerves that disinhibit integrative nuclei of the central nervous system can activate efferent sympathetic pathways and raise blood pressure. In addition, limited renal injury without any change in renal function, induced by intrarenal injection of phenol in the rat, raises blood pressure, increases the secretion of norepinephrine from the posterior hypothalamic nuclei, and increases renal efferent sympathetic nerve activity. Therefore, an injury to a limited portion of one kidney causes a permanent elevation of noradrenergic activity and blood pressure, irrespective of glomerular filtration rate.

Other mechanisms potentially responsible for the increase in sympathetic nerve activity in uremic patients include reduced central dopaminergic tone, reduced baroreceptor sensitivity, abnormal vagal function, increased $[Ca^{2+}]_i$ concentration, and increased plasma β-endorphin and β-lipotropin levels.

Role of the vascular endothelium.
Endothelial cells cause vasodilation in part through formation of nitric oxide (NO) from endothelial nitric oxide synthase (NOS), and impaired endothelium-dependent vasodilation has been observed in patients with ESRD and those with CKD. In rats, chronic inhibition of NO synthesis by N^{ω}-nitro-L-arginine methyl ester causes systemic hypertension, marked renal vasoconstriction and hypoperfusion, a fall in glomerular filtration rate, an increase in filtration fraction, a rise in plasma renin levels, focal arteriolar obliteration, and segmental fibrinoid necrosis of the glomeruli. Administration

of N^g-methyl-L-arginine (an NO synthase inhibitor) increased renal sympathetic nerve activity and systemic blood pressure in male Wistar rats. *In vitro* and *in vivo* NO synthesis can be inhibited by an endogenous compound, N^G,N^G-dimethylarginine (asymmetrical dimethylarginine, ADMA). Significantly higher plasma levels of ADMA and significantly lower plasma arginine:dimethylarginine ratios have been observed in some uremic patients on chronic hemodialysis. This raises the possibility that hypertension in the uremic patient might be due to NO synthesis inhibition caused by increased levels of this circulating endogenous inhibitor.

In addition, stimulation of the endothelin-a (ET-A) receptor on vascular smooth muscle cells by ET-1 causes vasoconstriction, and a correlation exists between blood pressure and serum ET-1 levels in patients with renal disease. Hypertensive patients with ESRD and those with CKD exhibit higher plasma levels of ET-1 and ET-3 than normotensive subjects. Furthermore, ET receptor antagonists have been shown to reduce blood pressure and proteinuria in patients with CKD. In two cases of hemangioendothelioma, a rare malignant vascular neoplasm, plasma levels of ET were 10-fold to 15-fold greater than that of normal or essential hypertensive subjects. Surgical removal of the tumor led to resolution of hypertension in both cases.

Role of erythropoietin. Recombinant human erythropoietin (rHu-EPO), which is currently widely used to treat anemia in patients with chronic renal failure, can worsen hypertension and increase the requirement for antihypertensive drugs. The rise in blood pressure during treatment with rHu-EPO has not been observed in patients receiving rHu-EPO for other reasons, suggesting that renal disease may confer a particular susceptibility to the hypertensive effect of rHu-EPO. The rise in blood pressure during rHu-EPO administration usually occurs within 2 to 16 weeks, although some patients may experience a rise in blood pressure several months after the initiation of therapy. Patients who are at greater risk for developing hypertension during rHu-EPO therapy are those with severe anemia, those whose anemia is corrected too rapidly, or those with preexisting hypertension.

Clinical and experimental studies have confirmed the importance of hematocrit in the regulation of both systemic and renal hemodynamics. Anemia causes a hyperdynamic state characterized by increased cardiac output and decreased total peripheral vascular resistance (TPR). Correction of the anemia with rHu-EPO leads to a decrease in cardiac output and a rise in TPR. Patients who become hypertensive or experience an exacerbation of hypertension during rHu-EPO therapy either have an exaggerated rise of TPR in response to the increase in hematocrit or do not suppress cardiac output to the same extent as patients who remain normotensive. The increase in blood viscosity during rHu-EPO therapy correlates with the increase in TPR but not with blood pressure changes. Hypertension induced by rHu-EPO therapy could also be a result of enhanced pressor responsiveness to norepinephrine and angiotensin II. Other potential mechanisms responsible for the rise in blood pressure during therapy with rHu-EPO are an increase in cytosolic free calcium, and an increase in ET-1 secretion.

Role of divalent ions and parathyroid hormone. Chronic renal failure is associated with secondary hyperparathyroidism and increased $[Ca^{2+}]_i$ in many organs, including the myocardium and circulating platelets. A relationship between platelet or lymphocyte $[Ca^{2+}]_i$ and blood pressure has been demonstrated in essential hypertension.

A study in 36 patients with chronic renal failure found that 10 had normal serum parathyroid hormone(PTH) levels, 17 had elevated serum PTH, and 9 had elevated PTH but were treated with nifedipine. A significant relationship was present between serum PTH and platelet $[Ca^{2+}]_i$ or between platelet $[Ca^{2+}]_i$ or PTH and mean blood pressure. In patients with high serum PTH receiving nifedipine, platelet $[Ca^{2+}]_i$ was not increased. Nine patients with hyperparathyroidism were restudied during treatment with alfacalcidol, a Vitamin D metabolite. In these patients, serum PTH, platelet $[Ca^{2+}]_i$, and mean blood pressure all decreased significantly. The changes in blood pressure during treatment with alfacalcidol were linearly related with the changes in serum PTH and $[Ca^{2+}]_i$. These studies suggest that increased serum levels of PTH may be responsible for both the rise in $[Ca^{2+}]_i$ and the increase in blood pressure in these patients.

Oxidative stress and hypertension

Considerable attention has been given to the effects of short-lived reactive oxygen species (ROS) and reactive nitrogen species on blood pressure and cardiovascular toxicity. ROS or oxygen free-radicals are O_2 molecules with an unpaired electron, and include superoxide anion (O_2^-), hydrogen peroxide (H_2O_2), and hydroxyl ion (OH). Reactive nitrogen species, including peroxynitrate, are chemically unstable and highly reactive molecules, and nicotinamide adenine dinucleotide phosphate (NADPH) oxidase, xanthine oxidase, and NOS enzymes regulate their concentration. NADPH oxidase is a multimeric enzyme responsible for the reduction of oxygen, electron transport, and superoxide production at the cell surface. The vascular isoform of NADPH is constitutively active and is a major source of vascular superoxide production. Although NOS is a major source of NO, under conditions of L-arginine deficiency, this enzyme may also generate the NO-scavenger superoxide. All three isoforms of NOS—the neuronal, inducible and endothelial—are capable of superoxide production.

Oxygen radicals and endogenous scavenging systems, such as superoxide dismutase, modulate vascular tone and function. In addition, ROS may stimulate vascular contraction directly or through quenching of the vasodilator NO and production of peroxinitrite $[O_2^- + NOO^- \rightarrow ONOO^-]$. Peroxinitrite may induce oxidative damage to DNA, lipids and proteins in vascular cells, and result in endothelial dysfunction.

ROS production is increased in several experimental models of hypertension including uremic hypertension. ROS are increased in uremic rats and they react with NO producing cytotoxic reactive nitrogen species capable of nitrating proteins and damaging other molecules. Antioxidant therapy ameliorated the CRF-induced hypertension, improved vascular tissue NO production, and lowered tissue nitrotyrosine.

However, the exact mechanisms through which oxidative stress may raise blood pressure, and the potential role of antioxidant therapy, have not been fully elucidated.

Suggested Readings

Baumgart P, Walger P, Gemen S, et al. Blood pressure elevation during the night in chronic renal failure, hemodialysis, and renal transplantation. *Nephron* 1991; 57:293–298.

Baylis C, Mitruka B, Deng A. Chronic blockade of nitric oxide synthesis in the rat produces systemic hypertension and glomerular damage. *J Clin Invest* 1992; 90:278–281.

Campese VM, Chervu I. Hypertension in dialysis subjects. In: Henrich WL, ed. *Principles and practice of dialysis.* Baltimore: Williams & Wilkins, 1994:148–169.

Campese VM, Mitra N, Sandee D. Hypertension in renal parenchymal disease: why is it so resistant to treatment? *Kidney Int* 2006;69:967–973.

Converse RL Jr, Jacobsen TN, Toto RD, et al. Sympathetic overactivity in patients with chronic renal failure. *N Engl J Med* 1992;327:1912–1918.

Katholi RE. Renal nerves and hypertension: an update. *Fed Proc* 1985;44:2846–2850.

Raine AEG, Bedford L, Simpson AW, et al. Hyperparathyroidism, platelet intracellular free calcium and hypertension in chronic renal failure. *Kidney Int* 1993;43:700–705.

Shichiri M, Hirata Y, Ando K, et al. Plasma endothelin levels in hypertension and chronic renal failure. *Hypertension* 1990;15:493–496.

Steffen HM, Brunner R, Müller R, et al. Peripheral hemodynamics, blood viscosity, and the renin-angiotensin system in hemodialysis patients under therapy with recombinant human erythropoietin. *Contrib Nephrol* 1989;76:292–298.

Vaziri ND, Oveisi F, Ding Y. Role of increased oxygen free radical activity in the pathogenesis of uremic hypertension. *Kidney Int* 1998;53:1748–1754.

Weidmann P, Maxwell MH, Lupu AN, et al. Plasma renin activity and blood pressure in terminal renal failure. *N Engl J Med* 1971;285:757–762.

Ye S, Ozgur B, Campese VM. Renal afferent impulses, the posterior hypothalamus, and hypertension in rats with chronic renal failure. *Kidney Int* 1997;51:722–727.

CHAPTER A51 ■ PATHOPHYSIOLOGY OF RENOVASCULAR HYPERTENSION

L. GABRIEL NAVAR, PhD AND DAVID W. PLOTH, MD

KEY POINTS

■ Reduced renal perfusion pressure resulting from arterial stenosis of one or both kidneys causes unilateral or bilateral renovascular hypertension through the interaction of increased activity of the renin-angiotensin-aldosterone system (RAAS) and impaired salt and water excretion with resultant volume retention.

■ In bilateral renal artery stenosis, reduced renal perfusion pressure causes early activation of the RAAS, impaired renal function and volume and sodium retention that leads to hypertension; these actions partially restore poststenotic renal perfusion pressure.

■ In unilateral renal artery stenosis, hypertension is primarily due to persistence of systemic and renal angiotensin (Ang) II–dependency, coupled with impairment of pressure natriuresis in the nonstenotic kidney due to the effects of raised intrarenal Ang II levels.

■ Drugs that block the RAAS can reduce glomerular filtration in patients with renal artery stenosis; this phenomenon is reversible upon discontinuation of the offending agent and offers a clinical clue to the presence of renovascular hypertension.

See also Chapters A50, **C116,** and **C168**

Increased arterial pressure caused by stenosis, constriction, or lesions of the renal arteries involving one or both kidneys is categorized as renovascular hypertension. The derangements may be quite variable, ranging from overt renal arterial stenosis of one or both renal arteries to subtle intrarenal microvascular lesions that are not usually detectable clinically.

Subtypes and animal models

There are two main categories of renovascular hypertension in conditions in which two kidneys are present: unilateral and bilateral renovascular disease. In animals, these conditions are represented respectively by models in which a constricting clip is applied to one or both renal arteries to create the two-kidney,

one-clip (2K-1C) (Goldblatt) model and the two-kidney, two-clip (2K-2C) model. A third model that corresponds to renovascular hypertension in a single kidney, as in patients who had undergone renal transplantation, is the one-kidney, one-clip (1K-1C) model, which shares many features of the 2K-2C model.

Renal artery stenosis is most commonly caused by atherosclerotic disease of the renal artery, fibromuscular dysplasia, or stenosis at the anastomotic site of a transplanted kidney. Microvascular lesions resulting from diffuse atherosclerosis or arteritic occlusions within the intrarenal vasculature can be causes of renovascular hypertension but are difficult to detect other than for their form of clinical presentation and/or progression. Because of the autoregulatory capacity of the renal vascular bed and other compensatory alterations in intrarenal hemodynamics, there is

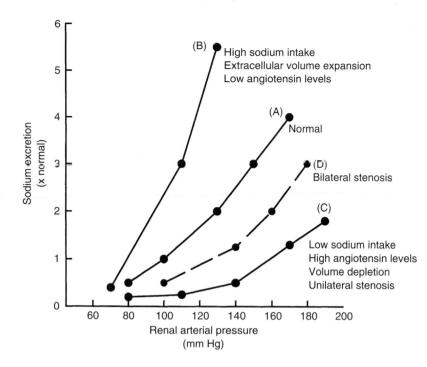

Figure A51.1 Relationship between renal arterial pressure and sodium excretion for normal conditions, high angiotensin (Ang) states, and reduced Ang states. The increase in sodium excretion in response to an increase in renal arterial pressure is referred to as *pressure natriuresis* and serves as the critical link between the regulation of arterial pressure and the renal regulation of sodium balance and extracellular volume. In bilateral renal vascular hypertension, the curve is shifted to the right (*curve D*) because of the reduced intrarenal perfusion pressure. In unilateral renovascular hypertension, the curve for the stenotic kidney is shifted to the right (*curve D*), and the relationship in the nonstenotic kidney becomes markedly less sensitive because of elevated intrarenal Ang II levels (*curve C*).

not a tight relationship between the degree of luminal narrowing of the main renal arteries and any ensuing decrease in glomerular filtration rate (GFR).

Mechanisms of hypertension

There are two main mechanisms of hypertension in renovascular disease: activation of the renin-angiotensin-aldosterone system (RAAS) and impaired salt and water excretion as a result of reduced pressure beyond the stenosis. The extent to which these two mechanisms contribute to the chronic blood pressure (BP) elevation of renovascular hypertension depends on the specific characteristics of the condition. Hypertension resulting from bilateral renal artery stenosis (2K-2C model) or stenosis of the artery to a solitary kidney (1K-1C model) share the same fundamental mechanisms. Although there is activation of the RAAS in these conditions, impaired salt and water excretion [leading to sodium (Na+) and volume retention] is the most prominent mechanism for chronic hypertension.

Renin-angiotensin-aldosterone system activation (early phase). The critical initiating event is the decrease in renal perfusion pressure, with or without marked or sustained reductions in renal blood flow and GFR. Release of renin occurs in response to (a) decreased perfusion pressure at the juxtaglomerular apparatus of the afferent arterioles and (b) decreased Na+ and chloride delivery to the macula densa segment of the ascending loop of Henle. Increased intrarenal and systemic concentrations of renin lead to increased systemic and intrarenal generation of angiotensin (Ang) I and subsequent conversion to Ang II by angiotensin-converting enzyme (ACE) with the latter being a potent vasopressor substance. Over time, the hyperreninemia subsides, at least in part because the volume-mediated elevation in systemic arterial pressure to a degree restores poststenotic perfusion pressure.

Salt and water retention (late phase). With time, Ang II-dependency of the systemic hypertension becomes attenuated because of progressive retention of salt and water, leading to

a relative expansion of extracellular fluid/blood volume and an increase in cardiac preload and stroke volume. Reductions in mean renal arterial pressure (probably down to the range of approximately 60 mm Hg, even less in some situations) do not generally cause sustained decreases in renal blood flow and GFR because renal autoregulatory mechanisms are still able to maintain renal hemodynamic function. Nevertheless, the reduced intrarenal perfusion pressure in these models markedly compromises maximal Na+ excretory capability because of the characteristic relationship between renal artery pressure and Na+ excretion (pressure natriuresis, **Figure A51.1**). When the degree of stenosis results in marked lowering of intrarenal perfusion pressure, the kidneys are no longer able to adequately excrete water and electrolytes. As a result, Na+ retention and expansion of extracellular fluid volume and cardiac preload occur not dissimilar to the pattern observed in chronic renal insufficiency. The resultant increase in systemic arterial pressure partially restores the post stenotic renal perfusion pressure thereby reestablishing Na+ balance.

Bilateral renal artery stenosis or stenosis in a solitary kidney

Because functional renal mass is subjected to reduced perfusion pressure, there is a direct reduction in pressure-dependent Na+ excretion, referred to as *resetting* of the pressure-natriuresis phenomenon (**Figure A51.1**). For any given hormonal and neural setting, there is a direct relationship between arterial pressure and the rate of Na+ excretion. In the presence of bilateral renal arterial stenosis (2K-2C) or stenosis in a solitary kidney, the reduced renal perfusion pressure diminishes Na+ excretion; moreover, it minimizes Na+ excretory responsiveness to natriuretic stimuli ordinarily activated by volume expansion. Furthermore, increased intrarenal Ang II activity promotes renal vasoconstriction, directly stimulates tubular Na+ reabsorption, and further contributes to Na+ retention by way of increased aldosterone levels. These changes are additive to synergistic with the direct effects of reduced perfusion pressure to cause Na⁺ and water retention, expansion of the extracellular and intravascular compartments, and, ultimately, an increased cardiac output. Chronically, salt and water balance is restored at the expense of systemic hypertension. Even if the pressure-natriuresis relationship is returned to a more normal profile, the entire relationship is shifted to a higher systemic pressure because of the pressure gradient derived from the stenotic lesions (curve A of **Figure A51.1**). This situation is represented by curve D in **Figure A51.1**; the extent of the shift is dependent on the degree of stenosis.

Two kidney, unilateral renal artery stenosis (Goldblatt hypertension)

In experimental two-kidney, single artery stenosis (2K-1C) renovascular hypertension, early changes in renal function and arterial pressure are due to the systemic and neural actions of Ang II. The elevated systemic Ang II activity results in sympathetic nervous system activation that also contributes to Na⁺ and volume retention.

Persistent renin-angiotensin-aldosterone system dependency. The important difference between hypertension caused by unilateral versus bilateral renal arterial stenosis is the persistent Ang II-dependency in unilateral stenosis. Although the elevated arterial pressure partially restores renal perfusion pressure, the pressure distal to the stenosis is never completely restored, thereby resulting in a continued stimulus to renin release and elevated circulating Ang II levels (**Figure A51.2**). In response to relatively subtle but sustained increases in circulating Ang II concentrations, there is accumulation of Ang II in the nonstenotic kidney by an AT₁ receptor–mediated internalization mechanism. In addition, the chronically elevated circulating and intrarenal Ang II levels augment angiotensinogen messenger RNA levels and angiotensinogen production, thereby causing increased or maintained local production of Ang II despite reduced renin content in the juxtaglomerular apparatus. There is also an increase in the angiotensinogen secreted into the tubules and spilling over into the distal nephron segments. Renin present in collecting duct cells can then lead to increased formation of Ang I and Ang II in distal nephron segments.

Role of the nonstenotic kidney. Although a single normal kidney is sufficient to maintain fluid and electrolyte balance at normotensive arterial pressures, the contralateral (nonstenotic) kidney cannot prevent hypertension in the case of unilateral renal arterial stenosis. The pathophysiology of hypertension in this model (2K-1C) depends on progressive changes in hormonal, neural, and hemodynamic factors originating from the stenotic kidney (**Figure A51.1**). Although the nonstenotic kidney is not an initial causative factor, it inappropriately resorbs Na⁺ in such a manner that extracellular fluid volume expands, which can only be counteracted by elevated arterial pressure. Reduced perfusion pressure in the stenotic kidney causes increased unilateral renin production and release, resulting in elevated circulating levels of Ang I and more importantly Ang II. Unlike the situation in bilateral stenosis, however, the nonstenotic kidney remains exposed to the elevated systemic arterial pressure and should therefore be able to increase Na⁺ excretion as long as the pressure-natriuresis mechanism remains intact. However, increased circulating and intrarenal Ang II levels and the ensuing rise in aldosterone levels blunts the natriuresis expected from increased renal perfusion pressure.

In the presence of sustained elevations in intrarenal Ang II and/or plasma aldosterone levels, the pressure-natriuresis relationship of the nonstenotic kidney is markedly attenuated, as depicted in curve C of **Figure A51.1**. Elevated intrarenal Ang II levels influence the nonstenotic kidney through multiple mechanisms, including (a) vasoconstrictor effects on both afferent and efferent arterioles that reduce renal plasma flow and GFR; (b) enhanced proximal and distal tubule Na⁺ reabsorption; and (c) over the long term, afferent arteriolar hypertrophy and proliferation. Furthermore, prolonged elevations of intrarenal Ang II levels in the presence of hypertension activate proliferative, oxidative and inflammatory factors, and cytokines that further exacerbate the pressure-related injury leading to arteriosclerosis. Once this occurs, repair of the vascular stenosis or even nephrectomy of the stenotic kidney may not return arterial pressure to normal,

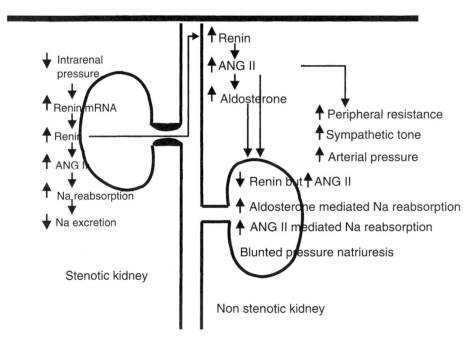

Figure A51.2 Effects of unilateral arterial stenosis on the responses from the stenotic kidney and on the changes in the systemic circulation and on the contralateral nonstenotic kidney. ANG II, angiotensin II; mRNA, messenger RNA.

probably because of damage to the nonstenotic kidney from the combination of hypertension and nephrosclerosis. Therefore, it is essential to detect and treat (or surgically correct) the hypertension due to single kidney renal artery lesions at the earliest possible time.

Antihypertensive drug effects

Pseudotolerance mechanisms. Having both volume and Ang II-dependent components of hypertension in the setting of bilateral renal artery stenosis inherently limits the effectiveness of single drug antihypertensive regimens. Vasodilator, ACE inhibitor, or angiotensin-receptor blocker (ARB) therapy reduces systemic arterial pressure but also lowers renal perfusion pressure and results in additional volume retention and doing so furthers the volume-dependency of the circumstance. Diuretic therapy enhances Na^+ excretion but any ensuing volume depletion can be expected to further activate the RAAS. These "pseudoresistance" or "pseudotolerance" effects can be minimized by combining diuretics with anti-RAAS drugs to treat the hypertension associated with renovascular disease.

Effects on glomerular filtration. In the extreme circumstance, diuretic therapy can render renal function extremely sensitive to reductions in arterial pressure. Therefore, patients with renal artery stenosis may respond to BP-lowering drugs with a reduction in GFR (increase in serum creatinine). Depending on the level of stenosis bilaterally, treatment with ACE inhibitors or ARBs may cause temporary deterioration in renal function. If the GFR decreases with RAAS blockade in a patient with Goldblatt hypertension, there must be substantial small vessel disease in the nonstenotic kidney.

If renal perfusion pressure is at or below the lower limit of the autoregulatory range, maximal constriction of the efferent arterioles becomes critical for the maintenance of glomerular capillary pressure and thereby glomerular filtration. If Ang II levels are decreased by ACE inhibitors or AT_1-receptors blocked by ARBs, maximal efferent arteriolar constriction cannot be maintained and glomerular capillary pressure and GFR will fall. Subsequent withdrawal of the anti-RAAS agent typically results in the rapid return of GFR, urine output, and BP. This demonstrates that the "apparent renal failure" associated with RAAS blockade reflects a hemodynamic alteration rather than progressive renal disease.

Suggested Readings

Cervenka L, Horacek V, Vaneckova I, et al. Essential role of AT1A receptor in the development of 2K1C hypertension. *Hypertension* 2002;40:735–741.

Crowley SD, Gurley SB, Herrera MJ, et al. Angiotensin II causes hypertension and cardiac hypertrophy through its receptors in the kidney. *Proc Natl Acad Sci U S A* 2006;103:17985–17990.

Imamura A, Mackenzie HS, Lacy ER, et al. Effects of chronic treatment with angiotensin converting enzyme inhibitor or an angiotensin receptor antagonist in two-kidney, one-clip hypertensive rats. *Kidney Int* 1995;47:1394–1402.

Kobori H, Ozawa Y, Suzaki Y, et al. Young scholars award lecture: intratubular angiotensinogen in hypertension and kidney diseases. *Am J Hypertens* 2006;19:541–550.

Mitchell KD, Navar LG. Intrarenal actions of angiotensin II in pathogenesis of experimental hypertension. In: Laragh JH, Brenner BM, eds. *Hypertension: pathophysiology, diagnosis, and management.* New York: Raven Press, 1995:1437–1450.

Navar LG, Hamm LL. The kidney in blood pressure regulation. In: Wilcox CS, ed. *Atlas of diseases of the kidney. Hypertension and the kidney,* Vol. 3. Philadelphia:Current Medicine, 1999:1.1–1.22.

Navar LG, Harrison-Bernard LM, Nishiyama A, et al. Regulation of intrarenal angiotensin II in hypertension. *Hypertension* 2002;39:316–322.

Ploth DW. Renovascular hypertension. In: Jacobson HR, Striker GE, Klahr S, eds. *The principles and practice of nephrology,* 2nd ed. St. Louis: Mosby-Year Book, 1995:379–386.

Pohl MA. Renal artery stenosis, renal vascular hypertension and ischemic nephropathy. In: Schrier RW, ed. *Diseases of the kidney,* 7th ed. Philadelphia: Lippincott Williams & Wilkins, 2001:1399–1457.

Textor SC. Ischemic nephropathy: where are we now? *J Am Soc Nephrol* 2004;15:1974–1982.

CHAPTER A52 ■ COARCTATION OF THE AORTA

ALBERT P. ROCCHINI, MD

KEY POINTS

■ Coarctation is suspected when blood pressure (BP) is higher in the arms than in the legs.
■ Coarctation can be corrected either with surgery or interventional catheterization.
■ Despite successful repair of coarctation, many individuals have persistent cardiovascular problems, including hypertension, coronary artery disease, aneurysms of the aorta, and stroke.

See also Chapter A51

Coarctation, the fourth most frequent (7.5%) form of congenital heart disease, requires either cardiac catheterization or surgery during the first year of life. Coarctation affects males more often than females (1.74:1). Coarctation of the aorta usually occurs sporadically but there are at least two reports of monozygotic twins concordant for this anomaly and there is a report of at least one family in which coarctation occurred in an autosomal dominant pattern. Finally, 35% of children with Turner's syndrome have coarctation of the aorta.

Mechanisms of hypertension

There are three different types of hypertension associated with coarctation of the aorta: prerepair hypertension, postrepair paradoxical hypertension, and postrepair hypertension that appears late.

Prerepair hypertension. The hypertension associated with coarctation of the thoracic aorta prerepair is relatively poorly understood. The three main theories used to explain the hypertension have included: the mechanical theory, the neural theory, and the Goldblatt-type phenomenon.

Mechanical theory. The mechanical theory was first proposed in 1948. The basis for this theory is that the increased blood pressure (BP) proximal to the coarcted segment is a function of the high impedance to left ventricular emptying. The findings that many patients with coarctation have hypertension both below and above the narrowing, together with the fact that hypertension persists despite the presence of large collateral channels, has cast doubt on this theory.

Neural theory. The neural theory proposes that hypertension is the result of readjustment of the baroreceptors in the aortic arch, such that an increased proximal pressure becomes necessary to ensure an adequate blood supply to the organs distal to the obstruction. There are no objective data to either support or refute this theory.

Goldblatt-type phenomenon. The third and most likely explanation for the hypertension observed in patients with coarctation of the aorta is that the changes are similar to those observed in renal artery stenosis (Goldblatt-type phenomenon). This theory suggests that the narrowed segment causes renal underperfusion with stimulation of the renin-angiotensin-aldosterone system and relative impairment of salt and water excretion. The studies of Scott and Bahnson strongly support this theory. These investigators created coarctations in dogs and showed that hypertension could be prevented if they transplanted one kidney above the coarctation and removed the other kidney. Until recently the major criticism of the renal underperfusion theory was that hypertensive children with coarctation did not have either elevated plasma renin activity (PRA) or decreased renal blood flow. However, when patients with coarctation are volume depleted, PRA is dramatically increased and BP becomes very responsive to antagonists of the renin-angiotensin system. A similar situation has been documented in experimental models of one-kidney one-clip Goldblatt hypertension.

Postrepair paradoxical hypertension. Severe "paradoxical" hypertension, which frequently occurs during the first week after surgical repair of coarctation, involves activation of the sympathetic nervous and renin-angiotensin systems. Since dilatation of a coarctation using balloon angioplasty does not tend to cause paradoxical hypertension, some other aspect of the surgical repair process may be involved. It has been postulated that disruption of cardiopulmonary baroreflex afferent fibers may lead to loss of the normal balance of excitatory and depressor sympathetic mechanoreceptors and thereby a net increase in sympathetic activity. This increased sympathetic activity in turn stimulates renin release and results in paradoxical hypertension. Paradoxical hypertension can be prevented with β-blocker pretreatment, with blockade of the renin-angiotensin system, or with the use of balloon angioplasty.

Late postrepair hypertension. Many individuals with good hemodynamic repairs (and no resting gradients) develop significant upper extremity hypertension with treadmill exercise but not with arm exercise. These patients have increased vascular reactivity to exogenous norepinephrine in the arm, normal vascular reactivity in the legs, and also have abnormal aortocarotid baroreceptor activity. It has been postulated that the resting and exercise-induced systolic hypertension in the late postoperative condition is due to different patterns of arterial remodeling (size and wall composition changes), either caused by the coarctation or by the different patterns of upper and lower extremity postoperative vascular remodeling that occur after the gradient is repaired. Children or adults who have both no or minimal resting arm-leg gradients who demonstrate resting or exercise-induced hypertension should probably be treated with antihypertensive medications such as angiotensin-converting enzyme (ACE) inhibitors or calcium antagonists.

Diagnosis

The physical findings diagnostic of coarctation are diminished femoral pulses and an abnormal systolic pressure gradient (or low ankle-brachial index) between the right arm and leg. A grade 2 or 3 over 6 systolic murmur, heard best in the posterior left interscapular area is frequently present and the particular location of this murmur is important in localizing the coarctation to the thoracic aorta. Among patients with well-developed collateral blood flow, systolic or continuous murmurs may be heard over the left and right sides of the chest.

Noninvasive confirmation of the diagnosis can be made by chest x-ray and echocardiogram. On the frontal projects of the chest x-ray, a discrete thoracic coarctation may show a "3 sign" whose outline is the result of the respective outlines of the proximal aorta, the coarcted segment, and the area of poststenotic dilatation. A barium swallow may reveal indentations by the same structures on the esophagus in a "reverse 3" configuration. Echocardiogram and Doppler determinations are extremely useful in localizing the site of the coarcted segment, in assessing the anatomy of the aortic arch, and in estimating the pressure gradient across the coarctation. Cardiac catheterization is now reserved for those infants and children in whom the echocardiogram or physical examination suggest: (i) abnormal location of the coarctation (i.e., abdominal aorta), (ii) the presence of other associated cardiac lesions, (iii) abnormal aortic arch anatomy, or (iv) to assess nonsurgical treatment with either balloon angioplasty or aortic stent placement (**Figure A52.1**).

Management

The poor prognosis of untreated patients with coarctation of the aorta is well known: 20% of patients die between the first and second decade of life and 80% expire before 50 years of age. Therefore, coarctation of the aorta should be treated as early in childhood as possible.

The two current approaches used to treating coarctation of the aorta are surgery and balloon angioplasty, with or without placement of an intravascular stent. Although balloon angioplasty has become a widely accepted therapy, in some patients it may be unsuccessful because of elastic recoil of the vessel or unfavorable anatomy such as long-segment narrowing or arch hypoplasty. Expandable stents have been used successfully in adults or older adolescents, individuals who have failed balloon angioplasty, or those with a hypoplastic aortic arch. Surgical treatment varies on

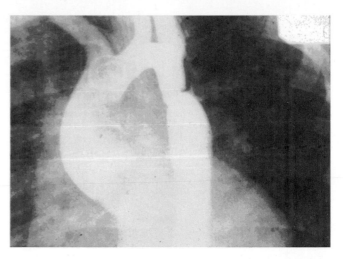

Figure A52.1 This is a left anterior oblique angiogram of a 12-year-old boy with a discrete thoracic coarctation of the aorta. There is also mild hypoplasia of the transverse arch. This patient also has a Gothic type of arch. This type of arch configuration has been associated with the presence of exercise hypertension post repair.

a case-by-case basis and may include resection and extended end-to-end anastomosis, left subclavian flap angioplasty, synthetic patch angioplasty, or rarely the use of a tube interposition graft.

The incidence of restenosis depends more on the age at the time of repair than the type of surgical repair (occurring in up to 20% of children younger than 1 year and only occurring in 3% of children older than 3 years). Balloon angioplasty is the treatment of choice in patients who develop restenosis after surgical repair.

Prognosis

On the surface it would appear that if the coarctation is successfully treated, then long-term survival should approach that of the general population. However, on the basis of recent reports, many individuals with a repaired coarctation do not have a normal life expectancy. These individuals often have other cardiovascular problems, including ischemic heart disease, cerebral hemorrhage, aortic aneurysms, and persistent hypertension. We have evaluated the long-term results of 254 survivors of coarctation repair performed between 1948 and 1976. After excluding the 20 individuals who died during the initial repair in an estimated survival analysis, 95% of patients were alive at 10 years, 89% at 20 years, 82% at 30 years and 79% at 40 years after operation, the mean age of the 45 individuals who died late after repair was 34 ± 22 years. Age at the time of initial surgical repair significantly affected long-term survival. The 30-year survival rates in individuals repaired before the age of 5, and in the group repaired between the ages of 5 and 10 were, $93 \pm 2.7\%$ and $91 \pm 2.4\%$, respectively. In contrast, the corresponding survival rate in those older than 10 years at operation was only $76 \pm 3.6\%$ ($p < .001$). Most common causes of death were coronary artery disease (10 patients, mean age at death 53 years, all >10 years old at initial surgery), death at reoperation (7), sudden death (7, of whom 6 were >10 years old at surgery), and a ruptured ascending aortic aneurysm (7). Predictors of survival were age at operation ($p = .004$), and the BP at the first postoperative visit ($p < .001$).

Suggested Readings

Cambell M. Natural history of coarctation of the aorta. *Br Heart J* 1970;32: 63–69.
Clarkson P, Nicholson M, Barratt-Boyes BG, et al. Results after repair of coarctation of the aorta beyond infancy. A 10 to 28 year follow-up with particular reference to late systemic hypertension. *Am J Cardiol* 1983;51:1481–1488.
Cohen M, Fuster V, Steele P, et al. Coarctation of the aorta. Long-term follow-up and prediction of outcome after surgical correction. *Circulation* 1989;80:840–845.

Gidding SS, Rocchini AP, Beekman RH, et al. Therapeutic effect of propranolol on paradoxical hypertension after repair of coarctation of the aorta. *N Engl J Med* 1985;312:1224–1228.
Markel H, Rocchini AP, Beekman RH, et al. Exercise-induced hypertension after repair of coarctation of the aorta: arm versus leg exercise. *J Am Coll Cardiol* 1986;8(1):165–171.
Salazar O, Steinberger J, Carpenter B, et al. Predictors of hypertension in long-term survivors of repaired coarctation of the aorta. *Am J Cardiol* 2002;89:541–547.
Scott HW, Bahnson HT. Evidence for a renal factor on the hypertension of coarctation of the aorta. *Surgery* 1951;30:206–217.
Stewart A, Ahmed R, Travill C, et al. Coarctation of the aorta life and health 20–44 years after surgical repair. *Br Heart J* 1993;69:65–70.

CHAPTER A53 ■ HYPERTENSION CAUSED BY THYROID AND PARATHYROID ABNORMALITIES, ACROMEGALY, AND ANDROGENS

YORAM SHENKER, MD

KEY POINTS

- Hypothyroidism is often associated with diastolic hypertension, increased catecholamine levels, and increased vascular resistance; replacement of thyroid hormone usually normalizes these parameters.
- Thyrotoxicosis is often associated with systolic hypertension due to increased cardiac output and decreased peripheral resistance; treatment of thyrotoxicosis normalizes blood pressure (BP).
- Hypertension in hyperparathyroidism is multifactorial and may be related to cellular effect of calcium, effects of parathyroid hormone (PTH), renal insufficiency, or changes in the renin-angiotensin-aldosterone system.
- Approximately 50% of acromegalic patients are hypertensive with increased cardiac output and left ventricular hypertrophy induced by a direct effect of growth hormone (GH).

See also Chapters A19, C106, and C170

THYROID AND HYPERTENSION

Demographic aspects

Hypothyroidism. The reported prevalence of hypertension in hypothyroidism is highly variable (0%–50%) although hypothyroidism has been identified as a reversible cause of hypertension in no more than 3% of hypertensive patients. Many patients with hypothyroidism and hypertension have diastolic blood pressure (BP) elevations to predominate. The level of hypothyroidism seems to be correlated with diastolic BP; however, a recent study found no increase in the prevalence of hypertension in geriatric patients with hypothyroidism when compared with a geriatric population that was euthyroid, and no association between thyroid-stimulating hormone (TSH) levels and diastolic BP. Thyroid hormone replacement decreases systolic and diastolic BP in patients with hypertension and hypothyroidism (including patients with subclinical hypothyroidism) but normalization of BP is less likely in older patients and in those with long-standing hypertension.

Hyperthyroidism. The prevalence of hypertension in thyrotoxicosis is probably in the range of 20% to 30%. Systolic hypertension is the predominant finding because of the increased cardiac output and decreased peripheral resistance seen with this disease; high diastolic BP is uncommon in thyrotoxicosis. The prevalence of hypertension in thyrotoxic patients is particularly increased in patients younger than 50 years. Treatment of thyrotoxicosis with return to a euthyroid state usually results in normalization of systolic BP, particularly in younger patients.

Mechanisms of hypertension

Cellular effects of thyroid hormone. Most of the effects of thyroid hormones are mediated through activation of specific nuclear receptors targeted by thyroid hormones, which increase transcription of a specific messenger RNA and heighten production of various proteins in different organ systems. Some of the effects of thyroid hormones, including cardiovascular effects, occur very rapidly and appear to be directly related to their nongenomic effects (**Table A53.1**).

Hemodynamic variations. Thyrotoxicosis or excess administration of thyroid hormones is associated with increased cardiac output, stroke volume, heart rate, and contractility. It also leads to increased blood volume, decreased peripheral vascular resistance, and a widened pulse pressure (increased systolic BP and decreased diastolic BP). Conversely, hypothyroidism is associated with a low cardiac output and increased total peripheral resistance, which may be partially related to acceleration of structural changes in vascular tissue caused by thyroid hormone deficiency. Total blood volume is also decreased in hypothyroidism.

Sympathetic nervous system interactions.

Hyperthyroidism. The cardiovascular manifestations of thyrotoxicosis closely resemble those caused by infusion of epinephrine, and many of the symptoms of thyrotoxicosis (especially tachycardia and tremor) are controlled by β-adrenergic-blockers. Yet, catecholamine levels in thyrotoxicosis are either low or normal. One possible explanation is increased sensitivity to catecholamines, which may be related to increased density of β-adrenergic receptors, as has been found in heart tissue and leukocytes. β-Adrenergic receptor density is controlled at least partially by the level of thyroid hormones. The absence of an increased response to exogenous adrenergic agonists in thyrotoxicosis, however, casts some doubt on the receptor sensitivity hypothesis.

Hypothyroidism. Patients with hypothyroidism have high plasma norepinephrine levels, particularly when they are hypertensive, along with high muscle sympathetic nerve activity. The number of β-adrenergic receptors in patients with hypothyroidism is decreased, leading to decreased β-adrenergic

responses. Diminished opposition to the α-adrenergic effects of catecholamines remains a possible explanation for the increase in peripheral vascular resistance and hypertension of hypothyroidism.

Renin-angiotensin system. Plasma renin activity (PRA) is low in hypothyroidism; it increases when thyroxine is replaced. This pattern would be predicted by the parallel changes in β-adrenergic receptor density. Yet aldosterone secretion rate and the response of aldosterone to various nonrenin secretagogues is diminished. PRA is increased in thyrotoxicosis, which may be related to thyroid hormone–induced hepatic synthesis of renin substrate (angiotensinogen). This pattern is similar to the effects of estrogen and cortisol, which can stimulate the entire renin-aldosterone system. Administration of angiotensin II antagonists in thyrotoxic patients does not necessarily reduce BP, which casts doubt on the role of the renin-aldosterone system in thyrotoxic hypertension.

PARATHYROIDS AND HYPERTENSION

Demographic aspects

Hypertension is frequently associated with primary hyperparathyroidism (caused by an adenoma or hyperplasia of the parathyroid gland), pseudohypoparathyroidism [caused by resistance to parathyroid hormone (PTH)], or secondary hyperparathyroidism, most often caused by advanced chronic kidney disease (CKD). The reported prevalence of hypertension in select groups with primary hyperparathyroidism varies from 10% to >70%; patients with pseudohypoparathyroidism have a 40% to 50% prevalence rate of hypertension.

Mechanisms of hypertension in hyperparathyroidism

Hypertension in different forms of hyperparathyroidism is probably multifactorial. The possibility that essential hypertension and hyperparathyroidism coexist cannot be ignored, considering the high prevalence of both conditions in the elderly population and in those with CKD.

Serum calcium. Acute infusion of calcium into normotensive patients usually leads to small increases in peripheral vascular resistance. Conditions of non–PTH-dependent hypercalcemia are also quite frequently associated with hypertension. These observations have led to the hypothesis that hypercalcemia increases free intracellular calcium, which increases vascular smooth muscle contractility and therefore leads to hypertension. Conversely, other studies do not support any hypertensive effects of hypercalcemia. Hypocalcemia has also been associated with hypertension, and multiple studies have shown the beneficial effects of calcium supplementation on systolic BP in essential hypertension.

Parathyroid hormone. Patients with pseudohypoparathyroidism (who are hypocalcemic with high PTH levels) have hypertension as frequently as patients with primary hyperparathyroidism, suggesting that increased PTH itself may be responsible for the hypertension. Moreover, patients with pseudohypoparathyroidism and hypertension not uncommonly remain hypertensive after correction of hypocalcemia. In a long-term study, PTH

TABLE A53.1

ENDOCRINE AND CARDIOVASCULAR CHANGES IN THYROID DISORDERS

Endocrine/cardiovascular functions	Hypothyroidism	Thyrotoxicosis
Catecholamine levels	Increased	Normal/ decreased
Density of β-adrenergic receptors	Decreased	Increased
Plasma renin activity levels	Decreased	Increased
Aldosterone levels	Decreased	Increased
Blood volume	Decreased	Increased
Cardiac output	Decreased	Increased
Stroke volume	Decreased	Increased
Heart rate	Decreased	Increased
Peripheral vascular resistance	Increased	Decreased

infusion in normotensive subjects resulted in an increase in BP possibly related to adrenocorticotropic hormone–stimulated cortisol and aldosterone secretion. Conversely, other acute studies have shown vasodilatory and hypotensive effects in the setting of high PTH levels.

Primary hyperthyroidism is also associated with left ventricular hypertrophy. A possible explanation for this would be ligand binding to PTH or PTHrP receptors, which would be expected to increase intracellular levels of calcium and activate protein kinase C and subsequent growth pathways that cause vascular and cardiac hypertrophy. In the long run (months to years), ventricular hypertrophy seems to regress following parathyroidectomy.

Parathyroid hormone–renal disease interaction. Most studies have shown that the prevalence of hypertension is higher in patients with hyperparathyroidism and renal insufficiency than that found in hyperparathyroidism without coincident renal dysfunction.

Renin-angiotensin-aldosterone system in hyperparathyroidism. Many studies have shown increased PRA and aldosterone levels in hyperparathyroidism. In a recent small study, patients with both hypertension and hyperparathyroidism were compared with normotensive patients with hyperparathyroidism and normotensive control subjects. PRA and plasma aldosterone levels were higher in the hypertensive patients with hyperparathyroidism, who also had a greater pressor response to infused norepinephrine. Parathyroidectomy normalized BP, PRA, plasma aldosterone, and pressor responsiveness to norepinephrine in 8 out of 10 subjects.

Response of hypertension to parathyroidectomy

According to different reports, at least 20% of patients with hypertension and hyperparathyroidism experience normalization or improved BPs after undergoing parathyroidectomy. Unfortunately, no known factor predicts which patient with hypertension will respond favorably to parathyroidectomy. Some studies suggest that the effect of decreased BP after such surgery usually does not last more than 3 years. At present, the consensus is that hypertension alone is not a reason to perform parathyroidectomy.

ACROMEGALY AND HYPERTENSION

Clinical features

Acromegaly is a disease of adults caused by chronic excess of growth hormone (GH). Gigantism is a similar condition associated with increased height that develops before puberty and closure of the epiphyses. The vast majority of cases of acromegaly are due to GH-producing pituitary adenomas, usually macroadenomas (which by definition are larger than 1 cm). Another cause of acromegaly is an excess of GH-releasing hormone secreted either eutopically by a hypothalamic tumor or ectopically by a carcinoid or islet cell tumor. Ectopic GH secretion is extremely rare, with only a single well-documented case of a GH-producing pancreatic islet cell tumor. Hypertension is very common in acromegaly, affecting one of three to one of two patients.

Mechanisms of hypertension

Cardiac stroke volume and plasma volume are increased in active acromegaly before the onset of high BP. Acromegalic patients with hypertension also have a reduction in end-systolic ventricular stress, an index of afterload. These changes result in increased cardiac output, which may be involved in the development of hypertension. Increased left ventricular mass, apparently due to a direct trophic effect on cardiomyocytes, is a very frequent finding in acromegaly.

Recently, an impaired circadian BP profile was found in acromegalic patients with and without hypertension. This nondipping profile was associated with higher GH levels and also with a greater degree of insulin resistance. The structural and functional cardiovascular abnormalities of acromegaly respond to treatment when GH levels are successfully controlled. In many cases, such treatment also leads to cure or at least amelioration of hypertension, particularly if patients are diagnosed and treated relatively early in the course of the disease.

ANDROGENS AND HYPERTENSION

The fact that young and middle-aged men are at greater risk for cardiovascular disease and have higher BPs than their premenopausal females raises questions about the possible role of androgens (or lack of estrogens) in hypertension. Hormone replacement therapy does not usually cause a significant reduction in BP, suggesting that loss of estrogen in postmenopausal women is not the predominant factor in their hypertension. It remains possible, however, that the relative hyperandrogenic state may play a role in postmenopausal hypertension, similar to polycystic ovary (Stein-Leventhal) syndrome or virilizing tumors, which are also associated with hypertension. On the basis of rat models, androgens blunt the pressure-natriuresis relationship and increase production of angiotensinogen, which together would be expected to raise BP.

Suggested Readings

Akpunonu BE, Mulrow PJ, Hoffman EA. Secondary hypertension: evaluation and treatment: thyrotoxicosis and hypertension [Published correction appears in *Dis Mon* 1997;43:62]. *Dis Mon* 1996;42:689–703.

Andersson P, Rydberg E, Willenheimer R. Primary hyperparathyroidism and heart disease–a review. *Eur Heart J* 2004;25:1776–1787.

Biondi B, Klein I. Hypothyroidism as a risk factor for cardiovascular disease. *Endocrine* 2004;24(1):1–13.

Colao A, Ferone D, Marzullo P, et al. Systemic complications of acromegaly: epidemiology, pathogenesis, and management. *Endocr Rev* 2004;25(1):102–152.

Gennari C, Nami R, Gonnelli S. Hypertension and primary hyperparathyroidism: the role of adrenergic and renin-angiotensin-aldosterone systems. *Miner Electrolyte Metab* 1995;21:77–81.

Pietrobelli DJ, Akopian M, Olivieri AO, et al. Altered circadian BP profile in patients with active acromegaly. Relationship with left ventricular mass and hormonal values. *J Hum Hypertens* 2001;15:601–605.

Reckelhoff JF, Fortepiani LA. Novel mechanisms responsible for postmenopausal hypertension. *Hypertension* 2004;43:918–923.

SaitoI, Saruta T. Hypertension in thyroid disorders. *Endocrinol Metab Clin North Am* 1994;23:379–386.

CHAPTER A54 ■ PATHOPHYSIOLOGY OF PREECLAMPSIA

ELLEN W. SEELY, MD AND MARSHALL D. LINDHEIMER, MD

KEY POINTS

■ Preeclampsia, classically characterized by *de novo* hypertension and proteinuria after midgestation, is a multisystem disorder that can also affect coagulation, liver function, and the central nervous system.
■ Hypertension in preeclampsia is primarily caused by marked increases in systemic vascular resistance.
■ The etiology of preeclampsia may be multifactorial.

See also Chapter **C160**

Preeclampsia is a hypertensive condition limited to pregnancy which, along with its convulsive phase (eclampsia), remains a leading cause of maternal and fetal morbidity and death. There are still no definitive means for its prevention, and the approach to its treatment remains controversial.

Epidemiology

Preeclampsia complicates >3% of all pregnancies and approximately 7% of nulliparous gestations in the United States. The disorder is more apt to occur in "high-risk" populations, including diabetes, twin gestation, chronic hypertension, underlying renal disease, previous preeclampsia (in which the incidence of recurrence is 20%–25%), and obesity (~10%). The disorder may also occur more frequently in patients with thrombophilias, including factor V Leiden, protein C and S deficiencies, increased antiphospholipid antibody syndromes, and hyperhomocystinemia. It may also be associated with genetic variations including those of the angiotensinogen gene. Chronic hypertension, in the absence of superimposed preeclampsia, and when not due to several forms of secondary hypertension, of which pheochromocytoma is the most dangerous, has a relatively benign course in pregnancy.

Etiology and pathophysiology

Preeclampsia is a complex disorder whose etiology and pathophysiology are not fully understood. Several candidate hypotheses have been advanced.

Abnormal placentation. Placentation gone awry is currently considered the most plausible causal hypothesis. Linked events culminate in failed remodeling of the spiral arteries due to the absence of trophoblastic invasion of these vessels. The failure of spiral arteries to dilate leads to restriction of placental blood flow

and a relatively hypoxic uteroplacental environment. Subsequent events mediated through hypoxemia-induced genes then result in the release of factors that may enter the maternal circulation and initiate the maternal syndrome. Presence of the angiotensinogen gene variant T235 suggests that there are abnormalities of the renin-angiotensin system in placental vessels that lead to inappropriate angiogenesis and possibly to clotting in very small vessels. Other areas of investigation include factors affecting apoptosis, the role of natural killer cells, human leukocyte antigen G (which may play a role in maternal tolerance to the placenta), alterations in the production of trophoblast growth factors, and synthesis of other placental proteins. Excessive trafficking of fetal DNA, cells, and trophoblastic debris across the placenta into the maternal circulation may occur as a result of alterations in the placental maternal–fetal barrier.

Altered production of antiangiogenic factors. *In vitro* studies have demonstrated both antiangiogenic and dysfunctional endothelial effects of sera from preeclamptic women. Angiogenic and antiangiogenic factors are important in placental development. Placentas of women destined to develop preeclampsia overproduce two antiangiogenic proteins that enter the maternal circulation; high maternal levels of these proteins are detectable months before overt disease. One, soluble Fms-like tyrosine kinase 1 (sFlt-1), is a receptor for placental growth and vascular endothelial growth factors (VEGFs), [placental growth factor (PlGF) and VEGF]. Increased levels of sFlt-1 in the mother decrease levels of free PlGF and VEGF and induce endothelial dysfunction. The second, soluble endoglin (sEng) may impair the binding of TGF-$\beta 1$ to endothelial receptors; thereby, decreasing endothelial nitric oxide (NO)-dependent vasodilatation. Simultaneous introduction of adenoviruses encoding both sFlt1 and sEng produces severe hypertension, heavy proteinuria, elevated liver-enzyme levels, and circulating schistocytes, in essence creating a powerful model that simulates most of the protean manifestations of preeclampsia in humans. This finding has obvious implications for the study of mechanisms and subsequent therapy of this disease.

Insulin resistance and sympathetic overactivity. Insulin resistance is postulated to play a role in the pathophysiology of essential hypertension. Insulin resistance is a hallmark of normal pregnancy but some studies have shown further increases in insulin resistance preceding preeclampsia and in postpartum women with preeclamptic pregnancies. The increase in sympathetic nervous tone in preeclampsia may be mediated by hyperinsulinemia and could explain the vasoconstriction seen in this disorder.

Immunologic changes. One explanation for the absence of or deficiency in trophoblastic invasion is that there is an abnormal maternal immune response to the trophoblast. It is postulated that in normal pregnancy, trophoblast cells interact with uterine natural killer cells altering cytokine production and stimulating vascular remodeling. In preeclamptic pregnancy, it is postulated that the uterine natural killer cells are inhibited and as a result, do not stimulate trophoblastic remodeling.

Genetic factors. Despite clear evidence for the heritability of preeclampsia, the search for a single susceptibility gene has not been successful. Studies searching for specific allelic substitutions associated with preeclampsia have generally been unsuccessful and when an association has been shown, it is not clear whether the association is with preeclampsia or with another disorder, itself a risk factor. Such examples include gene variants associated with essential hypertension, thrombophilia, endothelial function, and vasoactive hormones. Of interest are reports of a decreased incidence of preeclampsia with prophylactic doses of low-molecular weight heparin in populations harboring thrombophilia genes.

The failure to find a single gene for preeclampsia may stem from the possibility that preeclampsia is a final common pathway for multiple genetic abnormalities. It is also possible that some genetic predispositions to preeclampsia have been overlooked because of insufficient power of prior studies due to small case numbers. As a result, genomewide expression screening is now taking place in large populations. Recently, studies have suggested that the genetics of preeclampsia may be better understood with an epigenetic approach.

Abnormal vascular reactivity and renin-angiotensin activity. There is an increased response to all pressor hormones in preeclamptic women, ascribed primarily to increased vascular reactivity. Best known is the increased responsiveness to angiotensin II (Ang II). In normal gestation, all elements of the renin-angiotensin-aldosterone axis are upregulated but paradoxically, levels of all components are lower in preeclampsia. Explanations for the increased reactivity to Ang II include: upregulation of receptor sensitivity, circulating autoantibodies agonistic to the angiotensin type 1 receptor, and decreases in the level of circulating vasodilator Ang 1–7. Ang 1–7 levels are high in normotensive pregnancy and low in preeclampsia; antagonistic effects of this peptide may explain why pressor sensitivity in normotensive gravidas is low despite markedly increased Ang II levels.

Inflammation and oxidative stress. Another theory is that preeclampsia occurs when there is an exaggeration of the already increased systemic inflammatory status of normal gravidas. This results in higher levels of circulating cytokines and eventually endothelial damage. Still other views include alterations in the balance between circulating oxidants and antioxidants, as well as in the balance between vasodilating prostanoids and thromboxane, or other pressor substances such as endothelin.

Other substances. There may be impairment of NO synthase production resulting in decreased production of vasodilating NO, and NO-independent vasodilation may likewise be impaired. Finally, rounding out these theories are, alterations in autocoid systems, vitamin and/or mineral deficiencies.

These hypotheses have provided the theoretic basis for a number of expensive preventive trials that have generated findings that were either negative or of marginal importance as judged by the very large number needed to treat for minimal benefit. These trials have studied low dose aspirin (to alter the balance of prostacyclin/thromboxane), calcium supplementation (to correct calcium deficiency) and supplementation with large doses of the antioxidants vitamin C and E. Of note, some of the vitamin supplementation trials have in actuality yielded more adverse effects in the treatment arm.

Effects on target organs

Cardiovascular system. Hypertension in overt preeclampsia is primarily due to a marked reversal of the systemic vasodilation and resistance to the pressor effects of infused angiotensin characteristic of normal gestation. Even when peripheral edema is marked, most investigators find cardiac output to be decreased or normal and pulmonary capillary wedge pressure low or low normal. Plasma volumes are decreased compared to normal gestation, as reflected in a rise in hematocrit. Vascular compliance, normally markedly increased throughout gestation, is reduced in preeclampsia. The decrement in vascular compliance is related to the preeclampsia *per se* in that it exceeds what might be anticipated with increased blood pressure (BP) alone.

Kidney. Renal plasma flow (RPF) and glomerular filtration rate (GFR) normally increase from 30% to 50% by midgestation. With preeclampsia, GFR and RPF then decrease approximately 25%; therefore, these renal functional parameters may actually be similar to or slightly above those seen in the nonpregnant state. The decrement in RPF is attributable to vasoconstriction, whereas the fall in GFR relates both to the decrement of RPF as well as to morphologic changes in the kidney, marked by swelling of the capillary endothelial cells (occasionally mesangial cells, too) that produces a characteristic lesion termed *glomerular endotheliosis*. Scanning electron microscopic studies show that these changes (and other lesions) result in a reduction in the density and size of endothelial fenestrae, and lower the ultrafiltration coefficient (K_f). The severity of these vascular lesions correlates best with the magnitude of proteinuria and hyperuricemia. Despite even marked proteinuria, the epithelial foot-processes (podocytes) that control protein filtration appear intact. However, recent evidence suggests that these podocytes are also affected as considerable podocyturia accompanies the proteinuria.

Brain. The greatest clinical concern in managing women with preeclampsia is that their disease may progress to a convulsive phase termed eclampsia. These convulsions are frequently preceded by premonitory symptoms and signs, including hyperreflexia, visual disturbances, and severe headaches but may also occur suddenly and without warning. Fatal cases of preeclampsia demonstrate various degrees of cerebral bleeding from microscopic petechiae to gross hemorrhage. A coagulopathic state may occur with preeclampsia, as fibrin deposition has been noted in the brain at autopsy. Other researchers have suggested similarities to hypertensive encephalopathy, a view contested in the older literature. Using Doppler techniques some have suggested two forms of eclampsia: one characterized by cerebral underperfusion (consistent with severe vasoconstriction) and the other by over-perfusion (suggesting loss of autoregulation, as in hypertensive encephalopathy). Recently magnetic resonance imaging (MRI) studies that differentiate "vasogenic" and "cytotoxic" edema have suggested that some of these lesions may persist.

Liver. The liver involvement found in preeclampsia is characterized by periportal lesions with cell necrosis, a finding at times associated with infarction and fibrin deposition. There are also periportal hemorrhages, which may become confluent and develop into frank hematomas. Subcapsular bleeding that leads to hepatic rupture is a catastrophic complication of preeclampsia.

Placenta. The characteristic feature in placentas from pre-eclamptics is failure of the uterine spiral arteries to undergo normal remodeling and dilate, as noted when discussing abnormal placentation in the preceding text. Another change in the arterioles is acute *atherosis*, but this lesion is seen with other forms of hypertension, too. Preeclampsia is associated with intrauterine growth restriction attributed to decreased placental perfusion, but surprisingly as many as one-fourth of preeclamptics deliver babies that are large for gestational age. Preeclampsia is associated with increased incidences of both spontaneous, and provoked (i.e., induction or cesarean section because of the disease status) preterm delivery, making preeclampsia a leading cause of premature delivery in the United States.

Clinical correlation

Diagnosis. Preeclampsia typically presents after gestational week 20, most cases occurring in nulliparas and presenting late in the third trimester. It is a multisystem disease, affecting primarily the cardiovascular system, kidneys, brain, and placenta. Preeclampsia is diagnosed by the appearance of *de novo* hypertension ($\geq$140/90 mm Hg) and proteinuria ($\geq$300 mg/day, or a protein/creatinine ratio $\geq$0.3) after midgestation. In addition to the hallmark finding of proteinuria, other clinical and laboratory manifestations may include the rapid occurrence of facial and upper extremity edema, hemoconcentration, thrombocytopenia, hypoalbuminemia, hyperuricemia, and liver-enzyme abnormalities. Of importance, the National High Blood Pressure Education Program's working group recommends if the clinical circumstances are suggestive of preeclampsia it is best to manage a patient as if she had preeclampsia even in the absence of proteinuria.

Clinical course. Regardless of its severity, preeclampsia resolves postpartum, and BP usually normalizes within 10 days. Most of the morbidity occurs when this disease presents before gestational week 36, called *early preeclampsia* or *preeclampsia remote from term*. Left untreated, preeclampsia can progress to a life-threatening convulsive form termed *eclampsia*. A particularly dangerous form of preeclampsia is the HELLP syndrome (*h*emolysis, *e*levated *l*iver function tests and *l*ow *p*latelets). This variant is characterized by the sudden appearance of a microangiopathic hemolytic anemia, a rapidly falling platelet count, and sizable increments in bilirubin and liver enzymes. The HELLP syndrome is a medical emergency that often requires interruption of the pregnancy to avoid progression to frank hepatic or renal failure, sepsis, eclampsia with cerebral hemorrhage, and death. Of note, there is increasing evidence that women with a history of preeclampsia have an increased long term risk for hypertension and perhaps other cardiovascular diseases as well.

Suggested Readings

Bdolah Y, Sukhatme VP, Karumanchi, SA. Angiogenic imbalance in the pathophysiology of preeclampsia: newer insights. *Semin Nephrol* 2004;24:548–556.

Davison JM, Lindheimer MD. Introduction and guest editors. New Development in Preeclampsia. *Semin Nephrol* 2004;24:537–625.

Lindheimer MD, Roberts JM, Cunningham FG, eds. *Chesley's hypertensive disorders in pregnancy*, 2nd ed. Stamford: Appleton & Lange, 1999.

Matthiesen L, Berg G, Ernerudh J, et al. Immunology of preeclampsia. *Chem Immunol Allergy* 2005;89:49–61.

McMaster MT, Zhou Y, Fisher SJ. Abnormal placentation and the syndrome of preeclampsia. *Semin Nephrol* 2004;24(6):540–547.

Moffet A, Hiby SF. How does the maternal immune system contribute to the development of preeclampsia? *Placenta* 2007;21:S51–S56.

National High Blood Pressure Education Program Working Group. Report of the National High Blood Pressure Education Program Working Group on high blood pressure in pregnancy. *Am J Obstet Gynecol* 2000;183:S1–S22.

Oudejans CB, van Dijk M, Oosterkamp M, et al. Genetics of preeclampsia: paradigm shifts. *Hum Genet* 2007;120(5):607–612.

Redman CW, Sargent IL. Latest advances in understanding preeclampsia. *Science* 2005;308(5728):1592–1594.

Solomon CG, Seely EW. Hypertension in pregnancy. *Endocrinol Metab Clin North Am* 2006;35(1):157–171.

CHAPTER A55 ■ PATHOPHYSIOLOGY OF SLEEP APNEA

BARBARA J. MORGAN, PhD

KEY POINTS

- Apnea and hypopnea during sleep result in sleep fragmentation, intermittent hypoxemia and hypercapnia, sympathetic nervous system (SNS) activation, and marked transient blood pressure (BP) elevations.
- A direct relationship exists between severity of sleep-disordered breathing and the degree of daytime BP elevation.
- Intermittent hypoxia (rather than hypercapnia, sleep disruption, or intrathoracic pressure oscillations) is the most important prohypertensive factor associated with sleep-disordered breathing.
- Sleep-disordered breathing may be an important cause of drug-resistant hypertension.

See also Chapters A43, A46, and **C165**

In middle aged adults, the estimated prevalence of obstructive sleep apnea syndrome (OSAS, defined as ≥15 apneas or hypopneas/hour of sleep plus complaints of daytime sleepiness) is 4% for women and 9% for men. Although daytime hypersomnolence is the predominant symptom, frequent traffic accidents, declines in cognitive function, and an increased incidence of psychiatric disorders have also been reported. OSAS is associated with long-term cardiovascular morbidity from systemic and pulmonary hypertension, myocardial infarction (MI), stroke, and also with metabolic disorders such as glucose intolerance and insulin resistance.

Pathophysiology of airway obstruction and hypoxia

The onset of sleep is associated with a decrease in neural drive to the muscles of the respiratory pump and to those that stiffen and maintain patency of the upper airway. Loss of muscle tone can cause partial airway collapse and increased transpulmonary resistance. In individuals with anatomic compromise (e.g., peripharyngeal fat deposition, enlargement of the soft palate or tongue, or craniofacial abnormalities), sleep-induced loss of muscle tone predisposes to complete collapse of the upper airway, or apnea. Both apnea and hypopnea (episodes of partial airway collapse) produce transient hypoxemia, hypercapnia, respiratory acidosis, and, in most cases, arousal from sleep. Each event also triggers a marked increase in sympathetic nervous system (SNS) activity and blood pressure (BP) (**Figure A55.1**). Individuals with OSAS may experience hundreds of these events throughout the course of a single night's sleep. In these patients and also in

individuals with less severe sleep-disordered breathing, the normal sleep-related decline in BP and heart rate is greatly attenuated or on occasion absent.

Obstructive sleep apnea syndrome–hypertension mechanisms

Sympathetic nervous system. Enhanced SNS activity is a major component of the hypertension associated with OSAS. Augmented sympathetic activity is evident, not only during sleep, but also during wakefulness when breathing is stable. A rat model that produces intermittent hypoxia during sleep causes persistent daytime hypertension in as few as 5 weeks, but only when the SNS is intact. Alterations in both peripheral (carotid chemoreflex) and central neural regulation of sympathetic outflow contribute to diurnal elevations in arterial pressure in this model.

Renin-angiotensin-aldosterone system. The renin-angiotensin-aldosterone system (RAAS) contributes importantly to hypertension in rats exposed to intermittent hypoxia. In this model, renal nerve denervation, angiotensin II receptor blockade, and suppression of the RAAS by a high salt diet all prevent the rise in BP. Elevated angiotensin II and aldosterone levels have been observed in humans with OSAS. Excessive aldosterone release may contribute to drug-resistant hypertension in these individuals.

Vascular dysfunction. Exposure to intermittent hypoxia interferes with endothelial function. In rats exposed to hypoxia and in patients with OSAS, plasma endothelin levels are increased and nitric oxide levels are depressed. Endothelium-dependent vasodilatation is impaired in rats exposed to chronic intermittent

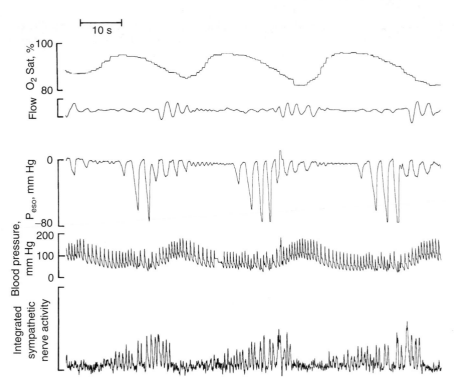

Figure A55.1 Mixed (central and obstructive) sleep apneas produce marked sympathoexcitation and transient BP elevations in a patient with sleep apnea syndrome. BP, blood pressure; P_{eso}, esophageal pressure; Sat, saturation. (From Skatrud JB, Badr MS, Morgan BJ. Control of breathing during sleep and sleep-disordered breathing. In: Altose M, Kawakami Y, eds. *Control of breathing in health and disease.* New York: Marcel Dekker Inc, 1999:379–422, with permission.)

hypoxia and in humans with OSAS (**Figure A55.2**). Increased circulating markers of inflammation, increased 8-isoprostane in breath condensate, and increased production of superoxide have been observed in such patients. Therefore, potential mediators of OSAS-related vascular dysfunction are inflammation and oxidant stress.

Vascular remodeling. Sleep-disordered breathing may alter arterial structure and biomechanics. Increases in carotid intima-media thickness and arterial stiffness have been observed in individuals with OSAS. Putative mechanisms for this vascular remodeling include hypoxic stimulation of mitogenic factors such as platelet-derived growth factor, endothelin-I, and vascular

endothelial growth factor; altered balance between extracellular matrix metalloproteinases and their inhibitors induced by chronic inflammation; stimulation of the local vascular renin-angiotensin system through cyclical stretch of vascular smooth muscle cells; and the trophic effects of chronic sympathetic activation.

Sleep apnea and hypertension

Established hypertension. Most clinical investigations linking sleep-disordered breathing and elevated BP have focused on the high prevalence of long-standing hypertension ($\geq 50\%$) in individuals with OSAS. Although some of the BP elevation may

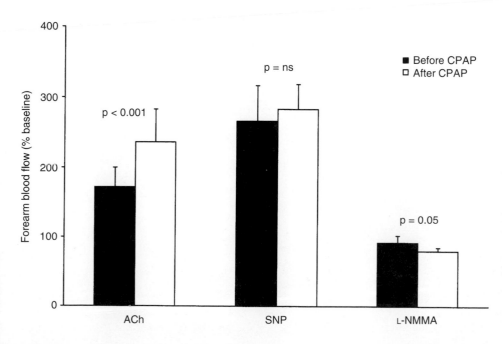

Figure A55.2 Acetylcholine (ACh)-induced (endothelium-dependent) increases in forearm blood flow were improved after 3 months of continuous positive airway pressure (CPAP) treatment in ten patients with obstructive sleep apnea, whereas endothelium-independent increases evoked by sodium nitroprusside (SNP) were not altered by CPAP (mean ± standard error). Decreases in forearm blood flow elicited by L-NMMA (N^G-monomethyl-L-arginine), a competitive antagonist of nitric oxide synthesis, were enhanced after CPAP treatment. These findings suggest that sleep apnea causes a reversible decrease in nitric oxide bioavailability. (Adapted from Lattimore JL, Wilcox I, Skilton M, et al. Treatment of obstructive sleep apnoea leads to improved microvascular endothelial function in the systemic circulation. *Thorax* 2006;61:491–495.)

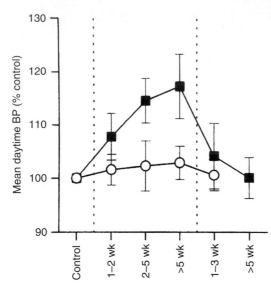

Figure A55.3 Mean daytime blood pressure (BP) in four dogs exposed to intermittent tracheal occlusions during sleep (*filled squares*) and sleep fragmentation (*open circles*) (mean ± standard error). The vertical dashed lines represent the durations of the exposures. (From Brooks D, Horner RL, Kozar LF, et al. Obstructive sleep apnea as a cause of systemic hypertension. *J Clin Invest* 1997;99:106–109, with permission.)

be attributed to comorbid obesity, several lines of evidence suggest that the relationship between OSAS and hypertension is causal. First, BP decreases in some individuals when sleep apnea is successfully treated. Second, a dose–response-type relationship with the appropriate temporal sequence has been observed between sleep-disordered breathing and daytime BP elevation in a large, population-based study. Finally, persistent daytime hypertension has been produced by frequent tracheal occlusions during

nocturnal sleep in a canine model (**Figure A55.3**). In parallel experiments, sleep fragmentation produced by acoustic stimuli failed to affect daytime BP, suggesting that the chemical or mechanical consequences of the occlusions contributed more importantly to the hypertensive effect of this intervention.

Intermittent hypertension and prehypertension. Marked fluctuations in arterial pressure often accompany mild to moderate sleep-disordered breathing. Hypopneas and infrequent apneas are very common in the undiagnosed population, and they contribute to small but statistically significant elevations in daytime BP. The health risks associated with mild to moderate sleep-disordered breathing and the effects of early intervention in this group of individuals remain to be more fully elucidated.

Suggested Readings

Carlson JT, Hedner J, Elam M, et al. Augmented resting sympathetic activity in awake patients with obstructive sleep apnea. *Chest* 1993;103:1763–1768.

Fletcher EC. Physiological consequences of intermittent hypoxia: systemic BP. *J Appl Physiol* 2001;90:1600–1605.

Goodfriend TL, Calhoun DA. Resistant hypertension, obesity, sleep apnea, and aldosterone: theory and therapy. *Hypertension* 2004;43:518–524.

Møller DS, Lind P, Strunge B, et al. Abnormal vasoactive hormones and 24-hour BP in obstructive sleep apnea. *Am J Hypertens* 2003;16:274–280.

Morgan BJ, Dempsey JA, Pegelow D, et al. BP perturbations caused by subclinical sleep disordered breathing. *Sleep* 1998;21:737–746.

Peppard P, Young T, Palta M, et al. Prospective study of the association between sleep-disordered breathing and hypertension. *N Engl J Med* 2000;342:1378–1384.

Phillips C, Hedner J, Berend N, et al. Diurnal and obstructive sleep apnea influences on arterial stiffness and central BP in men. *Sleep* 2005;28:604–609.

Phillips SA, Olson EB, Morgan BJ, et al. Chronic intermittent hypoxia impairs endothelium-dependent dilation in cerebral and skeletal muscle resistance arteries. *Am J Physiol Heart Circ Physiol* 2004;286:H388–H393.

Schulz R, Schmidt D, Blum A, et al. Decreased plasma levels of nitric oxide derivatives in obstructive sleep apnoea: response to CPAP therapy. *Thorax* 2000;55:1046–1051.

Young T, Palta M, Dempsey J, et al. The occurrence of sleep-disordered breathing among middle-aged adults. *N Engl J Med* 1993;328:1230–1235.

CHAPTER A56 ■ BLOOD PRESSURE VARIABILITY AND REACTIVITY

JOSEPH L. IZZO, Jr., MD

KEY POINTS

■ Variations in an individual's blood pressure (BP) depend on several factors, including the ability of baroreflexes to buffer sympathetic nervous output, physiologic and behavioral stimulus–response characteristics, and the reactivity of peripheral vessels.

■ Experimental BP reactivity is relatively reproducible within individuals but highly variable between individuals; increased BP reactivity is independent of resting (basal) BP and may signal higher cardiovascular risk in hypertension.

■ Hemodynamic responses are stimulus-specific and are modified by disease; for example, mental stress causes increased cardiac output in normotensive patients but in hypertensive patients, vascular resistance increases as well.

■ Exaggerated BP variability confounds the diagnosis of hypertension and presents a challenge to clinicians because standard antihypertensive drugs do little to reduce BP variation, whether due to pathophysiologic changes or behavioral factors.

See also Chapters A38, A39, A64, **B89, C104, C105, C117, C154** and Figures on back cover

Blood pressure (BP) is intrinsically variable because acute and chronic adjustments in pressure and flow are necessary for the organism to respond to its environment while still conserving cardiovascular energy expenditure. BP variability has been commonly viewed as "background noise" in the diagnosis of chronic hypertension but a closer view reveals that BP variability and reactivity have distinct pathophysiologic patterns and clinical significance.

Modulation of sympathoadrenal output

A mammal's ability to respond to acute stressors was attributed by Bernard to the "sympathetic" activation of multiple organ systems coordinated by the central nervous system (CNS). Selye believed that sympathetic nervous responses were essentially "all or nothing" or "fight or flight" responses. Today, it is recognized that the sympathoadrenal system guides a variety of different patterns of organ-specific responses that also involve other neurohormones. These specialized responses allow precise, energy-conserving adaptations to a broad range of environmental stimuli.

Systemic sympathoadrenal responses. Because there are separate nerves controlling the heart and blood vessels, BP and heart rate responses can vary independently to meet a variety of environmental challenges. Certain stimuli cause predictable changes in hemodynamics: increased cardiac output during mental stress or hypoglycemia, or cold-induced vasoconstriction. Disease states can modify these stimulus-specific patterns; whereas aerobic exercise or mental stress increase cardiac output in normotensive individuals, in hypertension there is a combined flow-resistance increase. Concomitant stimulation of other hormones (e.g., vasopressin or angiotensin II) causes further modulation of systemic responses and helps redirect blood flow to the organs most directly involved in the response.

Differential responses to stimuli. Life-threatening stimuli (e.g., cardiogenic shock) cause a generalized sympathoadrenal response that is characterized by a massive release of catecholamines from both sympathetic nerve terminals and the adrenal medulla. Less threatening stimuli promote more modest differential responses within the sympathoadrenal system, such as hypoglycemia-induced adrenal epinephrine release or pain-induced neuronal norepinephrine release. Different environmental stimuli also have intrinsically different relative durations, so the total and organ-specific responses or amounts of catecholamine released per stress episode can differ widely. Pathologic conditions (and heterogeneity within these conditions) also influence response patterns; in hypertensive patients, the cold pressor test usually (but not always) causes exaggerated catecholamine release and a supranormal BP response compared to normotensive patients.

Baroreflexes. Acute BP increases in normotensive patients are truncated by activation of aortocarotid (and to a lesser extent cardiopulmonary) baroreflexes, which directly limit further sympathetic outflow. Blunting of the aortocarotid baroreflexes occurs in hypertension and in older individuals with carotid arteriosclerosis and is associated with increased BP variability. Classic experiments in dogs demonstrate that variation increases while mean pressure remains constant. In man, it is believed that impaired baroreflex sensitivity may play some role in chronic hypertension as well. In those with marked baroreflex dysfunction (long-standing diabetes, autonomic insufficiency, carotid sinus hypersensitivity), BP swings can be wildly exaggerated, sometimes symptomatic, and always therapeutically problematic.

Hypothalamic control centers. Emotional responses and some conscious behaviors are integrated at the level of the posterior hypothalamus, which in turn modulates activity of the cardiovascular control centers in the rostral ventrolateral medulla that govern sympathetic nerve firing rates and neuronal catecholamine release. Through these pathways, cognitive and behavioral influences can modulate BP reactivity.

Hemodynamics and vascular reactivity

Aging and hypertension. In normotensive patients and younger hypertensive patients, acute responses to mental stress or dynamic exercise are characterized by increased cardiac output (both heart rate and stroke volume increase, as does pulse pressure). In contrast, hypertensive patients (especially those with insulin resistance or dyslipidemia) demonstrate a balanced increase in cardiac output and systemic vascular resistance to the same stimuli. In older people or hypertensive patients who have poorly compliant central arteries (arteriosclerosis), variations either in stroke volume or vascular resistance tend to increase systolic BP with little effect on diastolic BP. Exercise conditioning tends to blunt BP reactivity and heart rate responses.

Endothelial dysfunction. Conditions associated with endothelial dysfunction, including hypercholesterolemia and insulin resistance, are associated with modestly exaggerated vasoconstrictive and BP responses to mental arithmetic or isometric exercise. In these populations, treatment of dyslipidemia with statins (**Figure A56.1**) or insulin resistance with thiazolidinediones (insulin sensitizers) proportionally decreases endothelial dysfunction and in parallel, the degree of BP reactivity. It is possible that improved nitric oxide bioavailability is the underlying mechanism for the beneficial effect of these drugs on the pattern of heightened vasoreactivity.

Behavioral aspects

Anger and hostility. Several studies have found a correlation between anger or hostility (which are closely related parameters) and BP reactivity to various stressors. In addition, those with high anger or hostility scores demonstrate persistence of stress-induced BP elevations for a significantly longer period of time than normotensive patients (prolonged stress-decay). Other chronic environmental stressors may affect resting or reactive BP change. For example, adolescents with high scores for exposure to violence have a carryover effect for daytime sympathetic activation such that their overnight BP averages do not fall normally (nondipping pattern).

Stress perception, coping, and locus of control. An individual's perception of a given stimulus and that individual's

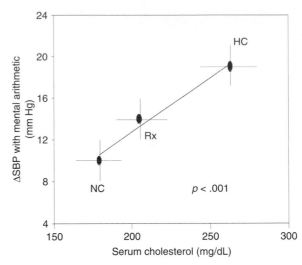

Figure A56.1 Relationship of serum cholesterol to systolic blood pressure (SBP) reactivity to mental stress. Despite similar baseline blood pressure (BP) values, hypercholesterolemic (HC) subjects have greater BP reactivity than normocholesterolemic (NC) controls. Treatment of HC with a statin (Rx) for 6 weeks proportionally lowered BP reactivity and total cholesterol. Error bars are 1 SD. SD, standard deviation. (Modified from: Sung BH, Izzo JL Jr., Wilson MF. Effects of cholesterol reduction on BP response to mental stress in patients with high cholesterol. *Am J Hypertens* 1997;10:592–599, with permission.)

ability to cope with a particular challenge significantly influences BP reactivity. A prevalent theory of stress modulation involves the concept of *coping ability,* which is a measure of an individual's ability to use available resources to neutralize the impact of stressful situations, sometimes termed *locus of control.* An example of the power of enhanced locus of control to blunt stress responses was found in patients undergoing ambulatory cataract extraction who were allowed to listen to music during the procedure (**Figures A56.2** and **A56.3**). The "no-music" group demonstrated significant BP reactivity to the stress of surgery, whereas the music group had virtually no BP elevations. Music recipients also reported less stress and greater coping ability than those who were not exposed to music (**Figure A56.3**).

Social support. Closely related to coping ability is the positive impact of adequate social support, which typically enhances coping. If resting BP is affected by physiologic mechanisms and reactive BP is more heavily dependent on level of social support level, then the effects of standard antihypertensive therapy may be independent of social support mechanisms. This pattern was observed in a small study where hypertensive patients were randomized to angiotensin-converting enzyme (ACE) inhibition alone or ACE inhibition plus pet acquisition (a form of stress-buffering "nonevaluative" social support). ACE inhibitors lowered resting at-home BPs equally well in both groups but had no effect on acute mental stress-induced BP increases. In contrast, presence of the pet during mental stress markedly diminished BP reactivity.

Cultural aspects of blood pressure reactivity. Differences in BP reactivity have been attributed to race and societal acculturation or "urbanization." Responses to mental stress in blacks are greater than those of white controls and BP tends to increase in individuals who move from primitive or rural settings to cities. Apparent racial differences in BP reactivity may represent different genetic traits, but it seems more likely that variations in stress responses are more dependent on "environmental maladaptations" that include aspects of diet,

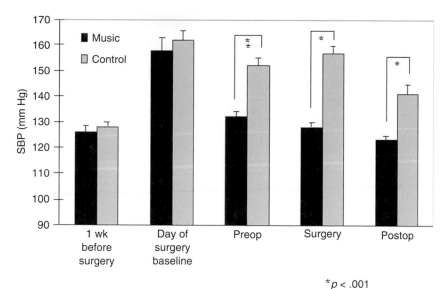

*p < .001

Figure A56.2 Blood pressure (BP) responses to ambulatory ophthalmologic surgery in individuals provided access to music and controls without music access. SBP, systolic blood pressure. (Modified from: Allen K, Golden LH, Izzo JL Jr., et al. Normalization of hypertensive responses during ambulatory surgical stress by perioperative music. *Psychosom Med* 2001;63:487–492.)

weight gain, decreased physical activity, differences in levels of anger/hostility, reduced social support, and a general imbalance between the amount of environmental stress and an individual's coping skills.

Blood pressure variability and risk

Dissociation of resting blood pressure and reactive blood pressure.

It has been erroneously assumed that BPs within a given individual are proportional to that individual's resting level of BP. Although there is a trend toward increased BP variability in those with the highest resting BP levels, an individual's BP response to stress is largely *independent* of resting BP level, with extremely wide variation from individual to individual. In a revealing study, Mancia et al. examined the hemodynamic effects of cuff BP measurement in hospitalized subjects; compared to unstimulated baseline values, the cuff technique increased intraarterial BP in the contralateral arm by an average of 27/15 mm Hg. What was most striking, however, was the wide range of reactive increase in systolic BP: from 4 to 75 mm Hg. Heart rate increases were not strongly correlated with BP changes, demonstrating the differential stimulation of cardiac

and vascular sympathetic nerves. In other studies, substantial variation in the time required for stress-induced BP increases to return to baseline has been found.

Morning blood pressure surge. Some individuals exhibit marked morning surges in BP coincident with the daily peak in incidences of myocardial infarction and stroke. Exaggerated morning BP responses are mediated by acute neurohumoral activation and are accompanied by enhanced platelet aggregation and reduced fibrinolytic capacity, all of which favor thrombosis in the early morning hours. Treatment with α blockers ameliorates the morning surge in BP.

Integrated risk model. The independent nature of resting BP elevations and reactive BP changes to predict higher levels of cardiovascular disease (CVD) risk are presented in an integrated model (**Figure A56.4**). In this model, either white-coat hypertension or sustained hypertension confers some degree of CVD risk increase; when the two coexist, CVD risk increases dramatically. BP variability itself may be cause and effect of organ damage (arteriosclerosis) and may also reflect the presence

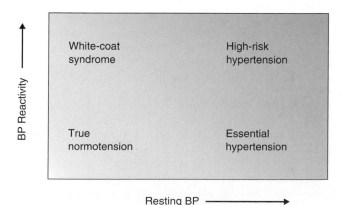

Figure A56.3 Self-reported perceptions of stress and coping levels in individuals provided headphone music compared to controls. (**See Figure A56.2.**)

Figure A56.4 An integrated model of hypertension and blood pressure (BP) reactivity. Resting BP is controlled by different factors than those that affect BP reactivity (neurogenic factors, vascular factors, and behavioral). Coexistence of exaggerated BP reactivity and resting hypertension leads to high-risk hypertension (*gray shading*), whereas increased BP reactivity alone causes the "white-coat syndrome," a condition of low cardiac risk.

TABLE A56.1

PATTERNS AND MECHANISMS OF INCREASED BLOOD PRESSURE (BP) VARIABILITY

Variability pattern	Region(s)/tissue(s) involved	Clinical examples
Increased resting variability (no obvious stimulus)	Baroreflex afferent nerves Brainstem control centers	Autonomic dysfunction Old age (arteriosclerosis) Morning BP surge
Enhanced vasoreactivity	Endothelium Vascular smooth muscle	Dyslipidemia Insulin resistance Hypertension
Behavioral BP response (anger, anticipation, etc.)	Hypothalamus Brainstem control centers	Stress-induced hypertension White-coat hypertension

of additional risk factors. For example, arterial stiffness and endothelial dysfunction are markers of diffuse vascular disease that may predispose to increased BP reactivity during stress.

Practical implications

Limitations of office blood pressure measurement. BP is a highly complex physiologic variable, so it is not surprising that casual BP measurements are only loose surrogates for subclinical or clinical CVD. Usual techniques of BP measurement in clinical settings reflect some degree of environmental stress and therefore would be expected to exhibit greater variability than corresponding home BP values. In the typical office setting, BP is measured after a few minutes in the seated position. For the vast majority of individuals, office BP reflects a "low-stress" state (the mild orthostatic stimulus of sitting plus behavioral "anticipatory" factors). Different levels of perceived and unperceived stress interact with variability in "stress-decay" time. These confounders enhance BP variation and make it difficult to establish an optimal standardized protocol for office BP determinations. Accordingly, the dependability of a given set of BP determinations in the physician's office is limited.

Placebo and antihypertensive drug responses. It is instructive to reflect on why placebo effects in antihypertensive drug trials occur with office BP but not 24-hour ambulatory BP readings. This phenomenon strongly suggests that the placebo effect involves attenuation of the low-grade stress response that is part of the standard office visit. In parallel with this observation, antihypertensive drugs (including β blockers) typically do not have much effect on home-office BP differences and therefore do not treat the "white-coat effect".

Therapeutic implications. There are substantial consequences of exaggerated BP variation, including confusion in diagnosis and management of individual patients. A summary of the different mechanisms and clinical situations associated with increased BP variability is presented in **Table A56.1.**

Currently there are no prospective data to give the clinician guidance on optimal strategies to manage patients with extreme BP variability. Since no current antihypertensive drug can directly improve baroreflex function, the clinician is left to try to manage the extremes of BP variation (especially in the elderly or those with autonomic dysfunction) with drugs ill-suited for this purpose. In those with exaggerated BP variability due to

baroreflex dysfunction or dysautonomia, antihypertensive drugs are indicated if average BPs are high but it is best to avoid drugs that cause significant volume depletion or venodilation (α blockers, nitrates, phosphodiesterase inhibitors) because they may promote hypotension. Similarly, individuals with white-coat hypertension are not the ideal candidates for standard antihypertensive drugs, whereas those with elevated resting BP and white-coat *effect* should be treated. It is attractive to speculate that improvement in hypercholesterolemia or insulin resistance may reduce BP reactivity but no studies have directly addressed this issue. Whether behavioral therapy or drugs with CNS effects are useful for management of reactive hypertension also remains to be proven.

Research implications. The greater variability of systolic compared to diastolic BP, especially in older subjects, has been an important hidden barrier to the study of systolic hypertension because larger sample sizes are needed to effectively offset the increased variability. This is especially problematic for systolic hypertension, which has a far greater disease burden than diastolic hypertension.

Suggested Readings

Allen K, Golden LH, Izzo JL Jr, et al. Normalization of hypertensive responses during ambulatory surgical stress by perioperative music. *Psychosom Med* 2001;63:487–492.

Allen K, Shykoff BE, Izzo JL Jr. Pet ownership, but not ACE inhibitor therapy, blunts home BP responses to mental stress. *Hypertension* 2001;38(4):815–820.

Fredrickson BL, Maynard KE, Helms MJ, et al. Hostility predicts magnitude and duration of BP response to anger. *J Behav Med* 2000;23:229–243.

Head GA. Baroreflexes and cardiovascular regulation in hypertension. *J Cardiovasc Pharmacol* 1995;26(Suppl 2):S7–S16.

Kario K, Pickering TG, Hoshide S, et al. Morning blood pressure surge and hypertensive cerebrovascular disease: role of the alpha adrenergic sympathetic nervous system. *Am J Hypertens* 2004;17:668–675.

Mancia G, Bertinieri G, Grassi G, et al. Effects of blood-pressure measurement by the doctor on patient's BP and heart rate. *Lancet* 1983;2:695–698.

Mancia G, Grassi G. Mechanisms and clinical implications of BP variability. *J Cardiovasc Pharmacol* 2000;35:S15–S19.

Sung BH, Izzo JL Jr, Dandona P, et al. Vasodilatory effects of troglitazone improve BP at rest and during mental stress in type 2 diabetes mellitus. *Hypertension* 1999;34:83–88.

Sung BH, Izzo JL Jr, Wilson MF. Effects of cholesterol reduction on BP response to mental stress in patients with high cholesterol. *Am J Hypertens* 1997;10(6):592–599.

van Rooyen JM, Huisman HW, Eloff FC, et al. Cardiovascular reactivity in black South-African males of different age groups: the influence of urbanization. *Ethn Dis* 2002;12:69–75.

CHAPTER A57 ■ EXPERIMENTAL MODELS OF HYPERTENSION

RALPH E. WATSON, MD, FACP AND DONALD J. DIPETTE, MD

KEY POINTS

- Because human hypertension (HTN) is heterogeneous, several animal models have been developed to mimic its many facets.
- HTN can be produced by various vascular, renal, adrenal, neural, and genetic manipulations.
- Newer molecular techniques have become increasingly important in the development of animal models to determine the involvement of a particular gene or genetic locus in HTN.

See also Chapters A37, A46, A50, A51, A52, A70, and A71

The difficulty in studying a disease process such as hypertension (HTN) begins with the fact that the etiology of HTN is heterogeneous. HTN can be primary ("essential") or secondary to a defined process, such as renal artery stenosis. The pathophysiology of essential HTN is also heterogeneous and varies by age, renin status, sodium (Na^+) dependency, and other characteristics. Therefore, a spectrum of experimental animal models of HTN has been developed to aid in the investigation of essential HTN and secondary forms of HTN.

Inbred rat models

Genetic models of experimental HTN that have been developed to approximate the pathogenesis of human essential HTN include the spontaneously hypertensive rat (SHR), the SHR-stroke-prone (SHR-SP) substrain, Dahl salt-sensitive and salt-resistant rat strains, the Sabra model, Milan hypertensive and normotensive rat strains, Lyon hypertensive and normotensive rat strains, fawn-hooded and Prague hypertensive rats. Although these inbred strains may differ in genetics, cellular alterations, or neurohumoral mechanisms, under appropriate conditions they all share a common feature: the spontaneous development of an elevation of blood pressure (BP) as the animals mature. The two most commonly studied animal models of HTN are the SHR and the Dahl salt-sensitive and salt-resistant strains.

Spontaneously hypertensive and stroke-prone rats.

Both SHR and SHR-SP rat strains develop HTN and target-organ damage similar to human essential HTN. The pathogenesis of HTN in the SHR appears to be heterogeneous; cellular, central nervous system (CNS), neurohumoral, and renal abnormalities have been proposed. The SHR is a "normal-renin" model, and its BP is relatively Na^+-independent. More recently, a substrain of SHR has been developed that is salt-sensitive.

There has been intense debate over the applicability of the SHR to human essential HTN. Part of this debate revolves around the appropriate normotensive control for the SHR strain. Most investigators use the normotensive Wistar-Kyoto (WKY) rat, as the SHR was originally derived from a WKY colony. However, normotensive WKY rats vary genetically among differing colonies and suppliers and exhibit different degrees of phenotypic expression of a given trait. The model remains useful in studies of the target-organ complications of HTN, in screening of potential pharmacologic antihypertensive agents, and in the investigation of genetic determinants of high BP. The stroke-prone SHR is often used to investigate the pathophysiology of cerebrovascular disease. For example, in this model, dietary potassium (K^+) supplementation has been shown to decrease the frequency of stroke, independently of BP.

At least three major gene loci are involved in the early development of HTN in this model, one of which may be in close association with the angiotensinogen gene. An additional gene on chromosome 10 contributes to the development and maintenance of HTN during aging in SHR. It has been speculated that a similar multiple gene interaction is involved in human essential HTN.

Dahl rats. In contrast to the SHR, the Dahl salt-sensitive strain requires administration of increased dietary Na^+ for the rapid and full development of any BP elevation. When the Dahl salt-sensitive and salt-resistant strains are placed on a high-salt diet (8% NaCl in the drinking water), the resistant strain develops only a small elevation of BP, whereas the sensitive strain exhibits a substantial BP rise within 4 to 6 weeks. Interestingly, even on a relatively low-salt diet (0.5% NaCl), Dahl salt-sensitive rats develop HTN, albeit over a longer period of time. This indicates that there is a genetic component of this model of HTN that may convey salt sensitivity.

Other models. Other important models exhibit HTN along with comorbidities, as frequently is the situation in clinical medicine. The Lyon rat strain has elevated plasma cholesterol. Other models have accompanying obesity and often type 2 diabetes, including the obesity prone Sprague-Dawley, the obese Zucker, and Wistar fatty rats.

Renal artery stenosis

Two classic animal models of renovascular disease have been developed in multiple species by constriction of one or both renal arteries. These models are named after the pioneering work of Goldblatt et al. and are classified as *two-kidney, one-clip* (2K-1C), *two-kidney, two-clip* (2K-2C), or *one-kidney, one-clip* (1K-1C) Goldblatt HTN models; the latter two are quite similar in their features.

Two-kidney, one-clip model. In the 2K-1C model, both native kidneys are intact, but a constricting clip (to resemble a clinical stenosis) is placed on one renal artery (usually the left renal artery in the rat model). In the absence of damage to the contralateral nonclipped kidney, this model represents the classic renin (or angiotensin)-dependent model, at least in its early phases. The closest analogous human circumstance is probably unilateral fibromuscular hyperplasia.

One-kidney, one-clip model. In the 1K-1C model, unilateral nephrectomy is followed by placement of a constricting clip on the renal artery of the remaining kidney. This model resembles patients who have only a solitary kidney and a significant renal artery stenosis in that kidney. The reduction in renal mass in this model may also contribute to the chronicity of the hypertensive state. This model most closely mimics the HTN accompanying renal artery stenosis in a transplanted kidney but may also approximate the pathophysiology of bilateral renal artery stenosis.

In contrast to the 2K-1C model, in which plasma renin activity (PRA) is significantly elevated and the HTN is clearly renin dependent, in the 1K-1C model, the PRA is increased only in the first few days after renal artery constriction. After this initial phase, PRA returns to the normal range. Furthermore, during this chronic phase, blockade of the renin-angiotensin system (RAS) does not significantly lower BP. Aggressive diuresis with accompanying Na^+ depletion renders the model renin dependent again. Therefore, in this model, there is clear interplay between early activation of the renin-angiotensin-aldosterone system (RAAS) and Na^+ retention in that both are required for the full development and maintenance of HTN.

Two-kidney, two-clip model. This approach is less often used than the other models. It differs relatively little from the 1K-1C model in hemodynamic and neurohumoral features and parallels bilateral renal artery stenosis in humans. The greater renal mass compared to the 1K-1C model may provide a greater ability to excrete a Na^+ load.

Renal parenchymal hypertension

Renal mass reduction salt-induced model. Clinically, the most common secondary cause of HTN is a loss of renal function from any cause. The animal model that most closely approximates this clinical condition is the renal mass reduction salt-induced model, most commonly studied in the rat and dog. In this model, a renal mass reduction of >85% is required. To accomplish this, a unilateral nephrectomy is followed by surgical removal of two thirds of the remaining kidney. By itself, this degree of renal mass reduction results in only a slight BP increase compared to sham-operated, normotensive control animals. A further increase in BP is provoked when excess salt is administered in the drinking water or in the diet.

In the renal mass reduction salt-induced hypertensive model, PRA is low and HTN is salt-dependent. Nevertheless, blockade of the RAAS with angiotensin-converting enzyme (ACE) inhibitors or AT_1 receptor antagonists results in a lowering of BP. Explanations for this apparent paradox include blocking effects of anti-RAAS drugs on tissue RAAS, decreased sympathetic nervous system activity by attenuation of CNS Ang II effects, suppression of vasopressin, or an increase in vasodilators, such as calcitonin gene-related peptide or substance P.

Other renal models. Although not as commonly used for experimental purposes, there are many other renal animal models of experimental HTN, such as renal ischemic models, perinephric fibrosis ("renal wrap" or Page) HTN, and the chronic administration of angiotensin II (angiotensin-induced HTN). Page HTN limits renal pulsatility and may mimic the intense fibrosis and HTN that occurs in the occasional posttransplantation patient.

Adrenal steroid models

Mineralocorticoid hypertension. The most common adrenal model studied is the mineralocorticoid-salt or deoxycorticosterone-salt model. This model resembles the clinical situation of aldosterone excess. HTN is produced by a surgical uninephrectomy followed by administration of a mineralocorticoid (usually deoxycorticosterone, DOC) along with excess salt (usually 0.9% NaCl drinking water). BP then rises into the hypertensive range within a few weeks. If left untreated, the HTN progresses and the animals lose weight and develop target-organ damage. If a more gradual BP rise is desired, the kidneys can be left intact.

This is a Na^+-dependent, low-renin model. As in other models, non-Na^+ mechanisms have been suggested to play a role in the full development of the HTN, including activation of the sympathetic nervous system, local renin-angiotensin production, and vasopressin activation. This model, in conjunction with the renin-dependent 2K-1C Goldblatt model, is useful in studying the dependency on the RAS of a therapeutic agent. The Yucatan miniature swine model of DOC-induced HTN involves increased sympathetic nervous activity; it also differs from the rodent models in that excess dietary salt is not required for the development of sustained HTN.

Glucocorticoid hypertension. Excess production of glucocorticoids, such as cortisol (Cushing's syndrome or disease), also clinically leads to secondary HTN. The glucocorticoid-induced HTN model is produced by the administration of excess glucocorticoid to normotensive animals usually rats. Unlike some of the other models, no other manipulation (surgery or salt administration) is necessary. The mechanism of the BP elevation is most probably multifactorial and is extremely difficult to treat pharmacologically, often requiring blockade of multiple pressor systems.

Neurogenic models

The brain is a major target organ of the hypertensive process, and it also plays a major role in BP regulation and the pathophysiology of HTN. Neurogenic models of experimental

HTN involve the surgical manipulation of specific brain areas, such as the periventricular (AV3V) region, or peripheral sinoaortic deafferentation. Recently, a model for borderline HTN has been developed.

Molecular models

A great deal of recent investigation of HTN has been devoted to dissecting the molecular basis of HTN. Human essential HTN is clearly polygenic (i.e., caused by small phenotypic effects of common genetic variations found throughout the population). Any one of these variations may not be sufficient to result in a BP increase, but their additive effect may produce HTN.

Gene titration. Using gene titration, the expression of a chosen gene product is varied by generating animals with different numbers of copies of the gene coding for the specific protein. This model of genetic overexpression allows determination of causation by testing the effects on a phenotype of changes in expression of the altered gene and can be performed in a variety of animal species. Reduplication of the angiotensinogen gene in rodents causes HTN. An example of this approach is the work of Smithies et al. demonstrating parallelism between chronic BP and the number of angiotensinogen gene duplications in the animal.

Transgenic and knockout models. There has been a rapid development of transgenic manipulations and specific gene knock-outs, both permanent and conditional, in the mouse. Transgenic animals have foreign DNA introduced into their genome using embryonic stem cell methodology, thereby creating a new strain that expresses the gene of interest. Examples of transgenic rat strains are those in which the mouse and human renin gene and the human angiotensinogen gene were incorporated into the rat genome, and the mouse that overexpresses the renin gene (Ren-2 mouse). There is also a knockout mouse model of the angiotensin AT$_2$-receptor. The latest developments in knockout technology allow for the control of the spatial and temporal onset of the gene modification of interest.

Congenic models. Congenic methodology uses repetitive inbreeding, resulting in a generation of animals that is almost entirely devoid of or exclusively contains a certain genetic locus. Therefore, the BP phenotype can be correlated with the presence or absence of a certain locus. For example, manipulation of nitric oxide, particularly its inhibition with $N^{[\omega]}$-nitro-L-arginine methyl ester, has led to newer models of experimental HTN, including one, which is pregnancy induced.

Suggested Readings

Bohr DF, Dominiczak AE. Experimental hypertension. *Hypertension* 1991;17 (Suppl I):I39–144.

DiPette DJ, Simpson K, Rogers A, et al. Haemodynamic response to magnesium administration in mineralocorticoid-salt and two-kidney, one-clip renovascular hypertension. *J Clin Hypertens* 1988;6:413–417.

Gavras H, Brunner HR, Thurston H, et al. Reciprocation of renin dependency with sodium volume dependency in renal hypertension. *Science* 1975;188:1316–1317.

Kreutz R, Higuchi M, Ganten D. Molecular genetics of hypertension. *Clin Exp Hypertens* 1992;14:15–34.

Lerman LO, Chade AR, Sica V, et al. Animal models of hypertension: an overview. *J Lab Clin Med* 2005;146:160–173.

Mockrin SC, Dzau VJ, Gross KW, et al. Transgenic animals: new approaches to hypertension research. *Hypertension* 1991;17:394–399.

Phillips MI. Gene therapy for hypertension: the preclinical data. *Hypertension* 2001;38(Pt 2):543–548.

Sun Z, Zhang Z. Historical perspectives and recent advances in major animal models of hypertension. *Acta Pharmacol Sin* 2005;26:295–301.

Takahashi N, Smithies O. Gene targeting approaches to analyzing hypertension. *J Am Soc Nephrol* 1999;10:1598–1605.

Tobian L. Salt and hypertension: lessons from animal models that relate to human hypertension. *Hypertension* 1991;17(Suppl I):I52–I58.

Yagil Y, Yagil C. Genetic models of hypertension in experimental animals. *Exp Nephrol* 2001;9:1–9.

Yamori Y. Overview: studies from spontaneous hypertension: development from animal models toward man. *Clin Exp Hypertens* 1991;13:631–644.

SECTION V ■ MECHANISMS OF TARGET ORGAN DAMAGE

CHAPTER A58 ■ AGING, HYPERTENSION, AND THE HEART

AQ1   EDWARD G. LAKATTA, MD AND SAMER S. NAJJAR, MD

KEY POINTS

■ The incidence of hypertension and resultant heart failure (HF) increase dramatically with age.
■ Human, animal, cellular, and molecular perspectives indicate that hypertension and aging both cause similar patterns of altered heart structure and function and gene expression.
■ The interaction of mechanisms that underlie cardiac and vascular aging with those that cause hypertension substantially modifies the hypertensive phenotype as organisms age.

See also Chapters **A44, A45,** A59, A60, C109, C110, C150, and C151

Hypertension, aging, and heart failure

It is estimated that by the year 2035, approximately one in four individuals in the United States will be 65 years of age or older. Hypertension and resultant complications, including chronic heart failure (HF), reach epidemic proportions among older persons. In older individuals, specific pathophysiologic mechanisms that underlie hypertension and HF become superimposed on heart and vascular substrates that are modified by an aging process, *per se*. Therefore, an understanding of how aging modifies cardiovascular structure and function is critical to an understanding of hypertension, particularly in the geriatric population.

Aging-hypertension continuum

A unified interpretation of cardiac changes that accompany advancing age in otherwise healthy persons without clinical hypertension suggests that the observed changes are at least in part adaptations to age-related arterial changes (**Figure A58.1**), which are increasingly recognized as potent risk factors for cardiovascular morbidity and mortality. In some works, this interaction is characterized as abnormal "ventricular–vascular coupling."

Large vessel changes. The major age-related change affecting the heart is large artery stiffening, which leads to increased pulse wave velocity and enhancement of early reflected pulse waves. There is also increased late-systolic augmentation of central systolic pressure, with a reduced or maintained diastolic pressure due to loss of aortic elasticity. There is usually no change or a mild increase in systemic vascular resistance (SVR) that accompanies the increased pulse pressure. Aortic dilatation, aortic wall thickening and endothelial dysfunction are also present. Increased left ventricular (LV) wall thickness, largely due to an increase in ventricular myocyte size, results in part from increased

vascular impedance and acts to moderate the increase in LV wall tension. Deterioration of the elastin network and modest focal increases in wall collagen content also occur with aging.

Cardiac changes. Prolonged contractile activation of the thickened LV wall maintains a normal ejection time in the presence of early (forward wave-related) and late (reflected wave-related) increases in aortic impedance; this adaptation preserves cardiac pump function at rest. A downside of prolonged contractile activation is that at the time of the mitral valve opening, myocardial relaxation is less complete in older than in younger individuals, which then reduces the early diastolic LV filling rate. Structural changes and functional heterogeneity occurring within the LV with aging may also contribute to this reduction in peak LV filling rate. However, concomitant age-related cardiac adaptations, especially left atrial enlargement and an enhanced atrial contribution to ventricular filling, attempt to compensate for the reduced early diastolic filling and act to maintain sufficient end-diastolic volume to optimize Starling forces.

Potential age-associated changes in the concentrations or sensitivities to pressor hormones, growth factors, and cytokines, (catecholamines, angiotensin II, endothelin, transforming growth factor β, and fibroblast growth factor) that influence myocardial or vascular cells or their extracellular matrices, may also have a role in the cardiac adaptive changes as depicted in **Figure A58.1**.

Impaired cardiovascular reserve. At peak exercise, impaired LV ejection, heart rate, and reserve capacity are accompanied by an acute modest increase in LV end-diastolic volume in healthy, community-dwelling persons (**Table A58.1**). Mechanisms that underlie the age-associated reduction in maximal ejection fraction are multifactorial and include (a) a reduction in intrinsic myocardial contractility, (b) an increase in afterload, (c) a diminished effectiveness of the autonomic modulation of

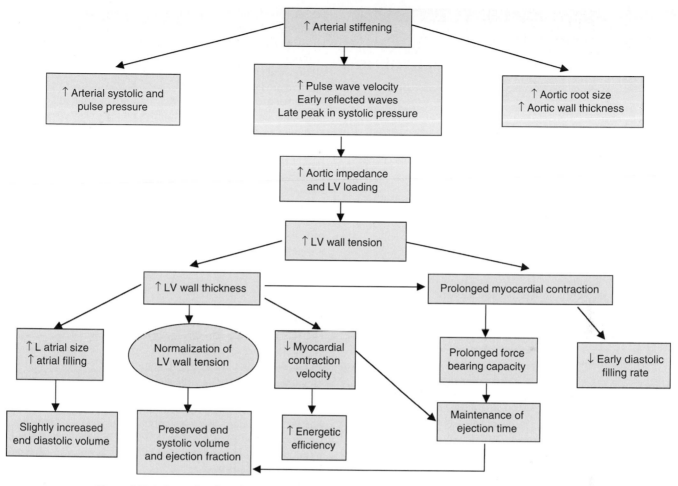

Figure A58.1 Arterial and cardiac changes that occur with aging in healthy humans. One interpretation of the constellation (*flow of arrows*) is that vascular changes lead to cardiac structural and functional alterations that maintain cardiac function. ↓, decrease; ↑, increase; LV, left ventricular. (Reproduced with permission from Lakatta EG. Cardiovascular regulatory mechanisms in advanced age. *Physiol Rev* 1993;73:413–465.)

LV contractility and arterial afterload, and (d) mismatching of arterial-ventricular loading. Although these age-associated changes in cardiovascular reserve, *per se*, are insufficient to produce clinical HF, they do affect the clinical presentation of HF by modifying the threshold for symptoms, signs, severity, and prognosis of HF.

Altered responses to sympathetic stimulation. Sympathetic nervous activity increases with aging and hypertension. Yet the efficiency of postsynaptic β-adrenergic signaling declines with aging, most likely due in part to reduced β-receptor density and desensitization of the β-receptor signaling cascade. Many other factors aggravate the deficient response to sympathetic stimulation and decreased cardiovascular reserve with aging, including reduced heart rate, prolonged filling time, increased afterload (cardiac and vascular), reduced myocardial contractility, and redistribution of blood flow.

Chronic hypertension versus accelerated aging. Parallel structural and functional changes in the large arteries (stiffness), cardiac mass (hypertrophy), and myocardial relaxation and filling (diastolic dysfunction) occur in normotensive aging and also with hypertension at any age. This continuum of age-related change is simply accelerated in individuals with chronic hypertension, so that the same changes occur at an earlier age or to an exaggerated

degree. In this regard, the traditional clinical distinction between normotension and hypertension is quite arbitrary, although it may be useful with regard to cardiovascular risk stratification. In fact, the similarities between aging and hypertension are so striking that aging can be considered to be "muted hypertension," whereas hypertension can be considered to be "accelerated cardiovascular aging."

Some differences exist, however, between hypertension and aging. For example, in contrast to a modest increase in SVR in normotensive aging, in hypertension, SVR and wave reflection increase more substantially. Increased SVR therefore plays a greater role in vascular loading of the ventricle in hypertensives. Additionally, in older hypertensives, resting stroke volume and cardiac output are progressively less well maintained than in younger hypertensives.

Cellular mechanisms of cardiac aging in animal models

Many age-associated changes in cardiac structure and function observed in humans also occur across a wide range of species. The vast majority of studies of cardiac cellular aging have employed rodent models (**Table A58.2**).

EXHAUSTIVE UPRIGHT EXERCISE: REDUCTION IN
AEROBIC CAPACITY AND CARDIAC REGULATION
BETWEEN AGES OF 20 AND 80 YEARS IN HEALTHY MEN
AND WOMEN

Oxygen consumption	↓ (50%)
(Arteriovenous) O_2	↓ (25%)
Cardiac index	↓ (25%)
Heart rate	↓ (25%)
Stroke volume	No change
Preload	
End-diastolic volume	↑ (30%)
Afterload	↑
Vascular (pulmonary vascular resistance)	↑ (30%)
Cardiac (end-systolic volume)	↑ (275%)
Cardiac (end-diastolic volume)	↑ (30%)
Contractility	↓ (60%)
Ejection fraction	↓ (15%)
Plasma catecholamines	↑
Cardiac and vascular responses to β-adrenergic stimulation	↓

↓, decrease; ↑, increase.

Left ventricular structure. Even in the absence of hypertension, the hearts of senescent rats (24–30 months of age) exhibit moderate LV hypertrophy (25%) compared to hearts from young and middle-aged animals. Matrix and myocyte volume increase. The average LV collagen content doubles between adulthood and senescence and the level of fibronectin is also markedly increased. The average volume of individual cardiomyocytes approximately doubles over the adult range, whereas the number of myocytes generally decreases with aging, due primarily to apoptosis with some increase in necrosis.

Excitation–contraction–relaxation. The kinetics of cellular reactions that underlie cardiac automaticity are reduced in senescent versus younger adult rodent hearts. There is prolongation of the action potential, the transient increase in cytosolic Ca^{2+} evoked by the action potential, and the ensuing contraction (**Table A58.2**). This altered pattern of Ca^{2+} regulation allows the myocardium of older hearts to generate force for a longer time after excitation. The prolonged isovolumic relaxation period in the healthy human heart may with aging, in part, be attributable to extended contractile protein Ca^{2+} activation, enabling the continued ejection of blood during late systole, a beneficial adaptation with respect to enhanced vascular stiffness and early reflected pulse waves (**Figure A58.1**).

Ca^{2+} loading. Excess cardiomyocyte Ca^{2+} loading can lead to dysregulation of Ca^{2+} homeostasis, impaired diastolic and systolic function, arrhythmias, and cell death. In the senescent heart during high pacing rates, the excess of cytosolic Ca^{2+} promotes incomplete relaxation and favors increased diastolic tone. The senescent heart also exhibits a reduced threshold for pathologic manifestations of excess Ca^{2+} loading during conditions (physiologic and pharmacologic) that increase Ca^{2+} influx such as neurotransmitter stimulation, postischemic reperfusion, or oxidative stress. Causes of reduced Ca^{2+} tolerance of the older cardiocytes, compared to those of the younger adult heart, include (a) changes in Ca^{2+} regulatory protein levels (**Table A58.2**) and

(b) alterations in the composition of membranes in which Ca^{2+} regulatory proteins reside, including an increase in membrane $\omega_6{:}\omega_3$-polyunsaturated fatty acids with aging. It is believed that ω_3-polyunsaturated fatty acid promotes cardiac calcium dysregulation and enhances the likelihood of intracellular generation of reactive oxygen species.

Adrenergic responsiveness. Studies in isolated LV muscle in individual rat ventricular cardiomyocytes, similar to recent studies in humans, indicate that a reduced response to β-adrenoceptor (βAR) stimulation occurs with aging. The most remarkable change within the βAR system with aging appears to be the decrease in the efficacy of coupling of the βAR receptor to the postreceptor signal transduction system that generates the contractile response. Aging is also accompanied by a striking increase in ventricular messenger RNA and protein levels of atrial natriuretic peptide, proenkephalin, and adenosine. Negative effects of opioid peptides and adenosine on cardiac contraction parameters may also contribute to age-associated reduction in the βAR responsiveness of the heart.

Integrated view

Coordinated changes in several key steps of excitation–contraction coupling and its regulation by cell-surface receptors occur with aging. These changes at the structural, biochemical, biophysical, and molecular levels, result in prolonged Ca^{2+} transients and contraction. The resultant altered Ca^{2+} homeostasis permits prolonged and efficient force-bearing capacity in the older heart, but renders it more prone to spontaneous Ca^{2+} oscillations and Ca^{2+}-dependent arrhythmias. These mechanisms act in concert with impaired β-adrenergic modulation of excitation–contraction coupling mechanisms.

Pressure overload versus normotensive aging. Many of the age-associated changes in structure, function, and gene expression that occur with aging also occur in the hypertrophied myocardium of younger animals with experimentally induced chronic hypertension. Additionally, similar reductions in cellular RNA concentration and the rate of protein synthesis are observed with aging and chronic myocardial overload in the rat model. It is tempting to speculate that this nearly identical pattern of change in gene expression in young hypertensive and older normotensive rodents may indicate that a common set of transcription factors regulates cardiac cellular adaptation during pressure-overload hypertrophy and aging. This particular constellation of shifts in gene expression appears to be adaptive, in that it allows for an energy-efficient and prolonged contraction. In the hypertensive rodent heart, it can be inferred that these changes in gene expression permit functional adaptations in response to an increased vascular "afterload." Specifically, the capacity for molecular adaptation to hemodynamic overload, ischemia, or both is diminished in aged hearts.

Aging and heart failure in hypertension. With advancing age in the spontaneously hypertensive rat (SHR), chronic hypertension and cardiac hypertrophy eventually give way to HF and normotension. Young adult and middle-aged SHRs exhibit compensated cardiac hypertrophy. Depressed contractile function and increased fibrosis are observed with aging, beginning at approximately 18 months. The transition from compensated hypertrophy to failure with aging in the SHR seems to demonstrate quite well the consequences of interactions between "normal aging" and disease. This transition is characterized by a

TABLE A58.2

MYOCARDIAL CHANGES WITH ADULT AGING IN RODENTS

Structural Δ	Functional Δ	Ionic, Biophysical/Biochemical mechanism(s)	Molecular mechanisms
Myocyte size Myocyte number	Prolonged contraction	Prolonged cytosolic Ca^{2+} transient	
		$\downarrow$ Sarcoplasmic reticulum Ca^{2+} pumping rate	$\downarrow$ Sarcoplasmic reticulum Ca^{2+} pump mRNA
		$\downarrow$ Pump site density	No Δ calsequestrin mRNA
	Prolonged action potential	$\downarrow$ Calcium influx inactivation	$\uparrow$ Na–Ca exchanger mRNA
		$\downarrow$ Transient outward K^+ current density	
	Diminished contraction Velocity	$\downarrow$ α MHC protein	$\downarrow$ α MHC mRNA
		$\uparrow$ β MHC protein	$\uparrow$ β MHC mRNA
		$\downarrow$ Myosin ATPase activity	No Δ Actin mRNA
		$\downarrow$ RXRβ1 and γ mRNA	$\downarrow$ RXRβ1 and γ mRNA
		$\downarrow$ RXRβ1 and γ protein	
		$\downarrow$ Thyroid receptor protein	
	Diminished β-adrenergic contractile response	$\downarrow$ Coupling β-adrenergic receptor-acylase	$\downarrow$ β_1AR mRNA
		No Δ inhibitory G protein activation	No Δ β-adrenergic receptor kinase mRNA
		No Δ β-adrenergic receptor kinase activity	
		$\downarrow$ Troponin-I phospholamban	
		$\downarrow$ Phospholamban phosphorylation	
		$\downarrow$ Calcium influx augmentation	
		$\downarrow$ Intracellular calcium transient augmentation	
		$\uparrow$ Enkephalin peptides	$\uparrow$ Proenkephalin mRNA
$\uparrow$Y Matrix connective tissue	$\uparrow$ Myocardial stiffness	$\uparrow$ Hydroxyproline content	$\uparrow$ Collagen mRNA
		$\uparrow$ Activity of myocardial renin-angiotensin system	$\uparrow$ Fibronectin mRNA
			$\uparrow$ Angiotensin AT-1 receptor mRNA
		$\uparrow$ Atrial natriuretic peptide	$\uparrow$ Atrial natriuretic peptide mRNA
	$\downarrow$ Growth response		$\downarrow$ Induction of immediate early genes
	$\downarrow$ Heat shock response		$\downarrow$ Activation of heat shock factor

Δ, change; $\downarrow$, decrease; $\uparrow$, increase.
MHC, myosin heavy chain; ATPase, adenosine triphosphatase; RXR, retinoid X-receptor; mRNA, messenger RNA.

progressive impairment of LV function and ventricular dilatation in the absence of an additional increase in LV mass. The pattern of altered gene expression that accompanies the transition to HF during advanced age in the SHR supports the notion that total contractile protein decreases whereas total connective tissue protein increases and suggests that these processes are regulated at a pretranslational level. Although the accumulated effects of long-term hypertension and the genetic nature of the model cannot be dismissed, it seems appropriate to hypothesize that the effects of normal aging reduce the reserve capacity of the heart for adaptation in the SHR and conspire with hypertension to decrease the chances of survival.

Therapeutic implications

Alterations in cardiovascular function that exceed the identified limits for age-associated changes in healthy elderly individuals are most likely manifestations of the interaction of "normal" aging with a variety of age-associated changes, including severe physical deconditioning and other cardiovascular diseases. Specific accelerated cardiovascular changes that occur during apparently healthy aging perhaps should be construed as risky because they are so similar to those seen with hypertension and other risk factors that merit intervention. Lifestyle changes such as regular vigorous exercise have already been shown to be effective in retarding the speed of cardiovascular aging, including preservation of ventricular ejection capacity and lower cardiac afterload, arterial stiffness, and blood pressure (BP). Efforts are underway to evaluate whether screening programs for accelerated cardiovascular aging could help identify normotensive individuals who are high risk for developing hypertension and its complications. By extrapolating from the worldwide metaregression studies, doubling of systolic BP (from 120 to 240 mmHg) is identical to a doubling of age (40–80 years); the risk of death from cardiovascular disease is increased by 64-fold. Therefore, it remains attractive to postulate that interventions targeting accelerated cardiovascular aging will prevent or retard the adverse outcomes associated with the most potent risk factors for cardiovascular diseases: aging and hypertension.

Suggested Readings

Lakatta EG. Cardiovascular regulatory mechanisms in advanced age. *Physiol Rev* 1993;73:413–465.

Lakatta EG. Age-associated cardiovascular changes in health: impact on cardiovascular disease in older persons. *Heart Fail Rev* 2002;7:29–49.

Lakatta EG, Levy D. Arterial and cardiac aging: major shareholders in cardiovascular disease enterprises: Part I: aging arteries: a "set up" for vascular disease. *Circulation* 2003;107:139–146.

Lakatta EG, Levy D. Arterial and cardiac aging: major shareholders in cardiovascular disease enterprises: Part II: the aging heart in health: links to heart disease. *Circulation* 2003;107:346–354.

Lakatta EG, Schulman SP, Gerstenblith G. Cardiovascular aging in health and therapeutic considerations with respect to cardiovascular disease in older patients. In: Fuster V, Alexander RW, King S, et al. eds. *Hurst's the heart*. New York: McGraw-Hill, 2001:2329–2355.

Lakatta EG, Sollott SJ, Pepe S. The old heart: operating on the edge. In: Bock G, Goode JA, eds. *Aging vulnerability: causes and interventions, Novartis foundation symposium 235*. Chichester: John Wiley and Sons, 2001:172–201.

Najjar SS, Schulman SP, Gerstenblith G, et al. Age and gender affect ventricular-vascular coupling during aerobic exercise. *J Am Coll Cardiol* 2004;44:611–617.

Najjar SS, Scuteri A, Lakatta EG. Arterial aging: is it an immutable cardiovascular risk factor? *Hypertension* 2005;46:454–462.

CHAPTER A59 ■ PATHOGENESIS OF HYPERTENSIVE LEFT VENTRICULAR HYPERTROPHY AND DIASTOLIC DYSFUNCTION

EDWARD D. FROHLICH, MD

KEY POINTS

■ Left ventricular hypertrophy (LVH) is an independent risk factor for premature cardiovascular morbidity and mortality that is associated with impaired coronary hemodynamics, increased predisposition to cardiac dysrhythmias, sudden death, systolic or diastolic dysfunction, cardiac failure, and angina pectoris.

■ LVH is associated with increased wall tension and myocardial oxygen demand, endothelial dysfunction of the myocardium and coronary arteries, reduced coronary blood flow and flow reserve, and angina pectoris with or without occlusive atherosclerotic epicardial coronary artery disease.

■ LVH is a heterogeneous condition in which individual myofibrils are increased in their circumferential diameter (concentric hypertrophy) or length (eccentric hypertrophy).

■ Histologically, LVH is characterized by increased myocytic mass (hypertrophy), increased fibrosis in the extracellular matrix, perivascular fibrosis, and apoptosis, which may be at least partially reversed by effective antihypertensive therapy.

See also Chapters **A58**, A65, B78, **C150,** and **C151**

Natural history

As the left ventricle progressively hypertrophies in response to increased afterload and aging, its contractile (systolic) pumping reserve becomes diminished. Eventually, cardiac failure supervenes unless arterial pressure is effectively controlled. Even before systolic dysfunction becomes evident clinically, the hypertrophic left ventricle becomes "stiffer" (less distensible), and diastolic filling becomes impaired as a result of ventricular fibrosis.

In response to the increased ventricular stiffness, the left atrium enlarges and thickens to provide a "booster pump" that acts to maintain diastolic filling. Increased left atrial size is notable by the development of a fourth heart sound (i.e., the atrial diastolic gallop), P wave electrocardiographic (ECG) changes, and corresponding echocardiographic findings that predispose to the development of atrial dysrhythmias.

Hypertensive patients with left ventricular hypertrophy (LVH) [especially those who are elderly, black, diabetic, or with ischemic heart disease (IHD)] may develop diastolic dysfunction and experience cardiac failure despite apparent normal systolic function. Angina pectoris may occur in response to the increased wall tension and myocardial oxygen demand. Endothelial dysfunction, increased collagen deposition, perivascular fibrosis, hypertensive coronary arteriolar disease, or concomitant occlusive atherosclerotic disease of the epicardial coronary arteries also occur in varying proportions. Further, apoptosis (programmed myocardial cell death) accelerates the development of cardiac failure.

Etiology

The primary factors responsible for development of LVH are pressure and volume overload, but nonhemodynamic factors also contribute, including a variety of humoral mechanisms and growth factors (e.g., catecholamines, angiotensin II, endothelin) that promote vascular and cardiac myocytic growth. Other clinical considerations include the stage of hypertensive disease, demographic factors (e.g., age, gender, race), comorbid diseases (e.g., obesity, diabetes mellitus, atherosclerotic coronary artery disease), and coincident pharmacologic therapies.

Eccentric versus concentric hypertrophy

LVH is characterized by changes in individual myofibrils that increase in circumferential diameter (concentric hypertrophy), length (eccentric hypertrophy), or both. Left ventricular (LV) end-diastolic volume tends to increase with eccentric hypertrophy, as in the athlete's heart, with asymmetric septal hypertrophy and, of course, volume overload. Concentric hypertrophy occurs most commonly in hypertension or aortic stenosis and tends to be associated with normal or reduced LV end-diastolic volume. A mixed pattern of LVH may result from combined chronic pressure and volume overload.

When hypertension is associated with increased preload, the structural changes may be more eccentric, especially in patients with obesity or chronic renal insufficiency. In untreated hypertension, progression from LVH to cardiac failure is associated with eccentric or concentric hypertrophy (individually or together), ischemia, increased fibrosis and ventricular stiffness, apoptosis, and eventually systolic ventricular failure. However, in those patients effectively treated with antihypertensive therapy, concentric hypertrophy (associated with ischemia, fibrosis, and apoptosis) may be manifested by impaired diastolic function and preserved systolic function.

Systolic versus diastolic dysfunction

Impaired LV systolic function is a common consequence of LVH, particularly in the untreated patient. Diastolic dysfunction can occur in the absence of systolic dysfunction but also occurs in almost all situations where systolic dysfunction already exists. When diastolic dysfunction exists in the absence of impaired systolic function, it usually occurs in elderly patients with ventricular collagen deposition, fibrosis, and ischemia.

Pathogenesis of increased cardiovascular risk

The precise explanations for the increased risk associated with LVH are not completely known, but a number of mechanisms are currently being clarified. Therefore, LVH is associated with progressively impaired coronary blood flow and flow reserve and increased minimal coronary vascular resistance, fibrosis of the extracellular matrix and perivascularly, as well as endothelial dysfunction and programmed myocytic cell death (apoptosis). Epicardial and microvascular arteriolar disease are frequently exacerbated by the atherogenic process.

Progressive contraction of intravascular (plasma) volume and cardiac preload, in conjunction with increasing arterial pressure and vascular resistance, may further alter the rheology and

viscosity of the coronary microcirculation in patients with LVH. Any or all of the foregoing changes contribute to development of cardiac failure, coronary arterial insufficiency, angina pectoris, cardiac dysrhythmias, and sudden death. Compounding these factors is increased deposition of collagen and fibrosis that increases ventricular stiffness, promotes apoptosis, and enhances the ischemia and likelihood of developing ventricular dysfunction and eventual cardiac failure. Moreover, several clinical studies have indicated that if diabetes mellitus complicates the LVH of hypertension, cardiac mass is greater at any level of arterial pressure; this increased mass may be related to increased deposition of hyaline and other substances.

Clinical correlation

Comparison of diagnostic techniques. Detection of LVH may be accomplished by various techniques. The chest x-ray is not nearly as sensitive as the ECG and may be associated with changes that not only reflect LVH but ventricular chamber dilation as well. For routine clinical evaluation, the ECG has relatively high specificity and remains the most useful and cost-effective method, but it also falls short of detecting early LVH. The most useful and sensitive clinical means for detecting early LVH and associated changes in LV function is the echocardiogram. A less costly limited echocardiography has been suggested in carefully selected patients, particularly those with stage I blood pressure (BP) levels without other evidence of LVH. It provides an accurate index of LV mass and chamber measurement as well as an index of ventricular function and should not be used routinely in all patients with hypertension, because increased LV mass can be detected by the less costly ECG. Other more costly techniques that provide a more clear-cut definition of LVH are magnetic resonance and positron emission imaging techniques.

Electrocardiogram criteria. There are 30 or more indices that have been proposed for ECG diagnosis of LVH. The most common are the Sokolow–Lyons criteria (sum of the negative deflection in V_1 and positive deflection in V_5 or V_6 >35 or 38 mV) and the Cornell voltage (product of the QRS duration and the sum of the positive deflection in aVL and negative deflection in V_3 >2,440 mV/msecond) criteria. Highly sensitive are the McPhee index (sum of the tallest precordial R wave and deepest S wave $\geq$4.5 mV) and the LV strain pattern (i.e., the QRS complex and T wave vectors are 180 degrees apart) that cause few false-negative diagnoses. The latter strain pattern is associated with severely diminished vascularity of the hypertrophied ventricle and with coronary arteriography evidence of ischemic disease. Enhancing the diagnostic ability of the ECG, particularly in early LVH, are left atrial (P wave) abnormalities. Among these latter criteria are the following: P wave $\geq$0.12 second in duration, bipeak interval "notched" P waves $\geq$0.04 second, P wave duration to PR segment ratio of $\geq$1.6 in lead II, and terminal atrial forces (V_1) $\geq$0.04 second. Presence of two or more of these criteria is highly concordant with the presence of cardiac dysrhythmias, echocardiographic evidence of left atrial enlargement, and LVH.

Echocardiogram. The M-mode, two-dimensional (2D) echocardiogram (with or without Doppler flow measurements) provides a highly precise clinical means of detecting LVH. Interventricular septal hypertrophy ($\geq$1 cm) may be the first finding, and increased width of the LV free wall to $\geq$1.1 cm indicates LVH. Increased LV mass suggests LVH, but this index takes into consideration LV diastolic volume, which is different between men and women (<100 and ≥131 g/m², respectively) and even varies with intravascular and ventricular volume (which change with weight reduction). Also important are changes in early and late ventricular filling (E-A wave reversal) that correlates strongly with increased left atrial pressure.

Treatment

The best treatment for LVH is prevention; this means early and effective treatment of hypertension and the attendant systolic and diastolic dysfunction, Effective therapy results in reduction of arterial pressure and LV mass along with improved diastolic distensibility and relaxation. Treatment of systolic functional impairment may also improve to some degree the diastolic dysfunction. The major objective in treatment is the fastidious control of systolic and diastolic pressure, at least to <140/<90 mm Hg. Given the common occurrence of LVH with IHD, a lower target of <130/<80 mm Hg may often be warranted, as recommended by the American Heart Association (AHA)/American College of Cardiology (ACC) 2007 guidelines for treatment of IHD. Despite some concern about reducing diastolic pressure to levels <80 to 85 mm Hg for fear of impairing coronary arterial blood flow in diastole (the so-called J-curve), prospective trials (i.e., SHEP, STOP-Hypertension, MRC, SAVE, SOLVD) have not demonstrated increased risk at therapeutically lower diastolic pressures. To this end, the AHA/ACC guideline suggests careful monitoring when diastolic BP is <60 mm Hg.

All forms of antihypertensive therapy reduce LV mass in animals and man. The effectiveness of angiotensin-converting enzyme (ACE) inhibitors, angiotensin-receptor blockers (ARBs), and calcium antagonists are most clearly documented in clinical trials. Therapy with agents that inhibit the renin-angiotensin system appear to reduce LV hydroxyproline and collagen content and fibrosis. No single trial, however, has yet demonstrated benefit that reversal of LVH by itself improves morbidity and mortality. Diminished risk from LVH reduction must be disassociated from the pharmacologic actions of reducing pressure, improving coronary blood flow and flow reserve, or even preventing dysrhythmias.

Suggested Readings

Devereux R, Wachtell K, Gerdts E, et al. Prognostic significance of left ventricular mass change during treatment of hypertension. *JAMA* 2004;292:2350–2356.

Dunn FG, Pringle SD. Sudden cardiac death, ventricular arrhythmias, and hypertensive left ventricular hypertrophy. *J Hypertens* 1993;11:1003–1010.

Fortuño MA, González A, Ravassa S, et al. Clinical implications of apoptosis in hypertensive heart disease. *Am J Physiol Heart Circ Physiol* 2003;284:1495–1506.

Frohlich ED. Is reversal of left ventricular hypertrophy in hypertension beneficial? *Hypertension* 1991;18(Suppl I):33–38.

Frohlich ED. Risk mechanisms in hypertensive heart disease. *Hypertension* 1999;34:782–789.

Frohlich ED, Apstein C, Chobanian AV, et al. The heart in hypertension. *N Engl J Med* 1992;327:998–1008.

López B, González A, Querejeta R, et al. The use of collagen-derived serum peptides for the clinical assessment of hypertensive heart disease. *J Hypertens* 2005;23:1445–1451.

Roman MJ, Pickering TG, Schwartz JE, et al. Relation of arterial structure and function to left ventricular geometric patterns in hypertensive adults. *J Am Coll Cardiol* 1996;28:751–756.

Sheps SG, Frohlich ED. Limited echocardiography for hypertensive left ventricular hypertrophy. *Hypertension* 1997;29:560–563.

de Simone G, Pasanisi F, Contaldo F. Link of nonhemodynamic factors to hemodynamic determinants of left ventricular hypertrophy. *Hypertension* 2001;38:13–18.

Siscovick DS, Raghunathan TE, Psaty BM, et al. Diuretic therapy for hypertension and the risk of primary cardiac arrest. *N Engl J Med* 1994;330:1852–1857.

Strauer BE. Repair of coronary arterioles after treatment with perindopril in hypertensive heart disease. *Hypertension* 2000;36:220–225.

Vasan R, Larson MG, Benjamin E, et al. Left ventricular dilatation and the risk of congestive heart failure in people without myocardial infarction. *N Engl J Med* 1997;336:1350–1355.

CHAPTER A60 ■ PATHOGENESIS OF CHRONIC HEART FAILURE

THIERRY H. LE JEMTEL, MD AND PIERRE V. ENNEZAT, MD

KEY POINTS

■ Heart failure (HF) due to left ventricular systolic dysfunction (LVSD) is most common in aging patients with more than one classical risk factor (hypertension, coronary artery disease, or diabetes mellitus). Less commonly HF due to LVSD occurs as a result of substance/alcohol abuse, valvular disease, myocarditis, or infiltrative diseases.

■ A new paradigm describes the evolution of HF due to LVSD in three stages: (i) asymptomatic LV remodeling, (ii) appearance of progressively worsening symptoms, and (iii) a state of low cardiac output and tissue perfusion.

■ HF associated with preserved LV systolic function is a heterogeneous clinical entity, which includes prolonged diastolic relaxation, LV hypertrophy, and reduced functional myocardial reserve.

See also Chapters **A45, A58, A59,** B78, C150, and C151

Preexisting conditions in heart failure

The incidence of clinical heart failure (HF), whether associated with left ventricular systolic dysfunction (LVSD) or preserved LV systolic function, increases with the number of classical cardiovascular risk factors present in the individual.

Hypertension. As demonstrated most clearly in the Framingham Heart Study, hypertension is the predominant preexisting condition in patients with HF. A history of hypertension is present in 65% to 85% of patients with HF. The HF syndrome can occur in patients with reduced LV systolic function and in those with preserved LV systolic function and diastolic relaxation abnormalities. Patients with a history of hypertension who develop HF with preserved LV systolic function may have an impaired capacity to excrete salt and water in addition to LV hypertrophy and impaired relaxation.

Coronary artery disease. Coronary artery disease is more prevalent in patients with reduced than preserved LV systolic function. In this condition, segmental wall motion abnormalities due to ischemia or infarction impair ventricular emptying and lead to ventricular remodeling that can be marked by increased end-diastolic diameter and a reduced ejection fraction.

Obesity and diabetes. Diabetes mellitus is more prevalent in the instance of HF with preserved LV systolic function. The greater occurrence of diabetes mellitus in patients with HF and preserved LV systolic function probably relates to the increased prevalence of obesity in diabetics and may be a late manifestation of the cardiovascular dysmetabolic syndrome (insulin resistance).

Other causes of heart failure. For the most part, patients with HF have more than one of the major preexisting conditions

that predispose to HF (coronary artery disease, type 2 diabetes mellitus); however, alcohol/substance abuse, valvular heart disease, myocarditis, or infiltrative diseases can also cause HF.

Progression to left ventricular systolic dysfunction

HF due to LVSD is a progressive syndrome marked by cardiac, renal, and somatic abnormalities of varying severity.

Left ventricular concentric hypertrophy. Left ventricular (LV) wall thickness increases in response to chronic pressure overload ("increased afterload") to normalize LV wall tension according to the law of Laplace (Wall tension = Pressure × LV radius/LV wall thickness). The resulting LV concentric hypertrophy has been viewed historically as a "normal" adaptive compensatory process in patients with systemic hypertension but is more appropriately viewed as a maladaptive response because there is a two to fourfold increase in cardiovascular events in humans with increased LV mass. There is a short-term hemodynamic improvement that occurs after reversal of cardiac hypertrophy in small rodents exposed to pressure overload, suggesting that pharmacologic reversal of LV hypertrophy may decrease the prevalence of HF due to LVSD or prevent the development of symptoms in patients with preserved LV systolic function.

Transition from left ventricular hypertrophy to left ventricular systolic dysfunction. Over the last 50 years, the transition from LV concentric hypertrophy (with normalized workload/mass ratio) to LV dilatation (and a decline in LV systolic function) has been thoroughly documented in experimental models of pressure overload. Despite the high prevalence of LVSD, the transition from LV concentric hypertrophy to systolic dysfunction has rarely been documented in patients with hypertension alone, that is, in the absence of coexisting coronary artery disease, type 2 diabetes mellitus or alcohol/substance abuse. A hastened loss of cardiac myocyte by apoptosis could be responsible for the transition from LV hypertrophy to LV dilatation and systolic dysfunction but current estimates of the rate of myocyte apoptosis are highly inconsistent. The uncertain relevance of myocyte apoptosis as a pathway to LV dilatation and dysfunction argues in favor of a multifactorial etiology of HF due to LVSD in patients with a history of hypertension.

The progression of HF due to LVSD and the development of symptoms are classically imputed to a steady deterioration in LV systolic performance. Yet data from the Study of Left Ventricular Dysfunction (SOLVD) do not support this view; LV ejection fraction was not markedly different in asymptomatic and symptomatic patients with HF. Furthermore, LVSD severity (ejection fraction) and functional capacity are extremely poorly correlated.

A paradigm shift in heart failure

Given the disparities in the classical model of HF, the syndrome may be better understood by dividing its progression into three separate stages (**Figure A60.1**): The three stages of clinical HF parallel the paradigm shift that has occurred in modeling HF: the remodeling stage corresponds to the model of neurohumoral activation, the clinical stage to the cardio-renal model, and the low output stage to the older hemodynamic model. The three stages of HF also provide clear therapeutic targets: reversal of the remodeling process, control of excess volume, and restoration of a normal cardiac output, respectively. Specific therapeutic interventions for the three stages of HF are summarized in **Figure A60.1**.

Left ventricular remodeling. The first stage, LV remodeling, is most often clinically silent and patients rarely experience symptoms during routine daily activities. Resting stroke volume and cardiac output are preserved but the ventricular chamber dilates; resting LV end-diastolic volume steadily increases and ejection fraction steadily declines. In contrast, the maximal cardiac output response to exercise is markedly blunted, declining from a fivefold increase over the resting value to a twofold increase. Reduced cardiac output responses to exercise fully explain the low peak aerobic capacity of patients with LV remodeling when compared to age and gender-matched healthy subjects. Somatic alterations are minimal, as evidenced by preserved skeletal muscle (SM) mass and normal exercise-induced vasodilation of SM vessels. Glomerular filtration rate also remains normal.

Clinical symptom development. The second stage of HF is characterized by the development of symptoms including dyspnea, fatigue, and salt and water retention. Ejection fraction continues to decline at rest and in response to exercise and cardiac output begins to decrease at rest. Owing to physical inactivity and possibly the systemic inflammatory state associated with HF, SM mass and vasodilatory responses to exercise are markedly abnormal. At this stage of clinical HF, SM alterations are primarily responsible for the reduced functional capacity. Renal function also begins to decline, mainly during episodes of clinical decompensation.

Low output phase. The third stage of HF is characterized by a profound reduction in resting cardiac output and the lack of cardiac output response to exercise and other stimuli. Ejection fraction may further decline. Loss of SM mass progresses to cachexia but functional capacity is primarily limited by the lack of cardiac output reserve. Renal function deteriorates markedly and takes on an important prognostic value.

Heart failure with preserved left ventricular systolic function

HF with preserved LV systolic function is particularly common in elderly women with preexisting hypertension, type 2 diabetes mellitus and obesity, conditions that also predispose to concentric

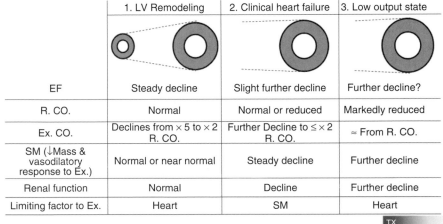

	1. LV Remodeling	2. Clinical heart failure	3. Low output state
EF	Steady decline	Slight further decline	Further decline?
R. CO.	Normal	Normal or reduced	Markedly reduced
Ex. CO.	Declines from × 5 to × 2 R. CO.	Further Decline to ≤ × 2 R. CO.	≈ From R. CO.
SM (↓Mass & vasodilatory response to Ex.)	Normal or near normal	Steady decline	Further decline
Renal function	Normal	Decline	Further decline
Limiting factor to Ex.	Heart	SM	Heart

TX
LVAD
ICD/CRT
Digitalis
Loop diuretics
Aldosterone blockade
Beta adrenergic blockade
ACE Inhibition

Figure A60.1 The syndrome of heart failure due to left ventricular systolic dysfunction (LVSD) progresses through three separate states: 1. LV remodeling, 2. Clinical heart failure, and 3. low output state. The changes in ejection fraction (EF), resting and exercise cardiac output (R.CO, Ex. CO), skeletal muscle (SM) and the treatment are summarized for each separate state (ACE for Angiotensin converting enzyme, ICD for implantable cardiac defibrillator, CRT for cardiac resynchronization therapy, LVAD for left ventricular assist device and TX for cardiac transplantation).

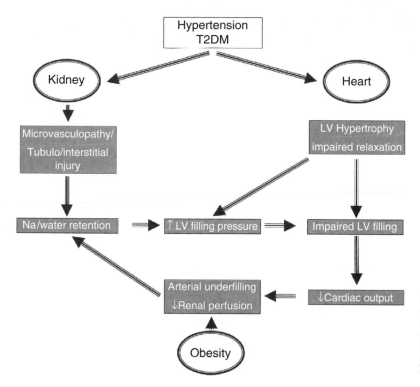

Figure A60.2 Pathogenesis of heart failure with preserved left ventricular (LV) systolic function. Systemic hypertension and type 2 diabetes mellitus are responsible for renal and LV structural and functional alterations that promote salt and water retention, increase LV filling pressure and reduce cardiac output. These alterations are compounded by the presence of obesity.

LV hypertrophy. Impaired diastolic relaxation can occur in the absence of hypertrophy and HF with preserved LV systolic function remains a poorly understood clinical entity. Intrinsic LV diastolic dysfunction, combined ventricular and arterial stiffening, and concomitant alterations in LV systolic function have been held primarily responsible for the development of the symptoms and signs of this form of HF. The pathogenesis of this condition may also involve the kidneys, because hypertension and type 2 diabetes mellitus commonly affect this organ.

Cardio-renal interactions.
Figure A60.2 suggests that the heart, the kidneys, and obesity interact in the pathogenesis of HF with preserved LV systolic function. There is currently little evidence to support the dual role of the heart and the kidneys in this condition in humans, LV structural and functional alterations are prominent in aged dogs with renal hypertension. Underestimation of renal dysfunction by measurement of serum creatinine level may be in part responsible for the lack of recognition of the role of the kidney in the genesis of HF, especially when systolic function is preserved. Renal microvasculopathy involving preglomerular arterioles and tubulointerstitial injury occur in long-standing hypertension, resulting in salt and water retention. The exact mechanism(s) that mediate the effect of hypertension on the kidneys are unclear although systemic endothelial dysfunction appears to play a role.

Left ventricular diastolic function.
Owing to the coupling of LV hypertrophy, prolonged LV relaxation, and increased LV stiffness, the left ventricle cannot accommodate the rise in intravascular volume. As a result, LV filling pressure increases, perhaps as a maladaptive attempt to maintain optimal Starling forces to sustain efficient systolic function. Eventually, impaired LV filling lowers cardiac output and thereby promotes arterial underfilling, thereby increasing cardiac preload, compromising renal perfusion, and aggravating salt and water retention.

Obesity.
Obesity may further compromise renal perfusion as an increasing fraction of cardiac output is shunted away from the kidneys to the abundant adipose tissue. Myocardial mechanics are subsequently altered.

Hypertension and progression to clinical heart failure.
Besides initiating LV hypertrophy and contributing to LV remodeling, systemic hypertension directly affects vascular endothelial and renal function. Long-standing hypertension is associated with a steady decrease in vascular endothelial and renal function that affects the transition from LVSD to clinical HF and from clinical HF to the low output state (**Figure A60.3**). HF and a low output state further worsen the decline deterioration in vascular and renal function.

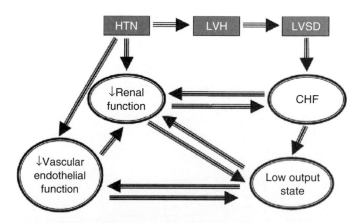

Figure A60.3 The pressure overload associated with hypertension (HTN) promotes left ventricular hypertrophy (LVH) that leads to left ventricular systolic dysfunction (LVSD), clinical heart failure (CHF) and the low cardiac output state. Hypertension also promotes vascular endothelial and renal dysfunction that directly impact on the progression of heart failure that, in turn, affects vascular endothelial and renal function. When considering therapeutic options at the low output stage of heart failure one needs to assess carefully the reversibility of renal and vascular alterations.

Early recognition and heart failure management

Early recognition of LV remodeling by cardiac imaging is a prime consideration in the management of HF. LV remodeling often progresses without symptoms in elderly patients with hypertension, coronary artery disease, type 2 diabetes mellitus or alcohol abuse. LV remodeling in elderly patients is most often recognized at a late stage of the process when the appearance of symptoms triggers invasive or noninvasive cardiac imaging. In young patients, LV remodeling is recognized earlier than in elderly patients if cardiac imaging is performed during a persistently symptomatic viral illness, in the peripartum or in the context of familial cardiomyopathies and valvular heart disease.

Delayed recognition of on-going LV remodeling compromises the likelihood of therapeutic success with β-adrenergic blockade, the only pharmacologic intervention shown to reverse the LV remodeling process. In HF with preserved systolic function, angiotensin receptor blockers have been shown to reduce the incidence of HF hospitalizations, although no major mortality benefit has been proven with these or other drugs, perhaps due to the short duration of most clinical trials and the relatively low death rate in this group compared to those with LVSD.

The challenge when considering therapeutic options such as LV assist device implantation in the late stages of the syndrome of HF is to assess the reversibility of renal impairment and correctly gauge the risk of cardiovascular events. Renal dysfunction may be irreversible in advanced HF necessitating permanent dialysis, whereas a rapidly evolving diffuse vasculopathy may compromise life expectancy despite restoration of cardiac output.

Suggested Readings

Devereux RB, Dahlof B, Gerds E, et al. Regression of hypertensive left ventricular hypertrophy by losartan compared with atenolol: the losartan intervention for endpoint reduction in hypertension (LIFE) trial. *Circulation* 2004;110:1456–1462.

Drazner MH. The transition from hypertrophy to failure. How certain are we? *Circulation* 2005;112:936–938.

Frey N, Katus HA, Olson EN, et al. Hypertrophy of the heart a new therapeutic target? *Circulation* 2004;109:1580–1589.

Levy D, Larson MG, Vasan RS, et al. The progression from hypertension to congestive heart failure. *JAMA* 1996;275:1557–1562.

Mann DJ, Bristow MR. Mechanisms and models in heart failure. The biomechanical model and beyond. *Circulation* 2005;111:2837–2849.

Munagala VK, Hart CY, Burnett JC Jr, et al. Ventricular structure and function in aged dogs with renal hypertension. A model of experimental diastolic heart failure. *Circulation* 2005;111:1128–1135.

O'Rourke MF, Safar ME. Regression of hypertensive left ventricular hypertrophy by losartan compared with atenolol. The losartan intervention for endpoint reduction in hypertension (LIFE) trial. [Comment]. *Circulation* 2005;111:e377.

Rosen BD, Edvardsen T, Lai S, et al. Left ventricular concentric remodeling is associated with decreased global and regional systolic function: the multi-ethnic study of atherosclerosis. *Circulation* 2005;112:981–984.

Wang TJ, Evans JC, Benjamin EJ, et al. Natural history of asymptomatic left ventricular systolic dysfunction in the community. *Circulation* 2003;108:977–982.

Wong CY, O'Moore-Sullivan T, Leano R, et al. Alterations of left ventricular myocardial characteristics associated with obesity. *Circulation* 2004;110:3081–3087.

Yusuf S, Pfeffer MA, Swedberg K, et al. Effects of candesartan in patients with chronic heart failure and preserved left-ventricular ejection fraction: the CHARM-Preserved Trial. *Lancet* 2003;362:777–781.

CHAPTER A61 ■ MECHANISMS OF VASCULAR REMODELING

GARY L. BAUMBACH, MD

KEY POINTS

■ The term *vascular remodeling* describes a variety of changes in vascular dimensions and composition, including hypertrophy.
■ Hypertrophic inward remodeling describes a decrease in lumen diameter associated with an increase in vessel wall material that is more dependent on increased pulse pressure than mean pressure.
■ Eutrophic inward remodeling describes a decrease in lumen diameter without an accompanying change in the composition or amount of vessel wall material.
■ Many of the factors that play a role in hypertrophy of cerebral arterioles (such as arterial pulse pressure, sympathetic nerves, and endothelial factors) do not appear to contribute to eutrophic remodeling.
■ Hypertrophic remodeling involves cell division and enlargement, whereas eutrophic remodeling involves cell migration and rearrangement. Integrins and oxidative stress are probably involved in remodeling.

See also Chapters A28 and A62

Mechanisms and terminology

Study of the alterations in vascular structure that occur during chronic hypertension has been ongoing for approximately two centuries. These structural changes can be characterized by several different parameters.

Wall to lumen ratio. A common approach to the study of arterial wall pathophysiology has been to measure the wall to lumen (W/L) ratio. The W/L ratio, however, describes both functional and structural change because a vessel that dilates acutely exhibits an increase in lumen diameter and a slight attenuation of wall thickness that leads to a marked decrease in W/L ratio. The opposite pattern accompanies physiologic vasoconstriction. Therefore, the W/L ratio by itself cannot reliably describe chronic structural changes in peripheral vessels; other concepts and terminology are required.

Definitions of hypertrophy and remodeling. *Hypertrophy* of the vessel wall was thought to be the primary structural change underlying altered vascular responses in chronic hypertension until the 1980s, when the concept of remodeling was introduced. *Remodeling* was initially defined as a reduction in arteriolar diameter during chronic hypertension that could not be attributed to altered distensibility. It soon became apparent, however, that a further refinement in terminology was needed because the term *remodeling* has been used in a more general sense to describe nonspecific changes in vascular structure, including hypertrophy of the vessel wall. Consequently, appropriate modifiers have been added to more precisely define the meaning of

remodeling. *Eutrophic inward remodeling* refers to a decrease in lumen diameter without a change in the thickness of the arterial wall or the characteristics of the material within the vessel wall. In contrast, *hypertrophic inward remodeling* is defined as a decrease in lumen diameter associated with an increase in wall thickness and vessel wall material. In the context of this review, *hypertrophy* refers to hypertrophic inward remodeling and *remodeling* refers to eutrophic inward remodeling (**Figure A61.1**).

Mechanisms of hypertrophy

Intravascular pressure. Pharmacologic studies using responses to BP-lowering drugs have inherent limitations in the study of vascular pathology, not only because the drugs cause physiologic changes in vascular dimensions but also because they often affect hormones and other potential determinants of vascular hypertrophy. An approach that avoids the limitations of antihypertensive drugs is to reduce arterial pressure locally by ligation of upstream vessels. After arterial ligation, neurohumoral factors are similar in blood vessels downstream from the ligation and in control vessels. On the basis of arterial ligation studies, increases in arterial pressure during chronic hypertension contribute directly to vascular hypertrophy. An unanticipated outcome of these studies is the finding that hypertrophy depends more on pulse pressure than mean pressure, systolic pressure, or wall tension. This conclusion is supported by the finding that cyclic stretching increases DNA synthesis and rate of growth of cultured vascular smooth muscle cells.

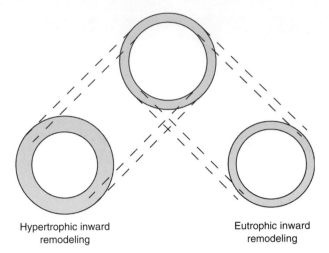

Hypertrophic inward
remodeling

Eutrophic inward
remodeling

Figure A61.1 Hypertrophic and eutrophic inward remodeling of small resistance arteries and arterioles. *Inward remodeling* refers to a structural reduction in the vascular lumen. When lumen reduction is due to encroachment on the lumen by an increase in vessel wall mass (i.e., hypertrophy), it is referred to as *hypertrophic inward remodeling*. When, on the other hand, lumen reduction is owing to an overall decrease in vessel caliber (i.e., reduced external diameter) without an increase in wall mass, it is referred to as *eutrophic inward remodeling*.

Sympathetic nerves. Sympathetic nerves play an important role in the development of cerebral vascular hypertrophy during chronic hypertension. W/L ratio and cross-sectional areas of the vessel walls in cerebral arterioles of spontaneously hypertensive stroke-prone rats (SHRSP) can also be reduced by sympathetic denervation. Denervation reduces the content of all components in the arteriolar wall (smooth muscle, elastin, collagen, basement membrane, and endothelium) but its effect is greatest on smooth muscle. Sympathetic denervation also reduces, rather than increases, the external diameters of cerebral arterioles in SHRSP. Therefore, in contrast to their contribution to vascular hypertrophy, sympathetic nerves do not appear to contribute to cerebral vascular remodeling during chronic hypertension.

Angiotensin II. In cultured vascular smooth muscle cells, angiotensin II (Ang II) stimulates hyperplasia and hypertrophy. In experimental Goldblatt hypertension in rats, hypertrophy of cremaster muscle arterioles is attenuated by doses of an angiotensin-converting enzyme (ACE) inhibitor that do not reduce arterial pressure. Therefore, vascular hypertrophy may be stimulated by Ang II independent of its pressor effect. This hypothesis, however, is not without controversy because there is evidence that ACE inhibitor effects on vascular structure also depend on their effects on blood pressure (BP).

Genetic factors. A genetic predisposition to increased sympathetic nerve activity and hypertrophy of peripheral resistance vessels may exist. Increases in W/L ratio in mesenteric arteries, increases in tissue norepinephrine, and elevated hind limb minimal resistance all precede development of hypertension in spontaneously hypertensive rats (SHR). Therefore, genetic factors may influence development of vascular hypertrophy in chronic hypertension. On the other hand, vascular hypertrophy has been found in a variety of models of secondary hypertension, which suggests that genetic factors are not required for the development of hypertrophy.

Endothelin-1. Studies relating endothelin-1 (ET-1) to alterations in vascular structure in chronic hypertension have yielded conflicting results. Treatment of SHR with the dual endothelin

antagonist bosentan does not inhibit hypertrophy in small mesenteric, coronary, renal, or femoral arteries. In contrast, bosentan prevents hypertrophy in cerebral arterioles of SHRSP. Several factors may account for these different findings. First, ET-1 may contribute to hypertrophy of cerebral vessels but not other vessels. Second, the contribution of ET-1 to vascular hypertrophy may vary with vessel size. Third, ET-1 may contribute to hypertrophy only when arterial pressure increases above a critical threshold. This possibility is suggested by observations that arterial pressure is somewhat higher in SHRSP than in SHR and by the related observation that the ET-1 blocker bosentan lowers arterial pressure in SHRSP but not in SHR.

Nitric oxide. Nitric oxide (NO) suppresses mitogenesis and proliferation of vascular smooth muscle cells in tissue culture. Yet inhibition of nitric oxide synthase (NOS) has no effect on serum-stimulated DNA synthesis in organ cultures of carotid and renal arteries. Hypertension in Sprague-Dawley rats induced by administration of L-nitroarginine methyl ester (L-NAME), an inhibitor of NOS, results in hypertrophy of cerebral arterioles that is not prevented by carotid ligation. Therefore, NO deficiency may be a determinant of cerebral vascular hypertrophy during chronic hypertension. Alternative interpretations include indirect effects of NOS inhibition such as altered production of endothelin or increased activity of the renin-angiotensin system.

Oxidative stress. Evidence of increased superoxide (O_2^-) production in hypertension has been obtained from indirect measurements (e.g., reduction of nitroblue tetrazolium) in animals infused with vasoconstrictors. Interestingly, endothelium-dependent vasorelaxation was found to be markedly impaired at the same time. These observations have led to the suggestion that O_2^- may play a key role in pathologic changes of vascular reactivity induced by hypertension. Consistent with this hypothesis, superoxide dismutase prevents vascular damage and increases survival in hypertensive rats. A mechanism by which oxidative stress may influence vascular growth is by reducing availability of NO in the vessel wall, which would be expected to blunt NO-dependent growth inhibition in cultured vascular smooth muscle cells. The bioactivity of NO depends, in part, on its interaction with reactive oxygen species, particularly O_2^-.

Because O_2^- inactivates NO *in vivo*, it has been suggested that inactivation of NO by O_2^- contributes to impaired vascular function under several pathophysiologic conditions. Oxidative stress during chronic hypertension may contribute to hypertrophy by inactivating NO and thereby diminishing its growth inhibitory influence (**Figure A61.2**). O_2^- may also contribute to vascular growth through alterations in cell signaling. Hydrogen peroxide in particular has been shown to mediate Ang II-induced activation of epidermal growth factor–receptors, p38 mitogen-activated protein kinase, and protein kinase β. In addition, exposure of vascular smooth muscle cells to hydrogen peroxide results in increased cell volume and intracellular incorporation of amino acids. Furthermore, inhibition of hydrogen peroxide by overexpression of human catalase inhibits vascular smooth muscle proliferation.

Mechanisms of remodeling

Intravascular pressure. Antihypertensive treatment with hydralazine or carotid ligation normalizes l arteriolar pulse pressure in cerebral arterioles of SHRSP, but neither treatment prevents arteriolar remodeling. Importantly, both treatments fail to normalize cerebral arteriolar mean pressure in SHRSP. Therefore,

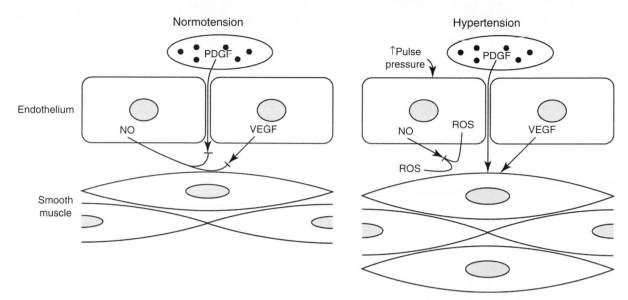

Figure A61.2 Possible roles of reactive oxygen species and nitric oxide (NO) in development of vascular hypertrophy in response to increases in arterial pulse pressure during chronic hypertension. Under normotensive conditions, NO may prevent hypertrophy by inhibiting trophic responses of vascular muscle to growth promoters, such as platelet-derived growth factor (PDGF) and vascular endothelial growth factor (VEGF). Chronic hypertension increases oxidative stress in the vessel wall. Reactive oxygen species (ROS), and in particular superoxide, react with NO to yield peroxynitrite ($ONOO^-$), thereby reducing levels of available NO. Reduced levels of NO may contribute to hypertrophy owing to removal of its growth inhibitory influence. In addition to an indirect role through inactivation of NO, recent evidence now points to a more direct role for superoxide in the development of hypertrophy.

although pulse pressure can be excluded as a mechanism of cerebral vascular remodeling, a role for mean pressure cannot be ruled out.

Angiotensin II. Treatment with an ACE inhibitor or a selective AT_1-receptor antagonist, but not hydralazine, attenuates remodeling of cerebral arterioles in SHRSP. Therefore, in contrast to increased sympathetic nerve activity or pulse pressure, Ang II may be a determinant of cerebral vascular remodeling and hypertrophy during chronic hypertension. Several provocative concepts have recently emerged that may lead to a greater understanding of mechanisms through which the renin-angiotensin system promotes eutrophic remodeling. First, a large body of recently accumulated evidence suggests that reactive oxygen species, such as O_2^- and hydrogen peroxide, may play an important role in alterations of vascular structure induced by Ang II. Second, numerous investigations suggest that Ang II may alter vascular structure through transactivation of receptor tyrosine kinases by Ang II type 1 (AT_1) receptors. Third, the peroxisome proliferator activated receptor, PPARγ, may exert protective effects in the vessel wall by preventing Ang II-induced alterations in vascular structure.

Genetic factors. In contrast to the questionable role of genetic factors in the development of vascular hypertrophy, two lines of evidence suggest that there are genetic factors that contribute to vascular remodeling in chronic hypertension. First, remodeling occurs in several types of genetic hypertension, including SHR, SHRSP, and Dahl salt sensitive (S/JR) hypertensive rats. Remodeling rather than medial hypertrophy is responsible for reductions in lumen diameter and increases in media to lumen ratio that occur in renal afferent arterioles in SHR and small subcutaneous arteries from human essential hypertensives. The second line of evidence is that vascular remodeling has not been observed in models of secondary hypertension such as renal

hypertension or hypertension secondary to inhibition of NO synthesis. Therefore, remodeling does not appear to be secondary to hypertension *per se* and may involve genetic factors.

Endothelin. ET-1 influences eutrophic remodeling in small mesenteric arteries in deoxycorticosterone acetate–salt hypertensive rats. However, treatment with bosentan has no effect on remodeling of cerebral arterioles, suggesting that ET-1 probably does not contribute to remodeling of cerebral arterioles in SHRSP.

Nitric oxide and eutrophic outward remodeling. Treatment of Sprague-Dawley rats with L-NAME does not result in a reduction of external diameter in cerebral arterioles; rather, it results in an increase in external diameter. In other words, treatment with L-NAME produces eutrophic outward remodeling in cerebral arterioles rather than inward remodeling. This finding suggests that reductions in NO availability do not play a role in eutrophic inward remodeling of resistance arteries during chronic hypertension.

Integrins. Eutrophic inward remodeling of small mesenteric arteries in TGR (mRen2)27 rats (transgenic rats harboring the human renin and angiotensinogen genes) is associated with an increase in αvβ3 integrins. Administration of an αvβ3 peptide antagonist prevents arterial remodeling in TGR (mRen2)27 rats. These findings suggest an important role for αvβ3 integrins in eutrophic inward remodeling.

Suggested Readings

Baumbach GL, Didion SP, Faraci FM. Structure of cerebral arterioles in mice deficient in expression of the gene for CuZn superoxide dismutase. *Stroke* 2006;37:1850–1855.

Baumbach GL, Heistad DD. Remodeling of cerebral arterioles in chronic hypertension. *Hypertension* 1989;13:968–972.

Folkow B. Physiological aspects of primary hypertension. *Physiol Rev* 1982;62: 347–504.

Heerkens EH, Izzard AS, Heagerty AM. Integrins, vascular remodeling, and hypertension. *Hypertension* 2007;49:1–4.

Intengan HD. Vascular remodeling in hypertension: roles of apoptosis, inflammation, and fibrosis. *Hypertension* 2001;38:581–587.

Lassegue B, Griendling KK. Reactive oxygen species in hypertension; an update. *Am J Hypertens* 2004;17:852–860.

Mulvany MJ, Baumbach GL, Aalkjaer C, et al. Vascular remodeling. [See Comments]. *Hypertension* 1996;28:505–506.

Schiffrin EL. Peroxisome proliferator-activated receptors and cardiovascular remodeling. *Am J Physiol* 2005;288:H1037–H1043.

Ungvari Z, Wolin MS, Csiszar A. Mechanosensitive production of reactive oxygen species in endothelial and smooth muscle cells: role in microvascular remodeling? *Antioxid Redox Signal* 2006;8:1121–1129.

CHAPTER A62 ■ MICROVASCULAR REGULATION AND DYSREGULATION

ANDREW S. GREENE, PhD

KEY POINTS

■ Microvascular abnormalities in hypertension are functional (increased vascular sensitivity and constriction) and structural (increased vessel wall thickness and loss of capillaries, rarefaction).

■ Microcirculatory rarefaction is associated with metabolic abnormalities such as insulin resistance and altered organ function.

■ Long-term normalization of blood pressure (BP), especially with renin-angiotensin blocking drugs, ameliorates arteriolar hypertrophy.

See also Chapters A41, A42, A44, and A61

The microcirculation is involved in the genesis and maintenance of hypertension and plays a major role in many of the functional changes observed in hypertensive individuals. Because the microcirculation provides the vast majority of systemic resistance to flow, as well as virtually all of the oxygen and nutrient exchange, changes in microcirculatory function and structure are of great interest in the syndrome of hypertension and its target organ consequences (**Figure A62.1**).

Basic microcirculatory structure and function

The microcirculation begins with small arteries/arterioles (internal diameter <0.5 mm) and also involves the capillary-venous plexus (**Figure A62.2**). Under physiologic conditions, most of the resistance to flow is generated in arterioles with internal diameters of 0.1 to 0.3 mm. There are two major subdivisions within the microcirculation: metarterioles, or bypass channels (30–100 μ) and true or "nutritive" capillaries (<10 μ in diameter) that cross-link with each other and connect arterioles with venules. White cells, by virtue of their size cannot enter true capillaries; instead they must flow through the metarteriolar arches (that are always "open") to return to the heart.

Precapillary "sphincters" at entrances to the capillary bed are located at right angles to the arteriolar/metarteriolar vessels;

these smooth muscle fascicles are the principal sites of action of vasoconstrictors such as norepinephrine or angiotensin II. The anatomic characteristics of these different microcirculatory vessel types, which differ with the organ and its functional need, are rarely considered when terms such as *systemic vascular resistance* are discussed. In clinical extremes such as endotoxic shock, metarteriolar bypass channels may be widely patent, whereas true capillary flow is virtually abolished. Conversely, increased total organ blood flow does not necessarily mean that true capillary flow is equivalently increased.

Microcirculatory structural changes in hypertension

Blood pressure and remodeling. In response to a chronic elevation in blood pressure (BP), there is dramatic remodeling of the microcirculatory architecture, including the vascular connections and the blood vessels themselves. Increased growth of the media of arterioles, owing primarily to vascular smooth muscle hypertrophy (rather than hyperplasia), results in an increased wall to lumen ratio. When the muscular wall is hypertrophic, peripheral resistance tends to increase because thicker-walled vessels tend to have reduced luminal diameters, especially during neurogenic or humoral vasoconstriction. Medial hypertrophy is

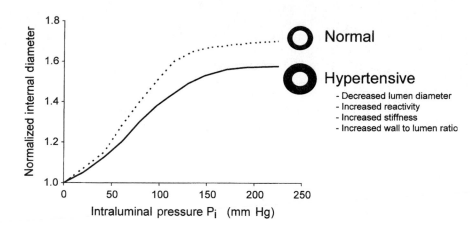

Figure A62.1 Hypertension results in thickening of vascular wall, which shifts pressure-diameter relationship of arterioles in such a way that internal diameter is reduced. This hypertrophic response to increased pressure results in decreased lumen diameter, increased vascular reactivity, and decreased compliance. Recent studies suggest that only through aggressive long-term normalization of blood pressure can these structural changes be reversed. P_i, intraluminal pressure.

thought to develop as a response to increased flow velocity and shear stress: This mechanical signal is transduced by intracellular kinases and allows for arteriolar remodeling. In this capacity, the hypertrophic response acts to normalize shear stress in arterioles. Increased shear forces in the microcirculation appear to be vasodilatory and angiogenic and may serve to protect endothelial cells from cytokine stimuli. In normal situations, neoformation of capillaries restores normal shear forces. In prehypertension and hypertension, reverse angiogenesis of small arterioles and capillaries (rarefaction) may occur.

Rarefaction. Rarefaction, resulting in a vessel loss of up to 50% of microvessels, may be due either to hemodynamic factors or to the action(s) or depletion of locally acting trophic or growth factors such as angiotensin II, insulin, vascular endothelial growth factor (VEGF), fibroblast growth factor, transforming growth factor-β, platelet-derived growth factor, or others. Ultimately, rarefaction in chronic hypertension is thought to be mediated through degenerative changes in microvessels, such as atrophy of vascular smooth muscle cells (VSMCs) and attenuation of the endothelium through apoptosis. Some evidence exists that microcirculatory rarefaction precedes the development

of chronic hypertension in certain vascular beds and therefore may play a role in causality.

Cellular changes. In addition to the postgrowth remodeling of established microvascular networks, a series of other morphologic abnormalities can be seen. VSMCs may be retracted or atrophic with extensive rough endoplasmic reticulum and other organelles, suggesting transformation of some VSMCs toward a secretory phenotype. Vessels undergoing hypertrophy have an increased number of polyploid VSMCs. Endothelial cells may be attenuated, separated from VSMCs, or detached from their basement membrane, whereas pericytes are frequently absent from capillaries. These changes in endothelial cell morphology may impact dramatically on the permeability of the microvasculature, resulting in alterations in the transport of metabolites, interstitial matrix injury, and end-organ damage. Thrombi, neutrophils, and prephagocytic cells may also be present in the microcirculatory vessels during the early stages of some experimental forms of hypertension. Interestingly, many degenerative structural changes associated with arteriolar rarefaction are similar to those that occur during ischemic injury; however, no inflammatory phagocytic response is observed during the development of hypertension compared with such a response that is normally seen with ischemic injury. Stimuli associated with microvascular rarefaction increase the appearance of apoptotic endothelial cells.

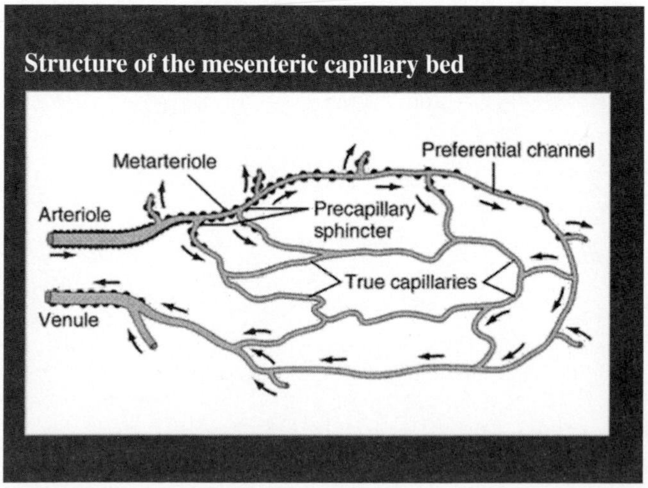

Functional consequences of microcirculatory damage

Functional impact of structural changes. Functional abnormalities of the microcirculatory vessels arise in part from anatomic changes. Microvascular compliance and capacity are reduced because of an increased collagen to elastin ratio in microvessels as well as a reduced number of vessels. Increased myogenic tone, which contributes to reduced capacity, is due in part to vascular wall hypertrophy.

Role of the autonomic system. Damage to the blood–brain barrier, which occurs primarily in capillaries and small venules (rather than on the arterial side), may be linked to increases in central sympathetic drive. In addition to increased autoregulatory tone, microvascular diameters may also be decreased because of elevated sympathetic nerve activity. Although much of the evidence for participation of a neural component in high systemic resistance has been obtained by indirect approaches such as neural ablation, experimental evidence suggests that a primary genetic abnormality may exist in control of the peripheral sympathetic outflow, resulting in increased sympathetic drive in many

Figure A62.2 Idealized view of the microcirculation showing the sites of preferential pathways and precapillary sphincters. Sites of active constriction by smooth muscle are indicated. Reproduced with permission from Textbook of Medical Physiology by Arthur Guyton and John Hall, 11th ed. WB Saunders, Philadelphia, 2006.

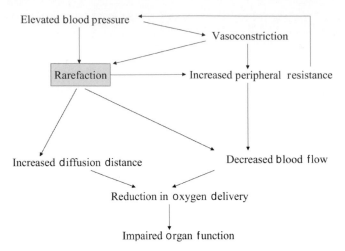

Figure A62.3 Elevated blood pressure and associated neuroendocrine changes cause vasoconstriction and a reduction in microvessel density, both of which increase peripheral resistance and decrease tissue blood flow. Rarefaction further compounds this decreased perfusion by increasing diffusion distance and further reducing oxygen delivery, resulting in impaired organ function.

forms of hypertension. Increased levels of adrenergic stimulation and of circulating pressor hormones contribute to increased peripheral resistance during the development of essential hypertension.

Other changes. Abnormal responses to constrictor and dilator stimuli are exacerbated by impairment in endothelial function. Permeability of capillaries is increased throughout the body, with a resulting redistribution of protein and water from plasma to the interstitial space. Changes in the population of hormone receptors on VSMCs and endothelial cells can augment the constrictor and hypertrophic effects of endocrine, paracrine, and autocrine factors. In addition to the enhanced sensitivity to vasoconstrictor agents, the arterioles of hypertensive individuals appear to be more sensitive to increased levels of oxygen and less responsive to vasodilatory stimuli, including hypoxia, than those of normotensive control subjects. The enhanced constriction of arterioles in response to increased oxygen availability may indicate heightened autoregulatory responsiveness, whereby small increases in total blood volume or decreases in vascular compliance could result in chronic elevation of systemic resistance **(Figure A62.3)**.

Suggested Readings

Cannon RO III. The heart in hypertension: thinking small. *Am J Hypertens* 1996;9:406–408.

Draaijer P, Le Noble JL, Leunissen KM, et al. The microcirculation and essential hypertension. *Neth J Med* 1991;39:158–169.

Drexler H. Endothelial dysfunction: clinical implications. *Prog Cardiovasc Dis* 1997;39:287–324.

Hutchins PM, Lynch CD, Cooney PT, et al. The microcirculation in experimental hypertension and aging. *Cardiovasc Res* 1996;32:772–780.

Kobayashi N, DeLano FA, Schmid-Schonbein GW. Oxidative stress promotes endothelial cell apoptosis and loss of microvessels in the spontaneously hypertensive rats. *Arterioscler Thromb Vasc Biol* 2005;25(10):2114–2121.

Petersen MC, Munzenmaier DH, Greene AS. Angiotensin II infusion restores stimulated angiogenesis in the skeletal muscle of rats on a high-salt diet. *Am J Physiol Heart Circ Physiol* 2006;291(1):H114–H120.

Rieder MJ, Roman RJ, Greene AS. Reversal of microvascular rarefaction and reduced renal mass hypertension. *Hypertension* 1997;30:120–127.

de Resende MM, Amaral SL, Munzenmaier DH, et al. Role of endothelial cell apoptosis in regulation of skeletal muscle angiogenesis during high and low salt intake. *Physiol Genomics* 2006;25(2):325–335.

Schiffrin EL. The endothelium of resistance arteries: physiology and role in hypertension. *Prostaglandins Leukot Essent Fatty Acids* 1996;54:17–25.

Sullivan JM, Prewitt RL, Josephs JA. Attenuation of the microcirculation in young patients with high-output borderline hypertension. *Hypertension* 1983;5:844–851.

CHAPTER A63 ■ OXIDATIVE STRESS AND HYPERTENSION

DAVID G. HARRISON, MD AND KATHY K. GRIENDLING, PhD

KEY POINTS

■ Reactive oxygen species (ROS), produced as a by-product of numerous cellular metabolic pathways, influences normal and abnormal cellular processes including cellular growth and hypertrophy, inflammation, remodeling, lipid oxidation and modulation of vascular tone.

■ Increased vascular production of superoxide ($O_2^{\cdot-}$) in various diseases modulates the bioactivity of nitric oxide (NO).

■ Vascular nicotinamide adenine dinucleotide (NAD)(P)H oxidases produce ROS; expression and activity of these enzyme systems are modulated by a variety of pathophysiologic stimuli.

■ Production of $O_2^{\cdot-}$ by NAD(P)H oxidases may mediate angiotensin (Ang) II-dependent hypertension through mechanisms involving the central nervous system (CNS), the vasculature and the kidney; ROS produced by nicotinamide adenine dinucleotide phosphate (NADPH) oxidases can further promote oxidative stress by activation of other oxidative enzymes and impairing antioxidant defenses.

■ ROS have been implicated in the pathogenesis of many human disorders including cancer, aging, dementia, and arthritis. In the cardiovascular system, there is substantial evidence to support a role for ROS in both hypertension and atherosclerosis.

See also Chapters **A9,** A25, and A64

Sources of reactive oxygen species

Reactive oxygen species (ROS) are produced by numerous enzymes that donate electrons to reduce oxygen and include the superoxide anion ($O_2^{\cdot-}$), hydrogen peroxide (H_2O_2), hypochlorous acid (HOCL), the hydroxyl radical (OH), reactive aldehydes, lipid peroxides, lipid radicals, and nitrogen oxides (**Figure A63.1**). Several ROS, including $O_2^{\cdot-}$, OH$^\cdot$, and nitric oxide (NO), are radicals with unpaired electrons in their outer orbitals. Others such as H_2O_2 and HOCl are biologically active oxidants but are not radicals. Sources of ROS include mitochondrial electron transport, xanthine oxidase, cyclooxygenase, lipoxygenase, nitric oxide synthase (NOS), heme oxygenase, peroxidases, and nicotinamide adenine dinucleotide phosphate (NADPH) oxidase. In phagocytes, such as neutrophils and macrophages, NADPH oxidases can produce very large cytotoxic amounts of radicals in bursts. A major source of ROS in blood vessels is a membrane-associated NADPH oxidase expressed by endothelial cells, vascular smooth muscle cells (VSMCs) and fibroblasts that bears some similarity to phagocytic oxidase.

Oxidative stress

The term *oxidative stress* was first employed to refer to a condition in which there is an imbalance between the cellular levels of oxidants and antioxidants. The production of ROS can be very localized (e.g., at the cell membrane, within the nucleus or mitochondria); these local concentrations might be functionally important and yet not greatly affect the overall cellular level of oxidants. Moreover, it has become clear that disorders of electron transfer (through enzymes such as NOS, prostaglandin synthases, or the mitochondrial electron transport system) affect cell function by increasing ROS generation; increased ROS also alter enzyme function.

Vascular effects of reactive oxygen species

Normal cell function. ROS can be cytotoxic but also serve important signaling roles and affect proteins in ways that are crucial for normal function and survival. Growth of vascular smooth muscle is stimulated by H_2O_2, a process that is dependent on the expression and binding of the transcription factors c-Fos and c-Jun. More importantly, hormone- and growth factor-stimulated proliferation and hypertrophy are mediated by and require intracellular H_2O_2. There are multiple molecular targets of ROS that mediate growth responses, including Ras, calcium calmodulin kinase II, c-Src, Akt, p38 mitogen-activated protein kinase, and protein tyrosine phosphatases. Recently, efforts have been made to create mice that lack p22^{phox}, a crucial docking

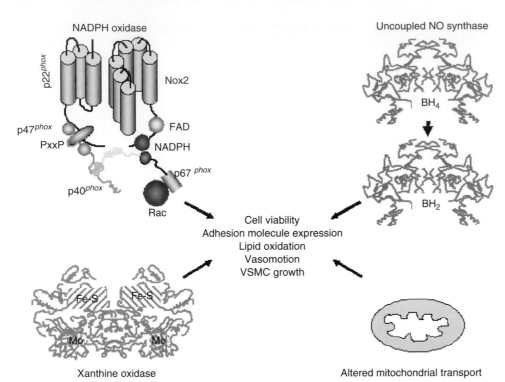

Figure A63.1 ROS in the vessel wall. Increased production of oxidants may alter vasomotor tone, gene expression, inflammatory responses, and remodeling through the mechanisms depicted, thereby contributing to hypertension and atherosclerosis. ROS are generated by Nox enzymes (illustrated here as the NADPH oxidase Nox2), uncoupled nitric oxide synthase, altered mitochondrial electron transport, and xanthine oxidase. There is interplay between these enzymes and ROS produced by one can activate others. NADPH, nicotinamide adenine dinucleotide phosphate; FAD, flavin-adenine dinucleotide; PxxP, proline rich domain of a Src homology region; NO, nitrix oxide; BH4, tetrahydrobiopterin; BH2, dihydrobiopterin; VSMC, vascular smooth muscle cell.

subunit for all of the mouse NADPH oxidases. This knockout proved to be embryonically lethal, demonstrating the critical role of these enzymes and their products in development.

Regulation of gene expression. ROS modulate gene expression, including expression of proinflammatory molecules such as vascular cell adhesion molecule-1 and monocyte chemotactic protein-1, which are critical in atherosclerosis lesion development. An important mediator is the transcription factor nuclear factor-κB, which exists in the cytoplasm as a heterotrimer and is stimulated by ROS through dissociation of an inhibitory subunit (IkB) from a p50–p65 complex that translocates to the nucleus to mediate gene transcription. ROS also modulate gene expression through transcription factors binding to activating protein 1 (AP-1), stimulatory protein 1 (SP-1), antioxidant response elements, and other *cis*-acting elements.

Modulation of extracellular matrix. A critical component of both vascular growth and remodeling is degradation and resynthesis of extracellular matrix. Specialized enzymes known as *matrix metalloproteinases* (MMPs) mediate the degradation and remodeling process. Several MMPs, including MMP-2 and MMP-9, involved in degradation of basement membrane and elastin respectively, are converted from inactive zymogens to their active form by ROS-mediated oxidation at a cysteine residue in the inhibitory domain. This process appears to cause matrix degradation in regions of vessels exposed to high levels of oxidant stress, such as the shoulder regions of vulnerable plaques.

Oxidation of lipoproteins. Under normal circumstances, native low-density lipoprotein (LDL) cycles in and out of the vessel wall; its uptake may be enhanced under certain conditions. Changes in the oxidative environment in the vessel wall favor oxidation of LDL particles and promote an inflammatory response, in part by acting on Toll-like receptors. Extensive oxidation of LDL leads to formation of oxLDL, which is no longer recognized by the LDL receptor but is avidly taken up by scavenger receptors. Oxidation of LDL leads to formation

of several biologically active molecules. For example, oxLDL contains phospholipase A2-like enzymatic activity, and within the LDL particle, active conversion of phosphatidylcholine to lysophosphatidylcholine causes numerous untoward biological effects on the endothelium. Linoleic acid and other fatty acids are oxidized to their respective hydroperoxides, which participate in radical chain reactions, resulting in transfer of electrons to other molecules and the formation of additional radicals.

Modulation of the biological activity of nitric oxide. Of particular importance to the subject of hypertension and vascular biology is the interaction between $O_2{}^{.-}$ and NO.

Radical interactions. Because $O_2{}^{.-}$ and NO radicals contain highly reactive unpaired electrons in their outer orbitals, they undergo a nonenzymatic, diffusion-limited, radical–radical reaction with extremely high reaction rates—10,000 to 100,000 times faster the reactions between $O_2{}^{.-}$ and the available antioxidants (e.g., vitamins A, E, and C). Given this stoichiometry, it is not at all surprising clinical trials of antioxidants have been completely unsuccessful in lowering cardiovascular disease rates.

Peroxynitrite. A major product of the spontaneous reaction of NO and $O_2{}^{.-}$ is peroxynitrite anion ($OONO^-$). Peroxynitrite is a weaker vasodilator than NO, so this reaction leads to less net vasodilation. Likewise, many of the other beneficial effects of NO [e.g., inhibition of platelet aggregation, prevention of smooth muscle cell growth, reduction of vascular cell adhesion molecule (VCAM)-1 expression] are lost when NO is oxidized by $O_2{}^{.-}$. The rapidity of the reactions between $O_2{}^{.-}$ and NO and between $O_2{}^{.-}$ and superoxide dismutases (SODs) suggest that in compartments where these three entities coexist, their interactions could markedly alter levels of NO. Indeed, this seems to be the case; in the normal vessel, the balance between NO and $O_2{}^{.-}$ favors the net production of NO, which counteracts the opposing vasoconstrictive forces.

Endothelial function. The critical balance between NO and $O_2{}^{.-}$ is altered in the setting of numerous common disease states including atherosclerosis, hypertension, diabetes, and in conditions such as cigarette smoking and aging. In all of these conditions, increased vascular levels of $O_2{}^{-}$ lead to impaired endothelium-dependent vascular relaxation. Treatment of isolated vessel preparations or intact animals with membrane-targeted forms of SOD markedly improves endothelium-dependent vascular relaxations. Likewise, infusions of high amounts of antioxidant vitamins can improve endothelium-dependent vasodilation of forearm vessels in human diabetics or cigarette smokers. It is not possible to achieve adequately high concentrations of antioxidant vitamins with oral doses.

NADPH oxidases

Numerous cell types other than phagocytes possess NADPH oxidase-like enzyme systems with catalytic subunits (Nox proteins) that contain binding sites for NADPH, flavin-adenine dinucleotide (FAD), and heme. Electrons transferred from NADPH to FAD, and ultimately to heme, reduce oxygen to $O_2{}^{-}$ (**Figure 63.1**).

Nox proteins. Seven Nox proteins exist. Nox1 was first cloned from colon carcinoma cells, but can be induced in vascular cells by pathophysiologic stimuli. Nox2 is the previously identified gp91^{phox} of the phagocytic oxidase, but also exists in endothelial cells and adventitial fibroblasts. Nox3 is present in the inner ear and is responsible for development of otoconia, and thereby regulates balance. Nox4, first identified in the kidney, is highly expressed in all cells of the vessel wall. Nox5, not present in rodents, is a novel enzyme that contains calcium binding (EF-hand) domains, such that increases in intracellular Ca^{2+} stimulate $O_2{}^{-}$ production by these enzymes in endothelial cells and VSMC. The Duoxes are the most distantly related Nox homologs, and are important in thyroid function, but have not been found in the vasculature.

Vascular nox. Vascular Nox proteins differ from the phagocytic Nox2 in many respects. The phagocytic enzyme releases massive bursts of $O_2{}^{-}$, whereas vascular oxidases constitutively and continuously produce low levels of $O_2{}^{-}$. $O_2{}^{-}$ generated in VSMC appears to be mostly intracellular, with only a limited amount of $O_2{}^{-}$ released to the exterior of the cell. In endothelial cells, $O_2{}^{-}$ is released both intra- and extracellularly.

Nox localization and signaling differences. The various Nox enzymes also vary in their requirements for cytosolic subunits and in the manner in which they are signaled. An important difference is their subcellular distribution, which markedly affects the role of ROS produced by these enzymes. For example, Nox1 is present in caveolae, whereas Nox4 is present in focal adhesions, on stress fibers and is highly expressed in the nucleus. Nox4 seems to play a role in cell differentiation whereas Nox1 is important and cell growth and migration. Nox2, which has a perinuclear distribution in endothelial cells, regulates gene expression and NO bioavailability. Endothelial Nox enzymes have also been implicated in host defenses against infection.

Physiologic stimulation. A particularly important aspect of the NADPH oxidases is that pathophysiologic stimuli, including angiotensin (Ang) II, cytokines and physical forces, increase NADPH activity and over the long-term, stimulate subunit messenger RNA (mRNA) and protein expression. A number of commonly employed drugs inhibit NADPH oxidases, likely contributing to their beneficial effects. Because Ang II activates these enzymes, both angiotensin-converting enzyme (ACE) inhibitors and Ang II receptor antagonists lower $O_2{}^{-}$

in experimental models of diseases such as hypercholesterolemia, diabetes, and hypertension. Likewise, the HMG–CoA reductase inhibitors inhibit activation of the small G protein rac-1 by preventing production of the isoprenoid geranyl–geranyl pyrophosphate, crucial for rac-1 membrane association.

Nitric oxide synthase uncoupling and tetrahydrobiopterin. NOSs produce large amounts of $O_2{}^{-}$ when deprived of their critical cofactor, tetrahydrobiopterin, or their substrate, L-arginine. In this state of "NOS uncoupling", electron flow through the enzyme results in reduction of molecular oxygen (to $O_2{}^{-}$ at the prosthetic heme site rather than formation of NO.

Recent evidence suggests that NOS uncoupling occurs in several models of hypertension. In aortas of mice with deoxycorticosterone acetate (DOCA)-salt hypertension, $O_2{}^{-}$ production by NOS is markedly increased and tetrahydrobiopterin oxidation is evident. In this setting, there is increased ROS production from NADPH oxidase, leading to oxidation of tetrahydrobiopterin and uncoupling of endothelial nitric oxide synthase (eNOS). Treatment with oral tetrahydrobiopterin reduces vascular $O_2{}^{-}$ levels, increases NO production, and blunts the increase in blood pressure (BP). There is also evidence of eNOS uncoupling in Ang II-induced hypertension, insulin resistance, Dahl salt-sensitive rats, and in rats with reduced renal mass. These studies suggest that therapeutic increases in tetrahydrobiopterin or prevention of its oxidation may lower BP.

Other effects. $O_2{}^{-}$ and other ROS can affect vascular reactivity independent of NO. In vascular smooth muscle, ROS increase intracellular calcium by blocking calcium reuptake by the sarcoplasmic reticulum. Oxidation of membrane fatty acids and in particular arachidonate can lead to formation of 8-isoprostanoids, which are present the blood of humans in whom oxidative stress is increased (e.g., patients with hypercholesterolemia, diabetics, and cigarette smokers). These oxidatively modified fatty acids act on prostaglandin H/thromboxane receptors to enhance vasoconstriction.

NADPH oxidase and hypertension

Animal models. A role of ROS in the pathogenesis of chronic hypertension is supported by a variety of animal studies. Nakazono et al. initially showed that bolus administration of a heparin binding form of SOD acutely lowered BP in hypertensive rats. Membrane-targeted forms of SOD blunt Ang II-induced hypertension. The SOD-mimetic tempol lowers BP and decreases renovascular resistance in hypertensive rats; it also lowers BP and improves acetylcholine-induced vasodilatation in rats with reduced renal mass hypertension. There is also ample evidence that NADPH oxidase is the major source of ROS. For example, Ang II-induced hypertension is substantially blunted in mice lacking p47^{phox} and also in rats treated with small interfering RNA (siRNA) against p22^{phox}.

At first glance, a compelling explanation for these findings is that increased $O_2{}^{-}$ production causes hypertension by rapid inactivation of NO, with reduced NO-mediated vasodilatation and increased systemic vascular resistance. This scenario has been supported by the fact that Ang II augments hypertension in mice with targeted overexpression of vascular smooth muscle NADPH oxidase.

Renal mechanisms. All NADPH oxidase subunits are present in the kidney and ROS can modulate renal function. There is upregulation of p47^{phox} and p67^{phox} in the kidneys of spontaneously hypertensive rats and chronic Ang II-infusion increases expression of Nox1 and p22^{phox} and decreases in expression of renal extracellular superoxide dismutase (ecSOD). Superoxide and reduced NO in tubular cells increase sodium reabsorption and alter tubuloglomerular feedback. In the renal medulla, NO produced by the tubular cells of the medullary thick ascending limb maintains medullary perfusion by dilating vasa recta and may be important in pressure-induced natriuresis; excess $O_2{}^{\cdot-}$ in the renal medulla could limit this antihypertensive mechanism.

Central nervous system mechanisms. In the brain, increased NADPH activity and ROS excess in the circumventricular organs and the nucleus tractus solitarius could affect sympathetic outflow. Inhibition of the NADPH oxidase in the circumventricular organs prevents hypertension. A renal-central nervous system (CNS) interaction is also likely; if activation of CNS oxidases promotes sympathetic outflow to vessels and the kidney, increased renal vasoconstriction may contribute to hypertension.

Fukui T, Ishizaka N, Rajagopalan S, et al. p22^{phox} mRNA expression and NADPH oxidase activity are increased in aortas from hypertensive rats. *Circ Res* 1997;80:45–51.

Griendling KK, Sorescu D, Lassegue B, et al. Modulation of protein kinase activity and gene expression by reactive oxygen species and their role in vascular physiology and pathophysiology. *Arterioscler Thromb Vasc Biol* 2000;20:2175–2183.

Halvey PJ, Watson WH, Hansen JM, et al. Compartmental oxidation of thiol-disulphide redox couples during epidermal growth factor signalling. *Biochem J* 2005;386:215–219.

Harrison, DG, Dikalov, S. Oxidative events in cell and vascular biology. In: Re R, DiPette D, Schiffrin E, et al. eds. *Molecular mechanisms in hypertension.* Abingdon, UK: Taylor & Francis Medical Books, 2006:297–320.

Irani K. Oxidant signaling in vascular cell growth, death, and survival: a review of the roles of reactive oxygen species in smooth muscle and endothelial cell mitogenic and apoptotic signaling. *Circ Res* 2000;87:179–183.

Laursen JB, Rajagopalan S, Galis Z, et al. Role of superoxide in angiotensin II-induced but not catecholamine-induced hypertension. *Circulation* 1997;95:588–593.

Madamanchi NR, Vendrov A, Runge MS. Oxidative stress and vascular disease. *Arterioscler Thromb Vasc Biol* 2005;25:29–38.

Mori T, Cowley AW Jr, Ito S. Molecular mechanisms and therapeutic strategies of chronic renal injury: physiological role of angiotensin II-induced oxidative stress in renal medulla. *J Pharmacol Sci* 2006;100:2–8.

Peterson JR, Sharma RV, Davisson RL. Reactive oxygen species in the neuropathogenesis of hypertension. *Curr Hypertens Rep* 2006;8:232–241.

Suggested Readings

Channon KM. Tetrahydrobiopterin: regulator of endothelial nitric oxide synthase in vascular disease. *Trends Cardiovasc Med* 2004;14:323–327.

CHAPTER A64 ■ ENDOTHELIAL FUNCTION AND CARDIOVASCULAR DISEASE

JULIAN P.J. HALCOX, MA, MD, FRCP AND ARSHED A. QUYYUMI, MD, FACC, FRCP

KEY POINTS

■ Endothelial dysfunction is a precursor of atherosclerotic vascular disease and future adverse cardiovascular events.
■ Risk factors for atherosclerosis and other novel risk factors contribute to endothelial dysfunction.
■ Improvement of endothelial dysfunction may improve cardiovascular risk.

See also Chapters A9, **A25,** A47, **A63, A65, B76,** C149, and C152

The endothelium

The vascular endothelium is the largest "organ" in the body, comprising >14,000 sq ft of surface area and weighing 2 to 3 kg. Vascular endothelial cells are extremely active and play a critical role in the regulation of blood vessel tone and cellular activity in the vascular wall. Endothelial cells modulate underlying blood vessel tone by secreting a variety of dilator and constrictor substances. Dilator substances include nitric oxide (NO), prostacyclin, endothelium-derived hyperpolarizing factor (EDHF), and carbon monoxide; constricting agents include endothelin, superoxide anions, vasoconstrictor prostanoids, and locally generated angiotensin II (Ang II) (**Figure A64.1**). In addition to their influence on vascular tone, these agents and other factors produced by the endothelium, may also modify platelet aggregation, thrombogenicity of the blood, vascular inflammation and oxidative stress, and more importantly, over

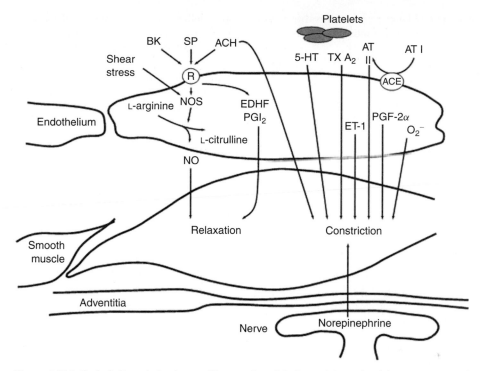

Figure A64.1 Endothelium-derived vasodilators. Acetylcholine (ACH), bradykinin (BK), and substance P (SP) stimulate endothelial cells to release vasodilator substances through activation of specific receptors on the endothelial cell surface. ACH binds to M_1 or M_3 muscarinic receptors, BK binds to B_2 kinin receptors, and SP binds to NK1 neurokinin receptors. Shear stress activates nitric oxide synthase (NOS), but does not release prostacyclin. Nitric oxide (NO) and prostacyclin also have inhibitory effects on platelet aggregation and adhesion. Endogenous vasoconstrictors. Angiotensin generated in circulating blood and by tissue-bound angiotensin-converting enzyme causes vasoconstriction through activation of smooth muscle AT_1 receptors. Endothelin vasoconstricts by activating ET_A and ET_B receptors on vascular smooth muscle. Platelet-derived serotonin and thromboxane A_2, and norepinephrine from sympathetic nerve terminals stimulate smooth muscles through 5-HT, TxA_2 and α_1 adrenergic receptors, respectively. AT I, angiotensin I; AT II, angiotensin II; EDHF, endothelium-derived hyperpolarizing factor; PGI_2, prostacyclin; PGF-2α, prostaglandin F-2α; R, receptor; ACE, angiotensin-converting enzyme; ET-1 = endothelin-1; 5-HT= 5-hydroxytryptamine (serotinin); TxA_2, thromboxane-A_2, O_2^-, superoxide ion.

the long-term, influence cell migration and proliferation with subsequent development and progression of atherosclerosis and its complications.

Endothelial function

Vasorelaxation. Furchgott and Zawadski first described the action of a labile substance secreted from endothelial cells and vasodilated rabbit aortic rings that was termed *endothelium-derived relaxing factor* (EDRF). EDRF was subsequently identified as NO, a diatomic molecule produced from L-arginine by the constitutive action of the enzyme endothelial nitric oxide synthase (eNOS). Under healthy conditions, tonically released NO modulates underlying cellular functions by diffusion into vascular smooth muscle cells (VSMCs), activation of G protein bound guanylyl cyclase, increasing intracellular cyclic guanosine monophosphate (cGMP) levels, and causes VSMC relaxation. NO inhibits platelet adhesion and, to a lesser extent, suppresses aggregation. In addition, NO modulates transcription of several genes that are involved in inflammatory processes in the vascular wall, including inhibition of P-selectin and monocyte chemoattractant protein 1 (MCP-1) gene expression, thereby suppressing inflammatory activity. Furthermore, endothelial NO attenuates

the generation of endothelin, a potent vasoconstrictor polypeptide which also possesses proinflammatory and proproliferative activity.

Thrombosis. NO diffuses from the endothelium toward the smooth muscle cell, and also into the lumen, where by stimulating platelet cGMP activity, it acts to prevent platelet aggregation and adhesion to the blood vessel surface. The inhibitory effect of endothelium-dependent inhibition of platelet cGMP generation and aggregation is attenuated in patients with endothelial dysfunction. Increased platelet adhesiveness to the vascular wall, observed in endothelial dysfunction, would ultimately be expected to promote inflammation and atherosclerosis by the local activity of platelet-derived growth factors.

Similarly, the vascular endothelium is also important in maintaining the balance of the fibrinolytic system. Release of tissue-plasminogen activator, which helps protect against endogenous thrombosis, is depressed in conditions associated with endothelial dysfunction, whereas generation of its endogenous inhibitor plasminogen-activator inhibitor (PAI-1) is increased. The mechanisms underlying this relationship have not yet been clearly elucidated; however bradykinin (BK) and Ang II appear to play an important role. Therefore, endothelial dysfunction leads to an increase in platelet activation and aggregability and a shift in the intrinsic fibrinolytic balance toward a prothrombotic state which may predispose to acute thrombotic cardiovascular events.

Endothelial dysfunction

Traditional cardiovascular risk factors such as hypertension, hyperlipidemia, insulin resistance/diabetes, and tobacco use are associated with endothelial dysfunction. Several cellular processes modulate endothelial function.

Nitric oxide synthase. In certain disease states such as renal failure, eNOS activity may be attenuated by naturally occurring L-arginine analogs [e.g., asymmetric dimethyl L-arginine, (ADMA)] that compete for L-arginine binding sites, or reduced cofactors, such as tetrahydrobiopterin that help to uncouple eNOS so that it can generate superoxide anion.

Nitric oxide release modulators. Basal release of NO from the vascular endothelium is also closely regulated by other endothelial-derived peptides and mediators. Therefore, BK, a polypeptide that is tonically synthesized in the vascular wall from kininogen by the action of kallikreins, appears to modulate vascular NO activity at rest and on stimulation. Inhibition of BK B2 receptors causes constriction and inhibits flow-mediated vasodilation indicating its crucial role in modulating resting coronary vascular tone and function. Similarly, endogenous endothelin, the most powerful constrictor polypeptide produced by the endothelium, is responsible for maintenance of vasoconstrictor tone through endothelin ET-A receptors. Blockade of this receptor also improves endothelial dysfunction in patients with risk factors for atherosclerosis. Other local modulators of endothelial NO are probably Ang II, substance P (SP), and hyperpolarizing factor.

Superoxides and nitric oxide bioavailability. Reduced bioavailability of NO is a function of increased superoxide anion levels [largely due to increased nicotinamide adenine dinucleotide (NADH)/nicotinamide adenine dinucleotide phosphate (NADPH) activity], a common underlying abnormality in high risk conditions. Free radicals oxidize NO to nitrite, nitrate, and peroxynitrite that leads to further generation of free radicals and cytokine activation.

NO bioavailability can be enhanced by administration of antioxidants, such as ascorbic acid, probucol, or vitamin E which scavenge oxygen free radicals, and agents such as superoxide dismutase, Ang II receptor antagonists, angiotensin-converting enzyme (ACE) inhibitors, and endothelin receptor antagonists have the potential to reduce superoxide generation.

Transcription factors. As NO bioavailability decreases, transcription factors such as NFκB, which are in an inactive state in normal endothelial cells, become activated and translocate to the nucleus where they transcribe genes that generate a cascade of events characterized by activation of cytokines such as interleukin-1 and TNF-α, proceeding to expression of adhesion molecules [e.g., E-selectin, vascular cell adhesion molecule (VCAM-1) and intercellular adhesion molecule (ICAM-1)] on the surface of the endothelial cells. These processes stimulate inflammatory activity in the vessel wall by enhancing initially the binding and subsequent transendothelial migration of leukocytes, thereby initiating and facilitating the progression of atherogenesis.

Endothelial repair and regeneration

When endothelial denudation and apoptosis occur, repair and regeneration of the endothelial lining depends on the release and delivery of bone marrow-derived stem cells of endothelial lineage, called *endothelial progenitor cells* (EPCs), which can be cultured from peripheral blood. EPCs contribute to postnatal neovascularization and may play a key role in ongoing endothelial repair. The numbers of EPCs in peripheral blood are reduced in patients with coronary artery disease and correlate inversely with the number of risk factors to which patients are exposed. Endothelial dysfunction and low EPC counts are correlated; this relationship is independent of individual risk factors. Finally, exercise, statins, and Ang II receptor antagonists increase EPC counts. These observations raise the intriguing possibilities that bone marrow-derived EPCs repair damage to the endothelium and that endothelial dysfunction occurs as a result of a combination of exposure to risk factors as well as dysunction and depletion of reparative EPCs.

Clinical assessment of endothelial function

The most commonly employed techniques for assessing endothelial function are measurements of vasomotor response to pharmacologic agents, including acetylcholine (ACH), BK, and substance P, or the measurement of flow-mediated vasodilator response of the brachial artery in response to increased shear stress. Studies that have examined the relationship between peripheral and coronary endothelial vasodilator function have shown a reasonable but not perfect correlation between the two.

Coronary endothelial function. In human studies, the integrity of the endothelium is defined by the presence of a preserved vasodilator response to ACH. Abnormal function is characterized by either a reduced dilator or a constrictor response, resulting from direct smooth muscle muscarinic receptor stimulation, overwhelming the depressed or absent dilating effect of endothelium-derived NO. Although stimulation of NO release accounts for most of the observed epicardial dilation and part of the coronary microvascular dilation with ACH, SP, and BK, the remainder appears to be secondary to release of a hyperpolarizing factor (an epoxide generated from arachidonic acid by the action of cytochrome P450), stimulation of potassium channels, activation of gap-junctions or hydrogen peroxide release.

Patients with angiographically normal coronary arteries and one or more conventional atherosclerotic risk factors exhibit depressed responses to ACH and other endothelium-dependent relaxing factors. The degree of depression correlates with the number of risk factors, implying that combined or repeated injury to the vascular endothelium results in greater dysfunction.

Peripheral endothelial function. Conduit vessel endothelium-dependent vasodilator function can be assessed using two-dimensional (2D) ultrasonography to measure vasodilation of the brachial artery in response to increased flow and shear stress induced by hyperemia (phase of reperfusion following a 5-minute period of forearm ischemia). Microvascular endothelium-dependent vasodilator function is measured by assessing the increase in forearm blood flow in response to endothelium-dependent probes (ACH, BK, or SP). Newer techniques, that may offer practical advantages include assessing changes in the pulse-waveform in response to endothelium-dependent agonists and also measuring changes in digital pulse-volume amplitude following hyperemia with digital pulse applanation tonometry (PAT).

As in the coronary circulation, conduit artery endothelium-dependent vasodilation is largely NO-dependent and is depressed in the presence of conventional atherosclerotic risk factors. In the periphery, EDHF plays a larger role in resistance vessel dilation.

Circulating markers. Conventional risk factors for atherosclerosis, including diabetes, hyperlipidemia and smoking, along with infection and novel putative risk factors, are associated with activated cytoplasmic transcription factors (e.g., NFκB), expression of cell surface adhesion molecules (e.g., VCAM), activation of cytokines and chemokines [e.g., Interleukins, MCP-1, regulated on activation normal T cell expressed and secreted (RANTES)] and markers of vascular inflammation (LpPLA-2, TNF-α) Alteration in endothelial cell function may result in the generation and release of endothelial microparticles and even loss of entire endothelial cells which can be detected and quantified in blood.

Cardiovascular risk factors and endothelial dysfunction

Gene-environment interactions. The contribution of family history to coronary artery disease can now be appreciated by understanding the interaction of the individual's genotype and vascular phenotype. Polymorphisms in several genes (**Table A64.1**) are likely to modulate protein expression in diverse molecular pathways, can modulate endothelial function, and in turn, alter the risk of development of atherosclerosis and its complications.

Risk factors.

Conventional risk factors. The correlation between the number of conventional risk factors and endothelial dysfunction by no means accounts for the full range of population variability observed. A recent analysis of 2,883 Framingham study participants revealed that in the older population (mean age of 61), mean flow-mediated vasodilation was 3.3% in women and 2.4% in

men. Among the conventional risk factors, age, systolic blood pressure (BP), lipid lowering medication use, and smoking were independent predictors of endothelial function but together they accounted for only 16% of the variability observed.

Novel risk factors. Novel risk factors for endothelial dysfunction (**Table A64.1**) include hyperhomocysteinemia, sedentary lifestyle, and exposure to multiple pathogens including *Chlamydia pneumoniae*, cytomegalovirus, herpes simplex viruses, *Helicobacter pylori*, and hepatitis virus. Mediators of endothelial activation and inflammation can be measured in the circulation and have been studied as indicators of increased risk of future cardiovascular events. In the Framingham cohort of 2,113 participants several biomarkers were measured including neurohumoral [N-atrial natriuretic peptide (N-ANP), brain natriuretic peptide, renin, aldosterone], inflammatory [C-reactive protein (CRP)], hemostatic (plasminogen-activator inhibitor 1), and urinary (albumin/creatinine ratio). Of these, only N-ANP and renin positively correlated with endothelial function. When CRP and myeloperoxidase levels were measured in comparison to endothelial function in 298 patients with coronary artery disease, the latter were more predictive of endothelial function. Finally, in 120 healthy subjects, biomarkers of oxidative stress, including cysteine redox and lipid hydroperoxide levels correlated with flow-mediated vasodilation.

Cardiac consequences of endothelial dysfunction

Coronary vessels. The L-arginine analog, L N^G monomethyl arginine (L-NMMA), a competitive inhibitor of eNOS, elevates systemic BP, reduces coronary blood flow and constricts epicardial coronary arteries, indicating that tonic basal release of NO in the normal human circulation importantly contributes to resting coronary and peripheral vasodilator tone. However, this effect is significantly attenuated in subjects with atherosclerosis or its risk factors, consistent with reduced bioavailability of NO in these individuals.

Physiologic coronary vasomotion and myocardial ischemia. Physiologic vasodilation in response to stimuli such as exercise, pacing and cold-pressor testing, is depressed in the circulation of subjects with atherosclerosis and its risk factors, in part secondary to reduced NO bioavailability. This limitation may result in myocardial ischemia even in the presence of normal epicardial coronary arteries. Constriction of epicardial coronary arteries during physical or psychological stress can worsen lesion severity during these maneuvers and precipitate myocardial ischemia more readily. Although this phenomenon was appreciated for several decades, the mechanisms underlying the paradoxical coronary arterial constriction during stress remained unknown until the critical role of the vascular endothelium and of shear-mediated release of NO became known. Shear stress provokes release of NO by activating the AKT kinase pathway in the endothelial layer. Therefore, endothelial dysfunction appears to play an important contributory role toward precipitation of ischemia in atherosclerosis.

Endothelial dysfunction and ischemic heart disease (IHD) prognosis. Unstable angina, myocardial infarction, acute thrombotic stroke and sudden cardiac death usually occur as a result of accidental plaque rupture or fissuring that exposes the lipid rich contents of the atherosclerotic plaque to the bloodstream, triggering thrombosis. Although systemic factors are important contributors, local events that affect plaque morphology and particularly the integrity of the fibrotic plaque

TABLE A64.1

RISK FACTORS FOR ENDOTHELIAL DYSFUNCTION

Conventional risk factors	
Sedentary status/obesity	
Men	
Hypertension	
Hypercholesterolemia	
Type 1 and type 2 diabetes	
Smoking	
Aging	
Postmenopausal status	
Heart failure	
Novel risk factors for endothelial dysfunction	
Insulin resistance	
Homocysteine	
Lipoprotein (a)	
Asymmetric dimethylarginine	
Depression	
Chronic Infections	
Inflammatory factors	C-reactive protein
	Interleukin-1
	Interleukin-6
	Tumor necrosis factor α
Genetic factors	Endothelial nitric oxide synthase
	Angiotensin-converting enzyme I/D
	Angiotensinogen
	Interleukin-6 promoter
	Chemokine receptors
Impaired repair	Low endothelial progenitor activity

cap appear to play a crucial role in determining the site of plaque rupture. Increasing shear stress and vasoconstrictor tone may also help trigger rupture of such a "vulnerable" plaque. The severity of either coronary or peripheral vascular endothelial dysfunction appears to be an independent predictor of adverse long-term cardiovascular prognosis in several studies. Moreover, in postmenopausal women, those who had endothelial dysfunction were four to five times more likely to develop hypertension and diabetes during a 5-year follow-up period.

Strategies to improve endothelial function

Numerous therapeutic strategies may improve endothelial dysfunction. Physical exercise reliably improves endothelial dysfunction in the coronary and peripheral circulations of sedentary individuals. Substitution of ω-3-fatty acids in the diet and adoption of a "Mediterranean style diet" improves vascular dysfunction, whereas a high fried-fat meal transiently impairs endothelial function. L-arginine 5 to 9 g/day has shown promise in some studies, particularly if there is a high level of asymmetric dimethyl arginine, an endogenous antagonist of L-arginine. Statin therapy trials have demonstrated significant and sustained improvement of endothelial dysfunction and an increase in endothelial progenitor cell activity. Similarly antihypertensive therapy can partially restore normal endothelial function in hypertensives, particularly if ACE inhibitors or Ang II receptor antagonists, and perhaps calcium antagonists are used. Thiazolidinediones may improve endothelial dysfunction in diabetics and those with insulin resistance, whereas sulfonylureas do not. Antioxidant vitamins such as vitamin C and E, although able to improve dysfunction when given systemically in high concentrations, are not effective as long-term oral therapy. In contrast, novel antioxidants such as tetrahydrobiopterin show greater promise. Phosphodiesterase inhibitors that decelerate metabolism of cGMP produced as a result of NO release may also improve endothelial dysfunction.

Suggested Readings

Barnes PJ, Karin M. Nuclear factor-kappaB: a pivotal transcription factor in chronic inflammatory diseases. *N Engl J Med* 1997;336:1066–1071.

Cai H, Harrison DG. Endothelial dysfunction in cardiovascular diseases: the role of oxidant stress. *Circ Res* 2000;87:840–844.

Deanfield JE, Halcox JP, Rabelink TJ. Endothelial function and dysfunction: testing and clinical relevance. *Circulation* 2007;115:1285–1295.

Diodati JG, Dakak N, Gilligan DM, et al. Effect of atherosclerosis on endothelium-dependent inhibition of platelet activation in humans. *Circulation* 1998;98(1):17–24.

Halcox JPJ, Schenke WH, Zalos G, et al. Prognostic value of coronary vascular endothelial dysfunction. *Circulation* 2002;106:653–658.

Halcox JPJ, Quyyumi AA. Coronary vascular endothelial function and myocardial ischemia: why should we worry about endothelial dysfunction? *Coron Artery Dis* 2001;12:475–484.

Hill JM, Zalos G, Halcox JPJ, et al. Circulating endothelial progenitor cells as novel determinants of vascular dysfunction and risk. *N Engl J Med* 2003;348:593–600.

Ludmer PL, Selwyn AP, Shook TL, et al. Paradoxical vasoconstriction induced by acetylcholine in atherosclerotic coronary arteries. *N Engl J Med* 1986;315:1046–1051.

Quyyumi AA, Dakak N, Andrews NP, et al. Nitric oxide activity in the human coronary circulation. Impact of risk factors for coronary atherosclerosis. *J Clin Invest* 1995;95:1747–1755.

CHAPTER A65 ■ ATHEROGENESIS AND CORONARY ARTERY DISEASE

THOMAS D. GILES, MD

KEY POINTS

■ Atherosclerosis is a complex degenerative condition initially characterized by endothelial dysfunction and lipid accumulation in the endothelium and media, followed by wall thickening and outward remodeling, and later by luminal encroachment, thrombosis, and occlusion.

■ Atherosclerotic plaque formation involves the interaction of genetic predisposition and environmental risk factors (e.g., dyslipidemia, hypertension, insulin resistance, smoking, infections) with diffuse vascular injury caused by hemodynamic (shear) stress, cellular proliferation, chronic low-grade inflammation, and thrombosis. Many of these factors are also involved in the pathogenesis of chronic hypertension.

■ Increased blood pressure (BP) promotes or accelerates all phases of the development of atherosclerotic lesions, from plaque formation to rupture.

■ Plaque instability and deterioration lead to sudden events such as erosion, fracture, or thrombosis, with or without vessel occlusion, that can then result in acute myocardial infarction and/or sudden death.

See also Chapters **A63, A64, B77,** C109, C110, and **C149**

Atherosclerosis is a degenerative disorder that includes vascular cell proliferation, medial expansion of conduit arteries, ischemia, and, ultimately, ischemic necrosis of myocardium. This major disease is a dominating worldwide source of morbidity and mortality, expressing itself not only as coronary heart disease, but also as cerebrovascular and peripheral arterial disease. The risk of atherosclerosis is significantly amplified by the presence of hypertension, insulin resistance, smoking, and lack of exercise.

Metabolic factors in atherogenesis

Low-density lipoprotein and apolipoproteins. Epidemiologic studies have established that elevated total cholesterol, increased low-density lipoprotein (LDL), and decreased high-density lipoprotein (HDL) are major risk factors associated with atherosclerosis and its major consequences. The chain of events increasing blood lipids begins with intestinal hydrolysis to form triglycerides and accumulation into chylomicrons in the portal circulation. The liver loads triglycerides into verylow-density lipoprotein (VLDL), which interacts with apoproteins, LDL and HDL to allow transport of lipids to and from peripheral tissues.

LDL particles consist of a phospholipid coat enclosing cholesterol and carrying a unique protein apolipoprotein B-100 (Apo-B). In industrialized societies, circulating LDL increases dramatically in the first two decades of life. Abnormalities of other components, including lipoprotein (a), which surrounds the lipid center and serves as a transport mechanism, also exist in individuals with coronary disease.

Low-density lipoprotein metabolism and receptor action. The N-terminal domain of apoprotein B (Apo-B) is recognized by specific LDL receptors that allow hepatic uptake. Approximately 75% of LDL is removed from the circulation by LDL receptors in the liver that are regulated by specific genes controlled by transcription factors sensitive to circulating LDL levels. Decreased blood or tissue LDL leads to upregulation of LDL receptors and enhanced LDL removal and turnover. Apo-B is also recognized by LDL receptors on endothelial cells and hepatocytes. The removal rate of LDL from the circulation depends on the number and availability of LDL receptors. LDL can accumulate in the arterial wall when serum concentrations are high. Upregulation of LDL receptors is a major part of the beneficial effects of hydroxymethylglutaryl coenzyme A reductase inhibition (statins).

High-density lipoprotein metabolism. HDL is a unique protein secreted into the plasma by the liver and intestines that binds to circulating cholesterol. HDL prevents the oxidation of LDL by binding to transitional metal ions in the intima. HDL serves as a reservoir for apolipoproteins and is the major factor controlling cholesterol uptake by the liver. When HDL interacts with cell membranes, lecithin cholesterol acyltransferase combines cholesterol and phosphatidyl choline to make cholesteryl ester, which is then transported to the liver. HDL contains a phospholipid coat with an Apo-E protein, which affects reverse cholesterol transport and can also function as an antioxidant that controls subsequent inflammatory responses. Therefore, in contrast to LDL, high HDL levels help prevent atherosclerosis.

Oxygen radicals and nitrate metabolism. Oxidation and oxidized LDL (oxo-LDL) itself lead to a continuous local excess of oxygen free radicals that play an important pathogenic role in atherosclerosis. Excess free radicals bind to nitric oxide (NO) to produce peroxynitrite. When free radicals are generated in conjunction with peroxynitrite formation, there is a reduction in the activity of endothelial NO synthase (eNOS). The appearance of abnormal substrates that compete for eNOS, including asymmetric dimethylarginine (ADMA), impairs the ability of DNA and messenger RNA to code for the production of eNOS and also cause abnormal binding of eNOS and caveolin, a membrane-bound protein that further disables the enzyme. All of these mechanisms lead to impairment of endothelium-dependent dilation and other vascular protective properties.

Low-density lipoprotein oxidation and vascular scavenger pathways. LDL is protected from oxidation in the blood, but if it is present in sufficient excess to penetrate the extracellular matrix in the vessel wall, it is subsequently oxidized by a variety of enzymatic and nonenzymatic mechanisms, including myeloperoxidase, 15-lipoxygenase, and nicotinamide adenine dinucleotide phosphate oxidase. Lipid oxidation is amplified in diabetes, insulin resistance, smoking, and hypertension.

In atherogenesis, the lysine component of the LDL particle is modified so that it is no longer recognized by the classic LDL receptor. At the same time, lipoprotein scavenger receptors appear on vascular and inflammatory cells. Oxo-LDL is taken up by macrophages and foam cells through the scavenger receptors at a rate up to ten times faster than LDL receptors can process. Therefore, activation of vascular scavenger receptors leads to preferential accumulation of oxo-LDL within cells, a process that is central to the progression of atherosclerosis. Oxo-LDL is also a potent chemoattractant for circulating macrophages, and when ingested by macrophages, inhibits their motility, leads to sequestration of macrophages in the intima of arterial wall, and exhibits cytotoxicity in endothelial cells. Glycated LDL is highly immunogenic and LDL-immune complexes are rapidly phagocytized by macrophages. The unique Apo-B protein associated with LDL also becomes fragmented and immunogenic.

Vascular susceptibility to atherosclerosis

There is wide variation in the clinical expression of atherosclerosis that is explained in part by differences in individual blood vessels.

Endothelial dysfunction. The healthy endothelium maintains adequate constitutively produces NO locally, which maintains optimum lumen area, limits the impact of shear forces, and contributes to the local defense against coagulation. Early impairment of endothelium-dependent, NO-dependent vasodilation appears in young relatives of patients with arterial disease. This clinical observation is consistent with outcomes from a wide range of genetic knockout experiments involving LDL receptors, interleukin-10, Apo-A1 receptors, and other receptors that lead to impairment of the protective mechanisms in the arterial wall and amplify atherosclerosis. The endothelium normally exhibits a slow turnover rate, and maintains adequate anticoagulant defenses, including production of tissue plasminogen activator (tPA) and

heparans and limited production of PAI-1 and thrombomodulin. Turnover of endothelial progenitor cells (EPCs) is also impaired.

Hemodynamic factors and shear stress. Local physical forces are important in the pathogenesis and location of initial fatty streak development and early atherosclerotic lesions. Atherogenesis appears to be heightened at branch points and at flow dividers in conduit arteries. There is clinical evidence of early endothelium-dependent vasodilator dysfunction at these sites. There is also experimental evidence of the augmented activation of transcription factors such as nuclear factor κB (NFB) that code for genes that initiate inflammation at susceptible branch points. Typically, the outer walls of arterial bifurcations and inner walls of arterial curvatures are most affected. Low shear stress alters Akt signaling, promotes vasoconstriction, inhibits vasodilation, and promotes clotting. These processes are probably mediated through release of growth factors such as platelet-derived growth factor, transforming growth factor β, and fibroblast growth factor 2, as well as through local release of inflammatory mediators such as vascular cell adhesion molecule-1 (VCAM-1), intercellular adhesion molecule-1 (ICAM-1), and monocyte chemotactic peptide (MCP-1). At the same time, vascular synthesis of NO and tPA are reduced and thrombosis is promoted through the release of thrombomodulin.

Cellular elements.

Vascular smooth muscle cells. During atherogenesis, vascular smooth muscle cells (VSMCs) alter their phenotypic state. They migrate and proliferate locally, while accumulating oxo-LDL. VSMCs exhibit proinflammatory mechanisms and secrete additional matrix that contributes to intimal–medial thickening and vascular stiffness.

Mononuclear cells. Abnormal and immunogenic protein epitopes on oxo-LDL provoke a response that resembles the normal reaction to infective agents. The expression of adhesion molecules, at first E-selectin and then ICAM and VCAM, attract and then bind mononuclear cells to endothelial cell membranes. The bound monocytes are then subject to enhanced LDL oxidation through expression of ligands that bind MCP-1, which permits bound monocytes to take up more oxo-LDL through scavenger pathways. MCP-1 also impairs cholesterol efflux and binds to proteoglycans, subintimal collagen, and fibrin. Local inflammation is further enhanced when bound monocytes produce tumor necrosis factor α, MCP-1, interleukins (ILs), chemoattractants, and chemokines. Monocyte-macrophages also present oxo-LDL antigens to T lymphocytes, contributing to the appearance of circulating antibodies to these altered proteins.

Inflammation and infection. The presence of excess oxidant stress leads to activation of transcription factors such as NFκB, which cause upregulation of genes that initiate inflammation. Inflammation is exacerbated by the presence of certain intermediates of cholesterol synthesis, including mevalonate and geranyl-pyrophosphate, which interact with oxo-LDL to facilitate the isoprenylation (activation) of small proteins [e.g., rho geranyl–geranyl pyrophosphate (GGP) and geranyl rho-kinase] that regulate the inflammatory processes leading to atherogenesis and plaque formation. The processes mentioned in the preceding text lead to impairment of endothelium-dependent dilation, in part because of the loss of available NO, as well as propagation of chronic low-grade inflammation, with the further differentiation of monocytes into macrophages in the blood vessel wall. Inflammation plays a role in every stage of atherosclerosis, including increased serum C-reactive protein (CRP), a marker of inflammation.

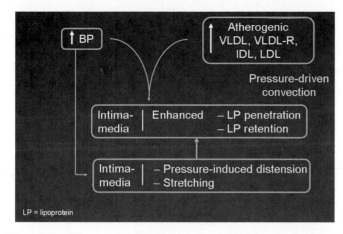

Figure A65.1 The relationship between pressure-driven convection of lipoproteins and pressure-induced distension of the arterial wall is shown. BP, blood pressure; VLDL, very low-density lipoprotein; VLDL-R, very low-density lipoprotein receptor; IDL, intermediate-density lipoprotein; LDL, low-density lipoprotein; LP, lipoprotein. (Reproduced with permission from: Sposito AC. Emerging insights into hypertension and dyslipidaemia synergies. *Eur Heart J Suppl* 2004;6:G8–G12.)

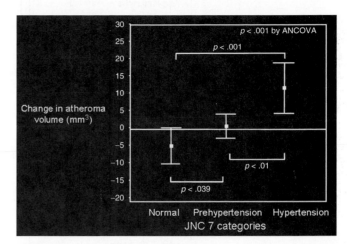

Figure A65.2 The influence of levels of blood pressure on the progression of coronary atherosclerosis as assessed by serial intravascular ultrasonography is shown. This study suggests that in patients with coronary artery disease, the optimal blood pressure is <120/80 mm Hg. JNC 7, Joint National Committee on the Prevention, Detection, Evaluation, and Treatment of High Blood Pressure; BP, blood pressure; ANCOVA, analysis of covariance. (Reproduced with permission from: Sipahi I, Tuzcu EM, Schoenhagen P, et al. Effects of normal, prehypertensive, and hypertensive blood pressure levels on progression of coronary atherosclerosis. *J Am Coll Cardiol* 2006;48:833–838.)

Evidence continues to mount that infectious agents may contribute to atherogenesis. In particular, *Chlamydia pneumoniae* and cytomegalovirus exacerbate lesion development in animal models of atherosclerosis and restenosis. The risk of atherosclerosis related to infections is probably additive to other atherogenic stimuli to which an individual is exposed.

Coagulation. The proinflammatory mediators that cause inflammation also lead to the development of a procoagulant endothelial vascular interface that favors thrombosis. A deficiency of tPA relative to the available amount of plasminogen-activator inhibitor 1 (PAI-1) enhances these procoagulant tendencies.

Interaction of hypertension and atherogenesis. The increase in blood pressure (BP) associated with hypertension may also influence the movement of atherogenic lipoproteins into the arterial wall. The relationship of this pressure-related convection of lipids into the vasculature is illustrated in **Figure A65.1**. Therefore, as would be expected from processes involving BP and atherosclerosis, the progression of coronary atherosclerosis (as assessed by intravascular ultrasonography) is directly related to the level of systemic arterial BP. Longitudinal studies have associated normal (<120/80 mm Hg) BP with slower progression (or even regression when BP is lowered by drugs; **Figure A65.2**).

Hypertension, itself a prominent risk factor for atherosclerosis, is sometimes associated with a high levels of inflammatory markers such as CRP. These associations, however, are relatively weak. Some investigators believe that a major link between BP and atherogenesis is angiotensin II, which is thought to promote hypertensive end-organ damage through enhanced production of superoxide anion, increased expression by arterial smooth muscle cells of proinflammatory cytokines (e.g., interleukin-6 and MCP-1) and adhesion molecules (e.g., VCAM-1, ICAM, and P-selectin) by endothelial cells.

Progression of coronary atherosclerosis

Angioscopic and pathologic studies in humans have clearly shown that patients with clinically manifest coronary artery disease almost always have multiple plaques at different stages of development throughout their epicardial coronary arteries, with many exhibiting the features of instability and high risk. Each plaque has its own history of growth, activation, erosion, fracture, thrombosis, and healing.

Early lesions. The early lesions (**Figure A65.3**) can be described morphologically as fatty dots or streaks associated histologically with the presence of isolated macrophage foam cells and multiple foam cell layers within the arterial intima. Accumulation of lipid in the arterial intima occurs when levels of oxo-LDL and BP exceed threshold levels. Oxidized lipoproteins are then internalized by macrophages and intimal smooth muscle cells that change into characteristic foam cells. The integrity of the endothelium plays a key role in the rate at which lipids accumulate in the intima. When the endothelium is functionally impaired, as in dyslipidemia or insulin resistance, atherogenesis proceeds faster. Typically, smooth muscle cells and macrophages accumulate with some preference for the outer edges of branch points and flow dividers.

Arterial remodeling. Arterial remodeling is the result of the response of the arterial wall to the atherosclerotic process. In the past, atherosclerosis was thought to cause only progressive luminal encroachment. However, intravascular ultrasonographic studies have confirmed the model of progression proposed by Glagov et al.; accumulation of lipid in the arterial wall initially causes adventitial ("eutrophic outward") remodeling, with preservation of the arterial lumen. Only in advanced stages of atherogenesis does arterial narrowing occur. Therefore, the focal stenoses seen in conventional coronary angiography underrepresent the degree of intimal thickening and plaque formation that occurs in susceptible coronary arteries.

Advanced lesions. The connection between minimal and advanced atherosclerosis resides principally in the formation of pools of extracellular lipid and the local fibrotic responses to the associated chronic inflammation (**Figure A65.4**). Local oxidant

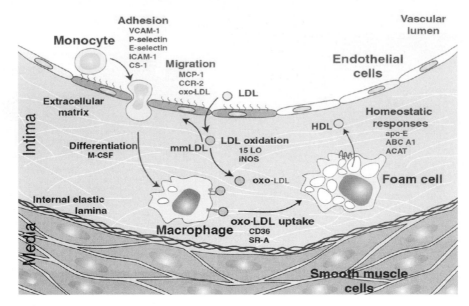

Figure A65.3 Early cell biology of atherosclerosis. Low-density lipoprotein (LDL) passes into the subintimal space and becomes oxidized. This leads to activation of the endothelium, where chemoattractants such as macrophage chemoattractant protein-1 serve to attract inflammatory cells. Activation of the endothelial surface includes expression of adhesion molecules such as vascular cell adhesion molecule-1 (VCAM-1), P-selectin, E-selectin, and intercellular adhesion molecule-1 (ICAM-1). These initiate monocyte transport into the subintima where macrophage colony stimulating factor facilitates transformation into a macrophage. Further uptake of oxidized LDL (oxo-LDL) occurs under the influence of specific receptors (CD36 and SR-A) in foam cell formation. (Reproduced with permission from: Glass CK, Witzum JL. Atherosclerosis: the road ahead. *Cell* 2001;104:503–516.) CS-1, connecting segment 1; MCP-1, monocyte chemotactic peptide 1; CCR-2, CC chemokine receptor 2; LDL, low-density lipoprotein; M-CSF, macrophage colony-stimulating factor; LO, lipoxygenase; iNOS, inductible NO synthase; HDL, high-density lipoprotein; apo-E, apolipoprotein-E; ABC A1, adenosine triphosphate binding cassette A1; ACAT, acyl-coenzyme A:choesteryl acyltransferase.

stress maintains continuous monocyte activation and results in production of tissue factor, impairment of cholesterol efflux, and appearance of several mechanisms mediating apoptosis (death receptors, protooncogenes, and tumor suppressor genes). These mechanisms may also be responsible for increased collection of debris in an expanding plaque. Extracellular lipid is mostly

derived from macrophage foam cells that have died. As the lesions advance, the central core of the atheroma lesion is replaced by lipid, and there is disruption of the plaque surface layer ("fibrous cap"), with local hematoma and thrombus formation and, often, distal embolization. Disruption occurs where the shear forces are greatest, at the shoulder of the fibrous cap of the plaque.

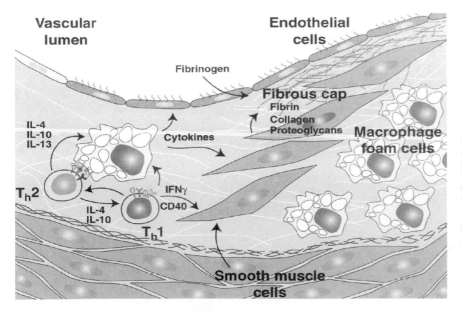

Figure A65.4 Plaque formation in atherosclerosis. The activated endothelium under the influence of oxidized low-density lipoprotein continues to permit the subintimal collection of inflammatory cells. In concert with T lymphocytes (T_H2) and local production of chemokines [interleukin (IL)-1, IL-6, and IL-10], this chronic low-grade inflammation attracts activated smooth muscle cells that deposit collagen in the intima. The collection of the macrophage, foam cells, smooth muscle cells, matrix, and collagen as shown make up the development of the plaque. IFNγ, interferon gamma; T_H1, T helper cell 1. (Reproduced with permission from: Glass CK, Witzum JL. Atherosclerosis: the road ahead. *Cell* 2001;104:503–516.)

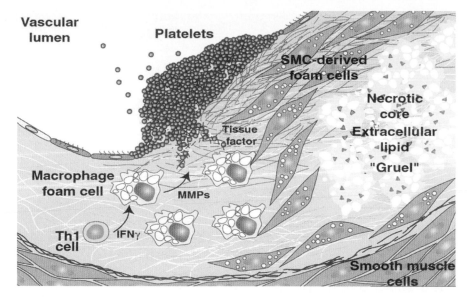

Figure A65.5 Advanced atherosclerosis: ruptured plaque. Advanced activation and dysfunction of the endothelium results in a procoagulant surface that attracts platelet and fibrin thrombi. In the atherosclerotic plaque, foam cells undergo programmed cell death to form a necrotic core. At the edge of the plaque, activated macrophages and foam cells continue to propagate low-grade inflammation and produce matrix metalloproteinases (MMPs) and tissue factor that enhance plaque rupture, hemorrhage, and thrombosis. IFNγ, interferon γ; SMC, smooth muscle cell; T_H1, T helper cell. (Reproduced with permission from Glass CK, Witzum JL. Atherosclerosis: the road ahead. *Cell* 2001;104:503–516.)

Activated cellular processes result in the formation of new connective tissue matrix, but these lesions do not narrow the arterial lumen until the process is far advanced. Activated macrophages at these sites produce matrix metalloproteinases (MMPs) that are capable of digesting collagen-1, leaving behind weak and fragmented collagen fibers. Neovascularization in the intima appears to be another late phenomenon, likely in response to repeated cycles of local rupture, hemorrhage, thrombosis, and healing, which all appear to be characterized by local accumulation of proteases.

Vulnerable plaques. Any plaque that is susceptible to disruption is said to be vulnerable (**Figure A65.5**). With further progression of the atherosclerotic process, calcification occurs. When 50% or more of the cross-sectional area of an atherosclerotic lesion is mineralized, the lesion is termed *calcified*. Narrowing may occur abruptly with plaque disruption. The vulnerability of a plaque does not correlate well with its appearance at angiography. The most vulnerable plaques are usually those with large lipid cores, thin fibrous caps, and less calcium, so the determination of the degree of calcification (often obtained by semiquantitative measurement using computerized tomography) may mislead one into underestimating the severity of the atherosclerotic plaque.

Clinical correlations: coronary syndromes

Occlusive coronary disease and stable angina. With plaques of the stable variety, stenoses grow slowly without sudden deterioration. The progressive lumen narrowing impairs laminar flow and stress-induced increases in blood flow velocity. A pressure gradient eventually appears, there is progressive failure to increase flow on demand, and finally, episodic decreases in flow, in part due to the loss of endothelium-dependent dilation and abnormal reflex constriction. Transient decreases in coronary blood flow contribute to episodes of regional myocardial ischemia and a pattern of relatively stable angina pectoris that appears predictably at a given level of myocardial work.

Unstable angina and infarction. In contrast to stable angina, unstable angina (progressive or Prinzmetal's angina) is caused by vulnerable plaques, which have episodic local inflammatory flares, erosion, rupture, and thrombosis (with

or without occlusion). Often, the acute event is minor and is followed by a degree of healing. When an unstable plaque suddenly deteriorates, major consequences are also common and acute alterations in regional coronary blood may lead to unstable angina, acute myocardial infarction, or death. The same pathogenic risk factors that cause chronic inflammation in each plaque remain actively involved throughout the development of the disease. Vulnerable plaques and complex lesions that acutely degenerate are often not visible with conventional angiography.

Atherosclerotic markers

The appreciation of the relationship between the cell biology and clinical syndromes in atherosclerosis has encouraged the exploration of markers or surrogates to detect disease activity, estimate risk, and monitor therapies. These efforts include the imaging of atherosclerosis by optical coherence tomography or magnetic resonance. Blood tests to assess insulin resistance, CRP, PAI-1, and ICAM-1 have been employed in clinical studies, but none of these promising biomarkers has been shown to be uniquely sensitive or specific in primary or secondary prevention.

Suggested Readings

Epstein SE, Zhou YF, Zhu J. Infection and atherosclerosis: emerging mechanistic paradigms. *Circulation* 1999;100:e20–e28.

Fuster V, Badimon L, Badimon JJ, et al. The pathogenesis of coronary artery disease and the acute coronary syndrome. *N Engl J Med* 1992;326:242–250.

Glagov S, Weisenberg E, Zarins CK, et al. Compensatory enlargement of human atherosclerotic coronary arteries. *N Engl J Med* 1987;316:1371–1375.

Glass CK, Witzum JL. Atherosclerosis: the road ahead. *Cell* 2001;104:503–516.

Kinlay S, Selwyn AP, Delagrange D, et al. Biological mechanisms for the clinical success of lipid-lowering in coronary artery disease and the use of surrogate end-points. *Curr Opin Lipidol* 1996;7:389–397.

Lee RT, Libby P. The unstable atheroma. *Arterioscler Thromb Vasc Biol* 1997;17:1859–1867.

Libby P, Ridker PM, Maseri A. Inflammation and atherosclerosis. *Circulation* 2002;105:1135–1143.

Malek AM, Alper SL, Izumo S. Hemodynamic shear stress and its role in atherosclerosis. *JAMA* 1999;282:2035–2042.

Selwyn AP, Kinlay S, Libby P, et al. Atherogenic lipids, vascular dysfunction, and clinical signs of ischemic heart disease. *Circulation* 1997;95:5–7.

Stary HC. Evolution and progression of atherosclerotic lesions in coronary arteries of children and young adults. *Arteriosclerosis* 1989;9:119–132.

CHAPTER A66 ■ PATHOGENESIS OF STROKE

J. DAVID SPENCE, BA, MBA, MD, FRCPC, FAHA

KEY POINTS

- Blood pressure (BP)-related strokes are caused by hyaline degeneration (lipohyalinosis) of the arteries at the base of the brain, which can be reduced markedly by good BP control.
- Atherosclerotic strokes are usually due to emboli consisting of atheromatous debris, platelet aggregates (white thrombus), but may be due to an occlusion with *in situ* (red) thrombus.
- Emboli may arise from an artery, the aorta, the heart, or the venous system by way of a patent foramen ovale; identification is important because treatment depends on the specific cause of stroke.
- Cerebral ischemic injury is not an "all-or-none" phenomenon, and the degree and duration of cerebral hypoperfusion are important in determining the severity of a stroke.
- Clinical features may help localize the cerebral ischemic injury but are not reliable indicators of underlying pathogenesis; imaging studies are important for the appropriate management of a stroke patient.
- Dementia is commonly preceded by cerebrovascular disease and stroke.

See also Chapters A41, A45, A61, A67, **B79,** and **C153**

There are important pathogenetic differences between stroke and heart attacks, most notably the stronger association of stroke with hypertension. Atheromatous diseases and coagulation disturbances also cause strokes.

Pathogenesis

Hypertension is the most potent risk factor for cerebrovascular disease and contributes directly to the occurrence of stroke in two major ways (lacunar infarction, and intracerebral hemorrhage). It also contributes indirectly to stroke by exacerbating atherosclerosis (**Table A66.1**).

Lacunar infarcts and cerebral hemorrhage. Hypertension is associated with focal damage to small resistance arteries at the base of the brain, through lipohyalinosis or fibrinoid necrosis. When these vessels occlude, the result is lacunar infarction; when they rupture, the result is intracerebral hemorrhage (ICH). The most vulnerable areas at the base of the brain have been called the *vascular centrencephalon* (basal ganglia, thalamus, internal capsule, brain stem, and cerebellum). In this territory, short straight arteries with few branches transmit the pressure load directly to the resistance vessels, which can be mechanically damaged. In contrast, the arteries to the cortex are relatively long and have many branches, so the pressure load is dissipated to a greater degree. BP control reduces stroke by 40% and virtually eliminates strokes due to hypertensive small vessel disease.

Embolism. Emboli arise either from the heart, from proximal arteries, or from the venous system in patients with a right-to-left shunt such as a patent foramen ovale. High-risk and medium-risk sources of embolism were identified as part of the Trial of ORG 10172 in acute stroke treatment (TOAST) study.

Cardiac embolism. Cardiac emboli arise from cardiac thrombi in the left side of the heart secondary to myocardial infarction (MI) with endocardial damage (acutely), ventricular dyskinesia or aneurysm, or left atrial enlargement with atrial fibrillation. Paradoxical emboli due to thrombi arising in the systemic veins and traversing to the left side of the heart through a patent foramen ovale account for approximately 4% of ischemic strokes.

Arterial embolism. Arterial emboli are dislodged fragments of atherosclerotic debris or platelet aggregates (white thrombus) arising from an area of carotid injury/ulceration, or red thrombus from a dissection. Arteriogenic emboli frequently arise from the internal carotid artery near the carotid bifurcation and from the vertebral artery near its origin or termination. Measuring the surface area or volume of plaque in the carotid artery can be used to predict future stroke. Embolization of atheromatous debris from a site of severe carotid stenosis can be prevented by endarterectomy.

Coagulation disorders. Coagulation disorders, including hyperhomocysteinemia and factor V Leiden, predispose to cardioembolic stroke; in atrial fibrillation an elevated level of homocysteine increases stroke risk three- to fourfold. Factor V Leiden probably

TABLE A66.1

PATHOPHYSIOLOGY OF STROKE

Definition:
  Acute onset of a central nervous system (CNS) deficit from a
    vascular etiology
Ischemic (80%)
  Occlusive
      Large-vessel occlusion
        Intraplaque hemorrhage, plaque rupture, dissection
      Small vessel disease ("lacunar")
        Fibrinoid necrosis, hyaline degeneration
  Embolic
      Artery-to-artery
        Carotid stenosis, vertebral, intracranial
        Aortic arch
      Cardiogenic
        Atrial fibrillation, SBE, ventricular aneurysm
          Paradoxical, atrial myxoma, recent MI
      Unusual
        Air, fat, amniotic fluid
  Stasis
      Watershed ischemia with ipsilateral carotid occlusion
      Blood constituents
        WBC, RBC, platelets, sickle, immunoglobulins
      Venous infarction
  Vasculitis
      Giant cell, syphilis, SLE, etc.
Hemorrhagic (20%)
  Intracerebral hemorrhage (ICH)
    Hypertensive
    Amyloid angiopathy
    Arteriovenous malformation, cavernous angioma
  Subarachnoid hemorrhage (SAH)
  Cerebral vein thrombosis

Note that "cerebral thrombosis" does not occur in arteries until they have
been occluded by another process.
SBE, subacute bacterial endocarditis; WBC, white blood cells; RBC, red
blood cells; SLE, systemic lupus erythematosus.

underlies the early excess of thromboembolic events in women treated with hormone replacement therapy.

Atherosclerosis. Cerebral atherosclerosis may become symptomatic by any of three major mechanisms: hypoperfusion, embolization or occlusion. *In situ* thrombosis is secondary to the occlusion.

Hypoperfusion. Occlusion of an artery secondary to plaque rupture or intraplaque hemorrhage causes hemodynamic obstruction and produces distal cerebral hypoperfusion. The term *cerebral thrombosis* is often used for this process but is misleading if it is assumed that cerebral arteries are typically occluded by primary thrombus formation. In actuality, the high blood flow velocity in cerebral arteries does not allow sufficient time for polymerization of fibrin to produce red thrombus.

Thrombosis. Arterial thrombosis occurs after the artery occludes. The distinction between white and red thrombus is clinically useful: white thrombus is treated preventively with antiplatelet agents, red thrombus with anticoagulants.

Cortical hemorrhage. Hemorrhages in the cerebral cortex itself or in subcortical areas are much more commonly due to amyloid

angiopathy or vascular malformation rather than hypertension, or in the setting of thrombosis of cerebral dural sinuses or cerebral veins.

Clinical aspects

Figure A66.1 gives the relative frequency of ischemic stroke subtypes. With current levels of BP control, lacunar strokes are approximately equal in frequency to embolic and large-vessel strokes. In elderly Western populations, stroke incidence often exceeds MI rates.

Ischemic stroke disease spectrum. Ischemic stroke is not an all-or-none phenomenon as was once thought. Reduction of cerebral blood flow due to arterial stenosis or occlusion may produce any degree of tissue injury, varying from isolated neuronal dropout to rarefaction of all tissue elements to complete cavitary necrosis. The two factors that appear to be most important in determining the severity of injury secondary to arterial occlusion are the efficiency of the collateral circulation and cerebral blood flow, which is related to perfusion pressure.

Acute stroke and the ischemic penumbra. Moderate reduction of cerebral blood flow may not produce injury if reversed quickly but will progress to infarction if it persists for >2 to 3 hours (**Figure A66.2**). Many strokes have a central core of severe reduction of blood flow and permanent infarction that is surrounded by a rim of tissue with moderate reduction of blood flow, in which the dysfunction is potentially reversible: the *ischemic penumbra*. Restoration of normal flow to the penumbra within a few hours can result in restoration of function and clinical improvement.

The ability of anticoagulants and fibrinolytics and neuroprotective therapies (drugs, hypothermia) to improve outcome after a stroke appears to depend on the presence of an ischemic penumbra. Methods for assessing the ischemic penumbra, including MRI, computed tomography (CT) cerebral blood flow studies and positron emission tomography (PET)-CT are now being investigated for their usefulness in the management of ischemic stroke.

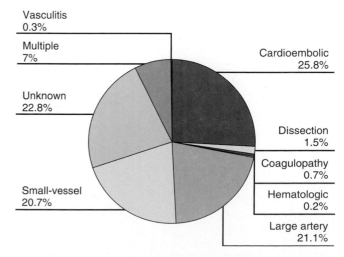

Figure A66.1 Frequency of subtypes of ischemic stroke. (Adapted from Grau AJ, Weimar C, Buggle F, et al. Risk factors, outcome and treatment in subtypes of ischemic stroke. *Stroke* 2001;32:2559–2566.)

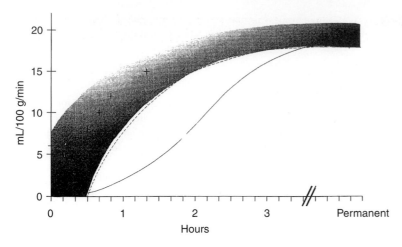

Figure A66.2 Graph showing time-intensity relationship of ischemia and incomplete infarction. *Area above curves* represents combination of duration and intensity of ischemia that is tolerated without development of infarction, whereas *points below curves* result in infarction. *Shaded area* represents ischemic injury without infarction. (From Helgason CM, Wolf PA. American Heart Association Prevention Conference IV: prevention and rehabilitation of stroke. *Stroke* 1997;28:1498–1526, with permission.)

Clinical manifestations. The clinical manifestations of occlusion of a specific artery vary according to how the interplay of these factors affects local brain perfusion. A spectrum of clinical syndromes therefore exists, although a minor degree of hypoperfusion is often asymptomatic (**Figure A66.2**). More severe ischemia results in a reversible symptomatic loss of function (transient ischemic attack) but not tissue injury. Marked hypoperfusion and prolonged ischemia causes tissue necrosis with persistent clinical sequelae (irreversible stroke). Imaging techniques [magnetic resonance imaging (MRI), single-photon emission computed tomography, or transcranial Doppler] help define lesion extent and degree of cerebral perfusion, thereby improving therapy.

Stroke and dementia

The Nun Study showed a strong interaction between stroke and expression of Alzheimer's disease. Among some 700 nuns followed prospectively with testing of cognitive function, those with Alzheimer's disease at autopsy were 20 times as likely to have been demented in life if they had even one or two small lacunar infarcts. The Syst-Eur trial showed that treating isolated systolic hypertension reduced Alzheimer's dementia by half.

Suggested Readings

Adams H, Adams R, Del ZG, et al. Guidelines for the early management of patients with ischemic stroke: 2005 guidelines update a scientific statement from the Stroke Council of the American Heart Association/American Stroke Association. *Stroke* 2005;36(4):916–923.

Adams HP Jr, Bendixen BH, Kappelle LJ, et al. TOAST Investigators. Classification of subtype of acute ischemic stroke: definitions for use in a multicenter clinical trial. *Stroke* 1993;24:35–41.

Barnett HJ, Taylor DW, Eliasziw M, et al. Benefit of carotid endarterectomy in patients with symptomatic moderate or severe stenosis. North American Symptomatic Carotid Endarterectomy Trial Collaborators [See Comments]. *N Engl J Med* 1998;339(20):1415–1425.

Forette F, Seux M-L, Staessen J, et al. Prevention of dementia in the Syst-Eur trial. *Lancet* 1998;352:1347–1351.

Goldstein LB, Adams R, Alberts MJ, et al. Primary prevention of ischemic stroke: a guideline from the American Heart Association/American Stroke Association Stroke Council. *Stroke* 2006;37(6):1583–1633.

Grau AJ, Weimar C, Buggle F, et al. Risk factors, outcome and treatment in subtypes of ischemic stroke. *Stroke* 2001;32:2559–2566.

Harrer JU, Wessels T, Franke S, et al. Stroke recurrence and its prevention in patients with patent foramen ovale. *Can J Neurol Sci* 2006;33:39–47.

SHEP Cooperative Research Group. Prevention of stroke by antihypertensive drug treatment in older persons with isolated systolic hypertension. Final results of the Systolic Hypertension in the Elderly Program (SHEP). *JAMA* 1991;265:3255–3264.

Snowdon DA, Greiner LH, Mortimer JA, et al. Brain infarction and the clinical expression of Alzheimer disease. The Nun Study. *JAMA* 1997;277:813–817.

Spence JD. Cerebral consequences of hypertension. In: Laragh JH Brenner B, eds. *Hypertension: pathophysiology, diagnosis, and management*. New York: Raven Press, 1995:741–753.

CHAPTER A67 ■ PATHOGENESIS OF ACUTE HYPERTENSIVE ENCEPHALOPATHY

DONALD D. HEISTAD, MD; FRANK M. FARACI, PhD AND WILLIAM T. TALMAN, MD

KEY POINTS

- Hypertensive encephalopathy, a medical emergency characterized by hypertension, headache, and other neurologic symptoms, usually in the setting of severe hypertension, responds clinically to blood pressure (BP) reduction.
- Hypertensive encephalopathy is apparently due to marked cerebral vasodilatation and disruption of the blood–brain barrier, particularly in postcapillary venules.
- "Breakthrough" of autoregulation may be, in part, an active process, mediated by potassium channels and activation of parasympathetic nerves to cerebral vessels. Sympathetic nerves and local myogenic tone protect the cerebral microvasculature from hypertensive damage.

See also Chapters **A42**, A66, and **C147**

Hypertensive encephalopathy is a syndrome of severe hypertension, cerebrovascular dysfunction, and neurologic impairment. The diagnosis may be in doubt until neurologic improvement occurs after reduction of arterial pressure. However, that improvement may not be immediate and may, in fact, only occur several days after reduction of arterial pressure (**Table A67.1**).

Pathophysiology

Vasospasm versus vasodilation. It was thought in the past that hypertensive encephalopathy is produced by cerebral ischemia that results from spasm of cerebral blood vessels. This suggestion was based in part on the finding that, during acute hypertension in experimental animals, cerebral arterioles may resemble a "sausage string," with alternating segments of constricted and dilated blood vessels. A similar sausage-string appearance may be seen in retinal and cerebral vessels of patients with hypertensive encephalopathy. There is now considerable evidence that constricted portions of the sausage string represent normal segments of the arterioles.

Hypertension and cerebral autoregulation. The normal response of cerebral arterioles to acute increases in blood pressure (BP) is constriction. This "autoregulatory response" prevents increased blood flow during periods of increased BP. Acute hypertension, with BP beyond the autoregulatory range, leads to dilatation of small arteries and arterioles, to an increase or "breakthrough" of cerebral blood flow, and to increased microvascular pressure.

In most patients with hypertensive encephalopathy, arterial pressure is extraordinarily high (often >250/150 mm Hg), but

because the effectiveness of autoregulation is related to basal BPs, the level of BP associated with encephalopathy varies between individuals. Other metabolic, disease, vascular, and age-related differences between individuals may also contribute to the clinical heterogeneity of this entity.

In patients with chronic hypertension, there is a shift in the autoregulatory curve, and encephalopathy occurs only at

TABLE A67.1

HYPERTENSIVE ENCEPHALOPATHY

Triad
Severe hypertension
Encephalopathy
Rapid resolution with treatment
Usually associated with malignant hypertension
Pathophysiology
Cerebral vasodilatation
Disruption of blood–brain barrier
Etiology
Untreated essential hypertension
Renal disease
Renal vascular disease
Pheochromocytoma
Intravenous cocaine or amphetamines
Differential diagnosis
Central nervous system lesion, including tumor and stroke
Drugs, vasculitis, uremia

very high levels of BP. In contrast, in patients with rapid development of hypertension, such as occurs during acute glomerulonephritis or eclampsia, there is not sufficient time for a shift in the autoregulatory curve to evolve. In these circumstances, encephalopathy may occur during acute but otherwise quantitatively modest elevations of arterial pressure, especially in children.

Venules and the blood–brain barrier. With breakthrough of autoregulation, the blood–brain barrier may be interrupted. During an acute episode of hypertension the initial site of disruption of the blood–brain barrier appears to be cerebral venules, not capillaries or arterioles. Cerebral arterioles are protected by a layer of smooth muscle cells, and wall stress in capillaries may not increase greatly because their diameter is small. In contrast, cerebral venules may be most vulnerable to increases in wall stress during acute hypertension, because their diameters are rather large and they do not have a layer of smooth muscle cells. As cerebral blood flow increases during acute hypertension and the blood–brain barrier is disrupted, focal cerebral edema follows. Edema and local changes in ions and neurotransmitters probably contribute to impaired neuronal function and encephalopathy.

Sympathetic vasoconstriction. Sympathetic neural discharge, which normally has little effect on cerebral blood vessels, constricts cerebral vessels during acute hypertension, and may shift autoregulation and the breakthrough point to higher levels of arterial pressure. Therefore, activation of sympathetic nerves may attenuate increases in cerebral blood flow during acute hypertension and protect against disruption of the blood–brain barrier in downstream vessels.

Potassium channels and parasympathetic nerves. Recent evidence suggests that activation of calcium-dependent potassium channels may contribute to "breakthrough" of autoregulation. The finding suggests that "breakthrough" of autoregulation may involve an active vasodilatory process, with activation of potassium channels, and may not be simply a passive phenomenon that occurs when arterial pressure exceeds the autoregulatory capacity of cerebral blood vessels. This process may, in part, be mediated by parasympathetic innervation of cerebral vessels; interruption of these nerves attenuates "breakthrough" at very high levels of BP. Therefore, a balance between sympathetic and parasympathetic influences may modulate cerebral blood flow during acute hypertension. During chronic hypertension, hypertrophy and inward "remodeling" of vessels (augmented by a trophic effect of sympathetic nerves) reduce vascular wall stress and afford vascular protection.

Angiotensin II and oxidative stress. A key mechanism that likely contributes to hypertensive encephalopathy involves angiotensin II generation and subsequent promotion of oxidative stress within the vasculature and brain. As in other vascular beds, increased levels of reactive oxygen species produce abnormal vascular function and altered vascular growth. Both acute and chronic hypertension increase reactive oxygen species in brain and in cerebral blood vessels. Oxidative stress and disruption of the blood–brain barrier in models of hypertensive encephalopathy are inhibited by angiotensin receptor antagonists.

Clinical features

Hypertensive encephalopathy occurs in the setting of acute increases in arterial pressure and consists of a triad of hypertension, signs of diffuse, or multifocal cerebral dysfunction, and resolution

of cerebral signs some time after effective treatment of hypertension.

Signs and symptoms. Headache, sometimes with restlessness, typically occurs early in the syndrome. Nausea, projectile vomiting, and visual blurring or blindness may be followed by drowsiness, confusion, and seizures. Papilledema, usually with retinal hemorrhages and exudates, may be observed, and retinal arteries may exhibit a sausage-string appearance. Papilledema, however, is not a *sine qua non* of hypertensive encephalopathy.

Risk factors. The most common underlying cause of hypertensive encephalopathy in adults is untreated essential hypertension. In many patients, however, and especially in children, hypertensive encephalopathy and malignant hypertension are due to underlying treatable diseases such as parenchymal renal disease, renal vascular hypertension, pheochromocytoma, and eclampsia. Patients should be evaluated for these conditions once they have become clinically stable.

Drugs. Drugs, especially intravenous amphetamines and cocaine, can produce intense vasoconstriction and occasionally vasculitis (with prolonged use) and thereby hypertension with a symptom profile consistent with hypertensive encephalopathy. In patients who are taking monoamine oxidase inhibitors with foods that contain tyramine (such as cheddar cheese) acute hypertension with stroke or hypertensive encephalopathy may occur. Oral contraceptives have been associated with malignant hypertension. Withdrawal from clonidine treatment may produce acute rebound hypertension and symptoms and signs consistent with hypertensive encephalopathy, as may treatment with cyclosporine or tacrolimus in transplant patients.

Imaging findings. Compression of the lateral ventricles on computed tomographic (CT) scans or magnetic resonance imaging (MRI) suggests cerebral edema, and the presence of cerebellar and brain stem edema may indicate hypertensive encephalopathy. Hypodense areas of white matter, presumably secondary to edema, have been observed during hypertensive encephalopathy and typically clear after treatment. The propensity for edema in the occipital lobes, with associated cortical blindness in hypertensive encephalopathy, has led to the use of the term *posterior leukoencephalopathy syndrome.*

Associated findings. Patients with hypertensive encephalopathy usually have other findings that are suggestive of malignant hypertension. In addition to papilledema, they may have left ventricular hypertrophy, heart failure, and/or renal insufficiency. Urinalysis may reveal hematuria, proteinuria (sometimes >3 g protein), and cellular casts. Microangiopathic hemolytic anemia may also be present.

Differential diagnosis. Intracerebral hemorrhage, subarachnoid hemorrhage, brain tumor, subdural hematoma, cerebral infarction, acute nephrotic syndrome, herpes simplex encephalitis, or seizures may produce hypertension and generalized or multifocal cerebral symptoms. These disorders often manifest characteristic neurologic findings and, with the exception of acute stroke or seizures, can generally be distinguished from hypertensive encephalopathy by MRI studies. Vasculitis from lupus erythematosus or polyarteritis may be associated with moderate to severe hypertension and cerebritis, but the clinician must be cautious in making a diagnosis of vasculitis, because angiographic changes of encephalopathy (sausage-string appearance, as discussed in the preceding text) may mimic those of central nervous system (CNS) vasculitis. Uremic encephalopathy may occur when renal function is substantially reduced (glomerular filtration rate <15 mL /minute). Its clinical presentation, in that it is often accompanied by hypertension, may be difficult to distinguish from hypertensive encephalopathy. Lumbar puncture is probably not necessary in these cases, unless infectious or inflammatory causes of encephalopathy are being considered. Lumbar puncture should not occur if a mass lesion is suspected.

Management

Reduction in BP usually produces rapid clinical improvement. Resolution of symptoms should not be expected immediately, but may instead occur over several days. Antihypertensive therapy should not be delayed for brain imaging if the diagnosis of hypertensive encephalopathy is being strongly considered. However, if a stroke is acutely evolving or the neurologic findings cannot be distinguished from hypertensive encephalopathy, any reduction in BP should occur cautiously. Approaches to antihypertensive therapy include intermediate target values for BP and use of appropriate immediate-acting pharmacologic agents given parenterally, as discussed elsewhere. Seizures in patients with hypertensive encephalopathy are not a primary disturbance. They typically cease with normalization of BP, making anticonvulsant therapy unnecessary.

Suggested Readings

Baumbach GL, Heistad DD. Cerebral circulation in chronic arterial hypertension. *Hypertension* 1988;12:89–95.

Faraci FM, Lamping KG, Modrick ML, et al. Cerebral vascular effects of angiotensin II: new insights from genetic models. *J Cereb Blood Flow Metab* 2006;26:449–455.

Healton EB, Brust JC, Feinfeld DA, et al. Hypertensive encephalopathy and the neurologic manifestations of malignant hypertension. *Neurology* 1982;32:127–132.

Mayhan WG, Heistad DD. Permeability of blood-brain barrier to various sized molecules. *Am J Physiol Heart Circ Physiol* 1985;17:H712–H718.

Paterno R, Heistad DD, Faraci FM. Potassium channels modulate cerebral autoregulation during acute hypertension. *Am J Physiol Heart Circ Physiol* 2000;47:H2003–H2007.

Poulet R, Gentile MT, Vecchione C, et al. Acute hypertension induces oxidative stress in brain tissues. *J Cereb Blood Flow Metab* 2006;26:253–262.

Schwartz RB, Feske SK, Polak JF, et al. Preeclampsia-Eclampsia: clinical and neuroradiographic correlates and insights into the pathogenesis of hypertensive encephalopathy. *Radiol* 2000;217:371–376.

Strandgaard S, Paulson OB. Hypertensive disease and the cerebral circulation. In: Laragh JH, Brenner, BM, eds. *Hypertension: pathophysiology, diagnosis, and management.* New York: Raven Press, 1990;399–416.

Talman WT, Nitschke Dragon D. Parasympathetic nerves influence cerebral blood flow during hypertension in rat. *Brain Res* 2000;873:145–148.

Vaughan CJ, Delanty N. Hypertensive Emergencies. *Lancet* 2000;356:411–417.

CHAPTER A68 ■ PATHOGENESIS OF MILD COGNITIVE IMPAIRMENT AND DEMENTIA

LINDA A. HERSHEY, MD, PhD

KEY POINTS

- Systolic blood pressure (BP) is a stronger predictor of future dementia than pulse pressure or diastolic pressure.
- *Mild cognitive impairment* (MCI), a transitional state between normal aging and mild dementia, occurs more frequently when BP is poorly controlled in midlife and progresses to dementia in 12% to 18% of patients with MCI each year.
- *Midlife BP elevations* predict several other brain conditions in addition to MCI, including diffuse small vessel disease (cerebral arteriolosclerosis), mesial temporal atrophy, vascular dementia (VD), and Alzheimer's disease.
- *Use of any antihypertensive medication* in midlife lowers the incidence of Alzheimer's disease in older adults; diuretic use is associated with the greatest risk reduction.

See also Chapters A66 and C153

Hypertension and cognitive decline

Several recent epidemiologic studies have shown that midlife BP elevation is a predictor for cerebral arteriosclerosis, subcortical demyelination, vascular dementia (VD), mesial temporal atrophy, mild cognitive impairment (MCI), and Alzheimer's disease (AD) in later years. Risk of dementia is proportional to systolic, diastolic, and pulse pressure but the strongest association exists for systolic BP. These findings are independent of age, educational level,

TABLE A68.1

SYMPTOMS OF MILD COGNITIVE IMPAIRMENT

- Memory complaint is present
- Memory impairment can be validated by neuropsychological tests
- Unlike dementia, other cognitive functions are normal
- Unlike dementia, independence is maintained in instrumental activities of daily living
- There are no disturbances of consciousness

TABLE A68.2

SYMPTOMS OF PROBABLE ALZHEIMER'S DISEASE

- Memory impairment is present
- There is at least one other cognitive symptom in addition to poor memory
- Cognitive losses are sufficient to interfere with some instrumental activities of daily living
- Onset of symptoms is insidious and unassociated with stroke
- Progression of cognitive impairment occurs gradually over time
- There are no disturbances of consciousness

or baseline level of cognition. Diabetes and hyperlipidemia are the other two major vascular risk factors other than hypertension (HTN) that are associated with MCI, VD, and AD. Smoking status does not appear to appreciably influence cognitive decline. The risk of cognitive deterioration and demyelination of subcortical white matter in hypertensive individuals can be reduced by normalizing BP with antihypertensive medications. A recent prospective epidemiologic study among elderly patients in Cache County, Utah, showed that potassium-sparing diuretics were more strongly associated with a reduced incidence of AD than any other class of antihypertensive medications.

Mild cognitive impairment

Mild cognitive impairment refers to a transitional state between the memory changes of normal aging and those of mild dementia (**Table A68.1**) Patients with MCI not only complain of memory problems, but they also have impaired memory function on neuropsychological tests. Nevertheless, they do not meet standard criteria for dementia (they can still perform instrumental activities of daily living such as driving, balancing a checkbook, preparing meals, shopping, and remembering to take their medicines). Both cerebrovascular disease and neurodegenerative changes can contribute to the symptoms of MCI. Positron emission tomography (PET) studies have demonstrated that patients with MCI who are at greatest risk of conversion to AD are those with bilateral hypometabolism in the inferior parietal, posterior cingulate, and mesial temporal cortices. Patients with MCI are at higher risk than normal for developing AD and other dementia illnesses (12%–18% per year become demented). New studies have shown that patients with HTN and those with the metabolic syndrome are at greater risk than normal for developing MCI. Treating HTN can delay the conversion from MCI to AD; up to 44% of patients with MCI have been shown to return to normal function in a year's time.

Alzheimer's disease

Pathogenesis. Brains from patients with "pure" AD (~45% of all dementia) show histopathologic evidence for neuronal loss, accumulation of extracellular amyloid plaques, and intracellular neurofibrillary tangles. These changes are particularly apparent in the basal forebrain, hippocampus, and amygdala. If there are any cerebral infarcts in "pure" AD brains, they are considered too small to contribute to the dementing process. On the other hand, 25% of dementia brains show evidence at autopsy of both AD and VD. The Rotterdam Study (a large population-based cohort study of older adults from the Netherlands) has demonstrated that untreated high diastolic pressure 5 years

before magnetic resonance imaging (MRI) predicts accelerated hippocampal atrophy. In a different population of older adults (the Honolulu-Asia Aging Study), elevated systolic pressure was the most significant of all BP predictors of incident dementia (either AD or VD) over a 5-year period.

Differentiating clinical symptoms. Table A68.2 outlines the clinical symptoms of probable AD. In addition to memory deficit, at least one other area of cognition (visuospatial function, executive abilities, or language function) must be impaired to support the diagnosis of AD, with limitation of at least one instrumental activity of daily living, such as managing finances, performing hobbies, preparing meals, or driving. Patients with AD do not usually have sudden onset of cognitive decline, early focal neurologic findings, gait disorders, postural instability, or urinary incontinence; these features suggest VD.

Therapy. Clinical trials have demonstrated the efficacy of cholinesterase inhibitors in treating the cognitive and behavioral changes of mild to moderate AD. These drugs include donepezil (Aricept), galantamine (Reminyl), and rivastigmine (Exelon). Agitated patients with moderate to severe stages of AD often respond to the addition of memantine (Namenda).

Vascular dementia

Pathogenesis. Brains from patients with "pure" VD (5%–10% of all dementia illnesses) show histopathologic evidence for cortical or subcortical infarcts, arteriosclerosis (small vessel disease) and subcortical demyelination. In "pure" VD, there are insufficient numbers of plaques and tangles for the brains to meet pathologic criteria for AD but 25% of brains of patients with dementia show pathologic evidence for both VD and AD. The most common form of "pure" VD, Binswanger's disease (*subcortical arteriosclerotic encephalopathy*), is strongly associated with chronic HTN. The pathologic hallmark of Binswanger's disease, medial necrosis of small penetrating arterioles, is identical to the afferent arteriolar lesions (nephrosclerosis) found in the kidneys of these same individuals. Single photon emission computed tomography (SPECT) and PET imaging studies of patients with Binswanger's disease show diffuse hypoperfusion of subcortical white matter that correlates with cognitive decline and gait instability. Demyelination of subcortical white matter is thought to be the result of chronic hypoperfusion and is represented on computed tomography (CT) by periventricular lucencies; these same areas show hyperintensity on T2-weighted images in MRI studies. Increased numbers of white matter lesions are found in individuals with postprandial hypotension. Nevertheless, in the

TABLE A68.3

SYMPTOMS OF PROBABLE VASCULAR DEMENTIA

- Memory impairment is present
- There are at least two other cognitive symptoms in addition to poor memory
- Cognitive losses are sufficient to interfere with some instrumental activities of daily living
- Onset of symptoms occurs within 3 mo of a stroke
- Progression of cognitive impairment may plateau over time
- Gait disturbances and postural unsteadiness may develop early on
- Evidence of cerebrovascular disease is present on CT or MRI

CT, computed tomography; MRI, magnetic resonance imaging.

Rotterdam study of older adults, diastolic BP correlated directly with the severity of subcortical white matter changes and inversely with cognitive performance.

Differentiating clinical symptoms. Patients with VD differ from those with AD in that they are more likely to have early gait problems, postural instability, and focal neurologic deficits. The frontal subcortical white matter changes in the brains of patients with Binswanger's disease are likely to explain the symptoms of urinary incontinence, emotional lability, depression, lower-extremity hyperreflexia, postural instability and wide-based gait. **Table A68.3** emphasizes that symptoms of VD develop more acutely than in AD but the progression of VD is more likely to plateau over time, whereas there is a progressive decline in patients with AD.

Therapy. Future strokes and the progression of dementia can be prevented in patients with VD by using antiplatelet agents (for stroke prophylaxis) and antihypertensive drugs (diastolic BP of 70-80 mm Hg). When there are signs of both VD and AD, cognitive decline may be stabilized and behavior improved with the addition of a cholinesterase inhibitor.

Suggested Readings

Anchisi D, Borroni B, Franceschi M, et al. Heterogeneity of brain glucose metabolism in mild cognitive impairment and clinical progression to Alzheimer's disease. *Arch Neurol* 2005;62:1728–1733.

Den Heijer T, Launer LJ, Prins ND, et al. Association between blood pressure, white matter lesions, and atrophy of the medial temporal lobe. *Neurology* 2005;64:263–267.

Dufouil C, deKersaint-Gilly A, Besancon V, et al. Longitudinal study of blood pressure and white matter hyperintensities. *Neurology* 2001;56:921–926.

Freitag MH, Peila R, Masaki K, et al. Midlife pulse pressure and incidence of dementia. *Stroke* 2006;37:33–37.

Gauthier S, Reisberg B, Zaudig M, et al. Mild cognitive impairment. *Lancet* 2006;367:1262–1270.

Khachaturian AS, Zandi PP, Lyketsos CG, et al. Antihypertensive medication use and incident Alzheimer's disease. *Arch Neurol* 2006;63:686–692.

Knopman D, Boland LL, Mosley T, et al. Cardiovascular risk factors and cognitive decline in middle-aged adults. *Neurology* 2001;56:42–48.

Peterson RC, Doody R, Kurz A, et al. Current concepts in mild cognitive impairment. *Arch Neurol* 2001;58:1985–1992.

Van der Flier WM, van Straaten CW, Barkhof F, et al. Small vessel disease and general cognitive function in nondisabled elderly. *Stroke* 2005;36:2116–2120.

Yaffe K, Kanaya A, Lindquist K, et al. The metabolic syndrome, inflammation, and risk of cognitive decline. *JAMA* 2004;292:2237–2242.

CHAPTER A69 ■ PATHOGENESIS OF NEPHROSCLEROSIS AND CHRONIC KIDNEY DISEASE

SHARON ANDERSON, MD

KEY POINTS

- Hypertension is both a cause and consequence of chronic kidney disease (CKD).
- Elevated glomerular capillary pressure and glomerular ischemia lead to focal glomerulosclerosis, glomerular capillary dropout, and progressive nephron loss, the pathogenetic features that underlie most forms of CKD.
- Diabetes is associated with early increases in glomerular capillary pressure, whereas greater afferent arteriolar constriction in hypertension may limit glomerular capillary pressure increases; CKD in hypertension is more commonly associated with glomerular ischemia.
- Elevated cholesterol, cigarette smoking, and hypertension act synergistically to accelerate glomerulosclerosis and CKD progression.

See also Chapters A50, A62, **B80,** C115, and C156

Progressive sclerosis of glomeruli is the final common pathway of a number of otherwise dissimilar forms of chronic kidney disease (CKD). The gross and microscopic appearance of the end-stage kidney in most forms of CKD is that of a shrunken and scarred mass of sclerotic glomeruli with tubulointerstitial fibrosis. At end stage, the initial renal insult often cannot be identified. Hypertension is integrally related to progressive CKD, and hypertensive nephrosclerosis cannot be readily distinguished from other forms of glomerulosclerosis.

Hypertension and progressive chronic kidney disease

The vicious cycle. Hypertension is a consequence of renal disease and systemic hypertension is one of the most important risk factors for progressive CKD. Previously normotensive patients usually develop systemic hypertension as renal function deteriorates. Therefore, a vicious cycle of worsening hypertension and progressive renal injury accelerates the development of end-stage renal disease (ESRD) (those requiring dialysis or transplantation) in patients with intrinsic renal disease, accelerating the age-related loss of renal function. Although hypertension may initiate renal disease, the incidence of "pure" hypertensive nephropathy, in which hypertension is the only known etiologic factor, is difficult to quantify. Often, the coexistence of hypertension and CKD leads to a presumptive diagnosis of hypertensive nephropathy although the underlying problem may be renovascular or parenchymal renal disease.

High-risk individuals. The incidence and prevalence of ESRD, presumed to be secondary to essential hypertension, are considerable (**Figure A69.1**) and are particularly high in African Americans (**Figure A69.2**). The incidence of CKD is increasing, particularly in the elderly and African American populations. The impressive reductions in morbidity and mortality from stroke and coronary artery disease resulting from modern antihypertensive therapy have not been reflected in commensurate reductions in ESRD. Although ESRD has long been recognized as a risk in patients with malignant hypertension, three large cohort studies have confirmed that more modest elevations in blood pressure (BP) can predict the remote onset of CKD and ESRD. In CKD and in diabetic nephropathy, higher waking BPs and the absence of the usual nocturnal decline in BP ("nondipping" pattern) increase the overall hypertensive burden.

Morphology of hypertensive renal injury

Malignant nephrosclerosis. Malignant nephrosclerosis is characterized by fibrinoid necrosis and myointimal hyperplasia. If left untreated, progressive renal insufficiency typically occurs. This form of renal injury is relatively uncommon in the modern era of hypertension therapy.

Nephrosclerosis. More common is a simpler form of nephrosclerosis, in which histopathologic features include microvascular changes with hyalinosis of the preglomerular vessel walls and thickening of the intima and reduplication of the internal elastic lamina of the arcuate and interlobar arteries. These changes may lead to glomerular damage, glomerulosclerosis,

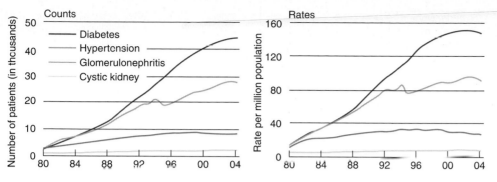

Figure A69.1 Incident rates of end-stage renal disease by primary diagnosis and first modality, adjusted for age, gender, and race. (Reproduced with permission from USRDS 2006 Annual data report: *atlas of end-stage renal disease in the United States*. National Institutes of Health, National Institute of Diabetes and Digestive and Kidney Diseases. Bethesda. Available at: http://www.usrds.org/adr_2006.htm.   Accessed on February 25, 2007.)

patchy tubular atrophy, and interstitial fibrosis. Glomerular injury is initially focal in nature and consists of tuft shrinkage with loss of cellularity. Eventually, global sclerosis occurs with accompanying atrophy and fibrosis of tubules.

Mechanisms of hypertensive renal injury

Hemodynamics and ischemia. Hypertension causes renal damage by multiple mechanisms, which may differ somewhat in various forms of renal injury. One mechanism is ischemia, with glomerular hypoperfusion causing glomerulosclerosis and subsequently tubulointerstitial fibrosis. This mechanism likely predominates in patients with renovascular hypertension and diffuse intrarenal small vessel disease, and may occur in patients with hypertensive renal disease as well. In contrast, in hypertension secondary to other forms of CKD (including diabetes), glomerular capillary hyperperfusion and hypertension (rather than ischemia) appear to be the major early pathogenetic mechanisms.

Protective role of afferent arteriolar constriction. The degree of afferent arteriolar constriction determines transmission of systemic and pulsatile pressure into the glomerular capillary network. The autoregulatory response of the normal kidney to increased perfusion pressure is an increase in afferent arteriolar (preglomerular) resistance, so that the increased systemic pressure

is not fully transmitted to the glomerulus. However, if reflex afferent arteriolar constriction is impaired by disease or drugs, increases in systemic pressure can be freely transmitted into the glomerular capillary network, resulting in glomerular capillary hypertension. Clinically, high systemic pressures with normal intraglomerular capillary pressures may explain the relatively low incidence of CKD in essential hypertension, particularly if BP elevations are minimal.

In the spontaneously hypertensive rat (SHR), despite very high systemic BP, afferent arteriolar vasoconstriction prevents excessive transmission of pressure into the glomerular capillary network, and glomerular capillary pressure (P_{GC}) remains nearly normal. Despite high pressures, renal injury is modest and late to develop. The importance of afferent arteriolar vasoconstriction in protecting the glomerular microvasculature is clearly demonstrated by uninephrectomy in the SHR, which results in lowering of afferent arteriolar resistance in the remaining kidney and elevation in P_{GC}. This latter hemodynamic alteration is associated with a large increase in proteinuria and an acceleration of glomerular sclerosis.

Afferent arteriolar dilation and glomerular capillary hypertension. Some forms of CKD are characterized by primary afferent arteriolar vasodilation and elevation of P_{GC} with coexisting systemic hypertension. This persistent afferent vasodilation can lead to glomerular hypertension, even when

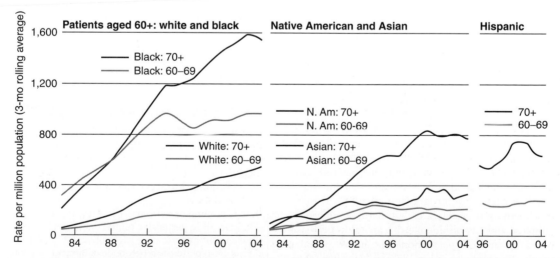

Figure A69.2 Adjusted incident rates of end-stage renal disease due to hypertension, by age and race/ethnicity: age 60+. (Reproduced with permission from USRDS 2006 Annual data report: *atlas of end-stage renal disease in the United States*. National Institutes of Health, National Institute of Diabetes and Digestive and Kidney Diseases. Bethesda. Available at: http://www.usrds.org/adr_2006.htm. Accessed on February 25, 2007.)

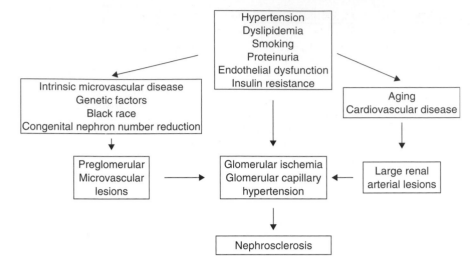

Figure A69.3 Factors influencing the development of nephrosclerosis. Initiators could be genetic, an intrinsic abnormality of preglomerular microvasculature, and/or a congenital reduction in nephron number. In the elderly, the aging process could be accelerated by concomitant cardiovascular disease and/or atherosclerotic aortorenal changes. (Adapted from Marín R, Gorostidi M, Fernández-Vega F, et al. Systemic and glomerular hypertension and progression of chronic renal disease: the dilemma of nephrosclerosis. *Kidney Int* 2005;68 (Suppl 99):S52–S56.)

systemic BP is normal, as in early diabetes. In diabetic animals with CKD, afferent and efferent arteriolar resistances are reduced. Because the reduction in afferent resistance exceeds that of efferent resistance, there is a net increase in P_{GC} and persistent glomerular capillary hypertension. Reduction of P_{GC} by dietary protein restriction or pharmacologic intervention [angiotensin-converting enzyme (ACE) inhibition or angiotensin receptor blockade (ARB)] slows the rate of loss of renal function and limits development of proteinuria and glomerulosclerosis.

Indirectly, clinical studies are consistent with the notion that afferent arteriolar vasodilation and consequent glomerular capillary hypertension are present in diabetes and other forms of progressive CKD. Increased glomerular pressures or renal plasma flow rates affect the growth and activity of glomerular component cells, inducing the elaboration or expression of cytokines and other mediators, which then stimulate mesangial matrix production and promote structural injury.

Other mechanisms of injury

Additional mechanisms of injury act in concert with high systemic and glomerular capillary pressures to accelerate glomerulosclerosis (**Figure A69.3**).

Endothelial dysfunction. Fibrinoid material is found within the glomerulus in many forms of injury, suggesting that glomerular injury is promoted by endothelial cell dysfunction, a process similar to systemic atherosclerosis. Abnormal hemodynamic stresses and intracapillary thrombosis also occur and may be triggered by endothelial dysfunction. The vascular endothelial cell is an important source of vasoactive peptides (e.g., endothelin and nitric oxide), which modulate the tone of subjacent vascular smooth muscle, affect vascular reactivity, and influence cellular injury.

Cholesterol oxidation. It is increasingly recognized that hypercholesterolemia, which is also associated with endothelial dysfunction, is a risk factor for progression of CKD. Dietary cholesterol supplementation accelerates glomerular injury in experimental animals, and hypolipidemic therapy slows disease progression. When systemic hypertension and hyperlipidemia coexist, the combination induces more glomerular injury than with either risk factor alone. It is widely postulated that reactive oxygen species contribute to glomerulosclerosis. As with atherosclerosis, oxidation of low-density lipoprotein appears to be a critical injury-promoting step.

Cigarette smoking. Epidemiologic studies confirm that cigarette smoking is a risk factor for progressive CKD, particularly in patients with diabetes. Mechanisms and risk factors relevant to atherosclerosis appear to be equally relevant to glomerulosclerosis and comparably aggravated by smoking.

Proteinuria. Elevated P_{GC} leads to enhanced traffic of macromolecules into the mesangial region and the urinary space. Increased macromolecular flux into the mesangium may stimulate the synthesis of matrix components by these cells. It has been suggested that persistent proteinuria may accelerate glomerular and tubular cell injury, consequently accelerating glomerulosclerosis. Indirect evidence in support of this notion derives from intervention trials in which antiproteinuric therapy is associated with slowing of CKD progression.

Diagnosis of hypertensive nephropathy

Several clinical features are consistent with hypertensive nephrosclerosis (**Table A69.1**) but this diagnosis can seldom be made with absolute confidence. Prospective clinical follow-up, with observed progression from normal to impaired renal function over many years, improves diagnostic accuracy. Urinalysis is helpful to exclude other conditions. A low degree of proteinuria (usually <1.5 to 2 g/day) may be found, but there should not be evidence of active renal disease (cells or casts). Recently, it has been recognized

---

TABLE A69.1

CLINICAL FEATURES CONSISTENT WITH HYPERTENSIVE NEPHROSCLEROSIS

Black race
Positive family history; onset of hypertension between ages 25 and 45 yr
Long-standing or very severe hypertension
Evidence of hypertensive retinal damage
Evidence of hypertensive left ventricular hypertrophy
Onset of hypertension before development of proteinuria
Absence of any cause for primary renal disease
Biopsy evidence: degree of glomerular ischemia and fibrosis compatible with degree of arteriolar and small arterial vascular disease

that a subset of patients (perhaps 15%) with essential hypertension exhibit microalbuminuria (e.g., >20 mg/day), which is not detectable with a standard dipstick and requires a different analytic technique. Microalbuminuria, considered to be a reflection of generalized endothelial dysfunction, predicts increased cardiovascular risk in all populations studied. However, its prognostic value in essential hypertension is not yet known, and its presence does not confirm the diagnosis of hypertensive nephropathy. Renal imaging studies are also not helpful, other than to exclude alternative causes, such as obstruction, nephrolithiasis, and renal artery stenosis. Even renal biopsy may not confirm the diagnosis because the morphologic findings are not pathognomonic. Accordingly, the diagnosis of hypertensive nephropathy is usually only presumptive, and can be made with reasonable confidence only when other causes of CKD are excluded.

Antihypertensive therapy and chronic kidney disease progression

Given that hypertension hastens loss of kidney function, aggressive antihypertensive therapy is mandatory. There is strong evidence that lowering BP slows disease- and age-related loss of renal function. The Hypertension Detection and Follow-up Program Cooperative Group and the Multiple Risk Factor Intervention Trial (MRFIT) studies found accelerated loss of renal function in patients with persistent hypertension. As outlined in the *Seventh Report of the Joint National Committee on Prevention, Detection, Evaluation, and Treatment of High BP*, CKD mandates more aggressive treatment and lower target BP: ≤130/80 mm Hg in patients with diabetes or CKD, and ≤120/75 mm Hg in patients with proteinuria >1 g per day. Patients with CKD tend to be resistant to treatment, and often require three or more antihypertensive agents to achieve goal BPs. Antihypertensive drug classes differ in their ability to lower proteinuria and slow the progression of CKD. Drugs that block the renin-angiotensin system (ACE inhibitors and ARBs) are the most potent antiproteinuric

agents and have also been shown to be highly effective in slowing the progression of CKD. As is noted in the National Kidney Foundation KDOQI Guidelines, the evidence basis supporting the preferential use of ACE inhibitors or ARBs in nonproteinuric CKD is not as strong as in patients with proteinuria, but the high cardiovascular risk in such patients makes these drugs reasonable first-line therapy. Dihydropyridine calcium antagonist–based therapy was not renoprotective in the African American Study of Kidney Disease and Hypertension (AASK) study and dihydropyridines are not generally antiproteinuric. There is controversy as to the degree to which nondihydropyridine calcium antagonists exert a favorable effect on proteinuria.

Suggested Readings

Campese VM, Mitra N, Sandee D. Hypertension in renal parenchymal disease: why is it so resistant to treatment? *Kidney Int* 2006;69:967–973.

Casas JP, Chua W, Loukogeorgakis S, et al. Effect of inhibitors of the renin-angiotensin system and other antihypertensive drugs on renal outcomes: systematic review and meta-analysis. *Lancet* 2005;366:2026–2033.

Chobanian AV, Bakris GL, Black HR, et al. Seventh report of the joint national committee on prevention, detection, evaluation, and treatment of high blood pressure (JNC 7). *Hypertension* 2003;42:1206–1252.

Marin R, Gorostidi M, Fernández-Vega F, et al. Systemic and glomerular hypertension and progression of chronic renal disease: the dilemma of nephrosclerosis. *Kidney Int* 2005;68(Suppl 99):S52–S56.

National Kidney Foundation. K/DOQI clinical practice guidelines on hypertension and antihypertensive agents in chronic kidney disease. *Am J Kidney Dis* 2004;43(Suppl 1):1–290.

Sarafidis PA, Khosla N, Bakris GL. Antihypertensive therapy in the presence of proteinuria. *Am J Kidney Dis* 2007;49:12–26.

Smith MC, Rahman M, Dunn MJ. Hypertension associated with renal parenchymal disease. In: Schrier RW, ed. *Diseases of the kidney*, 7th ed. Philadelphia: Lippincott Williams & Wilkins, 2001:1363–1397.

Textor S. Ischemic nephropathy: where are we now? *J Am Soc Nephrol* 2004;15:1974–1982.

U.S. Renal Data System. *USRDS 2006 Annual data report: atlas of end-stage renal disease in the United States*. National Institutes of Health, National Institute of Diabetes and Digestive and Kidney Diseases, Bethesda. Available at: http://www.usrds.org. Accessed on February 25, 2007.

Wiederkehr M, Toto R, Fenves AZ, et al. Hypertension and the kidney. *Semin Nephrol* 2005;25:236–245.

CHAPTER A70 ■ THE EYE IN HYPERTENSION

ROBERT N. FRANK, MD

KEY POINTS

- The three circulations of the posterior portion of the eye (retinal, choroidal, and optic nerve) are all affected by hypertension.
- Diabetes and other diseases also affect the ocular circulations, often in ways similar to hypertension.
- Clinical descriptions of ophthalmoscopic changes in hypertension are important and should include specific observations about the three ocular circulations rather than a nonspecific grade.
- Although the classic changes of severe hypertension in the retina, choroid, and optic nerve have become less common, hypertension may accelerate other retinal disease processes, including diabetic retinopathy, retinal vein occlusions, and neovascular age-related macular degeneration.

See also Chapters A61 and A62

The retina is the only tissue in the body in which blood vessels can be observed directly. Examination of the ocular fundi therefore provides an opportunity to observe the effects of hypertension in a unique vascular bed. In humans and other species with vascularized retinas, the rates of retinal glucose consumption and oxygen use are threefold higher than in any other tissue in the body. The retinal circulation is therefore highly sensitive to local tissue metabolic needs and is susceptible to damage from circulatory dysfunction.

Ocular circulations and hypertensive changes

The retina and optic nerve in humans are supplied by three circulations, all of which derive from branches of the ophthalmic artery.

Retinal circulation. The retinal circulation is composed of the central retinal artery, the central retinal vein, and their respective branches.

Normal anatomy and physiology. The central retinal artery supplies the inner retinal layers and usually divides into four principal branches at the anterior surface of the optic nerve. Anterior to the lamina cribrosa of the optic nerve head, the retinal arteries and veins have no autonomic innervation but are controlled by autoregulation in response to local metabolic signals, especially partial pressure of oxygen, partial pressure of carbon dioxide, and intraocular pressure. Tight junctions between adjoining endothelial cells in the retinal vessels form one part of the blood–retinal barrier, which strictly governs the passage of molecules into the neural tissue of the retina. Breakdown of this barrier is an important pathologic change.

Changes in hypertension. Changes in the retinal blood vessels are the most common vascular lesions of systemic hypertension in the eye. There have been a number of classifications of hypertensive retinopathy, of which the best known are those of Keith, Wagener, and Barker, first proposed in 1939 and those of Scheie proposed in 1953. Although these classifications are of historic interest, they are less useful clinically than a careful description of the lesions existent in the eye. Hypertensive retinopathy is actually a continuum, and certain types of lesions may be found in various combinations. Some lesions are relatively specific for hypertensive retinopathy [e.g., "copper wiring" of arterioles, "arteriovenous (A-V) nicking" and related crossing changes, and arterial macroaneurysms]. Other "hypertensive" lesions found in a number of disorders include the "cotton-wool spots" of diabetic retinopathy, systemic lupus erythematosus, retinal vein occlusions, and acquired immune deficiency syndrome. Flame-shaped intraretinal hemorrhages also occur in diabetic retinopathy, retinal vein occlusions, profound anemia, the leukemias, and other blood dyscrasias. Arterial "silver wiring" may occur in diabetic retinopathy, collagen-vascular diseases, and arterial occlusive diseases.

Choroidal circulation. The choroidal circulation includes the short posterior ciliary arteries and their branches in the choroid.

Normal anatomy and physiology. In humans, there are two external layers of arteries and veins and an inner layer, the choriocapillaris, which lies just outside the pigment epithelium of the retina. The portion of the choriocapillary endothelium immediately adjacent to the pigment epithelium is thin and fenestrated, and small molecules and even larger proteins readily pass in and out of these vessels. However, tight junctions connecting the cells of the retinal pigment epithelium form the second part of the blood–retinal barrier, governing the ingress of nutrient molecules and the egress of waste products. The choroidal vessels have an autonomic nerve supply that can regulate choroidal blood flow, which is substantially greater than that of the retina. The choroidal circulation supplies the retinal pigment epithelium and the photoreceptor layers of the retina, which are rich in mitochondria and are therefore responsible for the very active metabolism of the retina.

Changes in hypertension. Hypertensive choroidopathy occurs most frequently in younger individuals with acute, severe hypertensive episodes such as malignant hypertension or toxemia of pregnancy. Hypertensive changes in the choroidal vessels are observed much less frequently than hypertensive changes in the vessels of the retina. In theory, hypertensive choroidopathy occurs because the short choroidal arteries, which are most commonly affected by hypertensive changes, feed at right angles into the choroidal capillaries, allowing direct transmission of systemic blood pressure to the capillaries. Initial changes may include focal regions of choriocapillary nonperfusion owing to fibrinoid necrosis of the vessels. Clinically, this may be recognized initially only by special techniques such as intravenous fluorescein angiography. Subsequently, the retinal pigment epithelium over these nonperfused regions may develop a yellowish coloration, the Elschnig spot, which later becomes a scar with a pigmented center and an atrophic surrounding halo.

Optic nerve circulation. The third circulation is that of the optic nerve.

Normal anatomy and physiology. Anteriorly, the optic nerve circulation is composed of branches of the central retinal artery, and posteriorly of branches of the short posterior ciliary vessels and of vessels supplying the pia mater. Blood flow in these vessels is highly influenced anteriorly by the intraocular pressure and posteriorly by intracranial pressure transmitted through the subarachnoid space.

Changes in hypertension. Hypertensive changes in the optic nerve are also relatively uncommon. The principal optic nerve lesion of hypertension is disc edema (**Figure A70.1**). The cause of this lesion is unclear because, as noted earlier, the optic nerve in the orbit receives a different blood supply in its anterior and posterior portions. Some investigators believe that a combination of ischemia (caused by vascular changes and increased intraocular or intracranial pressure) and diminished axoplasmic flow in the optic nerve fibers causes hypertensive optic nerve swelling.

Ophthalmoscopy in hypertension

Arteriolar changes. Arteriolar changes are the most common manifestations of hypertensive retinopathy.

Terminology. The central retinal artery and its four major branches are commonly called *arteries,* whereas smaller branches are termed *arterioles,* irrespective of the actual microscopic anatomy. However, this terminology is not used by all writers, and anatomically, the vessels that are visible in the retina by ophthalmoscopy are arterioles.

Arteriolar diameter changes. The initial visible change in the retinal vessels in hypertension is arteriolar narrowing. The median ratio of retinal arteriolar to venular diameters in nonhypertensive individuals has recently been determined, by an elaborate digital photographic method, to be 0.84. Owing to arterial remodeling, this ratio progressively decreases with increasing mean arterial blood pressure. Progressive arteriosclerotic changes also produce an increase in the central light reflex and a decrease in the width of the blood column seen on either side of the light reflex. As these changes progress, the normally yellowish-white light reflex becomes reddish-brown, giving rise to the term *copper-wire*

change. As thickening of the wall progresses, visibility of the blood column diminishes and eventually disappears, leading to the appearance of the artery as a white thread, the silver-wire change (**Figure A70.2**). Arterial silver wiring does not always mean that the vessel is no longer perfused, because blood flow can often be demonstrated by fluorescein angiography.

Arteriovenous nicking. An additional ophthalmoscopically visible change produced in the retinal vessels by hypertension and arteriosclerosis is A-V nicking. Ocular vessels are contained in an adventitial sheath. At those points where branch arteries cross over veins, the sheaths are essentially shared. The artery with its thickened wall and increased luminal pressure, together with proliferation of perivascular glia, externally compresses the low-pressure, thin-walled vein causing a tapered or "nicked" junction. In more long-standing hypertension, the vein changes direction where the artery crosses it, producing a right-angled bend. The most serious consequence of A-V nicking is actual occlusion of the vein.

Atherosclerosis versus arteriosclerosis. Changes in the retinal arterial wall in hypertension represent true arteriosclerosis, with thickening of the wall represented histopathologically by multiple internal elastic laminae and replacement of the muscle layer by collagen. By contrast, atherosclerosis is demonstrated in the retinal vessels only when cholesterol emboli lodge in the central retinal artery or one of its branches, where they may become visible ophthalmoscopically (**Figure A70.3**).

Central vein occlusion. Central retinal vein occlusion can occur at the point where the central retinal artery and vein come in continuity with one another within the substance of the optic nerve. It is characterized by sudden, severe loss of vision and a "blood-and-thunder" fundus appearance, with dilated and tortuous veins and extensive hemorrhages in all four quadrants around the nerve head (**Figure A70.4**). Branch vein occlusion may cause vision loss if the macular portion of the retina is affected. A wedge-shaped cluster of hemorrhages, with its apex pointing at the responsible A-V crossing, is always present. The size of the hemorrhagic area is related to the size of the retinal vein affected by the occlusion. In cases where the central retinal vein bifurcates into a superior and an inferior branch (rather than the usual division into four major branches), the entire superior or inferior half of the retina may be covered by hemorrhage, a so-called hemi-retinal vein occlusion, rather than the usual wedge-shaped area of hemorrhage. After diabetic retinopathy, retinal vein occlusion is the second most common vascular disorder of the retina and is an important cause of visual loss. Although several causal factors may be involved, systemic hypertension is one of the most important.

Cotton-wool spots. Reduced blood flow produced by sclerosis or fibrinoid necrosis of small retinal arterioles may lead to regions of infarction, which eventually become evident as round to oval white patches with soft borders, the so-called cotton-wool spots, or cytoid bodies (**Figure A70.5**). Because these lesions are the result of infarction, not exudation, they should not be termed *soft exudates.*

Aneurysms. Lesions induced by excessive transmural pressure in the retinal vascular wall in hypertensive retinopathy include capillary microaneurysms and arterial (or arteriolar) macroaneurysms. Capillary microaneurysms are fusiform or berry-shaped outpouchings of the retinal capillaries. Although capillary microaneurysms are usually considered to be classic lesions of diabetic retinopathy, they may also occur in hypertensive retinopathy, in retinal vein occlusions (even in the absence of hypertension), and in the retinopathy produced by leukemias and other blood dyscrasias. Arteriolar macroaneurysms, however, are characteristic of hypertension alone. They are berry-shaped dilations of a retinal artery or arteriole (**Figure A70.6**), which may be surrounded by hemorrhage or retinal edema with a circumferential ring of lipid exudate. Although macroaneurysms are dramatic in appearance, they are usually benign in behavior, because they often thrombose spontaneously. Evidence of hemorrhage or substantial retinal edema may be indications for laser photocoagulation.

Flame hemorrhages. Hypertensive retinopathy may also lead to a breakdown in the blood–retinal barrier, as demonstrated by intraretinal hemorrhages that are often flame-shaped. In the retinopathy of malignant hypertension, there is profound leakage of plasma from the capillaries within the macula. This condition may lead to loss of vision from the resultant macular edema and to the precipitation of lipid exudate in the form of radial deposits, the so-called macular star figure surrounding the fovea at the center of the macula.

Clinical significance

The ocular lesions of systemic hypertension convey important information about the duration and severity of the hypertensive state and the efficacy of treatment. Because several of these lesions may have adverse consequences, the clinician should carefully examine the ocular fundi of all hypertensive patients as a regular part of the initial examination and at periodic follow-up visits. Individuals with suspicious regions of the fundus, acute, severe hypertensive episodes, or accelerated or malignant hypertension merit consultation with an ophthalmologist. Classic hypertensive retinopathy in its malignant stages has become less frequent owing to more effective treatment of systemic hypertension. Yet systemic hypertension remains a major contributor to several other vision-threatening ocular disorders. In addition to the risk of retinal vein occlusion, diabetic retinopathy (at least in individuals with type 2 diabetes) progresses more rapidly in individuals whose blood pressures are not controlled. Several epidemiologic studies in the United States and in Europe suggest that hypertension is a risk factor for both early and late stages of age-related macular degeneration. The Macular Photocoagulation Study, a national randomized controlled clinical trial of laser photocoagulation for the neovascular form of age-related macular degeneration, showed better outcomes in normotensive patients than in hypertensives. However, laser photocoagulation of neovascular lesions in this disease is no longer widely used, being largely supplanted by the injection of antiangiogenic drugs directly into the vitreous cavity of the eye. Although this new treatment is of demonstrated success, there is as yet no data to indicate whether the presence of systemic hypertension has any influence on the therapeutic outcome.

Suggested Readings

Age-Related Eye Disease Study Research Group. Risk factors associated with age-related macular degeneration. A case-control study in the age-related eye disease study: age-related eye Disease Study report number 3. *Ophthalmology* 2000;107:2224–2232.

The Eye Disease Case-Control Study Group. Risk factors for branch retinal vein occlusion. *Am J Ophthalmol* 1993;116:286–296.

The Eye Disease Case-Control Study Group. Risk factors for central retinal vein occlusion. *Arch Ophthalmol* 1996;114:545–554.

Frank RN. Vascular disease of retina. In: Tso MOM, ed. *Retinal diseases.* Philadelphia: JB Lippincott Co, 1987:138–164.

Hubbard LD, Brothers RJ, King WN, et al. Atherosclerosis Risk in Communities Study Group. Methods for evaluation of retinal microvascular abnormalities associated with hypertension/sclerosis in the Atherosclerosis Risk in Communities Study. *Ophthalmology* 1999;106:2269–2280.

Keith NM, Wagener HP, Barker NW. Some different types of essential hypertension: their course and prognosis. *Am J Med Sci* 1974;268:336–345.

Klein R, Peto T, Bird A, et al. The epidemiology of age-related macular degeneration. *Am J Ophthalmol* 2004;137:486–495.

Knowler WC, Bennett PH, Ballintine EJ. Increased incidence of retinopathy in diabetics with elevated blood pressure: a six-year follow-up study in Pima Indians. *N Engl J Med* 1980;302:645–650.

van Leeuwen R, Ikram MK, Vingerling JR, et al. Blood pressure, atherosclerosis, and the incidence of age-related maculopathy: the Rotterdam Study. *Invest Ophthalmol Vis Sci* 2003;44:3771–3777.

Macular Photocoagulation Study Group. Laser photocoagulation for juxtafoveal choroidal neovascularization: five-year results from randomized clinical trials. *Arch Ophthalmol* 1994;112:500–509.

Scheie HG. Evaluation of ophthalmoscopic changes of hypertension and arteriolar sclerosis. *Arch Ophthalmol* 1953;49:117–138.

UK Prospective Diabetes Study Group. Tight blood pressure control and risk of macrovascular and microvascular complications in type 2 diabetes: UKPDS 38. *BMJ* 1998;317:703–713.

Wagener HP, Clay GE, Gipner IF. Classification of retinal lesions in presence of vascular hypertension: report submitted by committee. *Trans Am Ophthalmol Soc* 1947;45:57–75.

Retinal findings in hypertension

Figures A70.1 through A70.6 are found on the back cover of the *Hypertension Primer*

Figure A70.1 (*Upper left*) Edema of the optic disc in a severely hypertensive, 20-year-old woman. Note also the markedly dilated retinal veins.

Figure A70.2 (*Upper middle*) This photograph of the ocular fundus of a 48-year-old hypertensive woman shows several of the changes associated with hypertension and arteriosclerosis. The arteries and arterioles are severely narrowed, and there are "copper-wire" (*arrowhead*) and "silver-wire" (*arrow*) changes.

Figure A70.3 (*Upper right*) This fundus photograph of a 57-year-old woman shows a cholesterol plaque lodged in a branch retinal artery (*arrowhead*). This finding is evidence of atherosclerosis.

Figure A70.4 (*Lower left*) This 74-year-old man has had a central retinal vein occlusion, as demonstrated by multiple blot and flame-shaped hemorrhages surrounding his optic nerve head in all four quadrants and extending out into the retinal periphery. Central retinal vein occlusions are usually associated with profound and irreversible loss of vision.

Figure A70.5 (*Lower middle*) Multiple cotton-wool spots (*arrowheads*) surrounding the optic nerve head of a 57-year-old hypertensive man.

Figure A70.6 (*Lower right*) A retinal arterial macroaneurysm (*arrow*) presents as a large, berry-shaped, yellowish dilation of a retinal branch artery (*arrowhead*). The lesion is surrounded by hemorrhage.

CHAPTER A71 ■ GENETICS OF HYPERTENSION

ALAN B. WEDER, MD

KEY POINTS

- Essential hypertension is a heterogeneous disease with multiple phenotypic and genotypic subtypes; each gene has only a small effect on blood pressure (BP).
- Genes are permissive; environmental factors are also necessary for hypertension to develop.
- Advances in genotyping will lead to detailed examination of the entire human genome for genes that are related to hypertension.

See also Chapters **A57, A72,** and **A73**

Genetic studies in human essential hypertension are beginning to identify specific genes contributing to the risk of developing hypertension. Progress has been driven by technical advances in genotyping and in the statistical analysis of genotype information. Major challenges remain, the most vexing being the imprecision of the phenotypes employed for most studies. The complexity inherent in all studies of multigenic diseases and the limitations of our understanding of how the environment interacts with genes to promote hypertension also remain substantial barriers.

Genetic determinants of hypertension

Polygenic versus monogenic phenotypes. Many of the diseases we typically think of as "genetic" are the result of rare mutations of single genes. In contrast, diseases such as essential hypertension are genetically complex; multiple genes influence the final observed features (phenotype) of the disease. The standard model of complex diseases assumes that the action of the multiple genes is additive, with the hypertensive phenotype resulting from the cumulative burden of susceptibility genes. The genetic variants affecting blood pressure (BP) are referred to as alleles, that is, different versions of a gene with structural differences at the DNA or RNA levels that result in differences in gene expression or protein structure.

Evolutionary aspects. Because hypertension is common worldwide, it is likely that the mutations that produced the alleles now associated with hypertension occurred in the remote past of evolutionary time; many are likely to be ancestral to early human populations in Africa. Within the African diaspora, new variants arose and were retained in the human genome either because they improved reproductive success, that is, were favored by natural selection, or by the process of genetic drift, the random preservation of variants by chance. In either case, it is likely that many of the alleles associated with hypertension are common in all populations worldwide. Therefore, much of the gene-related variation in the prevalence of hypertension between populations is the result of differences in the prevalence of those alleles, as opposed to the action of completely novel variants. This is particularly true in the modern world, where mingling of populations is the rule.

Natural selection. Natural selection did not preserve genes promoting hypertension by operating directly on BP phenotypes. As evidenced by cross-cultural observations, hypertension is the product of the interaction of genes and environment. Therefore, it is probable that in preagricultural times, there were few if any individuals with high BP. Even if hypertension existed, it probably did not affect survival enough to be a factor in natural selection because of the short life expectancies of primitive peoples. Hypertension causes some morbidity and mortality during early adulthood from complications such as preeclampsia, but in general, its adverse consequences are confined to postreproductive years, and such postreproductive diseases are not typically subject to strong natural selection. Therefore, it is likely that the genes selected improved survival in a much different environment; now those genes promote hypertension because the environment changed. Exactly what was selected is subject to debate, but the ability to conserve sodium (Na^+) and water in response to sweat losses in hot environments and the ability to conserve calories in "feast-or-famine" Paleolithic times are prime candidates for natural selection forces.

Heterogeneity of hypertension phenotypes and genotypes

Essential hypertension is a disease defined by an arbitrary division of a continuous population distribution of BP. It is widely assumed that there are numerous physiologic and biochemical mechanisms contributing to increased BP and therefore many ways to become hypertensive. From a clinical standpoint, this is not a problem, because lowering BP decreases cardiovascular risk even when an individual's specific pathophysiology is obscure. However, in the identification of candidate genes, heterogeneity is extremely troublesome; the problem is further compounded by the imprecise nature of the phenotypes used to define the syndrome.

Phenotypic heterogeneity. The most common approach to minimizing heterogeneity is to define subsets of the hypertensive population based on measurable characteristics, termed *intermediate phenotypes*, more narrowly defined than the categories of hypertension and normotension. In almost all cases, the characteristics chosen to subdivide the hypertensive population are based in pathophysiologic processes believed to contribute to the development of hypertension. The level of BP itself can be used as a quantitative phenotype or to define a subgroup such as "prehypertension." Other measures of integrated cardiovascular function, such as hemodynamics, BP reactivity to psychological tasks or dietary Na^+ loading, have been used to define physiologic subtypes. Biochemical measures, for example, plasma renin activity, or cell membrane ion transport activities, are appealing ways of identifying subgroups, because the proteins and the genes encoding them are often well known. Some characteristics used to subdivide hypertensive individuals, for example, race and sex, are problematic because they are associated with a wide spectrum of social dimensions that have nothing to do with the pathophysiology of the disease.

Genetic heterogeneity. In addition to problems created by phenotypic heterogeneity there is a parallel problem of genetic heterogeneity. All available evidence supports the theory that multiple genes contribute to hypertension, and it is very likely that each of the genes provides a small contribution to the increased BP, with the resultant hypertension representing the additive effect of many genes. In different individuals, different subsets of genes act on BP, and yet the end product, hypertension, looks the same in all. Even the rare monogenic forms of hypertension would look alike if BP is the only criterion considered; the differences are in the other phenotypic features of the diseases. Genetic heterogeneity creates major problems for gene discovery, because in any population, no matter how carefully characterized for BP, many genotypes will contribute to BP elevation. Unfortunately, current gene discovery methods depend on detecting relationships between the transmission of genetic markers and phenotypes (hypertension) from generation to generation. This approach is seriously compromised by the presence of multiple sets of genes.

Population characteristics. One strategy that has helped to identify disease-related genes is studying populations of limited genetic diversity. Such populations are usually geographically or culturally isolated, with the result that genes contributing to a particular disease are fewer than those found in outbred populations and are therefore more amenable to identification by family-based strategies. Some, although not all, genes identified in such studies also have variants involved in the same disease in other populations.

Genetic background. Genes do not operate in isolation, and we are only beginning to grapple with the issue of how the rest of the genome, the genetic background, affects the action of genes involved in the predisposition to hypertension. Gene–gene interactions (known as *epistasis*), along with protein–protein interactions affect cellular, organ system, and whole-organism physiologic phenotypes, and genetic background effects will become an increasingly important problem as we try to translate allelic differences to pathophysiologic processes (**Figure A71.1**).

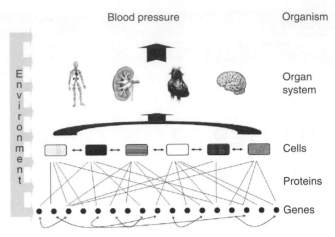

Figure A71.1 Genes that predispose to hypertension operate within a hierarchically ordered biological system. At each level, new properties emerge that were not predicted simply from the features of the levels below. Within the genome, gene–gene epistatic interactions modify the effects of individual alleles. Many cell types share multiple proteins; some gene products are unique to particular cells. At higher levels, organ systems have specialized functions (e.g., the cardiovascular system). Hypertension is the result of an increase in the set point of BP regulation about which the system functions. Environmental influences impact each level and modify the functions of genes, proteins, cells and organs to promote hypertension.

Strategies for genetic studies

Despite these difficulties, there has been real progress in identifying genetic determinants of human hypertension using two complementary strategies.

Genetic linkage. On the basis of observations dating back a century, many traits tend to be genetically transmitted together. This phenomenon is referred to as *genetic linkage* and forms the basis for gene identification in large multigenerational pedigrees (family-based linkage) and in populations (linkage disequilibrium mapping). The latter strategy has been widely adopted in recent hypertension studies and has allowed identification of numerous chromosomal regions likely to harbor genetic variants affecting BP.

Linkage disequilibrium mapping takes advantage of the fact that during the first phase of meiosis, after DNA strands are duplicated, sister chromatids can exchange segments to create new combinations of genetic variants. This process, known as *recombination* or *crossing-over*, is rare during any single meiosis, but over human evolutionary history it has occurred frequently. Since these new combinations are passed on to the offspring of successful matings, they are subject to natural selection and can therefore be preserved in future generations.

By genotyping any of several types of DNA variations of known location on the genome, "markers" are identified. By tracking how markers and phenotypes are passed from parents to offspring, it is possible to identify which genomic regions travel together with hypertension. Typing of additional markers further narrows the regions of interest, which are presumed to harbor genes predisposing to hypertension. Eventually, if small enough regions are identified, specific genes can be identified and their variants identified by sequencing.

Gene associations. The second major strategy for gene discovery, the association study, is appropriate once specific genes are identified, either by linkage or simply by choosing known genes based on *a priori* knowledge of gene function. Association studies are relatively straightforward and in simplest form involve comparisons of allelic variant frequencies in a case–control design.

Association studies can be confounded by both phenotypic heterogeneity and background effects as well as by population genetic stratification. This latter problem usually results from the mixing of two populations that differ in disease prevalence and the frequencies of multiple alleles, the vast majority of which have nothing to do with the disease. When cases and controls are identified, the two subpopulations may not be equally represented in each group, resulting in spurious associations of the disease with alleles not related to the problem under study.

Despite these drawbacks, association studies have the considerable appeal of directly identifying genetic variants causing disease. Recent advances in high-throughput genotyping and statistical methods for analyzing huge amounts of genetic information are rapidly shifting gene discovery from linkage-based to association approaches.

Genetic mapping: the HapMap project

The bellwether of the current era is the HapMap project, which is constructing a map of the human genome anchored by the positions of millions of single base pair variants, referred to as single nucleotide polymorphisms (SNPs). This map will be much more detailed than any whole-genome map previously created and will allow delineation of the genomic substructure created by the numerous meiotic recombination events that have occurred throughout human history.

Our genome is a mosaic of "blocks" of DNA spanning the intervals between recombination sites. These blocks have considerable conserved nucleotide sequence shared within and between populations. Because most of the DNA sequence in a block is the same in any two individuals, blocks can be characterized by the relatively small set of SNPs that differ. Unlike SNPs, these sets can be grouped into haplotypes, strings of SNPs representing their relative map locations in the genome. By comparing haplotypes in a case–control design, very small regions, often limited to as few as one gene, can be identified and examined for genetic variants associated with hypertension.

Although the technical and computational challenges to this "whole-genome association" approach are daunting, it is clear that sufficient progress is being achieved that its application to diseases such as hypertension will soon be feasible. One great advantage of the whole-genome approach is that once haplotypes have been defined in an individual, any number of phenotypes can be examined for association with other markers.

Characterizing genetic variants

Gene discovery is only the first step in proving that a gene causes hypertension. Once identified, genetic variants must be studied for associations with phenotypes. This involves epidemiologic studies of populations, either in case-controlled or interventional trials. Because of the potential problems related to population stratification and environmental differences, it is critical to confirm that an association in one population of a gene variant and disease can be generalized to other populations. Multiple population studies also yield estimates of the frequency of alleles in different groups, which may help to explain observed differences in disease frequency. Once a gene is known to be associated with a disease, case-controlled studies can be used to address its relationship to intermediate phenotypes, which may reveal relevant pathophysiologic pathways. Similarly, comparing the responses to interventions between groups defined by genotypes can reveal the importance of environmental factors, for example, Na$^+$ intake, in promoting disease. Finally, identification of genes may suggest targets for pharmacologic interventions.

Clinical impact

One of the great promises of understanding the genetics of hypertension is the possibility of developing individualized therapeutic approaches for patients or preventive strategies for those at risk to develop hypertension. Coupled with a better understanding of the genetic determinants of target organ susceptibility, it is possible that we may eventually be able to achieve much better outcomes than are currently possible. Fulfilling the promise of genetic studies will probably require systems analysis, an approach that has only recently been applied to genetic data.

Suggested Readings

Burton PR, Tobin MD, Hopper JL. Key concepts in genetic epidemiology. *Lancet* 2005;366:941–951.

Cooper RS. Gene-environment interactions and the etiology of common complex disease. *Ann Intern Med* 2003;139:437–440.

Meneton P, Jeunemaitre X, De Wardener HE, et al. Links between dietary salt intake, renal salt handling, blood pressure, and cardiovascular diseases. *Physiol Rev* 2005;85:679–715.

Tanira M, Balushi K. Genetic variations related to hypertension: a review. *J Hum Hypertens* 2005;19:7–19.

Teare MD, Barrett JH. Genetic linkage studies. *Lancet* 2005;366:1036–1044.

Turner ST, Boerwinkle E. Genetics of blood pressure, hypertensive complications, and antihypertensive drug responses. *Pharmacogenomics* 2003;4(1):53–65.

Weder AB. Pathogenesis of hypertension: genetic and environmental factors. In: Hollenberg NJ, Braunwald E, eds. *Atlas of hypertension*, 5th ed. Philadelphia: Current Medicine Group LLC, 2005:1–38.

CHAPTER A72 ■ MONOGENIC DETERMINANTS OF BLOOD PRESSURE

ROBERT G. DLUHY, MD

KEY POINTS

■ Monogenic (single-gene) forms of human hypertension involve gain-of-function mutations that result in overproduction of mineralocorticoids or increased mineralocorticoid activity.

■ Clinical phenotypes usually include severe hypertension from birth, apparent volume expansion, suppression of plasma-renin activity, and variable hypokalemia.

■ Autosomal dominant and recessive renal salt-wasting syndromes result from loss-of-function mutations in the renin-angiotensin system or renal ion transporters, with blood pressure (BP) dependent on intake of dietary sodium.

See also Chapters A19, A20, A70, and A73

Progress has recently been made in identifying the genetic mutations of Mendelian (single-gene) forms of human hypertension. The great majority of these monogenic hypertensive syndromes result in excessive renal sodium (Na^+) retention that arises from mutations in genes causing gain-of-function changes in transporters in the distal nephron or in components of the renin-angiotensin-aldosterone system (RAAS) (**Table A72.1**). Such genetic syndromes can be divided into (a) overproduction of mineralocorticoids, as with glucocorticoid-remediable aldosteronism (GRA), or (b) increased mineralocorticoid activity. Identification of these mutated genes has also permitted targeted antihypertensive therapies. Mendelian pheochromocytoma syndromes are also well known.

Mineralocorticoid overproduction

Glucocorticoid-remediable aldosteronism. GRA, an autosomal dominant disorder characterized by moderate to severe hypertension in affected patients from birth onward, is the most common form of monogenic human hypertension. Because most patients with GRA are not hypokalemic, serum potassium (K^+) lacks sensitivity as a screening test for this disorder. Early hemorrhagic stroke (mean age, 32 years) is characteristic of GRA pedigrees. In a recent study, 48% of all GRA pedigrees and 18% of all GRA patients sustained cerebrovascular complications.

In GRA, aldosterone secretion is positively and solely regulated by adrenocorticotropic hormone (ACTH), not by angiotensin II or K^+. As a consequence, exogenous low-dose glucocorticoid administration (which potently suppresses ACTH) profoundly suppresses aldosterone secretion in affected subjects, reversing

the syndrome. As in other causes of primary aldosteronism, plasma-renin levels are suppressed.

Aldosterone synthase gene duplication. Genetic analysis of GRA kindreds has revealed linkage of GRA to a mutation in the aldosterone synthase gene, which is closely related to steroid 11β-hydroxylase, a second gene involved in adrenal steroidogenesis. Both genes are 95% identical in DNA sequence, have identical intron–exon structures, and are located in close proximity on chromosome 8. In all GRA kindreds, affected subjects have two normal copies of genes encoding aldosterone synthase and 11β-hydroxylase. In addition, they have a novel gene duplication: a hybrid, or chimeric, gene duplication where the 5′ regulatory sequence conferring ACTH responsiveness of 11β-hydroxylase is fused to more distal coding sequences of aldosterone synthase. The result is an unequal crossing-over between these two homologous genes (**Figure A72.1A**).

In GRA kindreds, the crossover sites are variable, indicating that in different pedigrees, the gene duplications arise independently rather than from a single ancestral mutation. In addition, the crossover sites are all upstream of exon 5 of aldosterone synthase, suggesting that encoded amino acids in exon 5 are essential for aldosterone synthase enzymatic functions (**Figure A72.1B**).

The gene duplication appears to explain all of the known physiologic and biochemical features previously reported in GRA. First, the promoter region of this chimeric gene contains regulatory sequences of 11β-hydroxylase and is regulated by ACTH. In addition, the chimeric gene allows ectopic expression of aldosterone synthase enzymatic activity in the ACTH-regulated zona fasciculata, which normally secretes only cortisol. Finally, the sole regulation of aldosterone secretion by ACTH and the suppression of aldosterone secretion by glucocorticoids in GRA is explained

TABLE A72.1

MONOGENIC FORMS OF HUMAN HYPERTENSION

Disorder	Site of alteration in kidney or renin-angiotensin-aldosterone system	Genes mutated
Glucocorticoid-remediable aldosteronism	Adrenal (aldosterone)	Aldosterone synthase
11β-Hydroxylase, 17α-hydroxylase deficiencies	Adrenal (mineralocorticoids)	CYP11B1; CYP17
Hypertension exacerbated in pregnancy	Renal (MR)	MR
Liddle's syndrome	Renal epithelial Na$^+$ channel (ENaC)	β or γ subunit of ENaC genes
Syndrome of apparent mineralocorticoid excess	Renal (MR)	11β-Hydroxysteroid dehydrogenase (renal isoform) gene
Pseudohypoaldosteronism type II	Renal (distal nephron)	WNK kinases (WNK 1, WNK 4)

MR, mineralocorticoid receptor; ENaC, amiloride-sensitive epithelial sodium channel; WNK, with-no-lysine kinase.

by the fact that the aldosterone synthase gene is abnormally regulated by ACTH promoter sequences.

Direct genetic screening for the presence of the gene duplication in GRA is 100% sensitive and specific for diagnosing GRA and is recommended for patients with primary aldosteronism without radiographic evidence of tumors, for young hypertensive individuals with suppressed levels of plasma-renin activity (especially children), and for at-risk individuals in affected families.

Directed treatments with low-dose glucocorticoids, amiloride, or spironolactone effectively treats the elevated blood pressure (BP) of GRA.

Disorders of steroid hormone biosynthesis (congenital adrenal hyperplasia). Various abnormalities of hydroxylase enzymes of the P450 class have been identified. These include C21, C17, and C11 hydroxylases, which are important steps in steroidogenesis. Disordered volume regulation and hypertension

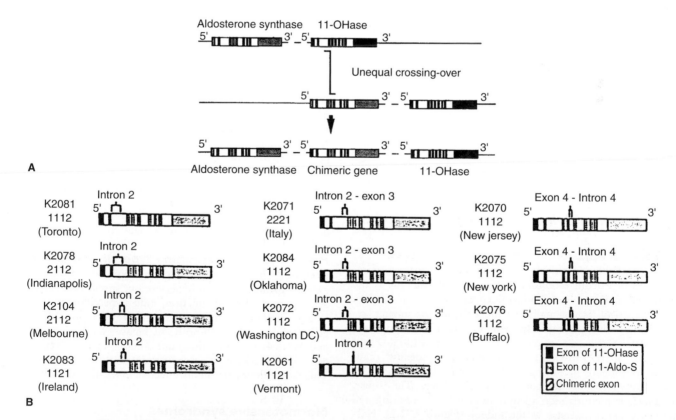

Figure A72.1 A: The chimeric gene duplication in glucocorticoid-remediable aldosteronism, a result of unequal crossing-over between the homologous 11β-hydroxylase and aldosterone synthase genes. The chimera fuses the 5′-regulatory sequences of the 11β-hydroxylase gene and the 3′-coding sequences of the aldosterone synthase gene. **B:** Crossover breakpoints in 11 glucocorticoid-remediable aldosteronism pedigrees. The sites of crossing-over are all upstream of exon 5 of aldosterone synthase. (From Lifton RP, Dluhy RG, Powers M, et al. Hereditary hypertension caused by chimeric gene duplications and ectopic expression of aldosterone synthase. *Nat Genet* 1992;2:66–74, with permission.)

are usually not the presenting symptoms in most patients with congenital adrenal hyperplasia (CAH). Rather, excessive androgenic effects in female patients or hypogonadism in male patients are more characteristic of the clinical phenotypes. 21-Hydroxylase deficiency, resulting from a mutated gene that encodes P450C21 and accounts for >90% of the CAH genetic disorders, is not associated with hypertension but rather with sodium (Na^+) wasting in the severe clinical variant presenting in childhood.

P450C11β deficiency. P450C11β deficiency causes a hypertensive variant of CAH, in which hypertension and hypokalemia variably occur because impaired conversion of 11-deoxycorticosterone to corticosterone results in the accumulation of 11-deoxycorticosterone, a potent mineralocorticoid. Increased shunting into the androgen pathway leads to ambiguous external genitalia at birth in girls (female pseudohermaphroditism) or hirsutism, virilization, or both in girls in the postnatal period. P450C11β deficiency is an uncommon cause of CAH in individuals of European ancestry but accounts for 15% of cases in Moslem and Jewish Middle Eastern populations. Mutations causing P450C11β deficiency cluster in exons 6 to 8 of the CYP11B1 gene.

P450C17α deficiency. P450C17α deficiency is characterized by hypogonadism, hypokalemia, and hypertension. This rare disorder causes decreased production of cortisol and shunting of precursors into the mineralocorticoid pathway; usually, 11-deoxycorticosterone production is elevated. Because P450C17α hydroxylation is required for biosynthesis of adrenal and gonadal testosterone and estrogen, this defect is associated with sexual immaturity, high urinary gonadotropin levels, and low urinary 17-ketosteroid excretion. Female patients have primary amenorrhea and lack of development of secondary sexual characteristics. Because of deficient androgen production, male patients have either ambiguous external genitalia or a female phenotype (male pseudohermaphroditism). A large number of random mutations can cause 17α-hydroxylase deficiency, making genetic diagnosis difficult.

Exogenous glucocorticoids can correct the hypertensive syndrome and treatment with appropriate gonadal steroids results in sexual maturation.

Hypertension with increased mineralocorticoid activity

Syndrome of apparent mineralocorticoid excess.

In vitro, cortisol and aldosterone are potent activators of renal mineralocorticoid receptors (MRs). Yet, aldosterone is the primary regulator of renal mineralocorticoid activity *in vivo*, because cortisol is normally excluded from occupying renal MRs by the enzyme 11β-hydroxysteroid dehydrogenase (11β-HSD). There are two isoforms of the 11β-HSD enzyme. The first, 11β-HSD1, is nicotinamide adenine dinucleotide phosphate–preferring and active primarily as a reductase of cortisone to cortisol in the liver. The other, 11β-HSD2, is nicotinamide adenine dinucleotide–requiring and active as a dehydrogenase in the kidney (**Figure A72.2**). Normally, cortisol is metabolized to biologically inactive cortisone by 11β-HSD2 in the kidney, a feature that "protects" the MR from activation by cortisol. In states of 11β-HSD deficiency, the enzyme deficiency allows cortisol to reach and activate the type I renal MR, causing sodium retention and suppression of the RAAS. The syndrome of apparent mineralocorticoid excess (AME) occurs as

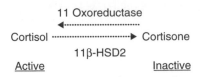

Glucocorticoid shuttle

Figure A72.2 The glucocorticoid shuttle whereby the two isoforms of the 11β-hydroxysteroid dehydrogenase (11β-HSD) enzyme act as a reductase in the liver (cortisone to cortisol, 11β-HSD1) or a dehydrogenase in the kidney (11β-HSD2).

an autosomal recessive (AR) disorder and is the result of mutations in the gene coding for the kidney-specific isoform 11β-HSD2.

Patients with congenital or acquired (licorice-ingestion) AME syndrome characteristically exhibit an increased ratio of cortisol to cortisone metabolites in the urine. The plasma half-life of cortisol is also prolonged in patients with AME.

Liddle's syndrome.
Liddle's syndrome, a rare autosomal dominant disorder with variable penetrance, is characterized by hypertension, excessive Na^+ retention, hypokalemia (usually), and low plasma-renin activity. Aldosterone levels are undetectable, and antagonism of the MR with spironolactone has no effect on BP or serum K^+. The defect in Liddle's syndrome results from constitutive activation of amiloride-sensitive epithelial Na^+ channels (ENaC) on distal renal tubules, which causes excess Na^+ reabsorption. This channel is composed of at least three subunits and is normally regulated by aldosterone. The mutations causing Liddle's syndrome have been localized to genes on chromosome 16 that encode the β and γ subunits of ENaC. These gain-of-function mutations prolong the half-life of ENaC at the renal distal tubule apical cell surface, resulting in increased channel number.

The syndrome is ameliorated by amiloride, which blocks Na^+ reabsorption and K^+ excretion by MR-independent mechanisms.

Activating mutations of the mineralocorticoid receptor.
An autosomal dominant mutation in the ligand-binding portion of the MR results in its activation by steroids lacking 21-hydroxyl groups, including progesterone and spironolactone. Normally spironolactone and progesterone are antagonists for the MR. Affected women exhibit early-onset hypertension that is exacerbated during pregnancy. Hypertension is accelerated during pregnancy by the elevated progesterone levels of the gravid state.

Pseudohypoaldosteronism type II (Gordon's syndrome).
The phenotype of pseudohypoaldosteronism type II patients includes familial hypertension, suppressed plasma-renin activity, normal renal function, mild hyperchloremic metabolic acidosis, and impaired potassium and H^+ excretion. Mutations in genes encoding the with-no-lysine kinase (WNK) family (WNK1 and WNK4) of serine-threonine kinases in the distal nephron cause overactivity of the thiazide-sensitive Na, Cl cotransporter. Thiazide diuretics are highly effective in treating this disorder.

Normotensive syndromes

A diverse group of loss-of-function mutations in ENaC, MR, and in renal tubule ion transporters results in Na^+ wasting and a tendency to hypotension unless compensated by a high Na^+ intake. Potassium levels are low or elevated depending on whether the mineralocorticoid activity of the elevated aldosterone levels is expressed (**Table A72.2**).

TABLE A72.2

LOSS-OF-FUNCTION MUTATIONS WITH RENAL SALT WASTING

Disorder status	Genes mutated	Potassium[a]
Autosomal dominant pseudohypoaldosteronism type I	Mineralocorticoid receptor	Hyperkalemia[a]
Autosomal recessive (AR) pseudohypoaldosteronism type I	Sodium epithelial channel	Hyperkalemia
Gitelman's syndrome (AR)	Thiazide-sensitive Na^+– Cl^- cotransporter in distal convoluted tubule	Hypokalemia[a]
Bartter's syndrome (AR)	Ion transporters in thick ascending loop of Henle	Hypokalemia

AR, autosomal recessive inheritance.
[a]In all of these disorders, aldosterone levels are markedly elevated as a result of activation of the renin-angiotensin system owing to salt wasting, but in the pseudohypoaldosteronism type I syndromes, increased mineralocorticoid action is blocked owing to loss-of-function mutations of the mineralocorticoid receptor and sodium epithelial channel.

Disorder of sympathetic regulation and pheochromocytoma syndromes

Hereditary brachydactyly and autosomal dominant hypertension. Affected individuals usually die of stroke before 50 years of age. The responsible gene is unknown but affected individuals exhibit severely impaired baroreflexes and a looping vessel in the posterior cerebral circulation that has been postulated to cause neurovascular compression of the sympathetic nervous control centers in the ventrolateral medulla. The RAAS is normal in this disorder.

Pheochromocytoma syndromes. Mendelian syndromes are seen in approximately 30% of patients with pheochromocytoma, including MEN2, von Hippel-Lindau disease, neurofibromatosis, and the paraganglioma syndromes, where mutations in succinate dehydrogenase subunits have been identified.

Suggested Readings

Curnow KM, Slutsker L, Vitek J, et al. Mutations in the CYP11β 1 gene causing congenital adrenal hyperplasia and hypertension cluster in exons 6, 7, and 8. *Proc Natl Acad Sci U S A* 1993;90:4552–4556.

Funder JW, Pearce PT, Smith R, et al. Mineralocorticoid action: target tissue specificity is enzyme, not receptor, mediated. *Science* 1988;242:583–585.

Geller DS, Farhi A, Pinkerton N, et al. Activating mineralocorticoid receptor mutation in hypertension exacerbated by pregnancy. *Science* 2000;289:119–123.

Lifton RP. Molecular genetics of human blood pressure variation. *Science* 1996;272:676–680.

Lifton RP, Dluhy RG, Powers M, et al. A chimeric 11β-hydroxylase/aldosterone synthase gene causes glucocorticoid-remediable aldosteronism and human hypertension. *Nature* 1992a;355:262–265.

Lifton RP, Dluhy RG, Powers M, et al. Hereditary hypertension caused by chimeric gene duplications and ectopic expression of aldosterone synthase. *Nat Genet* 1992b;2:66–74.

Luft FC. Mendelian forms of human hypertension and mechanisms of disease. *Clin Med Res* 2003;1:291–300.

Mune F, Rogerson FM, Nikkila H, et al. Human hypertension is caused by mutations in the kidney isozyme of 11β-hydroxysteroid dehydrogenase. *Nat Genet* 1995;10:394–399.

Shimkets RA, Warnock DG, Bositis CM, et al. Liddle's syndrome: heritable human hypertension caused by mutations in the β subunit of the epithelial sodium channel. *Cell* 1994;79:407–414.

Wilson FH, Disse-Nicodeme S, Choate KA, et al. Human hypertension caused by mutations in WNK kinases. *Science* 2001;293:1107–1112.

Yanase T, Simpson ER, Waterman MR. 17α-Hydroxylase/17,20 lyase deficiency: from clinical investigation to molecular definition. *Endocr Rev* 1991;12:91–108.

CHAPTER A73 ■ HERITABILITY OF HYPERTENSION AND TARGET ORGAN DAMAGE

DONNA K. ARNETT, PhD, MSPH

KEY POINTS

■ Hypertension and blood pressure (BP) levels aggregate in families, suggesting a genetic component.
■ Target organ damage to the heart and kidney is heritable, independent of hypertension.
■ Quantitative markers such as left ventricular (LV) mass and measures of cardiac and renal function are useful intermediate phenotypes for determining the genetic basis of the complex BP/hypertension phenotype.
■ Integrating findings from multiple studies suggest that regions on chromosomes 2, 3, 6, 16, and 17 may contain influential genes contributing to variation in BP-related phenotypes.

See also Chapters A71 and A72

Blood pressure (BP) and hypertensive target organ damage have a measurable genetic component, yet the identity of hypertension genes and the characteristics of the DNA variation within those genes are largely unknown. Multiple genetic pathways and environmental factors influence BP and its sequelae. This complexity provides a significant challenge to localizing genes with major effects on BP regulation that thereafter may affect target organ damage. Still, several genomic regions have been identified that are linked with BP and its consequences.

HYPERTENSION HERITABILITY

Familial aggregation

Family history. Family history of hypertension is a simple and commonly used index of familial aggregation. First-degree relatives of hypertensive persons are at a twofold greater risk of hypertension than the general population. This risk increases to fourfold when two or more family members have hypertension.

Both race and age strongly influence the risk of hypertension, and both interact with family history. For example, in blacks, parental history of hypertension confers a ninefold increased risk of hypertension. The strength of association between family history and incidence of hypertension is also dependent on the age of onset of hypertension in the family member and the age of the individual at risk for hypertension. An early parental history of hypertension (before age 60 years) invokes a greater risk of hypertension in offspring. Having two parents with hypertension before age 60 years increases the odds of hypertension to 5.3 in women and 7.8 in men. The older the individual, the less the impact of a positive family history of hypertension; at age older

than 70 years, the risk associated with a positive family history is equal to the risk of hypertension in the general population.

Correlation and heritability. Genetic correlation (the interdependence of relatedness and a given trait) and heritability (the proportion of a trait's variation that has a familial basis) are more sophisticated measures of familial aggregation of BP. Within-family correlation coefficients for systolic BP range from 0.15 to 0.60 across family studies; diastolic BP follows a similar pattern, with correlation coefficients ranging from 0.3 to 0.6. The correlation coefficient for sibling pairs (generally between 0.4 and 0.6) is higher than for parent–offspring pairs (generally ~0.2). Among monozygotic twins, the correlation for systolic and diastolic BP approaches 0.7. The overall heritability of BP estimated from family studies is approximately 20% compared to the 60% observed in twin studies.

Genes versus environment. Inferences regarding the role of genetics in family aggregation of BP are problematic because the shared genetic information within a family is confounded by the shared family environment. Studies incorporating measures of BP in spouses sharing similar environments often report small but significant spousal correlation. In fact, the spousal-pair correlation is quite similar to that of parent–offspring pairs (0.05 to 0.2 for systolic BP and 0.3 for diastolic BP). This finding supports the idea that the shared family environment also contributes to the BP level. A powerful method to assess the unique contribution of the genetic control of BP is to measure families with both natural and adopted children. There is a much stronger sibling correlation in natural compared to adoptive siblings. Likewise, the parent–natural child BP correlations are stronger than those observed in parents and adoptive children, suggesting the observed familial correlation of BP is at least partially determined by shared genes.

Chromosomal linkages to hypertension

To date, only rare monogenic mutations have been conclusively identified as causes of hypertension; all share a relationship to altered salt homeostasis and sodium-retaining steroids. Some progress has been achieved in identification of specific chromosomal regions or candidate genes for essential hypertension, leading researchers to speculate that multiple interactions among genes and environments contribute to the prevalence of hypertension in populations. Given the number of intermediate phenotypes that probably contribute to the overall hypertensive phenotype, variation in a multitude of genes and chromosomes can be expected.

Linkage studies have identified regions on all chromosomes that may contribute to BP-related traits but certain genomic regions appear to be most closely involved as determined from meta-analyses across multiple studies, populations, and ethnic groups. Table A73.1 summarizes regions showing suggestive or significant evidence of linkage for BP-related phenotypes in two or more meta-analyses. Using existing biological knowledge of gene and protein function, candidate genes around linkage regions can be identified and further scrutinized.

TARGET ORGAN DAMAGE HERITABILITY

Familial aggregation studies

Hypertension is associated with damage to the heart, kidney, and brain. Yet not all hypertensive persons manifest target organ damage and the damage appears to be more severe in some individuals. Understanding the genetic susceptibility to the target organ effects of hypertension is therefore a matter of intense interest.

Left ventricular hypertrophy and related cardiac phenotypes. There is considerable between-person variation in the response of the heart to hypertension. At equal BP levels, some individuals develop left ventricular hypertrophy (LVH), whereas others do not, suggesting a genetic susceptibility to its expression. LVH has a prevalence that ranges from 22% to 60% in hypertensive individuals. Within-family correlations of LV mass in first-degree relatives range from 0.05 to 0.44. Data from twin and cohort studies report LV mass heritability to be 22% to 70%, independent of body size, BP, gender, and age. The

heritabilities of LV functional and structural phenotypes are also high (Table A73.2).

Chronic kidney disease (CKD). Renal disease is a complex phenotype that is both a cause and consequence of hypertension. Sustained elevations in BP cause nephrosclerosis and glomerulosclerosis through hypertrophy, hyalinization, and sclerosis of the walls of the preglomerular (afferent) arterioles. Hemodynamic alterations in the kidney before the onset of hypertension also affect pressure-natriuresis relationships, thereby providing an additional mechanism for raising BP.

A growing body of evidence in humans and animal models supports the influence of genetic factors in the complex mechanisms affecting renal damage and suggests that the genetic basis for hypertensive nephropathy results from the interaction of BP genes and genes unique to renal damage. Familial aggregation of end-stage renal disease (ESRD) is observed in blacks and whites. Having one first-degree relative with renal disease increases the odds of ESRD by 1.3; having two or more affected first-degree relatives increases the odds of ESRD by 10.4. Cohort studies report the heritability of kidney function phenotypes to be 17%

TABLE A73.2

HERITABILITY ESTIMATES OF LEFT VENTRICULAR (LV) STRUCTURAL AND FUNCTIONAL TRAITS EVALUATED IN HYPERTENSIVE SIBLING PAIRS

LV structural measures	Blacks	Whites
LV mass	0.70	0.26
Relative wall thickness	0.23	0.45
Posterior wall thickness	0.27	0.39
LV internal dimension	0.60	0.37
Aortic root diameter	0.62	0.41
LV systolic functional measures		
Stress-corrected mid-wall shortening	0.31	0.26
Fractional shortening	0.24	0.30
LV diastolic filling indices		
Mitral E wave	0.56	0.75
Mitral A wave	0.60	0.66
Isovolumic relaxation time	0.28	0.30

TABLE A73.1

CHROMOSOMAL REGIONS SHOWING SUGGESTIVE OR SIGNIFICANT EVIDENCE OF LINKAGE FOR BLOOD PRESSURE (BP)-RELATED PHENOTYPES IN TWO OR MORE META-ANALYSES

Phenotype(s)	Race/ethnicity	Region	Candidate genes near region
HT, DBP, HT + SBP[a], HT + DBP	White	2p12-q22.1	ADRA2B, SLC9A2
HT, SBP, HT + SBP	Black + White	2p14-p13.1	ADD2, SLC4A5, ADRA2B,
HT, SBP, HT + SBP	Mixed	2p23.2-p12	ADD2, SLC8A1,
HT, DBP, HT + SBP[a], HT + DBP[a]	White	3p14.1-q12.3	CADPS, GPR15, GPR27
HT, HT + SBP	Mixed	6q25.3-qter	MAS1, LPA
DBP, HT + SBP, HT + DBP[a]	White	16p13-q12.2	SAH, SLC12A3, SCNN1G
HT[a], HT + DBP	Mixed	17p12-q21.33	NOS2A, HYT1

Candidate genes were identified on the basis of linkage evidence and existing biological knowledge of gene and protein function and can be targeted in future investigations
HT, hypertension; SBP, systolic blood pressure; DBP, diastolic blood pressure; +, compound phenotype.
[a]Phenotypes were suggestive or significant in all meta-analyses reporting linkage in the region.

to 75%, independent of effects of covariates such as age, body mass, and BP.

Chromosomal linkages

Left ventricular hypertrophy and related cardiac phenotypes. The genetic architecture of LV hypertrophy is likely structured by three separate pathways: genes that exert pleiotropic effects on hypertension and LV mass; genes that cause hypertension that, in turn, cause LVH; and unique LVH genes. Genetic mutations in sarcomeric proteins lead to severe, monogenic forms of hypertrophy. However, there is little information about the genetic contribution to the common, less severe form of LVH that occurs in most individuals with hypertrophy. Nevertheless, certain genomic regions on chromosomes 1, 4, 7, 9, 10, and 12 appear to contribute to LVH and related phenotypes. Variants of the angiotensin-converting enzyme (ACE), NOS3, GNB3, angiotensinogen (AGT), and other genes have been associated with particular LV phenotypes.

Chronic kidney disease. Evidence linking approximately 30 chromosomal regions to kidney function has been published. Unfortunately, very few of these findings have been replicated. Several studies have suggested variation in candidate genes, such as KLK1, IL2RA, IL15RA, are associated with renal disease.

Suggested Readings

Arnett DK, Devereux RB, Kitzman D, et al. Linkage of left ventricular contractility to chromosome 11 in humans: The HyperGEN Study. *Hypertension* 2001;38:767–772.

Arnett DK, Hong Y, Bella IN, et al. Sibling correlation of left ventricular mass and geometry in hypertensive African-Americans and whites: the HyperGEN study. Hypertension Genetic Epidemiology Network. *Am J Hypertens* 2001;14:1226–1230.

Doris P. Hypertension genetics, single nucleotide polymorphisms, and the common disease: common variant hypothesis. *Hypertension* 2002;39:323–331.

Freedman BI, Bowden DW. The role of genetic factors in the development of end-stage renal disease. *Curr Opin Nephrol Hypertens* 1995;4:230–234.

Leon JM, Freedman BI, Miller MB, et al. Genome scan of glomerular filtration rate and albuminuria: the HyperGEN study. *Nephrol Dial Transplant* 2006;22:763–771.

Levy D, DeStefano AL, Larson MG, et al. Evidence for a gene influencing blood pressure on chromosome 17. Genome scan linkage results for longitudinal blood pressure phenotypes in subjects from the Framingham Heart Study. *Hypertension* 2000;36:477–483.

Lifton RP, Gharavi AG, Geller DS. Molecular mechanisms of human hypertension. *Cell* 2001;104:545–556.

Mein CA, Caulfield MJ, Dobson RJ, et al. Genetics of essential hypertension. *Hum Mol Genet* 2004;13:R169–R175.

Thomas J, Semenya K, Neser WB, et al. Parental hypertension as a predictor of hypertension in black physicians: the Meharry Cohort Study. *J Natl Med Assoc* 1990;82:409–412.

Wu X, Kan D, Province M, et al. An updated meta-analysis of genome scans for hypertension and blood pressure in the NHLBI Family Blood Pressure Program (FBPP). *Am J Hypertens* 2006;19:122–127.

CHAPTER B74 ■ GEOGRAPHIC PATTERNS OF HYPERTENSION: A GLOBAL PERSPECTIVE

RICHARD S. COOPER, MD AND BAMIDELE TAYO, PhD

KEY POINTS

- Geographic patterns of hypertension primarily reflect the level of economic and social development, as mediated by local cultural practice, rather than climate or natural phenomena.
- Mass migrations over the last century demonstrate that the role of intrinsic (genetic) susceptibility is clearly secondary to social conditions.
- Interpreting cross-cultural variation in blood pressure (BP) is inherently difficult, given the problems of standardizing survey methods and the overlay of ethnicity and social factors.
- The primary determinants of geographic variation in hypertension that have been quantified are obesity, sodium, and fat intake.

See also Chapter **B75**

Hypertension accounts for 6% of adult deaths worldwide and is common to all human populations except those few thousand individuals surviving in cultural isolation. Unlike coronary heart disease, for which studies of "geographic pathology" were so instructive about the underlying cause, regional variation in blood pressure (BP) remains poorly understood. Global influences, such as a temperature gradient leading away from the equator, have been suggested, but BP patterns are determined primarily by social and cultural factors at the local level.

Population variation in blood pressure

Substantial problems confront attempts to sort out causal processes that determine BP variation among population groups. These include lack of standardization of BP measurements, potential bias introduced by variable treatment rates, and potential confounding effects of age. Despite these obvious problems, it is surprising that no databases exist that summarize in a standardized manner the prevalence of hypertension in the international context.

Genes versus environment

The interaction of race, ethnicity, and environmental factors has further limited our ability to extract meaningful etiologic insights. At the very least, mass migrations over the last century have demonstrated that the role of intrinsic (genetic) susceptibility is clearly secondary to social conditions. Several of the putative factors that lead to hypertension are also extremely difficult to measure, particularly physical activity and psychosocial stress.

Patterns of variation

Nonindustrialized societies. Populations can be separated into groups at four levels of risk (**Table B74.1**). Only a handful of "no hypertension" societies still exist, primarily confined to the Amazon basin. In these groups, BP does not rise with age and perhaps declines from age 18 years onward, following the pattern assumed to be "normal" for our species. In other regions of the tropics where subsistence agriculture remains the way of life, mean systolic pressure rises <10 mm Hg over the life course, and hypertension does occur. Moderate rates of hypertension also

TABLE B74.1

CATEGORIES OF HYPERTENSION PREVALENCE IN POPULATIONS

Category	Exemplary groups	Prevalence, %[a]
Absent	Yanomami, Xingu	0
Low	Rural Africa and South China	7–15
Usual	Europe, U.S. whites, Japan	15–30
High	U.S. blacks, Russia, Finland	30–40

[a]Assumes a population structure with even distribution among 10-year age groups from 25 to 74 years.

characterize most parts of Asia and the Indian subcontinent, with the notable exception of Korea and Japan where rates appear to be higher.

Industrialized societies. National survey data are available from only a small number of industrialized countries and lack of standardization makes comparisons difficult. The excess burden imposed by hypertension on U.S. blacks is well recognized. Surprisingly, however, little attention has been given to similar observations in Slavic countries and Finland. Local surveys, as well as a major U.S.–U.S.S.R. cooperative study that used a standardized methodology demonstrate virtually identical levels of BP and hypertension prevalence among Finns, Russians, Poles, and U.S. blacks. Recent analyses suggest that most people in European countries have BPs that are higher than those reported in North America (**Figure B74.1**). Hypertension at these levels has also been reported from northern rural areas in Japan. In these societies, the high prevalence of hypertension has been attributed to a high intake of sodium or of alcohol. Cardiovascular sequelae occur at similarly high rates among all these groups.

Latitude. At the global level, a north–south hypertension gradient is apparent, although this most likely reflects parallel economic and industrial development. Increasing hypertension with distance from the equator has also been documented in China. The cause is unlikely to be climate or temperature, given the reverse pattern in the United States.

United States. Geographic variation within the United States is limited. The primary exception has always been the rural South, particularly the Southeast, where during the 1950s and 1960s, both blacks and whites were found to have higher BPs than in other parts of the country. The regional variation in BP has left an indelible imprint on rates of cardiovascular disease. Specifically, migrants from the South carry with them a substantial excess risk. Although available survey data lack direct comparability, it appears that BP levels have declined in the United States over the last 3 decades and that this secular trend may have been most prominent in the rural South. No obvious amelioration of risk factors can explain this phenomenon, and for obesity the trends are in the opposite direction.

Role of covariation in risk factors

Geographic patterns in hypertension are modestly influenced by the overall variation in risk factors across the spectrum of economic development and specific local conditions. The high-fat diet of Finland and Russia, for example, has been suggested to be the cause of the exceptionally high prevalence of hypertension in that region. Blacks share the excess risk associated with lower socioeconomic status in industrialized societies and are exposed to additional psychosocial stressors. Given these complex patterns, it is virtually impossible to isolate variation in genetic predisposition across groups.

Intrinsic (genetic) factors have often been postulated as the cause of higher BPs among blacks. From the global perspective, however, populations of African origin are predominantly at low risk, given the level of economic development in most of Africa and the Caribbean. The recent International Collaborative Study on Hypertension in Blacks (ICSHIB) documents the wide variation in hypertension prevalence across the course of the African diaspora. Body mass index, a measure of obesity and a proxy for the industrialized lifestyle, is virtually colinear with hypertension prevalence in community samples from rural West Africa, the Caribbean, and the United States (**Figure B74.2**). A similar gradient in sodium and potassium intake exists across these populations, and, as shown by the International Study of Salt and Blood Pressure (INTERSALT), also explains some of

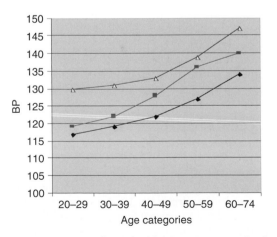

Figure B74.1 Comparison of systolic blood pressure—results from the Health Survey for England, 1998 and from the third National Health and Nutrition Examination Survey from 1991 in the United States. BP, blood pressure; ♦, U.S. white men; ■, U.S. black men; △, English men.

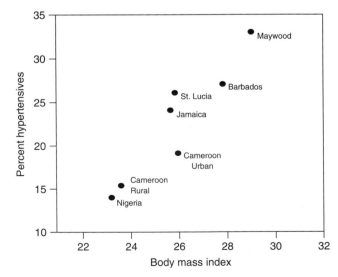

Figure B74.2 Prevalence of hypertension by body mass index in seven populations of the African diaspora.

the population variance. Factors that remain unaccounted for are psychosocial stressors and the direct effect of physical activity. Local variation among ethnic groups within a society may reflect various combinations of these risk factors.

Suggested Readings

Cooper R, Rotimi C, Ataman S, et al. The prevalence of hypertension in seven populations of West African origin. *Am J Public Health* 1997;87:160–168.

McDonough R, Garrison GE, Hames CG. Blood pressure and hypertensive disease among negroes and whites in Evans County, Georgia. In: Stamler J, Stamler R, Pullman TN, eds. *The epidemiology of hypertension.* New York: Grune & Stratton, 1967:167–187.

People's Republic of China–United States Cardiovascular and Cardiopulmonary Epidemiology Research Group. An epidemiological study of cardiovascular and cardiopulmonary disease risk factors in four populations in the People's Republic of China. *Circulation* 1992;85:1083–1096.

Primatesta P, Brooks M, Poulter NR. Improved hypertension management and control: results from the health survey for England 1998. *Hypertension* 2001;38:827–832.

Tyroler HA, Gasunov IS, Deev AD. *A Comparison of high blood pressure prevalence and treatment status in selected US and USSR populations.* First joint US-USSR symposium on hypertension. Bethesda: National Institutes of Health Dept. of Health, Education, and Welfare, 1972; Publication 79–1272.

Wolf-Maier K, Cooper RS, Banegas JR, et al. Hypertension and blood pressure level in six European countries, Canada and the US. *JAMA* 2003;289:2363–2369.

CHAPTER B75 ■ GEOGRAPHIC PATTERNS OF HYPERTENSION IN THE UNITED STATES

GEORGE A. MENSAH, MD

KEY POINTS

- Hypertension prevalence, associated stroke mortality, and all-cause mortality vary in a geographic pattern and are higher in the Southeast than in other regions of the United States.
- Contributors to this pattern include geographic variations in obesity, physical inactivity, and salt and nutritional intake, but not in hypertension treatment or control.
- Regional and within-state variation in income and other socioeconomic determinants may also contribute to geographic variation in stroke morbidity and mortality.
- Geography and race are confounded; as a result, some of the excess mortality attributed to race is instead a factor of geographic variation.
- The Stroke Belt includes states with stroke mortality >10% above the national mean; 10 of 11 states in the Stroke Belt are in the southeastern United States.

See also Chapter B74

There are important regional differences in the prevalence and impact of hypertension and its complications, especially stroke.

Geographic patterns of hypertension prevalence, incidence, and severity

Regions of the United States that feature prominently in discussions of geographic variation in hypertension include the South, Southeast, Stroke Belt, and the Stroke Belt "buckle". As used in this chapter, the South includes Alabama, Arkansas, Delaware, District of Columbia, Florida, Georgia, Kentucky, Louisiana, Maryland, Mississippi, North Carolina, Oklahoma, South Carolina, Tennessee, Virginia, and Texas. The Southeast includes the District of Columbia and all the states in the South as defined in the preceding text excluding Texas and Oklahoma. The Stroke Belt, defined as states with stroke mortality >10% above the national mean in 1990, originally included Alabama, Arkansas, Georgia, Indiana, Kentucky, Louisiana, Mississippi, North Carolina, South Carolina, Tennessee, and Virginia. The Stroke Belt "buckle" includes the coastal plain region of North Carolina, South Carolina, and Georgia.

The prevalence of hypertension in noninstitutionalized adults is higher in the South than in other regions of the United States (**Table B75.1**). Additionally, among hypertensive patients, the level of systolic blood pressure (BP) and the prevalence of severe hypertension are higher in the South than in other U.S. regions. Self-reported prevalence of hypertension in adults is also higher across the southeastern states. In 2005, 12 of the 15 highest ranked states for self-reported prevalence of hypertension were located in

TABLE B75.1

HYPERTENSION PREVALENCE AND MEAN SYSTOLIC BLOOD PRESSURE IN PERSONS AGED 40 TO 59 YEARS, BY RACE/ETHNICITY AND GENDER, NHANES-III, 1988–1994

Race/ethnicity	Hypertension prevalence, %			Systolic BP, mm Hg		
	South	Non-South	p	South	Non-South	p
Black women	45.6	39.4	.094	129.8	128.3	.376
Black men	44.1	36.7	.050	133.0	129.7	.033
Non-Hispanic white women	21.4	19.8	.617	120.6	119.6	.402
Non-Hispanic white men	33.1	23.0	.012	127.3	123.6	.002

(Source of data: Obisesan TO, Vargas CM, Gillum RF. Geographic variation in stroke risk in the United States. Region, urbanization, and hypertension in the Third National Health and Nutrition Examination Survey *Stroke* 2000;31:19–25.)

the South (**Figure B75.1**). In fact, with the exception of Texas, all 16 states and the District of Columbia in the South region had self-reported prevalence of hypertension ≥26.5% whereas only 4 of 34 states outside the South exceeded this prevalence. Analysis by geographic region and level of urbanization shows a statistically significant interaction in some, but not all racial/ethnic-gender groups. The 7-year incidence of elevated BP among young adults is also highest in the Stroke Belt and is most markedly so for black men, but is consistent for all race/sex groups.

Geographic patterns of hypertension-related morbidity and mortality

Circulatory diseases. Analysis of hospitalizations for circulatory diseases shows that geographic variation is highest for

hypertension. In 2000, hospitalization for hypertension in adults aged 18 years and older was significantly higher in the South than in the Northeast (57 vs. 44 per 100,000 population, *p* < .05) and was almost twice as high as in the West (57 vs. 29 per 100,000 population, *p* < .05). Hypertension-related target-organ damage, such as stroke, end-stage renal disease, and chronic heart failure, and other associated morbidity and mortality are also higher in the South than in other U.S. regions.

Stroke morbidity and mortality. Hypertension is the most common preventable cause of stroke and stroke mortality in adults. Of the 11 states that comprised the Stroke Belt, as defined in 1990, all the States except Indiana were in the Southeast. Among the ten highest ranked states for stroke mortality in 2003, all but one (Oregon) are in the South. Children in Stroke Belt states also have a higher risk of death from stroke than children

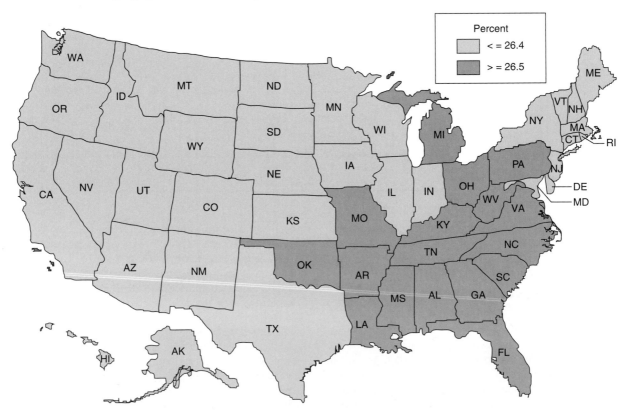

Figure B75.1 Percentage of adults aged 18 years and older who had been told they had high blood pressure (BP). (Source of data: Behavioral Risk Factor Surveillance System, 2005; www.cdc.gov/brfss.)

in other U.S. states, although regional variations in risk factors other than hypertension are suspected as contributory.

End-stage renal disease. End-stage renal disease and associated mortality are higher in the Southeast than other parts of the United States. Hypertension and diabetes are the two leading causes of end-stage renal disease; therefore, regional differences in hypertension prevalence and severity contribute to the variation in this disease.

Heart failure. Chronic heart failure, an important sequela of hypertension, is also more prevalent, and leads to more hospitalizations in the southern United States than in other regions. For example, in 2000, hospitalization for heart failure in adults aged 18 years and older was highest in the South and was approximately 65% higher than the rate in the West (603 vs. 366 per 100,000 persons).

All-cause mortality. During an average of 21 years of follow-up of 10,367 male hypertensive veterans (47% black), the 21-year mortality was higher for those who resided in the Stroke Belt; the unadjusted risk ratio of 1.27 was unchanged after adjustment for age, race, and BP. This finding confirmed the previously reported increased all-cause mortality in this cohort after a 15-year follow-up.

Contributors to hypertension prevalence and organ damage

Important regional differences in dietary patterns, lifestyle and behavioral choices, socioeconomic status (SES), income level, cultural factors, neighborhood characteristics, access to care, and response to antihypertensive medications may contribute to the observed differences in hypertension prevalence, related target-organ damage, hypertension-related mortality, and all-cause mortality.

Dietary patterns. Dietary patterns that may increase hypertension prevalence and associated morbidity include high sodium and low potassium consumption. Although no regional differences have been observed in the frequency of "adding salt on the table," the highest overall sodium consumption has been reported for the South. The lowest consumption of potassium, calcium, phosphorus, magnesium, copper, riboflavin, niacin, iron, and vitamins A, C, and B_6 has also been observed in the South. These dietary patterns are believed to contribute to the high prevalence of hypertension and associated cardiovascular complications not only in the Stroke Belt but also across the South.

Low birth weight. Although the precise pathophysiologic mechanisms are incompletely understood, low birth weight is associated with increased risk of hypertension and its associated renal and cardiovascular complications. Significant regional variation in low birth weight has been observed and tends to be higher in the "Deep South" (Mississippi, Louisiana, Arkansas, Tennessee, Alabama, Georgia, North Carolina, South Carolina, and Florida) than in other regions of the United States. In 2000, the South had the most low birth weights (62 per 100,000 neonates) whereas the West had the fewest (49 per 100,000 neonates).

Socioeconomic status. Studies in the 1970s, before the widespread implementation of high BP awareness and treatment programs, showed substantial inverse associations between hypertension and low SES, especially in the Southeast. Recent data suggest that low SES is not a major independent contributor to the excess hypertension prevalence and related mortality in the Southeast. In New York State, however, one study has shown that income is a nonlinear predictor of excess stroke and that income

alone explains a significant amount of the geographic variance in stroke prevalence within the state.

Geographic patterns in hypertension awareness, treatment, and control

Studies in the early 1960s and 1970s suggested that although hypertension awareness was good in the Southeast, treatment and control were poor. More recent data, however, show little regional difference in hypertension awareness and suggest treatment and control of hypertension may actually be better in the Stroke Belt states than elsewhere in the United States. For example, in the Reasons for Geographic And Racial Differences in Stroke (REGARDS) study, a national population-based longitudinal cohort of adult black and white men and women aged >45 years that began recruiting in 2003, hypertension awareness and treatment of aware persons did not differ between Stroke Belt and non–Stroke Belt states (**Figure B75.2**). However, control of hypertension in treated patients was significantly better in the Stroke Belt states (67.8% vs. 64.2%, $p = .0039$). These findings were unchanged after adjustment for demographic, socioeconomic, or risk factor measures.

Overall, there have been dramatic improvements in hypertension awareness and treatment in the United States over the last 3 to 4 decades in all regions, in both men and women, and in both black and white Americans, accompanied by important reductions in stroke mortality. Two additional points deserve emphasis. First, the excess morbidity and mortality associated with hypertension in the Southeast is preventable, and reinforces calls for increased national and regional efforts for the prevention and control of hypertension and associated risk factors. Second, elimination of regional differences in hypertension awareness, treatment and control does not necessarily imply concordant elimination in racial disparities. Black participants in REGARDS were more aware than whites of their hypertension and more likely to be on treatment when aware of their diagnosis but less likely than whites to have their BP controlled. As the REGARDS investigators correctly pointed out, continued efforts in the prevention and control of high BP in all patients, and especially among black patients, may play an important role in reducing excess morbidity and mortality associated with hypertension. It may

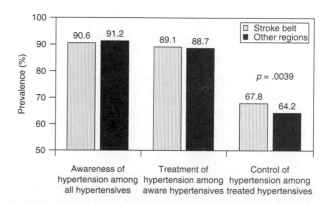

Figure B75.2 Prevalence of awareness, treatment, and control of hypertension in the Stroke Belt and other U.S. regions, the Reasons for Geographic And Racial Differences in Stroke (REGARDS). (Source of data: Howard G, Prineas R, Moy C, et al. Racial and geographic differences in awareness, treatment, and control of hypertension; the reasons for geographic and racial differences in stroke study. *Stroke* 2006;37:1171–1178.)

also contribute to the elimination of racial and ethnic disparities in health, an overarching goal of Healthy People 2010.

Importance of confounding in interpretation of geographic patterns

Confounding in geography and race is well established. Therefore, some of the excess mortality attributed to race is instead a factor of geographic variation. Similarly, low birth weight, which varies geographically, contributes to the regional variation in hypertension prevalence and severity as well as to regional variation in hypertension-related organ damage, such as renal disease. Hence, analyses of regional variation in hypertension and its independent contribution to regional variations in morbidity and mortality require cautious interpretation.

Suggested Readings

Fullerton HJ, Elkins JS, Johnston SC. Pediatric stroke belt: geographic variation in stroke mortality in US children. *Stroke* 2004;35(7):1570–1573.

Hajjar I, Kotchen T. Regional variations of BP in the United States are associated with regional variations in dietary intakes: the NHANES-III data. *J Nutr* 2003;133(1):211–214.

Han D, Carrow SS, Rogerson PA, et al. Geographical variation of cerebrovascular disease in New York State: the correlation with income. *Int J Health Geogr* 2005;4:25.

Howard G, Prineas R, Moy C, et al. Racial and geographic differences in awareness, treatment, and control of hypertension: the Reasons for geographic and racial differences in stroke study. *Stroke* 2006;37(5):1171–1178.

Kiefe CI, Williams OD, Bild DE, et al. Regional disparities in the incidence of elevated BP among young adults: the CARDIA study. *Circulation* 1997;96(4):1082–1088.

Kovesdy CP. Regional mortality differences in end-stage renal disease: how far can observational studies take us? *Kidney Int* 2007;71(1):11–12.

Kruzikas DT, Jiang HJ, Remus D, et al. *Preventable hospitalizations: a window into primary and preventive care, 2000.* Bethesda: Agency for Healthcare Research and Quality, 2004.

Lackland DT, Bendall HE, Osmond C, et al. Low birth weights contribute to high rates of early-onset chronic renal failure in the Southeastern United States. *Arch Intern Med* 2000;160(10):1472–1476.

Obisesan TO, Vargas CM, Gillum RF. Geographic variation in stroke risk in the United States. Region, urbanization, and hypertension in the Third National Health and Nutrition Examination Survey. *Stroke* 2000;31(1):19–25.

Ong KL, Cheung BM, Man YB, et al. Prevalence, awareness, treatment, and control of hypertension among United States adults 1999–2004. *Hypertension* 2007;49(1):69–75.

Yang D, Howard G, Coffey CS, et al. The confounding of race and geography: how much of the excess stroke mortality among African Americans is explained by geography? *Neuroepidemiology* 2004;23(3):118–122.

CHAPTER B76 ■ CARDIOVASCULAR RISK FACTORS AND HYPERTENSION

WILLIAM B. KANNEL, MD, MPH AND PETER W.F. WILSON, MD

KEY POINTS

- Hypertension generally doubles the risk of cardiovascular diseases (CVDs), of which coronary disease is the most common and lethal.
- Systolic and diastolic pressure are associated with a stepwise increase in cardiovascular events, even within the high-normal range.
- Elevated systolic blood pressure (BP) is strongly associated with CVD even in the presence of normal diastolic BP; high pulse pressure further enhances systolic pressure risk.
- Hypertension is usually accompanied by other risk factors and risk of CVD varies with the burden of associated risk factors.

See also Chapters **B77**, **B78**, and **B79**

Hypertension is an established risk factor for all clinical manifestations of atherosclerosis. It is a common and powerful independent predisposing factor for development of coronary heart disease (CHD), strokes, peripheral artery disease, and heart failure. The high prevalence of this condition, its powerful independent impact on the incidence of cardiovascular disease (CVD), and its controllability justify giving it a high priority for its detection and treatment.

Blood pressure and atherosclerotic hazards

Atherogenic CVD sequelae promoted by hypertension occur at a two- to fourfold increased rate compared with same-aged normotensive persons. Although the risk ratio it imposes is greatest for heart failure and least for coronary disease, CHD is the most common hazard of hypertension because of its greater prevalence in the general population. (**Table B76.1**).

TABLE B76.1

RISK OF CARDIOVASCULAR EVENTS IN SUBJECTS WITH HYPERTENSION: 36-YEAR FOLLOW-UP IN FRAMINGHAM HEART STUDY PARTICIPANTS 35 TO 64 YEARS OLD

Cardiovascular events	Age-adjusted biennial Rate per 1,000			Age-adjusted Excess Risk ratio per 1,000			
	Men	Women	Men	Women	Men	Women	
Coronary disease	45	21	2.0[a]	2.2[a]	23	12	
Stroke	12	6	3.8[a]	2.6[a]	9	4	
Peripheral artery disease	10	7	2.0[a]	3.7[a]	5	5	
Cardiac failure	14	6	4.0[a]	3.0[a]	10	4	
Cardiovascular events	65	35	2.2[a]	2.5[a]	36	21	

[a] $p < .001$.

In early trials, the lower-than-expected efficacy of antihypertensive therapy for prevention of CHD led to unjustified doubt about the etiologic role of hypertension in development of CHD. However, risk of all clinical manifestations of CHD is related to the severity of antecedent hypertension in population-based investigations. Blood pressure (BP) is critical in atherogenesis because atherosclerosis occurs less commonly in low-pressure segments of the circulation, such as the pulmonary vessels or systemic veins. Also, animal experiments indicate that lipid-induced atherogenesis can be accelerated or retarded by raising or lowering BP.

Elevated BP is related to development of CVD in a continuous graded manner, with no indication of a critical value. CVD mortality doubles with each 20/10 mm Hg increment in BP. CVD incidence increases with each increment in BP, even within the high-normal range (**Figure B76.1**). As compared with normal BP, high-normal (130–139/85–89 mm Hg) pressure is associated with a 2.5- and 1.6-fold hazard of CVD in women and men respectively. Stage 1 hypertension and even prehypertension, are substantial contributors to atherosclerotic CVD, and because they are so much more prevalent than severe stages of hypertension a large proportion of the CVD attributable to elevated BP derives from this seemingly innocuous elevation of BP.

Blood pressure components

Comparison of the impacts of systolic and diastolic BP components gives no indication of a greater influence of the diastolic BP for any sequela of hypertension. In fact, isolated systolic hypertension (systolic BP $\geq$140 mm Hg and diastolic BP <90 mm Hg) has been shown to be hazardous, particularly in the elderly (**Figure B76.2**).

Age and blood pressure components. With increasing age there is a gradual shift from diastolic to systolic BP and then to pulse pressure as dominant predictors of CHD. Only in those younger than 50 years is diastolic BP a stronger predictor. Systolic hypertension is a persistent risk factor even taking arterial compliance into account. Treatment of elevated systolic BP, whether isolated or accompanied by elevated diastolic BP, greatly reduces the risk of CVD. Overreliance on diastolic BP to assess hypertensive risk is misleading, particularly in advanced age when the predominant type of hypertension is of the isolated systolic variety. After age 60 diastolic BP is inversely related to CHD so that pulse pressure also predicts CVD in older persons. The relative importance of pulse pressure versus systolic BP is uncertain.

Low diastolic blood pressure (wide pulse pressure). Low diastolic BP has been alleged to impose an excess risk of CVD, impeding vigorous treatment of hypertension. However, most investigations incriminating low diastolic BP have not taken systolic pressure and pulse pressure into account and have (inappropriately) used or included all-cause mortality as the outcome. The Framingham Study found that in persons initially free of CVD, the upturn in CVD incidence at low diastolic BP is largely confined to persons with increased systolic pressure (**Figure B76.3**). While ignoring systolic BP, fatal and nonfatal CVD incidence increases with each increment in diastolic BP in both sexes.

An increasing tendency for a J-curve relation of CVD incidence to diastolic BP emerges with successive increments in accompanying systolic BP. In both sexes, a statistically significant excess of CVD events is observed at low diastolic BPs (<80 mm Hg) only when accompanied by an elevated systolic BP (>140 mm Hg) even after adjustment for age and associated CVD risk factors. The excess of CVD noted at low diastolic BP is therefore attributable to elevated pulse pressure. Persons with isolated systolic hypertension or increased pulse pressure have been shown to benefit from antihypertensive treatment.

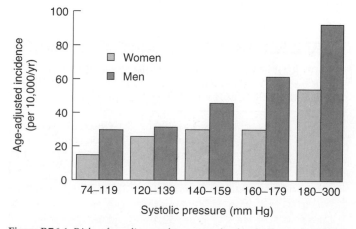

Figure B76.1 Risk of cardiovascular events by level of systolic blood pressure: 38-year follow-up for Framingham subjects aged 65 to 94 years.

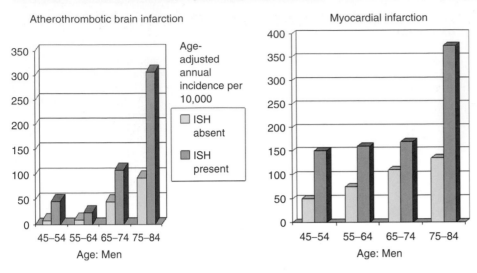

Framingham study 24-yr follow-up

Figure B76.2 Risk of myocardial infarction and stroke in isolated systolic hypertension (ISH). (Reproduced with permission from Kannel WB. Hypertension as a risk factor for cardiac events—epidemiologic results of long-term studies. *J Cardiovasc Pharmacol* 1993;21(Suppl 2):S27–S37.)

Risk factor clustering

Hypertension seldom occurs in isolation from other CVD risk factors; rather, it tends to occur in association with other atherogenic factors that promote its occurrence and greatly influence its CVD impact.

Population occurrences. Hypertension appears to be metabolically linked to dyslipidemia, glucose intolerance, abdominal obesity, hyperinsulinemia, and hyperuricemia, among others. Investigation of risk factor clustering with hypertension by the Framingham Study indicated that hypertension occurs in isolation less than 20% of the time; clusters of two or three major risk factors with hypertension occurs approximately 50% of the time, a rate twice that expected by chance (**Table B76.2**). Approximately 63% of CHD in hypertensive Framingham Study participants occurred in men with two or more additional risk factors. Hence, in evaluating patients with elevated BP, it is imperative that other atherogenic risk factors be anticipated and evaluated. This is important because the hypertensive risk of CVD varies widely depending on the burden of associated risk factors (**Figure B76.4**). The risk of coronary events in hypertensive

Framingham Study participants increased with the amount of risk factor clustering; 39% of the coronary events in men with elevated BP were attributable to having two or more additional risk factors.

Risk factor interactions. The influence of risk factor clustering is particularly important in stage 1 hypertension, where the average risk is modest, requiring that many be treated to prevent one CVD event. The same cluster of atherogenic risk factors that often accompanies hypertension also influences the hazard of developing a stroke, peripheral artery disease, or heart failure. Atrial fibrillation, CHD, and left ventricular hypertrophy (LVH) also play an important role in hypertensive stroke risk. For hypertensive heart failure candidates, CHD, heart murmurs, cardiomegaly, a low vital capacity, and a rapid heart rate are the additional risk factors. A rapid resting heart rate is more common in persons with hypertension and also predisposes to its occurrence. Hypertension associated with a rapid resting heart rate has a higher CVD mortality. A rapid resting heart rate, low vital capacity, proteinuria, LVH, and silent myocardial infarction often signify organ damage in hypertension and escalate a hypertensive person's risk of developing overt CVD by two- to threefold.

Determinants of clustering. Postulated causes of metabolic clustering of hypertension with dyslipidemia, glucose intolerance, hyperinsulinemia, obesity, LVH, and hyperuricemia include

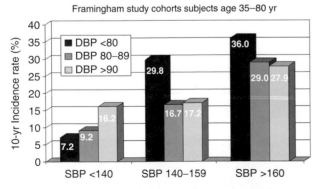

Figure B76.3 Systolic–diastolic blood pressure interactions in predicting cardiovascular disease (CVD). In adults aged 35 to 80, low diastolic blood pressure (DBP) predicts risk only in those with systolic blood pressure (SBP) >140 mm Hg. (Reproduced with permission from Kannel WB, Wilson PWF, Nam B-H, et al. A likely explanation for the J-curve of BP cardiovascular risk. *Am J Cardiol* 2004;94:380–384.)

TABLE B76.2

NUMBER OF OTHER RISK FACTORS: FRAMINGHAM HEART STUDY OFFSPRING WITH ELEVATED BLOOD PRESSURE IN SUBJECTS 18 TO 65 YEARS OLD

Number of risk factors	Percentage with risk factors		Observed/expected ratio	
	Men (%)	Women (%)	Men	Women
0	24.4	19.5	0.74	0.59
1	29.1	28.1	0.71	0.69
≥2	46.5	52.4	1.8	2.01

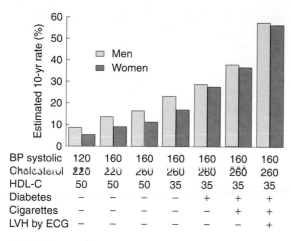

Figure B76.4 Estimated 10-year coronary heart disease risk in a hypothetical 55-year-old adult according to levels of various factors. BP, blood pressure; HDL-C, high-density lipoprotein cholesterol; LVH, left ventricular hypertrophy; ECG, electrocardiogram.

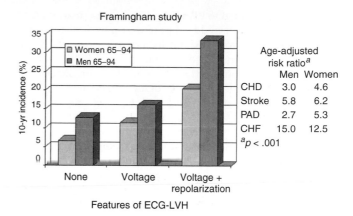

Figure B76.5 Risk of cardiovascular disease (CVD) in hypertension by features of ECG-left ventricular hypertrophy. CHD, coronary heart disease; PAD, peripheral artery disease; CHF, congestive heart failure; ECG, electrocardiogram. (Kannel WB. Cardiovascular risk in the hypertensive patient. In Hollenberg N, ed. *Atlas of Hypertension. Current Medicine.* Philadelphia, Pa, 2004;111–130.)

insulin resistance and sympathetic neuronal overactivity. Abdominal obesity promotes this syndrome in hypertensive persons. In the Framingham Study the tendency for these atherogenic traits to cluster with elevated BP was found to increase stepwise with the degree of obesity and the amount of weight gained on follow-up (**Table B76.3**). A 5-lb weight increase in hypertensive persons was associated with a 30% increment in the extent of atherogenic risk factor clustering.

Left ventricular hypertrophy

Hypertrophy of the left ventricle is no longer accepted as an incidental compensatory feature of hypertension and is now recognized as an ominous harbinger of CVD. Recent population-based investigation indicates that each 39 g increase in left ventricular mass per square meter confers a 40% increase in CVD events. Risk of heart failure, myocardial infarction, and

stroke increase when long-standing or severe hypertension induces LVH. It is a prominent feature of evolving heart failure increasing the hypertension-imposed risk two- to threefold. Approximately 20% of heart failure cases have antecedent electrocardiogram-left ventricular hypertrophy (ECG-LVH) and 60% to 70% on the more sensitive echocardiogram. ECG-LVH characterized by voltage alone carries only half the risk of adverse CVD outcomes of left ventricular hypertrophy also accompanied by repolarization abnormality (**Figure B76.5**).

Global cardiovascular risk

Hypertension is associated with greater risk of all atherosclerotic vascular disease outcomes compared with same-aged persons with nonhypertensive BP (<140/90 mm Hg). However, arterial pressure should not be considered in isolation, because age, sex, blood lipids, cigarette smoking, ECG-LVH and diabetes all further enhance hypertensive CHD risk (**Figure B76.4**). In both sexes, CHD risk rises with the burden of other risk factors. Hypertensive persons with multiple risk factors typically experience the highest CHD rates. Men or women with diabetes, who smoke cigarettes, have LVH and a low HDL-cholesterol in the presence of systolic BP of 160 mm Hg have an estimated 10-year CHD risk that exceeds 55%. Predicted CHD rates for men are typically greater than those for women by 1.3 to 1.5 times when only a few risk factors are present, but the male-to-female difference is small when risk factor levels including diabetes, smoking, and LVH by ECG, are all present.

Preventive implications

Hypertension and dyslipidemia are the most common remediable risk factors for atherosclerotic CVD. Apart from age, hypertension is the most common modifiable risk factor that accompanies dyslipidemia.

Age interactions. Aggressive BP control is required and of proven efficacy in reducing the CVD risk of dyslipidemia and diabetes. High-normal and normal BPs frequently progress to *definite hypertension* in Framingham Study subjects. Over a period of 4 years, 37.5% of those younger than 65 years developed hypertension and over that age 49.5%. Obesity and weight gain

---

TABLE B76.3

RISK FACTOR CLUSTERING IN THE FRAMINGHAM STUDY OFFSPRING WITH ELEVATED BLOOD PRESSURE ACCORDING TO THE BODY MASS INDEX: SUBJECTS 18 TO 74 YEARS OLD

Men		Women	
Body mass index	Average number of risk factors	Body mass index	Average number of risk factors
<23.7	1.68 ± 0.91	<20.8	1.80 ± 0.87
23.7–25.5	1.85 ± 0.95	20.8–22.3	2.00 ± 1.02
25.6–27.2	2.06 ± 1.05	22.4–23.9	2.22 ± 1.06
27.3–29.5	2.28 ± 1.09	24.0–26.8	2.20 ± 0.99
≥29.5	2.35 ± 1.08	≥26.8	2.66 ± 1.09

Elevated BP defined as systolic pressure ≥138 mm Hg (men) and ≥130 mm Hg (women). Other risk factors included the top quintiles for the factors total cholesterol, body mass index, triglycerides, and glucose and bottom quintile for HDL-cholesterol.

significantly contributed to BP progression to hypertension. A 5% weight gain increases the odds of progression by 20% to 30%.

Goal blood pressure. Many hypertensive patients do not achieve JNC 7 recommended goals of <140/90 mm Hg for most patients, and <130/80 mm Hg for diabetes or chronic kidney disease. Among diabetic patients, 81% are not at JNC recommended goals and 64% of uncomplicated hypertensive patients are not at recommended goals. Isolated systolic hypertension is the variety of hypertension least likely to be treated and when treated is not being brought to the recommended goal.

Risk profiling. Optimal CVD protection from hypertension requires more than simply lowering the BP. At the cellular level, CVD risk factors can promote vascular disease through the common pathway of endothelial dysfunction impaired by hypertension, dyslipidemia, and impaired glucose tolerance. The potential for development of CVD, the best choices for antihypertensive therapy, and the aggressiveness of therapy needed are best evaluated by determining the multivariable risk of the hypertension, taking into account commonly associated risk factors.

Risk calculations can be conveniently done for strokes and coronary disease using multivariable risk factor scoring profiles based on Framingham Study data. This requires only ordinary office procedures and simple laboratory tests for the multivariable assessment. In this way, hypertensive persons can be efficiently targeted for cost-effective treatment using more optimal therapy likely to maximize the benefit. In particular, the type and aggressiveness of antihypertensive therapy should be tailored to take into account the often associated dyslipidemia, glucose intolerance, and any associated cardiovascular condition as well as the severity and character of the BP elevation.

Suggested Readings

Chobanian AV, Bakris GL, Black HR, et al. Joint National Committee on prevention, detection, evaluation, and treatment of high BP. National heart lung and blood institute; National high BP education program coordinating committee. Seventh report of the Joint National Committee on prevention, detection, evaluation and treatment of high BP. *Hypertension* 2003;42:1206–1252.

Franklin SS, Larson MG, Kahn BS, et al. Does the relation of BP to coronary heart disease change with aging? The Framingham Heart Study. *Circulation* 2001;103:1245–1249.

Kannel WB. BP as a cardiovascular risk factor: prevention and treatment. *JAMA* 1996;275:1571–1576.

Kannel WB, Wilson PWF, Nam B-H, et al. A likely explanation for the J-curve of BP cardiovascular risk. *Am J Cardiol* 2004;94:380–384.

Reaven GM. Insulin resistance and compensatory hyperinsulinemia: role in hypertension, dyslipidemia, and coronary heart disease. *Am Heart J* 1991;121:1283–1288.

Vasan RS, Larson MG, Leip EP, et al. Impact of high-normal BP on the risk of cardiovascular disease. *N Engl J Med* 2001;345:1291–1297.

Vasan RS, Larson MG, Leip EP, et al. Assessment of frequency of progression to hypertension in non-hypertensive subjects in the Framingham Heart Study. A cohort study. *Lancet* 2001;358:1682–1686.

Verdecchia P, Carini G, Circo A, et al. Left vetricular mass in essential hypertension. The MAVI Study. *J Am Coll Cardiol* 2001;38:1829.

Wilson PWF, D'Agostino RB, Levy D, et al. Prediction of coronary heart disease using risk factor categories. *Circulation* 1998;97:1837–1847.

Wolf PA, D'Agostino RB, Belanger AJ, et al. Probability of stroke: a risk profile from the Framingham Study. *Stroke* 1991;22:312–318.

CHAPTER B77 ■ ISCHEMIC HEART DISEASE RISK

DONALD M. LLOYD-JONES, MD, ScM

KEY POINTS

- Ischemic heart disease (IHD) is the most common manifestation of cardiovascular disease (CVD) and IHD is the leading cause of morbidity and mortality in developed countries.
- Higher levels of blood pressure (BP) are associated with continuous, logarithmic increases in risk for IHD events, beginning at levels well below the traditional hypertensive range (normotension and prehypertension).
- In older individuals with hypertension, systolic blood pressure (SBP) predominates over diastolic and pulse pressures (PPs) in determining risk for IHD events.
- Treatment of hypertensive individuals with antihypertensive agents reduces risk for IHD in patients with and without known IHD.
- The presence of additional risk factors increases BP-associated IHD risks substantially and warrants additional management considerations.

See also Chapter B76

Ischemic heart disease (IHD), including myocardial infarction (MI) and chronic coronary disease, affects approximately 16 million adults in the United States, with approximately 1.2 million ischemic heart disease (IHD) events annually. In the United States in 2004, IHD was the leading cause of death (450,000) and hospitalization (~2 million). In 2007, estimated costs for IHD care exceed $150 billion. Hypertension, which currently affects 65 million Americans, is the most prevalent major risk factor contributing to morbidity and mortality due to IHD.

Blood pressure and ischemic heart disease risk

Individuals with hypertension have a two- to threefold increased relative risk for any cardiovascular disease (CVD) event compared with normotensive individuals at the same age. Hypertension increases the *relative* risk of any manifestation of CVD but it increases the relative risk of stroke and heart failure the most. Because IHD incidence is substantially greater than the incidence of stroke and heart failure in the U.S. population, the *absolute* impact of hypertension is greater for IHD than for other manifestations of CVD.

Continuity of the blood pressure–cardiovascular disease risk relationship. Much of the literature assessing risks associated with elevated BP has focused on the categorical presence of "hypertension," usually defined as systolic blood pressure (SBP) ≥140 mm Hg, diastolic blood pressure (DBP) ≥90 mm Hg, or ongoing antihypertensive therapy. Risk for IHD is not limited to subjects with definite hypertension, however; risk for IHD and other CVD outcomes is strongly associated with BP at all levels, beginning well within the range considered "optimal" or "normal" (<120/<80 mm Hg). In the Prospective Studies Collaboration, pooled worldwide data from prospective cohort studies in approximately 1 million individuals were used to study CVD outcomes. At any age in adulthood (40–90 years) an over SBP range of 115 to 185 mm Hg and a DBP range of 75 to 115 mm Hg, risk for IHD death and other outcomes doubled for each 20 mm Hg increase in SBP or each 10 mm Hg increase in DBP. For example, the risk for IHD death of a 60-year-old with an SBP 135 mm Hg is twice that of a 60-year-old with SBP 115 mm Hg.

Prevalence of events and blood pressure level. Most IHD events occurring in the population happen at modestly elevated levels of BP. In the cohort of more than 347,000 men screened for the Multiple Risk Factor Intervention Trial (MRFIT), the *relative* risks for IHD death were largest for men with the highest levels of SBP (i.e., ≥180 mm Hg) but there were only 3,000 men (~1%) in this group. Although relative risks were much lower for men with SBP of 130 to 159 mm Hg, this group included >40% of the sample and experienced >60% of the excess IHD deaths attributable to elevated BP. Therefore, levels of BP that are considered only modestly elevated cannot be ignored.

Further evidence for the importance of "prehypertensive" BP levels, in the range of 130 to 139 mm Hg systolic or 85 to 89 mm Hg diastolic, comes from the Framingham cohort. Compared with optimal BP levels of <120/<80 mm Hg, men and women with these levels had risks for CVD that were 1.6 to 2.5 times higher. Similar findings were recently reported by the Women's Health Initiative investigators.

Age effects. With advancing age, the impact of BP remains fairly constant in terms of relative risk for IHD events. Therefore, as shown in **Figure B77.1A**, in those with Stage 2 or treated hypertension at 80 years or older, the multivariable-adjusted *relative* risk for major IHD events is 2.2 compared with normotensive individuals at the same age, which is similar to the relative risk observed in those younger than 60 or those aged 60 to 79 years. However, *absolute* risks for IHD associated with higher BP stage increase markedly with advancing age. As shown in **Figure B77.1B**, 6-year rates of major IHD events for those with stage 2 or treated hypertension were 2.2% for those younger than

60 years, 5% for those 60 to 79 years of age, and 8.5% for those 80 years of age and older, indicating the combined effects of BP and age on absolute risk for IHD.

Natural history of ischemic heart disease and associated comorbidities

Hypertension increases risks for other fatal and nonfatal CVD outcomes, including stroke, heart failure, and peripheral arterial disease. Hypertension also increases risk for kidney failure and all-cause mortality. After the onset of hypertension, any of these potential outcomes is possible, but individual patient characteristics influence which outcome occurs first.

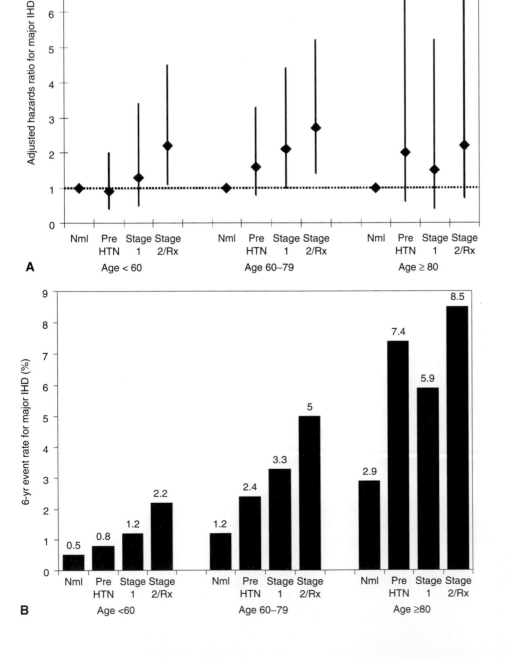

Figure B77.1 Relative risks (**A**) and absolute risks (**B**) for major ischemic heart disease (IHD) events in participants of the Framingham Study, by age and BP stage. Nml, normal BP (untreated BP <120/<80 mm Hg); PreHTN, prehypertension (untreated systolic 120–139 or diastolic 80–89 mm Hg); stage 1, untreated systolic 140 to 159 or diastolic 90 to 99 mm Hg; stage 2/Rx, untreated systolic ≥160 or diastolic ≥100 mm Hg, or treated hypertension. (Data from Lloyd-Jones DM, Evans JC, Levy D. Hypertension in adults across the age spectrum: current outcomes and control in the community. *JAMA* 2005;294:466–472.)

For men and women with new-onset hypertension at any age in the Framingham cohort, a CVD event was more likely to occur before a non-CVD death. The 12-year competing cumulative incidence of any CVD endpoint as a first event in men was 24.7%, compared with 9.8% for noncardiovascular death [heart rate (HR) 2.53, 95% confidence interval (CI) 1.83–3.50]; in women, the competing incidences were 16.0% versus 10.1%, respectively (HR 1.58, 1.13–2.20). The type and incidence of first CVD events varied by age, sex, and severity of hypertension at onset. Overall, the most common first major CVD events after hypertension onset were hard IHD events (MI or hospitalized unstable angina; 10.6%) in men, and stroke (5.8%) in women. For men with hypertension onset *before age 60*, hard IHD events were the most common first major event by far, with a 12-year incidence of 9.9%. Both hard IHD (incidence 12.5%) and stroke (11.3%) were common first events for men with hypertension onset *after* age 60. Conversely, for women, stroke predominated as the first event after hypertension onset at younger and older ages.

Viewed from a different perspective, hypertensive men and women at age 50 have a life expectancy that is approximately 5 years shorter than normotensive men and women. During that shortened overall lifespan, hypertensive men and women, compared with normotensive persons, live 7 fewer years free of CVD and 2 more years with CVD on average, including 1 more year with MI. Therefore, both morbidity and mortality from IHD and other causes are substantially increased with hypertension.

Blood pressure components and ischemic heart disease risk

Systolic versus diastolic blood pressure.
Historically, elevated DBP was believed to confer greater risk for cardiovascular events than elevated SBP. However, epidemiologic data suggest that elevated SBP is a stronger risk factor than elevated DBP for the development of CVD at all but the youngest ages. Data from more than 347,000 men free of IHD between the ages of 35 and 57 who were screened for the MRFIT indicate that the adjusted relative risk of IHD death for SBP was consistently higher than that for DBP when comparing each decile. For example, the relative risk for IHD mortality for men in the highest compared to those in the lowest decile of SBP was 3.82, as opposed to 2.90 for those in the highest versus lowest decile of DBP. When stratified by age, the relative risk for IHD mortality was greater for the top decile of SBP than for the top decile of DBP at every age, except for those aged 35 to 39 years.

In addition, elevated SBP appears to confer a greater *absolute risk* of IHD than does elevated DBP, especially with advancing age. As age increases, mean BP levels tend to rise and the prevalence of hypertension increases. Beyond age 60, however, DBP tends to plateau or fall, whereas SBP continues to increase. Since most of the IHD events and cardiovascular morbidity occur in older individuals, this trend leads to greater risk conferred by SBP elevation than by DBP elevation. Framingham and MRFIT data support this finding, with higher age-adjusted rates of IHD mortality for SBP compared with DBP in each BP stage.

Pulse pressure and mean pressure.
Controversy persists regarding the relative importance of SBP, DBP, and pulse pressure (PP) in prediction of IHD events. In the Framingham Heart Study, SBP and DBP were each directly associated with IHD risk when considered alone, as expected. However, when considered in the context of SBP level, DBP was inversely associated with IHD risk. For example, the multivariable-adjusted risk for IHD was approximately 15% lower for each increment of 10 mm Hg in DBP for any stratum of SBP. Conversely, at any level of SBP, the risk was approximately 15% greater for each 10 mm Hg increment in PP. These data suggest some added benefit to consideration of PP.

In the Prospective Studies Collaboration, the informativeness for prediction of IHD death was best for mid-BP [(SBP + DBP)/2] followed closely by mean arterial pressure [MAP = (SBP + DBP × 2)/3] and SBP. DBP was only moderately informative and PP was poorly informative in this large study of pooled cohorts.

An analysis of the Chicago Heart Association Detection Project in Industry cohort, including 36,314 adults across the age

---

TABLE B77.1

RISKS AND PREDICTIVE UTILITIES[a] BY DIFFERENT BLOOD PRESSURE (BP) CHARACTERISTICS AT BASELINE

BP measure	Hazards ratio (95% CI) per SD[b]	p value	Likelihood ratio χ^2	BIC	AUC
SBP	1.76 (1.71–1.81)	< .001	1177.75	56622	0.67
DBP	1.75 (1.69–1.81)	< .001	991.95	56808	0.66
PP	1.47 (1.42–1.52)	< .001	475.65	57324	0.60
MAP	1.79 (1.74–1.85)	< .001	1231.75	56568	0.68
Mid-BP	1.79 (1.74–1.84)	< .001	1258.83	56541	0.68

N = 2,812 for ischemic heart disease deaths.
AUC, area under the receiver-operating characteristic curve; BIC, Bayes' information criterion; CI, confidence interval; DBP, diastolic blood pressure; MAP, mean arterial pressure [(SBP + 2 × DBP)/3]; Mid-BP, mid–blood pressure [(SBP + DBP)/2]; PP, pulse pressure (SBP–DBP); SBP, systolic blood pressure; SD, standard deviation.
[a] Higher values of the likelihood ratio χ^2 and lower values of the BIC indicate better model fit, informativeness and predictive utility; higher values of the AUC indicate better discrimination.
[b] For each BP measure, the SD are as follows: SBP 18.5 mm Hg, DBP 11.6 mm Hg, PP 13.2 mm Hg, MAP 12.8 mm Hg, Mid-BP 13.9 mm Hg.
Adapted from Mosley WJ, Greenland P, Garside DB, Lloyd-Jones DM. Predictive utility of pulse pressure and other blood pressure measures for cardiovascular outcomes. *Hypertension* 2007;49:1256–1264.

spectrum, examined the actual predictive value of BP components, rather than just relative risks, in greater detail. In this cohort, SBP and DBP were positively associated with IHD risk. PP was positively associated as well, but it was consistently a weaker predictor (**Table B77.1**). When SBP and PP were considered simultaneously, SBP was positively and PP negatively associated with IHD death or hospitalization for MI. Among all of the BP components considered, mid-BP was the best predictor of IHD outcomes, followed by MAP. SBP provided predictive information that was similar to mid-BP and MAP, whereas PP had poorer model fit, was less informative for IHD outcomes, and provided poorer discrimination (as judged by the area under the receiver-operating characteristic curve).

Clinical impact. On balance, these studies reinforce the approach of the National High BP Education Program and Seventh Report of the Joint National Committee (JNC 7) in maintaining the focus of risk stratification and treatment on SBP and DBP, and particularly SBP in those older than 50 years. PP is an important marker of arterial stiffness and risk, but its clinical utility is lacking in comparison to SBP. Part of the issue with PP is that, although it combines information from both SBP and DBP, it is a "floating" parameter. For example, a PP of 60 mm Hg reflects measured BPs of either 190/130 mm Hg or 130/70 mm Hg. The risk for these two BP levels are clearly not equivalent. If summary measures are to be used, mid-BP appears to have the best predictive value for IHD events, but this measure has not been widely used in clinical practice.

Risk factor clustering

Elevated BP seldom occurs in isolation from other CVD risk factors. Among all Framingham subjects with high-normal BP or hypertension examined between 1990 and 1995, only 2% had no other risk factors, target organ damage or clinical CVD. In 59%, there was at least one other risk factor (not including diabetes), and 38% had diabetes, target organ damage, or clinical CVD.

Using the *Framingham Risk Score*, one can easily view the additive risk associated with increasing levels of other risk factors in the context of differing levels of BP. As shown in **Figure B77.2**, absolute levels of risk for IHD increase substantially with increasing risk factor burden, and are augmented still further by elevated BP at every level of other risk factors in men and women. Therefore, BP levels, and the risk they confer, must always be considered in the context of other risk factors and the patient's global risk for IHD. In addition, numerous studies have demonstrated the additional risk associated with target organ damage (e.g., evidence of left ventricular hypertrophy, renal dysfunction) in hypertensive individuals.

Treatment implications

Ischemic heart disease reduction. In both primary prevention trials of individuals without IHD and secondary prevention trials of patients with existing IHD, antihypertensive therapy has consistently been shown to lower subsequent IHD event rates compared with placebo. Data are most robust for primary prevention in older individuals with isolated systolic hypertension, especially those older than 65 years with SBP ≥160 and DBP <90 mm Hg.

Limitations of clinical trials. Antihypertensive therapy is associated with substantial reductions in overall CVD events, particularly stroke and heart failure, with somewhat less impressive (15%–25%) effects on the incidence of IHD events. A major reason why most trials did not show more impressive benefit on

IHD endpoints is that they have been based on relatively small reductions in DBP. In trials based on SBP, such as the Systolic Hypertension in the Elderly Program (SHEP) and the Systolic Hypertension in Europe (Syst-EUR) study, systolic BP reductions of 10 to 12 mm Hg lowered IHD event rates by approximately one third compared to placebo. Another important factor is that although hypertension is a major associated risk factor for IHD, it is more closely linked pathogenetically to stroke, ventricular hypertrophy, and heart failure. Therefore, it would be expected that antihypertensive treatment would cause greater reductions in relative risk for those outcomes than for IHD. Nonetheless, given the very large incidence of IHD, even modest reductions in risk translate to large absolute benefit. Other potential methodologic deficiencies in antihypertensive outcome trials include durations too short to demonstrate effects on coronary atherosclerotic progression. Less likely is that small sample sizes masked potential benefits. Confounding caused by adverse events has also been postulated but not proved. For example, it has been suggested that hypokalemia from thiazide diuretics may have increased risk for sudden cardiac death (which is often classified as an IHD endpoint), thereby decreasing the efficacy of antihypertensive therapy compared with placebo.

Blood pressure versus blood glucose changes. Some drugs are known to have adverse effects on glucose tolerance and other factors but little attention has been directed to whether the overall coronary risk profile (or Framingham risk score) has been improved by therapy. In the Antihypertensive and Lipid-Lowering Treatment to Prevent Heart Attack Trial (ALLHAT), the thiazide diuretic chlorthalidone was at least as effective as angiotensin-converting enzyme (ACE) inhibition or calcium channel blockade at preventing IHD events over 7 years, although it was associated with higher rates of incident diabetes. Fasting glucose levels increased in older adults regardless of treatment assignment, but rates of incident diabetes at 2 years were 25% to 50% lower with amlodipine or lisinopril compared with chlorthalidone. Incident diabetes was in turn associated with increased risk for IHD, but the excess risk for IHD was no greater in those taking chlorthalidone. Furthermore, the overall similarity in IHD outcomes over 7 years regardless of treatment assignment suggests that the superior SBP reduction associated with chlorthalidone may offset the adverse metabolic consequences.

Comorbidities and complications. Just as risk for IHD that is associated with BP is influenced by the burden of other risk factors, the choice of antihypertensive therapy for IHD prevention requires consideration of other factors. JNC 7 identifies certain "compelling indications" as reasons for selection of certain classes of medications for lowering BP in hypertensive patients. For patients with impaired ventricular function, ACE inhibitors, angiotensin receptor blockers (ARBs) or β-blockers are preferred. For patients with IHD, ACE inhibitors or β-blockers are preferable. It should also be noted that diuretics and some β-blockers may make management of blood glucose more difficult.

Overview. Therapeutic planning in hypertension must take into consideration associated risk factors, concomitant disease, and potential drug side effect profiles. Before starting drug therapy, and concomitant with its use, weight control, decreased intake of salt, alcohol, and fat, and comprehensive risk reduction are recommended. Recent clinical trial data suggest significant additional reductions in IHD risk through adjunctive treatment of hypertensive patients with aspirin or with a low-dose statin, even in hypertensive patients with relatively low cholesterol levels, as in the Heart Protection Study.

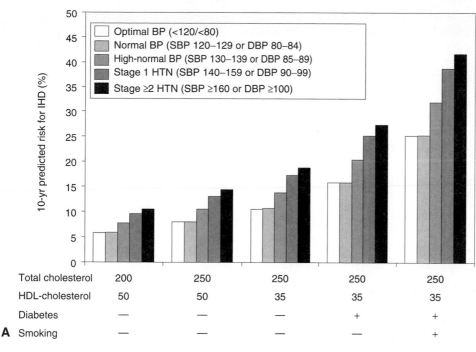

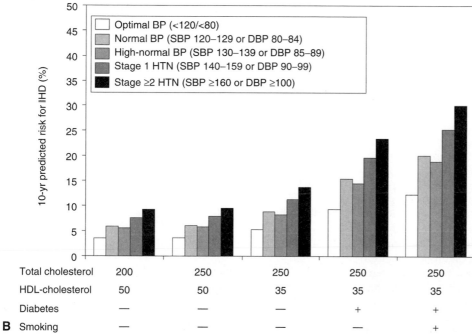

Figure B77.2 Ten-year predicted risk for major ischemic heart disease (IHD) event, defined as IHD death or nonfatal myocardial infarction, for men (**A**) and women (**B**) at age 50 years, by selected risk factor levels and BP stages. BP, blood pressure; SBP, systolic blood pressure; DBP, diastolic blood pressure; HTN, hypertension; HDL, high-density lipoprotein. (Adapted from the method of Wilson PW, D'Agostino RB, Levy D, et al. Prediction of coronary heart disease using risk factor categories. *Circulation* 1998;97:1837–1847.)

Suggested Readings

Franco OH, Peeters A, Bonneux L, et al. BP in adulthood and life expectancy with cardiovascular disease in men and women: life course analysis. *Hypertension* 2005;46:280–286.

Franklin SS, Khan SA, Wong ND, et al. Is pulse pressure useful in predicting risk for coronary heart disease? the Framingham heart study. *Circulation* 1999;100:354–360.

Kannel WB, Gordon T, Schwartz MJ. Systolic versus diastolic BP and risk of coronary heart disease: the Framingham study. *Am J Cardiol* 1971;27:335–345.

Lloyd-Jones DM, Evans JC, Larson MG, et al. Cross-classification of JNC VI BP stages and risk groups in the Framingham heart study. *Arch Intern Med* 1999;159:2206–2212.

Lloyd-Jones DM, Evans JC, Levy D. Hypertension in adults across the age spectrum: current outcomes and control in the community. *JAMA* 2005;294:466–472.

Lloyd-Jones DM, Leip EP, Larson MG, et al. Novel approach to examining first cardiovascular events after hypertension onset. *Hypertension* 2005;45:39–45.

Mosley WJ, Greenland P, Garside DB, Lloyd-Jones DM. Predictive utility of pulse pressure and other blood pressure measures for cardiovascular outcomes. *Hypertension* 2007;49:1256–1264.

Prospective Studies Collaboration. Age-specific relevance of usual BP to vascular mortality: a meta-analysis of individual data for one million adults in 61 prospective studies. *Lancet* 2002;360:1903–1913.

Vasan RS, Larson MG, Leip EP, et al. Impact of high-normal BP on the risk of cardiovascular disease. *N Engl J Med* 2001;345:1291–1297.

Wilson PW, D'Agostino RB, Levy D, et al. Prediction of coronary heart disease using risk factor categories. *Circulation* 1998;97:1837–1847.

CHAPTER B78 ■ LEFT VENTRICULAR HYPERTROPHY AND CARDIOVASCULAR DISEASE RISK

DANIEL LEVY, MD

KEY POINTS

- Hypertension increases cardiac workload and promotes left ventricular hypertrophy (LVH), which can be detected on the electrocardiogram (ECG), echocardiogram, and by other imaging methods.
- LVH is associated with an increased risk for heart failure, myocardial infarction, arrhythmias, sudden death, and stroke.
- LVH predisposes to heart failure by two mechanisms: systolic left ventricular dysfunction due to myocardial infarction and diastolic dysfunction as a consequence of increased left ventricular (LV) stiffness; the latter is especially common in older patients with long-standing hypertension.
- Aggressive hypertension treatment can regress LVH and reduce heart failure risk by approximately 50%.

See also Chapter **B76**

Etiology and diagnosis

Left ventricular hypertrophy (LVH) denotes increased left ventricular mass (LVM). In response to long-standing pressure overload, there is an increase in left ventricular (LV) wall thickness (concentric LVH); chronic volume overload promotes LV dilation (eccentric LVH).

The relation of long-term average blood pressure (BP) measured over a 30-year period to LVH prevalence on the echocardiogram is presented in **Figure B78.1**. In this investigation of healthy Framingham Heart Study participants, long-term average BP was more closely associated with LVH risk than was BP at the time of the echocardiogram, suggesting long-term burden of hypertension is most important. One fourth to one third of participants with long-term average systolic BP ≥140 mm Hg were found to have LVH compared to approximately 10% of those with long-term systolic BP <120 mm Hg. Other factors that promote LVH are increased age, obesity, valvular heart disease (producing LV pressure or volume overload), and increased neurohumoral factors. Genetic factors play a prominent role in some cases; rare familial forms of hypertrophic cardiomyopathy are due to genetic mutations, most notably in genes coding for sarcomere proteins.

Diagnosis

The diagnosis of LVH can be made in several ways but most commonly it is identified on the electrocardiogram (ECG), on the basis of increased voltage and repolarization abnormalities. A more sensitive indicator is the echocardiogram; measuring LV wall thickness and internal chamber dimensions allows calculation of

LVM. The greatest sensitivity is provided by magnetic resonance imaging, which permits the most precise characterization of LV wall thickness volume, and LVM.

Electrocardiographic left ventricular hypertrophy. The first studies to document the cardiovascular disease (CVD) hazards associated with LVH were based on its appearance on the ECG. The ECG hallmarks of LVH are increased R-wave and S-wave voltage, reflecting left ventricular forces; a widened QRS complex; a leftward frontal plane axis shift; ST- and T-wave repolarization abnormalities; and P-wave abnormalities reflecting left atrial enlargement. Individuals with ECG LVH are at increased

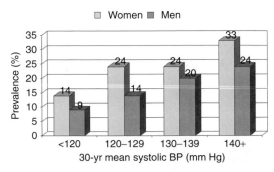

Figure B78.1 Prevalence of left ventricular hypertrophy (LVH) on the echocardiogram according to long-term average systolic BP in the Framingham Heart Study. (Adapted from Lauer MS, Anderson KM, Levy D. Influence of contemporary versus 30-year BP levels on left ventricular mass and geometry: the Framingham Heart Study. *J Am Coll Cardiol* 1991;18:1287–1294.)

risk for coronary heart disease (CHD), stroke, congestive heart failure, and sudden death. The CVD risks associated with LVH are greatest when increased QRS voltage is accompanied by repolarization abnormalities.

Echocardiographic left ventricular hypertrophy. Echocardiography provides a more sensitive tool for the detection of LVH than the ECG because, unlike the ECG, it provides precise anatomic characterization of LV structure and function. Whereas ECG LVH was present in only approximately 2% of subjects from the Framingham Heart Study, echocardiographic LVH was detected in approximately 15%. The echocardiographic diagnosis of LVH is based on the presence of increased LVM, which is calculated from an autopsy-validated formula that incorporates measures of LV wall thickness and cavity dimension. Therefore, LVH can occur as a result of increased wall thickness (as in hypertrophic cardiomyopathy) or LV dilation (as in dilated cardiomyopathy). LVH as a dichotomous variable (i.e., LVH present vs. absent), and LVM examined as a continuous variable are associated with increased risk for numerous forms of CVD including heart failure, myocardial infarction, arrhythmias, sudden death, and stroke. Of note, a Swedish study found that the prognostic information provided by the ECG and the echocardiogram were complementary; LVH detected by both approaches predicted increased mortality risk when considered jointly.

Left ventricular hypertrophy and cardiovascular disease risk

Electrocardiographic studies. More than 30 years ago, Framingham investigators reported that among >5,000 original study participants, new development of LVH on the ECG (increased voltage ECG evidence of LVH with accompanying major repolarization abnormalities) carried a relative risk for developing CHD of approximately twofold to fivefold in men and 1.5-fold to 2.5-fold in women. A subsequent investigation from Framingham examined the separate contributions of increased voltage and repolarization abnormalities to CVD risk in those with ECG LVH based on follow-up of 524 subjects who exhibited ECG LVH during approximately 40 years of observation. Among persons free of CVD at baseline, the relative risk for developing CVD, comparing subjects in the top quartile of Cornell ECG voltage (sum of R wave in augmented voltage unipolar left arm lead plus S wave in V_3) with those in the bottom quartile, was 3.08 [95% confidence interval (CI), 1.87–5.071] in men and 3.29 (95% CI, 1.78–6.09) in women. The presence of major repolarization abnormalities also identified individuals with LVH who were at increased risk for CVD.

Echocardiographic studies. An extensive body of literature has provided consistent evidence of the hazards associated with LVH on the echocardiogram. In a sample of 3,220 men and women from the Framingham Heart Study 40 years or older, 208 (6%) developed new CVD events and 124 (almost 4%) died within 4 years. As shown in **Figure B78.2**, LVM predicted the incidence of CVD and the association was continuous and graded. In multivariable models adjusting for age and traditional CVD risk factors (BP, antihypertensive treatment, lipids, diabetes, cigarette smoking, body mass index, and ECG LVH), in men a 50 g per m^2 increment in LVM was associated with a relative risk of 1.49 (95% CI, 1.20–1.85) for CVD events. The corresponding relative risk in women was 1.57 (95% CI, 1.20–2.04). Increased levels of LVM were also associated with increased risk for CVD death

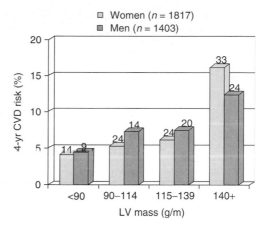

Figure B78.2 Risk of developing cardiovascular disease as a consequence of left ventricular mass (LVM) on echocardiogram in Framingham Heart Study participants free of cardiovascular disease (CVD) at baseline. (Adapted from Levy D, Garrison RJ, Savage DD, et al. Prognostic implications of echocardiographically determined left ventricular mass in the Framingham Heart Study. *N Engl J Med* 1990;322:1561–1566.)

and death from all causes. Increased LVM also increases risk for stroke or transient ischemic attack, suggesting that the target organ damage identified by echocardiography may be reflective of parallel damage throughout the cardiovascular system.

Hypertension, left ventricular hypertrophy, and heart failure

Hypertension substantially increases the risk of heart failure. In the Framingham Heart Study, during more than 20 years of follow-up, hypertension conferred a twofold hazard for heart failure in men and a threefold hazard in women. Of the 392 cases of heart failure that developed, 91% had a history of antecedent hypertension, making it by far the most common risk factor for heart failure. Among hypertensive men and women, myocardial infarction, diabetes, LVH, and valvular heart disease were all predictive of increased risk for heart failure. Although myocardial infarction carries the greatest relative risk for heart failure of all risk factors, the far greater prevalence of hypertension confers a greater population-attributable risk (i.e., the proportion of heart failure cases attributed to a given cause). Hypertension accounts for approximately 50% of heart failure cases, a finding closely matched by clinical trial results. In two placebo-controlled clinical trials of hypertension treatment in older people [the Systolic Hypertension in the Elderly Program (SHEP) and the Swedish Trial of Older Persons (STOP) hypertension], treatment of systolic hypertension in older men and women reduced heart failure risk by approximately 50% compared with placebo.

Dual mechanisms have been proposed for the association of hypertension with increased risk of heart failure (**Figure B78.3**). First, hypertension is a risk factor for myocardial infarction, which is associated systolic LV dysfunction and heart failure. Second, hypertension promotes LVH, which is associated with diastolic dysfunction and increased risk for heart failure.

Regression of left ventricular hypertrophy

In hypertensive patients, aggressive BP control can prevent the development of LVH and reverse or regress it. Numerous clinical trials of antihypertensive drug therapy have documented

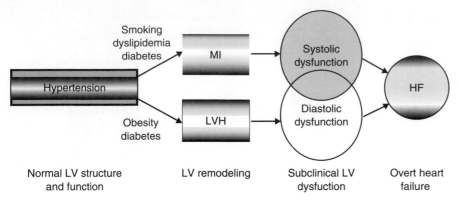

Figure B78.3 The progression from hypertension to heart failure. Dual mechanisms are present: (*upward arrow*) hypertension is a risk factor for myocardial infarction, which is associated systolic LV dysfunction and heart failure, and (*downward arrow*) hypertension promotes LVH, which is associated with diastolic dysfunction and increased risk for heart failure. MI, myocardial infarction; LVH, left ventricular hypertrophy; HF, heart failure; LV, left ventricular. (Adapted from Vasan RS, Levy D. The role of hypertension in the pathogenesis of heart failure. A clinical mechanistic overview. *Arch Intern Med* 1996;156:1789–1796.)

the occurrence of regression of LVH in response to lowering BP. It remains controversial whether, and to what extent, there are differential drug effects on reversing LVH related to hypertension and whether differences in clinical outcomes observed in comparative drug trials are dependent in part on drug mechanism differences.

Role of blood pressure. It is clear that the main determinant of the extent LVH regression in response to hypertension treatment is the magnitude of BP reduction. BP control, rather than LVH regression, should be the primary goal of therapy in patients with hypertension. Nevertheless, in light of the multiple risks associated with LVH, there has been great interest in determining the impact of LVH regression on CVD risk.

Observational data suggest an important role of LVH regression in determining CVD outcomes. A report from Framingham used serial ECGs to examine the implications of reversal of ECG LVH. In that study, individuals with a serial decline in ECG LVH voltage were at lower risk for CVD than were those with no serial change (men: odds ratio after adjustment for age and baseline voltage, 0.46; 95% CI, 0.26–0.84; women: odds ratio, 0.56; 95% CI, 0.30–1.04). The results of this investigation suggest that regression of LVH confers an improvement in risk for CVD. The benefits of LVH regression are also supported by studies of hypertensive patients undergoing repeat echocardiographic assessment

of LVM; these reports similarly have suggested that regression of LVH is associated with a reduction in CVD risk.

Specific drug effects. It is difficult to differentiate the effect of BP reduction from drug-specific effects on LVH regression.

Angiotensin-converting enzyme inhibition. The Heart Outcomes Prevention Evaluation (HOPE) trial examined whether treatment of >8,000 high-risk patients with the angiotensin-converting enzyme (ACE) inhibitor ramipril could prevent the development of LVH on ECG or promote its regression compared with placebo. The prevention or regression of LVH occurred more commonly in those receiving active therapy, whereas development or persistence of LVH were more frequent in those receiving placebo (*p* = .008). Prevention or regression of LVH was associated with a 25% reduction in CVD risk compared with the new development or persistence of LVH; of 7,539 patients with prevention/regression of LVH, 12% experienced a primary cardiovascular event (cardiovascular death, myocardial infarction, or stroke) compared with 16% of patients with development/persistence of LVH (*p* = .006). Risk of heart failure was especially reduced in those who experienced prevention or regression of LVH versus its development or persistence (9% vs. 15%; *p* < .0001). This placebo-controlled trial documented the feasibility of LVH regression and confirmed the benefits conferred by LVH regression (**Figure B78.4**).

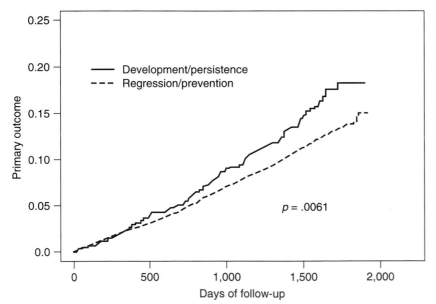

Figure B78.4 Reduction of cardiovascular risk by regression of electrocardiographic markers of left ventricular hypertrophy by the angiotensin-converting enzyme inhibitor ramipril. Heart Outcomes Prevention Evaluation (HOPE). Matthew J. et al. *Circulation* 2001;104:1615–1621.

Angiotensin receptor blockade. In the LIFE trial (Losartan Intervention for Endpoint Reduction in Hypertension), hypertensive patients with LVH on ECG were randomized to receive the angiotensin receptor blocker losartan or the β-blocker atenolol as their initial therapy. Reduction in LVM index by 25 g per m^2 was associated with a 22% reduction in risk for the primary CVD outcome of stroke, myocardial infarction, or CVD death over and above that predicted by changes in BP due to treatment.

Other drugs. A meta-analyses of multiple smaller studies suggested that LVH regression also occurs with use of thiazide-type diuretics and calcium-channel blockers, whereas less LVH reduction occurs with β-blockade. Given the dissimilar mechanisms of the drugs involved (diuretics and calcium blockers tend to increase renin-angiotensin-aldosterone system activity, whereas ACE inhibitors and β-blockers diminish it), BP reduction itself seems to be the critical factor in determining LVH regression.

Suggested Readings

Casale PN, Devereux RB, Milner M, et al. Value of echocardiographic measurement of left ventricular mass in predicting cardiovascular morbid events in hypertensive men. *Ann Intern Med* 1986;105:173–178.

Devereux RB, Roman MJ. Evaluation of cardiac and vascular structure and function by echocardiography and other non invasive techniques. In: *Hypertension: pathophysiology, diagnosis and management.* New York: Raven Press, 1995:1969–1985.

Koren MJ, Devereux RB, Casale PN, et al. Relation of left ventricular mass and geometry to morbidity and mortality in uncomplicated essential hypertension. *Ann Intern Med* 1991;114:345–352.

Lauer MS, Anderson KM, Levy D. Influence of contemporary versus 30-year BP levels on left ventricular mass and geometry: the Framingham Heart Study. *J Am Coll Cardiol* 1991;18:1287–1294.

Levy D, Garrison RJ, Savage DD, et al. Prognostic implications of echocardiographically determined left ventricular mass in the Framingham Heart Study. *N Engl J Med* 1990;322:1561–1566.

Levy D, Larson MG, Vasan RS, et al. The progression from hypertension to congestive heart failure. *JAMA* 1996;275:1604–1606.

Levy D, Salomon MS, D'Agostino RB, et al. Prognostic implications of baseline electrocardiographic features and their serial changes in subjects with left ventricular hypertrophy. *Circulation* 1994;90:1786–1793.

Mathew J, Sleight P, Lonn E, et al. The Heart Outcomes Prevention Evaluation (HOPE) Investigators. Reduction of cardiovascular risk by regression of electrocardiographic markers of left ventricular hypertrophy by the angiotensin-converting enzyme inhibitor ramipril. *Circulation* 2001;104:1615–1621.

Sundstrom J, Lind L, Arnlov J, et al. Echocardiographic and electrocardiographic diagnoses of left ventricular hypertrophy predict mortality independently of each other in a population of elderly men. *Circulation* 2001;103:2346–2351.

Vasan RS, Levy D. The role of hypertension in the pathogenesis of heart failure. A clinical mechanistic overview. *Arch Intern Med* 1996;156:1789–1796.

Schmieder RE, Messerli FH. Hypertension and the heart. *J Hum Hypertens* 2000;14:597–604.

CHAPTER B79 ■ CEREBROVASCULAR RISK

PHILIP A. WOLF, MD

KEY POINTS

- Hypertension is the key risk factor for stroke, including brain infarction and hemorrhage.
- Incidence of initial and recurrent stroke rises in proportion to increases in blood pressure (BP); older than 50 years, stroke risk is more strongly related to systolic rather than diastolic BP.
- Treatment of hypertension decreases stroke incidence and recurrence rates, especially in diabetics; approximately half of the 500,000 initial stroke events in the United States may be preventable by control of hypertension.

See also Chapter B76

Cerebrovascular disease is the third leading cause of death in the United States but stroke is four times more likely to produce disability than death, making it the leading cause of neurologic disability in the elderly. The American Heart Association has estimated that in 2006, 500,000 Americans sustained an initial stroke, 100,000 suffered a stroke recurrence, and 158,448 of them died from stroke, corresponding to 1 death every 3.3 minutes. However, death data do not portray the toll in human suffering experienced by stroke survivors and their families, whose lives are irrevocably altered by this neurologic catastrophe. There are approximately four million stroke survivors in the United States, many of whom require chronic care. Stroke is not limited to the elderly; approximately 20% occur in persons younger than 60 years, more than one third of whom will never work again. To many functionally independent persons, stroke represents a condition considered to be worse than death itself. To these stroke survivors, the loss of function and independence signals the end of worthwhile life.

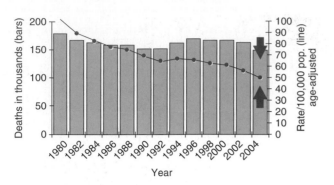

Figure B79.1 Mortality from stroke in the United States, 1980 to 2004. Pop., population. Data from Vital Statistics of United States, National Center for Health Statistics.

TABLE B79.1

FREQUENCY OF COMPLETED STROKE BY TYPE IN MEN AND WOMEN 35 TO 94 YEARS OLD

Completed stroke	Men	Women	Total	%
Atherothrombotic brain infarction	227	301	528	60.1
Cerebral embolus	87	131	218	24.8
Intracerebral hemorrhage	31	42	73	8.3
Subarachnoid hemorrhage	20	28	48	5.5
Other	4	7	11	1.3
Total	369	509	878	100

Data are from the Framingham Study: 50-year follow-up.

Secular trends

Since 1972, stroke death rates in the United States have fallen by <60% and rates of death from coronary heart disease (CHD) by 46%, whereas noncardiovascular death rates have remained unchanged. Similar improvement in stroke and CHD mortality has occurred in other industrialized nations. The 1% per year decline in stroke death rates from 1915 to 1965 accelerated to 5% per year from 1962 through the 1990s. Since then stroke mortality has continued to trend downward, although at a slower pace.

These trends highlight the role of modifiable environmental factors, particularly blood pressure (BP) control in stroke mortality. Despite the aging of the U.S. population, the total number of deaths attributed to stroke as well as death rates have continued to decline up through 2004 (**Figure B79.1**). In many populations, the incidence of stroke has also declined, with hemorrhage incidence declining more strikingly than that of brain infarctions. In other studies, no decline in incidence has occurred, although most found a decrease in stroke severity. Brain imaging has provided a dramatic increase in diagnostic sensitivity thereby documenting smaller brain infarcts with a briefer duration and lesser severity than were apparent previously. Even in the presence of such an increase in diagnostic sensitivity stroke incidence has apparently declined in men and women at most ages. However, with a growing number of elderly persons, it is likely that the number of persons who will die of or be disabled by stroke will increase during the next century.

Subtypes and incidence of stroke

Unlike CHD, in which atherosclerosis of the arteries supplying the myocardium is the underlying disease process, stroke is a heterogeneous condition. Hemorrhage is easy to distinguish from infarction by computed tomography (CT) scan of the brain, whereas it is often more difficult to determine the mechanism of infarction. Most brain infarctions result from atherothrombotic occlusions of large and small arteries in the intracranial and extracranial circulation, although cardiac embolic sources also occur, especially in individuals with atrial fibrillation.

In the Framingham Heart Study 50-year follow-up, the most frequent stroke subtype was atherothrombotic brain infarction (ABI) resulting from atherosclerosis and thrombosis without a cardiac source for embolism, accounting for 60% of cases (**Table B79.1**). The ABI category includes infarction resulting from

large-vessel atherothrombosis, lacunar infarction, and infarct of undetermined cause. Stroke from cerebral embolus occurred in 25%, chiefly from a left atrial clot in the presence of atrial fibrillation and from left ventricular thrombus after acute myocardial infarction (MI).

Stroke risk factors

Age. Death and disability from cardiovascular disease increase steadily with age, so that after age 65, cardiovascular disease accounts for approximately 50% of all deaths. Fully 20% of all cardiovascular disease deaths in the elderly are attributable to stroke. After 50 years of follow-up of a general population sample of 5,184 stroke-free individuals in Framingham, MA, stroke occurred in 878 persons, 369 men and 509 women. Stroke incidence increased with age, approximately doubling in each successive decade above age 55 (**Table B79.2**).

Age–gender interactions. Because the most common stroke type, ABI, may be considered to be analogous to MI, it is informative to compare the incidence, by age and sex, of these two manifestations of cardiovascular disease (**Figure B79.1**). Although both stroke and MI increase with age, approximately doubling in

TABLE B79.2

ANNUAL INCIDENCE OF COMPLETED STROKES IN MEN AND WOMEN AGES 35 TO 94 YEARS

Age (yr)	Men		Women	
	No.	Rate/1,000	No.	Rate/1,000
35–44	3	0.37	3	0.30
45–54	25	1.61	20	1.04
55–64	60	3.13	60	2.41
65–74	127	8.07	115	5.07
75–84	126	14.29	199	12.65
85–94	28	15.25	112	22.25
[a]Total	369	5.34	509	5.22

[a]Age adjusted, 35 to 94 years.
Data are from the Framingham Study: 50-year follow-up.

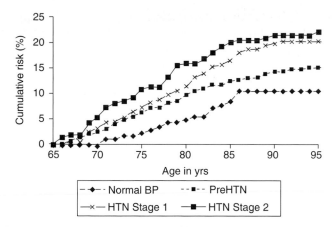

Figure B79.2 Men, age 65 years: risk of first-ever stroke by baseline blood pressure (BP); lifetime risk of all-stroke within four BP categories defined using systolic blood pressure (SBP) and diastolic blood pressure (DBP); subjects categorized using higher of two values.

1. Normal BP: SBP <120 and DBP <80
2. Prehypertension (PreHTN): 120 ≤ SBP <140 and/or 80 ≤ DBP <90
3. Stage 1 hypertension (HTN Stage 1): 140 ≤ SBP <160 and/or 90 ≤ DBP <100
4. Stage 2 hypertension (HTN Stage 2): SBP ≥160 or DBP ≥100.

successive decades, there are age–gender interactions in incidence rates. Below the age of 65, MI has a striking male predominance; the male-to-female ratio is 4:1. The incidence of MI in women lags 20 years behind that of men; the rate of MI in women 65 to 74 years old approximates that of men 45 to 54 years old. ABI incidence is approximately 30% higher in men, and this ratio is quite constant across the adult age span, without the striking male predominance at younger ages seen for MI.

Hypertension. Hypertension is the most common potent risk factor for hemorrhage and ischemic stroke; reduction of elevated BP clearly prevents stroke, regardless of subtype. Using the Joint

National Committee on Prevention, Detection, Evaluation, and Treatment of high blood pressure (JNC 7) classification, 10-year and lifetime risk of stroke increases in proportion to the severity of hypertension from normal BP to Stage 2 hypertension (**Figure B79.2, Table B79.3**). In the elderly, Stage 2 isolated systolic hypertension (BP ≥160/<90 mm Hg) becomes highly prevalent, affecting approximately 25% of persons older than 80 years. In Framingham, elderly subjects (65–84 years of age) with stage 2 isolated systolic hypertension, had twice the risk of stroke in men and 1.5 times increased risk in women.

Stroke risk predictions are generally based on measurement of current BP. Clearly the duration of the BP level, the height of the pressure, and host factors contribute to cardiovascular and stroke risk. From the Framingham Study, it is evident that elevated midlife BP (during the previous 10 years) increases the relative risk of stroke at age 60 by 1.68 [95% confidence interval (CI) 1.25–2.25] per SD increment in women and 1.92 (95% CI 1.39–2.66) per SD increment in men. Similar increases in relative risk by elevated antecedent pressures were also seen at age 70.

Left ventricular hypertophy. Other data from Framingham indicate that, at any level of pressure, persons with concentric left ventricular hypertrophy (diagnosed by electrocardiogram or echocardiogram) are at increased risk of stroke and other cardiovascular outcomes. Furthermore, clinical trials indicate that reduction in BP and left ventricular mass are associated with reduced stroke rates. Benefits of antihypertensive therapy also occurred in those with atrial fibrillation.

Stroke risk profile. At any level of BP, probability of stroke is strongly related to the presence and level of other risk factors. By using the Framingham Stroke Risk profile, a gender-specific model with points assigned for age, systolic BP level, antihypertensive drug usage, cigarette smoking, diabetes, atrial fibrillation, and other cardiovascular disease, it is clear the probability of stroke is strongly related to these associated risk factor abnormalities as well as level of BP.

TABLE B79.3

AGE- AND SEX-SPECIFIC, MORTALITY ADJUSTED, 10-, 20- AND 30-YEAR AND LIFETIME RISK ESTIMATES[a] FOR THE DEVELOPMENT OF STROKE (ALL TYPES) FOR SUBJECTS AGED 65 YEARS, DESCRIBED WITHIN SUBGROUPS DEFINED BY BLOOD PRESSURE (BP) AT AGE 65 YEARS

Gender	JNC 7 category[b]	First-ever stroke—all types			Lifetime risk
		Short- and intermediate-term risks			
		10-yr	20-yr	30-yr	
WOMEN	Normal	1.6(0–3.2)	5.7(2.8–8.6)	9.9(5.9–14)	**14.6(9.2–20.4)**
	Prehypertension	3(1.7–4.3)	10.8(8.5–13.1)	17.3(14.3–20.2)	**18.2(15.1–21.3)**
	Stage 1 hypertension	4.1(2.4–5.7)	15.8(12.7–18.9)	24.7(20.9–28.5)	**25.8(21.9–29.7)**
	Stage 2 hypertension	9.9(7.3–12.6)	19.9(16.3–23.5)	25.3(21.3–29.3)	**25.6(21.6–29.6)**
MEN	Normal	2.1(0.1–4.2)	8.2(4.2–12.1)	10.4(6–14.9)	**10.4(6–14.9)**
	Prehypertension	6.2(4.2–8.2)	12.3(9.6–15)	14.9(12–17.9)	**14.9(12–17.9)**
	Stage 1 hypertension	7.2(4.6–9.7)	16.3(12.6–20)	20(16–24.1)	**20.5(16.3–24.6)**
	Stage 2 hypertension	10.8(7–14.7)	19.9(14.9–24.9)	22.1(16.8–27.4)	**22.1(16.8–27.4)**

JNC 7, Joint National committee on Prevention, Detection, Evaluation, and Treatment of High Blood Pressure.
[a]Risks expressed in percentages over period of observation; values in parentheses are 95% confidence intervals.
[b]Blood pressure (BP) categories, all values in mm Hg, if categorization by systolic blood pressure (SBP) and diastolic blood pressure (DBP) varied, the higher value was used: Normal: SBP <120 and DBP <80; Prehypertension: 120 ≤ SBP <140 and/or 80 ≤ DBP <90; stage 1 hypertension: 140 ≤ SBP <160 and/or 90 ≤ DBP <100; stage 2 hypertension: SBP ≥160 or DBP ≥100.

Treatment trials

Primary stroke prevention. For stroke prevention, reduction of BP is key. Since 1967, a series of clinical trials has shown that treatment of Stage 2 hypertension reduces stroke incidence, regardless of age. The Systolic Hypertension in the Elderly Program (SHEP) and the Systolic Hypertension in Europe Trial (Syst-Eur) trials demonstrated reducing elevated systolic pressure significantly reduced stroke incidence. In these studies, isolated systolic hypertension was not as resistant to antihypertensive medications as had been previously thought and treatment did not precipitate increased numbers of adverse events (stroke, syncope, or produce an excess of confusion, falls, or depression) as feared by some.

Results from Antihypertensive and Lipid-Lowering Treatment to Prevent Heart Attack Trial (ALLHAT) demonstrate that the thiazide diuretic, chlorthalidone, and the calcium channel blocker, amlodipine, were particularly effective in preventing stroke. In African Americans, chlorthalidone was statistically significantly superior to the angiotensin-converting enzyme (ACE) inhibitor, lisinopril, at preventing strokes and not inferior to amlodipine. In non–African Americans, all of the intital therapy options were equally efficacious.

Stroke recurrence. There are fewer data for prevention of secondary stroke recurrence than for primary prevention. A recent meta-analysis of four trials of blood pressure–lowering drugs suggested that reduction of approximately 6 to 8 mm Hg systolic (3–4 mm Hg diastolic) was associated with approximately 20% fewer recurrent strokes. Stroke recurrence was reduced by the diuretic indapamide in the Poststroke Antihypertensive Study (PATS) and also by the combination of indapamide and ACE inhibitor (perindopril) in the Perindopril Protection against Recurrent Stroke Study (PROGRESS) trial. In the latter, the average BP reduction of 9/4 mm Hg was associated with a 28% relative risk reduction of stroke recurrence. In the Heart Outcomes Prevention Evaluation (HOPE) trial, the ACE inhibitor, ramipril, reduced initial stroke incidence and recurrence with only modest BP reduction of 3.8/2.8 mm Hg, although there remain questions of methodologic discrepancies in BP measurement in that study. Recently, the Anglo-Scandinavian Cardiac Outcomes Trial-Blood Pressure Lowering Arm (ASCOT-BPLA) trial found that the combination of amlodipine ± perindopril was superior to the combination of atenolol ± bendroflumethiazide for preventing fatal and nonfatal stroke (relative risk reduction 23%, $p = .0003$) in high-risk hypertensive patients. In this study as well as HOPE, the role of specific drug effects versus simple BP-lowering could not be easily differentiated. In both studies, the incidence of diabetes development was lower when ACE inhibitors were used compared to thiazide-β blocker combinations.

Prevention implications

The demonstration of the benefits of treatment and control of hypertension in stroke prevention in the elderly with diastolic and with isolated systolic hypertension suggests that considerable progress remains to be achieved. The American Heart Association estimated 59 million Americans, representing 32.3% of adults are hypertensive (≥140 mm Hg systolic or ≥90 mm Hg diastolic), only 49% had their BP controlled. In the elderly, control is less frequently achieved. In Framingham, only 38% of men and 23% of women had BP that met targets elaborated in the National High Blood Pressure Education Program's guidelines. It has been estimated that approximately half of all 500,000 new strokes in the United States could be prevented each year by treatment of elevated BP alone.

Optimal blood pressure

The optimal level to which BP should be reduced for stroke prevention remains undefined but the target is clearly lower than previously thought. Fears that overzealous BP reduction would reduce cerebral blood flow in persons with cerebral atherosclerosis and precipitate stroke have not been borne out. According to the JNC 7, optimal BP is ≤120 mm Hg systolic and ≤80 mm Hg diastolic. This threshold has been supported by a secondary analysis of the PROGRESS study, where those who achieved sustained systolic BP values <120 mm Hg had lower stroke recurrence rates than those whose systolic BPs were in the 120 to 140 range, who in turn had better outcomes than those whose systolic BPs remained >140 mm Hg. As >40% of the population has BP levels in the 120 to 160 mm Hg range (prehypertension and Stage 1 hypertension), a major effort in stroke prevention must be focused here.

Suggested Readings

The ALLHAT Officers and Coordinators for the ALLHAT Collaborative Research Group. Major outcomes in high-risk hypertensive patients randomized to angiotensin-converting enzyme inhibitor or calcium channel blocker vs diuretic: the Antihypertensive and Lipid-Lowering Treatment to prevent Heart Attack Trial (ALLHAT). *JAMA* 2002;288(23):2981–2997.

Bosch J, Yusuf S, Pogue J, et al. On behalf of the HOPE Investigators. Use of ramipril in preventing stroke: double blind randomized trial. *BMJ* 2002;324:1–5.

Carandang R, Seshadri S, Beiser A, et al. Temporal trends in incidence, lifetime risk, severity, and 30-day mortality of stroke over the past 50 years: the Framingham study. *JAMA* 2006;296(24):2939–2946.

Dahlöf B, Sever PS, Poulter NR, et al. The ASCOT Investigators. Prevention of cardiovascular events with an antihypertensive regimen of amlodipine adding perindopril as required versus atenolol adding bendroflumethiazide as required, in the anglo-scandinavian cardiac outcomes trial-blood pressure lowereing arm (ASCOT-BPLA): a Multicentre Randomised Controlled Trial. *Lancet* 2005;366:895–906.

Progress Collaborative Group. Randomised trial of a perindopril-based blood-pressure-lowering regimen among 6,105 individuals with previous stroke or transient ischaemic attack. *Lancet* 2001;358(9287):1033–1041.

Seshadri S, Wolf PA, Beiser A, et al. Elevated midlife blood pressure increases stroke risk in elderly persons: the Framingham study. *Arch Intern Med* 2001;161:2343–2350.

Seshadri S, Beiser A, Kelly-Hayes M, et al. The lifetime risk of stroke: estimates from the Framingham study. *Stroke* 2006;37(2):345–350.

SHEP Cooperative Research Group. Prevention of stroke by antihypertensive drug treatment in older persons with isolated systolic hypertension: final results of the systolic hypertension in the elderly program (SHEP). *JAMA* 1991;265:3255–3264.

Staessen JA, Fagard R, Thijs L, et al. The Systolic Hypertension in Europe (Syst-Eur) Trial Investigators. Randomised double-blind comparison of placebo and active treatment for older patients with isolated systolic hypertension. *Lancet* 1997;350:757–764.

Vasan RS, Massaro JM, Wilson PWF, et al. Antecedent blood pressure and risk of cardiovascular disease: the Framingham study. *Circulation* 2002;105:48–53.

CHAPTER B80 ■ RENAL RISK

LUIS M. RUILOPE, MD AND JOSEPH L. IZZO, Jr., MD

KEY POINTS

■ Chronic kidney disease (CKD) is a cause and a consequence of hypertension.
■ Hypertension is the most important etiologic factor in CKD; publications listing diabetic nephropathy as the most common cause of end-stage renal disease (ESRD) have assumed that diabetes and hypertension are independent; in reality, the rate of progression of diabetic nephropathy (like other renal diseases) depends on the blood pressure (BP) levels of the affected individuals.
■ ESRD likelihood is proportional to the level of BP (systolic or diastolic) or albumin excretion; race and gender also influence ESRD likelihood.
■ Stage 3 or greater CKD (defined as microalbuminuria or glomerular filtration rate (GFR) <60 mL/minute) is a coronary risk equivalent; in turn, the most common cause of death in ESRD patients is cardiovascular disease (CVD).
■ BP control to <130/<80 mm Hg or lower is paramount if any form of CKD is present.

See also Chapter B76

The kidney participates in the development of hypertension through different mechanisms, the most widely recognized is a defect in sodium excretion. The pressure–natriuresis relationship has been the focus of a great deal of research; resetting of this relationship can be the consequence of genetic differences or acquired defects in renal function that begin in intrauterine life and extend through growth and development to old age, as further modified by societal forces. Once blood pressure (BP) is elevated, it can relentlessly damage renal vessels and parenchyma and ultimately lead to the development of chronic kidney disease (CKD) and end-stage renal disease (ESRD).

Renal risk factors

Age, hypertension, and chronic kidney disease. After approximately the fourth decade of life, glomerular filtration rate (GFR) begins to decline in the general population at a rate (approximately 0.5 mL/minute/year) that varies with BP and other comorbidities. There is substantial heterogeneity in this age-related rate of renal deterioration, however, and some individuals "age" much faster than others, especially when intrinsic renal disease (such as diabetic nephropathy) is exacerbated by hypertension (**Figure B80.1**). The age-related decline in renal function is much more prominent in other organs with similar reserves of function (e.g., liver) that are not sensitive to BP, underscoring the importance of the interaction of hypertension with other comorbidities in causing CKD.

The overwhelming influence of BP on the development of renal damage has been amply demonstrated in observational studies that were originally limited to men but have now been extended to women. The risk of developing ESRD as a consequence of elevated BP is continuous, beginning at normal BP levels (>120/80 mm Hg) as can be seen in **Figure B80.2**.

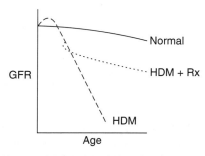

Figure B80.1 Glomerular filtration rate (GFR) and age. Normal aging includes a progressive fall in GFR that is markedly accelerated by hypertension/diabetes mellitus (HDM). Effective BP treatment (Rx) in HDM [goal BP<130/80 mm Hg, angiotensin-converting enzyme (ACE) inhibitor or angiotensin receptor blocker (ARB) included] normalizes the slope of the aging curve after an initial drop in GFR. Initial increase in GFR in HDM (glomerular capillary hypertension/hyperfiltration (causing microalbuminuria) is signal for preventive Rx; Rx remains important at any time for preservation of residual function.

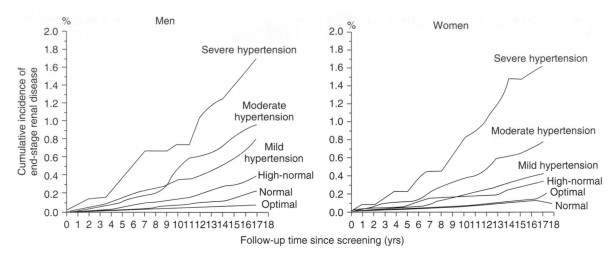

Figure B80.2 Cumulative incidence of ESRD in 46,881 men and 51,878 women, according to the six blood pressure categories. (Reproduced with permission from Tozawa M, Iseki K, Iseki C, et al. Blood pressure predicts risk of developing end-stage renal disease in men and women. *Hypertension* 2003;41:1341–1345.)

Systolic versus diastolic blood pressure. Elevations of systolic BP have a more robust relationship with the incidence of ESRD (dialysis or transplantation requirement, ESRD) than diastolic BP, especially in individuals older than 50 years, as demonstrated clearly by Klag et al. from the Multiple Risk Factor Intervention Trial (MRFIT). Increased diastolic BP elevation also confers substantial risk for ESRD development, especially because elevated diastolic BP is the most common form of hypertension in younger black men.

Race. Blacks (especially men) are at exceptionally high risk of ESRD as compared to whites (**Figure B80.3**). The rate of decline in renal function in blacks was closely related to the baseline level of albuminuria in the African American Study of Kidney Disease (AASK).

Proteinuria. Proteinuria or macroalbuminuria and uncontrolled BP are the two main factors facilitating the progression of CKD to ESRD. Proteinuria is not common in patients developing CKD as a consequence of elevated BP and age-related loss in renal function with time is significantly slower in those without albuminuria compared to those with albuminuria, especially in diabetic nephropathy. It may be that proteinuria is merely an indicator of more severe renal disease or alternatively, that another pathophysiologic process is present.

Hypertension–diabetes interaction. Hypertension is the most important etiologic factor in CKD and ESRD despite statements published by the U.S. Renal Data System that lists diabetic nephropathy as the most common cause of ESRD. This factual disparity arises from incorrect assumptions in the analysis: that diabetes and hypertension are independent. In reality, the rate of progression of diabetic nephropathy (like virtually all other renal diseases) depends most strikingly on the BP levels of the affected individuals. Three observations support this view: (1) normotensive diabetic patients (the few that exist) have very low rates of albuminuria and CKD, (2) longitudinal studies in diabetic patients have clearly identified the level of BP as the critical determinant of the rate of CKD progression, and (3) aggressive antihypertensive drug therapy markedly blunts the rate of development of ESRD. In fact, this concept is the basis for the advanced targets for BP control (<130/80 mm Hg) recommended by the guidelines of the American Diabetes

Association and National Kidney Foundation that were echoed in the Joint National Committee recommendations in the sixth and seventh reports.

Other risk factors. A series of conditions appears to contribute to the progression of CKD (**Table B80.1**). There is strong suspicion that hypercholesterolemia is an additional risk factor for CKD that accelerates the rate of decline in GFR but there is no strong clinical trial data to support this contention. It is also suspected that abnormal blood clotting or platelet function contributes to ischemic renal disease. Abnormalities of arterial structure and function such as pulse wave velocity (a measure of arterial stiffness) and augmentation index (a measure of wave

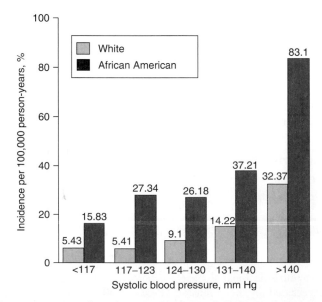

Figure B80.3 Age-adjusted 16-year incidence of all-cause end-stage renal disease by systolic blood pressure in 300,645 white men (*shaded bars*) and 20,222 African-American men (*solid bars*) screened for Multiple Risk Factor Intervention Trial. Numbers at the top of the bars are incidence rates. (Reproduced with permission from Klag MJ, Whelton PK, Randall BL, et al. End-stage renal disease in African-Americans and white men: 16-year MRFIT findings. *JAMA* 1997;277:1293–1298.)

TABLE B80.1

PERPETUATING FACTORS FOR CHRONIC KIDNEY DISEASE

African-American race
Low nephron number
Proteinuria
High dietary protein intake
Obesity (cardiometabolic risk)
Anemia
Dyslipidemia
Smoking
Nephrotoxins
Secondary hyperparathyroidism
Cardiovascular disease

(Adapted from Taal MW, Brenner BM. Predicting initiation and progression of chronic kidney disease: developing renal risk scores. *Kidney Int* 2006;70:1694–1705.)

reflection) are abnormal in ESRD but it is unclear that these indicators are useful in staging, prognosis, or management of the condition. Concomitant hyperparathyroidism is a factor that has gained much attention recently and may be important, at least in some individuals.

Staging chronic kidney disease progression

Recently, the progressive nature of CKD has been underscored by the Kidney Dialysis Outcomes Quality Improvement project (KDOQI) classification system (**Table B80.2**). There are two diagnostic elements in CKD: renal excretory function (estimated glomerular filtration rate or eGFR) and presence of microalbuminuria or albuminuria.

Estimated glomerular filtration rate. A simplified estimation of GFR can be derived from serum creatinine values (without urine collection) using a formula developed during the Modification of Diet in Renal Disease (MDRD) study. In essence, the most common application of the MDRD formula adjusts the reciprocal of serum creatinine by coefficients related to age and race. CKD has been staged by the level of eGFR. An eGFR <60 mL per minute signals clinically significant (stage 3) CKD.

Microalbuminuria and albuminuria. Like BP, progressive increases in the rate of albumin excretion (or leakage) herald the development of CKD. In general, the rate of albumin leakage parallels the loss of GFR. This relationship is not always tight, however, particularly in disorders that are predominantly glomerular in nature (e.g., systemic lupus or immunoglobulin A nephropathy). Accordingly, a parallel staging system for CKD is based on the degree of albuminuria. Of note, 24-hour urine collections are not recommended to quantitate albuminuria; rather, a spot urine specimen is used, with the urinary albumin concentration indexed to the corresponding urinary creatinine concentration. Microalbuminuria (30–300 mg albumin/g creatinine) occurs in very early (stage 1) in CKD; an albumin:creatinine ratio in excess of 300 mg per g creatinine heralds clinically significant (stage 3) CKD.

Risk assessment

Renal risk scores. The need to identify patients at risk of developing CKD has led to development of renal risk scores, analogous to the Framingham risk score for ischemic heart disease, for the general population and patients with CKD. **Table B80.2** contains a list of factors that promote the progression of CKD in patients with elevated (>130 mm Hg) systolic BP. The coexistence of many different factors contributes to enhance the progressive decay in renal function, most notably, arterial hypertension. As shown in **Figure B80.4**, the possibility of that either microalbuminuria (≥300 mg/day) or a diminished GFR

TABLE B80.2

STAGES OF CHRONIC KIDNEY DISEASE (CKD)

CKD stage	eGFR (mL/min)	Albuminuria	Comment
1	90–120	Microalbuminuria (>30 mg/d)	Early hyperfiltration
2	60–90	Increasing microalbuminuria (<300 mg/d)	Effects of aging and progressive disease
3	30–60	Macroalbuminuria (>300 mg/d) defines stage 3 CKD independent of eGFR	
4	15–30	Macroalbuminuria usually present	
5	<15	End-stage renal disease	Dialysis/ transplantation

eGFR, estimated glomerular filtration rate.
(Adapted from Levey, AS, Coresh J, Balk E, et al. National Kidney Foundation practice guidelines for chronic kidney disease: evaluation, classification, and stratification. *Ann Int Med* 2003;139:137–147.)

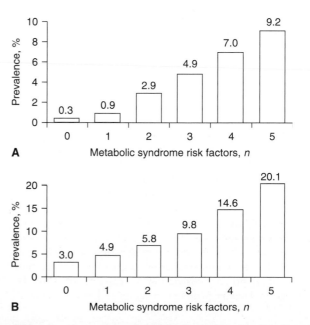

Figure B80.4 Prevalence of chronic kidney disease (**A**) and microalbuminuria (**B**) by number of the metabolic syndrome components. (Reproduced with permission from Chen J, Muntner P, Hamm L, et al. The metabolic syndrome and chronic kidney disease in US adults. *Ann Intern Med* 2004;140:167–174).

TABLE B80.3

THERAPEUTIC APPROACH TO TREATING A
HYPERTENSIVE PATIENT WITH CHRONIC KIDNEY
DISEASE

Lifestyle changes
　　Salt intake, body weight, and smoking
Strict blood pressure control (<125/75 mm Hg)
　　Combination therapy required in most cases
　　Blockade of angiotensin II effects is required
Control of associated risk factors
　　Lipids: statins, fibrates
　　Insulin resistance: insulin sensitizers (meltformin,
　　　glitazones?)
　　Platelet aggregation: aspirins, others?

will be present is proportional to the number of components of the metabolic syndrome that are found in the individual. This finding also indicates that prediabetes is an early risk factor for CKD, especially in hypertensive patients, many of whom will later develop overt diabetes mellitus.

Chronic kidney disease and cardiovascular disease risk. CKD (as a cause or consequence of hypertension) is accompanied by an increase in global cardiovascular risk that explains the elevated prevalence of myocardial infarction, stroke, and premature death in these patients. Stage 3 CKD can be considered to be a "coronary risk equivalent" (similar to diabetes or prior myocardial infarction). Rapid decline in renal function does not mean that the enhanced cardiovascular risk is less relevant. Both cardiovascular and renal risk run in parallel, the higher rate of progression in one is always accompanied by a parallel effect on the other.

Prevention of end-stage renal disease

Existing data indicate that a hypertensive patient with CKD requires a comprehensive treatment program to prevent premature CKD-ESRD, cardiovascular events, or death. **Table B80.3** summarizes the therapeutic approach to treating a hypertensive patient with CKD.

Lifestyle modifications. Early lifestyle intervention is recommended in high-risk individuals. Usual lifestyle modifications, such as increased physical activity, weight control and smoking cessation, are prudent given the increased prevalence of atherosclerosis; effect on CKD progression has not been established.

Diet. Dietary modifications are specific for CKD. Caloric restriction and reduction in dietary fat are reasonable but increased dietary potassium should only be entertained if kidney function is relatively normal (stages 1 and 2 CKD, and many patients with stage 3 CKD). Potassium restriction is necessary in stages 4 and 5 CKD. Another consideration is protein restriction. The MDRD study and smaller investigations offer the possibility that dietary protein restriction is capable of slowing CKD progression. Dietary protein restriction makes it difficult to follow usual dietary recommendations for CVD risk reduction; however, principally because it is difficult to restrict fat and carbohydrate composition if protein intake is reduced.

Antihypertensive therapy

Strict blood pressure control. The forgoing discussion has highlighted the overarching importance of fastidious BP control in preventing or blunting the progression of CKD. This recommendation is based on early studies of BP control that employed various antihypertensive drugs.

Type of antihypertensive drug. Blockade of the renin-angiotensin-aldosterone system (RAAS) is recommended in renal disease prevention and treatment and CKD is a "compelling indication" for the use of anti-RAAS drugs [angiotensin-converting enzyme (ACE) inhibitors and angiotensin receptor blockers (ARBs)] according to current worldwide guidelines. Whether CKD (microalbuminuria) can be prevented is currently being tested in the Randomized Olmesartan And Diabetes Microalbuminuria Prevention (ROADMAP) study. There is controversy whether calcium blockers are indicated for this purpose. In the AASK, amlodipine was said to accelerate the rate of renal deterioration in proteinuric, nephrosclerotic individuals. However, study design flaws limit interpretation and application of this observation. There is also controversy whether nondihydropyridines are superior to dihydropyridines in reducing proteinuria. β-Blockers do not appear to be beneficial in slowing the progression of CKD.

Other drugs. The presence of other cardiovascular risk factors and the increase in global risk requires that the components of the metabolic syndrome and hyperlipidemia be vigorously treated as well, both with lifestyle modification and drugs. Use of erythropoietin analogs is under increased scrutiny; although correction of anemia markedly improves functionality of ESRD patients, cardiovascular event rates may be increased.

Suggested Readings

Chen J, Muntner P, Hamm L, et al. The metabolic syndrome and chronic kidney disease in US adults. *Ann Intern Med* 2004;140:167–174.
Haller H, Viberti GC, Mimran A, et al. Preventing microalbuminuria in patients with diabetes: rationale and design of the Randomised Olmesartan and Diabetes Microalbuminuria Prevention (ROADMAP) study. *J Hyperten* 2006;24:403–408.
Joint National Committee on Prevention, Detection, Evaluation, and Treatment of High Blood Pressure. The seventh report of the Joint National Committee on Prevention, Detection, Evaluation, and Treatment of High Blood Pressure: JNC 7 express. *JAMA* 2003;289:2560–2572.
Klag MJ, Whelton PK, Randall BL, et al. Blood pressure and end-stage renal disease in men. *N Engl J Med* 1996;334(1):13–18.
Klag MJ, Whelton PK, Randall BL, et al. End-stage renal disease in African-Americans and white men: 16-year MRFIT findings. *JAMA* 1997;277:1293–1298.
Levey AS, Coresh J, Balk E, et al. National Kidney Foundation practice guidelines for chronic kidney disease: evaluation, classification, and stratification. *Ann Intern Med* 2003;139:137–147.
Taal MW, Brenner BM. Predicting initiation and progression of chronic kidney disease: developing renal risk scores. *Kidney Int* 2006;70:1694–1705.
Tozawa M, Iseki K, Iseki C, et al. Blood pressure predicts risk of developing end-stage renal disease in men and women. *Hypertension* 2003;41:1341–1345.
U.S. Renal Data System. *USRDS 1998 report.* Bethesda: NIDDK, NIH, 1998.
Wright JT Jr, Bakris G, Greene T, et al. Effect of blood pressure lowering and antihypertensive drug class on progression of hypertensive kidney disease: results from the AASK trial. *JAMA* 2002;288:2421–2431.

CHAPTER B81 ■ PERIPHERAL ARTERIAL DISEASE AND HYPERTENSION

EMILE R. MOHLER III, MD, MS AND MICHAEL H. CRIQUI, MD, MPH

KEY POINTS

- The 5-year risk of dying from a cardiovascular event is 20% for patients with peripheral arterial disease (PAD).
- The association of PAD with systolic blood pressure (SBP) appears to be stronger than the association with diastolic blood pressure (DBP).
- Compared to individuals without PAD, the prevalence of hypertension (HTN) is ≥50% higher in those with moderate PAD and approximately twice as high in those with severe PAD.
- HTN appears to be an important causal factor in the pathogenesis of PAD.

See also Chapters **B76** and **B77**

Peripheral arterial disease (PAD) is the systemic manifestation of generalized atherosclerosis. The lower extremity is a common target of progressive systemic atherosclerosis, with plaque formation and eventual obstruction of blood flow leading to the hallmark symptom, intermittent claudication (IC): ambulatory leg pain not present at rest and relieved by rest. The physical examination for PAD includes assessment of peripheral pulses, auscultation for bruits, and assessment of skin changes. The diagnosis is usually established by noninvasive testing.

Pathogenesis

PAD is a pathologic condition that may involve upper or lower extremities. Excessive deposition of oxidized lipids, inflammation, calcification, plaque rupture, thrombosis, and vascular occlusion follow the same pathophysiologic sequence as observed in coronary artery disease. Not surprisingly, PAD is commonly associated with coronary artery disease and cerebrovascular disease. These three conditions may arise in any sequence but it is not uncommon for PAD to appear after the others.

Risk factors and etiology

Cigarette smoking, dyslipidemia, diabetes, and hypertension (HTN) are major risk factors for PAD (**Table B81.1**). The most common cause of lower extremity PAD is atherosclerosis but rarer causes such as congenital anomalies, cystic adventitial disease, popliteal entrapment, and aneurysm should be considered in the diagnosis.

Association of hypertension and peripheral arterial disease

Claudication studies. Studies using IC as the basis for PAD have revealed variable associations with HTN. The data indicate that PAD is more strongly associated with systolic blood pressure (SBP) than diastolic blood pressure (DBP).

Framingham heart study. The surveillance of 5,209 subjects enrolled in the Framingham Heart Study identified 176 men and 119 women developing IC over 26 years. HTN increased the risk for IC 2.4 to fourfold, respectively in men and women. A steep, near-linear gradient was observed between the baseline level of SBP and the 26-year incidence of IC (**Figure B81.1**). When the data were examined for a threshold effect, the DBP at which level

TABLE B81.1

APPROXIMATE RANGE OF ODDS RATIOS FOR RISK FACTORS FOR SYMPTOMATIC PAD

Diabetes	3.0–3.7
Smoking	2.8–3.8
Hypertension	1.5–2.0
Dyslipidemia	1.4–2.1
Hyperhomocysteinemia	1.0–2.8
C-reactive protein	2.0–3.0
Renal insufficiency	1.25–2.5

(Modified from Norgren L, Hiatt WR, et al. Inter-society consensus for the management of peripheral arterial disease [TASC II]. *Eur J Vasc Endovasc Surg* 2007;33(Suppl 1):S1–S70 and *J Vasc Surg* 2007;45:1S–68S.)

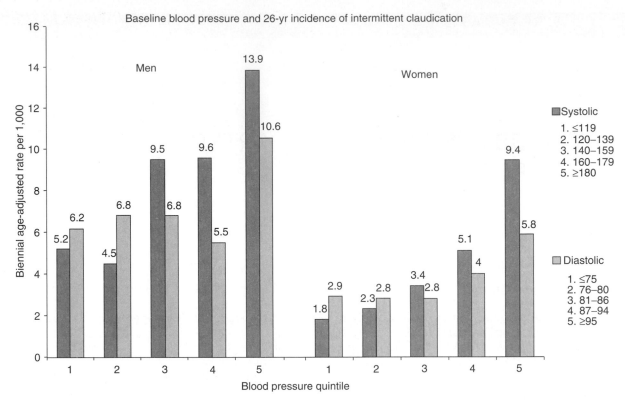

Figure B81.1 Risk of intermittent claudication by systolic and diastolic blood pressure. Subjects aged 35 to 84 years. Trends significant at p <.001. Data from 26-year follow-up of the Framingham Study. (Reproduced with permission from Kannel WB, McGee DL. Update on some epidemiologic features of intermittent claudication: the Framingham Study. *J Am Geriatr Soc* 1985;33:13–18.

there was an increased risk of developing IC was found at the fourth quartile (87–94 mm Hg) in women and at the fifth quintile (≥95 mm Hg) in men. When the fifth quintile of SBP (≥180 mm Hg) was compared to the first quintile of SBP (≤119 mm Hg), the relative risk in men was 2.7 and in women 5.2. Interestingly, the attributable (or excess) risk in men and women for the fifth versus the first quintile was the same in both men and women (8/1,000 biennial rate). The relative risk, although strong, may have even been more significant if less stringent criteria than the presence of IC were used as it is now known that a significant number of patients with an abnormal ankle-branchial index (ABI) do not have classic calf pain with ambulation.

National health and nutrition examination survey. The 1999 to 2000 National Health and Nutrition Examination Survey (NHANES) of 2,174 patients aged 40 and older reported the risk of PAD was significantly increased with HTN [odds ratio (OR) 1.75].

Methodological considerations. The relative weakness of associations in some studies could reflect the different pathogenetic mechanisms between HTN and atherosclerosis but could also arise from weaknesses in study methodology. First, IC is an imprecise endpoint for PAD. Although usually reflecting significant obstruction, approximately half the patients reporting IC in a population study had no demonstrable reduction in arterial flow with extensive noninvasive testing. Second, bias could also be introduced by diet, lifestyle, or pharmacologic interventions after the diagnosis of IC. Therefore, it is important to have a high degree of suspicion for PAD in patients with HTN although "classic" symptoms of claudication may not be present.

Ankle–brachial index studies

Ankle-brachial index measurement. A simple and reliable means to diagnose PAD is the ABI. Even when not measuring the ABI, it is important to measure blood pressure (BP) in both arms as a reduced pressure of >10 mm Hg in the left arm most likely indicates subclavian artery stenosis. Most reports and guidelines in the literature advocate the higher of the two posterior tibial and dorsalis pedis arteries in the foot for calculating the ABI. When a hemodynamically significant atherosclerotic lesion, usually >70% stenosis, occurs in the lower extremity arteries, the velocity of blood through the stenosis increases and may be accompanied by a decreases in limb pressure. An ankle pressure that is <90% of the brachial pressure is considered diagnostic for PAD although an ABI <1 but >0.90 is considered borderline. Studies using this criterion, or a more conservative criterion such as an ABI of <0.80 or even <0.75, have reported a significant association with elevated BP.

Cardiovascular health study. The Cardiovascular Health Study showed a gradation of effect, with an inverse relationship between ABI and prevalence of HTN [using the older World Health Organization (WHO) criteria of SBP >160 mm Hg or DBP >95 mm Hg], self-reported HTN, or self-reported use of antihypertensive medications. After adjustment for age and gender, strong inverse relations were observed for ABI and SBP and between ABI and relative risk of HTN. DBP did not differ significantly with varying levels of ABI.

Rotterdam study. The presence of HTN in the Rotterdam Study, where the definition was a pressure ≥160/95 or use of antihypertensive medications, was 60% for both men and women with an ABI <0.90. This association between ABI and HTN was reported in other studies but not all are concordant. One limitation of this type of cross-sectional studies is that the ABI is the only criteria and errors with this measurement may alter the sensitivity and specificity.

Noninvasive vascular testing

Rancho Bernardo study. A community-based study emanating from the Rancho Bernardo area of California of older individuals utilized noninvasive vascular testing to minimize the potential number of false-positive and false-negative cases. Moderate PAD cases had a somewhat higher SBP than normal individuals but the difference was not statistically significant. Severe PAD cases had a significantly higher SBP than normal individuals (11.7 mm Hg), but the increase in DBP (1.8 mm Hg) was not statistically significant (**Table B81.2**). HTN was defined either as an SBP $\geq$140 mm Hg or a DBP $\geq$90 mm Hg or use of hypertensive medications (**Table B81.3**). For both sexes, there was a stepwise increase in the proportion of hypertensive persons from normal individuals to persons with moderate PAD to people with severe PAD. For both sexes combined, with analyses adjusted for age and sex, individuals with moderate PAD had a 50% or greater prevalence of HTN. Individuals with severe PAD had approximately twice the prevalence of HTN as normal individuals.

San Luis Valley study. In the San Luis Valley Diabetes Study, two vessel criteria (both dorsalis pedis and posterior tibial artery meeting ABI criteria) was used to define PAD rather than the more conventional "highest of two" foot arteries. Hiatt et al. found that the odds ratio for HTN increased with worsening PAD percentiles. At the fifth percentile, the HTN odds ratio was 1.63; at the 2.5 percentile, it was 2.16; and at the first percentile, it was 3.12; all p values were <.05.

Angiographic studies. The evaluation of HTN as a risk factor when using angiographic data provides a highly reliable diagnosis for PAD. The results of these studies are mixed, ranging from no association to strong associations; similar to that reported when IC was used as diagnostic criteria. An Italian study found a statistically significant fivefold increase in the prevalence of HTN (SBP >160 mm Hg or DBP >95 mm Hg) among patients with PAD when compared with age- and gender-matched controls. In another study that matched patients with PAD and controls for mean arterial pressure, patients with PAD had increased SBP

TABLE B81.2

AGE-ADJUSTED MEAN LEVELS OF BLOOD PRESSURE BY PAD STATUS

PAD status	Men	Women	Men and women (sex adjusted)
Normal (N)	183	225	408
SBP	131.2	128.2	129.2
DBP	77.2	73.9	75.4
Moderate PAD (N)	22	27	49
SBP	138.9[a]	125.4	131.4
DBP	80.0	71.6	75.2
Severe PAD (N)	12	6	18
SBP	140.4[a]	141.9[a]	140.9[b]
DBP	78.2	74.8	77.2

DBP, diastolic blood pressure; SBP, systolic blood pressure.
[a]p < .05
[b]p < .01, compared to normal group.

TABLE B81.3

AGE- AND SEX-ADJUSTED PERCENTAGES OF HYPERTENSIVES BY PAD STATUS USING TWO DIFFERENT DEFINITIONS OF HYPERTENSION (HTN)

PAD status	Men	Women	Men and women (sex adjusted)
Normal (N)	183	225	408
% HTN1	39.5	46.6	41.6
% HTN2	24.3	32.8	26.9
Moderate PAD (N)	22	27	49
% HTN1	65.4[a]	58.5	60.3[b]
% HTN2	54.2[b]	43.8	46.5[b]
Severe PAD (N)	12	6	18
% HTN1	74.5[a]	90.0[a]	81.2[c]
% HTN2	53.8[a]	61.8	55.7[a]

HTN1 = (HTN DRUGS or SBP $\geq$140 or DBP $\geq$90)
HTN2 = (HTN DRUGS or SBP $\geq$160 or DBP $\geq$95)
[a]$p \leq .05$.
[b]$p \leq .01$.
[c]$p \leq .001$, compared to normal group.

and decreased DBP, and thereby increased pulse pressure. Pulse pressure inversely correlates with arterial compliance, owing to changes in viscoelastic properties of the arterial wall.

Peripheral arterial disease progression

The association of HTN with progression of disease was reported by Palumbo for 110 normal control subjects, 112 patients with PAD without diabetes mellitus, 240 patients with diabetes mellitus without PAD, and 100 patients with diabetes mellitus. PAD was defined by the rate of change in the postexercise ABI over 4 years, as well as the occurrence of clinical events, such as PAD surgery, including amputation. In multivariate analyses, SBP and smoking were independently and significantly predictive of PAD progression. Similar data exist in other studies.

Hypertension treatment and peripheral arterial disease

Symptoms of peripheral arterial disease. Although HTN is a risk factor for PAD, BP lowering does not conclusively improve IC, at least over the short term. Short-term trials using vasodilators such as calcium channel blockers have not proved effective in increasing pain-free walking distance. Although β-blockers have been alleged to worsen claudication symptoms, a meta-analysis did not support this. Furthermore, current National and International guidelines support the use of β-blockers in patients with PAD especially those undergoing vascular surgery. The Antihypertensive and Lipid Lowering treatment to prevent Heart Attack Trial (ALLHAT) reported atherosclerotic outcomes in high-risk patients but did not show differences in incident hospitalization for PAD or revascularization among groups assigned to diuretic, calcium-channel blocker, or angiotensin-converting enzyme (ACE) inhibitor therapy.

Limb loss. The prognosis regarding limb loss is relatively good with IC, as approximately 1% to 3.3% develop critical limb ischemia requiring a major amputation over 5 years.

Cardiovascular disease events. Mortality rate approaches 30% over 5 years in PAD, with approximately two thirds due to a cardiovascular event. In several studies of BP lowering that have included patients with PAD, strict BP control effectively reduces CVD events, particularly among those with diabetes.

Appropriate blood-pressure control in diabetes study. A *post hoc* analysis from the Appropriate Blood-Pressure Control in Diabetes (ABCD) trial reported on 447 diabetic patients with PAD that intensive BP control (<130/80 mm Hg) significantly reduced the risk for myocardial infarction (MI), stroke, or other vascular events compared with normotensive patients ($p = .009$), even at the lowest ABI levels. In the placebo group, ABI was inversely related to the event rate; BP treatment abolished this relationship, such that event rates in the treatment group were indistinguishable from those who had a normal ABI.

Heart outcomes prevention evaluation study. A *post hoc* analysis from the Heart Outcomes Prevention Evaluation (HOPE) study also showed that patients with an ABI <0.90 benefited somewhat more from treatment with an ACE inhibitor similar than those without PAD. A substudy using ambulatory BP monitoring in a subgroup of patients with PAD in HOPE demonstrated a large SBP reduction (>11 mm Hg) in contrast to the main study report (of SBP decrease of ~3 mm Hg).

Treatment guidelines

Current National [American College of Cardiology (ACC)/American Heart Association (AHA)] and International Transatlantic Inter-Society Consensus (TASC II) Guidelines advocate aggressive risk factor modification in patients with PAD along with SBP goal <140 mm Hg in general and <130 mm Hg in diabetes mellitus despite a relative lack of evidence in this area. However, the TASC II International PAD Guidelines recommend that thiazides and ACE inhibitors "should be considered as initial blood pressure lowering drugs in PAD to reduce the risk of cardiovascular events" based on well-conducted clinical trials but no good quality randomized clinical trials of antihypertensive agents in this population. National and International PAD Guidelines recommendations regarding treatment of HTN are in agreement with the Joint National Committee on Prevention, Detection, Evaluation, and treatment of High BP (JNC) 7th iteration. Given the high coprevalence with other atherosclerosis the JNC-7 suggests that "more intensive screening for these related cardiovascular disorders is appropriate in persons with [symptomatic] PAD." All groups caution that renovascular disease is more common in patients with PAD and therefore clinicians should consider the possibility of renovascular disease when encountering refractory HTN or when prescribing an ACE inhibitor or angiotensin receptor blocker (ARB).

Suggested Readings

Criqui MH, Fronek A, Klauber MR, et al. The sensitivity, specificity, and predictive value of traditional clinical evaluation of peripheral arterial disease: results from noninvasive testing in a defined population. *Circulation* 1985;71:516–522.

Fowkes FGR, Housley E, Riemersma RA, et al. Smoking, lipids, glucose intolerance, and BP as risk factors for peripheral atherosclerosis compared with ischemic heart disease in the Edinburgh artery study. *Am J Epidemiol* 1992;135:331–340.

Hiatt WR, Hoag S, Hamman RF. Effect of diagnostic criteria on the prevalence of peripheral arterial disease. The San Luis Valley diabetes study. *Circulation* 1995;91:1472–1479.

Hirsch AT, Criqui MH, Treat-Jacobson D, et al. Peripheral arterial disease detection, awareness, and treatment in primary care. *JAMA* 2001;286:1317–1324.

Kannel WB, McGee DC. Update on some epidemiologic features of intermittent claudication: the Framingham study. *J Am Geriatr Soc* 1985;33:13–18.

Meijer WT, Hoes AW, Rutgers D, et al. Peripheral arterial disease in the elderly: the Rotterdam study. *Arterioscler Thromb Vasc Biol* 1998;118:185–192.

Newman AB, Siscovick DS, Manolio TA, et al. CHS Collaborative Research Group. Ankle-arm index as a marker of atherosclerosis in the cardiovascular health study. *Circulation* 1993;88:837–845.

Norgren L, Hiatt WR, Dormandy JA, et al. Inter-society consensus for the management of peripheral arterial disease (TASC II). *J Vasc Surg* 2007;45:1S–68S.

Palumbo PJ, O'Fallon WM, Osmundson PJ, et al. Progression of peripheral occlusive arterial disease in diabetes mellitus. What factors are predictive? *Arch Intern Med* 1991;151:717–721.

Strano A, Novo S, Avellone G, et al. Hypertension and other risk factors in peripheral arterial disease. *Clin Exp Hypertens* 1993;15:71–89.

SECTION II ■ HYPERTENSION IN SPECIAL POPULATIONS

CHAPTER B82 ■ GENDER AND BLOOD PRESSURE

EDUARDO PIMENTA, MD AND SUZANNE OPARIL, MD

KEY POINTS

■ There is a sexual dimorphism in the relationship between age and systolic blood pressure (SBP): men have higher SBP levels than women during early and middle adult years, women tend to have higher SBP levels after the sixth decade.

■ Diastolic blood pressure (DBP) tends to be slightly higher in men than women, regardless of age.

■ Oral contraceptive or menopausal hormone therapy usually has only minimal effects on blood pressure (BP) but hypertensive postmenopausal women treated with estrogens and progestins may be at increased risk.

■ Antihypertensive therapy induces similar reductions in BP and cardiovascular disease outcomes in men and women.

See also Chapter **C160**

Age and blood pressure

Blood pressure patterns. Blood pressure (BP) manifests a sexually dimorphic pattern in humans, with mean BP being generally higher in men than women regardless of age. In the Third National Health and Nutrition Examination Survey (NHANES III), mean systolic blood pressure (SBP) increased progressively throughout adult life in both men and women but SBP was slightly higher in men during early adulthood. In contrast, the age-related rate of rise in blood pressure (BP) was steeper for women in all ethnic groups studied (non-Hispanic blacks, non-Hispanic whites, and Mexican Americans) and SBP in women was as high or higher than the corresponding values for men during and after the seventh decade of life.

In the overall population, diastolic blood pressure (DBP) increases progressively in both men and women until approximately the sixth decade of life, after which it decreases progressively. The consequence is a widening pulse pressure in men and women after the age of 60, probably due to loss of aortic and other large vessel elasticity. Wide pulse pressure independently predicts cardiovascular risk but yielded similar overall information to systolic BP in the large meta-regression reported by Lewington et al. Throughout adult life, men have a slightly higher average level of DBP than women. African American women have a higher mean DBP than white or Hispanic women. The same is true of men until the end of the fifth decade. Thereafter, mean DBP is similar in these three ethnic groups.

Prevalence of hypertension. The prevalence of hypertension increases progressively with age in men and women (**Figure. B82.1**). The prevalence of hypertension in NHANES 2003–2004 was 7.3% for people in the 18 to 39 age-group,

32.6% for people in the 40 to 59 age-group and 66.6% in the 60 years and older age-group. In early adulthood and in those aged 40 to 59 years, hypertension is more common among men than women. However, after the sixth decade of life, the incidence of hypertension increases more rapidly in women than men, with the prevalence of hypertension in women exceeding that in men. Data from the Framingham Heart Study showed that almost 80% of women 80 years of age or older have stage 1 or stage 2 hypertension or are on antihypertensive treatment based on the Seventh Report of the Joint National Committee on Detection, Evaluation, and Treatment of High Blood Pressure (JNC 7). African Americans tend to develop hypertension earlier than whites, such that most African American men and women are hypertensive by the age of 55.

Gender and blood pressure awareness, treatment, and control. Data from NHANES 2003–2004 showed no gender difference in awareness or treatment of hypertension. BP control is more difficult to achieve in older patients. Data from the Framingham Heart Study showed an age-related decline in BP control rate that was more pronounced in women than men (**Figure. B82.2**). The same study showed gender differences in the pattern of antihypertensive medications prescribed, that is, more frequent prescription of thiazide diuretics for women than men in all age-groups.

Menopause and blood pressure

The effect of menopause on BP is controversial. Longitudinal studies have not documented a rise in BP with menopause, whereas cross-sectional studies have found significantly higher

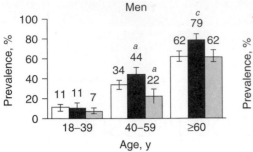

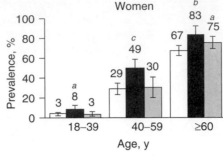

Figure B82.1 Prevalence of hypertension in the United States by age, gender, and race. National Health and Nutrition Examination Survey (NHANES) 2003–2004. [a]p < .05, [b]p < .01, [c]p <.001 for the difference within the same age-group (non-Hispanic whites as the referent for race/ethnicity).

SBP and DBP in postmenopausal versus premenopausal women. In NHANES III, the rate of rise in SBP tended to be steeper in postmenopausal women compared to premenopausal women until the sixth decade, when the rate of increase tended to slow. Staessen et al. reported a fourfold higher prevalence of hypertension in postmenopausal women than in premenopausal women (40% vs. 10%, $p < .001$). After adjustment for age and body mass index, postmenopausal women were still more than twice as likely to have hypertension as premenopausal women. In a recent prospective study of conventional and ambulatory BP levels in pre-, peri-, and postmenopausal women, the postmenopausal women had high SBP (4 to 5 mm Hg) compared to the pre- and perimenopausal controls. The increase in SBP per decade was 5 mm Hg greater in the peri- and postmenopausal women compared to the premenopausal group. Therefore, there is disagreement between longitudinal and cross-sectional studies as to the effect of menopause on BP but there is convincing evidence that at least part of the rise in BP (particularly SBP) seen later in life in women is related to menopause. Gender differences in the regulation of vascular function may partially explain the greater incidence of hypertension in men and postmenopausal women than in premenopausal women. A menopause-related increase in BP has been attributed to a variety of other factors, including estrogen withdrawal, overproduction of pituitary hormones, weight gain, or a combination of these, and other yet undefined neurohumoral influences.

Menopausal hormone therapy and blood pressure

Studies evaluating the effects of menopausal hormone therapy [also known as *hormone replacement therapy*, (HRT)] on BP have reported inconsistent findings due to differences in patient populations studied, routes of administration, methodologic differences in BP measurement, and hormone preparations administered. Most studies have described minimal BP effects of HRT in normotensive women. The Baltimore Longitudinal Study on Aging (BLSA) found that women receiving HRT (oral or transdermal estrogen and progestin) had a significantly smaller (1.6 mm Hg) increase in SBP over time than nonusers (8.9 mm Hg; **Figure B82.3**). DBP was not affected by HRT. The Postmenopausal Estrogen/Progestin Intervention (PEPI) trial followed 596 normotensive postmenopausal women, aged 45 to 64 years for an average of 3 years and found no significant effect of HRT (conjugated equine estrogen and native or synthetic progestin) on SBP or DBP. The Women's Health Initiative (WHI)'s cross-sectional analysis of almost 100,000 women aged 50 to 79 years indicated that current HRT use was associated with a 25% greater likelihood of having hypertension compared to past use or no prior use of HRT. However, the estrogen plus progestin arm of WHI, a placebo-controlled trial of HRT with 16,608 postmenopausal women, found a small (~1 mm Hg) increase in SBP in the HRT group compared to placebo.

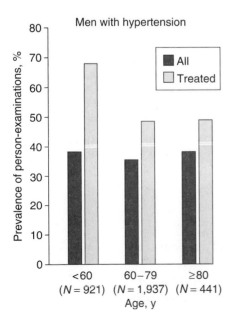

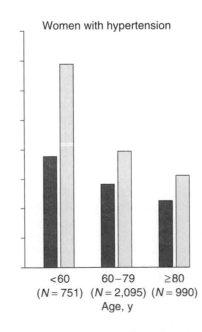

Figure B82.2 Prevalence of controlled blood pressure (BP) among all hypertensive and treated hypertensive men and women.

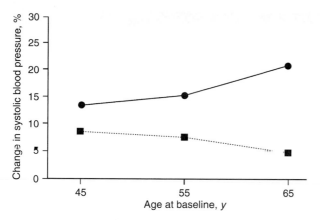

Figure B82.3 Systolic blood pressure (BP) effect in users (*dotted line*) compared to nonusers (*solid line*) of hormone replacement therapy in the Baltimore Longitudinal Study on Aging. Data are based on average 5.7-year follow-up of 226 normotensive postmenopausal women. (From Scuteri A, Bos AJ, Brant LJ, et al. Hormone replacement therapy and longitudinal changes in BP in postmenopausal women. *Ann Intern Med* 2001;135:229–238.)

A review of papers published since 1960 suggests that there is a very low risk of developing hypertension during HRT. In fact, BP was often lower in HRT-treated hypertensive women. Smaller studies using 24-hour ambulatory BP monitoring have yielded inconsistent results but overall, several of the studies suggest that HRT improves or normalizes impaired nighttime reduction ("dipping") in BP in postmenopausal women. Such an effect would tend to reduce total BP load and thereby reduce target organ damage. Overall, HRT-related change in BP is likely to be minor and should not preclude HRT use in either normotensive or hypertensive women. Nevertheless, all hypertensive women treated with HRT should have their BP measured initially and then at 3- to 6-month intervals depending on the difficulty of control.

Oral contraceptives and blood pressure

Combined agents. Combined oral contraceptive (COC) preparations that contain both estrogens and progestins tend to increase BP in all women. The BP increment is generally minor but a small percentage of COC users experience the onset of frank hypertension, which usually resolves with withdrawal of the drug. This is true even with modern preparations that contain lower doses (<30 μg) of estrogen. However, COCs occasionally precipitate accelerated, or even malignant hypertension. There appears to be increased susceptibility to COC-induced hypertension in those with a family history of hypertension, preexisting pregnancy-induced hypertension, occult renal disease, obesity, middle age (older than 35 years), and longer duration of COC use. **Table B82.1** summarizes contraindications for COC use based on World Health Organization recommendations.

The Nurses' Health Study found that current users of COCs had a significantly increased risk of developing hypertension [relative risk (RR), 1.8; 95% confidence interval, 1.5–2.3] compared with never-users. Absolute risk was small (41.5 cases/10,000 person-years) and risk decreased quickly with cessation of COCs. Controlled prospective studies have consistently demonstrated a return of BP to pretreatment levels within 3 months of discontinuing COCs. A cross-sectional survey (Health Survey for England) of 3,545 premenopausal women, 892 whom were current users of

oral contraceptives (815 COC, 77 progestin-only) demonstrated significantly higher mean BP among COC users than nonusers; this BP difference tended to increase with age.

Progestins. Progestins have mineralocorticoid receptor antagonist effects that may account for their BP reducing action. The fourth-generation progestin, drospirenone, when combined with estradiol, has been shown to reduce BP (**Figure B82.4**). In contrast to COCs, BP tends to be lower among the progestin-only users than nonusers. On the basis of these and other data, progestin-only contraceptives have been recommended for women with established hypertension and other cardiovascular risk factors.

Gender and therapeutic responses

Outcomes of antihypertensive trials. Recent outcome trials of antihypertensive treatment, including Antihypertensive and Lipid-Lowering Treatment to Prevent Heart Attack Trial (ALLHAT), Losartan Intervention For Endpoint Reduction (LIFE) and Anglo-Scandinavian Cardiac Outcomes Trial-BP Lowering Arm (ASCOT-BPLA), have generally shown comparable benefit in both men and women.

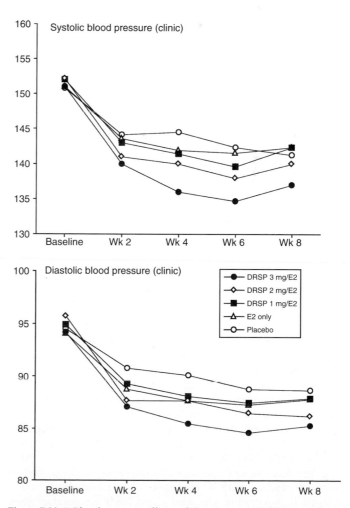

Figure B82.4 Blood pressure effects of drospirenone (DRSP) in different dosages associated with estradiol, versus estradiol only and placebo. Results of 750 postmenopausal women with stage 1 and 2 hypertension. (From White WB, Hanes V, Chauhan V, et al. Effects of a new hormone therapy, drospirenone and 17β-estradiol, in postmenopausal women with hypertension. *Hypertension* 2006;48:246–253.)

TABLE B82.1

CONTRAINDICATIONS TO COMBINED ORAL CONTRACEPTIVES

Contraindications	Risk-benefit grounds
Smoking in women older than 35 yr	
<15 cigarettes/d	Risk > benefit
>15 cigarettes/d	Risk unacceptable
Hypertension	
History of hypertension, current blood pressure (BP) unknown	Risk > benefit
Adequately controlled hypertension	Risk > benefit
Elevated BP levels	
Systolic 140–159 or diastolic 90–99	Risk > benefit
Systolic >160 or diastolic >100	Risk unacceptable
Vascular disease	Risk unacceptable
Multiple risk factors for cardiovascular disease	
Older age, smoking, diabetes, and hypertension	Risk > benefit: may be unacceptable
Deep venous thrombosis (DVT)/pulmonary embolism (PE)	
History of or current DVT/PE	Risk unacceptable
Major surgery	
With prolonged immobilization	Risk unacceptable
Known thrombogenic mutations (e.g., Factor V Leiden; prothrombin mutation; protein S, protein C, and antithrombin deficiencies)	Risk unacceptable
Ischemic heart disease	Risk unacceptable
Stroke	Risk unacceptable
Migraine	
Without aura in women >35 yr of age	Risk > benefit
With, at any age	Risk unacceptable
Diabetes	
Nephropathy/retinopathy/neuropathy	Risk > benefit/risk unacceptable
Other vascular disease or diabetes of >20-yr duration	Risk > benefit/risk unacceptable

Choice of antihypertensive drugs. Although women generally respond to antihypertensive drugs similarly to men, special considerations may dictate treatment choices for women. Angiotensin-converting enzyme (ACE) inhibitors and AT_1-receptor blockers should be avoided by women who are or intend to become pregnant due to the risk of fetal developmental abnormalities. Data from the Tennessee Medical database have shown that infants with first-trimester only exposure to ACE inhibitors had a (approximately symbol) 3-fold increased risk of major congenital malformations, including cardiovascular and central nervous system malformations, compared to infants who had no exposure to antihypertensive medications. In contrast, fetal exposure to other antihypertensive medications during the first trimester did not confer an increased risk. Diuretics are particularly useful in women, notably elderly women, because their use is associated with decreased risk of hip fracture.

Adverse event profiles. Antihypertensive drugs have gender-specific adverse effect profiles. In the Treatment of Mild Hypertension Study (TOMHS), women reported twice as many adverse effects as men. Biochemical responses to drugs may be gender dependent, with women more likely to develop diuretic-induced hyponatremia and men more likely to develop gout. Hypokalemia is more common in women taking a diuretic and ACE inhibitor–induced cough is twice as common in women as in men. Women are also more likely to complain of dihydropyridine calcium channel blocker–related peripheral edema and minoxidil-induced hirsutism.

In men, the effect of antihypertensive therapy on sexual function is a major obstacle to sustained treatment. In ASCOT-BPLA, men assigned to atenolol/bendroflumethoazide treatment had significantly more erectile dysfunction compared to those in the amlodipine/perindopril group. In LIFE, sexual dysfunction was significantly more frequent with atenolol than with losartan. Sexual dysfunction may be a problem in hypertensive women as well. However, additional evaluation is needed in this area, because sexual dysfunction in women is seldom assessed in clinical trials.

Suggested Readings

ALLHAT Collaborative Research Group. Major outcomes in high-risk hypertensive patients randomized to angiotensin-converting enzyme inhibitor or calcium channel blockers *vs* diuretic. The Antihypertensive and Lipid-Lowering Treatment to Prevent Heart Attack Trial (ALLHAT). *JAMA* 2002;288:2981–2997.

American College of Obstetricians and Gynecologists Practice Bulletin. Use of hormonal contraception in women with coexisting medical conditions: clinical management guidelines for obstetrician-gynecologists. *Obstet Gynecol* 2006;107:1453–1472.

Dahlof B, Devereux RB, Kjeldsen SE, et al. Cardiovascular morbidity and mortality in the Losartan Intervention For Endpoint reduction in hypertension study (LIFE): a randomised trial against atenolol. *Lancet* 2002;359:995–1003.

Dahlof B, Sever PS, Poulter NR, et al. Prevention of cardiovascular events with an antihypertensive regimen of amlodipine adding perindopril as required versus atenolol adding bendroflumethiazide as required, in the Anglo-Scandinavian Cardiac Outcomes Trial-BP Lowering Arm (ASCOT-BPLA): a multicentre randomised controlled trial. *Lancet* 2005;366:895–906.

Lloyd-Jones DM, Evans JC, Levy D. Hypertension in adults across the age spectrum: current outcomes and control in the community. *JAMA* 2005;294:466–472.

Mueck AO, Seeger H. Effect of hormone therapy on BP in normotensive and hypertensive postmenopausal women. *Maturitas* 2004;49:189–203.

Ong KL, Cheung BMY, Man YB, et al. Prevalence, awareness, treatment, and control of hypertension among United States adults 1999–2004. *Hypertension* 2007;49:69–75.

Scuteri A, Bos AJ, Brant LJ, et al. Hormone replacement therapy and longitudinal changes in BP in postmenopausal women. *Ann Intern Med* 2001;135:229–238.

Wassertheil-Smolller S, Anderson G, Psaty BM, et al. Hypertension and its treatment in postmenopausal women: baseline data from the Women's Health Initiative. *Hypertension* 2000;36:780–789.

World Health Organization. Low dose combined oral contraceptives. In: *Improving access to quality care in family planning: medical eligibility criteria for contraceptive use*, 3rd ed. Geneva, Switzerland: World Health Organization, 2004.

CHAPTER B83 ■ BLOOD PRESSURE IN CHILDREN

BRUCE Z. MORGENSTERN, MD AND ALAN R. SINAIKO, MD

KEY POINTS

■ Blood pressure (BP) is considerably lower in children than adults and increases steadily throughout the first 2 decades of life; pediatric BP tables are readily available. [http://www.nhlbi.nih.gov/guidelines/hypertension/child_tbl.htm]

■ Factors known to be associated with higher levels of BP in children and adolescents include greater weight, greater height, and a family history of hypertension.

■ Measurement of BP is recommended at least yearly after the age of 3 years.

■ The diagnosis of hypertension in children is based on the first and the fifth Korotkoff sounds to define BP as well as height, gender, and age.

See also Chapter **C161**

Arterial hypertension has a relatively low prevalence in children compared with adults but still has significant long-term morbidity. Because the adults of tomorrow with primary hypertension emerge in large part from the normotensive, seemingly healthy children of today, it is important from a disease prevention standpoint to consider elevated blood pressure (BP) as a risk factor in the pediatric age-group, well before clinical manifestations of the disease become apparent.

Prevalence and risks of hypertension in children

Prospective cohort data on the relationship between childhood BP and adult cardiovascular risk are not yet available. The prevalence of essential (primary) hypertension in the U.S. adult population has been estimated to be 25%, or >50 million Americans. Although the prevalence of clinical hypertension is far less in children, evidence suggests that the roots of primary hypertension extend from childhood. Familial patterns for BP have been established; children with BP in the higher distributional percentiles are more likely to come from families with histories of hypertension. Studies have shown that cardiac ventricular wall, arterial wall, and hemodynamic changes consistent with chronic hypertension are demonstrable before the third decade of life, as early as childhood in those with secondary hypertension. BP elevations are associated with the metabolic syndrome (hyperinsulinemia,

dyslipidemia, obesity) before adulthood, particularly during adolescence. Adolescents with high BP have a significantly greater clustering effect for metabolic syndrome factors when compared to adolescents with low BP. Therefore, elevation of BP during the first 2 decades of life is likely an early warning sign of overall future cardiovascular risk.

Age and blood pressure

BP is considerably lower in children than adults and increases steadily throughout the first 2 decades of life.

Infants. The average systolic blood pressure (SBP) at 1 day of age is approximately 70 mm Hg in full term infants and it increases to approximately 85 mm Hg by 1 month of age. BP increases at a greater rate in premature infants than full term infants during the first year of life. Among certain populations, there is a significant inverse relation between birth weight and the risk of hypertension in adulthood.

Tracking during growth and development. During the preschool years, BP begins to follow a tracking pattern in which children tend to maintain specific levels of BP relative to their peer group as they age. Tracking by a number of statistical methods, including percentile and raw BP data, tends to increase in significance for groups of subjects (as opposed to individuals) selected from the extremes of the BP distribution. Of particular importance is the documentation that BP tracking data, which provide indirect evidence of the early onset of a major adult cardiovascular risk factor, bridges the gap between childhood and early adulthood. Children who are even younger than 10 years of age who are in the higher distributions of BP show a tendency to become hypertensive adults. Tracking coefficients are higher in adolescents than in younger children.

Other risk factors for hypertension

A number of factors known to be associated with hypertension in adults have also been associated with higher levels of BP in children and adolescents.

Weight and height. A direct relation between current weight and BP has been documented as early as 5 years of age and is more prominent in the second decade. Height is independently related to BP at all ages.

Gender. BP in boys is slightly higher than in girls during the first decade of life. The difference between boys and girls widens around the onset of puberty, and BP is significantly higher in males by the end of the teenage years.

Race and ethnicity. Race does not have the same impact on BP in children as in adults. No significant differences have been found in comparisons of whites, blacks, Hispanics, and Southeast Asians until adolescence. Reference standards for BP in children do not distinguish between ethnic groups.

Family history. Primary hypertension is clearly polygenic in inheritance but children from hypertensive families tend to have higher BPs than children from normotensive families. The significant correlation of BP and cardiovascular risk factors between parents and children is widely recognized. The BP correlation is higher between mothers and their children than between fathers and their children, suggesting a prenatal influence. Siblings of children with high BP also have significantly higher BP than siblings of children with low BP.

Blood pressure measurement techniques

There are special features to the measurement and evaluation of BP in children that have been emphasized in the Fourth Report of the Task Force on BP Control in Children.

Oscillometry. Measurement by usual auscultation methods is difficult in infants and very young children. Therefore, automated oscillometric devices are recommended in this age group, and these devices are generally reliable. Measurement of BP is recommended yearly after the age of 3 years. In the Fourth Report, the use of oscillometric devices is only recommended for screening purposes for children older than 3 years, as these devices do not usually yield the same readings as the auscultatory technique, which is the technique used to develop the normal percentiles that appear in the Task Force reports. Pressures that have been determined by oscillometric devices and that exceed the 90th percentile in a given child should be repeated using a standard sphygmomanometer.

Cuff size. Use of an appropriately sized BP cuff is necessary to ensure accurate measurement and BP cuff sizes have been standardized. A wide array of pediatric cuffs, standard and large adult cuffs, and a thigh cuff should serve the needs of most practices. Using the manufacturer's suggested markings on the cuff or selecting a cuff size with a width approximately two thirds of the distance between the shoulder and elbow is recommended. In general, a cuff width meeting these criteria will also have a cuff bladder length that nearly encircles the arm.

Choosing an inappropriate cuff size may falsely elevate the BP, especially in the case of too small a cuff. Less commonly, a cuff that is too large will falsely reduce the BP. When choosing between two cuffs, both of which are close in size to the measured width of the arm, the larger cuff should be selected. It is uncommon for a slightly larger cuff to mask true hypertension, whereas use of a small cuff will often result in an elevated reading.

Korotkoff sounds. The onset of the first phase Korotkoff sound defines the SBP. The fifth phase Korotkoff sound is the diastolic blood pressure (DBP) for children of all ages.

Ambulatory pressures. Ambulatory blood pressure monitoring (ABPM) is being used increasingly in pediatrics but its role in complementing the casual office measurement has not been formally defined. ABPM enables computation of the mean BP during the awake time, the sleep interval at night, and over the full 24 hours. Measures to determine the degree to which BP exceeds the upper limit of normal, that is, the BP load, can also be calculated. ABPM is helpful in the evaluation of (a) white-coat hypertension, (b) the risk for hypertensive organ injury, (c) apparent drug resistance, and (d) apparent hypotensive symptoms with antihypertensive drugs. The Fourth Report recommends that only those experienced in its use and interpretation should use ABPM.

Evolution of guidelines

Historically, the initial orientation of health care providers toward BP in children and adolescents focused on the identification and pharmacologic or surgical treatment of secondary forms of hypertension. The incorporation of BP measurement into the routine pediatric examination during the last 20 years, the publication of national survey data on BP in children, and the increasing recognition of the long-term consequences of elevated BP in the young have confirmed that elevations in BP during childhood are more common than previously recognized, particularly in adolescents (i.e., beginning with the second decade of life). The First Task Force on BP Control in Children was convened in 1977 by the National Heart, Lung, and Blood Institute in response to the need to establish guidelines for the measurement and classification of BP and to develop recommendations for the treatment of childhood hypertension. The second Task Force report, published in 1987, revised and strengthened the norms for childhood BP Recommendations were further strengthened by an update of the 1987 report, published in 1996. The most recent update (the Fourth Report) in 2004 has refined BP norms, clarified issues regarding measurement of BP, and updated the approaches to investigation and treatment of hypertension in children and adolescents.

Current definitions and classification of high blood pressure

Definitions of hypertension in children and adolescents are, of necessity, based on clinical experience and consensus rather than on risk data. Categories are determined on the basis of percentile BP distribution within the pediatric population as follows: (a) normal BP: SBP and DBP <90th percentile for age and sex; (b) prehypertension: average SBP or DBP (or both) between the 90th and 95th percentiles for age and sex; (c) stage 1 hypertension: average SBP or DBP (or both) ≥95th but <the 99th percentile + 5 mm Hg, and (d) stage 2 hypertension: average SBP or DBP ≥the 99th percentile + 5 mm Hg for age and sex,

TABLE B83.1

REPRESENTATIVE SYSTOLIC AND DIASTOLIC BLOOD PRESSURE (BP) LEVELS FOR BOYS AND GIRLS 1 TO 17 YEARS OLD AT THE 50TH PERCENTILE FOR HEIGHT AT EACH AGE

| | Systolic BP centiles | | | | | | | |
| | Boys | | | | Girls | | | |
Age (yr)	50th	90th	95th	99th	50th	90th	95th	99th
1	85	99	103	110	86	100	104	111
4	93	107	111	118	91	104	108	115
8	99	112	116	123	98	111	115	122
12	106	120	123	131	105	119	123	120
17	129	132	136	138	111	125	129	126

| | Diastolic BP centiles | | | | | | | |
Yr	50th	90th	95th	99th	50th	90th	95th	99th
1	37	52	57	64	40	54	58	65
4	50	65	69	77	52	67	71	78
8	59	73	78	86	58	72	76	83
12	62	76	81	89	62	76	80	88
17	67	82	87	94	66	80	84	91

with measurements obtained on at least three occasions. The Fourth Report suggested the addition of 5 mm Hg to distinguish between stage 1 and stage 2 hypertension in an effort to make this distinction clearer and hopefully more clinically relevant. Prehypertension was adopted to be consistent with Joint National Committee on Prevention, Detection, Evaluation, and Treatment of high blood pressure (JNC 7).

Revised age–weight nomograms. Revised tables used to classify hypertension in children in the Fourth Report take into account the documented effect of body size and differential rates of growth in children by relating BP to age and height. The SBP and DBP values for boys and girls at the 50th percentile for height at selected ages and percentiles are provided in **Table B83.1.** For any given age, BP norms increase as height increases. Use of published norms helps prevent mislabeling of tall children who are not overweight as hypertensive, or missing the diagnosis of hypertension in shorter or heavier children, errors which occurred more frequently when BP level was related to age alone.

Surveillance and records

Except in cases of stage 2 or symptomatic hypertension, identifying children with high BP requires multiple BP measurements. Specifically, if the BP is above the 90th percentile, the child should be scheduled for repeat BP measurements over several visits. If the average BP is then below the 90th percentile, the child should return to continuing health care. If the average BP is between the 90th and 95th percentiles, the child has prehypertension and should remain under surveillance, with BP measurements at least every 6 months. If the average BP over time places the child ≥95th percentile, the child should undergo a diagnostic evaluation and

consideration should be given to therapy. In all cases, therapeutic lifestyle changes, including dietary modifications, increased physical activity, and weight loss should be instituted, optimally as a family-based endeavor.

Under optimal circumstances, children receive care from a continuing source, and good records are kept of their clinical progress. A record of the patient's BP should be maintained throughout the years and plotted against the age–weight nomograms. In this way, the health care provider is able to determine whether the child is trending in a favorable or an unfavorable direction. Such trends provide guidance for determining how closely the child should be monitored.

Suggested Readings

Butani L, Morgenstern BZ. Are pitfalls of oxcillometric BP measurements preventable in children? *Pediatr Nephrol* 2003;18(4):313–318.

Falkner B, Hulman S, Kushner H. Effect of birth weight on BP and body size in early adolescence. *Hypertension* 2004;43(2):203–207.

Ingelfinger JR. Pediatric antecedents of adult cardiovascular disease—awareness and intervention. *N Eng J Med* 2004;350(21):2123–2126.

Ingelfinger JR. The molecular basis of pediatric hypertension. *Pediatr Clin North Am* 2006;53(5):1011–1028. http://www.nhlbi.nih.gov/health/prof/heart/hbp/hbp_ped.pdf.

Lurbe E, Sorof JM, Daniels SR. Clinical and research aspects of ambulatory BP monitoring in children. *J Pediatr* 2004;144:7–16.

National High BP Education Program Working Group on Hypertension Control in Children and Adolescents. Update on the task force (1987) on high BP in children and adolescents: a working group from the National High BP Education Program. *Pediatrics* 1996;98:649–658.

National High BP Education Program Working Group on High BP in Children and Adolescents. The Fourth Report on the diagnosis, evaluation, and treatment of high BP in children and adolescents. *Pediatrics* 2004;114:555–576.

Rosenberg B, Moran A, Sinaiko AR. Insulin resistance (metabolic) syndrome in children. *Panminerva Med* 2005;47(4):229–244.

Sinaiko AR. Hypertension in children. *N Engl J Med* 1996;335:1968–1973.

CHAPTER B84 ■ ETHNICITY AND SOCIOECONOMIC STATUS IN HYPERTENSION

JOHN M. FLACK, MD, MPH; SAMAR A. NASSER, PA-C, MPH AND SHANNON M. O'CONNOR, BS

KEY POINTS

■ The age-adjusted incidence and prevalence of hypertension (HTN) is higher in blacks than whites and lowest in Hispanics.

■ Aggregate comparisons of mean blood pressure (BP) levels in various ethnic groups are confounded by differences in age, geographic factors, dietary patterns, socioeconomic status (SES), and other lifestyle attributes.

■ BP treatment rates are greatest in whites and higher in blacks than Hispanics; HTN control rates are higher in women compared to men, despite similar awareness rates.

■ BP and overall cardiovascular disease (CVD) burden are greater in women of lower SES of all three major ethnic groups.

See also Chapters B85, B86, B87, B88, and **C148**

Increasing blood pressure (BP), particularly systolic blood pressure (SBP) occurs commonly with advancing age in industrialized countries such as the United States, with the lifetime risk of hypertension (HTN) for most Americans probably exceeding 70%. Despite improvements in the treatment and control of HTN in recent years, ethnic disparities remain. There are persistent differences in health status experienced by ethnic minority and low socioeconomic status (SES) groups with an inverse relationship between SES and HTN prevalence.

Hypertension prevalence

Over the last decade, HTN incidence and prevalence has risen in the major race-ethnicity groups, with the largest increases among women.

United States. The most current age-adjusted prevalence of HTN according to National Health and Nutrition Examination Survey (NHANES) (2003–2004) in the U.S. population aged 18 years and older is 29.6%. Non-Hispanic blacks continue to have the highest age-adjusted HTN prevalence (39.1%), non-Hispanic whites are intermediate (28.5%), and Hispanics have the lowest at 27.8%. A multivariate analysis of the NHANES (2003–2004) data found that increasing age, higher body mass index (BMI), non-Hispanic black race, and lower education attainment were significantly and independently associated with HTN. However, gender was not independently associated with HTN.

Until recently, Native Americans had a relatively low prevalence of HTN. The Inter-Tribal Heart Project found a 31% prevalence of HTN in Chippewa and Menominee Indians older than 25

years of age, who were active users of the Indian Health Service clinics. The Strong Heart Study (SHS), the largest epidemiologic study of American Indians ever undertaken, confirmed this high prevalence of HTN. The SHS found a 27% to 56% prevalence of HTN in men and women between the ages of 45 and 75.

Europe and Africa. Blacks in the United States do not have the highest rates of HTN in the world. The age- and sex-adjusted prevalence of HTN at the standard threshold (i.e., BP ≥ 140/90 mm Hg or treatment with antihypertensive medication) was higher in Germany (55%), Finland (49%), and Spain (47%), than in U.S. blacks. The European average for HTN was 44.2% compared with 27.6% in North America. Nigerians, on the other hand, have much lower HTN prevalence rates than U.S. whites. One likely contributor to the lower prevalence of HTN in Nigerians compared to either whites or blacks in the United States is the very low prevalence of obesity within this population.

Asians. The age-adjusted prevalence of HTN in Koreans was 32%, a burden that was higher than in the general American population (24%). Asian American men were also more likely to have HTN (35%) than women (30%). The age-adjusted prevalence of HTN in Asian American (Chinese), according to the Multi-Ethnic Study of Atherosclerosis (MESA), was 39% which was similar to whites (38%) and Hispanics (42%) but less than in blacks (60%).

Hypertension awareness, treatment, and control

Over the last 2 decades, the number of Americans aware of their hypertensive condition has increased. NHANES (2003-2004) data indicate that overall HTN awareness is greatest among non-Hispanic whites (66.9%) and non-Hispanic blacks (66.4%) compared with the Mexican American population (63.5%). In all hypertensive persons, the NHANES BP control rates increased significantly from 29.2% in 1999-2000 to 36.8% in 2003-2004 (age-adjusted, $p = .006$).

Hispanics. Apart from Hispanics exhibiting lower awareness of their HTN than either non-Hispanic white or black adults, they also have a lower rate of antihypertensive medication use. Hispanic women are more aware of their HTN than men and the percentage of hypertensive women under treatment with controlled BP was greater than among men. Nevertheless, BP is not adequately controlled in the large majority of hypertensive persons of any racial/ethnic group. The most recent NHANES HTN treatment and control rates (all hypertensives <140/90 mm Hg) among non-Hispanic whites are 53.7% and 35.4%, non-Hispanic blacks are 55% and 28.9%, and are lowest overall among Mexican Americans (48.3% and 26.5%), respectively.

Blacks. In the Antihypertensive and Lipid-Lowering Treatment to Prevent Heart Attack Trial (ALLHAT) study, the largest difference in BP control was found in the black/non-black race comparison, where blacks were 31% less likely to be controlled [odds ratio (OR) 0.69; 95% confidence limits: 0.65–0.73] than non-blacks. Furthermore, from baseline through year 5, the highest control rate was in non-black men (70%) whereas the lowest control rate was in black women (58.8%). However, less intensive antihypertensive pharmacologic treatment likely contributed to the lower BP control rates in blacks compared to whites.

Asians and Native Americans. Fewer than 50% of Asian Americans with HTN were pharmacologically treated and approximately 14% appear to attain BP control with medication alone. According to the Inter-Tribal Heart Project only 58% of hypertensive Indians took antihypertensive medication and only 28% had BPs below recommended levels.

Geography and urbanization

United States demography. Geographic location influences HTN risk. The Coronary Artery Risk Development in Young Adults (CARDIA) Study (a cohort of >5,000 black and white men and women, aged 18 to 30 years, studied at four clinical centers located in different regions of the country) found that there was no initial difference in HTN prevalence. Over 7 years of follow-up, differences in HTN incidence and prevalence emerged; at the 7-year visit, HTN prevalence differed significantly by region. (Birmingham, AL, 14%; Oakland, CA, 11.2%; Minneapolis, MN, 7%; and Chicago, IL, 6.6%). Also at the 7-year visit, HTN prevalence in black and white men was 9% to 5%, respectively, in Chicago and 25% to 14%, respectively, in Birmingham. Among women, elevated BP did not differ significantly by regional center, but HTN prevalence was highest in black and white women in the Birmingham cohort. Regional dietary intake habits may contribute, at least in part, to these regional differences in HTN burden.

Southeastern stroke belt. Approximately one half of adult U.S. blacks reside in 13 southeastern states. Therefore, race/ethnic contrasts involving U.S. blacks are, to a degree, influenced by geography. Interestingly, the risk of stroke death among blacks varies by geographic region with rates being significantly higher in blacks residing in the Southeast compared to blacks residing in other regions of the country. Poor BP control, along with dietary factors (e.g., high sodium and low potassium intakes), may be an important factor contributing to the high rate of pressure-related complications among blacks in the southeastern United States.

Obesity and nutrition

Approximately 80% of people with HTN in the United States are overweight or obese (BMI ≥ 25 kg/m^2). Obesity is associated with HTN risk in all racial/ethnic populations and particularly in racial and ethnic minorities. There are multiple obesity-related physiologic effects that contribute to the intermediate BP phenotype, including salt sensitivity as well as resistance to hypertensive drug therapy. Additionally, obesity appears to be a plausible mediator of chronic renal injury.

Race–gender interactions. In black women, the prevalence of extreme obesity (BMI >40 kg/m^2) is almost one in six, a prevalence that is approximately three to fourfold higher than that of either white or Hispanic women. There are marked ethnic and age-based differences in the rates of weight accumulation. Relative to white women (reference group) the onset of obesity occurred sooner for black and Hispanic women. Hispanic men also develop obesity at younger ages than white men. After 28 years of age, black men develop obesity more rapidly than white men. Anthropometric measures, such as obesity, that correlate inversely with low SES, especially in women, can also influence biologic systems involved in BP regulation and the expression of pressure-related target organ damage. For example, obesity is a major anthropometric correlate of salt sensitivity in blacks and whites and is extremely prevalent among lower SES persons, particularly women.

Low birth weight. Maternal obesity increases the risk of preexisting maternal HTN, as well as pregnancy-induced HTN, preeclampsia, and eclampsia. All of these conditions increase the likelihood of preterm delivery and poor intrauterine growth resulting in low birth weight [(LBW) <2,500 g] infants. Accordingly, the risk of delivering an LBW infant is very high among black women. According to the 2003 Centers for Disease Control Pediatric Nutrition Surveillance System, the prevalence of LBW is higher for black infants (12.9%) than for white (8.5%), Asian or Pacific Islander (8.3%), Hispanic (7.3%), and American Indian or Alaska Native (7.1%) infants. LBW babies are not found evenly across all geographic locations in the United States; there is a higher proportion of LBW babies in the southeastern United States compared to other geographic regions.

Prematurity and LBW appear to contribute to adult cardiovascular disease (CVD) risk in several ways. LBW has been linked to central obesity and higher BMI later in life and to higher childhood BP. LBW has also been linked to having fewer nephrons at birth and to a relatively greater ratio of medullary to cortical glomeruli, the former being less able to autoregulate glomerular filtration rate and protect the glomeruli against transmission of systemic pressure into the glomerulus.

Caloric intake. During the past 3 decades, there has been little change in sodium intake, fat content and alcohol intake have declined, but total intake of calories and obesity prevalence have increased. Ethnic minority and low-income populations have some of the highest rates of CVD and the highest rates of physical inactivity, especially in lower SES women. In any population, potassium and calcium-rich and low sodium diets tend to favor lower BP levels. This type of diet would be rich in fresh fruits, vegetables, and low-fat dairy products while simultaneously being low in sodium; such a diet is similar, if not identical, to the Dietary Approaches to Stop Hypertension (DASH) diet.

Potassium. High levels of dietary potassium intake have been shown to modestly lower BP and to improve the nocturnal fall (dipping) in ambulatory BP studies. High dietary potassium intake enhances renal natriuresis, augments nitric oxide (NO) production, and prevents the sodium-induced rise in circulating asymmetrical dimethyl arginine (ADMA), a known inhibitor of NO synthesis. Dietary intake of potassium, which is found primarily in green leafy vegetables and fruit, is lower in blacks than in whites, probably due in part to the increasing cost of fresh fruits and vegetables compared to calorie-dense, high fat foods.

Calcium, vitamin D, and parathyroid hormone.
Calcium intake is lower in blacks than whites, and in lower income than higher income people. Lower intake of dairy products, which usually account for approximately 70% to 75% of total daily calcium intake, has been linked to HTN in blacks. Hypovitaminosis D coupled with low dietary calcium intake plausibly leads to transient reductions in ionized calcium, which in turn stimulate the reactive (and probably deleterious) rise in parathyroid hormone (PTH). In the United States, the prevalence of hypovitaminosis D (<37.5 nmol/L) is significantly more prevalent in black than white women (42.4% vs. 4.2%). A multiplicity of factors influences the striking excess prevalence of hypovitaminosis D in blacks, including darker skin and a higher prevalence of chronic kidney disease. Obesity is also strongly correlated with hypovitaminosis D and secondary hyperparathyroidism in blacks. In obese people, vitamin D production in the skin in response to ultraviolet light is normal but their greater sequestration of vitamin D in adipocytes leads to reduced circulating levels of 25(OH)D. The avoidance of dairy products that has been repeatedly identified in blacks probably relates to their relatively high prevalence ($\sim$80%) of lactose intolerance; Asian Americans are even more lactose intolerant than blacks. Calcium supplementation often modestly lowers BP in people with low dietary calcium intake, perhaps because of enhanced natriuresis as well as PTH suppression.

Socioeconomic status

SES indicators, especially education and income, function as surrogate markers for a constellation of lifestyle characteristics, including dietary patterns, physical activity, psychosocial and environmental stressors, social support, coping mechanisms, health-seeking behaviors, and access to health-related information and medical care.

Education. Data from all three NHANES revealed that the overall prevalence for HTN is higher among persons with less than a high school education compared to those with more than a high school education. Yet the trend of increased HTN prevalence has declined over time, in those with less than high school education (decrease of 15.9%) as well as those with more than high school education (decrease of 13.4%). An individual's attainment of durable goods has been related to education and BP among populations of African origin in the United States, Africa, and the Caribbean. Unlike previously reported associations between education and HTN in the United States, education level has been associated with a greater risk of HTN among Caribbean women (odds ratio 1.69, confidence interval, 1.15–2.48).

Income. The prevalence of black and Hispanic women with >12 years of education who were living in poverty was more than twice the rate observed in white women (18.9% and 18.6% respectively vs. 7.1%). These observations suggest a racial difference in the interface of education and income among women. According to the U.S. Department of Health and Human Services from 2001 to 2004, the age-adjusted prevalence of HTN was 34% for both poor and middle-income men and women. However, in those with high family incomes, there was a lower prevalence of HTN (28%).

Psychosocial factors

Psychosocial factors linked to lower SES also plausibly contribute to the excess risk of elevated BP and the disparity of HTN prevalence among blacks and whites. The relationships among social support, perceived stress, and BP have been studied in a cross-sectional, community-based sample (1,784 black men and women, aged 25–50 years, living in the southeastern United States). Differences in systolic BP associated with low social support/high stress ranged from 3.6 to 5.2 mm Hg in women and 2.5 to 3.5 mm Hg in men. There was an inverse association of BP with social support and a direct association of BP with perceived stress that was stronger for SBP than diastolic blood pressure (DBP); these correlations persisted after adjustment for age, obesity, waist–hip ratio, emotional support, instrumental support, and perceived stress. Therefore, chronic stress, low SES, and low social support may contribute to the development of HTN among blacks. In 4,086 blacks enrolled in the CARDIA study (age range: 25–37 years), black men and women who experienced no instances of racial discrimination tended to have lower systolic and diastolic BP ($\sim$7–10 mm Hg) than those who reported one or two instances of discriminatory or unfair treatment.

Suggested Readings

Bell AC, Adair LS, Popkin BM. Ethnic differences in the association between body mass index and hypertension. *Am J Epidemiol* 2002;155:346–353.

Flack JM, Neaton JD, Daniels B, et al. Ethnicity and renal disease: lessons from the multiple Risk Factor Intervention trial and the Treatment of Mild Hypertension Study. *Am J Kidney Dis* 1993;219:31–40.

Ganguli MC, Grimm RH Jr, Svendsen KH, et al. Higher education and income are related to a better Na:K ratio in blacks. Baseline results of the Treatment of Mild Hypertension Study (TOMHS) data. *Am J Hypertens* 1997;10:979–984.

Kanjilal S, Gregg EW, Cheng YJ, et al. Socioeconomic status and trends in disparities in 4 major risk factors for cardiovascular disease among US adults, 1971–2002. *Arch Int Neurol* 2006;166:2348–2355.

Kaufman IS, Tracy JA, Durazo-Arvizu RA, et al. Lifestyle, education, and prevalence of hypertension populations of African origin: results from the International Collaborative Study on Hypertension in Blacks. *Ann Epidemiol* 1997;7:22–27.

Kiefe CI, Williams OD, Bild DE, et al. Regional disparities in the incidence of elevated blood pressure among young adults: the CARDIA study. *Circulation* 1997;96:1082–1088.

Ong KL, Cheung BMY, Man YB, et al. Prevalence, awareness, treatment, and control of hypertension among US adults 1999–2004. *Hypertension* 2007;49:69–75.

Strogatz DS, Croft JB, James SA, et al. Social support, stress, and blocked pressure in black adults. *Epidemiology* 1997;8:482–487.

U.S. Department of Health and Human Services. *Health in America* 2006. Available at http://www.cdc.gov/nchs/hus.htm. Accessed on February 2, 2007.

Winkleby MA, Kraemer HC, Ahn DK, et al. Ethnic and socioeconomic differences in cardiovascular disease risk factors. *JAMA* 1998;280:356–362.

CHAPTER B85 ■ HYPERTENSION IN BLACKS

KEITH C. FERDINAND, MD

KEY POINTS

- Hypertension is more prevalent, begins earlier in life, and is of greater severity in U.S. blacks compared to non-blacks.
- Clinical trials have documented that U.S. blacks benefit from various lifestyle modifications and appropriate pharmacologic therapy.
- Thiazide diuretics are appropriate for most of these individuals as a first step; long-acting calcium channel blockers are also useful but most will require combination therapy to achieve sustained control of blood pressure (BP).
- Low sodium/high potassium diets, weight loss, physical activity, reduction in alcohol consumption, and psychologic stress reduction all have been shown to reduce BP in blacks.

See also Chapters **B84** and **C148**

Blacks in the United States, or African Americans, have one of the highest hypertension prevalence rates in the world, beginning earlier in life, with a higher prevalence of severe hypertension and target organ damage [heart failure (HF), end-stage renal disease, fatal and nonfatal stroke, and overall heart disease]. Hypertension is a predominant cause of the excess risk of premature mortality in this population.

Race as a social construct

Although medical researchers continue to use terms such as *race* and *racial differences*, the biologic basis for such classifications is uncertain and race remains primarily a social concept. Rates of hypertension in blacks of diverse African ancestry vary based on geography and risk factors.

Etiologic factors in blacks

In U.S. blacks, high blood pressure (HBP) is strongly associated with modifiable lifestyle factors: increased body mass index, physical inactivity, inadequate potassium intake, and increased sodium intake. Studies of patients of African descent, including native Africans, Afro-Caribbeans, and African Americans, have highlighted the importance of these lifestyle factors, with HBP being more prevalent in the U.S. black population, apparently related to increased body mass and a high ratio of sodium to potassium intake.

Lifestyle modifications

Lifestyle modifications (population-based and individual) would be expected to benefit U.S. blacks, considering the high prevalence of overweight/obesity, sedentary lifestyle, excess dietary sodium intake, and low potassium intake, along with excess consumption of alcohol. Several studies confirm the benefit of multiple lifestyle interventions. Potential opportunities for intervention include the traditional medical office for intensive counseling of high-risk patients, and population-based options utilizing community settings such as senior centers and churches for screening, education and referral.

Weight loss, physical activity, and stress reduction. In phase 2 of the Trial of Hypertension Prevention (TOHP), subjects in the black cohort (17% of 1,191 subjects, aged 30–54 years, with high normal BP on no antihypertensive drugs) tended to lose less weight than non-blacks, as has been found in previous trials. Nevertheless, BP reduction per kg of weight lost was significant (0.45 mm Hg reduction in systolic BP and 0.35 mm Hg reduction in diastolic BP per kilogram lost) and did not differ by race. Patients with high BP experience a reduction in left ventricular hypertrophy (LVH) and a decrease in BP with regular aerobic exercise of moderate intensity. Additionally, decreasing psychologic stress (a difficult indicator to measure) significantly reduced systolic and diastolic BP in another study of African Americans participating in transcendental meditation.

Sodium reduction and increased potassium intake. U.S. blacks tend to exhibit greater salt sensitivity of BP than whites. Therefore, although population surveys have not consistently demonstrated higher dietary sodium intake in U.S. blacks compared to whites, African Americans may experience greater BP reductions with lower sodium intake or increased potassium intake. In the initial Dietary Approaches to Stop Hypertension (DASH) trial, a diet rich in fruits, vegetables, and low-fat dairy products and limited total and saturated fat led to significantly greater BP reduction in blacks compared to whites (e.g., systolic BP −6.8 mm Hg vs. −3 mm Hg). In the subsequent DASH-Sodium trial, BP reductions from a lower sodium intake (∼65 mmol/day) were also consistently greater in blacks than whites. Additionally, the PREMIER trial (810 subjects, 34% black) demonstrated the health benefits of patient education to identify sodium levels in prepared foods, sources of potassium (including fresh fruits and vegetables), low-fat dairy products, calorie restriction, and increased physical activity.

Socioeconomic factors and health care quality

Generally, African Americans receive lower-quality health care than whites. Reviews of black Medicare beneficiaries have revealed a pattern of utilization of physicians with fewer qualifications and resources as compared to whites, potentially adversely affecting health outcomes in areas of low socioeconomic status. A trial of 309 African American men in inner-city Baltimore, Maryland over 36 months showed that comprehensive intervention by nurse practitioners and community health workers decreased BP and progression to LVH through the use of targeted educational, behavioral, and pharmacologic interventions. The Healthy Heart Community Prevention Project in New Orleans, Louisiana has used churches, barbershops, and beauty salons to increase awareness and education to improve hypertension control. Positive health behavior may be influenced by other community-based programs with favorable responses to health care outcomes.

Barriers to effective blood pressure control

Patient-related factors. Genetic factors may contribute to the increased prevalence, severity, and complications of hypertension in blacks. There are also many patient-related barriers to hypertension control: lack of patient awareness and education regarding hypertension and its consequences, delayed diagnosis, and distrust of medical professionals and medications.

Community factors. Resources in socioeconomically disadvantaged communities are often inadequate to support healthy lifestyle changes, with limited safe areas for walking or cycling and lack of fresh fruits, vegetables, whole grains, and low-fat protein sources at neighborhood grocery stores.

Health system-related factors. Additionally, local clinicians often fail to follow optimal treatment practices, do not treat HBP early and intensively, do not adhere to clinical guidelines, and have lower expectations for BP control in blacks. There is also reduced access to specialty care for patients with lower socioeconomic status who have comorbid diseases that require complex medical intervention.

Intervention. Implementing community screening, culturally sensitive education, and prescribing multiple medications, when needed, along with therapeutic lifestyle modifications should increase BP control and decrease morbidity/mortality in U.S. blacks.

Pharmacologic therapy

The National Heart, Lung, and Blood Institute–sponsored Antihypertensive Lipid-Lowering in Heart Attack Trial (ALLHAT),

was the largest antihypertensive trial ever (42,448) with patients from the United States, Canada, U.S. Virgin Islands, and Puerto Rico. This study included a significantly large black cohort (15,133), 35% of total subjects. Combination therapies based on chlorthalidone, lisinopril, and amlodipine showed similar outcomes in preventing major coronary events in blacks and whites. However, in blacks, chlorthalidone showed a greater fall in BP and stroke rate than lisinopril, and greater reduction in HF than either lisinopril or amlodipine.

Diuretics. In most individuals with uncomplicated hypertension, thiazide diuretics are appropriate first-step pharmacologic therapy, irrespective of race. However, a large proportion of individuals may require combinations of agents to achieve sustained BP control. Diuretics are also highly effective when added as a second step in combination with angiotensin-converting enzyme (ACE) inhibitors, angiotensin receptor blockers (ARBs), or β-adrenergic blockers. Of note, combining a diuretic with any of these other classes of antihypertensive drugs essentially removes any racial or ethnic subgroup differences in BP responses.

Other agents. In blacks, long-acting calcium channel blockers also effectively lower BP, more so than monotherapy with ACE inhibitors, ARBs and β-blockers. In general, because most of these individuals achieve better control with combination agents, calcium channel blockers can be combined with ACE inhibitors, ARBs or β-adrenergic blockers. In blacks, agents that modulate the renin-angiotensin-aldosterone system should be utilized primarily in individuals with stage 2 hypertension or "compelling indications" (chronic kidney disease, diabetes, ischemic heart disease, and left ventricular systolic dysfunction).

Suggested Readings

Appel LJ, Champagne CM, Harsha DW, et al. Effects of comprehensive lifestyle modification on blood pressure control: main results of the PREMIER clinical trial. *JAMA* 2003;289(16):2083–2093.

Chobanian AV, Bakris GL, Black HR. The Seventh Report of the Joint National Committee on prevention, detection, evaluation, and treatment of high BP: the JNC 7 report. *JAMA* 2003;289(19):2560–2572.

Clark L, Ferdinand K, Flack J, et al. Coronary heart disease in African Americans. *Heart Dis* 2001;3:97–108.

Cooper R, Rotimi C, Ataman S, et al. The prevalence of hypertension in six populations of West African origin. *Am J Public Health* 1997;87:160–168.

Douglas JG, Bakris GL, Epstein M, et al. Management of the high BP in African Americans consensus statement of the hypertension in African Americans working group of the international society on hypertension in blacks. *Arch Intern Med* 2003;163:525–534.

Ferdinand KC. Managing cardiovascular risk in minority patients. *J Natl Med Assoc* 2005;97(4):459–466.

Fields LE, Burt VL, Cutler JA, et al. The burden of adult hypertension in the United States 1999 to 2000: a rising tide. *Hypertension* 2004;44(4):398–404.

Sacks FM, Svetkey LP, Vollmer WM, et al. Effects on blood pressure of reduced dietary sodium and the dietary approaches to stop hypertension (DASH) diet. *N Engl J Med* 2001;344:3–10.

The Trials of Hypertension Prevention Collaborative Research Group. Effects of weight loss and sodium reduction intervention on BP and hypertension incidence in overweight people with high-normal BP. The Trials of Hypertension Prevention, Phase II. *Arch Intern Med* 2001;134:1–11.

Wright JT Jr, Dunn JK, Cutler JA. Outcomes in hypertensive black and nonblack patients treated with chlorthalidone, amlodipine, and lisinopril. *JAMA* 2005;293(13):1595–1608.

CHAPTER B86 ■ HYPERTENSION AMONG HISPANICS IN THE UNITED STATES

CARLOS J. CRESPO, DrPH, MS, FACSM AND MARIO R. GARCIA-PALMIERI, MD, FACC

KEY POINTS

- Hispanics constitute approximately 14% of the general population of the United States and are the largest minority groups in the United States.
- Hispanics are a heterogeneous group of subpopulations that share the common bond of the Spanish language; each group has racial, ethnic, and cultural characteristics that distinguish it from other Hispanic groups.
- Reduction in blood pressure (BP) control rates and heart disease mortality in the U.S. population has occurred to a much lesser extent among Hispanics, especially men, than in other ethnic groups.
- In elderly Mexican Americans, elevated BP continues to be an important predictor of heart attack and stroke, especially among diabetic patients.

See also Chapter B84

General demographics

Hispanics now constitute approximately 14% of the general population and are the largest minority groups in the United States. Because Hispanics are younger than non-Hispanic whites, efforts to prevent chronic diseases in this population are of public health significance. In general, the median age of Hispanics is 27.2 years, 9 years younger than the median (36.2 years) of the U.S. general population.

Socioeconomic status

Overall, Hispanics suffer disproportionately from higher unemployment rate, lower educational attainment, and income levels. These social and economic disadvantages, compounded with language barriers have made it very difficult for Hispanics to obtain comparable preventive and primary health care services.

Heart disease

Heart disease continues to be the leading cause of death in Hispanics and in the general population. Reduction in heart disease mortality rates have been observed in the total U.S. population; however, the decline in heart disease mortality rates observed in the general population in recent years has occurred to a much lesser extent among Hispanics. **Figure B86.1** shows the coronary heart disease (CHD) mortality rate among Hispanics 35 years and older by county. Furthermore, CHD and other chronic diseases are expected to increase among Hispanics over the next 20 years as this population ages. The relative young age

of Hispanics presents the opportunity to intervene with preventive measures to modify risk factors and reduce the development of cardiovascular diseases (CVDs) in this population. One of these modifiable risk factors is hypertension.

Hypertension mortality

Figure B86.2 shows the age-adjusted hypertension-related deaths among Hispanic adults in 2002 and shows that Hispanic subgroups differ in their hypertension-related mortality rates. Puerto Ricans living in the United States have the highest age-adjusted hypertension-related mortality, but the relative percentage change in hypertension-related mortality is highest among Mexican Americans (42.9%), and Central and South American subgroups (45.1%). This increase is alarming because these Hispanic subgroups had traditionally lower rates of hypertension-related mortality.

Hypertension prevalence

Hypertension among Hispanics varies by gender, country of origin, and geographic distribution. **Table 86.1** shows the prevalence and trends of high blood pressure (BP) among non-Hispanic whites, non-Hispanic blacks, and Mexican Americans. Despite a greater prevalence of obesity and diabetes, the prevalence of hypertension in Hispanics is lower than those of the general population. Most of the literature report hypertension rates in Mexican Americans and Puerto Ricans, with limited data among Cuban Americans.

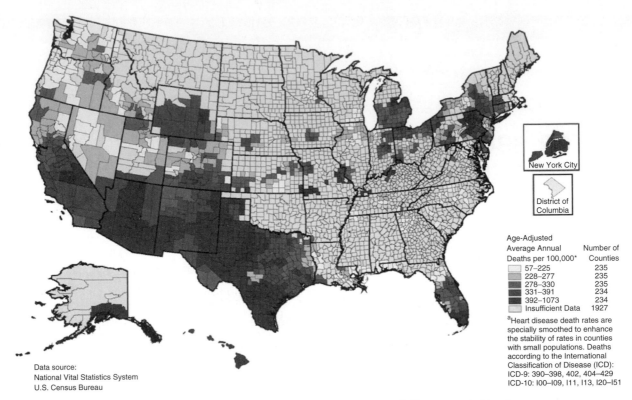

Figure B86.1 Heart disease[a] death rates, 1996–2000, Hispanics aged 35 years and older, by county. (Data from National Vital Statistics System. U.S. Census Bureau.)

The Hispanic Health and Nutrition Examination Survey (HHANES) conducted between 1982 and 1984 revealed that Hispanic men have higher prevalence rates of hypertension than Hispanic women. Hispanic women in the three ethnic groups were more aware of their hypertension status than men. Less than 9% of Hispanic men with hypertension had their high BP under control, whereas approximately 30% of Mexican American and Puerto Rican women had their BP under control.

Borrell et al. compared self-reported hypertension rates of U.S. Hispanic blacks, Hispanic whites, with those of non-Hispanic blacks and non-Hispanic whites from the National Health Interview Survey (NHIS), a national probability sample of the civilian noninstitutionalized adults. The NHIS is conducted yearly and permits the examination of time trends on selected conditions, such as hypertension. Because Hispanics can be of any race, the NHIS asked separate questions on race from those of Hispanic ethnicity. The prevalence of hypertension was higher among Hispanic blacks compared with Hispanic whites. Moreover, the "protective effect" against hypertension among Hispanics is disappearing as demonstrated by studies of the interaction between hypertension prevalence, race/ethnicity, and year of survey.

Subpopulations

Hispanics are a heterogeneous group of subpopulations that share the common bond of the Spanish language and each group has racial, ethnic, and cultural characteristics that distinguish it from other Hispanic groups. The largest Hispanic groups in the United States are Mexican Americans, followed by Puerto Ricans, and

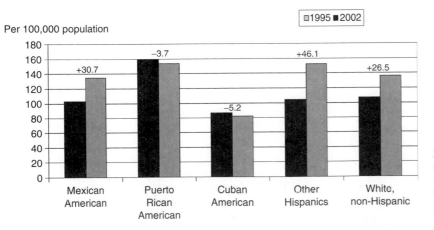

Figure B86.2 Age-standardized, hypertension-related mortality rates, and relative percentage changes among adults aged ≥25 years for non-Hispanic whites and selected Hispanic subpopulations—United States 1995 and 2000. (Adapted from Centers for Disease Control and Prevention, *MMWR* 2006;55(07):177–180.)

TABLE B86.1

AGE-ADJUSTED PREVALENCE OF HYPERTENSION; AWARENESS, TREATMENT, AND CONTROL OF HYPERTENSION; AND HIGH BLOOD PRESSURE DISTRIBUTION AMONG MEXICAN AMERICANS, CUBAN AMERICANS, AND PUERTO RICANS AGED 18 TO 74 YEARS FROM THE HISPANIC HEALTH AND NUTRITION EXAMINATION SURVEY

Race/ethnicity	Sex	Age (yr)	Sample size (N)	Prevalence[a] (%)	Aware[b] (%)	Treatment[c] (%)	Control[d] (%)	Stage 1[e] (%)	Stage 2–4[f] (%)
Mexican Americans	Men	35	1,554	22.7	40	16	8	15	6
	Women	37	1,964	19.2	76	55	34	11	3
Cuban Americans	Men	43	401	20.9	49	23	8	13	5
	Women	44	497	13.6	91	41	14	7	4
Puerto Ricans	Men	37	495	20.4	6	19	9	13	6
	Women	36	835	17.6	66	43	28	9	4

[a] *Hypertension* is defined as systolic or diastolic blood pressure $\geq$140/90 or currently on antihypertensive medication.
[b] *Aware* is defined as hypertensive patients who have been told by a physician or health professional that they have high blood pressure or hypertension.
[c] *Treatment* is defined as hypertensive patients who are currently on antihypertensive medication.
[d] *Control* is defined as hypertensive patients who are currently treated and who have mean blood pressures <140/90 mm Hg.
[e] *Stage* 1 is defined as mean systolic blood pressure distribution between 140 and 159 mm Hg or mean diastolic blood pressure between 90 and 99 mm Hg, regardless of medication.
[f] *Stage* 2 to 4 is defined as mean systolic blood pressure $\geq$160 mm Hg or diastolic blood pressure $\geq$100 mm Hg, regardless of medication.
(Adapted from Crespo CJ, Loria CM, Burt VL. Hypertension and other cardiovascular disease risk factors among Mexican Americans, Cuban Americans, and Puerto Ricans from the Hispanic Health and Nutrition Examination Survey. *Public Health Rep.* 1996; 111:7–10, with permission.)

Cuban Americans; persons with ethnic backgrounds from Central and South America, and the Dominican Republic combined contribute another 7% of the total Hispanic population. Hispanics live all 50 states and the District of Columbia but >90% live in only 10 states, in mainly urban areas. The observed disparity in awareness, treatment, and control of hypertension warrants attention and an educational campaign targeted at members of different gender and ethnic subgroups.

Mexican Americans. Progress in the percentage reduction in the prevalence of hypertension observed in non-Hispanic whites and non-Hispanic blacks has not been observed in Mexican Americans. Historically, Mexican American men and women have suffered from poor control of their hypertension (defined by the older World Health Organization (WHO) criteria as systolic BP $\geq$160 mm Hg or diastolic BP $\geq$95 mm Hg), with alarmingly higher BP levels than their non-Hispanic white counterparts. They have also had higher prevalence of hypertension than their counterparts in Mexico. The prevalence of hypertension in Mexican Americans in the San Antonio Heart Study were similar to HHANES, despite the higher frequency of obesity and type 2 diabetes mellitus. Results from Starr County, on the border between Texas and Mexico, are different: with >97% of the residents who report being of Mexican descent, the prevalence of hypertension by age and gender are elevated compared with the general population. These differences are not attributable to measurement problems but may be related to differences in population structure, employment, life style, diet, and socioeconomic status.

The Mexico City Diabetes Study examined diabetes and CVD in men and women, aged 35 to 64 years, living in Mexico City and San Antonio, Texas. Hypertension in Mexico City remains lower than prevalence rates observed in San Antonio. After careful analysis of social and economic indicators in these two groups, the authors identified a biphasic relationship to BP that was related to degree of modernization in men. Modernization and education among women were consistently inversely associated

with both systolic and diastolic BP. It therefore seems likely that modernization adversely affects male health until a second transition point is reached, after which it is beneficial.

The Hispanic Established Population for the Epidemiologic Study of the Elderly (H-EPESE) is a population-based study of noninstitutionalized Mexican Americans aged 65 years and older from five southwestern states (Texas, California, New Mexico, Colorado, and Arizona) for which older participants of Mexican ancestry were selected using probability-sampling procedures. In all, 3,050 Mexican-American elders (65+ years, representing an 83% response rate) completed in-home face-to-face interviews in Spanish or English. In this cohort of elderly Mexican Americans, elevated BP continues to be an important predictor of heart attack and stroke, especially among diabetic patients.

Puerto Ricans. Prevalence of hypertension in Puerto Rico is well documented: among persons <45 years of age, hypertension is twice (8.1%) as common as that of the mainland United States (4.2%). Deaths caused by heart disease have also been increasing in Puerto Rico by approximately 72% since 1960, whereas in the United States, mortality from CHD and stroke has been declining. Concomitantly, end-stage renal disease in Puerto Rico is higher than in any other Latin American country. Wide pulse pressure (systolic minus diastolic BP) is another emerging independent risk factor for CVD mortality in this population.

The Puerto Rico Heart Health Program has examined risk factors, morbidity, and mortality of CHD among Puerto Ricans living in Puerto Rico. They found that urban men had higher average BP levels than rural men and that systolic BP showed increasing mean values with increasing education in both the rural and urban areas; mean systolic BP increased by approximately 8 mm Hg in those with a high school education or higher compared to no education. This inverse relationship is not consistent with other findings from the United States and may imply that urban, educated Puerto Rican men (similar to their counterparts in Mexico City) have adopted lifestyles that were more conducive to increased CHD risk factors. Dark-skinned

Puerto Rican men had a higher prevalence than light-skinned men of both definite and "borderline" left ventricular hypertrophy [as assessed by electrocardiogram (ECG)].

Suggested Readings

Borrell LN. Self-reported hypertension and race among Hispanics in the National Health Interview Survey. *Ethn Dis* 2006;16(1):71–77.

Cooper R, Cutler J, Desvigne-Nickens P, et al. Trends and disparities in coronary heart disease, stroke, and other cardiovascular diseases in the United States: findings of the national conference on cardiovascular disease prevention. *Circulation* 2000;102(25):3137–3147.

Crespo C, Loria C, Burt V. Hypertension and other cardiovascular risk factors among Mexican Americans, Cuban Americans and mainland Puerto Ricans from the Hispanic health and nutrition examination survey. *Public Health Rep* 1996;111(Suppl 2):7–10.

Garcia-Palmieri MR, Crespo CJ, Mc Gee D, et al. Wide pulse pressure is an independent predictor of cardiovascular mortality in Puerto Rican men. *Nutr Metab Cardiovasc Dis* 2005;15(1):71–78.

Hazuda HP. Hypertension in the San Antonio Heart Study and the Mexico City Diabetes Study: sociocultural correlates. *Public Health Rep* 1996;111(Suppl 2):18–21.

Hypertension-related mortality among Hispanic subpopulations—United States, 1995–2002. *MMWR Morb Mortal Wkly Rep* 2006;55(7):177–180.

Lorenzo C, Williams K, Gonzalez-Villalpando C, et al. Lower hypertension risk in Mexico City than in San Antonio. *Am J Hypertens* 2005;18(3):385–391.

Ong KL, Cheung BM, Man YB, et al. Prevalence, awareness, treatment, and control of hypertension among United States adults 1999–2004. *Hypertension* 2007;49(1):69–75.

Otiniano ME, Ottenbacher KJ, Markides KS, et al. Self-reported heart attack in Mexican-American elders: examination of incidence, prevalence, and 7-year mortality. *J Am Geriatr Soc* 2003;51(7):923–929.

Ottenbacher KJ, Ostir GV, Peek MK, et al. Diabetes mellitus as a risk factor for stroke incidence and mortality in Mexican American older adults. *J Gerontol A Biol Sci Med Sci* 2004;59(6):M640–M645.

CHAPTER B87 ■ HYPERTENSION IN SOUTH ASIANS

PRAKASH C. DEEDWANIA, MD, FACC, FAHA AND RAJEEV GUPTA, MD, PhD

KEY POINTS

■ Hypertension is a major public health problem in the Indian subcontinent and among South Asians worldwide.

■ In South Asian residents, the prevalence of hypertension is low, especially in rural populations; in urban populations and in emigrant South Asians hypertension prevalence is high and similar to other populations in these countries.

■ There is an urgent need for a concerted public health response in South Asia for increasing awareness, treatment, and target-driven control of high blood pressure (BP).

See also Chapter B84

Hypertension is a major public health problem in the Indian subcontinent and among South Asians worldwide. Although large population-based prospective studies have not been conducted, available data indicate that the prevalence of hypertension is increasing substantially in these populations. Recent studies among Indians have shown a high prevalence of hypertension in urban and rural areas, with prevalence rates in urban subjects similar to those in the United States. Trends of hypertension prevalence in Indian urban and rural populations, aged 20 to 70 years, from several epidemiologic studies are displayed in **Figures B87.1 and B87.2**.

India

Urban populations. Indian urban population studies in the mid-1950s reported hypertension prevalence of 1% to 4%. Subsequent studies that used the standardized World Health Organization (WHO) guidelines for the diagnosis of hypertension [known hypertension, systolic blood pressure (BP) ≥160 or diastolic BP ≥95 mm Hg] show a steadily increasing trend in hypertension prevalence: 4% in Agra (1961), 6% in Rohtak (1975), 15% in Bombay (1980), 14% in Ludhiana (1985), 11% in Jaipur (1995), and 12% in Delhi (1997) (**Figure B87.1**). The prevalence of hypertension defined by Joint National Committee-5 criteria also shows a steep increase from 6% (Delhi, 1959) to 31% (Jaipur, 1995), 44% (Mumbai, 1999), 36% (Chennai, 2001), 38% (Jaipur, 2002), 40% (Jaipur, 2004) and 45% (Bangalore, 2005) (**Figure B87.3**).

Rural populations. Although the prevalence of hypertension is lower in rural compared to urban Indian populations (**Figure B87.2**), there has also been a steady increase in hypertension prevalence over time in rural regions: 0.5% in Bombay (1959), 2% in Delhi (1959), 4% in Haryana (1978), 5% in Delhi (1983), 6%

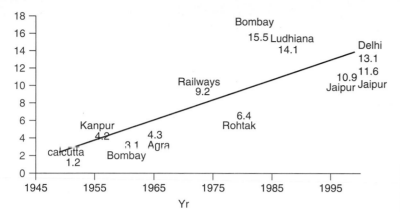

Figure B87.1 Hypertension prevalence (%) in urban Indian populations. Hypertension diagnosis is based on known hypertensives or blood pressure >160 mm Hg systolic, >95 mm Hg diastolic, or both.

in Rajasthan (1984), 3% in Punjab (1985), 4% in Maharashtra (1993), 3% in Maharashtra (1993), 7% in Rajasthan (1994), and 4% in Delhi (1998). In South Indian urbanized rural subjects, hypertension prevalence has been reported to be as high as 18% (1993) and 12% (1994). Overall, there is a significant increase in hypertension prevalence in rural areas, although the rise is not as steep as in urban populations. The increased prevalence of hypertension, along with the rising rates of diabetes and dyslipidemia, has dire public health consequences, including a potential epidemic of coronary artery disease in India.

Other South Asians populations

In other South Asian countries, urban–rural differences are similar to India. A study in Nepal in the early 1980s reported hypertension in 10% of urban subjects whereas in Bangladesh hypertension has been reported in <5% of rural subjects. The Pakistan National Health Survey reported large regional differences in hypertension prevalence with high prevalence in cosmopolitan cities such as Karachi and low prevalence in rural areas.

Emigration effects

Hypertension prevalence data in emigrant South Asians differs somewhat across three available studies. Bhatnagar et al. reported that mean systolic BP among emigrant South Asians as compared with Indian siblings was 146 ± 23 versus 132 ± 22 in men and 143 ± 28 versus 142 ± 23 in women. A review of various South Asian emigrant studies revealed that hypertension prevalence was not different in this group as compared with whites. Bhopal et al. compared hypertension prevalence rates in Indians,

Pakistanis, and Bangladeshis living in Britain and reported that the hypertension was more common in Indians as compared to other South Asian groups. In the Study of Health Assessment and Risk in Ethnic Groups (SHARE) Study in Canada, prevalence of self-reported hypertension in South Asians was 12.5%. This was almost similar to Europeans (11%) but lower than that of the Chinese (15.9%).

Reasons for the increasing prevalence of hypertension

Although the precise reasons for the increase in hypertension prevalence in South Asians are not established, several possibilities exist.

Acculturation. Studies in unacculturated societies have shown lower BP levels that are not influenced by age. Among the so-called unacculturated and less-cultured Indian rural populations, there is only a small increase in prevalence of hypertension over time. On the other hand, in urban populations that are exposed to acculturation and modernization, the hypertension prevalence rates have more than doubled in the last 30 years.

Socioeconomic factors and urbanization. Population demographic changes in India have caused increased life expectancy, urbanization, development, and affluence. In 1901, only 11% of the population was living in an urban area; this proportion was 17.6% in 1951, 18.3% in 1961, 20.2% in 1971, 23.7% in 1981, and 26.1% in 1991. There is a strong, direct association between urbanization and the increased prevalence of hypertension. Affluence as measured by per capita net domestic product, growth of production, or human development index has increased sharply

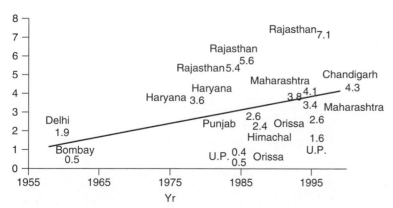

Figure B87.2 Hypertension prevalence trends in rural Indian populations.

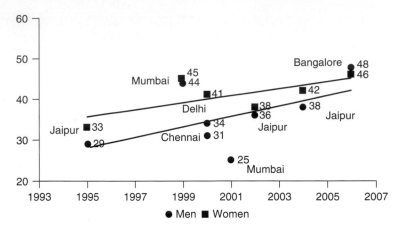

Figure B87.3 Recent Indian urban hypertension prevalence studies report a high prevalence (%) of hypertension diagnosed using JNC-5 criteria in both men and women in different urban populations.

in India in recent years and correlates positively with the BP increase.

Tobacco and diet. Tobacco production, which is a surrogate for its consumption, is also increasing at a very high rate in India. Per capita fat and oil consumption has also increased in the last 40 years. It was 5.79 kg/person/year in 1961, 5.85 in 1971, 6.48 in 1981, and 6.96 in 1987. Salt consumption was 10.7 g/person/day in 1971 and increased to 13 in 1981, 15.8 in 1991, and 16.9 in 1994. In this setting, it is reasonable to hypothesize that summation of these sociodemographic and lifestyle factors is accelerating the hypertension epidemic currently sweeping India and other parts of South Asia. Obesity, especially truncal obesity, is a powerful influence because of the associated insulin resistance and cardiovascular dysmetabolic syndrome, which is often associated with hypertension. Other important environmental factors that can contribute include excess alcohol intake, physical inactivity, high dietary intake of sodium, and deficiency of potassium.

Public health implications

There is an urgent need for a concerted public health response for hypertension control among South Asians to prevent its cardiovascular complications such as stroke, coronary artery disease, and renal and ocular complications. This should include an upscaling of the health services in South Asian countries to

tackle chronic diseases such as hypertension by enhancing skills of health care providers and equipping facilities for detection, treatment, and continued surveillance for hypertension.

Suggested Readings

Anand SS, Yusuf S, Vuksan V, et al. Differences in risk factors, atherosclerosis and cardiovascular disease between ethnic groups in Canada: the Study of Health Assessment and Risk in Ethnic Groups (SHARE). *Lancet* 2000;356:279–284.

Bhatnagar D, Anand IS, Durrington PN, et al. Coronary risk factors in people from the Indian subcontinent living in West London and their siblings in India. *Lancet* 1995;345:405–409.

Bhopal R, Unwin N, White M, et al. Heterogeneity of coronary heart disease risk factors in Indian, Pakistani, Bangladeshi, and European origin population: cross sectional study. *BMJ* 1999;319:215–220.

Deedwania P. The changing face of hypertension—is systolic blood pressure the final answer? *Arch Intern Med* 2002;162:506–508.

Gupta R. Trends in hypertension epidemiology in India. *J Hum Hypertens* 2004;18:73–78.

Gupta R, Al-Odat NA, Gupta VP. Hypertension epidemiology in India: meta-analysis of fifty-year prevalence rates and blood pressure trends. *J Hum Hypertens* 1996;10:465–472.

Nissinen A, Bothig S, Grenroth H, et al. Hypertension in developing countries. *World Health Stat Q* 1988;41:141–154.

Pappas G, Akhtar T, Gergen PJ, et al. Health status of the Pakistani population: a health profile and comparison with the United States. *Am J Public Health* 2001;91:93–98.

Reddy KS, Shah B, Varghese C, et al. Responding to the threat of chronic diseases in India. *Lancet* 2005;336:1744–1749.

CHAPTER B88 ■ HYPERTENSION IN EAST ASIANS AND NATIVE HAWAIIANS

KHIET C. HOANG, MD AND NATHAN D. WONG, PhD, MPH

KEY POINTS

■ The prevalence of hypertension has increased in developing Asian nations, is high among Native Hawaiians, and varies dramatically among Asian ethnic subgroups.

■ The prevalence of hypertension is lower in rural than urban Chinese, but rural Japanese demonstrate high prevalence rates of hypertension.

■ In clinical trials, pharmacologic therapy effective in white populations is also effective in East Asian populations, but drug side effects such as cough or flushing may be greater among certain Asian ethnic subgroups.

See also Chapter **B84**

Hypertension has become increasingly prevalent in developing East Asian populations and among immigrant East Asian and Pacific Islander populations living in the United States (**Table B88.1**). Hypertension is a major contributor to cardiovascular disease morbidity and mortality, which may even be higher among some Asian immigrants to the United States than among their white counterparts.

China

In 2001, the International Collaborative Study of Cardiovascular Disease in ASIA (InterASIA), after surveying 15,540 adults between 35 and 74 years old, found that 27.2% (130 million) adults in China have hypertension. When compared to data from the 1991 Chinese National Hypertension Survey, the prevalence of hypertension has increased from 20.2% to 28.6% in men and from 19.1% to 25.8% in women. Only 44.7% of those with hypertension were aware of their diagnosis, only 28.2% were taking prescribed medication, and only 8.1% had controlled hypertension. Hypertension is less common among those living in southern China, particularly in rural areas, where dietary and exercise patterns are substantially different from those in northern or urban areas.

The prevalence of hypertension in 346 Chinese older than 60 years living in the United States was 29.7% for men and 33.5% for women. More recently, the Multiethnic Study of Atherosclerosis (MESA) estimated that 39% of Chinese adults living in the United States have hypertension, a figure comparable to the prevalence in whites. However, after adjustment for risk factors [age, sex, body mass index (BMI), waist circumference, alcohol consumption, current tobacco use, presence of diabetes, education, income, and financial strain], Chinese ethnicity was associated with a significantly greater likelihood (odds ratio 1.30) of hypertension compared to whites.

Japan

Among native Japanese, a recent national survey of 12 rural communities (N = 11,302 subjects; mean age, 55 years) revealed a prevalence of hypertension of 37% for men and 33% for women. Only 7% of those who were hypertensive, however, had blood pressure (BP) controlled to <140/90 mm Hg. In Japanese 60 years and older, an overall prevalence of hypertension of 53% has been reported, with 11% having isolated systolic hypertension (defined in this study as a systolic BP of ≥160 mm Hg and diastolic BP <90 mm Hg). Among Japanese Americans, systolic and diastolic BP are the most important independent predictors of cardiovascular, coronary heart disease, stroke, and overall mortality.

In the Honolulu Heart Study, the prevalence of hypertension increased among men from 53% in those aged 60 to 64 years to 67% among those aged 75 to 81 years. Those who had isolated systolic hypertension, isolated diastolic hypertension, and systolic/diastolic hypertension at baseline were 4.8, 1.4, and 4.3 times more likely to experience a stroke over the next 20 years compared to normotensive subjects. A survey of 2,053 Japanese adults living in Hawaii, Los Angeles, and Hiroshima found a significantly higher prevalence of hypertension in Japanese Americans in Hawaii and Los Angeles than Native Japanese in

TABLE B88.1

PREVALENCE RATES OF HYPERTENSION AMONG EAST ASIANS AND NATIVE HAWAIIANS

Population	Prevalence (%) in men	Prevalence (%) in women	Reference
Chinese, aged 35–74 yr	28.6	25.8	Gu et al. 2003
Chinese Americans, aged 60 yr and older	29.7	33.5	Choi, 1990
Japanese, mean age 55 yr	37	33	Asai et al. 2001
Japanese Americans, men aged 60–81 yr	53 (60–64 yr), 67 (75–81 yr)	—	Curb et al. 1996
Japanese Americans, aged 34–75 yr	41.5	33.8	Fujimoto 1996
Korean, aged 18–92 yr	41.5	24.5	Jo et al. 2001
Korean Americans, aged 18 and older	35	30	Kim et al. 2000
Native Hawaiians, aged 20–54 yr	6 (20–24 yr), 37 (45–54 yr)	8 (20–24 yr), 41 (50–54 yr)	Curb et al. 1996

Hiroshima (42.6%, 37.2%, and 29.7% respectively). Of note, the prevalence of glucose intolerance, hyperinsulinemia, and dyslipidemia was also higher in Hawaii and Los Angeles than in Hiroshima.

Korea

In a large meta-analysis, hypertension was a strong risk factor in Koreans for ischemic, hemorrhagic, and overall stroke (odds ratios of 3.3–6.6). A Korean national BP survey among 21,242 persons older than 30 years showed 20% with hypertension, but only 25% aware, 16% treated, and 5% with controlled BP. Among >100,000 Korean workers, aged 35 to 59, the prevalence of hypertension was 28.9% in men and 15.9% in women. A more recent urban survey, which included older adults aged 18 to 92 (N = 4,226) revealed 41.5% of men and 24.5% of women to have hypertension.

A 1998 study of Korean Americans (N = 761) in Maryland showed that 32% of subjects (35% of males and 30% of females) had high BP, a figure that was higher than in other Americans and in their counterparts in Korea.

Native Hawaiians

Relevant data in Native Hawaiians is limited to one survey conducted among those aged 20 to 59 years in the Molokai Heart Study. Hypertension prevalence rates ranged from 6% in men and 8% in women, aged 20 to 24, to 37% of men and 41% of women, aged 45 to 54. Data also suggests an association of degree of Hawaiian ancestry with increasing prevalence of hypertension. In addition to hypertension, other aspects of the metabolic syndrome, including abdominal obesity and glucose intolerance/diabetes, are common among Native Hawaiians.

Benefits of hypertension control

Ethnic differences in response to antihypertensive agents have long been recognized but only recently have data become available in East Asian populations. Comparative efficacy and tolerability data are still lacking for Native Hawaiian and Pacific Islander populations. The Systolic Hypertension in China trial assigned 1,253 older patients with isolated systolic hypertension to receive the dihydropyridine calcium antagonist, nitrendipine with addition of captopril or hydrochlorothiazide, if needed. Active therapy reduced total strokes by 38%, a reduction comparable to similar American and European studies. All-cause mortality and cardiovascular mortality was each reduced by 39%, relative to

placebo. In another study, 7,443 Japanese patients were treated and followed for 5 years. A reduced cardiovascular event rate was seen with the use of diuretics and β-blockers, but calcium antagonists increased risk. The Perindopril pROtection aGainst REcurrent Stroke Study (PROGRESS) randomized 6,105 patients (25% Chinese, 13% Japanese, and 62% Caucasian) with prior cerebrovascular disease to perindopril ± indapamide or placebo. The treatment group had a 28% significant reduction in recurrent stroke, with Asian patients deriving significantly greater benefits than non-Asian patients in a multivariate model.

Specific treatment issues

Efficacy and tolerability of drugs. A review of hypertension management in 200 Asian patients and 196 white patients revealed that medication changes, dose reductions, and side effects were all more common in the Asian patients. Among 6,289 Japanese patients receiving antihypertensive treatment, calcium antagonists were most often prescribed, followed by angiotensin-converting enzyme (ACE) inhibitors, angiotensin receptor blockers, β-blockers, and diuretics. Hypertension control was similar regardless of class of agent. Among Chinese patients (in Hong Kong and Taiwan), similar effectiveness and tolerability of commonly used medications (amlodipine, atenolol, felodipine, and isradipine) have been observed, with some reports of higher side effect rates in those taking felodipine. Multiple studies have shown an increased cough in Asians with use of ACE inhibitors, with reported incidence rates as high as 48% and 17% in Chinese and Japanese patients, respectively. Flushing is also more common.

Herbal therapies. There is some evidence that Chinese and other Asian-based herbal therapeutic approaches may reduce BP. Among 50 well-matched patients with mild to moderate hypertension, reductions in BP were greater among those assigned to the Western therapy, including dihydrochlorothiazide and atenolol, but those assigned to the Chinese mixtures of nine herbs still showed modest control of BP from a mean systolic/diastolic BP of 168/96 mm Hg to 146/81 mm Hg.

Suggested Readings

Asai Y, Ishikawa S, Kayaba K, et al. Prevalence, awareness, treatment, and control of hypertension in Japanese rural communities. *Nippon Koshu Eisei Zasshi* 2001;48:827–836.

Choi E. The prevalence of cardiovascular risk factors among elderly Chinese Americans. *Arch Intern Med* 1990;150:413–418.

Curb JD, Aluli NE, Huang BJ. Hypertension in elderly Japanese Americans and adult native Hawaiians. *Public Health Rep* 1996;111:53–55.

Fujimoto W, Boyko EJ, Leonetti DL, et al. Hypertension in Japanese Americans: the Seattle Japanese-American Community Diabetes Study. *Public Health Rep* 1996;111(Suppl 2):56–58.

Gu DF, Jiang H, Wu XG, et al. Prevalence, awareness, treatment, and control of hypertension in Chinese adults. *Zhonghua Yu Fang Yi Xue Za Zhi* 2003;37:84–89.

Hui KK, Pasic J. Outcome of hypertension management in Asian Americans. *Arch Intern Med* 1997;157:1345–1348.

Jee SH, Appel LJ, Suh I, et al. Prevalence of cardiovascular risk factors in South Korean adults: results from the Korea Medical Insurance Corporation (KMIC) study. *Ann Epidemiol* 1998;8:1–2.

Jo I, Ahn Y, Lee J, et al. Prevalence, awareness, treatment, control and risk factors of hypertension in Korea: the Ansan study. *J Hypertens* 2001;19:1523–1532.

Kim MT, Kim KB, Juon HS, et al. Prevalence and factors associated with high blood pressure in Korean Americans. *Ethn Dis* 2000;10(3):364–374.

Kramer H, Han C, Post W, et al. Racial/ethnic differences in hypertension and hypertension treatment and control in the multi-ethnic study of atherosclerosis(MESA). *Am J Hypertens* 2004;17:963–970.

Liu L, Wang JG, Gong L, et al. Comparison of active treatment and placebo in older Chinese patients with isolated systolic hypertension. Systolic Hypertension in China (SYST-China) Collaborative Group. *J Hypertens* 1998;16:1823–1829.

Uchiyama M, Kondo T, Tsuzuki Y, et al. Difference in occurrence of cardiovascular events according to class of antihypertensive agent, based on a follow-up study of Japanese hypertension patients. *Jpn Heart J* 2001;42:585–595.

Wong ND, Ming S, Zhou HY, et al. A Comparison of Chinese traditional and Western medical approaches for the treatment of mild hypertension. *Yale J Biol Med* 1991;64:79–87.

SECTION III ■ LIFESTYLE FACTORS AND BLOOD PRESSURE

CHAPTER B89 ■ STRESS, WHITE COAT HYPERTENSION, AND MASKED HYPERTENSION

THOMAS G. PICKERING, MD, DPhill

KEY POINTS

- Stress is defined as a situation perceived as an uncontrollable threat to the individual's well-being, and can raise blood pressure (BP) both acutely and chronically; chronic stress, such as living in poverty or having a stressful job, is associated with hypertension.
- White coat hypertension (WCH), a special case where stress-induced hypertension is found only in medical settings, occurs in approximately 20% of stage 1 hypertension; prevalence increases with age and varies according to definitions and populations studied.
- WCH is relatively benign; with low risk of morbid events; risk may increase with long-term follow-up (6 years or more).
- Antihypertensive medication in white coat hypertension patients may decrease clinic BP but produces little or no change in ambulatory BP; thus drug treatment may not confer substantial benefit.
- Masked hypertension is the mirror image of WCH (clinic BP normal, ambulatory, or home measurements high), and is associated with high risk.

See also Chapters **A56, C104,** and C105

The stress response evolved because it is critical to survival in a dangerous and hostile environment, and prepares the organism for fight or flight. It involves both neural and hormonal activation, most prominently of the sympathetic nervous system. Acute stress, such as occurs during fear or anxiety, can cause a rapid and large increase of blood pressure (BP) and heart rate, but it is usually transient.

Acute stress and panic disorder

Hypertensive patients often complain of symptoms such as dizziness, palpitations, and headache, which are also symptoms of anxiety. Panic attacks are common in the general population but are more frequently seen in hypertensive patients than would be expected by chance. During an attack there is an acute rise of BP and heart rate.

Chronic stress and hypertension

The role of chronic stress in contributing to the development of sustained hypertension is less clear, partly because chronic stress is so hard to quantify. The perception of stress is largely subjective and what may be stressful for one person may be much less so for another.

Environmental stress. There is consistent evidence that "stressed" people in impoverished environments or who move from a traditional structured environment to a less secure urban lifestyle are likely to show an increase in BP. Personality factors such as time urgency and hostility may also be important. After the terrorist attacks of 9/11/2001, there was evidence for a nationwide increase of approximately 2 mm Hg in the United States during the month after the attack.

Job strain. One of the best-studied models of chronic stress is exposure to job strain, defined by a combination of high demands and low control or decision latitude at work. Men who work in high strain jobs have elevated BP not only during the hours of work, but also while at home and during sleep, suggesting that chronic stress can reset the diurnal profile of BP to a higher level. Women are less susceptible to this effect.

White coat hypertension

White coat hypertension versus white coat effect. White coat hypertension (WCH, also referred to as *isolated office hypertension* or *isolated clinic hypertension*) is the most commonly used term to describe patients whose BP is high only in a medical setting. Application of this term is generally reserved for those not on treatment and should be distinguished from the *white coat effect,* which is a measure of the BP response to the clinic visit and is generally defined as the difference between the average clinic BP and average daytime ambulatory pressure. The white coat effect is present to a greater or lesser degree in most hypertensive patients and is greatest in patients with the highest clinic BPs, perhaps because hypertension is identified primarily on the basis of an elevated clinic pressure. Accordingly, there may be a selection bias in the diagnosis of hypertension favoring individuals who tend to show a large white coat effect. The increase of BP that characterizes the white coat effect is not necessarily accompanied by any increase of heart rate.

Definition. Any definition of WCH is arbitrary. The most commonly used definition is a persistently elevated clinic or office BP (>140/90 mm Hg) together with a normal daytime ambulatory pressure (<135/85 mm Hg). As shown in **Figure B89.1,** this method of classification identifies four groups

of individuals: those who are hypertensive by both criteria (true hypertension), normotensive by both (true normotension), hypertensive only by clinic criteria (WCH), and hypertensive only by ambulatory criteria (masked hypertension). Home readings may be substituted for ambulatory readings, but they are less reliable.

It should be emphasized that WCH cannot be defined on the basis of a single clinic visit, especially the first visit. Many individuals have a relatively high BP when first seen, but BP tends to fall with repeated visits. A related question is whether WCH can be diagnosed by home BP monitoring, without the use of ambulatory BP monitoring. Although a high home BP excludes the diagnosis of WCH, normal home pressures (<135/85 mm Hg) do not establish the diagnosis because the pressure might be high under other conditions, especially at work.

Prevalence. Most studies have suggested that WCH occurs in 20% or more of the hypertensive population. Factors associated with WCH are female sex, increasing age, less severe hypertension by clinic measurement, and less frequent clinic visits and measurements. WCH should always be considered in the evaluation of elderly patients.

Natural history. At least three studies have included repeat ambulatory monitoring but have given very different estimates of how many patients make the transition from WCH to true hypertension (ranging from 12.5%–75%) or how long the process takes. The apparent transition of a patient from white coat to true hypertension could have several explanations. The one that has been most widely advocated is that WCH represents a prehypertensive state. An equally plausible explanation is that the transition is nothing more than regression to the mean, especially in a patient with more variable BP. Because WCH is defined by a relatively high clinic BP and a relatively low ambulatory BP, it is to be expected that some patients will have a lower clinic BP and higher ambulatory BP on repeat testing. In a study in which 90 patients were diagnosed with WCH, only 38 had the same diagnosis 3 months later when the ambulatory blood pressure monitoring (ABPM) was repeated; the other 52 showed higher ambulatory BPs and were subsequently diagnosed as having true hypertension. Therefore, all patients with a diagnosis of WCH must be followed indefinitely with both clinic and home or ambulatory readings.

Target organ damage. The extent to which WCH patients exhibit target organ damage is of interest for two reasons. First, absence of target organ damage supports the hypothesis that WCH is characterized by an elevation of BP only in the physician's office. Second, it would imply a benign prognosis. Although the bulk of studies have supported this view, the data have not been consistent, in some cases perhaps because of failure to match groups for demographic confounders. Some studies have showed increased left ventricular mass in WCH, but in these studies, the average daytime pressure has been significantly higher in white coat hypertensive patients than in normotensive patients. In general, left ventricular mass in WCH is closer to that found in true normotensive patients than true hypertensive patients. There is no correlation between the magnitude of the white coat effect and left ventricular mass, which is consistent with the idea that chronic BP burden is more important than increased BP reactivity in determining target organ damage. Other measures of target organ damage have also been investigated, but less extensively. In studies using carotid ultrasonography, white coat hypertensive patients generally have

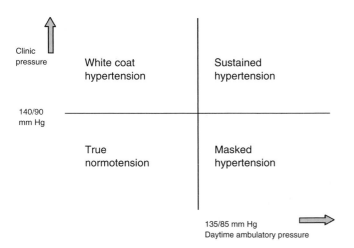

Figure B89.1 Classification of hypertension status according to clinic and ambulatory blood pressure (BP) criteria.

lower intimal-medial thickness ratios and less total atherosclerotic plaque than true hypertensive patients. Another index of target organ damage, microalbuminuria, which has been found to be an independent predictor of morbidity, is usually normal in WCH.

Morbidity and mortality. Several prospective studies have provided data consistent with the hypothesis that WCH is associated with a relatively low risk of morbidity, intermediate between truly normotensive and truly hypertensive subjects. Those subjects whose daytime ambulatory BPs are low in relation to their clinic BPs are at lower risk of morbidity. A good example is a substudy of the Systolic Hypertension in Europe (SYST-Eur) trial of treatment of isolated systolic hypertension in the elderly found that patients with WCH were at lower risk of strokes than patients with true hypertension. Other prognostic studies, although not defining a distinct group of white coat hypertensive patients, have concluded that ambulatory BP monitoring gives a better predictor of risk than clinic BP. Some recent studies have indicated that with longer follow-up the risk in patients with WCH may increase, to become similar to patients with sustained hypertension. These findings emphasize the importance of long-term follow-up with out-of-office monitoring.

Management. The most controversial issue in the management of WCH is whether antihypertensive drug treatment should be prescribed. Most experts favor the view that there is less need to initiate antihypertensive medication in WCH than patients with true hypertension. The principal rationale for this approach is that WCH appears to have a more benign prognosis than true hypertension; overall, WCH confers only slightly higher risk than true normotension. Several studies have analyzed the effects of antihypertensive medications in patients with true hypertension and WCH; drugs such as α-blockers and calcium channel blockers lower clinic BP, but have a negligible effect on the ambulatory BP. However, there are also reports that angiotensin-converting enzyme (ACE) inhibitors lower ambulatory BP, although clinic pressure is still affected to a greater extent. In most patients with true hypertension, treatment reduces but does not eliminate the white coat effect. The value of lifestyle modification in the management of WCH is unproven in clinical trials but because most WCH individuals have prehypertension (clinic BP 120–139/80/89 mm Hg), lifestyle modification is consistent with standard treatment guidelines.

Masked hypertension

In normotensive subjects and some hypertensive patients, the white coat effect may be absent or even reversed (i.e., the clinic pressure is lower than the daytime BP). This condition is the mirror image of WCH, and is defined as a normal clinic pressure and high ambulatory pressure.

In keeping with the fact that it is the ambulatory pressure that is most closely related to cardiovascular events, masked hypertension is not a benign condition. In untreated patients, it may be detected before a diagnosis of hypertension has been made but it is also seen in treated patients, where it is associated with poor prognosis. The role of stress in contributing to masked hypertension is not clear, but may be one of the factors that raises daytime BP. Although the prevalence of masked hypertension is low, perhaps only 6% of the normotensive population, the absolute number in the United States may approach 15 to 18 million.

Suggested Readings

Bjorklund K, Lind L, Zethelius B, et al. Prognostic significance of 24-h ambulatory BP characteristics for cardiovascular morbidity in a population of elderly men. *J Hypertens* 2004;22(9):1691–1697.

Fagard R, Staessen JA, Thijs L, et al. Response to antihypertensive therapy in older patients with sustained and nonsustained systolic hypertension. *Circulation* 2000;102:1139–1144.

Gerin W, Chaplin W, Schwartz JE, et al. Sustained BP elevation following an acute stressor: the effects of the september 11, 2001 attack on the New York City World Trade Center. *J Hypertens* 2005;23:279–284.

He J, Klag MJ, Wu Z, et al. Effect of migration and related environmental changes on serum lipid levels in southwestern Chinese men. *Am J Epidemiol* 1996;144(9):839–848.

Palatini P, Dorigatti F, Roman E, et al. White-coat hypertension: a selection bias? Harvest Study Investigators. Hypertension and Ambulatory Recording Venetia study. *Hypertension* 1998;16(7):977–984.

Pickering TG. Could hypertension be a consequence of the 24/7 society? The effects of sleep deprivation and shift work. *J Clin Hypertens (Greenwich)* 2006;8(11):819–822.

Pickering TG, Shimbo D, Haas D. Ambulatory blood-pressure monitoring. *N Engl J Med* 2006;354(22):2368–2374.

Pierdomenico SD, Lapenna D, Bucci A, et al. Cardiovascular outcome in treated hypertensive patients with responder, masked, false resistant and true resistant hypertension. *Am J Hypertens* 2005;18:1422–1428.

Schnall PL, Schwartz JE, Landsbergis PA, et al. A longitudinal study of job strain and ambulatory BP: results from a three-year follow-up. *Psychosom Med* 1998;60(6):697–706.

Yan LL, Liu K, Matthews KA, et al. Psychosocial factors and risk of hypertension: the Coronary Artery Risk Development in Young Adults (CARDIA) study. *JAMA* 2003;290(16):2138–2148.

CHAPTER B90 ■ OBESITY, BODY FAT DISTRIBUTION, AND INSULIN RESISTANCE: CLINICAL RELEVANCE

STEVEN M. HAFFNER, MD AND HENRY R. BLACK, MD

KEY POINTS

■ Obesity is widely recognized as a risk factor for the development of hypertension; abdominal (visceral) fat is associated with elevated blood pressure (BP) independent of body weight.

■ Increased visceral fat distribution is associated with insulin resistance, which may contribute to hypertension.

■ Persons who develop hypertension at an early age have an increased frequency of lipid disorders (familial dyslipidemic hypertension); many of these people have increased glucose and insulin concentrations and insulin resistance.

■ Diuretics and β-blockers tend to exacerbate glucose intolerance and induce diabetes, whereas α-blockers, angiotensin-converting enzyme (ACE) inhibitors, and angiotensin receptor blockers tend to have favorable effects.

See also Chapters A34, **B46,** and **B47**

Obesity

Obesity in clinical and epidemiologic studies is most often defined and assessed by body mass index (BMI) (BMI: weight in kg divided by the square of height in meters). Currently we define those with a BMI of <25 kg/m^2 as nonobese, those with a BMI of 25 to 29.9 kg/m^2 as overweight and those with a BMI of ≥30 kg/m^2 as obese. Obesity is widely recognized as a risk factor for the development of hypertension and as a strong predictor of cardiovascular (CV) and all-cause mortality. In the follow-up study of the First National Health and Nutrition Examination Survey (NHANES I), overall adiposity (BMI) strongly predicted the incidence of hypertension in blacks and whites. Weight loss has been shown to be associated with decreased blood pressure (BP) in many studies irrespective of age or ethnicity.

Body fat distribution

The pattern of body fat distribution itself is a major risk factor: upper body (central or visceral or "apple-shaped") obesity being associated with other CV risk factors [dyslipidemia, type 2 diabetes mellitus (DM), and hypertension] and increased CV risk. In contrast, peripheral (lower body or "pear-shaped") obesity may not be a reliable marker of insulin resistance or increased likelihood of premature morbidity and mortality. It also follows that BMI alone is less tightly associated with increased CV disease risk than visceral fat mass.

Assessment techniques. The most common clinical and epidemiologic assessments of body fat distribution use measures of central adiposity: subscapular skinfold thickness, the ratio of subscapular to triceps skinfolds, or the ratio of waist:hip circumferences (WHR). Unfortunately, there is no uniform practice for identifying waist or hip landmarks. Often, waist circumference is measured at the umbilicus or, alternatively, at the minimum diameter between the thorax and the hips. Hip circumference can be measured at the maximum diameter of the hips or, alternatively, at the level of the greater trochanter. There are also no internationally recognized standards for defining upper-body adiposity, although some authors have suggested a WHR >0.95 in men and a WHR >0.85 in women. The WHR and ratio of skinfolds are related to the general degree of adiposity. Central adiposity, as assessed by skinfolds, has been related to BP cross-sectionally in whites, blacks, and Hispanics. Waist-hip circumference has also been related to BP elevation in Hispanics and whites but the association between body fat distribution and levels of BP is independent of obesity or BMI in a number of studies.

Visceral fat. There are differences in metabolic activity of adipocytes in different fat depots; visceral fat (measured by computerized tomography) is much more metabolically active than subcutaneous fat. The ratio of visceral fat to subcutaneous fat is more closely correlated with the risk of type 2 DM than are assessments of fat distribution that use less sensitive methods (circumferences or skinfolds). Fewer data are available on the possible role of visceral fat in hypertension, although there is a high correlation between visceral and retroperitoneal adipose tissue mass and BP in normoglycemic humans. Waist circumference may be a better indicator of visceral fat than WHR but an update of the third Adult Treatment Panel (ATP III) guideline has noted that the degree of elevated waist circumference needed to define the metabolic syndrome varies by ethnicity. In whites and those of African descent, a waist circumference of $\geq$40 in. in men or $\geq$35 in. has been the standard cutoff, whereas in Asians, the definition of increased waist circumference must be lower ($\geq$35 in. for men or $\geq$31 in. for women).

Insulin resistance and hypertension

The mechanisms by which obesity and body fat distribution lead to increased BP are not well understood. An adverse body fat distribution is usually associated with insulin resistance, which may contribute to the development of hypertension. The clustering of CV risk factors, including dyslipidemia, DM, hypertension, obesity, and central adiposity (the metabolic syndrome to some), has long been recognized. Many studies have shown that lean, normoglycemic untreated hypertensive subjects are more insulin-resistant than comparable normotensive subjects. Furthermore, subjects who develop hypertension at an early age have an increased frequency of lipid disorders (familial dyslipidemic hypertension); a subset of these patients has increased glucose and insulin concentrations; insulin resistance may underlie this cluster of atherogenic changes. Multiple mechanisms have been proposed to explain a possible relationship between insulin resistance and hypertension, including increased sympathetic nervous system activity, vascular smooth muscle hypertrophy, altered cation transport, and salt sensitivity.

Racial differences. The association between insulin and hypertension is still somewhat controversial, in part because of inconsistent evidence. One reason for the discrepancy between studies is the possibility that the etiology of hypertension is different among ethnic groups. One cross-sectional study suggested a relationship between insulin resistance and BP in whites but not in blacks or Pima Indians, whereas another found a definite association between insulin resistance and hypertension in young, lean, black men with stage 1 hypertension. A relationship between insulin resistance and hypertension has been shown in lean type 1 diabetic subjects but not in obese type 2 diabetic subjects. Because the blacks in the later report were much leaner than those in the former study (BMI, 24 vs. 31 kg/m^2, respectively), the variable association of insulin resistance and hypertension may be due to differences in adiposity. Studies using the hyperinsulinemic euglycemic clamp showed that decreased insulin sensitivity is directly associated with BP in a large number of nonobese nondiabetic Europeans.

Insulin and blood pressure. The relationship between insulin and BP is extremely complex. Short-term insulin infusions (2 hours) raise catecholamines but not BP in normotensive men but short-term infusions of insulin are vasodilatory in humans and in dogs. The effect of chronic hyperinsulinemia (i.e., lasting months or years) is not known but it is generally agreed that patients with insulinomas are not hypertensive. Ecologic data also do not support a strong relationship between insulin and BP. Pima Indians and Mexican Americans have very high rates of type 2 DM, hyperinsulinemia, and insulin resistance and yet

have a lower prevalence of hypertension. Certain antihypertensive agents have been reported to increase insulin resistance and induce dyslipidemia. Many studies have avoided this problem by studying hypertensive subjects not currently on medications. However, another potential problem with cross-sectional studies is that the clustering of risk factors (including insulin resistance) could result from compensatory mechanisms that induce secondary metabolic changes such as increased catecholamines.

Risk factor clustering

In a prospective study in 1,440 nonhypertensive Mexican American and non-Hispanic white subjects over 8 years, obesity, glucose intolerance, and fasting insulin were each significantly related to the incidence of hypertension in univariate analyses. Subjects in the highest category of BMI ($\geq$30 kg/m^2) had an increased incidence of hypertension relative to subjects with lower BMIs [13.8% vs. 6.3%, respectively; relative risk (RR) = 2; $p < .001$]. Similarly, subjects in the highest third of insulin concentrations (>95 pmol/L) had an increased incidence of hypertension relative to subjects with lower insulin concentrations (13.4% vs. 6.9%, respectively; RR = 1.93; $p = .001$). Subjects with type 2 DM had an increased incidence of hypertension relative to subjects with normal glucose tolerance (17.1% vs. 7.8%, respectively; RR = 2.18; $p = .04$). None of the interactions of ethnicity with BMI, insulin, and glucose tolerance status were statistically significant ($p > .50$), suggesting that the effects of BMI, hyperinsulinemia, and glucose intolerance on hypertension incidence were similar in both ethnic groups. In nondiabetic populations, subjects demonstrated dyslipidemia (increased triglyceride and decreased high-density lipoprotein cholesterol levels) before the onset of hypertension. This observation supports the general concept of the clustering of the CV risk factors (the familial dyslipidemia-hypertension syndrome). Because the relative impact of insulin resistance may be greater in lean than in obese subjects, the incidence of hypertension was examined stratified simultaneously by BMI and fasting insulin concentrations. In nonobese (BMI <25 kg/m^2) but not obese subjects, the incidence of hypertension correlated with baseline fasting insulin concentrations. In lean subjects, the incidence of hypertension for those in the highest third of insulin concentration compared with those in the lowest two thirds was 10.1% versus 4.5%, respectively (RR = 2.24; $p = .0032$), in subjects with BMI between 25 and 30 kg/m^2, and the incidence in the corresponding insulin categories was 11.5% versus 15%, respectively (RR = 0.70; p = not significant). Therefore, the effect of fasting insulin on the incidence of hypertension decreased with increasing obesity.

Antihypertensive drugs and glucose intolerance

Whether particular antihypertensives are more likely than others to induce DM in hypertensive persons is a matter of debate. Antihypertensive agents that worsen insulin sensitivity might be expected to increase the risk of developing DM because hyperinsulinemia and insulin resistance are strongly related to the incidence of type 2 DM. This is important because hypertensive persons appear to be at increased risk of developing DM, as evidenced by the clustering of DM and hypertension.

Diuretics and β-blockers. In some studies, thiazide diuretics and β-blockers worsen glucose tolerance and insulin resistance.

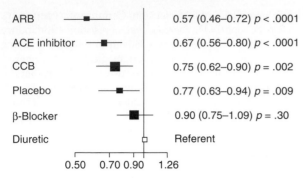

ARB		0.57 (0.46–0.72) p < .0001
ACE inhibitor		0.67 (0.56–0.80) p < .0001
CCB		0.75 (0.62–0.90) p = .002
Placebo		0.77 (0.63–0.94) p = .009
β-Blocker		0.90 (0.75–1.09) p = .30
Diuretic		Referent

0.50   0.70 0.90   1.26

Odds ratio of incident diabetes   Incoherence = 0.000017

Figure B90.1 Incident diabetes in clinical trials of antihypertensive drugs: a network meta-analysis. This figure uses thiazide diuretics as the referent point for comparison of other antihypertensive agents and placebo on the likelihood of causing new diabetes mellitus in currently available clinical trials. The technique of a network meta-analysis allows the investigator to compare the effects of drugs which have not been directly compared to each other in specific trials and derive a reasonable estimate of whatever would have happened had that comparison been done. ARB, angiotensin receptor blocker; ACE, angiotensin-converting enzyme; CCB, calcium channel blocker.

In a longitudinal study of Swedish women, it was observed that hypertensive women taking thiazide diuretics have a significant 3.4-fold higher risk of developing DM than untreated hypertensive women. Relative to hypertensive subjects not on therapy, the risk of developing DM was even higher in hypertensive subjects taking β-blockers and hypertensive subjects taking both thiazide diuretics and β-blockers. In a 10-year follow-up study, 12.7% of hypertensive men developed DM, as opposed to 3.6% of nonhypertensive men (p < .001). In another prospective study, subjects who were hypertensive at baseline had a higher 8-year incidence of type 2 DM (8.9% vs. 4.9%, p = .041) and impaired glucose tolerance (25.2% vs. 10%, p < .001) than subjects who were normotensive at baseline. After adjustment for age, sex, ethnicity, obesity, body fat distribution, fasting glucose, and insulin, this excess was present only for impaired glucose intolerance. Therefore, the excess risk of type 2 DM in hypertensive patients can be explained by their greater age, obesity, more unfavorable body fat distribution, and hyperinsulinemia, whereas their excess risk of impaired glucose intolerance is independent of these factors. Kostis, et al. reported a 14-year follow-up from the Systolic Hypertension in the Elderly Program (SHEP), where participants who developed DM on treatment (chlorthalidone with or without atenolol) had the same prognosis as those who remained normoglycemic, whereas those who entered the study with overt DM did considerably worse.

Other agents. Angiotensin-converting enzyme (ACE) inhibitors and angiotensin receptor blockers (ARBs) generally improve insulin sensitivity, although to a relatively small degree. In the Heart Outcomes Prevention Evaluation (HOPE) trial, ramipril was associated with a decreased risk of developing type 2 DM. A similar reduced incidence of new type 2 DM was observed in the Losartan Intervention for Endpoint (LIFE) trial in which a regimen beginning with an ARB (losartan) was compared to a β-blocker (atenolol). Calcium channel blockers (CCBs) (with the possible exception of nifedipine) do not affect insulin sensitivity and α-blockers tend to improve insulin sensitivity.

Direct drug comparisons. In the largest hypertension trial ever done, the Antihypertensive and Lipid Lower Trial to Reduce Heart Attack (ALLHAT) subjects whose regimen began with chlorthalidone had an increased likelihood of developing DM over a 4-year period (11.6%) compared to those who started with a CCB, amlodipine (9.8%) or an ACE inhibitor lisinopril (8.1%). In a network meta-analysis using all available clinical trial data, Elliott and Meyer found an increased risk of developing DM in those who receive both thiazide diuretics and to a lesser degree, β-blockers (**Figure B90.1**). Compared to thiazide diuretics, those receiving β-blockers had a nonsignificant 10% lower risk of developing DM, whereas those on placebo (−23%), CCBs (−25%), ACE inhibitors (−33%) and ARBs (−43%) were all significantly less likely to develop DM than those whose initial treatment was a thiazide diuretic; there was no statistically significant difference between any of these drugs or placebo.

Suggested Readings

ALLHAT Collaborative Research Group. Major outcomes in high-risk hypertensive patients randomized to angiotensin-converting enzyme inhibitor or calcium channel Blocker vs Diuretic: the antihypertensive and lipid-lowering treatment to prevent heart attack trial (ALLHAT). *JAMA* 2002;288:2981–2997.

Blair D, Habicht JP, Sims EA, et al. Evidence for an increased risk for hypertension with centrally located body fat and the effect of race and sex on this risk. *Am J Epidemiol* 1984;119:526–540.

Elliott WJ, Meyer PM. Incident diabetes in clinical trials of antihypertensive drugs: a network meta-analysis. *Lancet* 2007;369:201–207.

Ferrannini E, Natali A, Capaldo B, et al. Insulin resistance, hyperinsulinemia, and BP. *Hypertension* 1997;30:1144–1149.

Grundy SM, Cleeman JI, Daniels SR, et al. Diagnosis and Management of the Metabolic Syndrome. *Circulation* 2005;12:2735–2752.

Haffner SM, Ferrannini E, Hazuda HP, et al. Clustering of cardiovascular risk factors in confirmed prehypertensive individuals. *Hypertension* 1992;20:38–45.

Kostis JB, Wilson AC, Freudenberger RS, et al. SHEP Collaborative Research Group. Long-term effect of diuretic-based therapy on fatal outcomes in subjects with isolated systolic hypertension with and without diabetes. *Am J Cardiol* 2005;95:29–35.

Lorenzo C, Serrano-Rios M, Martinez-Larrad MT, et al. Prevalence of hypertension in hispanic and non-Hispanic white populations. *Hypertension* 2002;39:203–208.

Morales PA, Mitchell BD, Valdez RA, et al. Incidence of NIDDM and impaired glucose tolerance in hypertensive subjects: the San Antonio Heart Study. *Diabetes* 1993;42:154–161.

Saad MF, Lillioja S, Nyomba BL, et al. Racial differences in the relation between BP and insulin resistance. *N Engl J Med* 1991;324:733–739.

CHAPTER B91 ■ PHYSICAL ACTIVITY AND BLOOD PRESSURE

DENISE G. SIMONS-MORTON, MD, PhD

KEY POINTS

■ Epidemiologic studies have shown an inverse relationship between amount of physical activity and blood pressure (BP) level.

■ Clinical trials demonstrate that physical activity significantly decreases BP in all population groups studied.

■ Physical activity is a cornerstone therapy for preventing hypertension; 150 minutes per week of moderate-intensity aerobic activity (e.g., brisk walking) is recommended, divided into 30 minutes a day, accumulated or in one session.

See also Chapters **B97, C120,** and **C121**

Physical activity has an important influence on blood pressure (BP) as well as on overall cardiovascular disease (CVD) risk. Physical activity includes bodily movement during daily living and exercise that is purposeful activity to improve health or fitness.

Benefits

Cardiovascular. Physical activity (behavior that results in energy expenditure) and cardiorespiratory fitness (a physiologic attribute of the body's ability to use oxygen that is increased by physical activity) are inversely associated with BP level and hypertension incidence. Randomized trials have demonstrated that physical activity can lower BP in normotensive, prehypertensive, and hypertensive persons. A substantial body of evidence strongly supports the assertion that a physically active lifestyle can delay or prevent the development of hypertension and thereby the need for antihypertensive medication. Although more evidence is needed about biologic effects of physical activity, the implicated mechanisms include neurohumoral, vascular, and structural adaptations.

In addition to effects on BP and cardiorespiratory fitness, physical activity provides other benefits that reduce risk of CVD, including favorable effects on blood lipids, body weight, and blood glucose levels. Physical activity and cardiorespiratory fitness are inversely associated with CVD incidence and mortality as well as with total mortality.

Other. Physical activity also has favorable effects on other conditions, such as osteoporosis, risk of some cancers, depression, and physical functioning in the elderly. Therefore, physical activity should be promoted for a variety of benefits, including BP effects.

Physical activity and hypertension

Observational studies. Prospective epidemiologic studies have found that the incidence of hypertension is higher in those with lower physical activity levels or lower levels of cardiorespiratory fitness. The associations generally have held when age, sex, smoking, weight, body mass index, blood lipids, and other potentially confounding factors are controlled. Although the evidence from observational studies is strong for an inverse relationship between physical activity level and BP, these studies are limited by the inability to ensure that all other factors that affect BP are the same between active and nonactive groups. For this reason, randomized controlled trials provide more valid assessments of the effects of physical activity on BP.

Clinical trials. More than 70 randomized controlled trials have examined effects on BP of physical activity or exercise regimens. Most of the regimens tested have been *aerobic (endurance) exercise,* defined as rhythmic exercise that involves large muscle movements (e.g., running, walking, cycling, or swimming) and causes increases in heart and respiration rates (which results in increased oxygen consumption). The exercise regimens tested in most trials have used a frequency, intensity, and duration largely based on the American College of Sports Medicine (ACSM) exercise prescription for improving cardiorespiratory fitness. Fewer trials have examined BP effects of resistance exercise (weight training).

Numerous quantitative meta-analyses have been conducted to examine the effects of exercise on BP seen in the controlled trials. Trials have been testing effects on BP of aerobic exercise for several decades. A recent meta-analysis of trials examined effects of aerobic exercise on BP overall (72 trials), and in normotensive (28 trials), prehypertensive (46 trials), and hypertensive individuals (30 trials). The effects of resistance training (weight training) on BP has received more recent study, and another recent meta-analysis examined the effects on BP of resistance training (12 trials). The meta-analysis results show that aerobic endurance training reduces systolic BP from 2 to 7 mm Hg, with the greatest reduction in hypertensive participants, and that resistance training reduces systolic BP from 3 to 6 mm Hg (**Figure B91.1**). These and other meta-analyses on the topic have concluded that physical activity significantly decreases BP in all population groups analyzed and by all types of exercise examined. The BP-lowering effects of exercise are independent of weight changes. For aerobic exercise, the amount of BP lowering is significantly associated with the gain in cardiorespiratory fitness.

The average exercise regimen tested used 120 minutes of moderate-intensity exercise a week, resulting in a clinically relevant BP effect. Behavioral intervention studies provide evidence that people may be more successful in being regularly active if they pursue activity that is of moderate intensity (e.g., brisk walking) rather than of vigorous intensity (e.g., running).

National recommendations

Joint National Committee 7. The Seventh Report of the Joint National Committee (JNC 7) identified reduced physical activity as a causal factor for hypertension and recommended regular aerobic physical activity, such as brisk walking 30 or more minutes most days, for BP management. Physical activity is recommended as part of lifestyle treatment for all levels of BP. *Other guidelines.* Numerous organizations, including the U.S. Preventive Services Task Force, recommend that patients engage in physical activity to reduce cardiovascular risk factors. The ACSM gives an "A" level (the highest level) rating for evidence that "dynamic aerobic training reduces resting BP in

TABLE B91.1

EXERCISE PRESCRIPTION RECOMMENDED FOR PERSONS WITH HIGH BLOOD PRESSURE (BP)

Parameter	Description
Mode of activity	Primarily endurance physical activity supplemented by resistance exercise
Frequency	Most, preferably all, days of the week
Duration	≥30 min of continuous or accumulated physical activity per d
Intensity	40% to 60% of $\dot{V}O_2R$ (oxygen uptake reserve) (i.e., moderate-intensity)

[Adapted from American College of Sports Medicine, Exercise and Hypertension Position Stand. *Med Sci Sports Exerc* 2004;36(6):533–553.]

individuals with normal BP and in those with hypertension." For general health, the ACSM and the Centers for Disease Control and Prevention, as well as the Surgeon General's Report on Physical Activity and Health, recommend a minimum of 30 minutes of moderate-intensity physical activity on most days. These recommendations also state that additional activity, which can be achieved by increasing frequency, duration, intensity, or a combination of these, can result in additional health benefits.

Physical activity prescription

Aerobic activity. The ACSM exercise prescription to control hypertension, shown in **Table B91.1**, is for endurance activity of ≥30 minutes a day at a moderate intensity. The recommended intensity is 40% to 60% of oxygen update reserve ($\dot{V}O_2R$). However, prescriptions based on heart rate may be easier to calculate by physicians and to convey to patients. An intensity of 50% to 69% of maximum heart rate is considered to be moderate. Maximum heart rate can be roughly estimated by subtracting age from the constant 220. Moderate-intensity activity for most people is comparable to brisk walking at 3 to 4 miles per hour. *Other modes of activity.* All of the exercise recommendations for hypertension focus on aerobic exercise as the primary activity. Some of the recommendations include weight training as part of an overall fitness regimen, but none recommend weight training as a sole mode of exercise. The recent meta-analyses support this position. Initial changes in activity levels in sedentary or irregularly active people should employ moderate-intensity activities for both behavioral and safety reasons.

Suggested Readings

American College of Sports Medicine. Position stand: exercise and hypertension. *Med Sci Sports Exerc* 2004;36(6):533–553.

Cornelissen VA, Fagard RH. Effects of endurance training on BP, BP-regulating mechanisms, and cardiovascular risk factors. *Hypertension* 2005;46:66–675.

Cornelissen VA, Fagard RH. Effect of resistance training on resting BP: a meta-analysis of randomized controlled trials. *J Hypertens* 2005;23:251–259.

Thompson PD, Buchner D, Pina IL, et al. Exercise and physical activity in the prevention and treatment of atherosclerotic cardiovascular disease: a statement from the Council on Clinical Cardiology (Subcommittee on Exercise, Rehabilitation, and Prevention) and the Council on Nutrition, Physical Activity, and Metabolism (Subcommittee on Physical Activity). *Circulation* 2003;107:3109–3116.

Whelton SP, Chin A, Zin Z, et al. Effect of aerobic exercise on BP: a meta-analysis of randomized controlled trials. *Ann Intern Med* 2002;136:493–503.

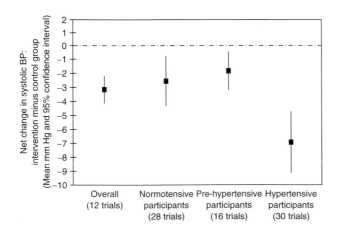

Figure B91.1 Results of a meta-analysis of 72 randomized controlled trials published through September 2003 that tested effects of aerobic (endurance) exercise on blood pressure (BP). (Based on data reported by Cornelissen VA, Fagard RH. Effects of endurance training on BP, BP-regulating mechanisms, and cardiovascular risk factors. *Hypertension* 2005;46:66–675.)

CHAPTER B92 ■ DIETARY PATTERNS AND BLOOD PRESSURE

FRANK M. SACKS, MD

KEY POINTS

- Populations eating mainly vegetarian diets have lower blood pressure (BP) levels and lesser BP rises with age than those eating omnivorous diets.
- The Dietary Approaches to Stop Hypertension (DASH) diet, which emphasizes fruits, vegetables, low-fat dairy products, whole grains, poultry, fish, and nuts, with only small amounts of red meat, sweets, and sugar-containing beverages, lowers BP.
- Further BP lowering occurs when DASH-type diets are combined with modest sodium restriction or caloric rebalancing, with reduced carbohydrate and higher unsaturated fat and protein content; the latter also improves lipid profiles.
- Relatively large doses of fish oil (Omega-3 fatty acid) are needed to demonstrate a significant BP-lowering effect.
- High fruit and vegetable consumption is associated with decreased stroke and ischemic heart disease.

See also Chapters **B97, C120, C121,** and C157

There are striking differences in the blood pressures (BPs) of populations worldwide. BP is higher and rises more steeply with age in industrialized than in nonindustrialized societies. A predominantly vegetarian dietary pattern is often present in those cultures that have generally low BP, and in industrialized countries vegetarians have lower average BP levels.

Epidemiologic surveys

The lowest average BPs in an industrialized country have been found in strict vegetarians in Massachusetts ("macrobiotics"), who consume almost no animal products of any kind (**Figure B92.1**). Their diets are very plentiful in whole grains, green leafy vegetables, squash, and root vegetables. The entire BP distribution of these vegetarians is shifted to lower levels than nonvegetarians residing in the same area, indicating that diet could have a population-wide effect on BP.

Less rigorous dietary restriction is also associated with lower BP; a dietary pattern high in potassium and polyunsaturated fats and low in starch, saturated fat, and cholesterol was inversely associated with BP in a large population of U.S. men. Prospective studies in the United States, one in women (Nurses' Health Study) and the other in men (Health Professionals Follow-Up Study), found that a high intake of fruits and vegetables was associated with lower BP and less change in BP with age. In a representative population sample of the United States (National Health and Nutrition Examination Survey Follow-Up Study), fruit and vegetable intake three times a day or more was associated with reductions in stroke and ischemic heart disease mortality of 25% to 40%.

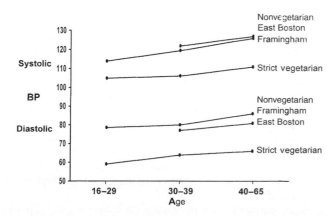

Figure B92.1 Blood pressure (BP) in a strict vegetarian population in Boston and in nonvegetarian populations in East Boston and Framingham, Massachusetts. (Adapted from: Sacks FM, Kass EH. Low BP in vegetarians: effects of specific foods and nutrients. *Am J Clin Nutr* 1988; 48:795–800.)

Dietary Approaches to Stop Hypertension trials

Dietary Approaches to Stop Hypertension (DASH), DASH-sodium, and Optimal Macronutrient Intake to Prevent Heart Disease (OmniHeart) were multicenter trials that tested dietary patterns that were considered to have potential to lower BP and improve dyslipidemia.

All diets were prepared centrally and given to the research participants for 1 to 2 months; body weight was kept constant to test diet type, not weight loss. The sample sizes of these trials were large enough (N = 160–459 participants) to provide precise estimates of the effects on BP and to analyze subgroups of the cohort, such as women, and blacks (who comprised approximately 50% of the study participants).

Dietary types

Fruit and vegetables diet. One diet, termed the *fruits-and-vegetables diet,* emphasized fruits and vegetables and included nuts and reduced amounts of sweets and sugar-containing beverages; it was otherwise similar in other nutrients to the control dietary pattern which resembled diets that Americans typically eat.

Dietary Approaches to Stop Hypertension diet. The diet now termed the *DASH diet,* emphasized fruits, vegetables, and low-fat dairy products, included whole grains, poultry, fish and nuts, and contained only small amounts of red meat, sweets, and sugar-containing beverages, with decreased amounts of total fat, saturated fat, and cholesterol. The DASH diet is low in total fat, 27% of daily energy intake.

Dietary Approaches to Stop Hypertension-low sodium diet. The DASH diet and the control diet were tested at three sodium levels, 3.5 g, 2.3 g, and 1.2 g daily intake.

Blood pressure effects. The DASH diet significantly reduced BP by 5.5 mm Hg systolic and 3.0 mm Hg diastolic. In contrast, the fruits-and-vegetables diet reduced BP by approximately half this amount, −2.8/−1.1 mm Hg. In hypertensive individuals, who comprised 29% of the group, the reductions in BP (−11.4/−5.5 mm Hg for the DASH diet and −7.2/−2.8 mm Hg for the fruits-and-vegetables diet) were much higher than in normotensive individuals (**Figure B92.2**). The effects of the dietary patterns were similar in men and women but the BP reductions in black participants were greater than those in whites. Therefore, the therapeutic effects of the DASH diet in hypertensive individuals were similar to those observed for angiotensin-converting enzyme (ACE) inhibitors, diuretics, or calcium channel blockers.

The combined effects on BP of lower sodium intake and the DASH diet are greater than either alone and are clinically relevant. The DASH diet lowered BP independent of sodium intake and sodium restriction can lower BP independent of dietary composition. The DASH diet and sodium restriction are also additive and have age-dependent effects. In those older than 45 years, DASH diet with low sodium reduced systolic BP by approximately 15 mm Hg in hypertensive individuals and 10 mm Hg in normotensive individuals (**Figure B92.3**), about twice the effect in those aged 45 years or younger.

Explaining the Dietary Approaches to Stop Hypertension diet effect

Potassium content. Comparing the BP lowering caused by the fruits-and-vegetables diet with the DASH diet, it may be surmised that high intake of fruits and vegetables, including nuts and reduced amounts of sweets and sugar-containing beverages can account for approximately 50% of the effect of the DASH diet. Fruits and vegetables are high in potassium, magnesium, fiber, and many other nutrients. Of these, potassium is the most well

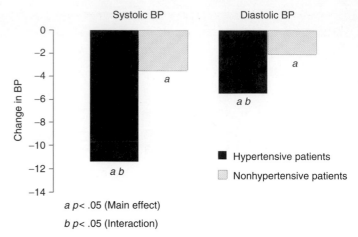

Figure B92.2 Effect of dietary patterns on blood pressure (BP) in the Dietary Approaches to Stop Hypertension (DASH) study. The DASH diet emphasizes fruits, vegetables, and low-fat dairy products; it includes whole grains, poultry, fish, and nuts and contains only small amounts of red meat, sweets, and sugar-containing beverages. The DASH diet contains decreased amounts of total and saturated fat and cholesterol. The fruits-and-vegetables diet was high in fruits and vegetables, included nuts, and reduced amounts of sweets and sugar-containing beverages but was similar in other nutrients to the control dietary pattern resembling average intake in the United States. There were 459 participants randomized to three diets—a control diet typical of that eaten in the United States, DASH, and fruits and vegetables. The diets were given to the participants for 8 weeks. Body weight was kept constant. Hypertensive individuals were included with SBP 140 to 160 mm Hg and DBP 90 to 95.

established for lowering BP, particularly in hypertensive patients, persons with low potassium intake, and in blacks. The DASH population included these subgroups and the magnitude of BP lowering in the fruits-and-vegetables group was similar to that observed for potassium supplementation. Therefore, a plausible explanation is that raising potassium intake from low (1,700 mg or 44 mmol) to high (4,100 mg or 105 mmol) contributed to the DASH effect on BP but it is also possible that reduced amount of sweets and sugar-containing beverages and other nutrients were also involved.

Limitations of interpretation. The DASH study was not designed to determine which foods or nutrients are responsible for the overall BP-lowering effect. Compared with the fruits-and-vegetables diet, the DASH diet had more low-fat dairy products, vegetables, poultry, fish, calcium, magnesium, potassium, protein, and cereal grains and was lower in saturated, monounsaturated, and total fat, as well as cholesterol, red meat, sweets, and high-carbohydrate snacks. Trials that have tested the BP impact of these nutrients individually (e.g., fat, fiber, calcium, or magnesium) have not found effects large enough to account for the overall DASH-diet response. Yet small individual BP-lowering effects of individual nutrients, even if not detected in a clinical trial or in a meta-analysis (e.g., 0.5 to 1.0 mm Hg), could combine to reduce BP.

OmniHeart study

The premise of OmniHeart was that partial replacement of carbohydrate with either unsaturated fat or protein will enhance the BP-lowering effect of the DASH diet and further improve dyslipidemic risk factors. High protein intake, especially plant protein, has been linked to lower BP in many populations in Asia,

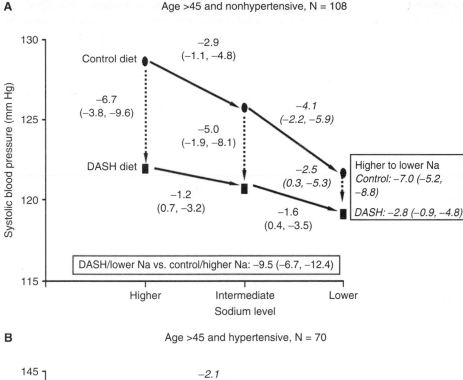

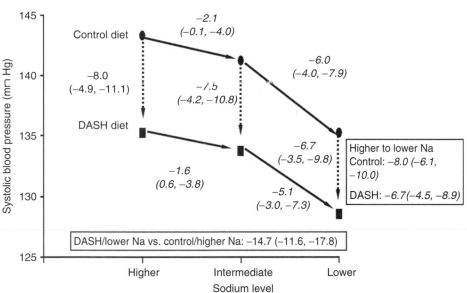

Figure B92.3 (A and B): Effect on systolic blood pressure (BP) of Dietary Approaches to Stop Hypertension (DASH) diet and reduced sodium. Participants were assigned to either a typical U.S. diet or the DASH diet given to them in three versions, high (150 mmol), intermediate (100 mmol), and low (50 mmol) sodium for 30 days each in a crossover design. Body weight was kept constant. (Reproduced with permission from: Bray GA, Vollmer WM, Sacks FM, et al. A further subgroup analysis of the effects of the DASH diet and three dietary sodium levels on BP. *Am J Cardiol* 2004;94:222–227.)

America, and Europe. Higher unsaturated fat diet is similar to the traditional Mediterranean diet.

The OmniHeart study tested a *higher unsaturated fat diet* (37% total fat, 48% carbohydrate, and 15% protein) and a *higher protein diet* (25% protein, 48% carbohydrate, 27% fat), and compared them to a DASH-like diet (27% fat, 58% carbohydrate, and 15% protein). Beans, nuts, whole grains, fish, and poultry were the main added-protein sources, and olive oil and canola (rapeseed) oil were the main added-unsaturated fats. The diets were modeled on the principles of the DASH diet and contained commonly consumed food items, so that the results could be conveniently implemented in dietary recommendations to the general public.

Either the added protein or unsaturated fat diets were superior to the high-carbohydrate, low-fat diet in lowering

BP and improving lipid risk factors (**Figure B92.4**). Estimated risk reductions from combined changes in BP and lipids were approximately 20% for the high-carbohydrate diet, and 30% for the protein and unsaturated fat diets.

Fish oil

Potential antihypertensive effects of fish oil derive from the ability of highly unsaturated fatty acids to stimulate the synthesis of vasodilating prostaglandins. Fish oil is often prescribed as capsules that contain 1 mL of purified oil or as crude cod liver oil. Large doses of fish oil (e.g., 30 to 45 mL daily) clearly lower BP levels in hypertensive patients but intervention trials of moderate, more practical amounts of fish oil have been inconsistent. Meta-analyses of these trials found a small BP-lowering effect (−3.0/−1.5 mm Hg) of 10 to 15 mL of fish oil daily, particularly in hypertensive

	Baseline	CARB	PROT	UNSAT
			Change from baseline	
SBP, All	131	−8	−10[a]	−10[a]
SBP, Hypertensive	146	146	−13[a]	−13[a]
LDL-C, all	129	−12	−14[a]	−13
LDL-C,≥130 mg/dL	157	−20	−24[a]	−22
HDL-C	50	−1.4	−2.6[a]	0[a]
Triglycerides	102	0	−16[a]	−9[a]

[a]$p < .05$ vs. CARB

Figure B92.4 Effect on systolic blood pressure (SBP) and lipid risk factors of Dietary Approaches to Stop Hypertension (DASH)-type diets that emphasize either carbohydrate (CARB), protein (PROT), or unsaturated fat (UNSAT): the OmniHeart study. Participants were given each diet for 6 weeks in a crossover design. Body weight was kept constant. Total group = 160 participants, 32 with stage 1 hypertension (140–159/90–99 mm Hg), 75 with low-density lipoprotein cholesterol (LDL-C) ≥130 mg per dL. HDL-C, high-density lipoprotein cholesterol.

patients. Smaller doses (e.g., six capsules daily) did not lower BP in either hypertensive or normotensive persons. The unpleasant taste of the fish oil and belching interfere with compliance, and fish oil is not considered a practical therapy for hypertension.

Public health and clinical implications

If the entire population shifted to a DASH or low-sodium type of diet, the BP distribution would shift to lower levels, thereby reducing the incidence of cardiovascular disease. For clinicians, the Joint National Committee on the Prevention, Detection, Evaluation, and Treatment of Hypertension (JNC 7) has endorsed the results of DASH and recommended the DASH diet with low sodium for the population and clinical practice. The higher protein and unsaturated fat versions of the DASH diet not only increase the reduction in BP but also offer attractive and healthy dietary alternatives to a low-fat diet.

Suggested Readings

Appel LJ, Moore TJ, Obarzanek E, et al. A clinical trial of the effects of dietary patterns on BP: DASH Collaborative Research Group. *N Engl J Med* 1997;336:1117–1124.

Appel LJ, Sacks FM, Carey VJ, et al. Effects of protein, monounsaturated fat, and carbohydrate intake on BP and serum lipids: results of the omniheart randomized trial. *JAMA* 2005;24:2455–2464.

Ascherio A, Hennekens CH, Willett WC, et al. Prospective study of nutritional factors, BP, and hypertension among US women. *Hypertension* 1996;27:1065–1072.

Bazzano KA, He J, Ogden LG, et al. Fruit and vegetable intake and risk of cardiovascular disease in US adults: the First National Health and Nutrition Examination Survey epidemiologic follow-up study. *Am J Clin Nutr* 2002;76:93–99.

Bray GA, Vollmer WM, Sacks FM, et al. A further subgroup analysis of the effects of the DASH diet and three dietary sodium levels on BP. *Am J Cardiol* 2004;94:222–227.

Morris MC, Sacks FM, Rosner B. Does fish oil lower BP: a meta-analysis of controlled trials. *Circulation* 1993;88:523–533.

Sacks FM, Kass EH. Low BP in vegetarians: effects of specific foods and nutrients. *Am J Clin Nutr* 1988;48:795–800.

Sacks FM, Svetkey LP, Vollmer WM, et al. Effects on BP of reduced dietary sodium and the Dietary Approaches to Stop Hypertension (DASH) diet. *N Engl J Med* 2001;344:3–10.

Stamler J, Caggiula A, Grandits GA, et al. The MRFIT Research Group. Relationship to BP of combinations of dietary macronutrients: findings of the Multiple Risk Factor Intervention Trial (MRFIT). *Circulation* 1996;94:2417–2423.

CHAPTER B93 ■ SALT AND BLOOD PRESSURE

MYRON H. WEINBERGER, MD, FAHA

KEY POINTS

- A direct relationship between dietary sodium intake and blood pressure (BP) has been demonstrated in basic science studies, epidemiologic observations, and interventional trials.
- Meta-analyses of interventional trials of sodium intake in humans have demonstrated statistically significant but small effects between salt intake and BP; effects have been inconsistent and dependent on the choice of study, magnitude and duration of change in sodium intake, susceptibility of the study population, and other confounding factors.
- Given the large excess of usual sodium intake above physiologic needs among individuals living in industrialized societies, a population-wide reduction in intake could be predicted to produce a significant decrease in population-wide BP and BP-related outcomes (stroke, myocardial infarction, heart failure, and renal failure).
- Benefits of sodium restriction would be expected to accrue to salt-sensitive individuals to a greater extent than those who are not salt sensitive.
- Education efforts must include the population and manufacturers of high salt-processed foods to achieve and maintain such a reduction.

See also Chapters **A49**, **B92**, and **C120**

A relationship between sodium intake and the cardiovascular system in humans has been documented since antiquity. In the last century, systematic studies have defined this interaction in greater detail. Basic studies in a variety of animal species have shown a relationship between dietary salt intake and blood pressure (BP), and in some species, there is heterogeneity in susceptibility.

Epidemiology

Early observations. Human population studies suggested that the prevalence of hypertension and its cardiovascular consequences are linearly related to the level of salt intake but early epidemiologic studies were often faulted on the basis of relatively imprecise measurements of BP and the use of crude techniques for the estimation of sodium intake in comparison to methods used currently. Additionally, population-based studies have suggested that the age-related increase in BP, previously thought to be a normal physiologic occurrence, is generally only observed among societies in which average sodium intake is >100 mmol per day and not among those groups with lower sodium intake. Criticism of these observations included the genetic homogeneity and cultural isolation, lifestyle differences, levels of physical activity and fitness, and increased potassium intake of the societies in which lower levels of BP were found to be associated with lower sodium intake.

International Study of Salt and Blood Pressure. The International Study of Salt and Blood Pressure (INTERSALT) was conducted among approximately 32 countries including more than 10,000 participants in 52 population samples. This study utilized more precise measures than earlier studies and demonstrated a highly significant relationship between sodium intake and BP as well as with the increase in BP with age. Some groups within the sampled populations had usual sodium intake <10 mmol per day. Although the minimal physiologic requirement for sodium in humans is not known, there appears to be no adverse physical effects from a lifetime consumption of such low levels. In most "acculturated" societies average dietary sodium intake exceeds 150 to 175 mmol per day and in some groups, average intake >250 mmol per day or more is usual.

Regional studies. There are many observational studies within groups of similar ancestral derivation (e.g., northern and southern Chinese; northern and southern Japanese) demonstrating a twofold or greater difference in average intake of sodium as well as a comparable difference in hypertension prevalence and, in some studies, stroke incidence. However, there are also similar differences in potassium intake, which may confound the sodium–BP relationship.

Meta-analyses. Several meta-analyses of interventional studies have been conducted purporting to show significant decreases in BP with dietary sodium reduction. The magnitude of these changes has been variable, presumably owing to the fact that the studies used differing levels of sodium intake, differing periods of time on the different diets, differing criteria for the assessment of dietary adherence, differing sample sizes and differing populations, particularly with respect to basal BP, age, and ancestry. Despite variable study designs and differences in the magnitude of changes in BP observed, the qualitative and directional nature of the change in BP with a change in sodium intake has been very consistent.

Metabolic balance studies

In the early 1970s, a series of studies was initiated to learn more about the effects of sodium on BP in humans. A group of healthy, normotensive young men participated in a metabolic ward study where dietary intake of sodium, potassium, calcium, and other components was controlled. After achieving balance following 7 days of a low (10 mmol per day) sodium intake, measurements of 24-hour urinary electrolytes and BP, as well as a variety of other factors were made. This was followed by 3 days of 300 mmol per day sodium intake, 3 days of 600 to 800 mmol per day, and 3 days of 1,200 to 1,500 mmol per day (with the other dietary components remaining the same).

Blood pressure effects. A progressive and significant rise in BP was observed comparing the observations at the end of the study to that at the end of the initial period of low sodium intake. In some individuals the increase was as little as 5 mm Hg mean arterial pressure (MAP), whereas in others it increased 35 mm Hg; the rise was statistically significant in all subjects. Half of the studied subjects were of declared African-American ancestry and the rest were whites. The threshold for a significant rise in MAP in the former group was lower (at the end of 600–800 mmol/day level) than for the latter who only demonstrated a significant rise in BP at the highest level of sodium intake. These observations suggested a difference in susceptibility to the BP-raising effect of salt on the basis of ancestry.

Potassium effects. Another observation made during these studies was that net potassium loss occurred at levels of sodium intake >300 mmol per day, where the daily urinary excretion of potassium was seen to exceed intake. To examine the relationship of potassium loss to the pressor effects of high salt intake, studies were repeated in the same subjects after potassium repletion was given daily to prevent potassium loss. In the subsequent study, the BP rise with sodium was blunted as compared to the initial study in which potassium loss occurred with salt loading. Other investigators have now confirmed that salt-sensitivity of BP among hypertensive men can be prevented with potassium supplementation.

Salt-sensitivity

Utilizing a protocol initially designed for the assessment of renin and aldosterone, responses to (i) intravenous administration of 2 L normal saline, (ii) sodium and volume depletion by a low-salt diet, and (iii) oral doses of furosemide (40 mg) in a large number of normal and hypertensive humans permitted the definition of salt-sensitivity and resistance of BP.

Blood pressure and salt. Hypertensive subjects were found to be significantly more salt sensitive than normotensive subjects.

Nonetheless, 25% of the normotensive subjects were defined as salt sensitive. Moreover, those salt-sensitive subjects who were normotensive when initially studied had a risk of death in a 25-year follow-up period that was indistinguishable from that of hypertensive subjects. In another smaller study, salt-sensitivity was found to be associated with a significantly greater rate of BP increase during follow-up than was seen in salt-resistant individuals, supporting the role of salt in the age-related increase in BP.

Ancestry and age. Hypertensive individuals of African-American ancestry were more often salt sensitive (75%) compared to only 52% of whites, yet the frequencies of salt sensitivity among normotensive individuals of both groups was the same (25%). The magnitude of salt sensitivity of BP with this protocol was shown to increase progressively with decades of age, from <20 to >60 years among hypertensive individuals, but was only observed in normotensive individuals older than 59 years.

Renin and aldosterone. Failure of renin to respond vigorously to sodium or volume depletion enhances salt sensitivity, that is, the magnitude of the fall in BP during a low-sodium diet or volume depletion. It is notable that most studies of salt sensitivity define this change in response to low sodium intake rather than by an increase in BP with sodium loading or a high-salt diet, presumably because individuals who are salt-sensitive already manifest the rise in BP on their ambient, already-elevated, sodium intake.

Intervention trials

Meta-analyses of intervention trials in humans have consistently shown decreases in BP with reduction of dietary sodium intake of variable magnitude depending on the level of baseline sodium intake and the amount of reduction, the length of the study and the degree of adherence, the basal BP and the characteristics of the subjects studied. Two recent trials [Dietary Approaches to Stop Hypertension (DASH) and DASH-Sodium] have provided additional information regarding the benefit of a complex dietary alteration involving sodium and other nutrients in a population enriched in susceptibility.

Dietary Approaches to Stop Hypertension study. These studies first compared a reduced sodium, increased fresh fruit, vegetable, legume, and low-fat dairy product diet to a control diet in prehypertensive and Stage I hypertensive subjects, including many who were older than 50 years and of African-American ancestry. This basic DASH diet demonstrated a reduction in BP in subjects taking it in comparison to those ingesting the control diet.

Dietary Approaches to Stop Hypertension–sodium study. In an attempt to identify the role of sodium reduction specifically in this response, the DASH-sodium study recruited a similar population to test the basic DASH diet modified at three levels of sodium intake: normal, modestly reduced, and low. There was a linear relationship between the magnitude of BP reduction and that of the reduction of sodium intake in this population enriched with salt-sensitive subjects. It was not possible to identify the specific components (decreased sodium, increased potassium, increased calcium, or other factors) in the diet or the interactions responsible for the BP responses in the DASH studies. Moreover, because the subjects received all of their food free of cost in the several months of the study, the ability to replicate these findings in free-living individuals responsible for purchasing and preparing their own food remains to be demonstrated.

Salt intake and cardiovascular disease risk reduction

It is generally conceded that BP reduction, when sustained, results in a decreased risk for cardiovascular and renal events in a population in whom such events are likely and that even a small reduction in BP on a population-wide basis can be expected to have dramatic benefit in reducing such events, if sustained. The intervention trials cited have demonstrated a significant reduction in BP with lowering of dietary sodium intake but have not yet provided convincing evidence of decreasing cardiovascular and renal events.

Observational studies. There are small studies, such as one from Finland, in which a direct association between urinary sodium excretion (a surrogate for intake) and subsequent heart disease was demonstrated. On the other hand, reports from a worksite hypertension program suggested that men with reduced urinary sodium excretion in a single-urine specimen, after being asked to decrease their salt intake modestly for estimation of plasma-renin activity, had a greater incidence of myocardial infarction during a subsequent, several-year follow-up period. However, it is curious that women participating in the same study had exactly opposite results. It is unlikely that cardiovascular outcome studies of dietary salt reduction will be feasible given the long-term period required for such demonstration and the likelihood that the greatest benefit can be anticipated among those in whom prevention of hypertension might occur, raising the potential harm of a nonintervention study arm.

Environmental influences. Attention has been called to the low-sodium, high-potassium diet of our hunter-gatherer ancestors, but these people had a very short life-span limited to their early reproductive years and therefore we know virtually nothing about their susceptibility to chronic and systemic diseases. The best evidence currently stems from the observations made in small populations in whom typical salt intake is low, including many living in tropical environments, among whom cardiovascular disease appears to be rare. For the average, healthy individual living in acculturated societies, there appears to be no apparent adverse effects from a habitual diet of moderately low

(<100 mmol/day) sodium intake and increased (100 mmol/day) potassium intake.

Population strategies

Achieving and maintaining a prudent diet poses many challenges now. Learning to purchase and prepare foods of low sodium and high potassium content requires both individual education and commercial cooperation. The use of sodium to enhance the taste of foods can be obviated by using other flavorings and condiments. However the use of sodium in the preservation of foods is a major factor because it extends the shelf life and storage of many items. Labeling of foods with respect to sodium and potassium content has provided an opportunity for the informed shopper to modify their diet. However, the selection of foods in restaurants still poses a major obstacle because the content of such foods is rarely provided.

Suggested Readings

Institute of Medicine. *Dietary reference intakes: the essential guide to nutrient requirements (sodium and potassium)*. Washington, DC: National Academies Press, 2006: 370–379, 386–396.

Luft FC, Rankin LI, Bloch R, et al. Cardiovascular and humoral responses to extremes of sodium intake in normal white and black men. *Circulation* 1979;60:697–703.

Sacks FM, Svetkey LP, Vollmer WM, et al. for The DASH-Sodium Collaborative Research Group. Effects on BP of reduced dietary sodium and the Dietary Approaches to Stop Hypertension (DASH) diet. *N Engl J Med* 2001;344:3–10.

Stamler J. The INTERSALT Study: background, methods, findings and implications. *Am J Clin Nutr* 1997;65:626s–642s.

Tuomilehto J, Joushilahti P, Rastenyte D, et al. Urinary sodium excretion and cardiovascular mortality in Finland: a prospective study. *Lancet* 2001;357:848–851.

Weinberger MH. Salt-sensitivity of BP in humans. *Hypertension* 1996;27:II481–II490.

Weinberger MH, Fineberg NS. Sodium and volume sensitivity of BP: age and BP change over time. *Hypertension* 1991;18:67–71.

Weinberger MH, Fineberg NS, Fineberg SE, et al. Salt-sensitivity, pulse pressure and death in normal and hypertensive humans. *Hypertension* 2001;37(Pt 2): 429–432.

Weinberger MH, Miller JZ, Luft FC, et al. Definitions and characteristics of sodium sensitivity and BP resistance. *Hypertension* 1986;8:II127–II134.

CHAPTER B94 ■ POTASSIUM AND BLOOD PRESSURE

PAUL K. WHELTON, MD, MS

KEY POINTS

- Many studies suggest that potassium intake is inversely related to systolic and diastolic blood pressure (BP); potassium deficiency may play a special role in the high incidence and prevalence of hypertension in blacks.
- Increased potassium intake reduces systolic and diastolic BP; this effect is more pronounced in hypertensive persons compared to normotensive persons, in blacks compared to whites, and in those consuming a high intake of sodium.
- Increased potassium intake in combination with weight loss, sodium restriction, moderation in alcohol consumption, and increased physical activity may provide the optimal means for prevention and treatment of hypertension.
- Increased potassium intake may reduce the risk of stroke independent of its effects on BP.

See also Chapters **B92** and **B97**

Evidence from a variety of sources, including interpopulation and migrant studies, suggests that diet and physical inactivity play an important role in the genesis of age-related increases in blood pressure (BP) and in the occurrence of hypertension. Weight gain, alcohol consumption, excessive intake of sodium, and insufficient dietary potassium are leading possibilities as dietary causes of hypertension. Interest in the potassium–BP relationship dates back to the early part of the twentieth century, when increased potassium intake was advocated as a treatment for hypertension. Numerous cross-sectional studies in economically developed and developing countries and meta-analyses of clinical trial results have rekindled interest in the role of increasing potassium intake as a means to prevent and treat hypertension.

Epidemiology

Cross-sectional studies conducted in the United States, Japan, England, Scotland, Sweden, Belgium, St. Lucia, Kenya, Zaire, and China have identified an inverse relationship between BP and various measures of serum, urine, total body, and dietary potassium.

International study of salt and blood pressure. The most precise estimates come from the International Study of Salt and BP (INTERSALT), a cross-sectional investigation conducted in 10,079 men and women aged 20 to 59 years from 52 populations around the world. In this study, a 50 mmol per day higher level of urinary potassium excretion was associated with a 3.4 [95% confidence interval (CI), 1.5–5.2] mm Hg lower level of systolic and 1.9 (95% CI, 0.7–3) mm Hg lower level of diastolic BP after

adjustment for the potentially confounding influences of age, sex, body mass index, alcohol consumption, and urinary sodium excretion and correction for regression dilution bias.

Race and culture. Epidemiologic studies are also consistent with the suggestion that potassium deficiency may play a special role in the strikingly high incidence and prevalence of hypertension in blacks and the elderly.

Isolated populations with a low prevalence of hypertension and a blunted age-related increase in BP almost uniformly consume a diet that is relatively high in potassium and low in sodium content (Table B94.1). Potassium intake is often lower in economically developed countries than in isolated rural societies because commercially prepared foods are an important part of the diet, and potassium is frequently removed during the manufacturing process.

Migration studies have identified a relationship between progressive diminution in potassium intake and increasing levels of BP and hypertension. Typically, these changes have been noted in a setting in which there is a concurrent increase in sodium, calorie, and alcohol consumption and a decrease in physical activity. It has been hard to separate the independent contribution of each of these changes to the concurrent change in BP. It is conceivable that they all play a role in the age-related increase in BP that is so common in the United States and most other societies.

Clinical trials

A critically important question is whether the inverse association between potassium intake and BP is causal or merely reflects

TABLE B94.1

URINARY EXCRETION OF POTASSIUM SODIUM/POTASSIUM RATIO IN FOUR LOW BLOOD PRESSURE POPULATIONS

Population	Urinary potassium, mmol/24 hr	Urinary sodium/ potassium ratio
Yanomamo Indians, Brazil	152	0.01
Kung bushmen, Botswana	70–103	0.28–0.44
Xingu Indians, Brazil	78–96	0.19–0.20
Asaro Valley, Papua New Guinea	62–79	0.53–0.70

(Data from He J, Whelton PK. Potassium, BP, and cardiovascular disease: an epidemiologic perspective. *Cardiol Rev* 1997;5:255–260.)

the presence of a confounding relationship between potassium and another variable. Clinical trials provide the most satisfactory study design for resolution of this question.

Early studies. Potassium was widely advocated as a means to lower BP during the 1920s and 1930s. The rice/fruit diet of Kempner, which received considerable attention during the 1950s, was characterized by a relatively high content of potassium and a low sodium to potassium ratio. Kempner's diet, however, also resulted in weight loss and a variety of metabolic changes. During the 1960s and 1970s, a series of animal experiments were conducted that suggested potassium administration could blunt the rise in BP after sodium loading in a variety of salt-sensitive rat models. Similar findings have been reported in humans who were exposed to extremely high and extremely low intakes of dietary sodium.

Meta-analyses. The first controlled trial of the efficacy of increased potassium intake in essential hypertension, however, was not reported until 1981. Since that time, a large number of randomized, controlled trials as well as many uncontrolled experimental studies have reported on the effect of increased and decreased potassium intake on BP in hypertensive and normotensive persons.

Whelton et al. identified 33 randomized, controlled trials (2,565 participants) in which the effects of an increased intake of potassium on BP were evaluated. Of these, 21 trials (2,565 participants) were conducted in hypertensive and 12 in normotensive (1,005 participants) persons. In all but two trials, the dose of potassium prescribed in the active intervention arm was >60 mmol per day. The weighted mean net change in urinary potassium excretion for the intervention versus control group was 53 mmol per 24 hours in the 31 trials in which such information was available. Overall, increased potassium intake was associated with a significant reduction in mean (95% CI) systolic and diastolic BP of 4.4 (2.5–6.4) and 2.5 (0.7–4.2) mm Hg, respectively (**Table B94.2**). After exclusion of one trial in which there was an extreme effect on systolic (−41 mm Hg) and diastolic (−17 mm Hg) BP, the overall mean (95% CI) reduction was 3.1 mm Hg (1.9–4.3) for systolic and 2 mm Hg (0.5–3.4) for diastolic BP. Subgroup analysis suggested that the treatment effect was enhanced in hypertensive individuals, blacks, and those consuming a high intake of sodium. In trials in which the participants were consuming a diet high in sodium content, there was a significant ($p < .001$) dose–response relationship between 24-hour urinary potassium excretion and treatment effect size.

In two subsequent trials, conducted in Japan and China, potassium supplementation resulted in a significant reduction in BP. In the Chinese trial, potassium supplementation resulted in a 5 mm Hg (95% CI, 2.1–7.9 mm Hg) reduction in systolic BP. Using randomized, cross-over design trials, Krishna, et al. have demonstrated that short-term potassium depletion produces an increase in BP in hypertensive and normotensive persons.

TABLE B94.2

POOLED ESTIMATES OF CHANGE IN BLOOD PRESSURE (BP) AFTER POTASSIUM SUPPLEMENTATION IN 33 RANDOMIZED CONTROLLED CLINICAL TRIALS

Trials in analysis	Systolic BP		Diastolic BP	
	Mean change	95% Confidence interval	Mean change	95% Confidence interval
All trials (N = 33)	−4.4	−2.53, −6.36	−2.5	−0.74, −4.16
Obel trial excluded (N = 32)	−3.1	−1.91, −4.31	−2.0	−0.52, −3.42
Hypertensive trials[a] (N = 20)	−4.4	−2.2, −6.6	−2.5	−0.1, −4.9
Normotensive trials (N = 12)	−1.8	−0.6, −2.9	−1.0	0.0, −2.1
Trials in blacks[b] (N = 6)	−5.6	−2.4, −8.7	−3.0	−0.7, −5.3
Trials in whites (N = 25)	−2.0	−0.9, −3.0	−1.1	−0.1, −2.1
Urinary Na, mmol/d[b]				
<140 (N = 10)	−1.2	0.0, −2.4	0.1	1.1, −1.0
140–164 (N = 10)	−2.1	−0.3, −4.0	−1.4	0.0, −2.8
≥165 (N = 10)	−7.3	−4.6, −10.1	−4.7	−1.1, −8.3

[a]Excludes outlier trial by Obel AO.
[b]Urinary sodium excretion during follow-up.
(Adapted from Whelton PK, He J, Cutler JA, et al. Effects of oral potassium on BP: meta-analysis of randomized controlled clinical trials. *JAMA* 1997;277:1624–1632.)

TABLE B94.3

REDUCTION OF BLOOD PRESSURE FROM POTASSIUM

Mechanism of action

  Direct natriuretic effect
    Suppression of the renin-angiotensin and sympathetic
      nervous systems
    Effect on kallikreins and eicosanoids
    Improvement of baroreceptor function
    Antagonism of the effects of natriuretic hormone
    Direct arterial vasodilatation

Antihypertensive drug effectiveness. Two randomized controlled trials have explored the efficacy of increased potassium intake in reducing the need for antihypertensive drug therapy in patients with well-controlled hypertension. In a dietary modification trial, an increased intake of potassium significantly reduced the need for antihypertensive drug therapy. In contrast, in a large and rigorously controlled trial of potassium chloride pill supplementation, Grimm et al. were unable to identify any apparent effect of potassium supplementation on BP. That the participants in this study were concurrently counseled to reduce salt intake may have blunted the effect of the potassium supplements.

Dietary Approaches to Stop Hypertension studies. Clinical trials have shown that consumption of a diet that is rich in fruits, vegetables, and low-fat dairy foods and with a reduced saturated and total fat content [Dietary Approaches to Stop Hypertension (DASH) diet] results in a substantial lowering of BP in hypertensive and normotensive persons. The high intake of dietary potassium in the DASH diet may contribute to its efficacy in lowering BP.

Pathophysiology

Various mechanisms have been proposed to explain the purported influence of potassium on BP (**Table B94.3**). Many studies have demonstrated short-term changes in sodium excretion, but it remains unclear whether any long-term effects on BP can be ascribed to a decrease in intravascular volume resulting from this initial and transient natriuresis.

Cardiovascular benefits

In addition to its BP-lowering effects, increased potassium intake may have independent vasculoprotective properties.

Animal models. In a series of animal models, including spontaneously hypertensive stroke-prone and Dahl salt-sensitive rats, Tobian reported that the addition of potassium chloride or potassium citrate markedly reduced stroke mortality despite a minimal effect on BP.

Cohort studies. An inverse relationship between 24-hour dietary potassium intake at baseline and subsequent stroke-associated morbidity and mortality has been noted in several population-based cohort studies. In the most generalizable and statistically powerful investigation, Bazzano et al. studied 9,805 U.S. men and women participants in the first National Health and Nutrition Examination Survey (NHANES I) who were followed for more than an average of 19 years, yielding 927 stroke and 1,847 coronary heart disease events (**Table B94.4**). After adjustment for a broad array of potential cardiovascular disease risk factors, those who had consumed a low potassium diet

TABLE B94.4

HAZARD RATIO AND CORRESPONDING 95% CONFIDENCE INTERVAL OF STROKE ASSOCIATED WITH A LOW DIETARY INTAKE OF POTASSIUM DURING 19 YEARS OF FOLLOW-UP OF 9,805 MALE AND FEMALE PARTICIPANTS IN THE NATIONAL HEALTH AND EXAMINATION SURVEY I EPIDEMIOLOGIC FOLLOW-UP STUDY

Adjustment model	Hazard ratio (95% confidence interval)	p value
Age-, energy-adjusted	1.37 (1.20–1.54)	<.0001
Age-, race-, sex-, energy- adjusted	1.26 (1.11–1.45)	.0007
Multivariate[a]	1.28 (1.11–1.47)	.0001

[a]Additionally adjusted for systolic blood pressure (BP), serum cholesterol, body mass index, history of diabetes, physical activity, education level, regular alcohol consumption, current cigarette smoking, vitamin supplement use, saturated fat intake, cholesterol intake, sodium intake, calcium intake, dietary fiber, vitamin C intake, and vitamin A intake (N = 9,244).
(Adapted from Bazzano LA, He J, Ogden LG, et al. Dietary potassium intake and risk of stroke in U.S. men and women. National Health and Nutrition Examination Survey I Epidemiologic Follow-Up Study. *Stroke* 2001;32:1473–1480.)

at baseline (first quartile, <34.6 mmol/day) experienced a 28% higher (95% CI, 11%–47%) risk of stroke compared to the remainder of the cohort.

Recognizing the limitations of observational studies in answering therapeutic questions, the accumulated experience from prospective analyses suggests that a high potassium diet reduces the risk of stroke. Evidence from a number of epidemiologic studies suggests that stroke mortality is inversely related to intake of vegetables and fruits. Although this evidence is indirect, these reports are consistent with a vasculoprotective effect from increased potassium intake.

Suggested Readings

Appel LA, Moore TJ, Obarzanek E, et al. DASH Collaborative Research Group. A clinical trial of the effects of dietary patterns on BP. *N Engl J Med* 1997;336:1117–1124.

Bazzano LA, He J, Ogden LG, et al. Dietary potassium intake and risk of stroke in US men and women. National Health and Nutrition Examination Survey I Epidemiologic Follow-up Study. *Stroke* 2001;32:1473–1480.

Gu D, He J, Wu X, et al. Effect of potassium supplementation on BP in Chinese: a randomized, placebo-controlled trial. *J Hypertens* 2001;19:1325–1331.

Institute of Medicine (U.S.). *Panel on dietary reference intakes for electrolytes and water. Dietary reference intakes for water, potassium, sodium, chloride, and sulfate. Chapter 5; Potassium.* Washington, DC: The National Academies Press, 2004:186–268.

INTERSALT Cooperative Research Group. INTERSALT: an international study of electrolyte excretion and BP: results for 24-hour urinary sodium and potassium excretion. *BMJ* 1988;297:319–328.

Joshipura KJ, Ascherio A, Manson MJ, et al. Fruit and vegetable intake in relation to risk of ischemic stroke. *JAMA* 1999;282:1233–1239.

Kawano Y, Minami J, Takishita S, et al. Effects of potassium supplementation on office, home and 24-h BP in patients with essential hypertension. *Am J Hypertens* 1998;11:1141–1146.

Klag MJ, He J, Coresh J, et al. The contribution of urinary cations to the BP differences associated with migration. *Am J Epidemiol* 1995;142:295–303.

Whelton PK, He J, Appel LJ, et al. The National High BP Education Program Coordinating Committee. Primary prevention of hypertension: clinical and public health advisory from the National High BP Education Program. *JAMA* 2002;288:1882–1888.

Whelton PK, He J, Cutler JA, et al. Effects of oral potassium on BP: meta-analysis of randomized controlled clinical trials. *JAMA* 1997;277:1624–1632.

CHAPTER B95 ■ BLOOD PRESSURE EFFECTS OF DIETARY CALCIUM, MAGNESIUM INTAKE, AND HEAVY METAL EXPOSURE

LAWRENCE J. APPEL, MD, MPH AND ANA NAVAS-ACIEN, MD, PhD

KEY POINTS

- In observational studies, an increased intake of calcium and magnesium is often associated with lower blood pressure (BP).
- In clinical trials, the BP effects of calcium and magnesium supplements are small and inconsistent; overall, available data do not support use of these minerals as pill supplements to lower BP.
- Environmental lead exposure increases BP; despite the modest association, there are implications for hypertension prevention.
- The relationship between mercury exposure and BP is uncertain.

See also Chapters B92 and C120

Reduced salt intake, increased potassium intake, weight loss, moderation of alcohol consumption among those who drink, and consumption of nutrients based on the "Dietary Approaches to Stop Hypertension (DASH) diet" are effective strategies to lower blood pressure (BP). An increased intake of calcium and magnesium and avoidance of heavy metal exposure have also been proposed as a means to lower BP.

CALCIUM

Basic physiology and nutrition

The adult body contains approximately 1,200 g of calcium, of which 99% is present in the skeleton. The remaining 1% is found in the intracellular space, cell membranes, and extracellular fluids, affecting numerous body functions, including nerve conduction, muscle contraction, blood clotting, and membrane permeability. Blood levels are tightly regulated within narrow limits through the effects of several hormones (vitamin D, parathyroid hormone, calcitonin, estrogen, testosterone, and perhaps others). These hormones control calcium absorption and excretion as well as bone metabolism.

Absorption and metabolism. Calcium absorption occurs through active transport and passive diffusion across the intestinal mucosa. Active transport, which accounts for the absorption of calcium at low to moderate levels, is dependent on vitamin D. Passive diffusion becomes more important at higher levels of calcium intake. Fractional absorption depends on several factors including age (greater in infants and during puberty), pregnancy

status (greater during the last two trimesters), and race (greater in blacks).

Calcium is lost through the body in feces, urine, and sweat. Urinary calcium excretion is typically 100 to 250 mg per day and varies as a function of the filtered load and the efficiency of reabsorption, which is regulated principally by parathyroid hormone. Increased intake of sodium, protein, and caffeine may increase calcium excretion. Other than a direct association between sodium intake and nephrolithiasis, the clinical relevance of these effects is unclear.

United States intake levels. According to the U.S. Department of Agriculture 1994 Continuing Survey of Food Intakes, the median dietary intake of calcium is less in women than in men and tends to decrease throughout adult ages (857 mg/day in men 31–50 years old and 708 mg/day in men older than 70 years, 606 and 571 mg/day in women at corresponding ages). Also, in both sexes and across all age-groups, blacks consume less calcium than whites. In terms of food sources, 73% of calcium in the food supply is from milk, 9% from fruits and vegetables, 5% from grain products, and the remaining 12% from all other sources. Milk products contain <300 mg of calcium per serving (e.g., 8 oz of milk, 1.5 oz of cheddar cheese). Other calcium-rich foods include kale, calcium-fortified orange juice, and broccoli. Use of calcium supplements is high among adult women (25% in 1986) and is probably rising as a result of efforts to prevent osteoporosis through increased calcium intake. In nutrition guidelines issued by the Institute of Medicine (IOM), an adequate intake of calcium for adults (men and women) is deemed to be 1 g per day at 19–50 years of age and 1.2 g per day at older ages; few people meet this guideline (e.g., among persons 70 years or older, <1% of women and <5% of men).

Clinical studies of calcium and blood pressure

Epidemiology. Ecologic studies suggesting an inverse association between drinking water hardness and mortality from atherosclerotic diseases have stimulated interest in the roles of calcium and magnesium intake on BP. Evidence of an effect of calcium intake on BP comes from a variety of sources including animal studies, observational studies, clinical trials, and meta-analyses of observational studies and controlled trials. In a meta-analysis of 23 observational studies, Cappuccio et al. documented an inverse association between BP and dietary calcium intake (as measured by 24-hour dietary recalls or food frequency questionnaires) but the size of the effect was relatively small and there was evidence of publication bias and heterogeneity across studies.

Clinical trials. Three meta-analyses of randomized trials have documented that calcium supplementation significantly reduces systolic BP (1.9 mm Hg in the most recent meta-analysis) but effects on diastolic BP have been inconsistent at doses of approximately 1 g per day. The unimpressive results of pill supplementation trials and the corresponding inverse relationships in observational studies have several possible explanations. First, calcium may have an effect but only in combination with a high intake of other nutrients. Yet a trial of combinations of cation supplements (calcium, magnesium, and potassium) in hypertensive patients found that none of the combinations reduced BP. Alternatively, some nutrients closely associated with calcium (e.g., protein, phosphorus, vitamin D, or an unknown nutrient) may be responsible for the BP-lowering effect attributed to calcium. One small trial demonstrated that increased milk consumption in the context of a low-calcium diet reduced systolic BP. Diets based on the DASH lower BP; these diets are rich in fruits, vegetables, and dairy products and are high in calcium.

Population response heterogeneity. One issue still unanswered is whether certain subgroups of the population are particularly sensitive to the effects of calcium. Such groups may include pregnant women at risk for preeclampsia and persons with a low dietary intake of calcium or sodium. In the meta-analysis by van Mierlo, there was a slight tendency toward greater BP reduction in persons with a relatively low calcium intake (**Figure B95.1**). In contrast, in a well-done trial in 300 female nurses with low dietary intakes of calcium, magnesium, and potassium, calcium supplementation did not lower BP. Likewise, in a trial of 4,589 pregnant women, calcium supplements had no effect on BP or the incidence of hypertension or preeclampsia. Surprisingly, the effects of calcium supplementation on BP in blacks have not been well studied, although they consume much less calcium than their white counterparts.

Although the effects of calcium supplementation on BP have been small and inconsistent, clinical trials have demonstrated that calcium supplementation in combination with vitamin D increases bone mineral density. Hence, pill supplements of calcium and vitamin D are commonly used as a means to prevent osteoporotic complications despite the fact that large-scale trials have not confirmed this potential benefit.

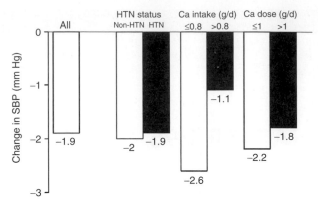

Figure B95.1 Mean systolic blood pressure (SBP) response to calcium supplementation, overall, and in subgroups. HTN, hypertension; Ca, calcium. (Adapted from the meta-analysis by van Mierlo LA, Arends LR, Streppel MT, et al. BP response to calcium supplementation: a meta-analysis of randomized controlled trials. *J Hum Hypertens* 2006;20:571–580.)

MAGNESIUM

Basic physiology and nutrition

The adult body contains <25 g of magnesium, of which 40% is in soft tissues, 60% in the skeleton, and only 1% in extracellular fluids. Magnesium is a cofactor in >300 enzyme systems and is required for aerobic and anaerobic energy production, glycolysis, membrane function, and DNA and RNA synthesis. It has been called *nature's physiologic calcium channel blocker* because it interferes with membrane calcium transport, particularly at L-type calcium channels. In magnesium depletion states, intracellular calcium rises and promotes contraction of smooth muscle and skeletal muscle along, with a rise in BP. Such findings raise the possibility that magnesium may be involved in BP homeostasis in healthy populations.

Absorption and metabolism. The mechanisms controlling blood levels and intestinal absorption of magnesium are poorly understood. The kidney has a predominant role in magnesium homeostasis, reabsorbing most filtered magnesium, particularly in magnesium deficiency states. As with calcium, fractional absorption is inversely proportional to the amount of magnesium ingested.

United States intake levels. According to data from the 1994 Continuing Survey of Food Intake, the median dietary intake of magnesium is approximately 330 mg per day in adult men and <230 mg per day in women. Magnesium intake decreases to a minor extent with age. Approximately 45% of dietary magnesium comes from fruits, vegetables, grains, and nuts and <30% from milk, meat, and eggs. According to recent IOM guidelines, the recommended dietary allowance of magnesium is 420 mg for adult men older than 30 years and 320 mg for adult women.

Clinical studies of magnesium and blood pressure

The body of evidence implicating magnesium as a major determinant of BP is inconsistent.

Epidemiologic studies. In observational studies, often cross-sectional in design, a common finding is an inverse association of dietary magnesium with BP. This relationship was seen in cross-sectional analyses of 15,248 participants in the Atherosclerosis Risk in Communities study, where hypertensive participants also had lower serum magnesium levels than did normotensive individuals. In a prospective observational study, dietary magnesium intake was inversely related to systolic and diastolic BP and change in BP; however, these relationships did not persist after adjustment for fiber intake.

Clinical trials. Evidence from clinical trials has been inconsistent. In phase 1 of the Trials of Hypertension Prevention, supplemental magnesium had no effect on BP in 461 persons with high normal BP. Magnesium in combination with either potassium or calcium had no effect on BP in a trial of 125 hypertensive patients. In a trial of 300 female nurses with low dietary intake of magnesium, potassium, and calcium, magnesium also had no effect on BP. In contrast, in a crossover, dose–response trial of only 17 hypertensive patients, oral magnesium resulted in a significant dose-dependent reduction in BP. In a meta-analysis of 20 clinical trials, there were nonsignificant reductions in systolic and diastolic BP of 0.6 and 0.8 mm Hg, respectively. A dose-dependent effect of magnesium was present for systolic but not diastolic BP. Overall, it appears that magnesium supplementation in nondeficient general populations has little impact on BP. However, as mentioned previously, the DASH diet and its variants, each rich in magnesium (>400 mg/day) and other nutrients, substantially lowered systolic and diastolic BP.

HEAVY METALS

Heavy metals such as lead, cadmium, and mercury may have direct and indirect effects on BP, the latter mediated through renal toxicity.

Lead

Exposure, absorption, and metabolism. Humans are exposed to lead from environmental sources, including air, food, and drinking water. With the elimination of leaded gasoline and soldered cans, lead exposure in the United States and in other countries has substantially decreased. Certain populations, however, continue to experience high lead exposure. In particular, inner city children and adults of low socioeconomic status remain disproportionately exposed to lead from paint, dust, and soils. Absorption through alveolar membranes is almost complete after lead inhalation. Gastrointestinal absorption ranges from 3% to 70%, depending on age, fasting, and nutritional calcium and iron status. In the human body, most lead (>95%) is stored in calcified tissues, predominantly bone. The half-life of lead in bone is in the range of years to decades depending on bone type, metabolic state, and subject age.

Epidemiologic studies of lead and blood pressure. Chronic lead poisoning can lead to cardiovascular-renal disease and hypertension. At environmental levels of exposure, the effect of lead exposure on BP levels has been controversial, partly because the observed association was modest. Meta-analyses combining data from >30 epidemiologic studies conducted in different settings, including prospective studies in approximately 60,000 participants overall have estimated increases in systolic BP ranging from 0.81 to 1.25 mm Hg for each two-fold increase in blood lead levels. Many studies adjusted for potential confounders, including alcohol intake, body mass index, and use of antihypertensive medication; several studies reported a dose–response relationship between blood lead levels and systolic BP levels or hypertension. A positive relation was also confirmed with bone lead levels as a marker of cumulative lead exposure.

Overall, although the strength of the association is modest, it may have been substantially underestimated by measurement error in lead and BP determinations.

Biologic plausibility and causal inference. Numerous experimental studies in animals have shown that chronic exposure to low lead levels results in arterial hypertension that persists after the cessation of lead exposure. Proposed mechanisms include enhanced oxidative stress, downregulation of nitric oxide and soluble guanylyl cyclase, stimulation of the renin-angiotensin system, stimulation of the sympathetic nervous system, activation of protein kinase C activity, and reduced renal function. Overall, the epidemiologic and experimental evidence support that lead exposure is causally related to increased BP levels and hypertension.

Cadmium

Exposure, absorption, and metabolism. Cadmium is a toxic and carcinogenic metal widely distributed in the environment. In the general population, the primary sources of cadmium exposure are cigarette smoke, food intake (shellfish, offal, certain vegetables), and ambient air particularly in urban areas and in the vicinity of industrial areas. After exposure, cadmium accumulates in target tissues, especially in the renal cortex that contain more than half of the body burden of cadmium. The biological half-life of cadmium is in the order of decades and consequently kidney cadmium concentrations increase with age.

Epidemiologic studies of cadmium and blood pressure. Cadmium is nephrotoxic, inducing tubular and glomerular dysfunction in occupationally and environmentally exposed populations. The relationship of cadmium exposure with hypertension, however, is unclear. Numerous epidemiologic studies have evaluated the association of cadmium exposure with BP levels. Their findings are inconsistent, but they are often limited by small sample sizes, lack of adjustment for potential confounders, lack of standardization of BP measurements, and other methodological limitations. No meta-analyses or systematic reviews have summarized the relationship of cadmium exposure with hypertension in epidemiologic studies.

Biologic plausibility and causal inference. Cadmium exposure has induced hypertension in animal models, although the mechanisms for cadmium-related hypertension remain unclear. Overall, the evidence is insufficient to evaluate the effect of cadmium on BP endpoints.

Mercury

Exposure, absorption, and metabolism. Humans are exposed to elemental mercury, inorganic mercury compounds, and organic mercury (primarily methylmercury). Exposure to elemental mercury may occur from mercury spillage from a thermometer or sphygmomanometer. At room temperature, elemental mercury vaporizes easily. The vapors can then be inhaled and subsequently absorbed through alveolar membranes. The major source of exposure to mercury in the population, however, occurs through consumption of fish and marine products that are contaminated with methylmercury.

Mercury and blood pressure. In children, toxic exposure to elemental mercury can simulate pheochromocytoma, with its markedly high BP and tachycardia. Occupational mercury exposure has been related to hypertension development. Chronic exposure to methylmercury and inorganic mercury increases BP levels in animal models. At environmental levels of exposure, the evidence is scarce. Overall, the evidence is insufficient to evaluate the relationship of chronic mercury exposure with BP levels and hypertension.

Suggested Readings

Appel LJ, Moore TJ, Obarzanek E, et al. DASH Collaborative Research Group. A clinical trial of the effects of dietary patterns on BP. *N Engl J Med* 1997;336:1117–1124.
Cappuccio FP, Elliott P, Allender PS, et al. Epidemiologic association between dietary calcium intake and BP: a meta-analysis of published data. *Am J Epidemiol* 1995;142:935–945.
Institute of Medicine. *Dietary reference intakes: calcium, phosphorus, magnesium, vitamin D, and fluoride.* Washington, DC: National Academy Press, 1997.

Jee SH, Guallar E, Singh VK, et al. The effect of magnesium supplementation on BP: a meta-analysis of randomized clinical trials. *Am J Hypertens* 2002;15:691–696.
Levine RJ, Hauth JC, Curet LB, et al. Trial of calcium to prevent preeclampsia. *N Engl J Med* 1997;337:69–76.
van Mierlo LA, Arends LR, Streppel MT, et al. BP response to calcium supplementation: a meta-analysis of randomized controlled trials. *J Hum Hypertens* 2006;20:571–580.
Navas-Acien A, Guallar E, Silbergeld EK, et al. Lead exposure and cardiovascular disease – a systematic review. *Environ Health Perspect* 2007;115:472–482.
Nawrot TS, Thijis L, Den Hond EM, et al. An epidemiological re-appraisal of the association between BP and blood lead: a meta-analysis. *J Hum Hypertens* 2002;16:123–131.
Sacks FM, Willett WC, Smith A, et al. Effect on BP of potassium, calcium, and magnesium in women with low habitual intake. *Hypertension* 1998;31:131–138.
Torres AD, Rai AN, Hardiek ML. Mercury intoxication and arterial hypertension: report of two patients and review of the literature. *Pediatrics* 2000;105:E34. Available at: http://www.pediatrics.org/cgi/content/full/105/3/e34. Accessed on October 28, 2002.

CHAPTER B96 ■ ALCOHOL USE AND BLOOD PRESSURE

WILLIAM C. CUSHMAN, MD

KEY POINTS

- Many epidemiologic studies have shown a direct relationship between alcohol intake and hypertension, especially above an average intake of two drinks (~28 g of ethanol) per day.
- Reduction in alcohol intake is associated with lowering of blood pressure (BP) in randomized controlled trials and meta-analysis: Each reduction by one drink per day lowers systolic and diastolic BP approximately 1 mm Hg.
- Although regular alcohol intake is associated with lower risk for atherothrombotic cardiovascular events, excessive intake increases the risk of many medical and psychosocial problems, including hypertension.
- For persons with hypertension or prehypertension who drink excessively, average maximum alcohol intakes of one drink per day in women and two drinks per day in men are reasonable goals if drinking is not otherwise contraindicated.

See also Chapter C120

Regular alcohol consumption can produce positive psychosocial effects and some beneficial effects on health, especially reduced atherothrombotic events and death. However, excessive alcohol intake causes many serious adverse psychosocial and health consequences, including increased mortality. One of the harmful effects of excess alcohol intake is its impact on blood pressure (BP); hemodynamic effects have been noted since the middle of the nineteenth century.

Epidemiology

The first population-based study of alcohol use and prevalence of hypertension was reported in 1915 by Lian, who found in French soldiers a linear relationship between the amount of wine regularly ingested and the prevalence of hypertension. Most studies on the relationship between alcohol intake and BP, however, have been reported in the last several decades.

Amount and type of alcohol. A standard drink in the United States is usually defined as 14 g of alcohol (ethanol). This amount of alcohol is in 12 oz of beer, 5 oz of table wine, or 1.5 oz of 80 proof (40% alcohol) distilled spirits. Some studies suggest that one type of alcoholic beverage, such as beer or liquor, is more strongly associated with high BP than other types of beverages, such as wine. However, when all studies are taken together, it appears that the relationship between alcohol and BP is primarily dependent on the amount of alcohol ingested, rather than the type of beverage. A recent crossover study in normotensive men showed similar elevations of awake ambulatory systolic BP and heart rate after 4 weeks of either beer or red wine (40 g ethanol equivalent per day) compared with a control abstinence period.

Epidemiologic associations. The relationship between the amount of alcohol consumed and BP is robust. Cross-sectional epidemiologic studies from many cultures have shown progressively higher BP levels or a higher prevalence of hypertension with increasing levels of alcohol intake. Alcohol intake also predicts future BP elevation and development of hypertension in prospective observational studies.

Above an average intake of two drinks per day, the higher the alcohol intake is, the higher the BP. This relationship is usually still present even when taking into account other factors, such as age, weight (or body mass index), sodium and potassium intake, cigarette smoking, and education. Alcohol has been found to increase BP in whites, blacks, and Asians (**Figure B96.1**). In the Atherosclerosis Risk in Communities (ARIC) study, it was estimated that in subjects drinking ≥30 g per day of alcohol, one in five cases of hypertension could be attributed to the consumption of alcohol.

Sometimes a J-shaped relationship is found, where the lowest BP levels are seen in those with low levels of alcohol intake (one to two drinks per day) compared with those who do not drink or those taking three or more drinks per day. Although low levels of alcohol intake are occasionally associated with higher BP levels than nondrinking, most often there is no meaningful BP difference between nondrinkers and those taking no more than two drinks per day.

Patterns of blood pressure elevation. Studies of the pattern of alcohol consumption and the temporal relationship of alcohol intake and BP suggest that acute BP elevations may be the result of the alcohol withdrawal syndrome, especially in episodic and predominantly weekend drinkers. In contrast, there is a sustained hypertensive effect of heavy daily drinking or alcoholism that is less reversible, even after subjects have become abstinent. There is some evidence that alcohol taken with a meal is less likely to elevate BP than that taken without a meal.

Drug resistance. Alcohol intake has also been associated with resistance to antihypertensive therapy but the mechanisms for this effect are not known. Some of the apparent resistance may be from poor medication adherence in heavy drinkers, but some resistance arises from true interference with the BP-lowering effects of medications.

Randomized controlled trials

Randomized controlled trials provide strong support of a direct causal link between chronic alcohol consumption and raised BP. They also provide a strong basis for public health and individual recommendations to reduce alcohol intake, if above two drinks per day, as part of a program to prevent or treat hypertension.

Reduction of alcohol intake. Most randomized controlled trials demonstrate a significant reduction in systolic BP, diastolic BP, or both; these were summarized in 2001 in a meta-analysis of 15 studies that included 2,234 participants (**Figure B96.2**). Alcohol reduction was associated with a significant reduction in systolic and diastolic BP means [95% confidence interval (CI)] of 3.3 (2.5–4.1) and 2 (1.5–2.6) mm Hg, respectively. A correlation was observed between percentage reduction in alcohol intake and mean BP reduction, suggesting a dose–effect relationship, and the effects of intervention were greater in those with higher baseline BP. Although most of these studies included relatively few subjects, were of short duration, and were not designed as effectiveness trials, overall results were consistent with the epidemiologic trends. The authors of this meta-analysis concluded that "alcohol reduction should be recommended as an important component of lifestyle modification for the prevention and treatment of hypertension among heavy drinkers."

Prevention and treatment of hypertension study. The largest and longest of the randomized controlled trials was the Prevention and Treatment of Hypertension Study (PATHS). The primary objectives of this National Institutes of Health-Veterans Affairs Cooperative Studies Program trial were to determine whether alcohol could be reduced for at least 6 months

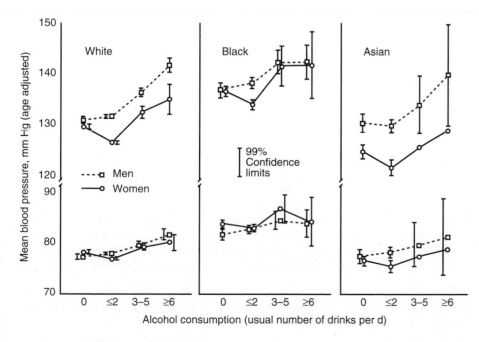

Figure B96.1 Mean systolic blood pressures (BPs) (*upper half*) and mean diastolic BPs (*lower half*) for white, black, and Asian men and women with known drinking habits. *Small circles* represent data based on fewer than 30 persons. (From Klatsky AL, Friedman GD, Siegelaub AB, et al. Alcohol consumption and BP. *N Engl J Med* 1977;296:1194–1200, with permission.)

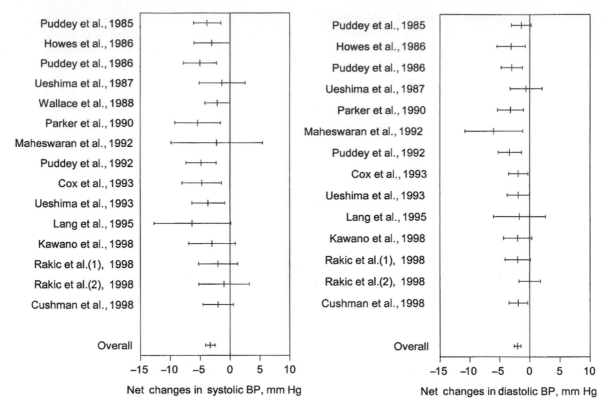

Figure B96.2 Average net change in systolic blood pressure (BP) (*left*) and diastolic BP (*right*) and corresponding 95% confidence intervals related to alcohol reduction intervention in 15 randomized controlled trials. (From Xin X, He J, Frontini MG, et al. Effects of alcohol reduction on BP: a meta-analysis of randomized controlled trial. *Hypertension* 2001;38:1112–1117, with permission.)

and whether BP was lowered by sustained reductions in alcohol intake in 641 moderate to heavy drinkers with diastolic BP 80 to 99 mm Hg. Anyone with evidence of alcoholism, complications of excess alcohol intake, or significant cardiovascular or psychiatric diseases was excluded. Differences in alcohol intake between randomized groups were highly significant over the 3 to 24 months of follow-up: 1.3 drinks per day. The study anticipated a difference of two drinks per day but the control group lowered its alcohol intake more than anticipated; BP differences were −0.9/−0.6 mm Hg. Although not statistically different, this BP difference is consistent with the approximately 1 mm Hg change in BP for each drink per day change in alcohol intake seen in controlled studies with larger alcohol intake differences. In most other controlled trials of alcohol reduction and BP, baseline levels of alcohol intake were higher and differences in alcohol intake larger than in PATHS.

Other trials. Short-term intervention trials have consistently demonstrated a decline in BP within 1 to 2 weeks of alcohol restriction, with further gradual declines in BP after 4 to 6 weeks. In an 18-week study in which alcohol restriction (by four to five standard drinks per day) was combined with caloric restriction (reducing weight by 7.5 kg), the two interventions had an additive effect and reduced BP by approximately 10 mm Hg. The studies from Perth, Australia, in normotensive and hypertensive participants are probably the best from which to estimate the expected change in BP with a change in alcohol intake. The investigators typically recruited middle-aged heavy-drinking men and randomized them to continue their usual beer or to low-alcohol beer, usually in a crossover design. Differences

in alcohol intake in the randomized groups averaged three to four drinks per day and 3.8–5.4/1.4–3.3 mm Hg decreases in BP, although most of the participants in these trials did not have hypertension or were normotensive on therapy. In the first two studies, a three-drink per day net reduction in alcohol intake produced a 4.4/2.2 mm Hg reduction in BP. Across all studies, for each one drink per day difference in reduction in alcohol intake, systolic or diastolic BP was reduced approximately 1 mm Hg.

Mechanisms of alcohol pressor effects

Several mechanisms have been proposed for the relationship between alcohol and elevated BP. An immediate effect of alcohol ingestion is vasodilation in some vascular beds. Sustained intake accompanied by high blood alcohol levels, however, results in short-term elevation of BP. BP levels usually correlate best with alcohol intake within the previous 24 hours, and BP levels fall within hours to days of cessation or reduction in intake. Therefore, it seems likely that the effect of alcohol on BP is not mediated by long-term structural alterations, but by neural, hormonal, or other reversible physiologic or vascular changes. Some evidence supports frequent episodes of alcohol withdrawal as the mechanism of hypertension in heavy drinkers but there is more evidence in favor of a direct effect of alcohol on BP. There are several suggested mediators for the direct effect of alcohol on BP (**Table B96.1**). There appears to be more evidence to support the role of the sympathetic nervous system, increased vascular endothelin-1 production, or cellular transport and electrolytes than the other mechanisms suggested, but this remains an open question.

TABLE B96.1

SUGGESTED MEDIATORS OF THE HYPERTENSIVE EFFECTS OF ALCOHOL

Neurohormonal (sympathetic nervous system, endothelin, renin-angiotensin-aldosterone system, insulin/insulin resistance, corticotropin or cortisol)
Inhibition of vascular relaxing substances (nitric oxide)
Calcium depletion
Magnesium depletion
Increased intracellular calcium or other electrolytes in vascular smooth muscle
Increased acetaldehyde

Alcohol and cardiovascular protection

Low to moderate levels of alcohol intake are associated with a lower incidence of atherosclerotic cardiovascular events, including myocardial infarction, atherothrombotic stroke, and peripheral and renal vascular disease, compared with no alcohol ingestion. These beneficial epidemiologic observations of alcohol may be related to increases in high-density lipoprotein and apolipoproteins A_1 and A_2, antioxidant effects, decreases in fibrinogen, and reduced platelet aggregation. However, higher intake levels are associated with increased risk of hypertension, cardiomyopathy and other cardiac complications, hemorrhagic and thrombotic strokes, certain kinds of cancer, hepatitis, cirrhosis, pancreatitis, gastritis, suicides, accidents, violence, and alcohol abuse and dependence.

The most recent study reporting cardiovascular outcomes associated with drinking in a hypertensive population was the Losartan Intervention For Endpoint (LIFE) reduction in hypertension study cohort; in drinkers there was no decrease in the composite cardiovascular outcome with losartan (compared with atenolol) because the lower incidence of myocardial infarction in the drinkers was offset by increased risk of stroke.

Clinical implications

Evaluation. All hypertensive patients and prehypertensive individuals should be asked about recent drinking, including quantity and frequency of drinking. Those who drink should be given appropriate screening for alcohol dependence.

Intervention. Effective interventions, such as the cognitive-behavioral technique used in the PATHS trial, have been developed to reduce alcohol consumption in nondependent heavy drinkers. Referral to alcohol treatment specialists is necessary in many cases, if there is evidence of alcohol dependence or more serious health consequences of drinking, but primary care physicians and other health care providers should routinely discuss alcohol consumption with their patients and recommend limitation of excessive intake whenever present.

Alcohol reduction and hypertension. Because of the association between heavy drinking and hypertension, other detrimental health and psychosocial effects, and the potential benefits of alcohol consumption, the current public health recommendation in the United States for those who drink is that average alcohol intake should not exceed two drinks per day in men and one drink per day in women, because women are generally smaller and have markedly reduced gastric alcohol dehydrogenase compared with men.

The reductions in BP from reducing alcohol intake in randomized controlled trials is similar to other effective lifestyle interventions. In the Trials of Hypertension Prevention, Phase I (TOHP-I), weight reduction was most effective in reducing BP (2.9/2.3 mm Hg), although sodium reduction also significantly reduced BP (1.7/0.9 mm Hg) and was comparable to the results of alcohol intervention in PATHS. Exercise has also produced reductions in BP at least of this magnitude. Therefore, reduction in alcohol intake should be considered along with weight reduction, limitation of sodium intake, exercise, and the Dietary Approaches to Stop Hypertension (DASH) eating plan as the primary lifestyle changes to encourage in patients with or at risk for hypertension. If alcohol intake exceeds an average of one to two drinks per day, then reduction in alcohol consumption should be included in the initial management plan.

Many persons should not drink at all, such as pregnant women or anyone with a history of problem drinking or alcoholism. Persons drinking more than one to two drinks per day should be encouraged to reduce their intake and thereby reduce BP as well as the risk of developing hypertension and of other alcohol-related problems.

Alcohol and cardiovascular disease risk. For those who are not in a high-risk category and who drink within the limits outlined in the preceding text, the risk of developing hypertension is probably not increased and beneficial effects of alcohol may predominate. Most medical authorities and consensus guidelines do not encourage initiation of alcohol consumption to reduce cardiovascular disease risk. However, for those who choose to drink and have no contraindications, low levels of drinking may be considered prudent.

Suggested Readings

Beilin LJ, Puddey IB. Alcohol and hypertension: an update. *Hypertension* 2006; 47:1035–1038.
Cushman WC, Cutler JA, Hanna E, et al. PATHS Group. The Prevention And Treatment of Hypertension Study (PATHS): effects of an alcohol treatment program on BP. *Arch Intern Med* 1998;152:1197–1207.
Di Castelnuovo A, Rotondo S, Iacoviello L, et al. Meta-analysis of wine and beer consumption in relation to vascular risk. *Circulation* 2002;105:2836–2844.
Marmot MG, Elliott P, Shipley MJ, et al. Alcohol and BP: the INTERSALT study. *BMJ* 1994;308:1263–1267.
Puddey IB, Beilin LJ, Vandongen R, et al. Evidence for a direct effect of alcohol consumption on BP in normotensive men: a randomized controlled trial. *Hypertension* 1985;7:707–713.
Reims HM, Kjeldsen SE, Brady WE, et al. Alcohol consumption and cardiovascular risk in hypertensives with left ventricular hypertrophy: the LIFE study. *J Hum Hypertens* 2004;18:381–389.
Suh I, Shaten BJ, Cutler JA, et al. Alcohol use and mortality from coronary heart disease: the role of high-density lipoprotein cholesterol: the Multiple Risk Factor Intervention Trial Research Group. *Ann Intern Med* 1992;116:881–887.
Thun MJ, Peto R, Lopez AD, et al. Alcohol consumption and mortality among middle-aged and elderly US adults. *N Engl J Med* 1997;337:1705–1714.
Xin X, He J, Frontini MG, et al. Effects of alcohol reduction on BP: a meta-analysis of randomized controlled trials. *Hypertension* 2001;38:1112–1117.
Zilkens RR, Burke V, Hodgson JM, et al. Red wine and beer elevate BP in normotensive men. *Hypertension* 2005;45:874–879.

CHAPTER B97 ■ TRENDS IN BLOOD PRESSURE CONTROL AND MORTALITY

THOMAS J. THOM, BA AND EDWARD J. ROCCELLA, PhD, MPH

KEY POINTS

■ Approximately 72 million Americans have hypertension; another 70 million have prehypertension, requiring lifestyle modifications to prevent hypertension and cardiovascular disease.

■ Hypertension prevalence declined from the 1960–1962 survey to the 1988–1994 survey in men, women, blacks and whites; rates increased by 1999–2004 but are still below earlier rates.

■ Aging of the population and the upward trend in obesity portend continued increases in the total numbers of Americans with prehypertension and hypertension.

■ Although the proportions of hypertensive patients treated and controlled increased markedly in 1999–2004, 39% of hypertensive patients were not being treated; in another 26%, treatment failed to lower blood pressure (BP) to values <140/90 mm Hg.

See also Chapters B74, B75 and **B98**

An estimated 72 million Americans have hypertension and another 70 million have prehypertension. For stroke and heart failure, the relationship between blood pressure (BP) and risk is stronger than the relationship between BP and coronary heart disease (CHD). Hypertension remains the major population-attributable risk factor for heart failure and stroke, the prevalence of which exceeds 5 million persons for each disease.

Data sources and definitions

Estimates of the national prevalence of hypertension are from BP measurements and health interviews of the following surveys of the National Center for Health Statistics (NCHS): The National Health Examination Survey of 1960–1962 and the National Health and Nutrition Examination Surveys (NHANES) of 1971 to 1974 (NHANES I), 1976–1980 (NHANES II), 1988–1994 (NHANES III), and 1999–2004 (NHANES). *Hypertension*, as defined for the prevalence table and figure, includes persons (a) with a systolic BP ≥140 mm Hg, or a diastolic BP ≥90 mm Hg; or (b) who responded "yes" when asked if they are on antihypertensive medication; and (c) who responded that on two or more occasions a physician or other health care providers told them that they had hypertension. The overall prevalence of hypertension, estimated as 72 million persons, is based on the definition given in the preceding text. On the basis of the interview questions and actual BP measurements, awareness of hypertension diagnosis, treatment, and control status can be ascertained. Mortality data in this paper are from the NCHS based on tabulation of U.S. death certificates coded according to

the International Classification of Diseases of the World Health Organization.

Trends and age-sex-race differences

Average blood pressure and prevalence of hypertension. National surveys show that among persons 18–74 years of age, average systolic and diastolic BPs have declined since the 1960s (**Table B97.1**). Declines were observed in men and women and in the white and black populations. Average systolic and diastolic pressures were higher in the black than in the white and Mexican-American populations, and higher in men than women. Men had higher average BPs than women at younger ages, but later in life, the reverse was true (data not shown). Between 1988–1994 and 1999–2004, average systolic and diastolic BP increased in women but not in men aged 18–74 years. The prevalence of hypertension for persons 20–74 years of age was essentially unchanged during the 1960s and 1970s for white and black men and women, followed by a large decline in 1988–1994, but then an increase in 1999–2004 (Table B97.2).

Hypertension awareness, treatment, and control. For persons aged 18–74 years, **Figure B97.1** shows the marked improvement between 1971–1974 and 1988–1991 in the proportion of individuals with hypertension (old cut points: 160/95 mm Hg) who were aware of their condition, were being treated, and had their BP under control. Increases are also seen for persons older than 18 years for the current BP cut points (140/90 mm Hg) used to define hypertension. Although improvement from 53% treated

TABLE B97.1

AVERAGE BLOOD PRESSURE IN PERSONS 18–74 YEARS OF AGE BY SEX
IN WHITES, BLACKS, AND MEXICAN AMERICANS, UNITED STATES,
1960–1962 TO 1999–2000 NATIONAL HEALTH EXAMINATION SURVEYS[a]

Years	White		Black		Mexican American	
	Men	Women	Men	Women	Men	Women
	Systolic BP, mm Hg					
1960–1962	130	127	135	137	NA	NA
1971–1974	133	129	138	136	NA	NA
1976–1980	129	121	130	127	NA	NA
1988–1994[b]	123	116	127	123	124	119
1999–2004[b]	123	118	128	125	124	121
	Diastolic BP, mm Hg					
1960–1962	78	77	83	83	NA	NA
1971–1974	85	81	89	86	NA	NA
1976–1980	82	77	84	81	NA	NA
1988–1994[b]	75	70	77	71	75	69
1999–2004[b]	73	71	75	73	72	70

NA, not available.
[a]Values are age-adjusted. BPs are based on 1, 2, or (usually) 3 seated measurements on one occasion.
[b]Non-Hispanic whites and blacks.

in 1988–1994 to 61% in 1999–2004 is gratifying, 39% are not being treated (28 million people). Similarly, although the percent of hypertensive patients treated and controlled increased to 35% in 1999–2004, for 26% (18 million), treatment did not lower BP to <140/90 mm Hg. The improvements in awareness, therapy, and control seen in 1999–2004 compared to 1988–1994 were only seen in men (data not shown).

Obesity. These survey data collected in separate time periods document the progress and regression during the more than 3 decades of national and community hypertension control efforts. Of concern is that a recent analysis of NHANES concluded that 70% of adult men (72,000,000) and 62% of adult women (68,000,000) are overweight or obese, with even higher proportions in the black population. The upward trend in overweight in Americans of *all* ages may slow future improvements in hypertension prevalence and control.

Prehypertension. The lifetime risk of hypertension (i.e., the probability of developing hypertension during one's lifetime) is calculated to be >90% for men and women not yet hypertensive at age 55 and 65 who survived up to age 80–89. Therefore, the vast majority of Americans who live long enough are destined to become hypertensive before death. Further, data from observational and clinical studies indicate that one third of stroke deaths occur before the onset of hypertension (defined as BP of ≥140/90 mm Hg) and before hypertension would traditionally have been treated. This information prompted the Joint National Committee on the Prevention, Detection, Evaluation, and Treatment of High Blood Pressure to develop

TABLE B97.2

PERCENT PREVALENCE OF HYPERTENSION IN PERSONS 20–74 YEARS OF AGE
BY SEX IN WHITES, BLACKS, AND MEXICAN AMERICANS, UNITED STATES,
1960–1962 TO 1999–2004 NATIONAL HEALTH EXAMINATION SURVEYS[a]

Years	White		Black		Mexican American	
	Men	Women	Men	Women	Men	Women
1960–1962	39.3	31.7	48.1	50.8	NA	NA
1971–1974	41.7	32.4	51.8	50.3	NA	NA
1976–1980	43.5	32.3	48.7	47.5	NA	NA
1988–1994[b]	29.8	24.3	39.3	40.3	28.7	26.9
1999–2004[b]	31.0	28.0	40.4	44.0	28.7	29.9

NA, not available.
[a]Either systolic BP ≥140 mm Hg or diastolic ≥90 mm Hg or taking antihypertensive medication. Values are age-adjusted.
[b]Non-Hispanic whites and blacks.

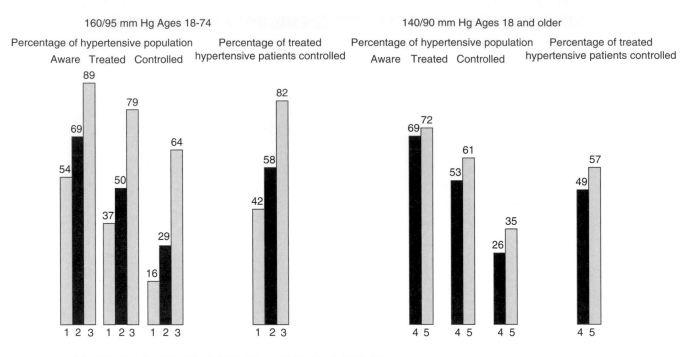

Survey period 1: 1971–74   2: 1976–80   3: 1988–91   4: 1988–94   5: 1999–04

Figure B97.1 Hypertension awareness, treatment, and control rates reported in the National Health and Nutrition Examination Surveys; 1971–1974 to 1999–2004.

the category of prehypertension in its seventh report (JNC 7). Prehypertension includes persons who are not on antihypertensive medication but have a BP of 120 to 139 mm Hg systolic and 80–89 mm Hg diastolic. Extrapolating from NHANES 1999–2004 to the total U.S. population in 2004 gives an estimate that 70 million Americans have prehypertension.

Mortality. Stroke is the third leading cause of death in the United States, accounting for approximately 150,000 deaths each year. Heart failure accounts for another 50,000 deaths and CHD for approximately 450,000 deaths. **Figure B97.2** shows the 1950 to 2004 age-adjusted death rates for all causes and major cardiovascular diseases. The death rate for stroke declined <1% per year before 1972 and 2.8% per year thereafter, a total decline of 66% from 1972 to 2004. Acceleration of the rate of decline occurred in all age, race, and sex groups (data not shown). **Figure B97.2** also shows the reduction in mortality from CHD. Not shown is the marked increase in the 1960s and 1970s in the death rate for heart failure and its level rates since the mid- 1980s. These trends demonstrate that mortality from hypertensive-related cardiovascular disease (CVD) improved considerably more than did the trend for all-cause mortality. Total prevalence and numbers of deaths from stroke and heart failure can be expected to increase further as the population ages and obesity increases.

Hospitalizations. Evidence of declining trends in incidence and immediate or long-term survival after stroke is not available on a national scale. Hospital discharge statistics for broad age-groups show modest increases in rates of hospitalization for stroke between 1970 and approximately 1988, followed by declines to 2004 (data not shown). They also show appreciable increases since 1970 in the percentage of stroke, heart failure, and patients with CHD discharged alive from hospitals and decreases in the length of stay since 1970. These statistics, however, are an incomplete

measure of incidence and case-fatality, and they are affected by repeat admissions and changes in hospital admission practices.

In addition, community-based studies conducted during the 1970s and 1980s (the Minnesota Heart *Survey,* the Honolulu Heart Program, the Framingham Study, and in Rochester, MN) also report substantial declines in stroke incidence and rates of hospitalizations for stroke as well as improved survival.

Role of education

National High Blood Pressure Education Program. In 1972, a large national effort was organized as the National High Blood Pressure Education Program (NHBPEP) of the National Heart, Lung, and Blood Institute. It was designed to educate the public, health professionals, and hypertensive patients about the health risks posed by hypertension and the health benefits of its detection, treatment, and control. Efforts of this group to define hypertension and propose standardized treatment strategies coincide with the beginning of the marked accelerated downward trend in age-adjusted stroke mortality in the United States.

Joint National Committee Guidelines. Since 1972, the NHBPEP and its partner organizations have built a national infrastructure that developed BP management guidelines under the Joint National Committee on the Prevention, Detection, Evaluation, and Treatment of High Blood Pressure (the JNC Clinical Guidelines) as well as numerous clinical advisory statements. The program has expanded its portfolio to include actions for the primary prevention of hypertension especially for those in the prehypertension range. The prehypertension category designation is intended to identify those individuals in whom early intervention by adoption of healthy lifestyles could reduce BP and decrease the rate of progression of BP with age to hypertensive levels.

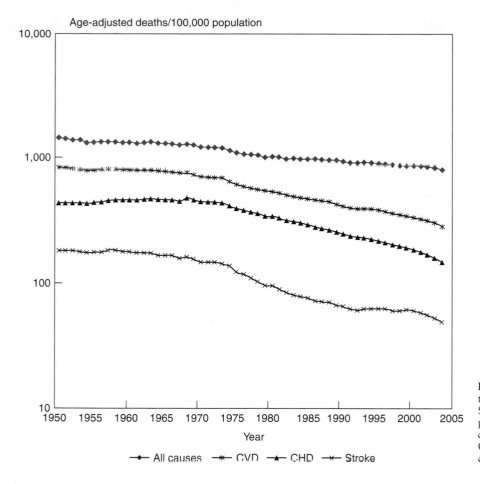

Figure B97.2 Death rates for total mortality and the major cardiovascular diseases in the United States, 1950 to 2004. Rates adjusted to U.S. population, 2000. Corrections made for changes caused by the Tenth Revision of the International Classification of Diseases. CVD, cardiovascular disease, CHD, coronary heart disease.

The sharp and accelerated rate of decline in stroke mortality that began after 1972 continues. As a result, the United States has one of the lowest death rates from stroke in the world. Many factors contributed to the decline in mortality from stroke and from CHD. These include the introduction of well-tolerated oral antihypertensive drugs and increased efforts to treat hypertension with these agents as well as changes in lifestyle as both adjunctive and definitive care. Improvements in the management of acute stroke and acute coronary disease also contribute to the decline in stroke and CHD mortality.

Suggested Readings

Chobanian AV, Bakris GL, Black HR, et al. Seventh Report of the Joint National Committee on prevention, detection, evaluation, and treatment of high BP: the JNC 7 Report. *JAMA* 2003;288:2560–2572.

Fields LE, Burt VL, Cutler JA, et al. The burden of adult hypertension in the United States, 1999 to 2000 a rising tide. *Hypertension* 2004;44:1–7.

Flegal KM, Carroll MD, Ogden CL, et al. Prevalence and trends in obesity among US adults, 1999–2000. *JAMA* 2002;288:1723–1727.

Hajjar I, Kotchen TA. Trends in prevalence, awareness, treatment, and control of hypertension in the United States, 1988–2000. *JAMA* 2003;290:199–206.

Kearney PM, Whelton M, Reynolds K, et al. Global burden of hypertension and analysis of worldwide data. *Lancet* 2005;365:217–223.

National Center for Health Statistics. *Health, United States, 2006 with chartbook on trends in the health of Americans with special feature on pain.* Hyattsville. http://www.cdc.gov/nchs/hus.htm, 2006.

Ong KL, Cheung BMY, Man YU, et al. Prevalence, treatment, and control of hypertension among United States adults, 1999–2004. *Hypertension* 2006;49:69–75.

Qureshi AI, Suri MFK, Kirmani JF, et al. Prevalence and trends of prehypertension and hypertension in the United States: National Health and Nutrition Examination Surveys 1976 to 2000. *Med Sci Monit* 2005;11(9):C403–C109.

Rosamond W, Flagel K, Friday G, et al. Heart Disease and Stroke Statistics – 2007 Update: a report from the American Heart Association Statistics Committee and Stroke Statistics Subcommittee. *Circulation* 2007;115:e69–e71.

Vasan RS, Beiser A, Seshadri S, et al. Residual lifetime risk for developing hypertension in middle-aged women and men: the Framingham heart study. *JAMA* 2002;287(8):1003–1010.

CHAPTER B98 ■ PREVENTION OF HYPERTENSION

JEFFREY A. CUTLER, MD, MPH AND JEREMIAH STAMLER, MD

KEY POINTS

- Epidemiologic and clinical trial evidence exists for hypertension prevention.
- Particularly important are prevention and control of the obesity epidemic, increased physical activity, moderation of sodium and alcohol intake, increased potassium intake, and a dietary pattern rich in fruits, vegetables, whole grains, legumes, low-fat and fat-free dairy products, fish, and shellfish.
- Both targeted (individual) and population-wide (public health) strategies are necessary for optimal hypertension prevention.

See also Chapters B97 and **C120**

Strategic challenge

In the United States, the prevalence of hypertension in adults is estimated at approximately three in ten, or 65 million persons. Each year, there are approximately 1 million new cases. Tens of millions of others have prehypertensive blood pressure (BP) levels—above normal, although not hypertensive (**Figure B98.1**). All these persons are at increased risk of cardiovascular and renal diseases. As large as this BP problem is overall, it is even more severe among those of lower socioeconomic status, regardless of race and ethnicity.

Public health strategies

From the 1970s to the 1990s, the approach to coping with the mass BP problem was primarily a "high-risk" strategy: detect, evaluate, and treat people with hypertension. This emphasis has accomplished much; it ended therapeutic nihilism in hypertension and has resulted in improved BP control for millions of Americans. It is a reasonable inference that this effort has been one of the most important factors contributing to the decades-long substantial declines in mortality rates from coronary heart disease and stroke and consequent increases in life expectancy for adult men and women.

But this high-risk strategy has serious limitations. It is late (i.e., defensive rather than proactive) and it relies primarily on drug treatment, with its mix of favorable and unfavorable effects and costs. In addition, millions of Americans with hypertension are treated inadequately or not at all, and tens of millions of other people with prehypertensive BP elevations are neglected despite their increased cardiovascular-renal risk. Above all, this high-risk strategy is never ending and offers no possibility of terminating the epidemic of high BP. Only primary prevention of this major risk factor is optimally proactive.

A pivotal fact is that elevated BP levels result from the rise in systolic and diastolic BP experienced by most people during the decades from youth through middle age, with a continuing rise in systolic BP in later years (**Figure B98.2**). Lifelong maintenance of the favorable BP levels that are common among young adults would end high BP as a mass problem. Recent research advances make achievement of this strategic goal possible.

Prevention of age-related blood pressure increases

Evidence is now clear on the relationship to BP of lifestyle, particularly adverse nutritional habits that are so common in the population. These include caloric imbalance with consequent obesity, habitual high salt (NaCl) intake, inadequate potassium intake, excess alcohol consumption, and sedentary habits. By the early 1990s, extensive data on these traits served as a scientific foundation for the first international and U.S. expert group reports on the prevention of high BP. Since the mid-1990s, new findings from observational studies, randomized trials, and animal experiments suggested other dietary factors in hypertension.

Observational studies of dietary factors and blood pressure of individuals

Salt intake. The International Study of Salt and Blood Pressure (INTERSALT) involved >10,000 men and women 20 to 59 years old, sampled at 52 centers in 32 countries. It tested both cross-population (ecologic) (N = 52) and within-population (N >10,000) prior hypotheses. To deal with the methodologic problem in assessing individual salt intake, it had a large sample size and one carefully collected 24-hour urine per person. Its

Blood pressure classification			
BP classification	SBP (mm Hg)		DBP (mm Hg)
Normal	<120	and	<80
Prehypertension	120–139	or	80–89
Stage 1 hypertension	140–159	or	90–99
Stage 2 hypertension	≥160	or	≥100

Figure B98.1 Systolic blood pressure (SBP) and diastolic blood pressure (DBP) criteria for classification of blood pressure (BP) as normal, prehypertensive, and hypertensive (stages 1 and 2) for adults aged 18 years or older. The recommendation is to classify on the basis of average BP for an individual from no less than two readings at each of two visits or more after an initial screening, with the individual not taking drugs and not acutely ill. Normal BP, with regard to cardiovascular risk, is SBP <120 mm Hg and DBP <80 mm Hg; however, unusually low readings should be evaluated for clinical significance. When systolic and diastolic BPs fall into different categories, the higher category should be selected to classify the individual's BP status (e.g., 138/78 mm Hg should be classified as prehypertension). (Reproduced with permission from Joint National Committee on Prevention, Detection, Evaluation, and Treatment of High Blood Pressure. *The Seventh Report of the Joint National Committee on prevention, detection, evaluation, and treatment of high blood pressure: complete report*. Bethesda: U.S. Department of Health and Human Services, National Institutes of Health, National Heart, Lung, and Blood Institute, National High Blood Pressure Education Program, 2004. NIH publication No. 04-5230.)

cross-population and within-population analyses gave concordant results. Results substantiated independent relationships of sodium and potassium excretion (direct and inverse, respectively) and the direct associations of body mass index and alcohol intake with BP levels, hypertension prevalence, and slope (rate of rise) of BP with age. INTERSALT also found an inverse relation between years of education and BP of individuals, with higher intake of sodium and alcohol and higher body mass among the less educated, as well as lower potassium intake. These dietary factors accounted significantly for higher BP levels of less educated persons.

Dietary protein and other factors. Subsequent analyses from INTERSALT, on the basis of measurement of urinary nitrogen excretion as a marker of dietary protein, provided evidence for an inverse association of total protein intake with BP. Additional support for this intriguing relationship has come from other observational studies, including analyses of data collected over 6 years from 11,342 middle-aged men in the Multiple Risk Factor Intervention Trial (MRFIT). The MRFIT results support the concept that multiple dietary factors influence BP independently and additively, including direct associations with overweight/obesity, sodium, and alcohol intake, possibly also with saturated fat intake, blood cholesterol, and inverse associations with potassium and protein intake.

This concept received further support from the International Population Study on Macronutrients and Blood Pressure (INTERMAP), involving 4,680 men and women aged 40 to 59 from 17 population samples in China, Japan, the United Kingdom, and the United States (2,195 Americans of diverse socioeconomic status and ethnicity). Nutrients were assessed by four standardized in-depth dietary recalls and two 24-hour urine collections; eight standardized BP measurements were made at four visits over 3 to 6 weeks. Significant direct independent associations with BP were found for body mass, alcohol intake, and 24-hour sodium excretion, as expected, and possibly for intake of arachidonic acid. In addition, inverse associations were recorded of BP with dietary vegetable protein, Omega-3 polyunsaturated fatty acids, phosphorus, magnesium, calcium, and potassium. Among American participants, intakes of several of these nutrients were less favorable for less educated individuals, and these factors considered together accounted significantly for the higher systolic BP levels of less educated persons (for both sexes and for African Americans, Hispanic Americans, and non-Hispanic white Americans). Multiple dietary variables also accounted significantly for the higher average BP of northern Chinese compared to southern Chinese.

Other studies. In the Chicago Western Electric Study of 1,714 middle-aged men examined annually for 9 years, usual dietary intake during the previous month was assessed by in-depth interview at years 0 and 1. Baseline dietary cholesterol,

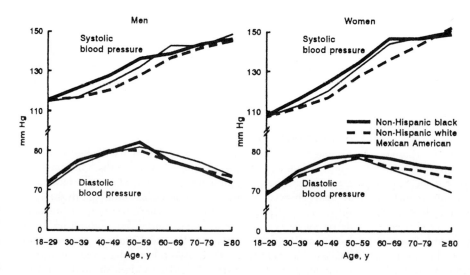

Figure B98.2 Mean systolic and diastolic blood pressures by age and race/ethnicity for men and women of U.S. population aged 18 years or older. (Reproduced from Burt VL, Whelton P, Roccella EJ, et al. Prevalence of hypertension in the US adult population: results from the Third National Health and Nutrition Examination Survey, 1998–1991. *Hypertension* 1995;25:305–313, with permission.)

alcohol intake, and Keys dietary lipid score were directly related to BP change over time; dietary vegetable protein and antioxidant intake (vitamin C and β-carotene) were inversely related. Change in weight over the years was directly related to BP change. (Sodium and potassium intake were not measured.)

Two large cohort studies of health professionals, conducted entirely by questionnaire, relied on self-report of usual post–baseline BP or diagnosis of incident hypertension. Usual intake of foods and nutrients was determined at baseline by food frequency questionnaire. Several of the expected variables—weight (body mass index) and alcohol intake—were found to be strong BP predictors. Dietary potassium, magnesium, and fiber were inversely related to BP change over time and incidence of high BP. Sodium intake was not, but salt intake is particularly difficult to measure accurately by questionnaire, and those health professionals with originally higher intake and high-normal BPs may have already reduced their dietary salt intake, with resultant confounding of the analysis.

These findings from epidemiologic studies on the relationship of several dietary variables to BP and BP change, along with previous reports on inverse relationships of vegetarian diets with BP and hypertension, gave impetus to the conduct of key randomized trials of lifestyle change, including the landmark Dietary Approaches to Stop Hypertension (DASH) trials.

Randomized lifestyle trials in adults and children with normal or prehypertensive blood pressures

Primary Prevention of Hypertension study. The 5-year Primary Prevention of Hypertension (PPH) study found that multifactor intervention (weight loss, reduction of sodium and alcohol intake, increased physical activity) significantly lowered average follow-up BP by 1 to 2 mm Hg and hypertension incidence by 54% (8.8% vs. 19.2% for intervention and control participants, respectively). This outcome was attributable to modest weight loss (average of approximately 3 kg) and, to a lesser extent, sodium reduction (approximately 20% on average).

Hypertension Prevention Trial study. The Hypertension Prevention Trial (HPT) studied sodium reduction and weight loss both separately and combined and tested increased dietary potassium as well. Again, weight loss lowered BP throughout the 3 years of the trial, with waning effect as weight was partially regained. Nevertheless, the data trended toward 27% lower incidence of hypertension. Low-order sodium reduction (10% at 3 years) did not significantly lower mean BP, although incidence of hypertension was apparently reduced.

Trials of Hypertension Prevention studies

Trials of Hypertension Prevention phase I. The Trials of Hypertension Prevention (TOHP) phase I tested a broad range of interventions aimed at factors thought to be related to BP levels. In addition to counseling overweight participants for weight reduction (with inclusion of an exercise component) or sodium reduction, a third lifestyle approach (stress management) was evaluated; also, four nutritional supplements (calcium carbonate, magnesium diglycine, potassium chloride, and fish oil) were tested in placebo-controlled, double-blind designs. During the first 6 months of intervention, only weight loss and sodium reduction produced significant BP reductions, by 2 to 4 mm Hg systolic and 1 to 3 mm Hg diastolic BP. By design, lifestyle groups were also followed for 18 months to assess maintenance of behavioral change. During this period, weight and sodium reduction each demonstrated tendencies to decrease hypertension incidence, by

51% and 24%, respectively. Stress management showed no such trend.

Trials of Hypertension Prevention phase II. This longer trial further evaluated weight loss and sodium reduction, singly and in combination. The most important additional finding of TOHP-II was that each of the interventions lowered incidence of hypertension significantly, by approximately 20% over 3 to 4 years. In addition, during the initial 6-month follow-up period, at the height of intervention adherence, effects of weight loss and sodium reduction on hypertension incidence were additive.

Trials of Hypertension Prevention phase III. This long-term observational follow-up of TOHP I and II combined has reported a significant one fourth reduction in cardiovascular morbidity/mortality in those assigned to sodium reduction during the trials compared to controls that were not exposed to this intervention. These findings, along with a similar trend in the Trial of Nonpharmacological Intervention in the Elderly (TONE) study, fill an important gap in the evidence on benefits of lowering dietary salt.

Trial of Nonpharmacological Intervention in the Elderly. A combination of weight loss and salt reduction was more effective than either one alone (although weight loss and sodium reduction were individually effective) in the 2.5-year TONE, which studied hypertensive participants aged 60 to 79 years.

Dietary Approaches to Stop Hypertension trials

Dietary Approaches to Stop Hypertension trial. The first DASH study was an 8-week outpatient feeding trial in adults with prehypertension or stage 1 hypertension. It found that a diet enriched in fruits, vegetables, whole grains, legumes, fat-free and low-fat dairy foods, with reduced total and saturated fat, dietary cholesterol, and sugars, plus modestly increased protein, lowered BP by 5.5/3.0 mm Hg. Body weight and sodium intake were maintained at constant levels in all participants, who consumed little or no alcohol. Also, in prehypertensive individuals evaluated separately, the diet reduced BP by 3.5/2.1 mm Hg.

Dietary Approaches to Stop Hypertension–sodium trial. In a second feeding trial (DASH-sodium), the same investigators reproduced the foregoing results at each of three levels of sodium intake, showed that lowered salt intake had independent stepwise effects on BP, and further documented that the greatest BP-lowering (e.g., by 7.1 mm Hg systolic in the nonhypertensive subgroup) was with the combination of the DASH diet and sodium intake reduced to approximately 65 mmol (approximately 3.8 g salt) per 24 hours.

The OMNIHEART feeding trial—with design and methods similar to those of the DASH trials—showed that BP reduction with the DASH-type diet was further enhanced by increased intake (as percent of total calories) of vegetable protein and monounsaturated fat.

Infants and children

Among newborns, consumption of formula with lower sodium content resulted in lower systolic BP at 6 months. Of potentially great significance, reexamination of 35% of these infants after 15 years showed maintenance of a 3.6/2.2 mm Hg advantage in BP levels for the group assigned to the lower sodium formula, despite little evidence of difference in current sodium intake or any other BP determinants at follow-up. Results of a recent meta-analysis that included this plus two other sodium reduction trials in infants and ten such trials in older children showed that 40%

to 50% lower sodium intake produced significant reductions in systolic BP.

Moving from clinical studies to public policy

Participants in clinical trials are volunteers and are therefore apt to be more highly motivated toward lifestyle change. They also enjoy socioeconomic circumstances more conducive to modifying behavior than other social groups. To achieve broad public health benefits, efficacious methods to prevent hypertension must be effective in representative populations. Reducing dietary salt should be one approach that is particularly amenable to a population approach, because more than 85% of dietary sodium comes from processed foods. Two community-intervention salt-reduction trials have been completed in Europe using "quasi experimental" designs (1 intervention, 1 control community).

Portuguese salt trial. In the Portuguese salt trial, two rural communities were compared, with random samples of residents 15 to 69 years old examined before intervention, then annually for 2 years. The health education program in the intervention community was facilitated by the fact that 50% of the very high salt consumption (360 mmol per day sodium) came from salt that was added in cooking at home, and another 33% was derived from one food item, salt-dried codfish. There was also a focus on reducing salt used in commercial bread baking. Results of this trial showed sodium excretion to be 42% lower in the intervention community at 1 year, and there were significant reductions of mean BPs of 4 to 5 mm Hg at years 1 and 2.

Belgian salt trial. In contrast, the Belgian salt trial was much less successful in its intervention; there were no net changes in sodium excretion or BP for men, sodium changes for women were modest (20%), and net mean BP reductions (2.9 mm Hg systolic and 1.6 mm Hg diastolic BP) were not significant. In contrast to the Portuguese trial, the same individuals were not examined at baseline and follow-up, leading to less precise estimation of BP change.

Other population interventions. Another community intervention experiment studied adolescents at two boarding schools. In a crossover design with each phase lasting 1 academic year, sodium intake was reduced 15% to 20% by changes in food purchasing and preparation, with a significant effect on systolic and diastolic BP of approximately 2 mm Hg. This study is encouraging because of simplicity of intervention and because prevention is theoretically most attractive when begun in childhood. Positive results have also been reported from a 3-year community trial in urban north China, which found significant reductions of systolic BP (5 mm Hg in men and 6 mm Hg in women aged 15 to 64 years) associated with net reductions in sodium intake estimated at 14% in men and 6% in women.

Current recommendations and future directions

Consistent recommendations for preventive medicine and public health have emerged from the World Health Organization/International Society of Hypertension Guidelines Committee and the U.S. Working Group Report on the Primary Prevention of Hypertension. The reports emphasize (a) weight control and increased physical activity, (b) no more than moderate alcohol intake [daily average of no more than two drinks (i.e., no more than 1 oz or 26 g of ethanol)] for men and half these amounts for women, (c) limitation of dietary sodium to ≤2.4 g per day (equivalent to 6 g of sodium chloride), and (d) increased dietary potassium. Largely based on results of the DASH-sodium trial, the 2005 *Dietary Guidelines for Americans* added a lower sodium goal of <1.5 g per day for middle-aged or older adults, all African Americans, and persons with hypertension. For these higher-risk groups, the *Guidelines* also added a quantitative goal of >4.7 g per day of dietary potassium. Regarding reduction of psychosocial stress, although some evidence is suggestive, more study is required. No specific roles for supplemental calcium or magnesium intake were recommended.

Recent results add to the extensive evidence on established lifestyle causes of rise in BP with age and resultant high incidence of prehypertension and hypertension. This evidence leads to the reasonable inference that most of the knowledge is in hand for the primary prevention of high BP. First and foremost is the substantial possibility for hypertension prevention and control, and progress in combating the obesity epidemic, through population-wide improved eating patterns (similar to DASH-sodium with caloric moderation) and increased physical activity. Needed research involves such issues as (a) the full potential of combined lifestyle approaches, (b) the effects in special population groups, (c) better methods for estimation of food and nutrient intake, and (d) potential for incorporation of hypertension prevention into primary medical care. Currently, given the societal will, widespread application of existing knowledge can make the rise in BP with age rare and optimal BP levels common in all population subgroups, thereby ending the epidemic.

Suggested Readings

Appel LJ, Brands MW, Daniel SR, et al. Dietary approaches to prevent and treat hypertension: a scientific statement from the American Heart Association. *Hypertension* 2006;47:296–308.

Appel LJ, Sacks FM, Carey VJ. OmniHeart Collaborative Research Group. Effects of protein, monounsaturated fat, and carbohydrate intake on blood pressure and serum lipids: results of the OmniHeart randomized trial. *JAMA* 2005;294:2455–2464.

Elliott P, Stamler J, Dyer AR, et al. INTERMAP Cooperative Research Group. Association between protein intake and blood pressure: the INTERMAP study. *Arch Intern Med* 2006;166:79–87.

Feng JH, MacGregor GA. Importance of salt in determining blood pressure in children: meta-analysis of controlled trials. *Hypertension* 2006;48:861–869.

Forte JG, Miguel JM, Miguel MJ, et al. Salt and blood pressure: a community trial. *J Hum Hypertens* 1989;3:179–184.

Sacks FM, Svetkey LP, Vollmer WM, et al. DASH-Sodium Collaborative Research Group. Effects on blood pressure of reduced dietary sodium and the Dietary Approaches to Stop Hypertension (DASH) diet: DASH-Sodium Collaborative Research Group. *N Engl J Med* 2001;344:3–10.

Stamler R, Stamler J, Gosch FC, et al. Primary prevention of hypertension by nutritional-hygienic means: final report of a randomized, controlled trial. [Published erratum appears in *JAMA* 1989;262:3132]. *JAMA* 1989;262:1801–1807.

Stamler J, Stamler R, Neaton JD. Blood pressure, systolic and diastolic, and cardiovascular risks: US population data. *Arch Intern Med* 1993;153:598–615.

The Trials of Hypertension Prevention Collaborative Research Group. Effects of weight loss and sodium reduction intervention on blood pressure and hypertension incidence in overweight people with high-normal blood pressure: the trials of hypertension prevention, phase II. *Arch Intern Med* 1997;157:657–667.

Whelton PK, He J, Appel LJ, et al. Primary prevention of hypertension: clinical and public health advisory from the National High Blood Pressure Education Program. *JAMA* 2002;288:1882–1888.

CHAPTER B99 ■ COMMUNITY-BASED MANAGEMENT PROGRAMS

DANIEL T. LACKLAND, DrPH AND BRENT M. EGAN, MD

KEY POINTS

■ The *community*, defined as places and groups in which people learn, work, worship, and play, can be approached to implement cost-effective lifestyle and health care delivery system changes.

■ The risk of cardiovascular disease (CVD) is likely to rise over the next 20 years given the increasing age and weight of the U.S. population and the growing numbers of high-risk ethnic groups; reliance on federal programs for an ever-increasing proportion of high-risk patients is costly and probably insufficient.

■ Strategies for implementing evidence-based guidelines in primary care settings can improve the efficacy of the high-risk strategy and reinforce lifestyle change.

See also Chapter **C124**

In the United States, truly impressive declines in cardiovascular disease (CVD) have occurred (see Chapter B97). From the 1960s through the early 2000s, age-adjusted death rates for heart disease and stroke in the United States fell by more than 50%, but relative disparities persist.

Rationale for community programs

Failure to reach goals. Despite advances, the population at risk for CVD remains too large. Approximately 60% of adults have a total cholesterol of >200 mg per dL. Moreover, one third of patients with coronary heart disease have a total cholesterol of <200 mg per dL. Many of them have low high-density lipoprotein and high triglycerides and dense low-density lipoprotein cholesterol. More than half of individuals older than 50 years have hypertension (according to the Joint National Committee, JNC 7) and many have hyperlipidemia, diabetes, or cardiometabolic syndrome. Only a minority of patients at risk are treated to evidence-based goals.

Despite long-standing evidence that treatment of hypertension reduces CVD morbidity and mortality, only one fourth of patients has a blood pressure (BP) <140/90 mm Hg with the more stringent goal of <130/80 mm Hg for hypertensive individuals with diabetes, renal disease, and ischemic heart disease, overall BP control rates are even lower. Control rates of hypercholesterolemia and diabetes are typically no better and often worse than corresponding rates for high BP. Prehypertension (BP 120–139/80–89 mm Hg) is found in one fourth of the adult population in the United States and should be treated primarily, if not exclusively, with lifestyle modification. Similarly,

interventions targeting emerging risk factors for high BP such as low birth weight, are most effective through community-based approaches.

Health system and patient barriers. Low rates of reaching goals reflect provider and system barriers. Adequate evidence-based interventions are often not prescribed. Treatment inertia and patient variables, such as adherence to appropriate therapy, lead to suboptimal population benefits. Despite decades of efforts to generate and disseminate treatment guidelines to providers and a plethora of studies to enhance patient adherence, the gap between potential and realized medical benefits remains wide.

Potential target populations

High-risk populations remain important targets for intervention because the number needed to treat to prevent morbid and mortal events is sufficiently low to warrant aggressive therapy. At the same time, prevention programs will need to target those most likely to derive benefit.

Elderly. The median age of the U.S. population is rising rapidly. In the next 20 years, the number of Americans aged 60 or older is projected to grow by more than 30 million, whereas the population within the age group of 30 to 49 years is expected to decline. Cardiovascular risk and disease advance sharply with increasing age, whereas the rates of those treated to goal, for hypertension in particular, decline. The major demographic changes are projected to place an extraordinary demand on financial and health care resources, including nursing homes.

Young. Cardiovascular risk among young Americans is rising even more rapidly than in older adults. The increasing risk among youth largely reflects the burgeoning obesity epidemic. More than half of the diabetes in children and teenagers in many areas is now type 2. The proportions of obesity and sedentary lifestyles are increasing in children.

Obese. More than 60% of U.S. adults are now overweight or obese, reflecting a major increase during the last 10 years. Compared to normal-weight individuals, overweight and obese subjects who are currently without cardiovascular risk factors are at two to fourfold greater risk for developing hypertension and CVD and 10 to 60 times more likely to develop diabetes mellitus in the next 10 years. The health risks of obesity are greater over longer periods of time. Consequently, the impact of the obesity epidemic in this country is likely to become more fully manifest in the next 20 years with devastating effects on public and individual health and finances.

Racial and regional groups. Individuals living in the southeast United States are 50% more likely to experience CVD. Given long-term trends, including lower birth weights, greater proportions of high-risk minorities, and preferential relocation of retirees, the Southeast disparities are likely to persist and grow. Moreover, blacks are twice as likely to die from a stroke and five times more likely to die from end-stage renal disease than whites, especially in the Southeast.

More than 20 years ago, the Hypertension Detection and Follow-Up Program showed that a systematic approach to treating high BP reduced the racial disparity in stroke mortality from >2:1 to 4:3 and also reduced the racial differential in total mortality. Despite the evidence, large ethnic disparities persist. Socioeconomic factors other than race appear to contribute significantly to health disparities. Evidence suggests that insurance and access to health care account for less than half of observed health disparities between ethnic groups.

Cost–benefit analyses: impact of risk level

The numerous problems currently encountered suggest that public health strategies should be reevaluated.

High-risk populations. The traditional Western approach to chronic disease prevention is to identify those at highest risk and implement an intensive strategy aimed at improving outcome for the individual. In hypertension, this means focusing on therapy for those who have had the condition for a relatively long time. Furthermore, when the cost (time and resource intensity) of an approach is high, it works best when the proportion of the population meeting the diagnostic criteria for intervention is relatively small (i.e., ±5% of the total). A BP of ≥180/110 mm Hg or total cholesterol ≥280 mg per dL, roughly define the upper 5% of the population. Initial clinical trials for hypertension and hypercholesterolemia focused on these high-risk patients and proved marked benefits of treatment.

Lower risk populations. Later hypertension trials demonstrated that treatment benefits extend well beyond the upper 5% to 10% of the distribution. These studies suggest that 50% or more of adults can benefit from a high-risk approach to CVD prevention. Nevertheless, attempts to apply the high-risk strategy on a mass basis have proved costly and have limited efficacy. Continued reliance on this model given the demographic changes cited may be intrinsically inefficient.

Very low-risk populations. Cardiovascular risk and disease are virtually absent in unacculturated peoples; however, these people develop CVD with acculturation. These observations strongly implicate a crucial role for lifestyle in the pathogenesis of CVD. The relationship between cardiovascular risk and disease is continuous. When a population is at high risk, small reductions in risk factor levels in the population (e.g., 2–3 mm Hg BP) can equal or exceed the life-saving potential of intensive treatment of a substantial number of low-risk individuals. This is especially true when considering the actual benefits of the high-risk approach, which includes provider, patient, and system failures.

Mass strategy: lifestyle modification

The mass strategies have suffered from perceptions that people are unwilling to change lifestyle sufficiently to obtain benefit and that genetic factors predominate in determining disease. Both notions minimize the role of individual responsibility for health outcomes. However, lifestyle changes have probably accounted for more than half of the 30% age-adjusted reduction of coronary heart disease in the United States from 1968 to 1976 and for a >50% reduction of CVD among the intervention group in the Oslo Diet and Heart Study. Lifestyle may account for up to 10 years of interindividual differences in longevity.

Lifestyle changes are probably easier to initiate and sustain when embraced by the community and supported by policy and insurance and tax law changes. For example, cigarette smoking cessation is one of the most difficult of all behavioral changes. Despite the tremendous challenges of smoking cessation for an individual, impressive reductions in the prevalence of cigarette smoking in the population occurred between the 1960s and 1980s. Evidence that cigarette smoking is deleterious and that smoking cessation is beneficial were reinforced by relevant public health messages, policy changes to limit smoking locations, and punitive taxes and court decisions. Incentives in insurance policies have not been explored adequately as a further incentive to reduce initiation and enhance cessation of tobacco use.

Community-based interventions

The traditional notion of community as a local neighborhood of people that care for each other has not disappeared entirely. However, as our society and family structure become more fluid, human relationships in the local neighborhood are being replaced by interactions in the places people learn, work, worship, and enjoy leisure time together. A growing body of studies documents that health care interventions in schools, worksites, and places of worship can have substantial and sustained beneficial impact on health behaviors and risk factors. Moreover, each of these locations addresses important issues raised earlier.

Principles of prevention in community health models. Three basic components define our overall strategy to any of the community-based interventions (**Table B99.1.**). The first and overall objective is to translate research into practice by extending the academic mission to the community. The second aim is to implement a successful intervention model. The third objective is to provide centralized data management for monitoring progress and providing reports to community leaders. This model allows for a dynamic structure that can be owned and modified by the community to best meet local needs.

School programs. School programs inside and outside the classroom can reach youth, raise awareness, and establish healthy lifestyle patterns early in life. Successful interventions in our nation's schools have tremendous potential for progressively reducing the burden of CVD risk over the long term. A primary area for improvement would be school lunch programs that provide far too much fat and caloric intake.

TABLE B99.1

MODEL FOR COMMUNITY INTERVENTION

Translate research into practice by extending the academic mission of patient care, education, and health care services research to the community.

Enhance and enlist local experts and leaders, then implement a proven model for intervention through the community leaders.

Provide administrative support for coordinating services together with ongoing monitoring of the intervention and relevant feedback to community leaders.

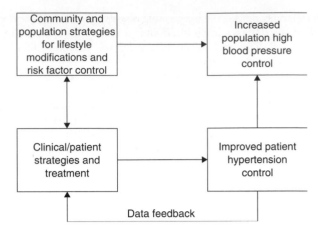

Figure B99.1 The importance of feedback in blood pressure (BP) control. Continuity of primary care with an effective therapeutic alliance between the patient and provider emerges as a critical component of chronic risk factor control. Relevant feedback to the provider appears to enhance the therapeutic alliance, improve adherence, and facilitate risk factor control.

Worksite programs. Health promotion in the workplace, especially programs that combine education with healthy lifestyle change and risk factor monitoring are highly cost effective. Moreover, the worksite is an ideal place to reach young adults and men who are less likely to receive crucial preventive services.

Faith-based programs. Health programs centered at sites of worship represent an excellent forum for risk factor screening and lifestyle interventions. In minority communities especially, the site of worship is often the heart of the community. Many individuals who do not access primary health care services can be reached at their site of worship with health messages and can be assisted in making important and sustained lifestyle changes.

Provider-based programs

No intervention will ultimately succeed without a major commitment from health professionals.

Primary care providers. In controlling risk factors for chronic disease, a regular source of primary health care is paramount. The therapeutic alliance between the patient and the provider is critical in obtaining and adhering to appropriate therapy (**Figure B99.1**). For example, the managed care program at the University of Pennsylvania School of Medicine nearly tripled hypertension control in 1 year, from 19% to 53% by monitoring BP control rates and giving comparative feedback to providers. This model has been adapted to the predominantly fee-for-service paradigm in rural and suburban Hypertension Initiative network in the Carolinas-Georgia region. Among 200,000 hypertension patients in the databank, control rates at <140/90 mm Hg improved from 49% to 65% from 2000 to 2005.

Pharmacists. Pharmacists can improve patient adherence with BP medications by providing information and monitoring. Effective strategies to improve communication between the patient's provider and pharmacist would probably be beneficial but are usually lacking.

Suggested Readings

Egan BM, Lackland DT. Strategies of prevention and the importance of public health and community programs. *Ethn Dis* 1998;8:143–154.

Egan BM, Lackland DT, Basile JN. American Society of Hypertension Regional Chapters: leveraging the impact of the clinical hypertension specialist in the local community. *Am J Hypertens* 2002;15:372–379.

Egan BM, Lackland DT, Igho-Pemu P, et al. Cardiovascular risk factor control in communities – Update from the ASH Carolinas-Georgia chapter, the hypertension initiative, and the community physician's network. *J Clin Hypertens* 2006;8:879–886.

Lackland DT. Population strategies to treat hypertension. *Curr Treat Options Cardiovasc Med* 2005;7:253–258.

Lackland DT, Egan BM. The dominant role of systolic hypertension as a vascular risk factor: evidence from the southeast. *Am J Med Sci* 1999;318:365–368.

Lackland DT, Egan BM, Syddall HE, et al. Associations between birth weight and antihypertensive medication in black and white medicaid recipients. *Hypertension* 2002;39:179–183.

Nissinen A, Kastarinen M, Tuomilehto J. Community control of hypertension—experiences from Finland. *J Hum Hypertens* 2004;18:553–556.

Oexmann MJ, Ascanio R, Egan BM. Preventing cardiovascular disease: efficacy of a church-based intervention on cardiovascular risk reduction. *Ethn Dis* 2001;11:817–822.

Plescia M, Groblewski M. A community-oriented primary care demonstration project: refining interventions for cardiovascular disease and diabetes. *Ann Fam Med* 2004;2:103–109.

Snella KA, Irons AE, Sleeper-Irons BK, et al. Pharmacy- and community-based screenings for diabetes and cardiovascular conditions in high-risk individuals. *J Am Pharm Assoc (Wash DC)* 2006;46:370–377.

CHAPTER B100 ■ ANTIHYPERTENSIVE TREATMENT TRIALS: OUTCOMES

WILLIAM J. ELLIOTT, MD, PhD

KEY POINTS

- Compared to placebo or no treatment, antihypertensive drugs significantly reduce all major types of cardiovascular events, strokes, and all-cause mortality; in meta-analyses against placebo, either an angiotensin-converting enzyme (ACE) inhibitor or an angiotensin receptor blocker (ARB) prevented doubling of serum creatinine or end-stage renal disease.
- Whether any specific drug or drug class has benefits "beyond blood pressure (BP) control" in preventing either cardiovascular or renal endpoints is controversial; most of the outcome benefits are directly correlated with systolic BP reductions, particularly in trials involving diabetic patients or those with chronic kidney disease.
- Traditional meta-analyses of outcome-based clinical trials comparing different classes of antihypertensive drugs (initial diuretic with or without β-blocker versus ACE inhibitor versus calcium channel blocker) show no major differences in reduction of ischemic heart disease endpoints; in network meta-analyses, low-dose diuretics are at least as good as other types of antihypertensive drugs in preventing cardiovascular events.
- Stroke reduction is prominent with diuretics and calcium channel blockers, whereas heart failure is prevented most reliably with diuretic or ACE inhibitor.

See also Chapters B101, **C119,** and C146

Drug treatment versus placebo or no treatment

Since the late 1960s, clinical trials comparing morbidity and mortality outcomes in hypertensive patients randomized to active drug treatment versus placebo or no treatment have demonstrated that the absolute benefits of treatment are generally proportional to the absolute risk of cardiovascular events in the treated population. In many cases, the relative benefits of treatment were often not significant, usually because only a small proportion of subjects suffered the endpoint of interest during the usual 5 years of follow-up. One method of overcoming the low statistical power in each individual trial is to combine the results of many trials using meta-analysis. This technique has demonstrated impressive benefits of drug treatment in reducing virtually all types of cardiovascular events, including all-cause mortality (**Table B100.1**). Meta-analyses of trials comparing placebo with either an angiotensin-converting enzyme (ACE) inhibitor or angiotensin receptor blocker (ARB) have shown a significant reduction in renal disease (doubling of serum creatinine, end-stage renal disease, or their composite) in nondiabetic renal disease or type 2 diabetic nephropathy.

Some classes of antihypertensive drugs have not been used as the initial drug in randomized outcome-based clinical trials (e.g., centrally-acting drugs, direct vasodilators). Only one outcome-based clinical trial [The Antihypertensive and Lipid-Lowering to prevent Heart Attack Trial, (ALLHAT)] has studied α-blocker-based therapy, which was inferior to diuretic-based therapy in preventing stroke, combined cardiovascular events, cardiovascular death, and heart failure.

Traditional meta-analyses

The most common way to obtain statistically significant estimates of the effects of one class versus another is to combine the results of several completed trials in a meta-analysis. The potential pitfalls involved in combining data from studies with different inclusion/exclusion criteria, treatment protocols, duration of follow-up, concomitant treatments, and definitions of outcomes are well known. Nevertheless, advocates of the "hierarchy of medical evidence" and "evidence-based medicine" inexplicably place such studies at the top of the list of robust scientific investigation. Results of meta-analyses of initial antihypertensive

TABLE B100.1

RESULTS OF TRADITIONAL META-ANALYSES OF CLINICAL TRIALS COMPARING ACTIVE ANTIHYPERTENSIVE DRUG TREATMENT VERSUS PLACEBO OR NO TREATMENT

Event	Number of trials	Active treatment	Placebo or no treatment	Summary odds ratio (95% confidence interval)[a]
All-cause mortality	42	4,986/72,473	5,321/71,144	0.91 (0.87–0.94)
Cardiovascular mortality	42	3,124/67,999	2,780/69,318	0.86 (0.81–0.91)
Stroke	43	2,310/72,473	3,107/71,144	0.71 (0.68–0.76)
Coronary heart disease	41	2,820/71,443	3,432/70.552	0.80 (0.76–0.84)
Major cardiovascular events[b]	39	5,424/65,328	6,505/63,104	0.78 (0.76–0.82)
Heart failure	28	937/40,898	1,195/40,114	0.72 (0.67–0.80)

[a]All p values for the summary odds ratios are <.0001, and all p values for homogeneity are >.05.
[b]Defined as first occurrence of myocardial infarction, stroke, or cardiovascular death, which was estimated for some trials. Updated from Elliott and Black.

drugs have been used to support clinical guidelines for "initial therapy."

Diuretic/β-blocker comparisons. Historically, diuretics (D) and beta-blockers (β) have been the "standards of comparison" because they were the first two classes of antihypertensives demonstrated in controlled trials to reduce morbidity and mortality compared to placebo- or no treatment. Traditional meta-analyses allowed the use of "D or β" as if it were a single class of agents because several of the protocols allowed the choice of *either* D or β after the subject was randomized to "conventional therapy" and also because the results of several such Scandinavian trials (Captopril Primary Prevention Project, Nordic Diltiazem Study, Second Swedish Trial in Old Patients with Hypertension) were never subanalyzed according to the initial drug class actually given. **Figure B100.1** shows the results of traditional (Mantel and Haenszel) meta-analyses of trials that compared initial D/β therapy with initial ACE inhibitor (ACE-I, top panel) or calcium channel blocker (CCB, bottom panel). With the exception of stroke and heart failure, the outcome differences

were small and statistically nonsignificant. Initial D/β was better in preventing heart failure than either an initial ACE inhibitor or initial CCB but the latter meta-analysis showed significant inhomogeneity mostly due to ALLHAT, but the conclusions would be little changed if a random-effects model were used. Stroke prevention was significantly better with initial CCB than with initial D/β but the latter was significantly better than initial ACE inhibitor.

β-Blocker comparisons. Several meta-analyses have compared outcomes in hypertensive patients randomized to initial β-blocker (especially atenolol) with either placebo or any other initial antihypertensive drug. These have generally suggested that, at least in older individuals, atenolol (or perhaps any β-blocker) is associated with significantly greater mortality, cardiovascular mortality, and stroke.

Angiotensin-converting enzyme inhibitors and angiotensin receptor blockers. Most trials in hypertension that compared an initial ARB with another class of drug used a diuretic as second-line treatment, sometimes in both randomized

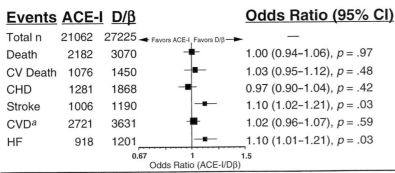

Events	ACE-I	D/β	Odds Ratio (95% CI)
Total n	21062	27225	—
Death	2182	3070	1.00 (0.94–1.06), p = .97
CV Death	1076	1450	1.03 (0.95–1.12), p = .48
CHD	1281	1868	0.97 (0.90–1.04), p = .42
Stroke	1006	1190	1.10 (1.02–1.21), p = .03
CVD[a]	2721	3631	1.02 (0.96–1.07), p = .59
HF	918	1201	1.10 (1.01–1.21), p = .03

Events	CCB	D/β	Odds Ratio (95% CI)
Total n	52596	59227	—
Death	4127	5147	0.97 (0.93–1.01), p = .18
CV Death	2343	2797	0.98 (0.93–1.04), p = .52
CHD	2297	2862	1.00 (0.94–1.06), p = .91
Stroke	1509	1990	0.88 (0.82–0.94), p = .0003
CVD[a]	4406	5539	0.96 (0.92–1.00), p = .049
HF	1457	1567	1.23 (1.14–1.33)[b], p < .0001

Figure B100.1 Results of traditional meta-analyses of clinical trials comparing an initial diuretic (D) or β-blocker with initial angiotensin-converting enzyme inhibitor (ACE-I, *top panel*) or an initial calcium channel blocker (CCB, *bottom panel*). CI, confidence interval; Total N, number of subjects; CV, cardiovascular; CHD, coronary heart disease; CVD[a], major cardiovascular disease events, estimated when necessary; HF, heart failure. [b]p (for homogeneity) = .005; all other p (for homogeneity) values were >.05. (Adapted from Elliott WJ, Jonsson MC, Black HR. It's NOT "Beyond the Blood Pressure," It IS the Blood Pressure. *Circulation* 2006;113:2763–2772.)

arms. Meta-analyses of ARBs, therefore, are more difficult to interpret than those involving ACE inhibitors or CCBs. Nonetheless, some meta-analyses have suggested that ARBs are less effective than, for example, ACE inhibitors in preventing myocardial infarction, but perhaps more effective in preventing stroke [due primarily to the Losartan Intervention For Endpoint reduction trial, (LIFE)]. Because only a few small trials directly compared an ARB with an ACE inhibitor, precise estimates of their relative effectiveness in preventing morbidity and mortality in hypertensive patients are not yet available.

Blood pressure lowering versus drug class. The most recent comprehensive prospective meta-analysis undertaken by the Blood Pressure (BP)-Lowering Treatment Trialists' Collaboration concluded that all BP-lowering regimens were broadly comparable (and similar) for reducing cardiovascular events in patients with and without diabetes. Lower BP goals resulted in larger reductions in major cardiovascular events in diabetic patients. A similar benefit of a lower-than-usual BP in patients with chronic kidney disease has been seen in some studies (Appropriate BP Control in Diabetes) and meta-analyses. In contrast, other trials (Second Ramipril Efficacy in Nephropathy and African American Study of Kidney disease and hypertension trials) specifically designed to examine renal endpoints suggested that there was no incremental value to BP-lowering to values <130/80 mm Hg compared to <140/90 mm Hg.

Network meta-analyses

This new type of meta-analysis not only allows direct comparisons of two drug types used as initial treatments in the same trial, but also incorporates "indirect comparisons" (e.g., ACE inhibitor vs. D vs. ARB). This strategy is particularly useful when the agents have not been compared in the same study (e.g., ACE inhibitor vs. ARB in the example mentioned in the preceding text). This strategy can include all the clinical trial data about each endpoint of interest and allows comparisons of all major drug classes, each versus an arbitrary standard (including placebo, if desired).

In 2003, the initial report of a network meta-analysis of antihypertensive drug treatment included 42 clinical trials involving 192,478 patients and seven major treatment strategies. Low-dose diuretics were significantly superior to placebo for all cardiovascular events studied, and no other strategy was significantly better than low-dose diuretics for any endpoint. Network meta-analysis has been used to compare antihypertensive drugs (and placebo) regarding incident diabetes mellitus in 24 clinical trials involving 143,153 subjects. Although not all subjects in the included studies were hypertensive, the results showed significantly higher rates of incident diabetes with an initial diuretic or β-blocker, compared to an ARB or an ACE inhibitor. Preliminary reports of network meta-analyses of antihypertensive drugs on cardiovascular events in 64 clinical trials involving 376,370 subjects have generally concurred with the results of traditional meta-analyses.

"Blood pressure-independent" benefits in clinical trials

Certain investigators have interpreted the results of specific trials [e.g., Heart Outcomes Prevention Evaluation (HOPE), LIFE, Irbesartan Diabetic Nephropathy Trial, Morbidity and Mortality after Stroke: Eprosartan vs. nitrendipine Study] as evidence that certain drugs may have "benefits beyond BP control" based on morbidity or mortality benefits in excess of those attributable

to BP differences between the randomized groups. On further investigation, however, it is unclear that there are actually BP-independent benefits.

Meta-regression studies. The Blood Pressure-Lowering Treatment Trialists' Collaborators used a meta-regression analysis to document a significant correlation between degree of reduction in morbidity/mortality endpoints (except heart failure) and degree of reduction in systolic BP. Most of the results of clinical trials completed after 1995 using various agents (circles in **Figure B100.2**) fall within the 95% confidence interval (CI) for the meta-regression equation (dotted lines in **Figure B100.2**), suggesting that no single antihypertensive drug class offers benefits beyond BP control. Casas et al. performed a set of meta-regression analyses of trials involving renal outcomes and concluded that the renal benefits of antihypertensive drugs could be attributed largely to BP lowering rather than specific effects of an ACE inhibitor or ARB. This conclusion contradicts the results of at least four trials designed prospectively to evaluate the benefits of ACE inhibitors or ARBs in renal disease.

Insensitivity of standard cuff blood pressure determinations. Two additional studies cast doubt on the concept that certain agents offer benefits beyond BP control, pointing to the insensitivity of standard office cuff BP determinations. A substudy of HOPE in patients with peripheral arterial disease demonstrated that mean 24-hour ambulatory BPs were 10/4 mm Hg lower in the ACE inhibitor–treated patients, whereas the difference was only 3/2 mm Hg using the clinic cuff BPs in the main study. This BP difference could fully account for all of the apparent benefits of ACE inhibition in HOPE.

Limitations of brachial cuff BP sensitivity have also been highlighted by the Conduit Artery Function Evaluation (CAFÉ) substudy of the Anglo-Scandinavian Cardiac Outcomes Trial

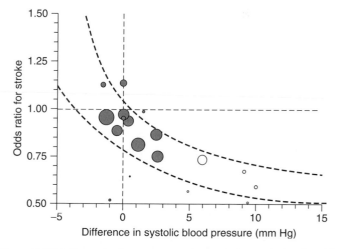

Figure B100.2 Example of a meta-regression analysis correlating the odds ratio for stroke (y-axis) with the difference in systolic blood pressure between randomized treatment groups (x-axis) for 170,139 hypertensive subjects enrolled in 24 clinical trials comparing an initial calcium channel blocker versus other treatment. Each circle represents a single comparison; the area of the circle is proportional to the number of strokes involved in the comparison. *Open circles* are placebo-controlled comparisons; *shaded circles* denote comparisons of antihypertensive drugs. The identities of the trials have been suppressed for clarity. The *curved dotted lines* are the 95% confidence intervals for a prior meta-regression line based on stroke outcomes involving 136,124 patients enrolled in 27 earlier studies. (Adapted from Elliott WJ, Jonsson MC, Black HR. It's NOT "Beyond the Blood Pressure," It IS the Blood Pressure. *Circulation* 2006; 113:2763–2772.)

(ASCOT), where arterial tonometry was used to estimate central aortic BP. Despite equal decreases in brachial cuff BP in the randomized groups, aortic systolic BP was approximately 4 mm Hg lower in the amlodipine-perindopril arm, potentially explaining an effect that some consider "beyond BP."

General pitfalls and limitations of antihypertensive drug trials

In the current hierarchy of "evidence-based medicine," randomized clinical trials and meta-analyses rank highest. Well-designed and executed clinical trials and meta-analyses generally yield the most reliable data on which to base treatment strategies, simply because the measures taken to reduce bias are not possible in cohort or case–control study designs. For this reason alone, the results of clinical trials are less likely than other study types to be confounded. Nevertheless, these studies all suffer from major flaws and their conclusions are rarely universally accepted.

Clinical trial problems. The largest sources of interpretative error are the narrow inclusion and exclusion criteria, which not only limit the pool of patients that might be enrolled, but also restrict the generalizability of the trial's conclusions. Most clinical trials use a composite primary endpoint, to reduce sample size, duration, and expense but often commingle outcomes with different pathophysiologic mechanisms, thereby diluting potentially important disease-specific benefits. Duration of study is another major deficiency of many trials; in hypertension, few clinical trials observe subjects for more than 5 years, whereas many complications (e.g., outcomes of higher blood sugar with thiazides) would not be expected to occur for 15 to 20 years. The total disease burden is also missed in studies that only include the time to the first adverse outcome rather than total disease prevalence (including multiple events per subject). Clinical trials typically employ a prespecified sequence of several drugs but the confounding caused by the additional drugs is typically ignored and differences in outcomes are usually attributed only to the first-line treatment. Most clinical trials have difficulty with subjects adhering to the protocol, which usually dilutes the overall effect. Use of other (typically newer) treatments differently across randomized arms after randomization can confound the overall results. Clinical trials are also traditionally analyzed by the "intent-to-treat" principle, which attributes an adverse event to a strategy that many participants never receive. Subgroup analyses, secondary endpoints, and *post hoc* comparisons are, by definition, subject to serious deficiencies in statistical power. Ethical principles sometimes prohibit a placebo as the comparator,

and choice of an appropriate "active control" treatment can be difficult and problematic. Randomization is the most effective way to reduce bias in assigning treatments, but occasionally it is unsuccessful. Single-blind trials can be biased because the investigator knows the identity of the randomized treatment; open-label trials may be even less reliable because the subject is informed of his/her treatment assignment.

Meta-analysis problems. Traditional meta-analyses ignore times-to-event, typically weighting equally those events that happen immediately after randomization and those that happen many years later. Meta-analyses can be unduly influenced by one study with a very high baseline risk of the outcome under study, which is one reason why testing for homogeneity is so important. Lastly, some meta-analyses compare one drug type with any and all other drug types, despite major intrinsic differences in the types of comparators.

Suggested Readings

Casas JP, Chua W, Loukogeorgakis S, et al. Effect of inhibitors of the renin-angiotensin system and other antihypertensive drugs on renal outcomes: systematic review and meta-analysis. *Lancet* 2005;366:2026–2033.

Elliott WJ, Black HR. The evidence-base for treatment of hypertension. In: McInnes GT, editor. *Handbook of hypertension, Volume 24: clinical pharmacology and therapeutics of antihypertensive drugs.* New York: Elsevier Science, 2007 (in press).

Elliott WJ, Jonsson MC, Black HR. It's NOT "Beyond the Blood Pressure," It IS the Blood Pressure. *Circulation* 2006;113:2763–2772.

Elliott WJ, Meyer PM. Incident diabetes in clinical trials of antihypertensive drugs: a network meta-analysis. *Lancet* 2007;269:201–207. Erratum: *Lancet* 2007;269:1518.

Lindholm LH, Carlberg B, Samuelsson O. Should β blockers remain first choice in the treatment of primary hypertension? A meta-analysis. *Lancet* 2005;366:1545–1553.

Mancia G, De Backer G, Dominiczak A, et al. 2007 Guidelines for the management of arterial hypertension. Task Force for the Management of Arterial Hypertension of the European Society of Hypertension and the European Society of Cardiology. *J Hypertens* 2007;25:1105–1187.

Psaty BM, Lumley T, Furberg CD, et al. Health outcomes associated with various antihypertensive therapies used as first-line agents: a network meta-analysis. *JAMA* 2003;289:2534–2544.

Staessen JA, Wang J-G, Thijs L. Cardiovascular prevention and blood pressure reduction: a quantitative overview updated until 01 March 2003. *J Hypertens* 2003;21:1005–1076.

Turnbull F. Blood Pressure Lowering Treatment Trialists' Collaboration. Effects of different blood-pressure-lowering regimens on major cardiovascular events: results of prospectively-designed overviews of randomised trials. *Lancet* 2003;362:1527–1535.

Turnbull F, Neal B, Algert C, et al. Blood Pressure Lowering Treatment Trialists' Collaboration. Effects of different blood pressure – lowering regimens on major cardiovascular events in individuals with and without diabetes mellitus: results of prospectively designed overviews of randomized trials. *Arch Intern Med* 2005;165:1410–1419.

CHAPTER B101 ■ ANTIHYPERTENSIVE TREATMENT TRIALS: QUALITY OF LIFE

RICHARD H. GRIMM, Jr., MD, PhD AND CARRIE L. SCHLEIS, MA

KEY POINTS

- *Quality of life* is defined as the patient's ability to function well in daily living, including psychologic and physical well-being, social and leisure activity, and satisfaction with life.
- Past clinical trials, including the Hypertension Optimal Treatment (HOT) study and the Treatment of Mild Hypertension Study (TOMHS), have shown better control of blood pressure (BP) was associated with enhanced quality of life.
- Both lifestyle modifications (especially weight loss) and antihypertensive drugs often improve quality-of-life measures.

See also Chapters B102 and **C119**

Historically, the treatment of hypertension with drugs was believed to diminish quality of life owing to side effects and adverse events. However, several large trials have now demonstrated that quality of life is not reduced with effective antihypertensive therapy. Often, "hidden" symptoms and overall quality of life are improved when effective blood pressure (BP) control is achieved with drugs or lifestyle modifications.

Quality of life: definition and measurement

Quality of life is a measure of a patient's ability to function well in daily living, including psychologic and physical well-being, social and leisure activity, and general satisfaction. It has been suggested that quality of life is the gap between patient expectations and achievements.

A wide variety of instruments has been used to measure quality of life, most of which are questionnaire based. These range from the Sickness Impact Profile, which comprises 136 questions, to the Battery-of-Scales Quality-of-Life Questionnaire, which has 22 questions. One of the most commonly used assessment tools is the Short Form 36 (SF 36), which consists of 36 questions. Seven domains have been identified as relevant to hypertensive patients: general health, psychologic well-being, sleep disturbance, social function, sexual function, cognitive function, and symptom control.

Clinical trials

Dietary Approaches to Stop Hypertension studies. The Dietary Approaches to Stop Hypertension (DASH) trial examined the effects of three dietary patterns on BP and quality of life. The

balanced combination diet, also termed the *DASH diet* (rich in fruits, vegetables, and low-fat dairy products, with reduced saturated and total fat) significantly reduced BP compared to a control diet, especially in elderly individuals. A diet rich in fruits and vegetables but otherwise similar to the control also significantly reduced BP. Quality of life was measured with the SF 36 questionnaire and showed improvement in all three treatment groups. When the subscales were summed into a total score, quality of life improved 4% in the control diet group, 5% in the fruits and vegetables diet group, and 5.9% in the DASH diet group.

Salt restriction. Two trials of nonpharmacologic therapies, the Trials of Hypertension Prevention (TOHP) and the Trial of Nonpharmacological Interventions in the Elderly (TONE), tested the effects of sodium reduction and weight loss. In each case, decreased BP was associated with improved quality of life. The Treatment of Mild Hypertension Study (TOMHS) compared medical therapies but also included a nonpharmacologic component to reduce weight, dietary sodium and alcohol intake, and to increase physical activity. Improved quality of life was measured by a 35-item questionnaire and included seven indexes: general health, energy or fatigue, mental health, general functioning, satisfaction with physical abilities, social functioning, and social contacts.

Weight loss. Almost all measures of quality of life improve significantly with greater weight loss. Overall, greater weight loss, increased physical activity, and improved BP control were each associated with improvements in quality of life.

Active drug comparisons. In TOMHS, quality of life improved in all active drug groups compared to placebo (**Table B101.1**). The most significant improvement among drugs was

TABLE B101.1

MEAN CHANGE FROM BASELINE IN QUALITY-OF-LIFE INDICES AVERAGED OVER ALL FOLLOW-UP VISITS FOR ALL ACTIVE DRUGS COMBINED (PLUS LIFESTYLE) AND PLACEBO (PLUS LIFESTYLE) IN THE TREATMENT OF MILD HYPERTENSION STUDY (TOMHS)

| Quality-of-life index | All active (N = 653) | | Placebo (N = 230) | | p value |
	Mean	SE	Mean	SE	Active vs. placebo
General health	1.26	0.16	0.98	0.25	.10
Energy or fatigue	0.95	0.1	0.67	0.17	.03
Mental health	2.14	0.23	1.43	0.43	.01
General functioning	−0.03	0.06	−0.32	0.1	.01
Satisfaction with physical abilities	0.38	0.03	0.25	0.05	.07
Social functioning	0.12	0.03	−0.12	0.06	.004
Social contacts	0.09	0.06	0.15	0.11	.75
Global quality-of-life statistic	450.10	5.65	420.31	9.39	.007

SE, standard error.
(Adapted from Grimm RH Jr, Prineas R1, Roel J, et al. The treatment of mild hypertension (TOMHS): design and additional analyses. In: Black HR, ed. *Clinical trials in hypertension.* New York: Marcel Dekker Inc, 2001.)

with thiazide diuretic (chlorthalidone) and β-blocker (acebutolol). Older studies demonstrated higher quality-of-life scores with angiotensin-converting enzyme (ACE) inhibition (captopril) than sympatholytic (methyldopa).

Adverse drug effects versus placebos. All drug treatments have the potential to produce bothersome side effects. A reportable adverse effect in drug development studies is considered by convention to be any symptom or complaint that occurs in any patient taking a particular drug, whether or not the symptom is causally related to the drug. In placebo-controlled studies, incidence rates of adverse effects in patients on placebo are frequently no higher than active drug-treated patients. Studies comparing angiotensin-receptor blockade (ARB) to placebo are interesting in that the adverse events on ARB therapy are usually lower than placebo.

Certain hypertension drugs have well-known side effects which have been observed in numerous trials. For instance, in the Swedish Trial in Old Patients with Hypertension-2 (STOP-2), the dihydropyridine calcium antagonist resulted in ankle edema in 25.5% of patients, whereas the ACE inhibitor was associated with dry cough in 30% of patients.

Blood pressure level. The Hypertension Optimal Treatment (HOT) study tested the impact of three different levels of diastolic BP control (<80 mm Hg, <85 mm Hg, and <90 mm Hg) on cardiovascular event rates in patients with stage 1 and 2 diastolic hypertension. In this trial, diastolic BP was reduced to <90 mm Hg in approximately 90% of patients and to <80 mm Hg in approximately 60% of patients with structured, stepped-care therapy in a general practice setting. There was a low incidence of side effects among all three treatment groups, indicating that antihypertensive drugs in combination can achieve target BP with minimal side effects.

Cognition. Cognitive function is an important contributor to quality of life especially in the elderly. With an increasing older population, much more attention is being given to cognitive function and dementia. Staessen et al. reviewed this topic and pooled results of five trials that assessed dementia. In the Systolic Hypertension in the Elderly Program (SHEP), the Systolic Hypertension in Europe (Syst-EUR) study, and in the ACE/diuretic combined subgroup of PROGRESS, there was a 25% reduction in incidence of dementia with BP reduction.

Suggested Readings

Fletcher A. Quality of life in the management of hypertension. *Clin Exp Hypertens* 1999;21:961–972.

Grimm RH Jr, Grandits GA, Cutler JA, et al. TOMHS Research Group. Relationships of quality of life measures to long-term lifestyle and drug treatment in the treatment of mild hypertension study (TOMHS). *Arch Intern Med* 1997;157:638–648.

Hansson L. The hypertension optimal treatment study and the importance of lowering BP. *J Hypertens Suppl* 1999;17:S9–S13.

Hansson L, Lindholm LH, Ekbom T, et al. Randomised trial of old and new antihypertensive drugs in elderly patients: cardiovascular mortality and morbidity in the Swedish trial in old patients with hypertension-2 study. *Lancet* 1999;354:1751–1756.

McInnes G. Integrated approaches to management of hypertension: promoting treatment acceptance. *Am Heart J* 1999;138:S252–S255.

Nunes MI. Quality of life in the elderly hypertensive. *J Cardiovasc Risk* 2001;8:265–269.

Plaisted C, Lin P-H, Ard J, et al. The effects of dietary patterns on quality of life: a substudy of the dietary approaches to stop hypertension trial. *J Am Diet Assoc* 1999;99:S84–S89.

Roel JP, Hildebrant CL, Grimm RH Jr. Quality-of-life with nonpharmacologic treatment of hypertension. *Curr Hypertens Rep* 2001;3:466–472.

Staessen JA, Richart T, Birkenhager WH. Less atherosclerosis and lower BP for a meaningful life perspective with more brain. *Hypertension* 2007;49:389–400.

Testa M. Methods and applications of quality-of-life measurement during antihypertensive therapy. *Curr Hypertens Rep* 2000;2:598–615.

CHAPTER B102 ■ ECONOMIC CONSIDERATIONS IN HYPERTENSION MANAGEMENT

WILLIAM J. ELLIOTT, MD, PhD

KEY POINTS

■ Cost-effectiveness calculations compute the cost per year of life saved, balancing the overall cost of treatment against its effectiveness in avoiding expensive adverse clinical outcomes.

■ Cost-utility analyses further incorporate quality-of-life data and adjust for disabilities from side effects of treatment and nonfatal adverse outcomes.

■ Beneficial cost-effectiveness ratios occur in patients at high risk of cardiovascular disease [e.g., diabetics or older patients with higher initial blood pressure (BP)] and when expensive outcomes are prevented (e.g., dialysis).

■ The cost-effectiveness ratio for treating hypertension may be improved by accurately diagnosing hypertension, assessing absolute risk for cardiovascular events, selecting treatments that minimize the total cost of care (although not adversely affecting quality of life), enhancing medication adherence, and avoiding unnecessary office visits or laboratory testing.

See also Chapter C119

Calculations of economic aspects of hypertension therapy

Cost-effectiveness and cost-utility. Cost-effectiveness calculations are a formalized method of comparing the cost of an intervention with the (discounted) benefits that presumably accrue to a population to whom it is administered. The cost-effectiveness ratio is the cost per year of extended life and depends on several factors (**Table B102.1**). Cost-utility analyses add a downward adjustment for the value of each year of extended life, using quality-of-life data for discomfort or disability owing to either side effects of treatment or nonfatal adverse events. Such analyses have units of cost per quality-adjusted life-year saved. Although there are wide regional and temporal variations in the cost of medicines and medical services, these calculations are being widely used to support treatment guidelines, both locally (by managed care organizations) and nationally (as in those provided in 2006 by the British National Institute for health and Clinical Excellence, NICE).

Figure B102.1 shows their results using the "base case" of a 65-year-old hypertensive man (left panel) or woman (right panel) with a 2% annual risk of cardiovascular events, a 1.1% annual risk of diabetes, and a 1% annual risk of heart failure. For each gender, the highest number of quality-adjusted life-years saved was attributable to initial calcium channel blocker therapy, although the lowest overall cost was seen with a thiazide diuretic. Similar results have been presented based on

the Antihypertensive and Lipid Lowering to prevent Heart Attack Trial (ALLHAT), despite a fivefold higher acquisition cost of amlodipine ($630/year) compared to $123 per year in the NICE analysis.

These types of analyses usually have their baseline parameters varied widely in "sensitivity analyses." **Table B102.2** shows the "incremental cost-effectiveness ratios" when baseline patient age or cardiovascular risk is altered in the computer model. In the NICE model, a higher baseline risk of diabetes or heart failure changes the most cost-effective initial strategy to an

TABLE B102.1

MAJOR DETERMINANTS OF THE COST-EFFECTIVENESS RATIO

The absolute risk for cardiovascular events for a given patient (which depends on age, BP stage, and concomitant diseases and comorbidities)
The efficacy of treatment in reducing the future risk of expensive adverse clinical events (e.g., stroke, myocardial infarction, heart failure, dialysis, or renal transplantation)
The (discounted) future cost of these adverse events
The total cost of treatment

BP, blood pressure.

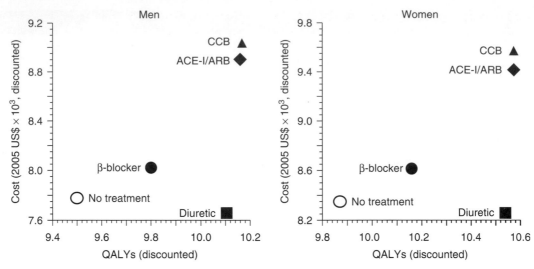

Figure B102.1 Results of cost-utility analyses by the British National Institute for Health and Clinical Excellence (NICE) regarding initial drug treatment for hypertension in a 65-year-old patient with an annual 2% risk of cardiovascular events, 1.1% risk of diabetes, and 1% risk for heart failure. Values on the x-axis represent quality-adjusted life-years (QALYs) saved; values on the y-axis represent lifetime cost of treatment (in thousands of US$), both of which are discounted at 3.5% per annum. The 2005 cost of amlodipine used in these calculations was approximately fivefold lower than its acquisition cost in the USA in 2005. CCB, calcium channel blocker; ACE-I, angiotensin-converting enzyme inhibitor; ARB, angiotensin receptor blocker. (Adapted, with permission, from the NICE partial update of Clinical Guideline 34.)

angiotensin-converting enzyme (ACE)-inhibitor (or angiotensin receptor blocker) or diuretic, respectively.

Effect of risk. Table B102.2 shows, as in many previous analyses, that higher-risk patients [e.g., older people with higher initial blood pressure (BP)] have lower (i.e., more beneficial) cost-effectiveness ratios. Negative (i.e., money-*saving*) ratios result when very high-risk patients (e.g., diabetic patients or those with a recent cardiovascular event) are treated with effective drugs, or when expensive events (e.g., dialysis) are prevented. These conclusions drawn from computer models are somewhat pessimistic compared to "real-world data" from Sweden, where the government carefully monitors both the costs and benefits of health care, and where drug treatment of older hypertensives *saves* money overall.

Improving the cost-effectiveness of hypertension therapy

Giving antihypertensive drugs to everyone with elevated BP costs money, overall. Judging the value of the return on that capital outlay is an important societal issue that requires a thorough and sober analysis. Nonetheless, there are several simple steps that can be easily incorporated into medical practice that could improve the cost-effectiveness ratio of hypertension treatment. These include (a) accurate diagnosis and classification of hypertension, (b) baseline risk assessment to determine whether costly medications should be prescribed, (c) choosing drug therapy that leads to the lowest overall cost, (d) maximizing patients' adherence to medications, and (e) reducing unnecessary office visits and laboratory testing.

TABLE B102.2

INCREMENTAL COST-EFFECTIVENESS RATIOS[a] FOR TREATMENT OF HYPERTENSION, ACCORDING TO BASELINE AGE AND ANNUAL CARDIOVASCULAR RISK IN GREAT BRITAIN

Annual CV risk (%)	Age (yr) for men				Age (yr) for women			
	55	65	75	85	55	65	75	85
0.5	$45,751	$27,454	$19,428	$18,491	$ 76,811	$35,975	$25,191	$20,524
1	$60,176	$28,868	$17,731	$17,360	$134,441	$41,031	$21,320	$18,580
2	$54,324	$21,656	$15,221	$15,521	$ 67,583	$23,848	$16,458	$15,663
3	$32,687	$17,660	$13,435	$14,072	$ 30,618	$17,271	$13,541	$13,577
5	$19,605	$13,400	$11,119	$12,003	$ 16,087	$11,721	$10,253	$10,819

CV, cardiovascular.
[a]In dollars per year of quality-adjusted life-year saved (compared to no treatment); exchange rate: 1 GB£ = US $1.7678 on 01 July 05. (Adapted, with permission, from the partial update of the NICE Clinical Guideline 34.)

Accurate diagnosis of hypertension. Approximately 20% of individuals with elevated BPs in the medical office setting have white coat hypertension and probably do not benefit from drug therapy to the same extent as people with sustained hypertension. Ambulatory BP monitoring is effective in documenting white coat hypertension, so selective use of ambulatory BP monitoring could lead to an overall reduction in costs. Medicare reimburses a nominal amount for this procedure in the United States but only when specific criteria are met. Home BP monitoring and multiple office visits to document the presence of sustained hypertension are more commonly used to avoid "wasting" treatment costs on patients who are at low cardiovascular risk.

Risk stratification before therapy. Most guidelines recommend formal risk stratification before prescribing drug therapy. For some patients with low baseline risk (without other risk factors, target organ damage, or cardiovascular disease), even with BPs as high as 159/99 mm Hg, lifestyle modifications are often recommended before initiating drug therapy. This practice may improve the cost-effectiveness ratio because it delays starting patients on drug therapy if they are at very low risk for cardiovascular events. At the other extreme, drug therapy should be intensified until the BP is below 130/80 mm Hg in patients with diabetes, chronic kidney disease, or ischemic heart disease. More intensive BP lowering saved lives *and money* in the United Kingdom Prospective Diabetes Study and in the diabetic patients in the Hypertension Optimal Treatment study. Compared to the usual target of <140/90 mm Hg, a BP goal of <130/85 mm Hg is also *cost saving* (due to reductions in expensive hypertension-related morbidity) in American diabetic patients older than 60, as long as the marginal annual cost of such treatment does not exceed $414.

Cost of lifestyle modifications. Lifestyle modifications are still routinely recommended for all hypertensives, although their efficacy in reducing cardiovascular events has never been proven and their true costs to patients are not really known. The Treatment of Mild Hypertension Study showed a slightly but significantly lower rate of cardiovascular events in hypertensive individuals randomized to receive drugs in addition to an excellent program of lifestyle modifications. Lifestyle modification programs are often expensive for individuals to implement and maintain, and long-term adherence among the general population to a low-salt diet, weight control, and physical activity is typically lower than adherence to antihypertensive drug therapy. Public health programs directed toward lifestyle modifications are, however, relatively cost effective, from the perspective of government agencies and health payers, because the cost of public service advertisements is relatively low and the potential for lower BPs across large at-risk populations is substantial.

Limiting costs of medicines. If efficacy were similar against all major adverse outcomes of hypertension, lower-cost medications could be easily recommended over higher-cost drugs. Yet the true lifetime cost of antihypertensive therapy is far more complex, and it is extremely difficult to compare one agent to another. According to estimates from the American Heart Association, antihypertensive medications are the largest part of the total cost of care for hypertension in the United States in 2007 (at $23 billion or 34.6% of the total). Pricing of medications is variable, particularly at pharmacies in large retail chains, where a few generic drugs are available for $4 per month. Costs of generic drugs also vary widely; despite having lower average wholesale prices, generic medications are only slightly less expensive than their branded counterparts in some pharmacies.

Some pharmacy benefits managers have implemented strategies that reduce pharmaceutical expenditures. Although some of these policies may be beneficial, worsened BP control and increased morbid events have been found in several studies. Some "innovations" [e.g., monthly bidding for an exclusive contract to dispense only one ACE inhibitor in a large health maintenance organization] may reduce the pharmacy budget but may also incur more office visits and lead to a higher total cost of care. Patient and physician satisfaction are also negatively affected. Usually, more than one medication is needed to control BP; a few pharmacy programs have begun to realize that certain fixed-dose combination products may cost less than two separate prescriptions, with a lower copayment.

Enhanced medication adherence. Long-term adherence to a medication (sometimes called *persistence*) is seldom considered when performing cost-effectiveness calculations. Yet persistence may be the most important factor in everyday medical practice. Patients who are prescribed antihypertensive medications, but fail to take them properly, incur the costs of therapy but derive little benefit from it, creating a very high cost/benefit ratio. Simple procedures to enhance adherence/persistence include educating the patient about the disease and the medication, prescribing once-daily pills that do not adversely affect quality of life, and minimizing out-of-pocket costs. Besides reducing pharmacy copayments and often having lower acquisition costs than two separate prescriptions, combination pills also limit the "pill burden," which is inversely proportional to long-term adherence.

Improved prescribing habits. Providers contribute to inefficiencies by failing to prescribe effective drugs and combinations. In general, drugs with complementary mechanisms of action (e.g., diuretic + ACE inhibitor) are quite effective. Drugs with similar or overlapping mechanisms of action (e.g., ACE inhibitor + angiotensin receptor blocker) are less effective overall in lowering BP. Because many drugs are relatively flat-priced across the dose range, prescribing 2 × 10 mg of a particular agent is often much more costly than a single 20-mg pill. Some health plans encourage physicians to prescribe "double-dose" pills that can be split by the patient, thereby saving money. Similarly, laboratory testing can often be minimized by choosing effective doses of drug therapy with few adverse metabolic effects.

Reducing health care provider–associated costs. Of the $66.4 billion spent on hypertension treatment in the United States in 2007, the American Heart Association estimates that 26% goes for indirect costs (transportation, time off work, and lost productivity), 19% goes to health care providers, and 18% goes to hospital and nursing home services. If patients were able to monitor home BPs and receive health care advice by telephone or Internet rather than making costly office visits, overall costs could be reduced. As more antihypertensive agents become generically available, the discussion about how to improve the cost-effectiveness of hypertension treatment is likely to shift from a focus on drugs to achieving target BPs and improving outcomes (about which there are few data). Cost-effectiveness analyses will continue to influence the development of "critical pathways" for hypertension treatment.

Suggested Readings

Elliott WJ. The economic impact of hypertension. *J Clin Hypertens (Greenwich)* 2003;5(Suppl 2):3–13.

Elliott WJ, Weir DR, Black HR. Cost-effectiveness of the lower treatment goal (of JNC VI) in hypertensive diabetics. *Arch Intern Med* 2000;160:1277–1283.

Heidenreich PA, Davis BR, Furberg CD, et al. Cost-effectiveness of chlorthalidone, amlodipine and lisinopril as first-line treatment for patients with hypertension: an ALLHAT analysis [Abstract 1028–128]. *J Am Coll Cardiol* 2006;47 (Suppl A):372A.

Jonsson B, Hansson L, Stalhammar NO. Health economics in the hypertension optimal treatment (HOT) study: costs and cost-effectiveness of intensive BP lowering and low-dose aspirin in patients with hypertension. *J Intern Med* 2003;253:472–480.

Montgomery AA, Fahey T, Ben-Shlomo Y, et al. The influence of absolute cardiovascular risk, patient utilities, and costs on the decision to treat hypertension: a Markov decision analysis. *J Hypertens* 2003;21:1753–1759.

Murray CJ, Lauer JA, Hutubessy RC, et al. Effectiveness and costs of interventions to lower systolic BP and cholesterol: a global and regional analysis on reduction of cardiovascular-disease risk. *Lancet* 2003;361:717–725.

National Collaborating Centre for Chronic Conditions. *Hypertension: management of hypertension in adults in primary care: partial update*. London: Royal College of Physicians, Found on the Internet at: http://www.nice.org.uk/guidance/CG34/guidance/pdf/English. Accessed 06 July 2006.

Osterberg L, Blaschke T. Adherence to medication. *N Engl J Med* 2005;353:487–497.

Raikou M, Gray A, Briggs A, et al. Cost-effectiveness analysis of improved BP control in hypertensive patients with type 2 diabetes: UKPDS 40. U.K. Prospective Diabetes Study Group. *Br Med J* 1998;317:720–726.

Rodriguez-Roca GC, Alonso-Moreno FJ, Garcia-Jimenez A, et al. Cost-effectiveness of ambulatory BP monitoring in the follow-up of hypertension. *Blood Press* 2006;15:27–36.

CHAPTER C103 ■ BLOOD PRESSURE MEASUREMENT

CARLENE M. GRIM, MSN, SpDN AND CLARENCE E. GRIM, MS, MD

KEY POINTS

- Hypertension detection, referral, and treatment guidelines are based on measurements by trained observers using the mercury sphygmomanometer, following standard techniques recommended by the American Heart Association (AHA).
- Regardless of the device used, blood pressure (BP) measurement accuracy requires initial standardized training and assessment. Accuracy can be improved with continued regular updates, and frequent performance evaluation for all observers.
- Readings from automated devices (particularly diastolic BP) may differ from standard measurements; automated devices are difficult to calibrate and do not fully eliminate human or technical errors.
- A protocol requiring regular maintenance and calibration of all BP measurement instruments should be the standard of care in all settings.

See also Chapters **C104, C105,** C161, and C163

Indirect blood pressure measurement

Blood Pressure (BP) measurement is safe, painless, and provides reliable information when performed accurately. Virtually all epidemiologic data used to determine hypertension detection, referral, and treatment guidelines are based on BPs obtained by the standardized indirect measurement method recommended by the American Heart Association (AHA). Health professionals base crucial clinical decisions on these measurements; therefore, the proven benefits of treating high BP can be accomplished only when BP measurement is performed accurately. Accurate BP measurement requires the ability to hear, interpret, and record Korotkoff sounds; and the ability to properly operate the equipment. *Failure to practice correct technique and the use of inaccurate equipment are the major reasons for inaccurate BP readings.*

Initial standardized training and lifetime performance monitoring

Lack of knowledge about accurate BP measurement technique can often be traced back to initial observer training. The most recent

AHA guidelines stress the importance of initial standardized training for all who are taught to measure BP with regular update and continued competency assessment throughout one's career. Updates should also include a review of clinic applications for recent advances in BP measurement.

Selecting and caring for blood pressure measurement equipment

Manometer. The manual pressure registering device (*manometer*) is a mercury or an aneroid instrument calibrated to the nearest 2 mm Hg. The mercury manometer, when read at the top edge (the meniscus) of the mercury column, is the most accurate measurement device available and is considered the primary standard for all BP measurements. Its accuracy is calibrated by observing whether the mercury meniscus rests at zero. The *aneroid* manometer consists of a metal bellows that expands as the pressure in the cuff increases and is read at the point indicated by a needle on its dial. The aneroid (usually a round gauge) is fragile, easily damaged during normal use, and is not always accurate even when the needle rests at "0". Portable aneroids should be fitted

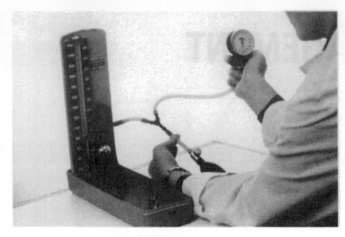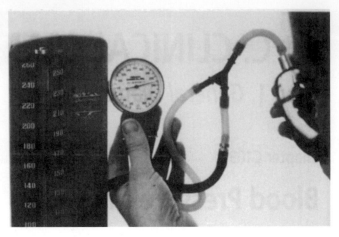

Figure C103.1 Aneroid instrument being tested by inserting a Y-tube connector or stopcock to create a communicating system with one pressure source, allowing simultaneous pressure application to both instruments. (Courtesy of Shared Care Research and Education Consulting, Inc., Milwaukee, WI.)

with a rubber gauge guard to help prevent mechanical damage. A "Y" connector must be used to connect and compare its pressure registering system to an accurate mercury manometer at least every 6 months (**Figure C103.1**). Recalibration is required if the difference between aneroid and mercury readings is ≥3 mm Hg. To improve and ensure accuracy, practice settings must institute a regular (at least every 6 months) calibration program for all instruments. When mercury-free settings are unable to keep one standard mercury instrument for calibrating aneroid and nonmercury devices, a nonmercury pressure calibration device must be purchased and used. All non-mercury calibration devices must be annually calibrated against a device that can be traced back to a mercury standard within the last year.

Stethoscope. The stethoscope head should have a low-frequency detector (bell) for listening to the low-pitched sounds. Earpieces should fit comfortably forward in the direction of the ear canal and block out external noise. For best sound transmission, the tubing should be thick and no longer than 15 in.

Automated blood pressure measurement devices

Automated devices should be checked in two ways before use. First, the observer must document accuracy by using a "Y-tube" to connect and compare the automated BP instrument to an accurate mercury device. Next, simultaneous (or sequential) digital and mercury readings should be compared in the individual patient. The use of automated devices is discouraged in most clinical settings because they are often difficult to calibrate, may fail to give accurate readings on many individuals, and do not eliminate technical and human errors due to poor preparation, environment, incorrect cuff size, and improper positioning.

Steps needed to obtain accurate and reliable readings

Standardized recording methods are necessary to correctly interpret and compare readings by different observers.

Step 1: Clinical setting. The setting should be private and quiet, with a comfortable room temperature. To get the best estimate of the patient's usual BP, one must control for environmental factors that may cause BP variation or interfere with one's ability to hear Korotkoff sounds.

Device positioning. Aneroid and mercury devices must be positioned at the observer's eye level (not necessarily the level of the heart or arm) because viewing the manometer above or below one's eye level reduces accuracy. The height of the table(s) should be such that the midpoint of the cuff while in place on the patient's right arm (or the arm known to produce the higher BP reading) is supported at heart level. It is important to minimize differences in hydrostatic pressure between the cuff and the point of artery compression at the center of the cuff. If the center of the cuff on the arm or leg is above heart level, the reading will be falsely low by 0.8 mm Hg for each 1 cm above heart level; if below heart level, it will be falsely high by a similar amount. Use adjustable tables, chairs, cushions, or phone books to elevate the patient or his arm to achieve the proper height.

Patient positioning. The room should be furnished with a straight-backed chair to provide back support, a table or desk to support the arm, a seat for the BP observer, and an adjustable table surface to support the arm during standing readings. When sitting, legs should not be dangling and a foot stool may be necessary. Foot and back support is important to avoid false high readings due to isometric muscle contraction; lack of back and foot support, such as occurs when the patient is seated on an examination table, causes diastolic BP elevation of approximately 5 mm Hg.

Step 2: Preparation and rest period. Proper preparation and a 5-minute rest before taking the first measurement help prevent elevated readings due to anticipation or anxiety about the measurement. Instruct patients to sit up straight with legs uncrossed, rest back against the chair, keep feet flat on the floor, and remain silent until after BP readings are completed. Talking or active listening during measurement causes BP elevation. Discuss the reason for repeated readings to achieve an average. Minimize biologic factors that may cause BP variation, such as pain, stress, full urinary bladder, and recent intake in order to get the best estimate of the patient's usual BP and note recent ingestion of prescription, over-the-counter or street drugs, caffeine, and nicotine that can affect BP readings. Place the cuff on a bare arm. Clothing interferes with cuff placement, pressure, and transmission of sound. Have patients with tight sleeves or multiple layers remove their arm(s) from the constricting sleeve(s) before placing the cuff.

Step 3: Proper cuff (bladder) size.

Using a bladder too narrow or too short for the limb is a common error that results in false high readings. To get an accurate reading, the *width* of the cuff bladder should encircle at least 40% of the limb circumference. The *bladder length* should be at least twice its width allowing the length of the bladder to encircle at least 80% of limb circumference. Determine and document arm circumference at the patient's first visit by measuring around the upper arm, midway between the olecranon and acromion processes. Do not rely on the manufacturer's marked cuff size until you have validated accuracy using the 40%/80% rule. When arm measurement is not practical, *estimate* correct cuff size by wrapping the width of the bladder around the arm at its midpoint, checking to see that it reaches almost halfway around the arm. *Chart* the appropriate cuff/bladder size for each patient.

Step 4: Cuff placement

Choice of arms. BP can differ by >10 mm Hg between arms. When unable to measure BP in both arms, the reading should be taken in the right arm. Diseases that cause BP differences between the arms are much more likely to cause a falsely low BP in the left arm. The higher pressure more accurately reflects intraarterial pressure. Arm choice should be noted prominently in the record; once chosen, it is not necessary to measure BP in both arms at each visit.

Cuff positioning. After choosing the arm, locate the patient's brachial artery at the midpoint of the upper arm by palpating between the biceps and triceps muscles on its inner surface. Wrap the cuff smoothly and snugly around the arm with its bladder center directly over the palpated artery and the lower edge of the cuff 2.5 cm (1 in.) above the antecubital fossa. Centering bladder pressure avoids false high readings that occur when cuff pressure is not equally distributed over the artery. Allowing enough space for the stethoscope avoids errors that result when the bell touches the cuff or tubing and causes extraneous sounds that mask and distort Korotkoff sounds.

Step 5: Two-step method for determining the maximum inflation level.

Optimal technique employs the minimum pressure needed to obtain an accurate systolic reading, decreases patient discomfort, and avoids errors that result from failure to inflate above the systolic BP reading. In some people, there is an "auscultatory gap" (disappearance of sounds) between the first and third Korotkoff phases. Therefore, an accurate systolic or diastolic reading is dependent on careful assessment of the maximum inflation level (MIL).

1. First, locate the radial pulse and note the heart rate and rhythm. When the heart rate is irregular, systolic BP may vary beat to beat, and additional readings are needed to get the best estimate of the systolic BP. Continue feeling the pulse while rapidly inflating the cuff. When cuff pressure reaches 60 mm Hg, begin inflating by 10-mm increments until the pulse is no longer palpable. Pulse obliteration is the first estimate of the palpated systolic. Begin deflation at 2 mm Hg per second, noting the pressure at which the pulse reappears. Pulse reappearance indicates the palpated systolic pressure and is usually within 10 mm Hg of pulse obliteration. Immediately release all pressure.

2. Wait 15 to 30 seconds. Add 30 mm Hg to the palpated systolic reading to obtain the MIL.

Step 6: Stethoscope placement.

Position the stethoscope earpieces pointing forward in the direction of the ear canal to allow unobstructed sound transmission. Locate the point where the brachial artery pulse is strongest, usually just above the antecubital fossa on the inner aspect of the arm, where the loudest sounds can be heard. The bell or a low-frequency detector is recommended to best hear the low-pitched Korotkoff sounds. Minimize errors in hearing and interpreting Korotkoff sounds by using light pressure to position the stethoscope below the cuff with all edges gently touching the skin surface. Too much stethoscope pressure may cause artery occlusion and distortion of BP sounds.

Step 7: Inflation and deflation.

Rapidly inflate the cuff to the MIL determined in step 5. Slow inflation traps venous blood in the arm and may result in pain and diminished or distorted sounds. If sounds are heard immediately, completely release all pressure and repeat step 5 to estimate the systolic pressure. Slow deflation is necessary to allow the observer to hear the systolic and diastolic pressures at the point of onset. A reading can be no more accurate than the rate of deflation (i.e., a deflation rate of 10 mm Hg/second results in a pressure accurate to only 10 mm Hg; if one beat is missed, to only 20 mm Hg). Release the air from the cuff so that the mercury falls at a rate of 2 mm Hg per second until Korotkoff sounds are heard and continue deflation at the rate of 2 mm Hg per beat. If unable to hear sounds clearly, quickly release all pressure, check and reposition the eartips and bell, and repeat the procedure.

Step 8: Systolic blood pressure.

Korotkoff sounds are designated as K1 through K5. Remember the systolic pressure (at

---

TABLE C103.1

PHASES OF THE KOROTKOFF (K) SOUNDS[a]

K1
The pressure level at which the first faint, consistent tapping sounds are heard. Sounds gradually increase in intensity as the cuff is deflated. The first of at least two of these sounds is defined as the *systolic pressure.*

K2
The time during cuff deflation when a murmur or swishing sounds are heard.

K3
The period during which sounds are crisper and increase in intensity.

K4
The time when a distinct, abrupt, muffling of sound (usually of a soft blowing quality) is heard. This is defined as the *diastolic pressure* in anyone in whom sounds continue to zero.

K5
The pressure level when the last regular BP sound is heard and after which all sound disappears. This is defined as the *diastolic pressure* unless sounds are heard to zero.

BP, blood pressure.
[a]*Variations.* The observer must recognize two normal Korotkoff sound variations associated with BP readings. An auscultatory gap is a period of silence between K1 and K3 where sounds disappear temporarily; it is usually short but can be as much as 40 mm Hg, often associated with higher systolic BP readings. An absent Korotkoff phase 5 occurs when sounds are heard to zero and should be recorded as K1/K4/K5, for example, 162/62/0 mm Hg; in this case, K4 is the best estimate of diastolic pressure.

the onset of Korotkoff phase 1 is the first of at least two regular "tapping" sounds (**Table C103.1**) read to the nearest 2 mm Hg mark). When the reading falls between two 2 mm Hg marks, round to the higher of the two. Forgetting the systolic reading is a very common source of error, often 8 to 10 mm Hg, especially when the pulse pressure (difference between the systolic and diastolic pressures) is wide. Improve memory and concentration by silently repeating the systolic number with every beat until you confirm disappearance (K5, the last regular sound). Observers must learn to rule out artifacts and recognize arrhythmias; single sounds that are inconsistent with heart rate are insignificant. Additional readings are needed to get the best estimate of the systolic BP when arrhythmias are present.

Step 9: Diastolic blood pressure.
Remember the point at which the last regular Korotkoff sound (K5, the diastolic BP) is heard. The onset of K5 (disappearance) is more reliably interpreted when observers listen for the last regular sound itself compared to the absence of sound. Immediately record systolic and diastolic BPs to minimize memory errors. When K5 is absent, the onset of K4 (the muffling of sounds) is the most accurate diastolic BP indicator. When the sounds continue to very low diastolic levels (or zero, i.e., absence of K5), remember and record the onset of K4 along with K5: for example, 162/72/0 mm Hg. If the diastolic BP is heard above 90 mm Hg, confirm disappearance after listening for an additional 40 mm Hg to avoid the inaccurately high diastolic readings that result when observers fail to listen through the period of silence (auscultatory gap) for sounds to reappear. Otherwise, confirm disappearance by listening for an additional 10 to 20 mm Hg.

Step 10: Recording.
Immediately record the reading to avoid recall errors. Also note the patient's position, cuff size, and arm used during measurement. Record the reading as K1/K5. If K4 is recorded, write the three numbers as K1/K4/K5. If sounds do not cease, record K5 as 0.

Step 11: Repeat the reading.
Make certain all air is out of the cuff, wait 1 to 2 minutes, then repeat steps 6 to 10. BP normally changes from minute to minute, especially during clinical measurements. The average of two or more BP readings in a single arm is more reliable and a better indicator of usual readings than is a single reading or 1 reading in each arm. Inform the patient. Discuss the results and explain the action needed.

Step 12: Additional readings.
Repeat the measurements in the opposite arm during initial workup. Perform standing or supine readings as dictated by the patient's situation. Postural changes in BP are measured after 1 and 3 minutes of standing.

Special situations

Absence of Korotkoff phase 5.
When cardiac output is high and the individual is vasodilated (in some children, with thyrotoxicosis, during fever, and in pregnant women) K5 is often absent. In this event, Korotkoff sounds are heard until the mercury column falls to zero and the BP is recorded as K5/K4/0.

Children.
The principles of measurement are the same in newborns, infants, and children. A most important consideration is the selection of a cuff that is appropriate for the arm circumference, as described in the preceding text. Normal values for children are related to the child's age, gender, and height.

Elderly.
In the elderly, the brachial arteries occasionally become very thickened and stiff. If the artery feels excessively thick when rolled back and forth under the finger, the BP reading measured with indirect techniques may be falsely high. When this happens, the indirect cuff pressure may overestimate intraarterial pressure, because higher cuff pressure is required to compress such a rigid vessel. The presence of a radial artery that is still palpable after the cuff is inflated above the systolic BP warns of this error. Recheck the pressure by palpation in the forearm. Rarely, the palpated systolic pressure differs by >15 mm Hg. When this happens, an alternative technique (arterial puncture for central BP) may be needed.

Very large, cone-shaped, or muscular arms.
If the patient's arm is >41 cm in circumference or if its shape prevents proper cuff placement, accurate BP measurement may be impossible. In this case, it may be necessary to substitute palpated brachial readings or forearm auscultated readings using a cuff of the appropriate size, for either the upper arm and forearm. When readings differ by >15 mm Hg, the palpated systolic pressure with the cuff on the forearm provides a better estimate of the patient's BP. If the upper arm circumference is >53 cm, take a forearm measurement using a cuff with *bladder width* 40% of the forearm circumference.

Suggested Readings

Bailey RH, Knaus VL, Bauer JH. Aneroid sphygmomanometers: an assessment of accuracy at a university hospital and clinics. *Arch Intern Med* 1991;151:1409–1412.

Grim CM, Grim CE. A curriculum for the training and certification of blood pressure measurement for health care providers. *Can J Cardiol* 1995;11:28H–42H.

Grim CE, Grim CM. Office BP measurement. In: Black HR, Elliott WJ, eds. *Hypertension: a companion text to Braunwald's heart disease*, Chapter 5. Philadelphia: WB Saunders, 2007:58–68.

Hayes MV. Managing mercury: simple, effective methods for cleaning up small spills. *Med Waste* 1993;1:3–7.

Jones DW, Frohlich ED, Grim CM, et al. Mercury sphygmomanometers should not be abandoned: an advisory statement from the Council for High BP Research, American Heart Association. *Hypertension* 2001;37:185–186.

O'Brien E, Pickering T, Asmar R, et al. Working Group on BP monitoring of the European Society of hypertension international protocol for validation of BP measuring devices in adults. *Blood Press Monit* 2002;7:3–17.

Pickering TG, Hall JE, Appel LJ, et al. Research. Recommendations for BP measurement in humans and experimental animals: part 1: BP measurement in humans: a statement for professionals from the Subcommittee of Professional and Public Education of the American Heart Association Council on High BP Research. *Hypertension* 2005;45:142–161. [Epub 2004 Dec 20.]

Pickering TG, Hall JE, Appel L, et al. Response to recommendations for BP measurement in human and experimental animals; part 1: BP measurement in humans and miscuffing: a problem with new guidelines: addendum. *Hypertension*. 2006 [Epub ahead of print].

Prisant LM, Alpert BS, Robbins CB, et al. American National Standard for nonautomated sphygmomanometers. Summary report. *Am J Hypertens* 1995;8:210–213.

Website regularly updated for BP devices: www.dableducational.org/sphygmomanometers.html. Accessed September, 2007.

CHAPTER C104 ■ AMBULATORY AND HOME BLOOD PRESSURE MONITORING

WILLIAM B. WHITE, MD

KEY POINTS

- Home or 24-hour ambulatory blood pressure (ABP) recordings are an integral part of the assessment and monitoring of hypertension.
- Important advantages of self-monitoring of blood pressure (BP) are multiple readings at different times of the day; avoidance of the "white coat" effect (15%–20% of stage 1 or 2 hypertensive patients in the doctor's office), and avoidance of placebo effects in drug trials.
- ABP monitoring can be useful in accurately identifying masked hypertension, those who truly require antihypertensive drug therapy, and lack of acceptable BP control in patients with excessive cardiovascular risk.
- Out-of-office BPs improve risk stratification and correlate better than office BPs with the consequences of hypertension (left ventricular hypertrophy, hypertensive cerebrovascular disease, renal disease, retinopathy, and alterations in vascular compliance).

See also Chapters **A56**, **B89**, C103, C125, and C145

Monitoring of blood pressure (BP) outside of the medical care environment is an important part of clinical hypertension assessment and management. There are two main forms of out-of-office BP monitoring: (i) self- or home-monitoring, usually performed by the patient with a semiautomatic oscillometric device (or aneroid manometer plus stethoscope) and (ii) ambulatory blood pressure (ABP) monitoring , which uses a portable automatic device for repeated determinations during an extended time period, typically 24 hours. Both techniques have been shown to substantially enhance the clinician's understanding of BP behavior in patients and aid in diagnosis and therapeutic decision making.

Self- or home-monitoring of blood pressure

There are several advantages of self-monitoring (home measurement) of BP. Patients may record multiple BP readings during different times of the day and these values and patterns can be reviewed by the physician along with office pressures to improve therapeutic decision making. A second useful feature is that self-monitoring usually avoids the pressor response ("white coat" effect) seen in approximately 15% to 20% of stage 1 and 2 hypertensive patients in the doctor's office. A third benefit is that with careful timing of measurements, patients may discover periods in which BP control is inadequate.

Device validation. Before they are used in practice by patients, any device must be independently validated against mercury manometry or another device validated by a rigorous standard, such as the American Association for Medical Instrumentation (AAMI) guidelines or the International Standard. Clinical calibration against a validated nonmercury pressure meter should be performed on a regular basis.

Issues in self-monitoring. Several types of BP monitors are available for use at home and work, including semiautomatic electronic sphygmomanometers (that generally use an oscillometric method of BP measurement) and aneroid manometers that require auscultation. Electronic devices are most convenient and have clearly become the device of choice for home- or self-monitored BP measurement during the last few years. Aneroid manometers with a stethoscope are relatively simple to use and are generally the most economical type of self-monitoring units available. However, in older patients lacking manual dexterity, or when hearing loss is an issue, an electronic device is preferable to a nonautomated sphygmomanometer. In rare patients or those with arrhythmias, oscillometric devices may not sense accurately. Patients are usually fairly accurate when transcribing their own pressures, but may tend to underreport high BP levels and monitor the BP at home, while relaxed, rather than during work or other stressful situations. For the diagnosis of hypertension based on an average of home BPs, 135/85 mm Hg is comparable to an office average of 140/90 mm Hg, but studies have demonstrated that a much lower home BP value (125/76 mm Hg) correlates with normotension as defined by ambulatory monitoring.

Clinical trials. Self-monitoring of BP has been utilized in clinical trials of antihypertensive therapy. The rationale for utilization of self-monitored BP in this setting includes the improved precision of the measurement compared to clinic measurements. Of particular interest is that there is no apparent white coat effect with self-monitored BPs and virtually no placebo effect in clinical studies (similar to what has been observed in ABP studies). In all there is greater accuracy and reproducibility compared to the measurements made by physicians or nurses in the clinical setting. Staessen et al. compared conventional clinic and automated self-monitored BP in the Treatment of Hypertension Based on Home or Office Blood Pressure (THOP) trial and showed that differences between the self-monitored BP and clinic BP were nearly the same as the differences between ABP and clinic BP. However, it is not clear that self-monitored BP will ever become a full surrogate for ABP in either research or clinical practice.

Organ damage and outcomes. Several cross-sectional studies have shown that self-monitored BPs correlate better with echocardiographically determined left ventricular mass than clinic pressures. One population study based in Ohasama, Japan has demonstrated that home BP is a better predictor of cardiovascular risk in older patients than BPs taken by clinicians. The self-monitored BP has the potential for reducing the bias and error in assessing the "true" average BP in a patient; office BPs can represent a highly atypical picture of a given individual, especially if a small number of readings in the doctor's office are used. In some studies, the self-monitored BP has been shown to be similar to the attenuated BP seen with repeated measurements over time (i.e., weeks and months) in the clinic. In addition, self-monitored BP may be more representative of the 24-hour BP than the clinic BP. In a study recently performed in Scotland, not only was the reproducibility of self-measurement twice as good as clinic BPs, it agreed with the results of an ambulatory recording in 81% of the patients.

Therapeutic decision making. Because self-monitored BP is more representative of the average daily BP of an individual, it is useful in therapeutic decision making. Once antihypertensive therapy has been initiated, self-monitoring of BP is an efficient way to evaluate the effectiveness of the therapy and may even preempt some clinic visits. Furthermore, the relationship between time of dosing of antihypertensive therapy and BP levels may be easier to assess with self-monitoring patients. As a final attribute, adherence to therapy and BP control have been shown to improve when patients (even previously noncompliant ones) self-monitor BP. Still, it must be recognized that despite the obvious theoretic advantages of self-monitoring, there are limited prognostic data comparing the prediction of cardiovascular risk by home BP versus doctor's office BP.

Ambulatory blood pressure monitoring

Over the last 30 years, noninvasive ABP devices have been developed for hypertension management and clinical research. ABP monitors have become relatively practical to use in patient care because the devices are small (less than 1 lb in most instances), simple to apply by a nurse or technician, and precise.

Ambulatory blood pressure, target organs, and cardio-vascular outcomes. Nearly all cross-sectional studies published to date have shown ABP to be superior to office BP in predicting target organ involvement. Most evidence has come from assessment of left ventricular hypertrophy and hypertensive heart disease. Additionally, ABP is superior to office BP in predicting hypertensive cerebrovascular disease, retinopathy, renal abnormalities, and alterations in vascular compliance. Older patients and those with severe hypertension have excessive BP variability and this may add to future cardiovascular events above and beyond the mean level of average daily pressure. Numerous studies have shown that ABP is an independent predictor of cardiovascular risk (**Table C104.1**). Many of these studies have also demonstrated that a loss of nocturnal decline in BP ("nondipping" pattern) conveys excessive risk for stroke and myocardial infarction. One recent study by Verdecchia et al. demonstrated that the stroke rate in white coat hypertensive patients began to increase and approach the rates of the sustained (i.e., non–white coat) hypertensive patients after 6 years of observation, (**Table C104.1 and Figure C104.1**).

Available devices. Fully automatic, programmable recorders are capable of 100 to 200 BP (systolic, diastolic, and mean)

TABLE C104.1

CLINIC AND AMBULATORY BLOOD PRESSURE AND CARDIOVASCULAR MORBIDITY IN PROSPECTIVE COHORT STUDIES

Study	Year	Population	N	Comments
Perloff	1983	Referred	1,076	Low risk if ABP < CBP
Verdecchia	1994	Referred	1,187	WCH at low risk
Imai	1996	Population	1,789	ABP and HBP predict, not CBP
Redon	1998	Refractory	86	Low risk if ABP < CBP
Khattar	1998	Referred	479	WCH at low risk (intraarterial)
Staessen	1999	Syst-Eur	808	ABP gives better prediction
Clement	2003	OvA	1,963	Elevated ABP predicts events in treatment hypertensives
Sega	2005	General	2,051	Home and ABP (systolic) best at predicting CV death

ABP, ambulatory blood pressure; CBP, clinical blood pressure; WCH, white coat hypertension; CV, cardiovascular.

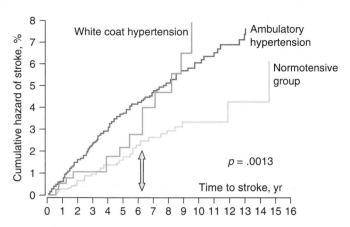

Figure C104.1 Time to stroke event in patients classified as normotensive, sustained hypertensive, and white coat hypertensive. Following 6 to 7 years of observation, patients with white coat hypertension began to have a marked increase in the stroke rate and in 8 to 10 years were similar to the rates seen in the sustained hypertensive patients. (From Verdecchia P, Reboldi GP, Angeli F, et al. Short- and long-term incidence of stroke in white-coat hypertension. *Hypertension* 2005;45:203–208, with permission.)

and pulse measurements from an energy source of two to four small (AA) batteries. Virtually all ambulatory devices measure BP by oscillometric technology, which depends on pulsatility in the brachial artery. A proprietary algorithm (different for each manufacturer) transforms the data from the BP cuff (amplitude of the oscillations) into standard BP values. Oscillometric methodologies have always been reasonably precise in patients who have mid-range BPs if the arm is motionless during cuff inflation and deflation. These techniques are less accurate at the extremes of systolic and diastolic BPs. In a few systems, auscultatory measurements (from microphone to detect Korotkoff sounds) are used but these devices are also subject to noise and motion artifact and are uncommonly used.

Ambulatory blood pressure technique. A standard monitoring period and sampling frequency must be established, usually 50 to 100 BP readings over a period of 24 hours. The first two to three recordings of the ABP should occur in the office with simultaneous sphygmomanometry for standardization. ABP monitoring is usually well tolerated by patients, especially because the technology has improved but a few technical problems are common. Approximately 10% to 15% of patients do not sleep well with the recorders. Experience has shown that BP values will not be much higher in those patients who do not sleep well unless they get out of bed and move about. Rarely, patients may develop erythema, ecchymoses, petechiae, or superficial phlebitis in the area distal to cuff placement. These soft tissue injuries are typically mild and self-limiting.

Interpretation. The 24-hour mean pressures should be established first. Most consensus groups, including the American Heart Association (**Table C104.2**) have used a 24-hour BP >130/80 mm Hg as abnormal based on new outcome studies comparing ABP versus clinic BP in patients with hypertension. In older analyses, a cutoff of 135/85 mm Hg was often used. Second, the diurnal pattern should be assessed. There is a reproducible diurnal/nocturnal pattern to BP during a 24-hour period of measurement in most (80%–85%) of patients. Typically, the pressure is highest while awake (especially during work) and lowest during sleep. Awake daytime and nighttime sleep BPs should be established. BP during

TABLE C104.2

SUGGESTED VALUES FOR THE UPPER LIMIT OF NORMAL FOR AMBULATORY PRESSURE

Time Period	Optimal (mm Hg)	Normal (mm Hg)	Abnormal (mm Hg)
Daytime	<130/80	<135/85	>140/90
Nighttime	<115/65	<120/70	>125/75
24-hour	<125/75	<130/80	>135/85

(From Pickering TG, Hall JE, Appel LJ, et al. Recommendations for blood pressure measurement in humans and experimental animals. *Hypertension* 2005;45:142–161.)

normal sleep is quite low compared to the office or clinic pressure, whereas BP during wakefulness is often similar to the values obtained in the office. Failure to observe a 10% decrease in BP during sleep ("nondippers") is suggestive of specific etiologies of hypertension (e.g., sleep apnea, steroid- dependent, salt-sensitive, chronic kidney disease).

Clinical decision making. Several subsets of hypertensive diagnoses have been elucidated as a result of ABP monitoring (**Table C104.3**). Clinical problems seen most often by practicing physicians that are appropriate for ABP monitoring include assessment for possible "white coat" hypertension, borderline hypertension (with and without evidence of target organ damage), evaluation of refractory hypertension in patients on complex antihypertensive regimens and assessment of 24 hour BP control in patients with increased cardiovascular risk (e.g., patients with cardiac and kidney diseases). A number of well-performed studies in these areas show that patients might benefit clinically when ABP is known in addition to the measurements made in the medical care environment.

It is not uncommon that resistant patients on antihypertensive drugs have a pressor response in the medical care environment that brings them into hypertensive ranges yet their out-of-office values are normal. Conversely, it is not unusual to perform ABP monitoring in a hypertensive patient with reasonably good office

TABLE C104.3

CLINICAL DIAGNOSES OR PROBLEMS IN WHICH NONINVASIVE AMBULATORY BLOOD PRESSURE MONITORING MAY BE USEFUL

Office- or white coat hypertension
Borderline hypertension with or without target organ involvement
Evaluation of patients refractory to antihypertensive therapy
Episodic hypertension
Hypotensive symptoms associated with antihypertensive medications
Autonomic dysfunction/nocturnal hypertension
Exclusion of placebo reactors when determining efficacy of antihypertensive drug therapy in controlled clinical trials

(Adapted from National High Blood Pressure Education Program Working Group. National High Blood Pressure Education Program Working Group report on ambulatory blood pressure monitoring. *Arch Intern Med* 1990;150:2270–2280.)

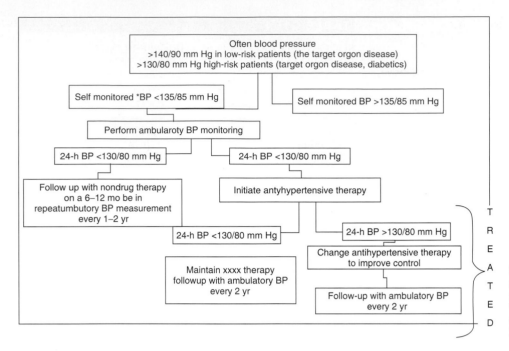

Figure C104.2 Algorithm for the use of ABP monitoring in the diagnosis and management of patients with hypertension. (From White WB. Ambulatory BP monitoring in clinical practice. *N Engl J Med* 2003; 348:2377–2378, with permission.)

pressures and find that BP levels are not normal late in the dosing period. Patients with so-called masked or hidden hypertension may be among those hypertensive phenotypes who benefit the most from the procedure. These types of findings have resulted in an algorithm for the utility of ABP monitoring in clinical practice (**Figure C104.2**).

Cost and coverage considerations. In 2002, the Center for Medicare Services independently evaluated ABP monitoring in clinical practice and approved a national policy that would pay for the study when it is used in the assessment of patients with white coat effect or white coat hypertension. The purpose of the ABP study from the insurance perspective is to verify the diagnosis of hypertension. Other diagnoses, such as episodic hypertension, refractory hypertension, and evaluation of antihypertensive therapy are not covered in the Medicare policy. Fortunately, many private insurance carriers have begun to provide improved coverage for ambulatory monitoring of the BP for patients with hypertension.

The cost to the patient of self-monitoring using a semiautomated recording device is relatively low (approximately $50–$150 for the instrumentation, $20–$60 for the training session by a nurse) and the data that it yields are helpful in hypertension management. Setting up of ABP monitoring may cost the physician, hospital, or heart station several thousand dollars to provide one

or two adequate recorders and software for data analysis and report generation. The patient charges range from $100 to $350 for 24-hour studies. Although more costly than self-monitoring, ABP monitoring is more useful because it may help identify those who truly require antihypertensive therapy as well as those who may be best managed with nonpharmacologic therapy.

Suggested Readings

Clement DL, De Buyzere ML, De Bacquer DA, et al. Prognostic value of ambulatory blood-pressure recordings in patients with treated hypertension. *N Engl J Med* 2003;348:2407–2415.

Peixoto AJ, White WB, Circadian BP. Clinical implications based on the pathophysiology of its variability. *Kidney Int* 2007;71:855–860.

Pickering TG, Hall JE, Appel LJ, et al. Recommendations for BP measurement in humans and experimental animals: part 1. BP measurement in humans. *Circulation* 2005;111:697–716.

Pickering TG, Shimbo D, Haas D. Ambulatory blood-pressure monitoring. *N Engl J Med* 2006;354:2368–2374.

Staessen JA, Celis H, Den Hond E, et al. Comparison of conventional and automated BP measurements: interim analysis of the THOP trial. *Blood Press Monit* 2002;7:61–62.

White WB. Ambulatory BP monitoring in clinical practice. *N Engl J Med* 2003;348:2377–2378.

White WB. Ambulatory BP monitoring as an investigative tool for characterizing resistant hypertension and its rational treatment. *J Clin Hypertens* 2007;9 (Suppl 1):25–30.

CHAPTER C105 ■ INITIAL WORKUP OF ADULTS WITH HYPERTENSION

JOSEPH L. IZZO, Jr., MD; DOMENIC A. SICA, MD AND HENRY R. BLACK, MD

KEY POINTS

- Objectives of initial evaluation are to establish the diagnosis and stage of hypertension [including office and nonoffice blood pressure (BP) readings], the likelihood of secondary hypertension, the presence of target organ damage, the level of global cardiovascular (CV) disease risk, and the plan for individualized monitoring and therapy.
- Basic components of the initial evaluation are: (a) thorough history and physical examination, including orthostatic BP change; (b) basic serum chemistries including serum potassium, creatinine, fasting glucose, and lipid profile; (c) urinalysis with microscopic evaluation and albumin:creatinine ratio; (d) electrocardiogram (ECG); and (e) nonoffice (home, workplace, or 24-hour ambulatory) BP determinations to establish the pattern of hypertension (sustained, "white coat," or "masked" hypertension).
- The initial evaluation is usually not complete at the end of the first office visit.
- Patient education and counseling should be prominent features of the initial evaluation.

See also Chapters **C103, C104, C119, C161**, and **C163**

Hypertension is the most common reason patients visit primary care providers and is the most important of all modifiable CV risk factors. For these reasons, an overall assessment of CV disease risk and careful definition of the pattern of blood pressure (BP) elevation is mandatory in all adults with elevated BP readings. The workup for children or athletes often differs slightly (See Chapters C161 and C163).

Objectives and specific aspects of the initial evaluation

The goals and objectives of the initial evaluation of a hypertensive patient are listed in **Table C105.1**. These include the need to establish the diagnosis and stage of hypertension (including office and nonoffice BP readings), the likelihood of secondary hypertension, the presence of target organ damage, the level of global CV disease risk, and a plan for individualized monitoring and therapy.

Specific aspects of the workup (**Table C105.2**) include thorough history and physical examination; basic chemistries, including serum potassium and creatinine, fasting glucose and complete lipid profile; urinalysis with microscopic evaluation and albumin: creatinine ratio; ECG; and home or ambulatory

BP readings. These recommendations expand on what has been suggested in the Seventh Report of the Joint National Committee on the Prevention, Detection, Evaluation, and Treatment of High Blood Pressure (JNC 7), most notably with respect to the requirement for nonoffice BP readings.

History

Family history. To determine the urgency of treatment, it is often helpful to establish whether there is a strong family history of hypertension, stroke, or coronary artery disease (CAD), especially if any of these events have occurred in close relatives younger than 55 years in men or younger than 65 years in women. The history should specifically include questioning regarding symptoms and any prior CV or renal disease such as stroke, CAD [especially premature myocardial infarction or angina, heart failure (HF), polycystic kidney disease, and diabetes].

General symptomatology. General well-being is difficult to assess on the initial visit but vague constitutional symptoms are common in hypertension, as demonstrated by the fact that quality-of-life measures improve consistently when BP is lowered by any of a number of different antihypertensive agents. Therefore, hypertensive individuals are not necessarily asymptomatic as has been previously believed.

Medication history. A careful and complete history of the use of other medications (prescribed, over-the-counter, herbal, and

TABLE C105.1

GOALS AND OBJECTIVES OF THE INITIAL EVALUATION

Specific objectives of initial workup	Indicators that affect prognosis, monitoring, and therapy
Diagnosis and pattern of hypertension	Hypertension duration and severity BP pattern (office and nonoffice BP determinations) JNC 7 BP staging (**Table C105.2**)

Assessment of target organs	Ischemic heart disease-equivalent: angina, prior MI
	  or revascularization, diabetes
	Chronic kidney disease: decreased glomerular
	  filtration rate, microalbuminuria
	Left ventricular hypertrophy
	Heart failure
	Stroke or transient ischemic attacks
	Peripheral arterial disease.

Cardiovascular disease risk assessment	Modifiable risk factors: fasting glucose and lipid
	  profile, serum creatinine, cigarette smoking
	Nonmodifiable risk factors (age, gender, family
	  history)

Likelihood of secondary hypertension	Refractory hypertension Various clinical signs and symptoms (**Table C105.3**)
Individualized planning for monitoring and therapy	Goal BP establishment Lifestyle modification counseling Medication choice Additional patient education

BP, blood pressure; JNC 7, Joint National Committee on the Prevention, Detection, Evaluation, and Treatment of High Blood Pressure; MI, myocardial infarction.

nutriceuticals) should be obtained because these medications may increase BP. Among such drugs are high-dose estrogens (especially when combined with progestogens), adrenal steroids, nonsteroidal anti-inflammatory drugs (NSAIDs), nasal decongestants, and appetite suppressants. The overall number of patients, however, who experience elevated BPs from these agents, is small.

Alcohol and street drugs. Both acute and chronic alcohol abuse raise BP. Use of stimulants such as amphetamines or cocaine can cause acute and dramatic and sometimes dangerous increases in BP. Abrupt withdrawal of alcohol, opiates, and other street drugs can be associated with "sudden" BP increases.

Sleep history. A thorough sleep history should be obtained in the newly hypertensive patient in that sleep apnea is commonly

TABLE C105.2

INITIAL LABORATORY TESTING

Source	Test	Purpose
Blood	Serum creatinine	Assess kidney status, CVD risk Plan therapy
	Serum potassium	Assess hyperaldosteronism, either primary or secondary (e.g., renovascular disease) Note: low K an inconsistent late finding Plan therapy
	Fasting glucose	Assess CVD risk
	Fasting lipid profile (high-density lipoprotein, low-density lipoprotein, and triglycerides)	Plan therapy for comorbidities
Urine	Microscopic examination	Assess glomerular function/disease, CVD risk
	Spot microalbumin:creatinine ratio	Plan therapy
Electrocardiogram	Voltage criteria	Assess LVH, prior IHD, CVD risk
	Prior myocardial infarction Rhythm disturbances	Plan therapy

CVD, cardiovascular disease; LVH, left ventricular hypertrophy; IHD, ischemic heart disease.

associated with the development of hypertension. Sleep apnea should be suspected in obese individuals with disrupted sleep patterns. Snoring is a frequent finding but is oftentimes more reliably reported by the sleep partner (or other family member) than by the affected individual. Daytime somnolence and fatigue are also common in this condition. Sleep apnea is probably the most common problem that goes unidentified during the routine evaluation of a hypertensive patient. Although patients with sleep apnea are usually obese, normal weight individuals may also have this syndrome. More recently, it is also recognized that distortion of sleep architecture, as may occur either on a primary or a secondary basis in association with comorbid conditions, can be associated with the onset of hypertension.

Physical examination

Blood pressure measurement. There are several very important subtleties to the office measurement of BP (**Table C105.3**). Adequate time for the patient to relax (usually 5–10 minutes) before BP measurement is important. Proper cuff size is extremely important; in very small or very large patients (obese or muscular individuals) use of an inappropriately sized BP cuff can lead to underestimation or overestimation of BP. BP should be measured in both arms at the initial visit; if one arm is higher than the other, the difference should be noted, with the higher arm used thereafter. BP readings should be within 10 mm Hg on repeat readings. Postural BP change must be evaluated, preferably by assessing supine and upright BP values; postural change from sitting to standing is less likely to identify orthostatic intolerance.

Before the diagnosis of hypertension is established, BP should be elevated on at least two occasions, except if the BP is very high (usually >180/110 mm Hg), where white coat hypertension is highly unlikely and therapy with at least two agents should be initiated promptly, certainly within days. It is common for follow-up readings to be lower than the initial reading, and some people may ultimately be classified at a lower stage of hypertension.

Funduscopic examination. Funduscopic examination is not grossly abnormal in most subjects with stage 1 hypertension (see Figures on back cover of book). The presence of significant arteriolar narrowing or the presence of hemorrhages and exudates indicates that BP has been elevated for a considerable length of time. Papilledema with a markedly elevated BP ("malignant hypertension") is a medical emergency with a poor prognosis unless therapy is instituted quickly.

TABLE C105.3

ASPECTS OF BLOOD PRESSURE (BP) MEASUREMENTS

Aspect	Comment
Ambient stress/anxiety	At least 5-min rest period
Accurate BP determination	Appropriate cuff size
	BP in both arms; higher arm is taken
Orthostatic homeostasis	Supine, sitting, and upright BPs and heart rates
Office BP reproducibility	Follow-up BP values
White-coat effect	Home or ambulatory BP determinations compared to office values

Cardiac examination. Heart rate and rhythm should be noted. Ectopic beats and atrial fibrillation are common findings, especially if left ventricular hypertrophy (LVH) is present. Signs of cardiomegaly (forceful, laterally displaced apical impulse) suggest LVH. An accentuated aortic second sound occurs frequently, especially with diastolic BP values >100 mm Hg. A fourth heart sound suggests atrial enlargement and increased ventricular stiffness (often with LVH); a third heart sound suggests dilated cardiomyopathy and reduced left ventricular function. Certain murmurs are associated with hypertension such as pulmonic flow murmurs in conditions of high cardiac output.

Peripheral pulses. Assessment of peripheral pulses is important to help rule out peripheral arterial disease or to confirm the diagnosis of aortic coarctation. The carotid arteries should be palpated and auscultated for the presence of bruits, which might indicate luminal narrowing or the presence of occlusive plaques. Even so, pulse palpation alone can be an unreliable physical sign and should be used in combination with objective measurements, such as determination of the ankle-brachial index or carotid Doppler, as a guide to clinical management.

Abdomen. Periumbilical or flank bruits may suggest the presence of renal artery stenosis, especially if there is a diastolic component. Active, forceful pulsations along the aorta may be a normal finding in young, thin people but suggest an abdominal aortic aneurysm in older individuals. Palpation of the abdomen, especially laterally, may trigger a BP surge in individuals with pheochromocytomas, so care must be taken performing an abdominal examination in a patient with a history suggestive of this rare tumor. Polycystic kidneys are usually palpable in the flanks and the related renal insufficiency may be the etiology of the patient's hypertension.

Neurologic examination. A basic screening examination for motor and cranial nerve function, gait, stance, and coordination is important to establish a baseline for therapeutic follow-up.

Laboratory evaluation.
The JNC reports have stressed that laboratory evaluation of hypertensive patients need not be extensive or costly and that the workup of secondary hypertension can be reserved for those with specific clinical signs or symptoms or those who do not respond to conventional therapy with one or two drugs (**Table C105.4**).

Basic studies. A general health screen should be performed, including automated blood chemistry, urinalysis with microscopic examination, fasting glucose and lipid profiles, and ECG. Complete blood count and chest x-ray are often performed during an initial health evaluation but are not specifically required for the workup of hypertension. An ECG is suggested to determine the presence or absence of arrhythmias, myocardial ischemia, and LVH, which may influence the choice of specific therapies.

Ancillary studies. Although an echocardiogram is a more sensitive and specific index of LVH than an ECG, a full echocardiogram is expensive and the information does not usually affect therapeutic decisions. An echocardiogram, chest radiograph, renal imaging studies, and plasma-renin activity or renin/aldosterone ratio are not recommended as routine procedures in the evaluation of the hypertensive patient. In the case of children and adolescents, however, additional testing is often warranted. Recent developments demonstrate that central systolic BP derived from radial pulse contour analysis may be quite different from arm cuff systolic BP due to marked clinical variation in pulse wave transmission and reflection; relevance to routine clinical practice is not yet established. Cardiac output profiling is at this time not recommended due to the wide

TABLE C105.4

SIGNS AND SYMPTOMS OF SECONDARY HYPERTENSION

Condition	Signs and symptoms
Obstructive sleep apnea	Refractory hypertension
	Obesity, somnolence, poor sleep duration, snoring, unexplained heart failure
Hyperaldosteronism	Refractory hypertension
	Hypokalemia, orthostatic BP drop
Renovascular hypertension	Sudden onset of severe hypertension in young women (fibromuscular disease)
	Severe coronary, peripheral arterial or cerebrovascular disease; cigarette smoking history (atherosclerotic disease)
	Holosystolic bruit with or without diastolic component
Drug-induced	Refractory or episodic hypertension
	Tachycardia, sweating, nausea (cocaine use or drug withdrawal)
	Liver function abnormalities, telangiectasias, macrocytic anemia (occult alcoholism)
	NSAID use
Pheochromocytoma	Refractory hypertension
	Anxiety, tremor, headaches, sweating, rapid pulse, recent weight loss, orthostatic BP drop
	Multiple endocrine neoplasia: thyroid or parathyroid enlargement, neurofibromas, *café au lait* spots
Cushing's syndrome	Obesity, unusual truncal distribution of fat and abdominal striae, excessive body or facial hair (Cushing's syndrome)
Aortic coarctation	Absent or diminished femoral pulses

BP, blood pressure; NSAID, nonsteroidal anti-inflammatory drug.

variation observed in the population and questionable relevance to therapeutic planning.

Target organ damage. Hypertensive target organ damage should be assessed directly or indirectly in all patients. In the initial evaluation, an ECG is used to screen for evidence of CAD or LVH. An elevated serum creatinine (reduced glomerular filtration rate) or the presence of microalbuminuria or albuminuria establishes the diagnosis of chronic kidney disease (CKD).

Out-of-office blood pressure determinations. Home or ambulatory BP monitoring is necessary to confirm the diagnosis of hypertension or to identify "white coat" or "masked" hypertension. The former is defined as persistently elevated BPs in a doctor's office with normal BPs at home or at work, whereas "masked" hypertension has the reverse pattern. Patients with white coat hypertension may develop LVH, CAD, and stroke but they do so at rates lower than those with sustained hypertension. Those with "masked hypertension" have risk profiles similar to those with sustained office and home BP elevations. Ambulatory BP monitoring has been approved for reimbursement by Medicare to establish the diagnosis of white coat hypertension. Home BP determinations can be used to establish the BP pattern but home devices require formal validation in the provider's office. There may be small but consistent differences in diastolic BP between the home (oscillometric) and office (sphygmomanometric) systems; if these occur, a correction factor may be applied. For systolic BP, differences between techniques are usually minimal. Wrist or finger devices should generally not be used as their accuracy has not been proved.

Clinical synthesis

At the end of the initial evaluation, the clinician should be able to address the individual objectives of the evaluation and convey them clearly to the patient. The initial evaluation may call for additional information, especially out-of-office BP readings, and therefore may not be complete at the end of the first office visit. Also important is the staging of hypertension (**Table C105.5**).

Initial counseling

Several factors make it problematic to make specific recommendations at the end of the initial visit, especially the likelihood that the clinician will not have sufficient knowledge of the nonoffice BP profiles, and may not have sufficient or current data

TABLE C105.5

STAGES OF HYPERTENSION (JNC 7)

Stage[a]	Systolic BP (mm Hg)	Diastolic BP (mm Hg)
Normal BP	<120	<80
Prehypertension	120–139	80–89
Stage 1 hypertension	140–159	90–99
Stage 2 hypertension	≥160	≥100

BP, blood pressure.
[a]Stage is higher category of systolic or diastolic BP.

regarding other risk factors or target organ damage studies. Much of the patient education must therefore be reserved for the second (or sometimes third) visit. Furthermore, as the patient becomes accustomed to the surrounding personnel, and potential diagnosis of hypertension, subsequent BP values may decrease. Therefore, it is not recommended to complete the BP staging at the first visit. Ideally, the clinician can use the opportunity to begin patient counseling.

Lifestyle modification. It is appropriate to initiate lifestyle counseling because virtually all patients benefit from the standard recommendations to lose weight if they are overweight, get sufficient physical activity, restrict sodium and alcohol intake, and refrain from smoking.

Risks of hypertension and goal blood pressure. The risks of untreated hypertension should be clearly identified at the first or second visit. Patients should be instructed to "know their numbers" and what they mean; particular attention should be paid to the systolic BP in adults: either <140/90 mm Hg as the general goal or <130/80 mm Hg in the presence of diabetes, CKD, or ischemic heart disease. It should be emphasized that the *average* BP should be below the specified targets, meaning that some values will be much lower than the nominal target. Lowest tolerable BPs are preferable.

Home blood pressure monitoring recommendations. Patients should be made aware that BP varies physiologically and that there are several facets of BP that will be scrutinized, including average values, morning and evening differences, and home–office differences. Specific instructions for home monitoring should include the number of readings to take per day, the times of measurement, and the need for a personal written log for home measurements that includes time of day, BP, heart rate (if feasible) and written commentary when appropriate. Those who measure their BPs at home should recognize that BP measurement is not like using a thermometer to establish the presence of fever and therefore should be done systematically, at times when they feel "bad" as well as when they feel "great." Patients must bring in their units for validation against a mercury sphygmomanometer (or other calibrated office device) to ensure that they have properly functioning instruments that yield accurate readings.

Suggested Readings

Chobanian AV, Bakris GL, Black HR, et al. Joint National Committee on Prevention Detection, Evaluation, and Treatment of High Blood Pressure. National Heart Lung, and Blood Institute, National High Blood Pressure Education Program Coordinating Committee. Seventh report of the Joint National Committee on Prevention, Detection, Evaluation, and Treatment of High Blood Pressure. *Hypertension* 2003;42:1206–1252.

Mancia G, de Backer G, Dominiczak A, et al. On behalf of the Task Force for the Management of Arterial Hypertension of the ESH and of the ESC 2007 guidelines for the management of arterial hypertension. *J Hypertens* 2007;25:1105–1187.

O'Brien E, Asmar R, Beilin L, et al. European Society of Hypertension Working Group on Blood Pressure Monitoring. Practice Guidelines of the European Society of Hypertension for Clinic, Ambulatory and Self Blood Pressure Measurement. *J Hypertens* 2005;23:697–701.

Pickering TG, Hall JE, Appel LJ, et al. Recommendations for blood pressure measurement in humans and experimental animals: part 1: blood pressure measurement in humans: a statement for professionals from the Subcommittee of Professional and Public Education of the American Heart Association Council on High Blood Pressure Research. *Circulation* 2005;111(5):697–716.

White W. Expanding the use of ambulatory blood pressure monitoring for the diagnosis and management of patients with hypertension. *Hypertension* 2006;47:14–15.

CHAPTER C106 ■ RESISTANT HYPERTENSION

NORMAN M. KAPLAN, MD AND DOMENIC A. SICA, MD

KEY POINTS

■ Resistant hypertension is defined as elevated office blood pressure (BP) values (>140/90 mm Hg for most hypertensive patients or >130/80 mm Hg for those with ischemic heart disease, diabetes, or renal insufficiency) despite use of approved maximal doses of three or more different antihypertensive classes, including a diuretic.

■ Resistant hypertension is present in approximately 10% of patients seen by primary care providers and >30% of patients referred to hypertension specialists.

■ Resistant hypertension falls into two broad categories: apparent resistance (e.g., medication doses too low or patient nonadherence) or true resistance (e.g., volume overload or secondary hypertension).

■ Causes of resistant hypertension can be identified by history, physical examination, and appropriate laboratory testing.

See also Chapters A56, B89, C103, C104, C119, C123, C124, C125, C128, C162, C166, and C167

Resistant hypertension is defined as the persistence of office blood pressure (BP) above the appropriate goal of therapy (140/90 mm Hg for most hypertensive patients or 130/80 for those with ischemic heart disease, diabetes, or renal insufficiency) despite use of three or more antihypertensive drugs from different classes at full doses, one of which is a diuretic. The condition is sometimes a clue to the presence of secondary hypertension but can be due to physician attitudes, medication nonadherence, or other pathophysiologic problems.

General approach to management

Resistant hypertension can be arbitrarily divided into two broad categories: apparent resistance or true resistance (**Table C106.1**). The prevalence of apparent resistance is considerably higher than that of true resistance. Within these general categories is a long list of possible specific causes, with most readily identified in the course of a thorough history and physical examination together with routine laboratory testing. Ancillary studies such as plasma-renin activity or plasma aldosterone are occasionally indicated to rule out identifiable causes of secondary hypertension that may be correctable. If resistance to therapy persists, referral to a hypertension specialist is a logical next step (see Chapter C125).

Apparent resistance

Patient nonadherence (see Chapter C123) and inadequate dosing (see Chapter C128) are the most common reasons for apparent resistance to treatment effect.

Cuff-related artifacts

Cuff too small. A common measurement error occurs with the use of a cuff that is too small for the arm. In general, the cuff should be large enough so that the bladder encircles at least 75% of the upper arm circumference and extends at least two thirds of its length (see Chapter C103).

Pseudohypertension. A rare cause of resistant hypertension is pseudohypertension due to noncompressibility of severely arteriosclerotic or calcified brachial and radial arteries. The presence of pseudohypertension is suspected when hypotensive symptoms arise without BP change, although this pattern is far more common in white coat hypertension. Oscillometric readings may be closer to intraarterial BP levels but direct invasive measurements are generally needed to confirm the presence of this condition.

Patient nonadherence. A common cause of apparent resistance is patient nonadherence (see Chapter C123). There are several nonadherence reasons for an apparent resistance pattern, including side effects of medications, lack of consistent and continuous primary care, inconvenient or chaotic dosing schedules, poor understanding of instructions, memory defects from organic brain syndrome, personality disorders, social and cultural barriers, and medication cost. Various educational tools or procedures can be used to reduce patient adherence problems, with strong physician motivation being a very important element.

Physician nonadherence

Failure to follow guidelines. As documented in a 2-year survey of physicians' behavior in treating hypertension, Berlowitz found

TABLE C106.1

CAUSES OF RESISTANT HYPERTENSION

Apparent drug resistance
    Cuff-related artifact
        Cuff too small
        Pseudohypertension (peripheral arterial
          calcification, rare)
    Patient non-adherence
    Physician nonadherence
        Goal nonadherence
        Underdosing, inappropriate combinations
True drug resistance
    Exaggerated BP reactivity or variability
        White coat hypertension
        Baroreflex failure
    Physiologic resistance (volume overload)
        Excess sodium intake
        Activation of BP homeostatic mechanisms by
          vasodilators
        Fluid retention from reduced renal perfusion
          pressure
        Inadequate diuretic therapy
    Drug effects and interactions
        Nonsteroidal antiinflammatory drugs
        Sympathomimetics (nasal decongestants, appetite
          suppressants)
        Cocaine, amphetamines, and other street drugs
        Caffeine
        Oral contraceptives
        Adrenal steroids
        Natural licorice (also in chewing tobacco)
        Cyclosporine, tacrolimus
        Erythropoietin
    Comorbidities
        Smoking
        Obesity/insulin resistance
        Sleep apnea
        Excess alcohol intake
        Anxiety-induced hyperventilation or panic attacks
        Chronic pain syndromes
        Intense vasoconstriction (arteritis)
    Secondary hypertension
    Genetic variation
        Racial/genetic differences in drug efficacy
        Rapid drug inactivation (hydralazine)

BP, blood pressure.

that doses of drugs were increased only 26% of the time despite clear chart documentation of inadequate control. Physician nonadherence to general principles of therapy may also be reflected in inconvenient and chaotic dosing schedules of multiple medicines without regard to synchronization and streamlining of therapy. With currently available formulations, each class of antihypertensive drugs has agents that can be given at convenient times, once or twice daily. Medications may cause side effects that previously asymptomatic patients are unwilling to tolerate. Fortunately, therapeutic options are available for patients who are side effect prone, especially angiotensin-converting enzyme (ACE) inhibitors (absent the development of cough), angiotensin receptor blockers (ARBs) and possibly direct renin inhibitors.

Prescription errors and underdosing. Perhaps the most common reason for apparent lack of control is inadequate antihypertensive drug doses or failure to titrate medications to reach goal

(see Chapter C128). The Antihypertensive and Lipid-Lowering Treatment to Prevent Heart Attack Trial (ALLHAT) study proved that community physicians could at least double their control rates (to approximately 68%) by following a specific titration algorithm. Another factor that might be considered as a form of prescription error is the failure to use optimal combinations of drugs.

True resistance

White coat hypertension. BP at rest does not predict the response an individual may manifest during physical or emotional stress (see Chapter A56). Approximately 20% to 25% of patients with persistent office BPs > 140/90 mm Hg do not have hypertension on home or ambulatory monitoring (average awake BP is <135/85 mm Hg), a phenomenon commonly called the *white coat effect* or *white coat hypertension* (WCH) (see Chapters B89, C104). Importantly, the office BPs in WCH are very unresponsive to standard antihypertensive drugs. At the same time, WCH-prone individuals often manifest a pattern of exaggerated sensitivity to antihypertensive drugs at home. WCH patients commonly self-discontinue their medications and may present considerable management difficulties. Therefore, out-of-office measurements (either home BP devices or automated ambulatory BP monitoring) should be obtained before additional testing or therapies are ordered in individuals suspected of having WCH. The exception to the recommendation for home self-measured or ambulatory BP monitoring is the presence of significant or progressive target organ damage, believed to be specifically related to hypertension. Under such circumstances, intensive drug therapy is mandated.

Baroreflex failure. Severe BP instability (increased lability) with wide excursions of BP and heart rate occur in individuals with impaired baroreflex function. This condition can go undetected for some time and as baroreflex function gradually declines, BP shifts become increasingly more volatile. Baroreflex failure can prove quite difficult to treat; frequent follow-up is important to enhance BP control (see Chapter C154).

Drug interference. The most common of these interactions is the interference by nonsteroidal anti-inflammatory drugs (NSAIDs) [including cyclooxygenase-2 (COX-2) inhibitors] with the antihypertensive efficacy of antihypertensive medications, which occurs with all classes of antihypertensives except calcium channel blockers (see Chapter C144). Even a single 300-mg tablet of aspirin can limit the effectiveness of a diuretic or an ACE inhibitor. Such interference can often be avoided if acetaminophen can be used. If NSAID is required, larger doses of antihypertensive drugs or more diuretic may be needed. Many drugs can raise BP (see Chapter C166); some have obvious pressor effects (e.g., sympathomimetic agents) whereas others raise BP by more subtle mechanisms (e.g., volume expansion linked to licorice-containing herbal remedies or chewing tobacco).

Physiologic resistance (volume overload). In most series of patients with resistant hypertension, volume overload is the most common cause of hypertension. Arising from multiple interacting factors, the usual scenario is that there is an initial medication-related fall in BP caused by a vasodilator (especially nonspecific vasodilators such as hydralazine and minoxidil, see Chapter C139), which activates counterregulatory pathways that "defend" arterial pressure (the sympathetic nervous and renin-angiotensin systems), which in turn cause sodium and water retention and volume overload. Marked volume expansion is the rule unless adrenergic inhibitors and large doses of potent diuretics are also given.

In the hypertensive patient receiving inadequate diuretic therapy, volume overload is the most common cause of resistance. Such volume overload may not manifest as edema and as such is unrecognizable on physical examination. Inadequate diuretic therapy may be a consequence of an inadequate dose of diuretic (dosage or potency) or because the frequency of administration is inadequate. The latter is often the case with furosemide, a short-acting loop diuretic. The 1- to 4-hour natriuresis that follows each dose of furosemide shrinks intravascular volume only until the episode of fluid ingestion, when the diuretic-activated renin system facilitates excess salt and water retention that may exceed the amount lost during the diuretic phase. In those with good renal function, substituting a morning dose of longer-acting agents (e.g., chlorthalidone 12.5–25 mg) may avoid this antinatriuretic cycle. In those with impaired renal function, metolazone (2.5–10 mg daily together with a loop diuretic) is usually effective. A longer-acting loop diuretic (e.g., torsemide) may also be effective under similar circumstances. Reduced dietary sodium intake is also usually beneficial.

Comorbidities. Correction of adverse lifestyle habits may allow patients with resistant hypertension to become more responsive. The pressor effect of each cigarette cannot be recognized by BP readings taken in the clinic because the pressor effect wears off within 15 to 30 minutes. Only by out-of-office readings taken while the patient is smoking can this pressor effect be recognized and used to further motivate the patient to quit smoking. Weight gain raises BP by several mechanisms, with or without the sympathetic nervous activation caused by obstructive sleep apnea, which affects as many as one third of resistant hypertensives who are usually obese, short-necked, and who fall asleep at various times of day. Excessive alcohol intake (usually more than three usual-sized portions a day) can raise BP both acutely and chronically.

Anxiety/panic attacks. Anxiety can interfere with therapy; patients who are appropriately concerned over the inability to have their hypertension controlled are often given more and more medication with little additional effect. The syndrome of anxiety/panic attack differs from WCH by virtue of the symptoms of dizziness, headache, paresthesias, fatigue, tachycardia, or atypical chest pain, which they commonly attribute to side effects of medications. Pain and fear with comorbid conditions such as migraine, transient ischemic attacks, or coronary disease, can further add to a patient's anxiety. Anxiety/panic attack can sometimes be diagnosed by voluntarily hyperventilating, which on occasion reproduces the symptoms and identifying a "hyperventilation" component to such a symptom profile can

avoid unnecessary diagnostic procedures. For some individuals, all that is needed is an explanation of the syndrome and instructions to rebreathe into a paper bag at the first appearance of symptoms. In others, anxiolytic therapy may be useful (see Chapter C162). Long-term management of such patients can prove challenging, oftentimes requiring adjunctive psychiatric care and frequent medication adjustments.

Secondary hypertension. The presence of any one of a large number of identifiable conditions may lead to resistant hypertension on a secondary basis. Progressive renal insufficiency is the most common and is easily recognized. Renovascular disease should be suspected in those patients with previously controlled hypertension that suddenly goes out of control, particularly if atherosclerosis is evident in other target organs. In the last few years, it has been suggested that there is a higher prevalence of primary aldosteronism than was previously noted; many of these patients are normokalemic (see Chapter C167).

Genetic variation. It is unusual for any genetic variation to interfere with the actions of approved antihypertensive drugs but in general, genetically "low renin" individuals have lesser responses to ACE inhibitors, ARBs, and direct renin inhibitors and enhanced responses to thiazides and calcium channel blockers. Genetic differences in acetylation kinetics can affect the amount of hydralazine necessary to lower BP.

Suggested Readings

Berlowitz DR, Ash AS, Hickey EC, et al. Inadequate management of BP in a hypertensive population. *N Engl J Med* 1998;339:1957–1963.

Hyman DJ, Pavlik VN. Characteristics of patients with uncontrolled hypertension in the United States. *N Engl J Med* 2001;345:479–488.

Kaplan NM. Anxiety-induced hyperventilation: a common cause of symptoms in patients with hypertension. *Arch Intern Med* 1997;157:945–948.

Knight EL, Bohn RL, Wang PS, et al. Predictors of uncontrolled hypertension in ambulatory patients. *Hypertension* 2001;38:809–814.

Logan AG, Perlikowski SM, Mente A, et al. High prevalence of unrecognized sleep apnea in drug-resistant hypertension. *J Hypertens* 2001;19:2271–2277.

Moser M, Setaro JF. Resistant or difficult-to control hypertension. *N Engl J Med* 2006;355:385–392.

Nuesch R, Schroeder K, Dieterle T, et al. Relation between insufficient response to antihypertensive treatment and poor compliance with treatment: a prospective case-control study. *BMJ* 2001;323:142–146.

Ouzan J, Pe'rault C, Lincoff AM, et al. The role of spironolactone in the treatment of patients with refractory hypertension. *Am J Hypertens* 2002;15:333–339.

Redon J, Campos C, Narciso ML, et al. Prognostic value of ambulatory BP monitoring in refractory hypertension. *Hypertension* 1998;31:712–718.

Sowers JR, White WB, Pitt B, et al. The effects of cyclooxygenase-2 inhibitors and nonsteroidal anti-inflammatory therapy on 24-hour BP in patients with hypertension, osteoarthritis, and type 2 diabetes mellitus. *Arch Intern Med* 2005;165:161–168.

CHAPTER C107 ■ DEFINING THE SYNDROME OF HYPERTENSION

JOSEPH L. IZZO, Jr., MD; THOMAS D. GILES, MD AND BARRY J. MATERSON, MD

KEY POINTS

- Hypertension is a complex syndrome that is separate from atherosclerosis and dysglycemia but interacts with these other processes to increase cardiovascular morbidity and mortality.
- Debate is growing whether a new definition of hypertension is needed that extends beyond arm cuff systolic and diastolic blood pressure (BP) cuff measurements.
- Any new definition of hypertension must be pathophysiologically accurate and also directly relevant to clinical practice; 3 different approaches are presented in this chapter.
- Validation will be needed for any new definition of the syndrome of hypertension.

See also Chapters C104 and C119

The challenge of defining hypertension

After two centuries of study, there is still no universal agreement on the definition of hypertension. Historically, the term *hypertension* has been synonymous with an elevation of arm cuff blood pressure (BP) beyond an arbitrary cutoff value. Yet it is increasingly clear that arm cuff systolic and diastolic BP measurements obtained in a medical office setting provide an inadequate database for optimal therapeutic recommendations in a large number of hypertensive patients because of the following:

- The failure to account for individuals with intermittent hypertension and exaggerated BP variability, including the "white coat syndrome"
- The pathophysiologic heterogeneity of sustained hypertension (e.g., isolated systolic hypertension due to large artery stiffness versus isolated diastolic hypertension due to arteriolar constriction and hypertrophy)
- The failure of currently available "vasodilator drugs" to be able to control BP adequately in all individuals
- The strong relationship between age, systolic BP, and pulse pressure (PP)
- The relative imprecision of cuff BP in predicting central systolic BP and cardiovascular events in a given individual
- The need to consider global cardiovascular risk in the management of BP

At the same time, it remains a practical necessity to provide a clear, reasonable definition so that meaningful practice guidelines can be constructed to achieve better overall BP control. Oversimplifying the definition of hypertension, with its many diverse aspects, diminishes our chances to provide optimal directed or "individualized" therapy. Hypertension is not simply a manifestation of insulin resistance or endothelial disease; anticholesterol or antidiabetic medications do not control BP and antihypertensive medications do not control blood glucose or cholesterol. Therefore, individual risk factor management remains essential. All individuals should have adequate global cardiovascular disease (CVD) risk factor assessment and control but in the end, what is needed is a meaningful roadmap to the treatment of these common conditions. A truly useful new definition of hypertension should remove some of the current empiricism and lead to more individualized therapy. It is even conceivable that the total number of medication-treated individuals could decrease if we were better able to identify individuals truly at risk for adverse events. Toward those ends, three independent views of these issues are presented.

Approach # 1: Application of current definitions and guidelines is best

Validity. Traditional methods for office BP evaluation have stood the test of time and have been extensively validated; any new definition will require extensive and expensive validation that is not needed. There are no large databases that unequivocally identify the risks associated with BP elevations determined outside the medical office setting and there is no validated outcome study identifying the value of a particular treatment for intermittent hypertension.

Acceptance. The size of the affected population is huge; using the standard definition of hypertension (>140/90 mm Hg), approximately one fourth of the U.S. population is hypertensive; using 120/80 mm Hg as the arbitrary BP norm, approximately half of the U.S. population has elevated BP (prehypertension or hypertension). The economic, cultural, and psychological implications of labeling half the population as diseased will assuredly be a major stimulus to strong "pushback" from practitioners, regulators, insurers, and the public at large. Any change in the definition of hypertension will require broad consensus to be truly useful.

Need for clear disease categories. Although BP and CVD risk are continuously related, discrete disease categories are a practical necessity to judge effectiveness of care. All of the worldwide guidelines recommend the use of BP categories as pioneered by the National High Blood Pressure Education Program (NHBPEP) in the reports of the Joint National Committee on the Prevention, Detection, Evaluation, and Treatment of High Blood Pressure (JNC). Disease stages are essentially platforms for therapy as recommended in JNC 7 (**Table C107.1**). This streamlined approach has aided overall BP control because of the clear path presented to clinicians.

Approach # 2. Subclinical disease markers improve risk stratification within disease categories

A new definition of hypertension. "*Hypertension is a progressive cardiovascular syndrome arising from complex and interrelated etiologies. Early markers of the syndrome are often present before BP elevation is sustained; therefore, hypertension cannot be classified solely by discrete BP thresholds. Progression is strongly associated with functional and structural cardiac and vascular abnormalities that damage the heart, kidneys, brain,* *vasculature and other organs and lead to premature morbidity and death*".

This definition from the Hypertension Writing Group attempts to identify the disease spectrum within which high BP and CVD coexist. What is substantially less clear is if there is a standard cause and effect relationship between hypertension and vascular disease. Does hypertension cause vascular disease or does vascular disease cause hypertension? Are both true or are hypertension and vascular disease parts of another larger process? The multiple pathophysiologic processes that lead to an increased BP have additional effects on morbidity and mortality. In this sense, BP measurements must be evaluated in the context of the patient's global cardiac risk (**Table C107.2**).

Blood pressure thresholds. CVD risk is continuously and logarithmically related to BP level from 115/75 to 185/110 mm Hg. In each successive JNC report, there was a significant change toward lower threshold values as a result of improvements in the evidence base. In JNC 7, BP levels <120/80 mm Hg are called *normal* and BP values ≥120/80 mm Hg and <140/90 mm Hg are classified as "prehypertension." But there is heterogeneity within groups; not everyone with BP >120/80 mm Hg is at equal risk and many may not require drug therapy. Some people with office BP levels <140/90 mm Hg have already had a stroke or a myocardial infarction, while those with modest BP elevations and no early markers of CVD are probably not at significantly increased risk and should not bear the stigma of a "predisease." Therefore, as has long been appreciated, hypertension represents a disease continuum and cannot easily be defined by a threshold level of BP.

TABLE C107.1

CLASSIFICATION AND MANAGEMENT OF BLOOD PRESSURE FOR ADULTS 18 YEARS OR OLDER

BP classification	Systolic BP, mm Hg[a]		Diastolic BP, mm Hg[a]	Management[a]		
					Initial drug therapy	
				Lifestyle modification	Without compelling indications	With compelling indications
Normal	<120	and	<80	Encourage		
Prehypertension	120–139	or	80–89	Yes	No antihypertensive drug indicated	Drug(s) for the compelling indications[b]
Stage 1 hypertension	140–159	or	90–99	Yes	Thiazide-type diuretics for most; may consider ACE inhibitor, ARB, β-blocker, CCB, or combination	Drug(s) for the compelling indications Other antihypertensive drugs (diuretics, ACE inhibitor, ARB, β-blocker, CCB) as needed
Stage 2 hypertension	≥160	or	≥100	Yes	Two-drug combination for most (usually thiazide-type diuretic and ACE inhibitor or ARB or β-blocker or CCB)[c]	Drug(s) for the compelling indications Other antihypertensive drugs (diuretics, ACE inhibitor, ARB, β-blocker, CCB) as needed

ACE, angiotensin-converting enzyme; ARB, angiotensin receptor blocker; BP, blood pressure; CCB, calcium channel blocker.
[a]Treatment determined by highest BP category.
[b]Treat patients with chronic kidney disease or diabetes to BP goal of <130/80 mm Hg.
[c]Initial combined therapy should be used cautiously in those at risk for orthostatic hypotension.

TABLE C107.2

HYPERTENSION WRITING GROUP DEFINITION AND CLASSIFICATION OF HYPERTENSION

Classification	Normal	Stage 1 hypertension	Stage 2 hypertension	Stage 3 hypertension
Descriptive category	Normal BP or rare BP elevations **AND** No identifiable CVD[c]	Occasional or intermittent BP elevations **OR** Early CVD[c]	Sustained BP elevations **OR** Progressive CVD[c]	Marked and sustained BP elevations **OR** Advanced CVD[c]
JNC 7 risk factors[a]	None or few	Several	Many	Many
Early disease markers (Table C107.3)	None	Usually present	Overtly present	Overtly present with progression
Target organ disease[b]	None	None	Early signs present	Overtly present ± CVD events

This approach recognizes the continuous nature of CVD Risk and suggests that hypertension is a late manifestation of a progressive series of changes that lead to organ damage.
BP, blood pressure.
[a]JNC 7 risk factors: Age (>55 years for men, >65 years for women), hypertension, cigarette smoking, obesity (BMI $\geq$30 kg/m^2), physical inactivity, dyslipidemia, diabetes mellitus, family history of premature CVD (men <55 years or women <65 years), estimated GFR <60 mL/min, microalbuminuria.
[b]Target organ disease = coronary artery disease, peripheral vascular disease, cerebrovascular disease, or chronic kidney disease.
[c]CVD = cardiovascular disease.

Global cardiovascular disease risk. Although BP remains one of the most important aspects of the clinical assessment of patients, the levels of BP must be evaluated in light of the total cardiovascular risk, particularly in individuals with lower BPs. For example, systolic BPs of 120 to 130 mm Hg are more problematic in individuals with diabetes mellitus or other components of the metabolic syndrome but may be much less so for people with no other cardiovascular risk factors.

Implementation. A definition is not the same as a guideline. BP categories may be necessary components of guidelines, clinical protocols, and certain insurance standards. The four categories used to classify hypertension in JNC 7 (normal, prehypertension, and stages 1 and 2 hypertension) need to be more closely associated with overall risk status. The Hypertension Writing Group proposed to classify patients as either normal or hypertensive, based on their cardiovascular status and BP above optimal (<120/80 mm Hg). The progression of hypertension—from early to advanced—can be represented as stages 1, 2, and 3 hypertension, with each stage of hypertension characterized by the presence or absence of cardiovascular risk factors, early markers of hypertensive CVD, and target organ damage (Table C107.3).

Optimal blood pressure. The optimal BP is the physiologic pressure at which the cardiovascular system is designed to operate most efficiently. When the BP is chronically elevated above the optimal value, the pressure itself damages the blood vessels and overloads the left ventricle. Alterations in either systolic or diastolic BP signal a disturbance in the circulation. When all components of BP are elevated, it is almost certain that the resistance arterial vessels will be narrowed, perhaps to protect capillary pressure at <25 mm Hg. On the other hand, because systolic BP is heavily dependent on the distensibility of the central arterial circulation, increased systolic BP may be present when constriction of resistance vessels is not present. Systolic and diastolic BP elevations must be considered separately and together.

Further evolution. The definition of hypertension will continue to evolve as more is learned about the pathophysiology of the various hypertension phenotypes. As that occurs, the classification of hypertension will also evolve. For example, the use of the term *primary* idiopathic (essential) does little to clarify for the clinician, or the researcher for that matter, the nature of the disease process. Hypertension NOS (not otherwise specified) is probably a better description until further clarification is known. The *International Classification of Diseases 10* still uses such arcane terms as *benign* and even has a classification of "benign hypertension with heart failure." Further, as we learn more about the various phenotypes of hypertension the number of secondary forms of hypertension will increase. The final result should be more accurate risk stratification and better prevention and treatment.

Approach # 3: Practical clinical phenotypes are necessary for realistic management

Rationale for clinical phenotyping. Subclassifying hypertension presents many challenges but it is no longer acceptable to ignore the diverse hemodynamic patterns of BP elevation because they have different prognoses and will require different therapies. A reasonable analogy is diabetes mellitus; without recognizing the fundamental differences between insulin deficiency (type 1) and insulin resistance (type 2) diabetes, little progress could have been made in treatment of the condition. As with diabetes, hypertension is neither a single disease process nor can it be defined effectively by the magnitude of a single variable (i.e., office cuff BP elevation) alone.

Hypertension is a heterogeneous hemodynamic syndrome resulting from abnormalities in one or more interacting physiologic processes that include central arterial stiffness (arteriosclerosis) that elevates pulse pressure (PP) and arteriolar constriction and hypertrophy that elevates mean arterial pressure (MAP). Furthermore, PP and systolic BP are not constant throughout the arterial

TABLE C107.3

EARLY MARKERS OF CARDIOVASULAR DISEASE

BP	Cardiac
Loss of nocturnal dipping Exaggerated response to exercise Salt sensitivity Widened pulse pressure	Left ventricular hypertrophy (mild) Increased atrial filling pressure Decreased diastolic relaxation
Vascular	**Renal**
Increased arterial stiffness Increased wave reflection and systolic pressure augmentation Increased carotid intima-media thickness Coronary calcification Endothelial dysfunction	Microalbuminuria Elevated serum creatinine Decreased estimated GFR
	Retinal
	Hypertensive retinal changes

GFR, glomelular filtration rate.

tree, so there are substantial methodological artifacts intrinsic to arm cuff BP measurements. BP is not a static variable; BP must change acutely to meet physiologic needs. The highly variable nature of BP, within and across individuals, becomes highly problematic unless it is recognized separately. Some people exhibit exaggerated responses to environmental stressors, whereas others have variations in circadian rhythms. These highly variable and interactive processes make it difficult, but not impossible, to provide a meaningful classification system based on practical home and office BP readings.

Hemodynamic subtypes of hypertension. There are three major hemodynamic mechanisms that can lead to clinically relevant BP elevations: (1) inappropriately high systemic vascular resistance (SVR), (2) elevated PP, and (3) intermittent hypertension (**Table C107.4**). All of these subtypes ("endophenotypes") of the syndrome (phenotype) of hypertension interact in various ways but can be relatively easily distinguished from one another by the patterns of systolic and diastolic BP elevations at home and in medical setting, without extensive laboratory testing.

TABLE C107.4

HEMODYNAMIC SUBTYPES OF HYPERTENSION

	Hemodynamics	Physiologic associations	Office BP[a]		Home or 24-hr BP[a]	
			DBP	SBP	DBP	SBP
Type 1: Diastolic hypertension	Inappropriately high systemic vascular resistance	Obesity Neurohumoral activation Microvascular remodeling	>90	>140 (variable)	>85	>135 (variable)
Type 2: Wide pulse pressure hypertension	2a. Increased aortic stiffness 2b. Decreased aortic diameter 2c. Very high stroke volume	High aortic impedance (relative or absolute) Age Gender	<90	>140	<85	>135
Type 3: Intermittent hypertension	3a. Exaggerated stress-related flow/resistance increase	"White coat hypertension"	SBP >140 or DBP >90		SBP <135 and DBP <85	
	3b. Exaggerated resting flow/resistance variation	Exaggerated AM BP surge Baroreflex impairment	Highly variable		Hypertension and hypotension	

[a]BP values in mm Hg. MAP = mean arterial pressure, DBP = diastolic BP, SBP = systolic BP, PP = pulse pressure. Note that reactive hypertension is also called *white coat hypertension*. See text for further explanation.

Type 1: diastolic hypertension. The simplest form of sustained hypertension and the one most prevalent in younger individuals is diastolic hypertension; both home and office BPs are elevated. The principal underlying hemodynamic abnormality in this condition is inappropriately increased SVR and therefore MAP, although it could be argued that without a corresponding inappropriate increase in cardiac output, there would be no sustained increase in diastolic BP. Systolic BP is commonly elevated as well but is the result of elevated diastolic BP. As in "prehypertension," these individuals tend to be obese and have inappropriate activation of the sympathetic nervous and renin-angiotensin systems; early pathologic changes in the microcirculation, such as arteriolar hypertrophy or microvascular rarefaction may also exist. Lifestyle modifications are indicated, as are vasodilator antihypertensive medications (diuretics, renin-angiotensin inhibitors, and calcium antagonists), all of which reduce SVR.

Type 2: wide pulse pressure hypertension. The most prevalent form of hypertension, particularly in older individuals, is "wide pulse pressure hypertension," which is always due to a relative or absolute increase in aortic impedance accompanied by a relatively high pulse volume. Both home and office systolic BPs are elevated and the PP is high (arbitrarily >50 mm Hg). In elderly individuals, wide PP is associated with arteriosclerosis and increased aortic stiffening (type 2a). In individuals with short stature (especially women), smaller aortic diameter is the principal abnormality (type 2b); aortic wall elasticity is usually normal. Also, in young individuals, particularly male athletes, wide PP can be the result of very high stroke volumes, with or without abnormalities in aortic stiffness (type 2c). The relevance of this condition is that the effects of "standard" antihypertensive drugs are somewhat different; treatment of this condition is undertaken with the realization that diastolic BP is relatively fixed and that systolic BP can be reduced by antihypertensive drugs only to the degree that SVR and MAP are reduced. Care should be taken to judge the degree of BP control in light of potential symptoms of hypotension, particularly orthostatic hypotension. At present, there are no approved agents that directly reduce aortic stiffness, although long-term BP control may allow a degree of favorable aortic remodeling.

Type 3: intermittent hypertension. Nonsustained BP elevations are extremely common and are differentiated by the patterns of intermittent BP elevation that occur at home and in the office and also by time of day. The condition can be divided into stress-induced (type 3a) and resting (type 3b) BP variation, which can be either systolic or diastolic depending on the underlying hemodynamic characteristics discussed for types 1 and 2 hypertension. The pathophysiology of intermittent hypertension is not well understood but likely involves a combination of exaggerated responses of neurohumoral systems and increased vasoreactivity. Diagnosis and monitoring of these conditions is currently not standardized but may include 24-hour ambulatory BP monitoring along with measures of target organ damage (e.g., microalbuminuria or ventricular hypertrophy). Therapy for intermittent hypertension syndromes is different from conditions of sustained hypertension: individuals with the white coat syndrome may not benefit from standard antihypertensive drugs because they do not tend to blunt stress-induced BP variability (see Chapters A56 and B89); marked early morning BP surges can be blunted with nighttime α-blocker therapy; baroreflex failure is extremely difficult to treat because of alternating hypertension and hypotension (see Chapter C154).

Suggested Readings

Chobanian AV, Bakris GL, Black HR, et al. National High BP Coordinating Committee. Seventh report of the Joint National Committee on Prevention, Detection, Evaluation, and Treatment of High BP. The JNC 7 Report. *Hypertension* 2003;42:1206–1252.

Giles TD. BP goals for hypertension guidelines: what is wrong with "optimal"? *J Clin Hypertens* 2006;8:835–839.

Giles TD, Berk BC, Black HR, et al. Hypertension Writing Group. Expanding the definition and classification of hypertension. *J Clin Hypertens* 2005;7:505–512.

The Joint National Committee on Prevention, Detection, Evaluation, and Treatment of High BP. *The sixth report of the Joint National Committee on Prevention, Detection, Evaluation, and Treatment of High BP.* Bethesda: National Institutes of Health, 1997. NIH Publication No. 98-4080.

Materson BJ. Commentary on "Expanding the definition and classification of hypertension". *J Clin Hypertens* 2005;7:540–541. Invited commentary.

Materson BJ. Prehypertension: an important preventive medicine concept—or marketing ploy? *J Clin Hypertens* 2006;8:729–730.

Moser M. Hypertension treatment guidelines: is it time for an update? *J Clin Hypertens* 2007;9:9–14.

Pickering TG. Do we really need a new definition of hypertension? *J Clin Hypertens* 2005;7:702–704.

Weber MA. Expanding the scope of hypertension: are we creating new diseases? *J Clin Hypertens* 2006;8:615–618.

SECTION II ■ EVALUATION OF TARGET ORGANS

CHAPTER C108 ■ EVALUATION OF ELECTROLYTE ABNORMALITES IN HYPERTENSION

JOHN W. GRAVES, MD, FACP, FACC

KEY POINTS

■ Disturbances in potassium are useful to screen for renal failure, hyperaldosteronism, renovascular hypertension, and Cushing's disease but serum K^+ is not always low in these disorders.

■ Disturbances in sodium in the hypertensive patient suggest underlying conditions such as kidney disease or heart failure (HF); mild changes in serum sodium also occur in thyroid and parathyroid disorders.

■ Electrolyte disturbances can influence the choice of antihypertensive drug therapies.

See also Chapters **C105,** C167, and C170

The evaluation of the patient with hypertension includes identifying secondary causes of hypertension, assessing evidence of target organ involvement, and uncovering additional factors that may influence the choice of antihypertensive treatment. A thorough history and physical examination should be complemented by a list of suggested laboratory tests according to the Joint National Committee (JNC 7): urinalysis, complete blood count, serum sodium (Na^+), serum potassium (K^+), serum creatinine, fasting blood glucose, and total and high-density lipoprotein (HDL) cholesterol measurements. Serum Na^+ and serum K^+ values at the time of diagnosis can aid the clinician in two ways: They may heighten suspicion of secondary forms of hypertension or they may be helpful in decisions about which drug to use.

Potassium and hypertension

Various clinical syndromes are associated with alterations in serum potassium.

Hypokalemia. The presence of hypokalemia is perhaps the most noteworthy aspect of screening blood tests performed in the hypertensive patient. In evaluating electrolyte abnormalities and hypertension, valuable clues are often obtained from a careful history and physical examination. Diseases marked by excessive activity of the renin-angiotensin-aldosterone system (RAAS) occasionally present with hypokalemia and hypertension.

Hyperaldosteronism. The most common RAAS abnormality seen in some centers is primary hyperaldosteronism, which may present with both hypokalemic alkalosis and hypernatremia. Of note, many cases of proven hyperaldosteronism do not present with hypokalemia and the diagnostic sensitivity of the test is low. Primary hyperaldosteronism is often associated with a significant orthostatic blood pressure (BP) decrease (supine to upright decrease that exceeds 20 mm Hg). Liddle's syndrome,

which mimics primary aldosteronism, is due to a specific mutation in the epithelial Na^+ channel in the collecting duct resulting in hypertension and hypokalemic alkalosis. It may be differentiated clinically from primary aldosteronism by the failure of hypokalemia and hypertension to respond to the mineralocorticoid receptor blockade.

Renovascular disease. A hypertensive patient with a history of previously controlled hypertension that becomes suddenly elevated or resistant to therapy should be considered for atherosclerotic renovascular disease, especially in the setting of heavy smoking, episodes of flash pulmonary edema, claudication, or angina. Hypokalemia is usually mild and transient. An abdominal bruit or bruit in any arterial circulation on physical examination are other signs of atherosclerotic disease.

Adrenal steroids. Another uncommon endocrine cause of hypertension with hypokalemia is Cushing's syndrome; the iatrogenic form is much more common than Cushing's disease (basophilic pituitary adenoma). Hypertension is typically a late manifestation of Cushing's syndrome, so diagnosis is often not inherently difficult.

Hypomagnesemia. Chronic significant alcohol ingestion can lead to hypertension and renal wasting of magnesium with resultant hypomagnesemia and hypokalemia.

Hyperkalemia. Hyperkalemia is a common occurrence in both acute and chronic renal insufficiency that is usually due to more than a single defect in K^+ homeostasis (**Table C108.1**) and is therefore more common in diabetic patients and the elderly in whom low aldosterone levels are coupled with some degree of renal insufficiency. Another common cause of hyperkalemia in diabetic patients is type IV renal tubular acidosis (hyporeninemic hypoaldosteronism). In such patients, anti-RAAS drugs may be deemed necessary for organ protection but BP responses may be lessened and combinations with

TABLE C108.1

ELECTROLYTE DISORDERS AND THEIR ASSOCIATED DISEASES

Disorder	Associated disease
Hypokalemia	Hyperaldosteronism Renovascular hypertension Cushing's syndrome Liddle's syndrome Hypomagnesemic syndromes
Hyperkalemia	Acute and chronic renal failure Type IV renal tubular acidosis Immunosuppressive drugs (cyclosporin, tacrolimus)

Hyponatremia	Acute and chronic renal failure
	Acute renal ischemia syndrome
	Malignant hypertension
	Renovascular hypertension
	Hypertensive heart disease
	Endocrine disease
	    Hyperparathyroidism
	    Hypothyroidism
	    SIADH and hypertension
	Increased intracranial pressure
	Medications (amitryptilene, etc.)

Hypernatremia	Water deprivation Hyperaldosteronism

SIADH, syndrome of inappropriate secretion of antidiuretic hormone.

diuretics required. With transplantation, even in the face of good allograft function, hyperkalemia and hypertension occur because of immunosuppressive medications such as cyclosporin and tacrolimus or most commonly as a result of the use of anti-RAAS drugs in the setting of underlying renal disease. Hyperkalemia may also be seen in postmenopausal women with primary hypertension, who are placed on hormone replacement therapy with a novel progestin drospirenone (YASMIN) which has spironolactone-like activity.

Sodium and hypertension

Hyponatremia. Hyponatremia may suggest the presence of a variety of diseases with hypertension as a feature (**Table C108.1**). Hyponatremia at the initial diagnosis of hypertension may be evidence for hypertensive target organ damage in the kidney or heart.

Renal failure. Renal insufficiency is a common cause of low serum Na$^+$ because when the glomerular filtration rate (GFR) falls below 30 mL per minute, patients with acute or chronic renal failure lose diuretic capacity. The timing of onset of hypertension can offer a clue to the etiology of the renal failure: In glomerular and vascular diseases of the kidney, hypertension occurs early in the course of renal disease; in interstitial renal disease, hypertension usually occurs late, when the renal insufficiency is more advanced. A hyponatremic-hypertensive syndrome has been reported with acute renal ischemia in malignant hypertension and also in the presence of chronic renal artery stenosis.

Heart failure. Hypertensive heart disease is also commonly associated with hyponatremia, particularly as heart failure

(HF) develops. In the setting of HF, there is marked volume dysregulation and renal hypoperfusion elicits a series of responses including increased renal vasoconstriction, activation of the RAAS, and excessive antidiuretic hormone (ADH) release, the sum of which cannot be overcome by increased levels of natriuretic peptides, nitric oxide, or prostaglandins. Excessive ADH release reduces the kidney's ability to excrete water and leads to hyponatremia.

Parathyroid and thyroid disease. Primary hyperparathyroidism may be associated with the development of hypertension and hyponatremia when far-advanced bone disease has developed. The advent of multichannel chemistry analyzers in clinical medicine has made early diagnosis of primary hyperparathyroidism common. Serum calcium is usually elevated and serum phosphorus depressed. The diagnosis is confirmed by simultaneous measurement of ionized calcium and serum parathyroid hormone. A second endocrine disease that may present with mild hyponatremia and hypertension is hypothyroidism. Thyroid hormone is required for maintenance of optimal GFR and normal handling of water in the distal tubule. Deficiencies of thyroid hormone may coincidently lead to both hyponatremia and hypertension, which typically develop at advanced stages of the disease and do not predict whether hypertension will occur.

Other. Other conditions or drugs may result in hyponatremia and hypertension, including the tricyclic antidepressant amitriptyline, which can acutely elevate BP and lead to hyponatremia due to inappropriate ADH release. Increased intracranial pressure from brain tumors, brain abscess, meningitis, or subdural hematoma may be associated with severe hypertension as well as ADH excess and hyponatremia.

Hypernatremia. Hypernatremia occurs most often as a result of water deprivation in institutionalized patients, many of whom have preexisting hypertension. The presence of hypernatremia, particularly when accompanied by hypokalemic alkalosis, should alert the physician to the possibility of primary hyperaldosteronism (**Table C108.1**). The diagnosis of primary aldosteronism should be confirmed by specific testing, including measurement of plasma renin activity and plasma aldosterone levels, or 24-hour urinary excretion of sodium and aldosterone after salt loading. The latter test is quite specific when urinary aldosterone excretion is not suppressed below 6 μg per day during salt loading. Hypernatremia in primary hyperaldosteronism has been shown to be due to a resetting of the osmostat to higher levels of plasma Na$^+$ (there is a normal response to water loading and to dehydration, but at a higher than normal serum sodium or osmolality).

Impact on therapeutic choices

Diseases that disrupt K$^+$ homeostasis can have a significant impact on choices of antihypertensive therapy (**Table C108.2**).

Hyperkalemia. The presence of hyperkalemia militates against the use of antihypertensive drugs that can affect distal tubular secretion of K$^+$ (spironolactone, amiloride, eplerenone, or triamterene), or lower serum aldosterone levels [angiotensin-converting enzyme (ACE) inhibitors, angiotensin receptor blockers (ARBs), and to a smaller degree, β-blockers]. If drugs in these classes are needed, as in the case of proteinuric renal disease or HF, reversible causes of hyperkalemia should be addressed and frequent monitoring of the serum K$^+$ considered. In these and other cases, especially HF, potassium homeostasis can be improved by additional recommendations. In addition to fastidious dietary K$^+$ restriction, modest liberalization of dietary salt can be

ELECTROLYTE DISORDERS THAT AFFECT THERAPY

Disorder	Drugs to avoid	Drugs to use
Hypokalemia	Diuretics	ACE inhibitors Angiotensin receptor blockers β-Blockers Potassium-sparing agents

Hyperkalemia	ACE Inhibitors
	Angiotensin
	  receptor blockers
	Potassium-sparing
	  agents
		Diuretics (1 or more)

Hyponatremia	Diuretics	ACE inhibitors Angiotensin receptor blockers

Hypernatremia	Diuretics (if
	  volume depleted
	  or K+ low)	

ACE, angiotensin-converting enzyme.

prescribed along with the combination of a loop diuretic and a distal tubular agent (thiazide) to enhance distal tubular sodium delivery, increase distal tubular sodium–potassium exchange, promote kaliuresis, and help normalize serum K^+.

Hypokalemia and hyponatremia. Diuretics may worsen preexisting hypokalemia or hyponatremia whereas use of ACE inhibitors or ARBs may help normalize serum Na^+ and K^+ values, particularly in HF. Elderly hypertensive patients (particularly women) are at a higher risk of developing hyponatremia with either thiazide diuretics or K^+-sparing agents (spironolactone, amiloride, eplerenone, and triamterene) and require frequent monitoring.

Suggested Readings

Agarwal M, Lynn KL, Mark RA, et al. Hyponatremic-hypertensive syndrome with renal ischemia: an under-recognized disorder. *Hypertension* 1999;33(4):1020–1024.

Friedler RM, Koffler A, Kurokawa K. Hyponatremia and hypernatremia. *Clin Nephrol* 1977;7(4):163–172.

Gennari FJ. Disorders of potassium homeostasis. Hypokalemia and hyperkalemia. *Crit Care Clin* 2002;18:273–228.

Joint National Committee on Prevention, Detection, Evaluation, and Treatment of High Blood Pressure. The Seventh Report of the Joint National Committee on Prevention, Detection, Evaluation, and Treatment of High Blood Pressure. *JAMA* 2003;289:2560–2572.

Miller M. Hyponatremia and arginine vasopressin dysregulation: mechanisms, clinical consequences, and management. *J Am Geriatr Soc* 2006;54(2):345.

Pacak K, Linehan WM, Eisenhofer G, et al. Recent advances in genetics, diagnosis, localization, and treatment of pheochromocytoma. *Ann Intern Med* 2001;134(4):315–329.

Palmer BF, Alpern RJ. Liddle's syndrome. *Am J Med* 1998;104(3):301–309.

Soupart A, Gross P, Legros JJ, et al. Successful long term treatment of hyponatremia in syndrome of inappropriate antidiuretic hormone secretion with satavaptan (SR121463B), an orally active non peptide vasopressin V2 receptor antagonist. *Clin J Am Soc Nephrol* 2006;1:1154–1160.

Young WF, Hogan MJ, Klee GG, et al. Primary aldosteronism: diagnosis and management. *Mayo Clin Proc* 1990;65:96–110.

CHAPTER C109 ■ BASIC CARDIAC EVALUATION: PHYSICAL EXAMINATION, ELECTROCARDIOGRAM, CHEST RADIOGRAPH, AND STRESS TESTING

CLARENCE SHUB, MD AND ANDREW J. LUISI, Jr., MD

KEY POINTS

■ Hypertensive heart disease can be detected by clinical examination, electrocardiogram (ECG), and cardiac imaging.

■ Left ventricular hypertrophy (LVH) is a manifestation of "target organ damage" and implies an adverse prognosis and the need for aggressive therapy in the hypertensive patient.

■ Although the ECG remains the traditional method for detecting LVH, its relative lack of sensitivity makes echocardiography the preferred modality for diagnosis and quantification.

■ Stress testing is appropriate for patients with a history of hypertension and provides prognostic data in the patient population.

■ An exaggerated blood pressure (BP) response during exercise stress testing may identify those subjects at risk for future hypertension and mortality from coronary artery disease.

■ In patients with left bundle branch block (LBBB) undergoing noninvasive evaluation of coronary disease, pharmacologic vasodilator stress should be used in conjunction with nuclear imaging to avoid imaging artifacts.

See also Chapters **C105, C110,** C111, C149, C150, and C151

Because the heart is one of the major target organs adversely affected by high blood pressure (BP), a careful and thorough evaluation of cardiac structure and function is an obligatory part of the examination of the hypertensive patient.

Physical examination

The presence of abnormalities on the cardiac and vascular physical examination affects choices in cardiac assessment and therapy and allows for more precise cardiovascular risk stratification, as recommended by the Seventh Report of the Joint National Committee on Prevention, Detection, Evaluation, and Treatment of High BP (JNC 7). The presence of "target organ" damage or clinical cardiovascular diseases [e.g., the detection of left ventricular hypertrophy (LVH) or peripheral vascular disease] should prompt more aggressive antihypertensive therapy and risk factor modification.

Palpation. One of the most important physical signs of LVH is a localized, sustained, and forceful apical impulse. This is best appreciated with the patient in the left lateral decubitus position, but it may be more difficult to elicit in obese patients and in those with chronic obstructive pulmonary disease. If the apical impulse in the supine position is laterally displaced, left ventricular (LV) dilatation should be suspected. In patients with hypertensive heart disease, LV dilatation is frequently associated with impaired ventricular function.

Auscultation

Heart sounds. A loud first heart sound (S_1) and brisk carotid upstroke in a hypertensive patient suggest a hyperdynamic circulatory state. The second heart sound (S_2) is usually narrowly split, and the aortic component may be accentuated. Although paradoxic splitting of S_2 may occur, it is uncommon and, in the absence of left bundle branch block (LBBB), suggests LV systolic dysfunction. A third heart sound (S_3) is unusual except when LV systolic failure occurs. In almost all patients, a fourth heart sound (S_4) develops before the S_3 is heard; when the S_3 is heard, the S_4 is almost always present. The incidence of an S_4 in hypertensive patients has been estimated to be between 50% and 70%, especially in the presence of LVH and in older patients. An S_4 is the auscultatory counterpart of a vigorous atrial contraction into a relatively noncompliant left ventricle. An S_4 may be associated with a palpable presystolic impulse or

A wave. The S_4 is best appreciated when the patient is in the left lateral decubitus position and the bell of the stethoscope is gently placed directly on the point of maximal apical impulse. Because of the difficulty in routine clinical assessment of an S_4, the presence of a palpable A wave appears to be more specific for the pathophysiologic mechanisms described earlier. An aortic systolic ejection sound (or click) is occasionally heard in hypertensive patients and appears to be related to forceful expansion of a dilated aortic root.

Systolic murmurs. A systolic murmur can frequently be heard in older hypertensive patients. This murmur is usually ejection in type, early in timing, and of low intensity (grade 1 or 2). It most often represents aortic outflow turbulence related to a sclerotic aortic valve. This murmur can be heard at both the apex and the base, but, occasionally, the murmur is localized to the apex alone and can be confused with mitral regurgitation. Some hypertensive patients with systolic murmurs may have LV outflow tract obstruction, a condition that has been referred to as *hypertensive hypertrophic cardiomyopathy.* Such patients often have a small LV cavity with hypertrophied walls and normal or hyperdynamic systolic function. Recognition of this disorder is important, because it may worsen with the administration of certain antihypertensive drugs, especially diuretics or direct-acting vasodilators. Bedside hemodynamic maneuvers, such as the Valsalva maneuver, that accentuate the systolic murmur may provide an important clue to the presence of LV outflow tract obstruction.

Diastolic murmurs. An early diastolic murmur of aortic regurgitation, which may be variable in intensity and duration, may occasionally be found in hypertensive patients. Unless there is a separate anatomic defect of the aortic valve, the aortic regurgitation represents a "functional" abnormality secondary to dilatation of the aortic ring. This abnormality is more common in older hypertensive patients and may lessen in severity or even disappear as BP is lowered.

Peripheral pulses. Examination of the carotid, femoral, and extremity arterial pulses is also important. Reduced volume of the femoral pulses or a delay in femoral pulse timing (especially in a young patient) compared with simultaneous palpation of the radial pulse suggests the possibility of coarctation of the aorta. The presence of femoral or carotid bruits and reduced arterial purses in the lower extremities suggests vascular obstructive disease, which, in older patients, is most commonly due to atherosclerosis. This process of vascular damage is enhanced and accelerated in the presence of systemic hypertension.

Electrocardiogram

Standard electrocardiography is a specific but poorly sensitive tool for the diagnosis of LVH. Compared with the chest radiograph, the routine scalar electrocardiogram (ECG) is more sensitive in detecting LVH in hypertensive patients. In the late stages of hypertensive heart disease, typical signs of LVH are almost always seen on the ECG. Therefore, when a patient presents with heart failure (HF) that is attributed to hypertension, in addition to other target organ involvement, he or she almost always has some evidence of LVH on the ECG; if not, other causes for HF should be considered. The ECG is the traditional and standard method for detecting LVH. However, it detects only 20% to 50% of instances of autopsy-proven LVH in patient populations and <10% of echocardiographic LVH in the general population. Despite this relative insensitivity, ECG-LVH is a strong predictor

of cardiovascular morbidity, including the risk of developing atrial fibrillation and HF, and mortality. The cost-effectiveness of the ECG may be questioned when detection of hypertensive LVH is the only goal and its prognostic value appears to be less than that of echocardiography. However, it does provide important information when other clinical abnormalities (e.g., myocardial ischemia or infarction, arrhythmias, or conduction defects) are sought.

Voltage criteria. Various ECG diagnostic criteria for diagnosing LVH exist [e.g., the scoring system recommended by Estes; the Sokolow-Lyon criteria; the criteria of McPhie (sum of tallest precordial R and S waves >45 mm); the sum of 12-lead QRS voltages; and the Minnesota code]. Conventional ECG criteria correlate with echocardiographic LV mass index (see Chapter C110) but do not predict specific geometric patterns very well (**Figure C109.1**). ECG evidence of left atrial enlargement may occur in the early stages of hypertension, is associated with LV diastolic dysfunction, and may precede abnormalities in the QRS complex. Improved diagnostic sensitivity with excellent specificity, especially in obese patients, is provided by sex-specific Cornell voltage criteria ($S_{V3} + R_{V1} \geq 20$ mm in women or ≥ 28 mm in men). Combining various ECG criteria improves sensitivity. With regard to QRS amplitudes, considerable overlap exists in normal and hypertensive patients. Factors such as age, sex, race, and body weight affect the QRS amplitude and may influence the predictive value of QRS criteria for the diagnosis of LVH. In the presence of LBBB, LVH is difficult to diagnose. Therefore, when precordial QRS voltages alone are used as criteria for LVH,

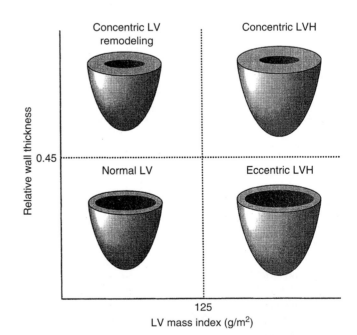

Figure C109.1 Diagram depicting relation between left ventricular (LV) mass index and relative wall thickness. An increase in LV mass index (defined as >125 g/m²) denotes development of left ventricular hypertrophy (LVH). If relative wall thickness (ratio of wall thickness/LV cavity radius) does not increase proportionately, chamber volume is increased and a more volume-dependent "eccentric" LVH occurs. However, if there is an increase in relative wall thickness along with LV mass index, a more "concentric" pressure-dependent LVH occurs. Conversely, if LV mass index does not increase but selective wall thickness increases, the more recently described "remodeling" phenomenon occurs. (Adapted from Frohlich ED, Apsten C, Chobanian AV, et al. The heart in hypertension. *N Engl J Med* 1992;327:998–1008.)

significant numbers of false-positive and false-negative results may occur.

Vectorcardiography. Vectorcardiographic analysis increases diagnostic sensitivity. The vectorcardiographic forces are shifted posteriorly and to the left. This is manifested in the scalar ECG as an increased R wave in leads I, aVL, V_5, and V_6. As anterior forces decrease (diminished R waves in precordial leads V_I through V_3), the pattern of anterior infarction may be simulated. Left axis deviation in the frontal plane may occur. Hypertensive patients with ECG-LVH are more likely to have impaired LV performance and greater LV mass.

Strain pattern. With increasing severity of hypertension, T-wave amplitude decreases, and T-wave inversion may occur, especially in ECG leads I, aVL, V_5, and V_6. The addition of J-point and ST-segment depression constitutes the pattern that has been called *LV strain*. Relative subendocardial ischemia may be responsible for these repolarization abnormalities. The ECG diagnosis of LVH is considerably strengthened in the presence of increased QRS voltages combined with typical repolarization abnormalities (LV strain). The LV strain pattern correlates with increased echocardiographic LV mass—especially when there is concomitant coronary artery disease.

QRS duration and Cornell product. The QRS duration has been reported to widen with increasing severity of hypertension, and the finding of ventricular conduction delay on the ECG has been correlated with certain histologic abnormalities (e.g., myocardial fibrosis). Increased QRS duration is a predictor of cardiovascular mortality. Inclusion of conduction abnormalities with voltage criteria further improves specificity. LVH can be reliably diagnosed with the Cornell voltage product, calculated as (R wave in aVL + S wave in V_3) × QRS duration ≥2,440. The ECG abnormalities may improve or even revert to normal with successful antihypertensive therapy (decreased QRS voltages and resolution of ST-T–wave abnormalities). Regression of ECG-LVH during antihypertensive therapy is associated with a lower likelihood of cardiovascular events.

QT changes. The QT interval may be prolonged in patients with LVH, and QT dispersion (difference between maximal and minimal corrected QT intervals) has been reported to be increased in elderly hypertensive patients and is associated with LVH, ventricular arrhythmias, and sudden death.

24-hour ambulatory electrocardiogram monitoring

Clinical investigations using 24-hour ambulatory ECG monitoring have shown a greater incidence of ventricular arrhythmias in hypertensive patients with LVH. Ventricular arrhythmias appear to worsen as the hypertrophy progresses, and LVH patients have an increased risk of sudden cardiac death. Atrial fibrillation, especially in the elderly, and other supraventricular tachycardias are more common in patients with hypertension than in the general population. Although it is not indicated for asymptomatic patients, 24-hour ambulatory ECG monitoring can be useful in assessing atrial and ventricular arrhythmias in patients with palpitations, near syncope, or syncope.

Chest radiograph

The chest radiograph of patients with uncomplicated hypertension is usually normal, although occasionally an abnormal cardiac contour suggesting LV enlargement or LVH may be found. However, one cannot rely on the routine chest radiograph to diagnose LVH. Subtle dilation of the ascending aortic shadow can be found in many patients with hypertension and no evidence of cardiac disease. In young patients and sometimes in adults, the presence of aortic coarctation as a cause of hypertension can be suspected on the chest radiograph.

Exercise stress testing

Exercise tolerance testing (ETT) has been used for decades to evaluate cardiorespiratory performance and inducible myocardial ischemia in patients with symptoms suggestive of coronary artery disease and in high-risk asymptomatic populations. The level of stress achievable during ETT and the ECG changes associated with exercise have long been used for risk stratification and prognosis, not only by medical providers but also life insurance underwriters. Severe systemic hypertension may cause exercise-induced ST depression in the absence of coronary atherosclerosis.

Blood pressure response to stress. Subjects with normal resting pressure who develop an abnormally high systolic blood pressure (SBP) with exercise (exaggerated BP response) have an increased risk of developing systemic hypertension in the future. The hypertensive response may be a predictor of future mortality from coronary artery disease. This finding may be a stronger risk factor than resting BP measurements for the eventual development of systemic hypertension.

Predisposition to myocardial ischemia in hypertension. When LVH is present, a coronary flow-demand mismatch may develop, with reduced myocardial blood flow per gram of tissue, decreased coronary flow reserve, myocardial ischemia, and symptoms of angina even without the presence of significant coronary artery disease.

Heart rate and electrocardiogram changes. The heart rate response to exercise is a rough measure of the degree of exercise stress [maximum predicted heart rate (MPHR), 220—age for men and 210—age for women is the formula used to calculate MPHR] when viewed in conjunction with the metabolic equivalents (mets) achieved. For example, deconditioned patients can reach target heart rates (85% MPHR) very quickly at low workload levels. Another marker of an adequate stress response is the double-product [rate-pressure product, HR × SBP at peak stress]; a value of ≥25,000 bpm·mm Hg is considered adequate.

ETT, when used in the evaluation of chest pain, relies on ECG changes associated with ischemia. These changes most commonly involve the ST segment; the more dramatic the ST abnormality, the more severe the magnitude of ischemic burden. If repolarization abnormalities are present, accurate interpretation of the stress-induced ECG changes is not possible leading to equivocal or nondiagnostic results. In this setting, radionuclide myocardial perfusion imaging (MPI) or stress echocardiography should be utilized in conjunction with ETT for an accurate estimation of stress-induced ischemia and ischemic burden. As with standard ECG stress testing, the sensitivity and specificity of MPI [single photon emission computed tomography (SPECT)] or stress echocardiography remains heavily dependent on the adequacy of physical stress as well as heart rate and rate-pressure product achieved during ETT.

Left bundle branch block. A special situation is the presence of LBBB, where the resulting repolarization abnormalities make the diagnosis of ischemia (both at rest and during exercise) very difficult. The presence of LBBB also causes perfusion abnormalities during nuclear imaging in the absence of obstructive

TABLE C109.1

CONTRAINDICATIONS TO EXERCISE TESTING

Absolute

- Acute myocardial infarction (within 2 d)
- High-risk unstable angina[a]
- Uncontrolled cardiac arrhythmias causing symptoms or hemodynamic compromise
- Symptomatic severe aortic stenosis
- Uncontrolled symptomatic heart failure
- Acute pulmonary embolus or pulmonary infarction
- Acute myocarditis or pericarditis
- Acute aortic dissection

Relative[b]

- Left main coronary stenosis
- Moderate stenotic valvular heart disease
- Electrolyte abnormalities
- Severe arterial hypertension[c]
- Tachyarrhythmias or bradyarrhythmias
- Hypertrophic cardiomyopathy and other forms of outflow tract obstruction
- Mental or physical impairment leading to inability to exercise adequately
- High-degree atrioventricular block

[a]ACC/AHA Guidelines for the Management of Patients with Unstable Angina/Non–ST-Segment Elevation Myocardial Infarction.
[b]Relative contraindications can be superseded if the benefits of exercise outweigh the risks.
[c]In the absence of definitive evidence, the ACC/AHA guidelines (2002) committee suggests systolic blood pressure of >200 mm Hg and/or diastolic blood pressure of >100 mm Hg. ACC/AHA 2002 Guideline Update for Exercise Testing, p. 5.

coronary disease when used either in conjunction with ETT or dobutamine infusion, probably due to ventricular dyssynchrony at higher heart rates. This artifact can be overcome with vasodilator imaging (i.v. dipyridamole or adenosine) that does not cause significant increases in heart rate but does adequately increase myocardial blood flow (approximately four times above baseline). Patients using negative chronotropic agents (i.e., β-blockers and calcium channel blockers) who are unable to attain a target heart rate during ETT are also candidates for pharmacologic vasodilator imaging in the evaluation of coronary disease. Alternatively, dobutamine stress echocardiography can be used in these circumstances.

Contraindications to exercise tolerance testing in hypertension

It has been assumed that an SBP >200 mm Hg or a diastolic BP >110 mm Hg is a relative contraindication to ETT (**Table C109.1**). Similarly, an exercise rise in SBP to values >200 mm Hg has been used as a reason to discontinue ETT by some practitioners. Newer work by Ellestad et al. does not support these restrictions, however, because there is little evidence of increased complications related to the acute BP elevations that occur. In fact, in patients with coronary disease and ST depression during ETT, those with a maximum SBP >200 mm Hg had fewer coronary events than those with "normal BP responses" possibly because better ventricular function is necessary to generate higher SBP values. Patients with known left main coronary disease or left main equivalent should not ordinarily undergo ETT, because the risk of ventricular fibrillation is higher in this population. Also, patients with severe aortic stenosis and symptoms secondary to this pathology are not candidates for stress testing.

Suggested Readings

Bulatov VA, Stenehjem A, Os I. Left ventricular mass assessed by electrocardiography and albumin excretion rate as a continuum in untreated essential hypertension. *J Hypertens* 2001;19:1473–1478.

Ellestad M. *Stress testing principles and practice*, 5th ed. New York: Oxford University Press, 2003.

Enstrom I, Burtscher IM, Eskilsson J, et al. Organ damage in treated middle-aged hypertensives compared to normotensives: results from a cross-sectional study in general practice. *Blood Press* 2000;9:28–33.

Gibbons RJ, Abrams J, Chatterjee K, et al. ACC/AHA Guideline update for exercise testing: summary article. A report of the American College of Cardiology/American Heart Association Task Force on Practice Guidelines. *Circulation* 2002;106:1883–1892.

Gryglewska B, Grodzicki T, Czarnecka D, et al. QT dispersion and hypertensive heart disease in the elderly. *J Hypertens* 2000;18:461–464.

Hsieh BP, Pham MX, Froelicher VF. Prognostic value of electrocardiographic criteria for left ventricular hypertrophy. *Am Heart J* 2006;150:161–167.

Okin PM, Devereux RB, Jern S, et al. Regression of electrocardiographic left ventricular hypertrophy during antihypertensive treatment and the prediction of major cardiovascular events. *JAMA* 2004;292:2343–2349.

Okin PM, Devereux RB, Nieminen MS, et al. Relationship of the electrocardiographic strain pattern to left ventricular structure and function in hypertensive patients: the LIFE study. *J Am Coll Cardiol* 2001;38:514–520.

Okin PM, Wachtell K, Devereux RB, et al. Regression of electrocardiographic left ventricular hypertrophy and decreased incidence of new-onset atrial fibrillation in patients with hypertension. *JAMA* 2006;296:1242–1248.

Verdecchia P, Dovellini EV, Gorini M, et al. Comparison of electrocardiographic criteria for diagnosis of left ventricular hypertrophy in hypertension: the MAVI study. *Ital Heart J* 2000;1:207–215.

Wachtell K, Rokkedal J, Bella JN, et al. Effect of electrocardiographic left ventricular hypertrophy on left ventricular systolic function in systemic hypertension (the LIFE study). Losartan intervention for endpoint. *Am J Cardiol* 2001;87:54–60.

CHAPTER C110 ■ CARDIAC IMAGING

CLARENCE SHUB, MD

KEY POINTS

■ Determination of left ventricular mass by echocardiography is the most commonly used noninvasive clinical method of diagnosing left ventricular hypertrophy (LVH).
■ Radionuclide angiography (RNA) can be used to assess the dynamic changes in the left ventricular blood pool but cannot directly evaluate the myocardium or the great vessels.
■ Magnetic resonance imaging (MRI) is a precise method to image the heart and great vessels, generally without need for contrast.
■ Choice of imaging modality depends on clinical presentation, availability, and local expertise.

See also Chapters **C109, C111,** C149, C150, and C151

Proper evaluation of the heart in hypertension often requires the use of imaging procedures.

Two-dimensional echocardiography

Overall, echocardiography is probably the most useful cardiac imaging technique for patients with hypertension and its complications.

Concentric versus eccentric hypertrophy. The type of overload to which the heart is subjected determines not only the specific chamber (or chambers) involved but also the pattern of left ventricular hypertrophy (LVH) (**Figure C110.1**). In concentric hypertrophy, the ratio of ventricular wall thickness to radius (relative wall thickness) is increased to >0.45. The ratio is decreased in eccentric hypertrophy. Eccentric hypertrophy should not be confused with the term *asymmetric hypertrophy*, in which a portion of the ventricle, usually the ventricular septum, is thicker than the other wall segments. *Eccentric* (or volume-overload) *hypertrophy* refers to a ventricle with an expanded cavitary volume in proportion to wall thickness, whereas *concentric hypertrophy* refers to a ventricle with thick walls relative to cavity volume. These specific geometric patterns appear to have prognostic implications.

Left ventricular mass determination. Increased ventricular septal and posterior wall thicknesses and left ventricular (LV) internal dimensions indicate LVH and LV chamber dilation, respectively. These parameters are more sensitive indicators of LVH, which has an adverse prognosis.

Calculations. LV muscle mass is calculated from standard M-mode echocardiographic measurements of the LV in necropsy-validated formulas. LV mass is directly related to body size and

should be indexed to body surface area or body height with use of sex-specific normative values. In addition, age appears to have a small but significant independent effect on LV mass in women but not in men. In comparison with autopsy-validated LVH, echocardiography has a specificity of 97%.

Accuracy. Echocardiographic LV mass has a sensitivity of 57% for mild, 92% for moderate, and 100% for severe LVH. In contrast, the sensitivity for the Romhilt-Estes electrocardiographic point score for LVH is only 7% in the general population and 54% in autopsied patients with relatively severe LVH. Therefore, echocardiography is more sensitive and specific (but also more expensive) than standard electrocardiogram (ECG) criteria.

Anatomy and function. LV dimensions, mass, and ejection fraction (EF) can also be measured by two-dimensional (2D) echocardiography, a technique that provides more complete global and regional information than M-mode echocardiography. Recent studies have shown that 3D echocardiography is more accurate and reproducible than M-mode or 2D echocardiography in the diagnosis of LVH. However, technical and feasibility issues need to be overcome before this modality becomes available for clinical purposes.

Left ventricular hypertrophy criteria. Partition values for detection of LVH by M-mode echocardiography, derived from apparently healthy subjects in the primarily white Framingham population, were an LV mass index in men >131 g per m^2 and in women >100 g per m^2. The upper-normal limits derived in a racially mixed normotensive population were >134 g per m^2 and 110 g per m^2, respectively.

Clinical correlations. Black hypertensive patients have higher LV mass and relative wall thickness than white hypertensive patients, even after controlling for clinical and hemodynamic

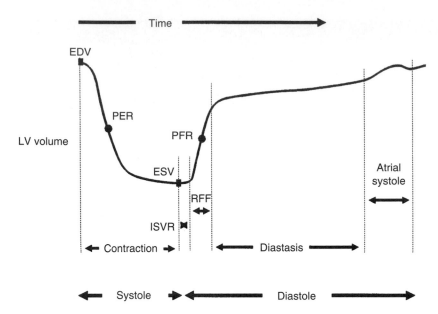

Figure C110.1 Dynamics of left ventricular (LV) volume and function as may be assessed by radionuclide angiography, computed tomography, and magnetic resonance imaging. Ejection fraction can be determined directly from the end-diastolic volume (EDV) and end-systolic volume (ESV). PER, peak systolic emptying rate; PFR, peak (early) diastolic filling rate; RFF, rapid (early) diastolic filling phase; ISVR, isovolumetric relaxation phase.

parameters. In obese subjects, identification of LVH is enhanced without loss of prognostic power by indexing LV mass to height. LV mass is best viewed as a continuous variable, and current partition values should ultimately be replaced by upper-normal limits that identify subjects with a more adverse prognosis. Echocardiographic LV mass is elevated in 20% to 50% of patients with stage 1 hypertension and up to 90% of hospitalized patients with stage 2+ hypertension. Regression of LV hypertrophy during antihypertensive therapy is associated with a reduction in cardiovascular (CV) risk. Echocardiography and, in selected circumstances, comprehensive echocardiography and Doppler assessment, would appear to be appropriate in the situations listed in **Table C110.1**. Limited, or focused, echocardiography has been proposed as a less costly screening method to detect LVH in hypertensive patients. Its clinical role in hypertensive patients needs to be further defined. Likewise, handheld echocardiography devices have become available and might prove to be useful in community-based screening for LVH in selected patients with hypertension.

Ventricular function

Systolic function. LV systolic function can be assessed by calculating systolic fractional shortening by M-mode echocardiography or EF by 2D echocardiography. The latter is preferable because it provides superior spatial resolution and is especially useful if LV shape or the pattern of wall motion is abnormal. 3D echocardiography is being increasingly used for this purpose, but is not yet considered a standard tool in clinical practice.

Diastolic function. Standard measurements of cardiac function in hypertensive patients show that although EF is preserved, mid-LV wall mechanics and diastolic filling are often impaired. These changes are better demonstrated using Doppler echocardiography.

Other diagnostic uses. Aortic valve sclerosis and mitral annular calcification are markers of atherosclerosis and both conditions can be easily imaged by 2D echocardiography. Hypertensive hypertrophic cardiomyopathy can be readily diagnosed by combined 2D and Doppler echocardiography and is especially important to consider in elderly patients with a systolic murmur. Echocardiography also allows imaging of the aorta, which can be useful in the evaluation of suspected aortic coarctation and aneurysm of the aortic root and ascending aorta. Transesophageal echocardiography is especially valuable for the rapid diagnosis of aortic dissection.

TABLE C110.1

INDICATIONS FOR USE OF ECHOCARDIOGRAPHY, COMPREHENSIVE ECHOCARDIOGRAPHY, AND DOPPLER ASSESSMENT

Possible cardiac involvement requires further confirmation (e.g., electrocardiographic diagnosis of left ventricular hypertrophy based on voltage criteria alone)[a]

Patient has a coexisting cardiac condition (e.g., valvular heart disease).

A child or adolescent has mild hypertension[a]

Etiology and significance of systolic murmurs need better definition

Hypertension occurs during exercise, but resting pressures are normal[a]

Dyspnea of unknown etiology (differentiate systolic vs. diastolic dys function and assess pulmonary artery pressures by Doppler)

[a]Limited or focused echocardiography to assess left ventricular hypertrophy only may be appropriate under these circumstances.

Doppler echocardiography and diastolic function

Doppler echocardiography allows separation of diastolic dysfunction into different patterns of LV filling abnormalities (e.g., delayed relaxation or restrictive filling patterns). Early myocardial relaxation (E' or Ea) can be assessed by Doppler tissue imaging and provides additional information about diastolic properties of the heart.

Delayed relaxation. Delayed myocardial relaxation is very common, especially in older patients, even in the absence of systolic dysfunction or LVH and can impair exercise capacity.

Restrictive filling. More advanced diastolic abnormalities, for example, pseudonormal or restrictive filling, may also represent impaired chamber compliance in LVH, with altered structure (e.g., collagen deposition), contractile proteins, or intracellular calcium flux. Restrictive filling patterns reflect a more severe diastolic abnormality and are more likely to be associated with clinical symptoms such as dyspnea. The compliance curve of the stiff, poorly compliant ventricle is shifted to the left and is steeper than normal in patients with LVH; for an equivalent increase in diastolic volume, diastolic blood pressure (BP) increases more abruptly in the hypertrophic than in the normal ventricle.

Correlated findings. Abnormal diastolic function in hypertensive patients has adverse prognostic implications. Left atrial enlargement is commonly found in hypertensive patients and is related to LV mass. Left atrial volume determination by echocardiography is a useful marker of chronic elevation of LV filling pressures and when increased has adverse prognostic implications. It is a marker of future CV events including atrial fibrillation.

Longitudinal LV function as assessed by Doppler tissue imaging or strain rate imaging may reveal abnormalities of myocardial performance, even when EF is normal. A global index of myocardial performance encompassing both systolic and diastolic parameters can also be obtained by Doppler tissue imaging. The incremental value of this information in clinical practice needs to be further defined.

Radionuclide angiography

Radionuclide angiography (RNA) is widely available, extensively used, and well validated for the assessment of cardiac size and function, especially dynamic changes in LV chamber volumes during the cardiac cycle. Because RNA examines the blood pool and not the myocardium directly, LV muscle mass cannot be quantified.

Ejection fraction. By registering externally the dynamic changes in the ventricular "blood pool," RNA measures relative changes in total LV chamber blood pool "counts" during the cardiac cycle. No assumptions regarding LV geometry are needed to quantify EF (as are necessary with echocardiography). As a result, RNA remains a very accurate clinical method to determine LV-EF, although imaging is suboptimal in very obese subjects.

Volume curves. By defining dynamic changes in the left ventricle during the cardiac cycle, the dynamics of contraction and relaxation can be defined (**Figure C110.1**). Radionuclide LV "volume" curves can be analyzed to determine relative rates

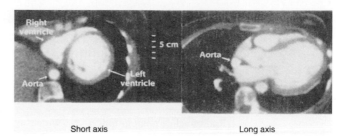

Short axis   Long axis

Figure C110.2 Ultrafast computed tomography scans at end diastole in the cardiac short-axis (transverse cardiac) and horizontal long-axis planes from the mid left ventricle in a patient with congestive heart failure. Note that this well-known complication of hypertension results in a dilated left ventricle that has poor contractile performance. Similar images can be obtained with magnetic resonance imaging.

of systolic contraction (peak emptying rate) and early diastolic relaxation (peak filling rate). Abnormalities of early diastolic filling are frequently observed in patients with hypertension before there is evidence of systolic dysfunction.

Electron beam (ultrafast) computed tomography

Methodology. Electron beam computed tomography (EBCT), also known as *ultrafast computed tomography* (CT) and *cine CT,* uses an electron beam and stationary target/detector pairing to replace the physical rotation of the X-ray source/detector pair required by conventional CT. Ultrafast CT can acquire tomographic images very rapidly. Ultrafast CT is used less commonly now than newer types of CT scanners. Methods for display and analysis of cardiac (50 microsecond) images derived from 2D echocardiography are used to quantify regional myocardial motion, EF, and chamber volumes (**Figure C110.2**); those developed from RNA define the dynamics of LV volumes during the cardiac cycle. Unlike RNA and magnetic resonance imaging (MRI), imaging by EBCT is "triggered" (as opposed to "gated") by the patient's ECG. Therefore, dynamic imaging of the entire heart can be completed in seconds.

Clinical use. Cardiac CT, like echocardiography and MRI, defines the cardiac chambers and myocardium and can also be used to define great vessel anatomy in hypertensive patients. CT scanning is extremely useful in assessing diseases of the aorta in severely ill patients and (because no sedation is necessary) in children. Calcium scores derived from EBCT identify individuals

TABLE C110.2

COMPARISON OF RADIONUCLIDE ANGIOGRAPHY, COMPUTED TOMOGRAPHY, AND MAGNETIC RESONANCE IMAGING METHODS TO DEFINE CARDIAC FUNCTION AND GREAT VESSEL ANATOMY

Imaging modality	Cardiac/vascular applications					
	Ejection fraction	Left ventricular mass	Left ventricular volume	Diastolic function	Regional wall motion (contraction) abnormalities	Great vessel anatomy
Radionuclide angiography	Yes	No	Yes	Yes	Yes	No
Conventional computed tomography	No	No	No	No	No	Yes
Computed tomography	Yes	Yes	Yes	Yes	Yes	Yes
Magnetic resonance imaging	Yes	Yes	Yes	Yes	Yes	Yes

TABLE C110.3

ADVANTAGES AND DISADVANTAGES OF RADIONUCLIDE ANGIOGRAPHY,
COMPUTED TOMOGRAPHY, AND MAGNETIC RESONANCE IMAGING
IN ASSESSING PATIENTS WITH HYPERTENSION

Imaging modality	Advantages	Disadvantages
Radionuclide angiography	Widely available in major medical centers	Radiation, limitations in large patients
Conventional computed tomography	Widely available in major medical centers	Radiation, contrast media
Computed tomography	Highly versatile and precise	Radiation, contrast media
Magnetic resonance imaging	Versatile, precise, no radiation	Limited availability[a], prolonged imaging[b]

[a]Although magnetic resonance imaging is widely available, currently there are limited facilities that can perform dynamic cardiac studies.
[b]See section Magnetic Resonance Imaging.

with atherosclerosis of the proximal coronary arteries. This test has been proposed to screen for coronary artery disease but its value remains to be established.

Magnetic resonance imaging

MRI provides exquisite tomographic images of the heart and great vessels that can be displayed from virtually any plane or orientation. Specific cine techniques (or magnetic resonance angiography) have been developed to allow quantification of EF, LV volumes, and LV muscle mass. Cine MRI can be used to assess the long-term effects of drug therapy on cardiac remodeling (i.e., regression of LVH, left atrial size, and improvement in diastolic function). MRI is used extensively to define aortic dissection and coarctation and to follow up such patients after surgical or pharmacologic therapy.

Advantages to MRI, in addition to the high-resolution imaging, include the absence of radiation or contrast-agent exposure to the patient, and the applicability with any level of renal function. MRI is useful to image the cardiac chambers or great vessels. A major disadvantage of MRI is the fact that the subject needs to remain still during image acquisition. Patients with claustrophobia or those with pacemakers or who are acutely ill cannot be imaged effectively with MRI. The method is safe for patients who have prosthetic (natural or metallic) valve replacements.

Comparison of imaging modalities

Echocardiography, RNA, CT, and MRI can all be used effectively to diagnose or quantify CV manifestations of hypertension (**Table C110.2**). Their relative utilities depend heavily on availability and the degree of local expertise with each technique and therefore, different diagnostic algorithms are found in different medical centers. Each modality has a role in defining specific complications of hypertension (LVH, diastolic dysfunction, reduced EF, heart failure, aortic aneurysm and dissection, or concomitant myocardial or valvular disease). Each has distinct advantages and disadvantages in clinical practice (**Table C110.3**) and accordingly, the clinician must choose carefully which method to apply to a specific patient. The decision is largely guided by individual clinical circumstances, the objectives of the study, relative costs of the various techniques, and the expertise of the local or referral laboratory or imaging center. Mere availability of a particular technique to image the heart and great vessels does not absolve the clinician of first establishing the necessity and objectives of the study. Although potentially useful in risk stratification, routine cardiac imaging in uncomplicated hypertensive patients is not a cost-effective strategy.

Suggested Readings

Cuspidi C, Lonati L, Macca G, et al. Cardiovascular risk stratification in hypertensive patients: impact of echocardiography and carotid ultrasonography. *J Hypertens* 2001;19:375–380.

Cuspidi C, Meani S, Fusi V, et al. Prevalence and correlates of left atrial enlargement in essential hypertension: role of ventricular geometry and the metabolic syndrome: the evaluation of target organ damage in hypertension study. *J Hypertens* 2005;23(4):875–882.

Hoffmann U, Globits S, Stefenelli T, et al. The effects of ACE inhibitor therapy on left ventricular myocardial mass and diastolic filling in previously untreated hypertensive patients: a Cine MRI study. *J Magn Reson Imaging* 2001;14:16–22.

Okin PM, Devereux RB, Jern S, et al. The Life Study Investigators. Baseline characteristics in relation to electrocardiographic left ventricular hypertrophy in hypertensive patients: the Losartan intervention for endpoint reduction (LIFE) in hypertension study. *Hypertension* 2000;36:766–773.

Rovner A, de las Fuentes L, Waggoner AD, et al. Characterization of left ventricular diastolic function in hypertension by use of doppler tissue imaging and color M-mode techniques. *J Am Soc Echocardiogr* 2006;19(7):872–879.

Rusconi C, Sabatini T, Faggiano P, et al. Prevalence of isolated left ventricular diastolic dysfunction in hypertension as assessed by combined transmitral and pulmonary vein flow Doppler study. *Am J Cardiol* 2001;87:357–360, A10.

Senior R, Galasko G, Hickman M, et al. Community screening for left ventricular hypertrophy in patients with hypertension using hand-held echocardiography. *J Am Soc Echocardiogr* 2004;17(1):56–61.

Verdecchia P, Carini G, Circo A, et al. Left ventricular mass and cardiovascular morbidity in essential hypertension: The MAVI Study. *J Am Coll Cardiol* 2001;38:1829–1835.

Wang M, Yip GWK, Wang AYM, et al. Tissue Doppler imaging provides incremental prognostic value in patients with systemic hypertension and left ventricular hypertrophy. *J Hypertens* 2005;23(1):183–191.

CHAPTER C111 ■ EVALUATION OF HEART FAILURE

KIRKWOOD F. ADAMS, Jr., MD

KEY POINTS

- Careful evaluation of systolic and diastolic function with echocardiography or other equivalent modalities (radionuclide ventriculography, magnetic resonance imaging) is routine to establish the type and severity of cardiac dysfunction present.
- Determination of heart failure (HF) etiology is a major part of the initial evaluation.
- Assessment of clinical severity based on standard metrics [New York Heart Association (NYHA) functional class] aids in prognosis and judging responses to therapy.

See also Chapters A59, **A60,** A73, **B78,** C109, **C110, C150,** and **C151**

Heart failure (HF) is a clinical syndrome characterized by edema, fatigue, and dyspnea, especially with exertion, that occurs primarily as a consequence of myocardial muscle dysfunction. It is often accompanied by characteristic abnormalities on physical examination that have important implications for staging and management. Although commonly referred to as *congestive HF,* the more restrictive term *HF* is preferred because (a) many patients with fatigue and exertional dyspnea have no obvious signs of fluid overload and (b) cardiac dysfunction in HF may be systolic or diastolic in nature. HF is the only major cardiovascular (CV) disease whose prevalence is increasing, a trend likely to continue as the population ages and patients survive longer with various cardiac diseases. In the last decade, this syndrome has emerged as a major public health problem now afflicting approximately 5 million patients in this country alone and accounting for >1 million hospitalizations a year. Patients with HF continue to experience a high death rate and 5-year survival rates in many groups is <50%, worse than many cancers.

Pathophysiologic considerations

Systolic dysfunction. The classic hemodynamic consequences of systolic dysfunction are reduced cardiac output and elevated ventricular filling pressure. Low cardiac output results in inadequate delivery of blood to meet the metabolic demands of body organs, particularly the kidney and skeletal muscle. Reduced blood flow to the kidneys impairs the ability to maintain normal sodium (Na^+) excretion and water balance; pedal edema is a characteristic finding. In more severe cases, fluid overload produces hepatic congestion, ascites, and anasarca. Inadequate cardiac output to meet the metabolic demands of exercise results in lethargy, easy fatigability, and exercise intolerance (see Chapter A60).

Left ventricular (LV) filling pressure rises in many patients as the result of impaired ventricular compliance and emptying. As filling pressure increases, pulmonary venous pressure rises, resulting in interstitial and alveolar edema and decreased pulmonary compliance. These alterations are the basis for orthopnea and paroxysmal nocturnal dyspnea (PND) and contribute to exertional dyspnea. Right ventricular failure often develops late in the course, with increased right-sided filling pressure evidenced by pleural effusions, hepatomegaly, a positive hepatojugular reflux, and abdominal congestion, which may be present even after pedal edema has resolved with diuretic therapy.

Diastolic dysfunction. Many patients with HF have "preserved systolic function" with normal LV ejection fraction. The pathophysiology of this syndrome is not fully understood but many patients with this condition have evidence of diastolic dysfunction by tissue Doppler (see Chapters A59, C150) or ventricular volume curves in addition to renal dysfunction and abnormal vascular compliance. LV diastolic dysfunction is especially characteristic of patients with left ventricular hypertrophy (LVH) due to hypertension or hypertrophic cardiomyopathy but occurs commonly in long-standing hypertension in the absence of LVH. Diastolic dysfunction results from poor intrinsic myocardial relaxation or abnormal chamber compliance, which increase ventricular filling pressure and may limit ventricular filling. Patients with coronary artery disease (CAD) may experience significant transient diastolic dysfunction during periods of angina or with a myocardial infarction (MI). Left ventricular end-diastolic pressure (LVEDP) is elevated, often in the absence of volume overload; symptoms of exertional dyspnea and orthopnea may result and episodic frank pulmonary edema can occur. These patients are very sensitive to Na^+ loads, which may rapidly precipitate an episode of HF.

Diagnostic evaluation of heart failure

HF is frequently misdiagnosed because it may cause only subtle complaints or may be confused with other conditions that cause similar symptoms and signs (e.g., severe obstructive lung disease with secondary right ventricular failure, obesity, or venous insufficiency). The essential elements in the evaluation of the patient for HF include a careful history, assessment of the presence or absence of specific physical signs, evaluation of systolic and diastolic function, and identification of the primary and secondary etiologic factors responsible (see Chapters C109, C110).

History

Congestive symptoms. Congestion due to volume overload is a characteristic of HF and is associated with the symptoms of orthopnea and PND. These symptoms may cause patients to sleep sitting up or to seek air from an open window. As fluid overload progresses, patients are often unable to recline more than a few degrees before difficulty in breathing ensues but patients may not always report orthopnea in association with PND. Accumulation of abdominal fluid is a subtle but relatively common finding and some patients characteristically become volume expanded in this way. Changes in body weight are more helpful in the assessment of the patient than generally recognized. On close questioning, patients will often give an accurate description of recent changes in weight and may report symptoms of fluid accumulation that are difficult to detect by physical examination.

Exercise intolerance. Dyspnea on exertion is an important complaint to elicit in patients with HF and may occur in the absence of classical symptoms or signs of volume overload. Patients whose cardiac dysfunction has evolved gradually often adapt their activity and minimize symptoms related to exertion. Comparing current activity to exercise tolerance in the past may be helpful in detecting a decline in functional capacity. The patient's functional capacity should be judged with allowance for his or her age and level of conditioning.

Low output syndrome. Development of a "low output" syndrome, where symptoms are not related to congestion, is a very poor prognostic sign and must be treated aggressively. Generalized fatigue and dyspnea at rest or on minimal exertion in the absence of fluid overload are the major historical findings. Fatigue invariably occurs in severe HF and it, as well as dyspnea on exertion, may persist despite successful treatment of volume expansion. These patients evince other symptoms of poor organ perfusion including reduced mentation and a variety of gastrointestinal complaints including early satiety, abdominal pain, and nausea.

Chest pain. Chest pain is a surprisingly frequent accompaniment of moderate to severe HF even in the absence of obstructive CAD. The pain is often atypical of angina when a careful history is taken but may be exertional in nature.

Family history. HF due to familial causes is an uncommon disorder that is important to elicit because the course of genetic cardiomyopathy may be rapidly progressive. The prevalence of idiopathic cardiomyopathy varies but has been reported to be 20% to 25% in some referral centers but detailed characterization of the genetic defects involved is still not possible in all cases (see Chapter A73).

Physical examination

General assessment. The major aim of the physical examination is to determine the general condition and volume status of the patient and to look for signs of hypertension, ventricular dysfunction and valvular impairment.

Vital signs. A rapid pulse is characteristic of decompensated HF and is a poor prognostic sign especially when appearing late in the patient's course. Determination of orthostatic blood pressure (BP) changes (i.e., supine and standing BPs) gives important insight into the patient's current volume status and health of baroreflex control mechanisms. Volume depletion can become a vexing problem during chronic treatment of HF and lead to functional impairment, orthostatic dizziness, and fatigue in patients with very low sodium intake or individuals treated with high doses of diuretics.

Evidence of left ventricular dysfunction. A number of physical signs are characteristic of LV systolic dysfunction. In severe cases, the apical impulse is shifted to the left of the midclavicular line. A third heart sound (S3) is an important diagnostic and prognostic sign of advanced LV dysfunction that often goes undetected but may also be absent despite the presence of severe systolic dysfunction. A fourth heart sound (S4) may be present in association with an S3 to form a summation gallop or be the sole auscultatory finding in a patient with diastolic HF.

Congestive signs. Important and common physical signs of congestion include rales, pleural fluid, jugular venous distension, and pedal edema. Unfortunately, rales also occur in primary lung disease and may be indistinguishable in quality from those due to cardiac failure. Nevertheless, serial examination often reveals a change in the pattern of rales, which would suggest the accumulation of fluid. Hepatomegaly, positive hepatojugular reflux, and ascites are particularly ominous signs of fluid overload in long-standing HF.

Routine laboratory studies

Chest x-ray. A chest x-ray should be obtained when HF is suspected, both to provide an accurate estimate of cardiac size and to determine whether there is pulmonary vascular congestion or evidence of intrinsic pulmonary disease. Radiographic findings of congestion, such as pulmonary venous cephalization, interstitial edema, Kerley's B lines and pleural effusion may not be present when the patient is well compensated and intracardiac and pulmonary pressures are normal. An electrocardiogram may reveal evidence of prior MI or LVH. Detection of atrial fibrillation is important as is the determination of rate during atrial arrhythmia.

Chemistries. Standard clinical chemistries provide additional information on the severity of the condition and may alter pharmacologic management of HF. Determination of blood urea nitrogen (BUN) and creatinine to evaluate renal function and volume status, and serum Na^+ and potassium to investigate the electrolyte effects of the disease or therapy are important before and during treatment.

Other tests. Although not routinely performed, exercise testing with measurement of expired gases may be of use in estimating prognosis and distinguishing cardiac from noncardiac causes of exertional symptoms. Holter monitoring for arrhythmia may be useful in individual patients suspected of having clinically significant atrial or ventricular arrhythmia.

Assessment of ventricular function. Assessment of ventricular function is recommended routinely for the evaluation of patients with suspected or established HF (see Chapter C110, C150). Quantitation of LV function by noninvasive means has become an important part of the initial evaluation of patients with HF.

Echocardiography. In the vast majority of centers, echocardiography and Doppler measurements represent the standard of care. Studies should include analysis of chamber size, valve function, LV mass and wall thickness, parameters of LV systolic and diastolic function, and an assessment of the pericardium. Approximately 50% of patients with symptoms and signs of HF will have preserved systolic dysfunction (variably defined typically as an ejection fraction above 45%). Detection of ventricular dilatation is an important finding and serial changes in LV volume are an important marker of the extent of remodeling during treatment.

Nuclear studies. Radionuclide ventriculography is an alternative modality that can provide information about right ventricular function that may provide useful prognostic information in patients with severe systolic dysfunction.

Clinical synthesis

A thorough workup of HF allows the clinician a position to give the patient important advice regarding prognosis, everyday management, and therapy.

Differential diagnosis. The symptoms and signs of HF are nonspecific, which may result in misdiagnosis.

Dyspnea. Because pulmonary disease may frequently result in exertional dyspnea, a history of cigarette smoking, chronic sputum production, wheezing, or asthma should be sought. Asthmatic symptoms can be particularly difficult to distinguish from those related to HF; shortness of breath due to asthmatic attacks often occurs at night and may not be accompanied by audible wheezing, while bronchospasm in response to pulmonary congestion triggers attacks of "cardiac asthma."

Edema. Multiple etiologic factors may result in edema, including venous disease or vasodilator drug use that is often mistaken for cardiac dysfunction. A critical differential point concerns the effect of posture on the patient's edema. Noncardiac edema often resolves overnight when the patient is supine only to reoccur during the daytime when the patient is active. Primary valvular heart disease can present with a picture of fluid retention or dyspnea. Echocardiography is an essential tool to identify primary valvular disease and may identify patients for whom surgical correction is the best management.

Chest pain. The presence of chest pain or exertional dyspnea in the absence of congestive signs can suggest CAD. Additional noninvasive stress testing or coronary angiography should be considered to rule out ischemic heart disease (IHD) in these patients. Patients with advanced age and no apparent cause of HF should also be evaluated for the possibility of CAD. Stress nuclear imaging can aid in the identification of patients with CAD with persistent ischemia that should be considered for revascularization.

Insensitivity of the physical examination. As a cautionary note, the clinician should be aware that severe LV dysfunction is not always accompanied by classic signs and symptoms of HF. Some patients maintain adequate exercise capacity and are free of fluid retention despite significant cardiac dysfunction. Furthermore, even when symptoms are present, physical signs, including an S3 gallop or evidence of cardiac enlargement, may not be detected on examination. Right heart catheterization may be useful to clarify discordance between symptoms and examination and may reveal surprisingly abnormal hemodynamics despite minimal findings, especially in patients with long-standing severe systolic dysfunction.

Establishing etiology. Establishing a specific etiology of the patient's HF is important because certain causes require specific therapies in addition to routine treatments for HF. Patients may

have reversible forms of cardiac dysfunction that can benefit from specific interventions.

IHD is a common cause of HF in patients younger than 65 years, accounting for 60% to 70% of cases. Since the presence of IHD will require additional therapies, most guidelines recommend diagnostic testing to assess for the presence or absence of obstructive CAD. Although this evaluation may be restricted to noninvasive stress imaging, coronary angiography is often necessary, especially in younger individuals. In contrast, elderly women who frequently have HF associated with hypertension and preserved systolic function typically do not have evidence of obstructive CAD and do not generally require a specific CAD workup. Untreated hypertension provides an obvious therapeutic target with the suggestion that a BP goal of <130/80 mm Hg is reasonable. Alcohol is uncommon as a primary etiologic factor and may often be overlooked because patients typically lack findings of cirrhosis and the social consequences typical of alcoholism. Alcoholic cardiomyopathy may be reversible in its early stages, which enhances the importance of identifying this causal factor. Valvular heart disease and other cardiomyopathies must also be considered and managed as warranted for the specific condition.

Determining functional class. Assessment of the degree of HF present through clinical metrics like New York Heart Association (NYHA) functional class provide a simple yet effective strategy for determining global clinical status (**Table C111.1**). Functional class has been established in many prospective studies to provide prognostic information beyond that obtained by assessment of ventricular function, biomarkers, and other clinical assessments. This simple scale provides a rapid way to assess changes in clinical status in response to optimization of therapy or during the course of follow-up.

Prognosis. NYHA functional classification describes clinical status as a simple but very helpful way to estimate prognosis. NYHA class IV patients have a 50% 1-year mortality rate, especially when this degree of symptoms is present despite aggressive therapy. In contrast, the risk of death declines to <5% per year in asymptomatic patients (NYHA class I). Left ventricular ejection fraction is another important independent prognostic factor. The presence of severe cardiac dysfunction (ejection fraction $\leq 35\%$) increases risk two- to threefold compared to HF patients with preserved systolic function (diastolic dysfunction) and well preserved LV function (>45%), who may experience many episodes of pulmonary edema but have a relatively low mortality rate despite symptoms of HF. Follow-up within 3 to 6 months is useful to assess response to therapy and future prognosis in high-risk patients (ejection fraction $\leq 35\%$ and NYHA class III

TABLE C111.1

NEW YORK HEART ASSOCIATION FUNCTIONAL CLASS

Classification of clinical severity of heart failure	Symptoms
Class I	No symptoms during usual activity
Class II	Symptoms of dyspnea and fatigue during ordinary daily activity
Class III	Dyspnea and fatigue on minimal activity
Class IV	Dyspnea or fatigue at rest

or IV) but it is not necessary to repeat echocardiographic studies at these intervals in stable patients. Improvement in cardiac function over the first few months of treatment is a very positive sign, whereas continued decline in ventricular function bodes poorly for the success of medical therapy alone. Recent evidence indicates that a simple test of exercise capacity, the distance walked in 6 minutes (6-minute walk test), can provide important information concerning outcomes.

LV systolic dysfunction can be staged according to guidelines from the Heart Failure Society of America or the comprehensive system proposed by the joint statement of the American Heart Association/American College of Cardiology (see Chapter C151). These systems recommend specific therapies that evolve with the severity of the condition.

Suggested Readings

Ahmed A. A propensity matched study of New York Heart Association class and natural history end points in heart failure. *Am J Cardiol* 2007;99:549–553.

Bittner V, Weiner DH, Yusuf S, et al. Prediction of mortality and morbidity with a 6-minute walk test in patients with left ventricular dysfunction. *JAMA* 1993;270:1702–1707.

Brutsaert DL. Cardiac dysfunction in heart failure: the cardiologist's love affair with time. *Prog Cardiovasc Dis* 2006;49:157–181.

Maisel AS, Bhalla V, Braunwald E. Cardiac biomarkers: a contemporary status report. *Nat Clin Pract Cardiovasc Med* 2006;3:24–34.

Perloff JK. The jugular venous pulse and third heart sound in patients with heart failure. *N Engl J Med* 2001;345:612–614.

Shiber JR, Santana J. Dyspnea. *Med Clin North Am* 2006;90:453–479.

Stevenson LW, Perloff JK. Limited reliability of physical signs for estimating hemodynamics in chronic heart failure. *JAMA* 1989;261:884–888.

CHAPTER C112 ■ EVALUATION OF ARTERIAL STIFFNESS AND CENTRAL SYSTOLIC PRESSURE

JOSEPH L. IZZO, Jr., MD

KEY POINTS

- An arterial pressure wave can be deconstructed into a forward pressure wave in early systole and a reflected pressure wave in late systole/early diastole; wave reflection amplitude is affected by physiologic or structural changes in the distal circulation (e.g., vasoconstriction or anatomic narrowing).
- Pressure waves travel within arterial walls; pulse wave velocity (PWV) varies in proportion to arterial wall stiffness and inversely with diameter.
- Diastolic BP is relatively constant but systolic BP and pulse pressure (PP) are variable along the arterial tree due to differences in timing of wave arrival, peripheral PP amplification, and wave reflection amplitude.
- Central aortic systolic BP, which can be determined noninvasively using peripheral arterial tonometry, tends to be lower than cuff systolic unless there is increased wave reflection.
- All of the currently available techniques to estimate arterial wall properties are directly or indirectly dependent on (and must be corrected for) local or systemic BP.

See also Chapters **A44, A45,** A58, and C156

In hypertension, the shift in primary focus from diastolic to systolic BP has necessitated a reevaluation of the pathophysiology of normal and abnormal pulsatile blood flow. In contrast to the relatively simple relationship between systemic vasoconstriction and diastolic BP, systolic BP is dependent on a series of complex "ventricular–vascular interactions." Arterial properties such as diameter and wall stiffness modify systolic BP and pulse pressure (PP) by altering the timing and amplitude of forward- and backward-traveling pressure waves within the arterial tree. The

differences between peripheral and central BP are only now being recognized for their potential importance in BP measurement, risk stratification, assessment of therapeutic benefit, and clinical trial interpretation.

Functional compartments of the arterial tree

During systole, the heart interacts in sequential manner with progressively more distal compartments of the arterial tree (sequential "ventricular–vascular interactions"). The corresponding time-dependent changes in arterial pressure give important information about the function of the arterial system. For convenience, three major anatomic-functional divisions can be assigned: central elastic arteries, peripheral conduit arteries, and small arteries/arterioles.

The large central arteries (aorta and its proximal branches) are elastic vessels of large diameter that function as the "third chamber" of the cardiac pumping system, converting highly pulsatile proximal aortic flow into more continuous "damped pulsatile" flow distally. The principal pathogenetic abnormality in isolated systolic hypertension is stiffening of these vessels.

Conduit arteries (femoral, brachial, etc.) are less elastic and serve mainly to transmit blood to the periphery. The total cross-section, tapering, and arborizing functions of these vessels are widely different in different organs. In hypertensive patients, despite increased aortic stiffening, brachial arteries are somewhat dilated and tend to have normal wall properties.

The third compartment (small arteries and arterioles) affects systemic resistance, diastolic and mean arterial pressure, and various aspects of wave reflection. Control of vasomotor tone of vessels with diameters <0.5 mm alters diastolic BP and allows flow redistribution among organ beds according to systemic and local needs. The density of the microcirculation is reduced in some forms of hypertension.

Arterial pulse waves

Clinical assessment of arterial wall properties is based on several basic principles.

Pulse wave velocity and characteristic impedance. Pulse wave velocity (PWV), the speed of transit of an arterial pressure wave within an arterial wall (distance between measurement sites/transit time), is closely related to characteristic aortic impedance (Z_c). Z_c is the vascular component of the ventricular–vascular interaction in early systole that determines central PP; central PP is also dependent on the speed and force of ventricular emptying. Z_c and PWV both depend on arterial wall dynamics according to the following relationship:

$$Y \propto \sqrt{\frac{Eh}{r^x}}$$

where Y is either PWV or Z_c, Eh is the elastance-wall thickness product and r is arterial radius raised to a power x (for PWV, x = 1, for Z_c, x = 5). Therefore, PWV is much less sensitive than Z_c to differences in arterial diameter (often induced by reactive vasoconstriction or vasodilation). Aging and hypertension strongly affect the wall composition and stiffness of arteries; PWV is directly proportional to the stiffness of the arterial wall, and varies from <5 m/sec (50 cm/msec) in young healthy individuals to >30 m/sec (300 cm/msec) in elderly individuals with hypertension. PWV increases with distance from the heart as vessels become progressively smaller and stiffer; regional assessment of PWV is necessary because central and peripheral arteries behave differently in various disease states, including hypertension. PWV is an independent risk factor for cardiovascular (CV) disease mortality but the incremental value it provides for routine clinical practice is unclear. Z_c is also strongly affected by aging, hypertension, and changes in vasomotor tone and provides the most sensitive measure to assess flow–pressure relationships in the proximal circulation.

Pulse pressure amplification. Progressive decreases in arterial diameter (principally in the arm and leg) cause a gradual increase in impedance and PP because the total cross-sectional area of the arterial tree within the limbs decreases over a long distance before it increases in the microcirculation. This anatomic relationship is different than that found in the brain or kidney and causes progressive pulse pressure amplification (PPA) in the arm that causes cuff systolic BP to be higher than aortic systolic BP, usually by approximately 5 to 10 mm Hg in healthy individuals. The degree of PPA is greater in certain young males who have been labeled as having "spurious systolic hypertension" but is also reduced by the degree of wave reflection that occurs (**Figure C112.1**). In most publications, PPA is defined as the difference between peak central systolic BP and peak brachial BP and therefore most often compares the forward wave peak in the arm with the peak central systolic BP comprised of both forward and reflected wave peaks.

Wave reflection. Pressure waves traveling within the arterial wall are reflected at points of impedance mismatch (branch points, abrupt areas of narrowing, etc.). The degree by which the pressure–flow relationship is disturbed affects the amplitude of the reflected wave, whereas the arrival time is affected by the PWV and the distance between the heart and the reflection site. Any arterial pressure wave can be deconstructed into a forward pressure wave in early systole and a reflected pressure wave in late systole/early diastole; summation of forward and reflected pressure waves determines the morphology of the arterial pulse contour at any point along the arterial tree (**Figure C112.1**). Forward and reflected wave morphologies are affected by functional and structural changes in arterial wall properties, including the amplitude of the forward and reflected pulse waves and the PWV.

Central versus peripheral blood pressure

Central systolic pressure augmentation. Despite the substantial impact of PPA in younger individuals, cuff systolic BPs in many middle-aged or older individuals are approximately the same as their peak aortic systolic BPs because of central systolic pressure augmentation.

In late systole, as reflected pressure waveforms from proximal and distal sites return to the aortic root, they summate with the forward pressure wave, augmenting late systolic BP [augmentation pressure is the increment in systolic BP caused by the reflected pressure wave; augmentation index (AI) is the ratio of augmentation pressure to central PP]. Most of the reflected waves return to the central aorta well after the peak of the forward wave (**Figure C112.1**) but some arrive sufficiently early to overlap with the forward wave, especially if PWV is high. Central pressure augmentation may have some value in sustaining forward flow in the cerebral and renal circulations but it also increases ventricular afterload and promotes ventricular hypertrophy.

Pulse pressure. Clinically, wide PP is associated most commonly with isolated systolic hypertension due to aortic stiffness. Changes in central PP are often not identical to those in peripheral PP because they include a greater contribution from reflected waves (**Figure C112.1**), and are therefore more sensitive to changes in systemic hemodynamics and distal vasoconstriction. For the vast majority of hypertensive patients, especially those older than 50 years, wide central or peripheral PP is a reasonable surrogate for increased central arterial stiffness but increased PP can be caused by aortic insufficiency or states of increased cardiac stroke volume/contractility (hyperdynamic hypertension,

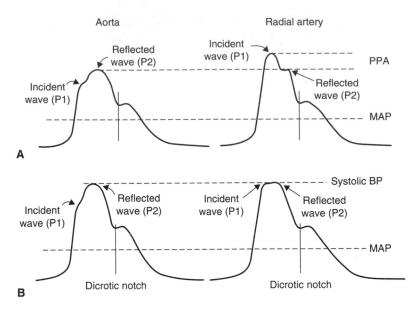

Figure C112.1 Central and peripheral pressure waveforms. Panel **A** depicts a healthy young individual with lower central than radial systolic blood pressure (BP) (pulse pressure amplification, PPA) due to decreasing diameter and increasing impedance in the arterial system of the arm. The reflected wave (P2) impacts differently on the aorta and radial arteries; centrally, it augments the systolic pressure increment caused by the forward pressure wave (P1); in the radial artery, P2 is a trailing shoulder peak that does not contribute to peak systolic BP. Panel **B** depicts typical changes with hypertension, where the amplitude of the reflected wave increases. In this example, there is no apparent PPA because the central augmentation index (pressure increment caused by wave reflection) is very high. Note that in both cases, P2 is representative of central systolic BP. MAP, mean arterial pressure, dicrotic notch, aortic valve closure.

thyrotoxicosis, vitamin deficiency, arteriovenous malformations, anemia, etc.).

Clinical application of central systolic blood pressure

Blood pressure measurement and risk stratification. In some healthy young people (more in men than women), the difference between central and peripheral systolic BP exceeds 20 mm Hg; this phenomenon has been called *spurious* systolic hypertension by some investigators because despite the isolated systolic hypertension measured by arm cuff, there is no apparent CV disease. The natural history of this condition has not been studied but the aggregate Framingham risk scores of this group are similar to normotensive individuals and it does not appear that antihypertensive drug therapy is warranted (see Chapter C163).

Clinical trial interpretation. In the Conduit Artery Function Evaluation (CAFÉ) Study, central systolic BP (from arterial tonometry) and peripheral systolic BP were compared between calcium antagonist-angiotensin-converting enzyme (ACE) inhibitor therapy and β-blocker-thiazide therapy. Despite identical cuff BPs, calcium antagonist therapy lowered central systolic pressure by approximately 4 mm Hg more than β-blocker therapy by virtue of a more marked effect on the reflected wave (central systolic pressure augmentation). This difference could explain most of the CV outcome improvements attributed to the calcium antagonist–ACE inhibitor combination.

Methods to study arterial properties

Limitations of arterial function parameters. There is no single parameter that can describe all clinically relevant arterial properties and all of the physical measurements share the common drawback of being directly or indirectly dependent on arterial pressure itself. It is usually quite difficult to obtain simultaneous BP values at the measurement site, so pressures obtained at a remote site are employed. This is problematic because of the variation in PP within the arterial circulation. Furthermore, extrapolation of the data obtained in one vascular bed may not be relevant to other parts of the circulation, owing to differences in arterial size, wall composition, and disease in different arteries. Therefore, in the purest sense, specific arterial properties only apply to the location being studied and not to the circulation as a whole. These points illustrate how difficult it is to ascertain

clinically useful information about local and integrated arterial function. Nevertheless, various techniques can provide useful information regarding specific scientific and medical questions.

Pulse wave velocity. Pulse transit time can be assessed noninvasively by a variety of techniques. The "QKD" measurement (time difference between the electrocardiogram (ECG) Q-wave and the systolic pressure peak at a distal site) is inadequate because of wide variability (mostly rate dependent) in the preejection period and because of variability in the morphology of the pressure peak. With most techniques, transit time is assessed noninvasively using arterial tonometry of the carotid, brachial, radial, or femoral arteries. The foot of the waveform (initial arrival time of the pressure wave) is taken as the index point. For convenience, PWV is calculated by measuring the differences in timing between two peripheral sites, even if they represent different parts of the circulation. The carotid-femoral PWV is most widely used parameter but this measurement has several theoretic drawbacks. First, it ignores the characteristics of the proximal aorta, the most important part of the arterial tree with respect to impedance and peak systolic BP. Second, it assumes that the characteristics of the carotid artery are similar to those of the lower aorta, which is not valid. Third, significant problems arise in estimating the exact timing of the pulse wave inflection point. Fourth, the distance between recording sites must be sufficiently large to allow for accurate assessment of the time delay. Fifth, the true transit distance often cannot be measured directly; by convention, carotid-femoral transit distance is estimated by measuring from the suprasternal notch to the carotid artery. Lastly, some devices are difficult to standardize (Complior), although newer developmental systems timed to the first heart sound (Colin-Omron) may prove useful.

Radial pulse contour analysis

Central systolic blood pressure. Central aortic pressure waveforms can be reconstructed from peripheral arterial waveform using an approved commercial device (SphygmoCor) that employs high fidelity radial or carotid tonometry and a generalized transfer function to construct an approximated central pressure waveform. The correlation between transfer function-derived central systolic BP and directly measured catheter-based pressures has been validated by at least three highly qualified academic laboratories. Yet there is ongoing debate whether a single generalized transfer function can be applied to all populations or whether it has sufficient fidelity to allow for analysis of critical waveform landmarks, including the timing of the reflected wave. Central pressure waveforms are roughly similar to carotid waveforms, potentially obviating the need for a transfer function but this technique requires further validation. It also appears that the radial arterial systolic shoulder peak (P2) is a reasonable approximation of central systolic BP in the vast majority of individuals. This convenient fact may prove useful in estimating central systolic BP directly from radial arterial tracings (see Figure C112.1).

Augmentation index. Use of a transfer function theoretically allows the estimation of central AI (the increment in central systolic BP caused by the reflected wave). Central AI (**Figure C112.1**) has been touted as a measure of arterial stiffness by some investigators but this claim is not justified because central AI is not proportional to PWV in systolic hypertension; in fact, the two are actually inversely related. Ability to quantify AI has theoretic value in assessing the increment to ventricular afterload caused by wave reflection and AI has been correlated in some studies (although weakly) with LV mass. At present, the direct clinical application of central AI is unclear. Radial AI appears to have limited value in assessing arterial properties but P2 appears to be generally equivalent to central systolic BP and may be useful in correcting for the artifact of peripheral PPA.

Characteristic impedance of the aorta. The most sensitive indicator of aortic stiffness, Z_c, can be determined noninvasively by combining Doppler flow and calibrated arterial tonometry if the carotid waveform is assumed to be similar to the aortic waveform and is scaled to cuff BP. Aortic flow is approximated by measuring the Doppler flow at the LV outflow tract. The best and most sensitive approach (Cardiovascular Engineering, Inc.) is a proprietary system that is expensive and technically demanding (requires specialized equipment and a specially trained echocardiographic technician) and depends on several independent assumptions regarding pressure scaling, wave morphologies, and the corresponding flow and diameter measurements. This technique has been used to identify important differences in mechanisms of action of different classes of antihypertensive medications, such as combined ACE-neutral endopeptidase inhibitors. Estimation or direct measurement of aortic diameter using this technique has also identified a new pathogenetic mechanism for isolated systolic hypertension in individuals of shorter stature (usually women): small aortic diameter with normal elastic properties. These individuals tend to have isolated systolic hypertension [and in other studies, a greater prevalence of concentric left ventricular hypertrophy (LVH)]. Z_c remains more applicable to research than clinical practice at present.

Other parameters

Older techniques are still occasionally useful but must be judged in light of the scientific or medical hypothesis being tested, the independence and heterogeneity of the compartments of the arterial tree, the diverse adaptations that occur in health and disease, and the specific populations being studied. Most of these techniques are extremely limited in the global insights they provide.

Compliance and distensibility. The term *arterial compliance* is very frequently misapplied; it relates to the "give" in the arterial wall [change in luminal volume (dV), diameter, or area caused by a corresponding change in distending pressure (dP) or

dV/dP, usually in mL/mm Hg]. Compliance is a local property that is strongly affected by arterial diameter and pressure and poorly describes the many different aspects of different sized arteries with intrinsically nonuniform characteristics. Furthermore, it is often difficult to simultaneously measure dP and dV at a single site. Distensibility is compliance adjusted for the initial arterial volume (V, therefore dV/VdP, expressed as 1/mm Hg). Although vessel geometry is taken into account to a greater degree, the parameter is still a local measure that is highly pressure sensitive with the all of the other major limitations of arterial compliance.

Stroke volume to pulse pressure ratio. Some studies have reported the stroke volume/PP ratio (SV/PP expressed in arbitrary units) as a measure of whole body compliance. The notion of whole body compliance is another highly hypothetical concept with questionable applicability because the advancing pressure wave has not yet been distributed to the entire arterial system. Use of SV/PP also assumes that the peripheral circulation is a single compartment where pressure waves arrive simultaneously, which is physiologically and pathophysiologically incorrect.

Arterial imaging. Vessel wall tracking and simple image-based (ultrasonography or magnetic resonance imaging) assessment of systolic and diastolic diameter have been coupled with remote BP measurements to derive local pressure-diameter relationships and the corresponding effective elastic modulus (Eh). An important limitation of the approach is that the pressure waveform is not usually obtained from the same site as the diameter waveform.

Diastolic pulse contour analysis (Windkessel model). In theory, the diastolic waveform contains information about distal runoff and elastic properties of distal vessels. The four-element Windkessel model, in which the main slope of the diastolic decay function was assumed to be related to the proximal (aortic) compliance (C_1) and a superimposed decaying sinusoid function (C_2) was believed to represent the damping (or compliance) coefficient of the distal arterial tree. This approach has been criticized for lack of reproducibility and physiologic significance (including the intrinsic dependence of C_2 on systemic vascular resistance.

Suggested Readings

Domanski MJ, Davis BR, Pfeffer MA, et al. Isolated systolic hypertension: prognostic information provided by pulse pressure. *Hypertension* 1999;34:375–380.

Izzo JL Jr, Gradman AH. Mechanisms and management of hypertensive heart disease: from left ventricular hypertrophy to heart failure. *Med Clin North Am* 2004;88:1257–1271.

Izzo JL Jr, Manning TS, Shykoff BE. Office blood pressures, arterial compliance characteristics, and estimated cardiac load. *Hypertension* 2001;38:1467–1470.

Izzo JL Jr, Mitchell GF. Aging and arterial structure-function relations. *Adv Cardiol* 2007;44:19–34.

Mitchell GF, Izzo JL Jr, Lacourciere Y, et al. Omapatrilat reduces pulse pressure and proximal aortic stiffness in patients with systolic hypertension: results of the conduit hemodynamics of omapatrilat international research study. *Circulation* 2002;105:2955–2961.

Mitchell GF, Lacourciere Y, Ouellet JP, et al. Determinants of elevated pulse pressure in middle-aged and older subjects with uncomplicated systolic hypertension: the role of proximal aortic diameter and the aortic pressure-flow relationship [See Comment]. *Circulation* 2003;108:1592–1598.

Takazawa K, Kobayashi H, Shindo N, et al. Relationship between radial and central arterial pulse wave and evaluation of central aortic pressure using the radial arterial pulse wave. *Hypertens Res Clin Exp* 2007;30:219–228.

Vyas M, Izzo JL Jr, Lacourciere Y, et al. Augmentation index and central aortic stiffness in middle-aged to elderly individuals. *Am J Hypertens* 2007;20:642–647.

Wilkinson IB, Franklin SS, Hall IR, et al. Pressure amplification explains why pulse pressure is unrelated to risk in young subjects. *Hypertension* 2001;38:1461–1466.

CHAPTER C113 ■ EVALUATION OF THE PERIPHERAL CIRCULATION

JEFFREY W. OLIN, DO

KEY POINTS

■ Evaluation of the entire vascular system is important because of the increased prevalence of extracranial carotid and peripheral arterial disease (PAD) in patients with hypertension.

■ Blood pressure (BP) should be measured in both arms to detect the presence of innominate or subclavian artery stenosis due to atherosclerosis.

■ The primary symptom of PAD is intermittent claudication, but many patients have atypical leg symptoms or no symptoms at all.

■ Evaluation of the peripheral circulation includes functional testing [ankle-brachial index (ABI), segmental BPs or pulse volume recordings] and imaging [duplex ultrasonography, computed tomographic (CT) angiography, magnetic resonance angiography, or catheter-based angiography].

See also Chapters B81 and **C152**

Evaluation of the peripheral circulation is extremely important in the hypertensive patient because hypertension is a strong risk factor for the development of peripheral arterial disease (PAD), carotid atherosclerosis, and aneurysmal disease. The Framingham Study showed a significant relationship between systolic and diastolic blood pressure (BP) levels and the 26-year incidence of intermittent claudication.

Signs and symptoms

Cold hands and feet are poor clues to the presence of arterial insufficiency because they also occur in patients who are anxious, have overactivity of the sympathetic nervous system, or have vasospastic disease. Some patients have *vasomotor instability* in which the hands and feet appear erythematous or cyanotic. In this condition, the blood vessels do not react (constrict or dilate) normally to exogenous stimuli such as changes in ambient temperature. There are several clues in a patient's history that suggest the presence of carotid atherosclerosis, PAD, or aneurysmal disease.

Transient cerebral ischemia. A history of transient ischemic attacks (focal neurologic deficit that usually resolves within 1 minute to 1 hour but may last up to 24 hours), including amaurosis fugax (monocular blindness), aphasia, dysphagia, hemiparesis, hemiplegia, focal sensory abnormalities, and stroke suggests the presence of cardiac disease, aortic arch atherosclerosis, or carotid artery atherosclerosis.

Claudication. The primary symptom of PAD is intermittent claudication, which is characterized as discomfort, pain,

cramping, tightness, heaviness, or tiredness in one or more muscle groups in the lower extremities. Most commonly, it occurs in the calf because of superficial femoral artery obstruction. However, thigh, hip, or buttock claudication may occur in patients with aortoiliac disease. Some patients with aortoiliac disease describe an overall heaviness, tiredness, or "power failure." The discomfort is brought on by exercise (usually walking) and is quickly relieved in the 2 to 5 minutes after the individual stops walking. Intermittent claudication can usually be differentiated from pseudoclaudication (neurogenic claudication) caused by spinal stenosis or disc disease on the basis of the history and physical examination (**Table C113.1**).

Only 10% to 20% of patients with PAD have classic claudication symptoms as discussed in the preceding text. Approximately 20% to 40% have atypical leg symptoms and approximately 50% are totally asymptomatic and the PAD is only detected by measuring the ankle-brachial index (ABI). Because even the asymptomatic patient with PAD is at increased risk for myocardial infarction and stroke, it has been suggested that ABI be measured in all patients older than 70 years or in patients between 50 and 69 years of age with a history of smoking or diabetes. In this at-risk population, the prevalence of PAD is close to 30%.

Critical limb ischemia. When vascular disease becomes advanced, the patient may experience pain at rest, or the development of ischemic ulcerations or gangrene on the toes, indicating that critical limb ischemia is present. It is not uncommon for individuals with rest pain to hang their leg over the side of the bed or sleep sitting in a chair so that gravity can

TABLE C113.1

DIFFERENTIATING (VASCULAR) CLAUDICATION FROM PSEUDOCLAUDICATION

	Claudication	Pseudoclaudication
Character of discomfort	Discomfort, pain, cramping, tightness, heaviness, tiredness, numbness	Same or tingling, weakness, or clumsiness
Location of discomfort	Buttock, hip, thigh, calf, foot	Same
Exercise induced	Always	May or may not be
Distance to claudication	Same each time	Highly variable
Occurs with standing	No	Yes or no
Relief	Stop walking. Discomfort usually disappears in 2–5 min	Often must sit, lean, or change body positions. Discomfort may take up to 15–20 min to disappear

(Adapted from Krajewski LP, Olin JW. Atherosclerosis of the aorta and lower extremities. In: Young JR, Graor RA, Olin JW, et al. eds. *Peripheral vascular diseases*. St. Louis: Mosby Year Book, 1991:183.)

improve the circulation to the lower extremity and thereby relieve the nocturnal pain. This may lead to significant edema, which may falsely lead the clinician to suspect venous or lymphatic disease.

Physical examination of the circulation

Blood pressure measurements. At the initial physical examination, BP should be measured in both arms. If the BP readings are different, the higher value should be used for subsequent BP readings. A discrepancy in BP readings between arms is usually indicative of innominate or subclavian artery stenosis on the side of the lower BP. The most common cause is atherosclerosis but BP differences between arms also occur in radiation-induced vascular disease, fibromuscular dysplasia, or inflammatory vascular diseases such as Takayasu's arteritis or giant cell arteritis. Occasionally, bilateral subclavian artery stenosis occurs; under these circumstances, the BP is higher in the legs than in the arms.

Neck

Palpation. In every hypertensive patient, the carotid artery should be palpated low in the neck, at the level of the thyroid gland, anterior to the sternocleidomastoid muscle. The carotid bifurcation (located at the angle of the jaw) should be avoided because palpation of this area may cause significant bradycardia or asystole in patients who have a hypersensitive carotid sinus. Although quite uncommon, palpation at the carotid bifurcation may also cause dislodgment of atheromatous material, producing a transient ischemic attack or a stroke. A fullness in the carotid pulsation in the elderly is most commonly due to a tortuous (kinked) carotid artery; carotid artery aneurysms are quite uncommon.

The subclavian artery pulse should be palpated in the supraclavicular fossa with the thumb while the fingers are placed behind the neck. The character of the pulsation as well as the presence or absence of an aneurysm should be noted. Next, the superficial temporal artery should be palpated. A decrease in the arterial pulsation may indicate stenosis of the common or external carotid artery.

Auscultation. After careful palpation, the examiner should listen to the cervical and supraclavicular regions for the presence of bruits. Bruits can be heard best with the bell of the stethoscope with the patient in the sitting position. The location, timing (a systolic bruit or a combined systolic and diastolic bruit), and quality of the bruit should be described. It is important to listen over the base of the heart to be certain that the bruit is not a transmitted murmur from the aortic or pulmonic valve.

A bruit that is heard during both systole and diastole indicates that there may be severe bilateral carotid artery disease. In fact, the artery on the contralateral side of the systolic/diastolic bruit is often more severely stenotic than the index vessel and may be totally occluded (**Figure C113.1**). Other conditions that cause a systolic/diastolic bruit include arteriovenous malformation, arteriovenous fistula, and a venous hum. A venous hum is usually heard at the base of the neck and can easily be detected by its disappearance on light compression of the external jugular vein.

Upper extremities. The axillary, brachial, radial, and ulnar pulses should be palpated. If there is evidence of ischemia of the hands or fingers or if there is any reason to believe that the arteries distal to the wrist are diseased, an Allen test should be performed. The patient is asked to make a tight fist, which causes most of the blood to empty from the hands and fingers. The examiners' thumbs then swipe over the thenar and hypothenar eminences to occlude the radial and ulnar arteries. When the patient opens his or her hand, it should be blanched. When the radial or ulnar artery is released, prompt return of color to the hand indicates that the artery is open, distal to the wrist. The maneuver is then repeated releasing the second artery. A positive test is failure of the hand to return to normal color promptly on release of the occluded artery.

Chest. The chest should be examined because occasionally a large aneurysm in the ascending aorta may be visualized or palpated as a pulsation high in the chest near the suprasternal notch. The bruit of aortic coarctation is best heard over the left subscapular area in most cases.

Abdomen. An attempt should be made to palpate the abdominal aorta during the physical examination. Infrarenal abdominal aortic aneurysms are not uncommon in the elderly hypertensive patient. By palpating the lateral border and the medial border of the aorta at the same time, the examiner can assess the size of the aorta. Gently rolling the aorta back and forth under the fingertips can help differentiate an aneurysm from a tortuous aorta. Careful auscultation of the epigastric region for the presence of bruits (systolic, systolic/diastolic) may reveal stenosis of the celiac artery, superior mesenteric artery, or renal arteries. A short systolic bruit

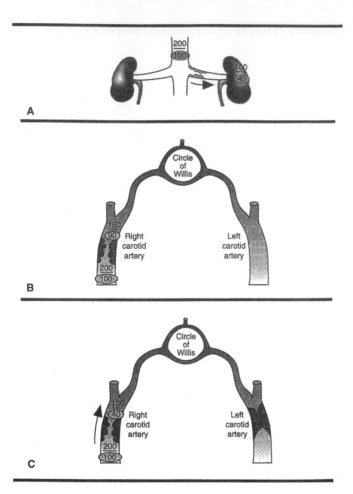

Figure C113.1 Systolic and diastolic bruits. **A:** Systolic/diastolic bruit in the renal artery. During systole, blood moves through a narrow arterial segment, turbulence is produced, and a bruit is heard. If the stenosis is severe enough, there is a significant pressure gradient during diastole as well (i.e., 100 vs. 40 mm Hg), blood continues to flow in a forward direction (*arrow*), and a systolic/diastolic bruit is heard. **B:** The right carotid artery is severely narrowed, turbulence is produced, and a systolic bruit is heard. Because the left carotid artery is patent, there is crossover flow from the left carotid through the circle of Willis maintaining pressure up in the distal right carotid artery. No forward flow occurs during diastole, and no diastolic bruit is heard. **C:** The left carotid artery is occluded, and there is no crossover from the left cerebral hemisphere. Pressure in the distal right carotid artery is very low, there is a substantial diastolic pressure gradient (*circled numbers*), blood flows forward (*arrow*) during diastole, and a systolic/diastolic bruit is heard, indicating severe stenosis or occlusion of the contralateral carotid artery.

is common in thin individuals and is generally not a cause for concern.

Lower extremities. Pulses in the lower extremities should be graded as normal, diminished, or absent. The femoral pulse should be palpated just below the inguinal ligament, with firm, constant pressure applied to feel the pulse, which is deep in most individuals. The size of the femoral artery should be noted, and an aneurysm should be considered if it is large. The amplitude and timing of the pulse should be compared with those of the radial artery, which may be diminished and delayed in coarctation of the aorta.

The popliteal pulse should be palpated in every individual. This pulse is often the most difficult for physicians to detect. Normally, the pulse can be found directly under the lateral aspect of the patella with the knee flexed <10 degrees. Firm pressure must be applied to allow the fingers to go deep into the popliteal space. The artery should be palpated with the pads of the fingers and not the fingertips. Popliteal artery aneurysms occur in 10% to 20% of patients with abdominal aortic aneurysms. The major complication of a popliteal aneurysm is thrombosis; when thrombosis occurs, the limb may become acutely ischemic, leading to limb loss in up to 50% of individuals.

Next, the posterior tibial, dorsalis pedis, and peroneal pulses should be palpated. The posterior tibial pulse can be detected posterior to the medial malleolus. The dorsalis pedis pulse is usually located over the second metatarsal bones. The dorsalis pedis pulse may not be palpable in some normal individuals because the anterior tibial artery dives deep at the level of the ankle. If the dorsalis pedis pulse cannot be detected, one should attempt to find the anterior tibial artery. If neither can be felt, the peroneal artery can often be detected in the lateral aspect of the ankle.

Imaging studies

If the patient has intermittent claudication, ischemic rest pain, or digital ulcerations, the circulation can be assessed noninvasively with segmental (Doppler) systolic pressures and pulse volume recordings (pulse waveform analysis). In severe arterial insufficiency (rest pain, ischemic ulcerations, or gangrene) or disabling claudication, the patient may require a magnetic resonance arteriogram, computed tomographic (CT) angiogram or a catheter-based angiogram to determine whether revascularization (endovascular or surgical) is feasible.

Ankle-brachial index. The least expensive way to screen for the presence of PAD is to measure the ABI, which is easily performed in any physician's office and predicts the severity of PAD and the risk of future cardiovascular events with reasonable accuracy. With a handheld continuous wave Doppler (5–8 MHz), the systolic BP should be measured in both arms, followed by the systolic BP in the right and left posterior tibial and dorsalis pedis arteries. A sample worksheet for measuring the ABI is shown in **Figure C113.2**.

Recent data have shown that 29% of primary care patients older than 70 years or between the ages of 50 and 69 years (with at least a 10-pack year history of smoking or the presence of diabetes) have PAD documented by measuring the ABI. More than 50% of patients identified with PAD on the basis of an abnormal ABI do not have typical claudication or leg pain at rest but nondescript leg pain, reduced ambulation, and a reduced quality of life. It has clearly been shown that the lower the ABI, the greater the risk of a cardiovascular death (myocardial infarction, stroke, vascular death). Patients with an ABI <0.40 and critical limb ischemia have a mortality of 25% per year. A useful algorithm for the evaluation of patients is shown in **Figure C113.3**. Patients with calcified blood vessels and a falsely elevated ABI should have a toe–brachial index measured.

Segmental pressures and waveforms. Segmental pressures can be measured by placing BP cuffs at the high thigh, calf, ankle, transmetatarsal region, and toe. Pressures and pulse volume waveforms are obtained at each level, and an ABI is obtained by comparing BPs in the ankle and in the arm. After this examination is performed in the resting position, the patient exercises on a treadmill and repeat BPs and pulse waveforms are obtained. Segmental pressure measurements help determine the location of the arterial obstruction or predict the level at which

Patient Name: _____

Date: _____ Patient Number: _____

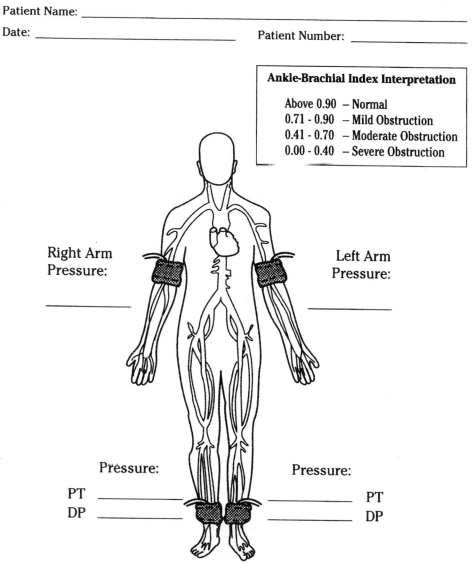

Ankle-Brachial Index Interpretation

Above 0.90 – Normal
0.71 - 0.90 – Mild Obstruction
0.41 - 0.70 – Moderate Obstruction
0.00 - 0.40 – Severe Obstruction

Right Arm Pressure: _____

Left Arm Pressure: _____

Pressure:

PT _____
DP _____

Pressure:

PT _____
DP _____

Right ABI

$$\frac{\text{Right Ankle Pressure}}{\text{Highest Arm Pressure}} = \frac{\text{mm Hg}}{\text{mm Hg}} = \_\_\_\_$$

Left ABI

$$\frac{\text{Left Ankle Pressure}}{\text{Highest Arm Pressure}} = \frac{\text{mm Hg}}{\text{mm Hg}} = \_\_\_\_$$

Example $\quad \dfrac{\text{Ankle Pressure}}{\text{Brachial Pressure}} = \dfrac{125 \text{ mm Hg}}{114 \text{ mm Hg}} = 1.09 \quad$ *See ABI Chart*

Figure C113.2 Sample ankle-brachial index (ABI) worksheet. (Reproduced from the Society for Vascular Medicine and Biology. *Peripheral arterial disease: marker of cardiovascular risk*, with permission.)

an amputation should occur. Although most patients with significant PAD demonstrate a decrease in the arterial pulsation, some have normal arterial pulses at rest. Therefore, it is important to perform pulse volume recordings and Doppler BPs not only at rest but also after the patient has walked on a treadmill until symptoms are reproduced. When arterial obstruction is present, the pressures in the ankles decrease after exercise.

Carotid imaging. If carotid artery atherosclerosis is suspected, a duplex ultrasonographic examination of the carotid arteries is warranted. The indications for carotid duplex ultrasonography are listed in **Table C113.2.** Carotid ultrasonography can determine the degree of stenosis of the common carotid artery, the external carotid artery, and the internal carotid artery. The

intracranial portion of the internal carotid artery cannot be adequately visualized with this technique. Although arteriography has been required in the past if carotid endarterectomy was to be performed, most centers now perform carotid endarterectomy on the basis of the results of carotid ultrasonography alone or after a confirmatory magnetic resonance or CT angiogram. Therefore, it is very important to be certain that the vascular laboratory is accredited and that appropriate quality control measures are followed. Carotid duplex ultrasonography is useful for following up patients after carotid endarterectomy or carotid stent procedure.

Abdominal imaging. An ultrasonography, multidector CT angiogram, or magnetic resonance angiogram can confirm the presence of an abdominal aortic aneurysm and give an

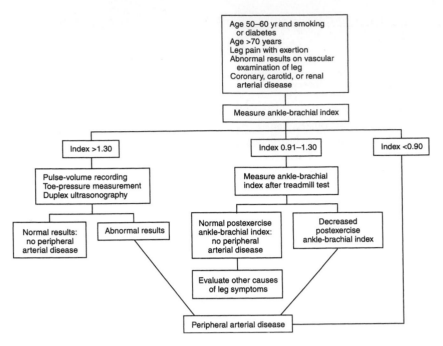

Figure C113.3 Evaluation algorithm for arterial disease. From Hiatt WR. Medical treatment of peripheral arterial disease and claudication. *N Eng J Med* 2001;344:1611.

accurate assessment of its size and location. An ultrasonographic examination is useful in determining the size of the femoral or popliteal arteries if aneurysms are suspected. Often, the vascular surgeon operates on the basis of a CT scan or magnetic resonance angiogram. Aortic stent grafting has replaced open aortic aneurysm reconstruction in many patients; therefore, an angiogram is obtained at the time of the stent graft placement.

TABLE C113.2

INDICATIONS FOR CAROTID ULTRASONOGRAPHY

Asymptomatic cervical bruit
Amaurosis fugax
Hemispheric transient ischemic attack
Stroke in a potential candidate for carotid endarterectomy or stent
Follow-up of a known stenosis (>20%) in asymptomatic individuals
Follow-up after carotid endarterectomy or stent
Intraoperative assessment of carotid endarterectomy
Unexplained neck pain (to evaluate for carotid dissection)
Pulsatile mass in the neck
Syncope
Trauma to neck
Vasculitis such as Takayasu's arteritis or giant cell arteritis

Suggested Readings

Hiatt WR. Medical treatment of peripheral arterial disease and claudication. *N Engl J Med* 2001;344:1608–1621.

Hirsch AT, Criqui MH, Treat-Jacobson D, et al. Peripheral arterial disease detection, awareness, and treatment in primary care. *JAMA* 2001;286:1317–1324.

Hirsch AT, Haskal ZJ, Hertzer NR, et al. ACC/AHA 2005 Practice Guidelines for the management of patients with peripheral arterial disease (lower extremity, renal, mesenteric, and abdominal aortic): a collaborative report from the American Association for Vascular Surgery/Society for Vascular Surgery, Society for Cardiovascular Angiography and Interventions, Society for Vascular Medicine and Biology, Society of Interventional Radiology, and the ACC/AHA Task Force on Practice Guidelines(Writing Committee to Develop Guidelines for the Management of Patients With Peripheral Arterial Disease). *J Am Coll Cardiol* 2006;47:1239–1312.

Kannel WB, McGee DL. Update on some epidemiologic features of intermittent claudication: the Framingham study. *J Am Geriatr Soc* 1985;33:13–18.

Norgren L, Hiatt WR, Dormandy JA, et al. TASC II Working Group. Inter-society consensus for the management of peripheral arterial disease (TASC II). *Eur J Vasc Endovasc Surg* 2007;33 (Suppl 1):S1–S75.

Sumner DS. Volume plethysmography in vascular disease. In: Bernstein EF, ed. *Vascular diagnosis*, 4th ed. St. Louis: Mosby, 1993:181–193.

Yao JST. Pressure measurement in the extremity. In: Bernstein EF, ed. *Vascular diagnosis*, 4th ed. St. Louis: Mosby, 1993:169–175.

Young JR. Physical examination. In: Young JR, Olin JW, Bartholomew JR, eds. *Peripheral vascular diseases*, 2nd ed. St. Louis: CV Mosby, 1996:18–32.

CHAPTER C114 ■ NEUROLOGIC EVALUATION IN HYPERTENSION

STEPHEN J. PHILLIPS, MBBS, FRCPC

KEY POINTS

■ Neurovascular evaluation is indicated in all hypertensive patients with focal or global cerebral dysfunction or with painless monocular vision loss.

■ In stroke, the clinical assessment is directed at localization, differentiation of infarct from hemorrhage, determination of cause, and treatment planning.

■ Computed tomography (CT) or magnetic resonance imaging (MRI) can be used to confirm localization and type of stroke.

■ Vascular imaging is a priority in patients with carotid-territory transient ischemic attacks (TIA) or minor ischemic strokes.

See also Chapters B79, **C105,** and C153

Among the principal aims of antihypertensive treatment is prevention of neurovascular complications such as subarachnoid hemorrhage, hypertensive encephalopathy, transient retinal ischemia, retinal infarction, anterior ischemic optic neuropathy, transient focal cerebral ischemia, cerebral infarction, and intracerebral hemorrhage. Neurovascular evaluation is indicated if the hypertensive patient presents with clinical features of acute global cerebral dysfunction, acute painless monocular vision loss, or acute focal cerebral dysfunction. In each of these situations, precise diagnosis is necessary to optimize subsequent management of the patient. The most important part of the evaluation is a careful history and neurologic examination.

Subarachnoid hemorrhage

Characterized by the sudden onset of excruciating headache that may be associated with reduced level of consciousness and focal neurologic findings, spontaneous subarachnoid hemorrhage is most often caused by rupture of an intracranial aneurysm. Prompt referral to a neurosurgical center is required for investigation and treatment.

Hypertensive encephalopathy

Clinical signs and symptoms. Although there is some disagreement as to how to diagnose and classify hypertensive encephalopathy, there is usually a marked elevation of blood pressure (BP), typically approximately 250/150 mm Hg, plus neurologic target organ damage characterized by severe headache, impaired consciousness (confusion, drowsiness, stupor, or coma), nausea and vomiting, vision disturbances, fleeting focal neurologic symptoms and signs, seizures, or retinopathy (papilledema, hemorrhages, and exudates). Rarely are all of these features present in the same patient, but usually three or more are noted. *Neuroimaging studies.* Computed tomography (CT) of the brain should be performed to exclude subarachnoid hemorrhage, cerebral infarction, and intracerebral hemorrhage. A magnetic resonance image (MRI) may show diffuse or multifocal cerebral edema or small focal ischemic infarcts. Neither is necessary for the emergency management of the patient, however, and appropriate treatment should not be delayed to obtain these tests.

Retinal ischemia

The retina and optic nerve head are supplied by branches of the internal carotid artery. Thromboembolic disease of the eye is an important cause of visual impairment and an indicator of increased risk of cerebral and myocardial infarction.

Clinical syndromes

Amaurosis fugax. Transient monocular blindness (amaurosis fugax) is the sudden loss ("like a curtain coming down" or "graying out") of vision in one eye, lasting minutes. This is highly correlated with carotid occlusive disease in patients older than 50 years but is usually due to migraine in younger patients.

Retinal artery occlusion. Retinal artery occlusion causes sudden, painless, permanent monocular vision loss associated with ophthalmoscopic evidence of retinal infarction. In cases of central retinal artery occlusion, the vision loss is complete, there is an afferent pupillary defect, and the entire retina (excluding the macula) loses its transparency and appears milky white. The macula remains red because its choroidal blood supply is preserved. In cases of branch retinal artery occlusion, the vision loss is incomplete, pupillary reactions are usually normal, and only a segment of the retina is infarcted.

Optic nerve disease. Anterior ischemic optic neuropathy (infarction of the optic nerve head) is sudden, painless, permanent, monocular vision loss accompanied by a nerve fiber bundle–type (arcuate) visual field defect, an afferent pupillary defect, and edema of the optic disc. The underlying lesion has been described as a lacunar infarct of the optic nerve head. Giant cell arteritis, lupus, or polyarteritis nodosa must be excluded by appropriate blood tests; for suspected giant cell arteritis, a temporal artery biopsy may be required.

Neurologic investigation

Brain imaging. Brain imaging is useful to look for coexisting silent cerebral infarct(s). The presence of any of these lesions indicates that the patient is at higher risk of subsequent cerebral reinfarction than a patient with an isolated retinal ischemic event.

Vascular imaging. The technique used depends on the clinical situation and the availability of resources and expertise. If the patient presents with a history of several recent episodes of amaurosis fugax and an ipsilateral neck bruit, the probability of finding severe carotid occlusive disease is high. Although the most definitive procedure to evaluate the extracranial and intracranial circulation remains cerebral angiography, MRI angiography and CT angiography provide high-resolution images without the risks of arterial catheterization. Duplex ultrasonography is often performed as an initial screening test; if a technically adequate study shows >50% stenosis of the suspected carotid artery, angiography usually need not be performed. Newer duplex carotid ultrasound systems allow quantification of plaque and measurement of carotid intimal-medial thickness (IMT). Increased IMT occurs in sustained hypertension and may have significant implications as a marker of progression of cardiovascular disease or response to antihypertensive therapy.

Transient focal cerebral ischemia

A transient focal cerebral ischemic attack (TIA) is an episode of focal cerebral dysfunction of sudden onset and offset, of presumed vascular cause, that usually lasts for a few minutes and never lasts more than 24 hours.

Diagnosis and implications. Diagnosis is often made on the basis of the patient's history and careful exclusion of other causes of transient focal cerebral dysfunction such as migraine or epilepsy. TIA is an indicator of increased risk of myocardial as well as cerebral infarction. The symptoms of an attack are variable and depend on the vascular territory involved (**Table C114.1**). Management of the patient also depends on the vascular territory involved; interventional treatment may be indicated for carotid-territory TIA but not vertebrobasilar-territory TIA. Carotid endarterectomy (CEA) substantially reduces the risk of stroke in patients who present with a carotid-territory TIA and an ipsilateral internal carotid artery stenosis ≥70%. The surgery is of less benefit in selected patients with symptomatic 50% to 69% stenosis. Carotid angioplasty and stenting may be appropriate for patients who are unfit for surgery. Vascular imaging is therefore a priority in patients with carotid-territory TIA.

TABLE C114.1

DIFFERENTIATION OF THE INVOLVED VASCULAR TERRITORY IN PATIENTS WITH TRANSIENT FOCAL CEREBRAL ISCHEMIC ATTACK OR STROKE

Vascular territory	Clinical features
Carotid	1. Unilateral motor or sensory abnormalities (or both) 2. Aphasia 3. Visuospatial dysfunction (neglect) 4. Combination of 1 and 2 or 3 5. Homonymous hemianopia plus 1, 2 or 3 6. Dysarthria with unilateral motor or sensory abnormalities, neglect, or hemianopia
Vertebrobasilar	1. Bilateral motor or sensory abnormalities 2. Bilateral limb or gait ataxia 3. Bilateral homonymous hemianopia 4. Any combination of 1 through 3 5. Dysarthria plus any combination of 1, 2, 3, 9, and 10 6. Homonymous hemianopia alone 7. Homonymous hemianopia plus any combination of 1, 2, 9, and 10 8. Unilateral motor or sensory abnormalities plus any combination of 2, 3, 9, and 10 9. Vertigo plus any combination of 1 through 8 10. Diplopia plus any combination of 1 through 9

Imaging. Brain imaging may be unrevealing in patients with TIA; CT scan shows evidence of acute cerebral infarction in only a small proportion of patients who present with early resolution of symptoms. A diffusion-weighted MRI shows the culprit lesion in a substantial minority of cases of hemispheric TIA when the scan is performed within 48 hours of the attack. Patients with TIA, who have imaging evidence of an acute ischemic brain lesion, have a higher risk of stroke recurrence.

Cerebral infarction and intracerebral hemorrhage

Cerebral infarction and intracerebral hemorrhage are considered together because they cannot be distinguished reliably on clinical grounds. They present as *stroke* (i.e., the sudden onset of a persistent focal neurologic deficit), by definition lasting >24 hours unless death occurs. The clinical picture depends on the part of the brain involved and the size of the infarct or hematoma. Diagnosis is a three-step process: (a) localization, (b) differentiation of infarction from hemorrhage, and (c) determination of the cause of the stroke.

Localization. Clinical evaluation and brain imaging allow localization of the lesion in most patients. Localization is important because it may indicate the need for urgent intervention such as surgical decompression of the posterior fossa in cerebellar

TABLE C114.2

PRESENTING CLINICAL FEATURES OF CEREBELLAR STROKE

Symptoms

    Dizziness or vertigo
    Nausea or vomiting
    Slurred speech
    Loss of balance

Signs

    Dysarthria
    Nystagmus
    Dysdiadochokinesis
    Intention tremor
    Heel-shin dysmetria
    Gait ataxia

TABLE C114.3

NONHYPERTENSIVE CAUSES OF SPONTANEOUS INTRACEREBRAL HEMORRHAGE

Arteriovenous malformation
Intraparenchymal rupture of a saccular or mycotic aneurysm
Neoplasm
    Primary (e.g., glioblastoma multiforme)
    Secondary (e.g., bronchogenic carcinoma, renal cell
        carcinoma, melanoma, or choriocarcinoma)
Cerebral amyloid angiopathy
Hemorrhagic transformation of an infarct
    Recanalization of an arterial occlusion
    Venous sinus thrombosis
Vasculitis
Bleeding diathesis
Anticoagulant therapy
Thrombolytic therapy
Sympathomimetic drugs (e.g., cocaine)

infarction or hemorrhage. Clinical features of a cerebellar stroke are shown in **Table C114.2**. Imaging studies may suggest specific treatment, such as carotid revascularization, aimed at reducing the risk of stroke recurrence. Imaging also helps predict the functional difficulties likely to be encountered by the patient, which is important for planning rehabilitation treatment. CT is most often used because it is relatively fast, inexpensive, and accessible. The disadvantages of CT are that it may not show an infarct in the brain stem or any infarct within the first few hours of a stroke. MRI is superior to CT in many respects and is finding increased application, though up to approximately 20% of patients with acute stroke cannot undergo MRI because of metallic implants, claustrophobia, or other comorbid conditions.

Differentiation of infarction from hemorrhage. Making this distinction is essential for decisions about acute therapy and secondary prevention treatment. For acute stroke, differentiation of infarction from hemorrhage can be achieved by CT or MRI with gradient echo and fluid attenuation inversion recovery (FLAIR) sequences. If the stroke occurred more than a few weeks before the diagnostic study, distinction can be made only by MRI. In a decision-analysis model, a policy of "scan all immediately" was more cost effective than "scan all within 48 hours" or "scan patients on anticoagulants or in a life-threatening condition immediately and the rest within 14 days".

Determining etiology

Intracerebral hemorrhage. The clinical evaluation and neurovascular imaging studies may be sufficient to diagnose the likely cause of the stroke and guide subsequent management. For example, cerebral amyloid angiopathy would be the most likely cause of a hemorrhage located superficially in the cerebral hemisphere of an 85-year-old patient. Such a patient could be spared cerebral angiography, might not require neurosurgical intervention, and should not be treated with antithrombotic drugs. Hemorrhages located in the basal ganglia, thalamus, pons, and cerebellum are usually a consequence of hypertension-induced rupture of small-diameter penetrating end-arteries. If the patient is young or does not have a history of hypertension, an alternative explanation should be considered (**Table C114.3**) and the appropriate investigations performed.

Cerebral infarction. Ischemic strokes are due to (a) thrombotic or embolic occlusion of precerebral or cerebral arteries or (b) hemodynamic compromise with relative or absolute hypotension. Emboli may arise from the heart or from arterial lesions between the heart and the brain. Rarely, emboli may arise from the venous side of the circulation and gain access to the arterial circulation through a pulmonary arteriovenous fistula, atrial septal defect, or patent foramen ovale. Therefore, determining the etiology of a cerebral infarct involves investigation of the heart, the precerebral and cerebral arteries, and the blood to determine if a prothrombotic state is present.

Factors affecting management decisions. The nature and extent of investigation should be guided by the patient's age, family history, timing of symptom onset, severity of the stroke, and the presence or absence of comorbid factors. Young patients tend to be more extensively investigated than older patients because there is a greater likelihood of finding an atypical cause. Certain comorbid factors may point to the cause of the stroke. For example, a recent large transmural anterior myocardial infarction or atrial fibrillation makes a cardioembolic mechanism likely. BP is elevated in most patients with acute stroke but the optimal management of hypertension in this setting remains controversial and the subject of ongoing clinical trials.

All patients with acute ischemic stroke should be evaluated to determine their eligibility for treatment with intravenous recombinant tissue-plasminogen activator (rt-PA) using the criteria from the National Institute of Neurological Disorders and Stroke (NINDS) rt-PA Stroke Study. Recombinant activated factor VII has shown promise in the treatment of intracerebral hemorrhage. The requirement that these therapies be administered within the first few hours of stroke onset remains a significant challenge.

Hypertension and dementia

High BP has a negative impact on cognitive function and poststroke dementia is a significant clinical problem occurring in up to one third of stroke patients within 3 months of the event. There is renewed interest in the role of vascular mechanisms in the pathogenesis of Alzheimer's dementia and trials are ongoing to specifically evaluate the effects of BP-lowering therapy on cognition in patients before and after stroke.

Suggested Readings

Adams HP Jr, del Zoppo G, Alberts MJ, et al. Guidelines for the early management of adults with ischemic stroke: a guideline from the American Heart Association/American Stroke Association Stroke Council, Clinical Cardiology Council, Cardiovascular Radiology and Intervention Council, and the Atherosclerotic Peripheral Vascular Disease and Quality of Care Outcomes in Research Interdisciplinary Working Groups: *The American Academy of Neurology affirms the value of this guideline as an educational tool for neurologists. Stroke* 2007;38:1655–1711.

Canadian Best Practice Recommendations for Stroke Care. Available at: www.canadianstrokestrategy.ca. 2006.

Giles MF, Rothwell PM. Prognosis and management in the first few days after a transient ischemic attack or minor ischemic stroke. *Int J Stroke* 2006;1:65–73.

International Society of Hypertension Writing Group. International Society of Hypertension (ISH): statement on the management of blood pressure in acute stroke. *J Hypertens* 2003;21:665–672.

Mayer SA, Rincon F. Treatment of intracerebral hemorrhage. *Lancet Neurol* 2005;4:662–672.

Suarez JI, Tarr RW, Selman WR. Aneurysmal subarachnoid hemorrhage. *N Engl J Med* 2006;354:387–396.

Warlow C, Sudlow C, Dennis M, et al. Stroke. *Lancet* 2003;362:1211–1224.

CHAPTER C115 ■ EVALUATION OF CHRONIC KIDNEY DISEASE

MICHAEL A. MOORE, MD, FACP, FAHA AND DOMENIC A. SICA, MD

KEY POINTS

■ Clinical presentation of glomerular, renal cystic, or renal interstitial disease in hypertensive patients virtually always includes an abnormal urinalysis or renal insufficiency.

■ Glomerular disease presents as one of five clinical syndromes: isolated proteinuria, isolated hematuria, nephrotic syndrome, nephritic syndrome, or renal insufficiency.

■ Nephrosclerosis is largely a diagnosis of exclusion that occurs in long-standing hypertension, often with mild renal impairment and some degree of proteinuria.

■ Evaluation of hypertensive patients for chronic kidney disease (CKD) should include a urinalysis, urine albumin/creatinine concentration, serum creatinine, estimated glomerular filtration rate (eGFR), and usually, a renal sonogram; percutaneous renal biopsy should be performed only when the information will contribute to the treatment of the patient.

See also Chapters A50, A69, B80, and **C156**

Chronic kidney disease (CKD), cystic renal disease, glomerular disease, interstitial nephritis, nephrosclerosis, and end-stage renal disease (ESRD) usually cause hypertension and are almost always associated with impaired renal function and an abnormal urinalysis.

Glomerular diseases

Glomerular diseases comprise five clinical syndromes: isolated proteinuria, idiopathic hematuria, nephrotic syndrome, nephritic syndrome, or ESRD.

Isolated proteinuria. These patients typically have <3.5 g (nonnephrotic range) of nonorthostatic proteinuria per day, with no hematuria. All proteinuric patients should have periodic (at least annually) measurement of urinary protein measurements and glomerular filtration rate (GFR) to determine if the underlying glomerular disease is progressing. Renal biopsy may be necessary if proteinuria quantity is increasing or renal insufficiency develops.

Idiopathic hematuria. Hematuria requires urologic evaluation. If no urologic disease is found and kidney function is normal, immunoglobulin A (IgA) nephropathy is probably present. Approximately half of all IgA patients will develop renal insufficiency, especially those with coexistent hypertension. If kidney function is decreased or if proteinuria is also present, further workup may be necessary, including a renal biopsy. Hypertension markedly accelerates the progression of CKD in IgA nephropathy.

Nephrotic syndrome. Proteinuria >3.5 g per day represents nephrotic range proteinuria; serum albumin drops below <3.5 g/dL when proteinuria is progressive and eventually produces edema. Approximately one fourth of nephrotic patients have secondary elevations in serum cholesterol, but the mechanisms of this anomaly are not well understood. Renal biopsy is usually done in patients with idiopathic nephrotic syndrome, but some centers first treat nephrotic adults and children with 6 to 8 weeks of corticosteroids, reserving renal biopsy for those with corticosteroid-resistant proteinuria. Cytotoxic agents are also employed in some cases. Hypertension in patients with nephrotic syndrome is oftentimes multifactorial relating to progressive renal disease and/or therapy with corticosteroids or cyclosporin.

Nephritic syndrome. Patients with the nephritic syndrome typically have proteinuria to a lesser degree than those with the nephrotic syndrome (<3.5 g/day), variable amounts of hematuria, and red blood cell (RBC) casts in the urine. RBC casts are pathognomonic of a nephritic syndrome and indicate glomerular arteritis. Serum complement components should be measured because a low level of one or more components is characteristic of several types of glomerulonephritis. Renal biopsy should be considered early in the course of nephritic patients who do not have postinfectious glomerulonephritis because disease may progress quickly and a tissue diagnosis is needed to correctly guide treatment selection.

End-stage renal disease. End-stage disease is characterized by significant azotemia, elevated serum phosphorus (>5.5 mg/dL) and hypocalcemia (<9.5 mg/dL), anemia, variable amounts of proteinuria, broad urinary casts, small echogenic unobstructed kidneys on renal sonogram, and a GFR <15 mL/minute/1.73 m^2. Hypertension is present in >85% of these patients, and the need for renal replacement therapy (dialysis or transplantation) is usually imminent.

Interstitial renal disease

Chronic interstitial disease presents with renal insufficiency (often nonoliguric), a history of exposure to a known cause of interstitial disease, and a normal urinalysis. Chronic interstitial disease typically has <1 g per day of proteinuria, reduced maximum urinary concentrating capacity, and bland urine sediment with minimal urinary cellular elements. The finding of eosinophiluria (>1% of all stainable white cells), although uncommon even in proven cases of interstitial nephritis, is strongly suggestive of "allergic" or drug-induced interstitial disease. A long list of drugs has been associated with interstitial renal disease of a nonallergic nature but nonsteroidal anti-inflammatory agents used in high doses for long periods of time are most widely recognized for causing this problem, especially in the elderly. Certain antibiotics are also capable of causing interstitial renal disease.

Cystic renal diseases

Cystic renal disease is readily diagnosed by ultrasonography. The prognosis of renal cystic disease varies with the etiology of the underlying condition. Simple, thin, smooth-walled renal cysts are usually asymptomatic and develop with age without any adverse effect on renal function or treatment requirement. Occasionally, decompression of fluid-filled cysts has been associated with reversal of hypertension. Hypertension is a common feature in medullary and polycystic kidney diseases. Medullary cystic disease in children usually presents with renal insufficiency. Polycystic kidney disease is usually an autosomal dominant inherited condition, but it can occur in an autosomal recessive pattern, and generations can be skipped. Polycystic disease can present in adults as back pain, hematuria, hypertension, or renal insufficiency. The anemia seen with progressive CKD is typically less so in patients with polycystic kidney disease.

Nephrosclerosis

Nephrosclerosis, characterized by thickening and hyalinosis of the walls of afferent renal arteries, is usually associated with hypertension and worsens with advancing age. In most cases, the diagnosis of nephrosclerosis is made by excluding other etiologies of CKD. Nephrosclerotic patients usually have some degree of renal insufficiency, a long-standing history of hypertension, <2 g per day proteinuria, and an otherwise unremarkable urinalysis. Renal sonography often demonstrates symmetrically sized kidneys, typically normal to small, and a uniform increase in echogenicity. Tight blood pressure (BP) control is needed if the progression of this particular form of CKD is to be slowed.

Recognizing and defining chronic kidney disease

Chronic kidney disease classification. A standard classification system for CKD has been developed by an advisory group to the Kidney Dialysis Outcomes Quality Improvement (KDOQI) initiative. A summary table is provided (**Table C115.1**).

Chemistries. Renal insufficiency is most commonly recognized by measurement of serum creatinine values. Serum creatinine is a more reliable measure than blood urea nitrogen (BUN) in detecting renal insufficiency, and it is inversely related to GFR. BUN is a relatively poor indicator of acute or chronic CKD because blood in the intestinal tract, dehydration, or high dietary protein intake can increase BUN, whereas overhydration, decreased dietary protein intake, or malnutrition lower BUN, irrespective of the GFR. Serum cystatin A is gaining popularity for estimating of GFR. Like creatinine, this protein is continuously secreted but its origin is epithelial cells rather than muscle and it is therefore somewhat less dependent on body size. It also has a lesser degree of tubular secretion than creatinine.

Creatinine clearance. Creatinine clearance (**Table C115.2**) approximates the GFR. Creatinine is a byproduct of the nonenzymatic dehydration of creatine and a fixed amount proportional to muscle mass is eliminated daily by the kidney. However, because creatinine is also secreted by the renal tubules, creatinine clearance overestimates the actual GFR and this discrepancy increases as renal function decreases. Determinations of 24-hour creatinine clearance are also notoriously inaccurate because of the difficulties in precise collection of urine samples. Collection difficulties are less problematic if shorter interval times (2 to 4 hour collections) are used. Creatinine clearance is calculated by a specific formula utilizing serum and urine creatinine as well as urine flow rate. Alternatively, urine-free formulae exist for estimation of creatinine clearance. The Cockcroft-Gault equation is most commonly used and is presented in **Table C115.2**.

There is always an inverse relationship between the serum creatinine and creatinine clearance; however, in renal disease the initial fall in creatinine clearance is oftentimes reflected in only a small change in serum creatinine (**Figure C115.1**). In an average-sized patient younger than 60 years, a serum creatinine level almost equal to 1.6 mg/dL usually reflects at least a 40% loss of GFR. In patients 60 years or younger with less muscle mass (hence an expected lower-than-normal serum creatinine), a serum creatinine level almost equal to 1.4 mg% may reflect a similar loss of renal function.

Estimated glomerular filtration rate. Most clinical laboratories now calculate estimated glomerular filtration rate (eGFR) based on a formula developed in the Modification of Diet in Renal Disease (MDRD) Study that modifies the reciprocal of the serum

TABLE C115.1

CLASSIFICATION OF CHRONIC KIDNEY DISEASE

Stage	Description	GFR (mL/min/1.73m^2)	Action[a]
	At increased risk	≥90 (with CKD risk factors)	Screening CKD risk reduction
1.	Kidney damage with normal or ↑ GFR	≥90	Diagnosis and treatment Treatment of comorbid conditions, slowing progression, CVD risk reduction
2.	Kidney damage with mild ↓ GFR	60–89	Estimating progression
3.	Moderate ↓ GFR	30–59	Evaluating and treating complications
4.	Severe ↓ GFR	15–29	Preparation for kidney replacement therapy
5.	Kidney failure	<15 (or dialysis)	Replacement (if uremia present)

Shaded area identifies patients who have chronic kidney disease; unshaded area designates individuals who are at increased risk for developing chronic kidney disease. Chronic kidney disease is defined as either kidney damage or GFR <60 mL/minute/1.73 m^2 for ≥3 months. Kidney damage is defined as pathologic abnormalities or markers of damage, including abnormalities in blood or urine tests or imaging studies. CKD, chronic kidney disease; GFR, glomerular filtration rate; CVD, cardiovascular disease.
[a]Includes actions from preceding stages.

creatinine by adjustment for ethnicity, gender, and age and does not rely on urine collection. The rationale for this approach was to increase the sensitivity of this screening test for CKD; largely because physicians tended to ignore small but meaningful changes in serum creatinine (a change in serum creatinine from 0.8 to 1.2 mg/dL represents a 33% reduction in GFR). The eGFR equation can be found on the web sites of the National Kidney Foundation (www.kidney.org) and the National Kidney Disease Education Program (www.nkdep.nih.gov).

Microalbuminuria. Proteinuria is first detected as microalbuminuria (30–299 mg/24 hours or roughly 200 mg albumin/g creatinine on spot urine); concentrations of albumin below 300 mg/dL are not detected by standard urinary dipsticks and their measurement requires more sensitive radioimmunoassay methods. Persistent microalbuminuria indicates increased risk for or the presence of cardiovascular (CV) disease, systemic endothelial dysfunction, the presence of CKD, and risk for progressive CKD patients with diabetes. Routine determination of microalbuminuria should be done in any type 2 and postpubertal type 1 diabetic patients or nondiabetic hypertensive patients for cardiovascular disease (CVD) risk stratification and CKD classification.

TABLE C115.2

CALCULATION OF CREATININE (Cr) CLEARANCE

General formula
[Urine Cr (mg/dL) × urine volume (mL)]/[serum Cr (mg/dL) × collection time (min)]
Modified Cockcroft-Gault formula
Men: [(140 − age) × weight (kg)]/[72 × serum Cr (mg/dL)]
Women: [(140 − age) × weight (kg)]/[72 × serum Cr (mg/dL)] × 0.85

Proteinuria detection methods. Standard urinary reagent dipsticks detect albumin (not globulin) when it is present at concentrations >150 mg%. Proteinuria should be quantified with a spot albumin to creatinine (A/C) from randomly voided urine or a 24-hour urinary protein collection. It is generally recommended that the presence of albumin in the urine in the range of microalbuminuria, is best determined by a urinary A/C ratio in a spot voided urine. The A/C correlates closely with a 24-hour urine albumin (normal A/C <0.2; 1.0–3.5 ratio correlates with 1.0–3.5 g/24 hours) and this measure has the advantage of avoiding inaccuracies in urine collection and the unpleasantness

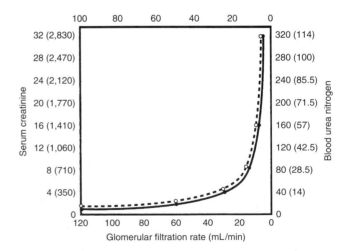

Figure C115.1 Percentage of normal glomerular filtration rate. Relation among serum creatinine, blood urea nitrogen, and glomerular filtration rate. *Dashed line*, blood urea nitrogen, mg/dL (mmol/L); *solid line*, serum creatinine, mg/dL (μmol/L). (Adapted from Kassirer JR. Clinical evaluation of kidney function-glomerular function. *N Engl J Med* 1971;285:385–389, with permission.)

TABLE C115.3

CLINICAL CLUES FOR RENAL PARENCHYMAL DISEASE

Medical history
Recurrent urinary tract infections, particularly in young patients Congenital bladder abnormalities or "reflux nephropathy" History of excessive analgesic use or use of any potential nephrotoxin Interstitial nephritis Previous renal failure; locate any previous renal function studies, such as blood urea nitrogen,   serum creatinine, urinalysis, or radiology studies A history of ingestion of moonshine or illicit alcohol suggests potential lead exposure

Physical examination	
Periorbital, back or leg edema	Expanded extracellular fluid volume
Rales	Expanded extracellular fluid volume
Pallor	Anemia of chronic renal failure
Systolic murmur	Increased cardiac output/anemia
Diastolic murmur	May precede pericarditis
Pericardial rub	Uremic pericarditis
Decreased tactile sense	Uremic neuropathy
Loss of muscle mass	Uremic myopathy

An abdominal bruit, particularly
    diastolic, suggests
	Renal artery stenosis or an arteriovenous
	    malformation.

Diabetic retinopathy	Diabetic nephropathy in a diabetic patient with proteinuria

Laboratory studies
Albuminuria indicates glomerular disease Red cell casts always indicate glomerular inflammation Renal disease should always be considered in the patient with unexplained anemia A urine test result negative for protein by dipstick (albumin) but positive for protein by   sulfosalicylic acid (any protein) suggests the presence of light chain dysproteinemia

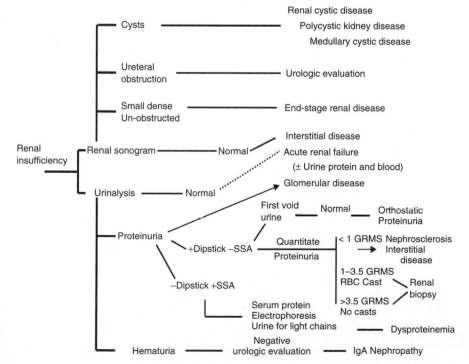

Figure C115.2 Algorithm for evaluation of chronic kidney disease. GRMS, grams; RBC, red blood cell; IgA, immunoglobulin A, SSA, sulfosalicylic acid.

of having to store urine during the collection process. Urine may be tested for total protein with sulfosalicylic acid (SSA) (one part SSA to nine parts urine), which precipitates all proteins including light chains (the predominant urine protein in dysproteinemic states).

Implications of proteinuria. The presence of proteinuria is always of clinical concern because albuminuria strongly predicts the risk of ESRD and CV disease. The exception is orthostatic proteinuria, which has a benign prognosis and is present if protein is negative from the first voided (overnight) urine but present in daytime samples. Differing amounts of proteinuria are present in the various types of CKD. Patients with persistent proteinuria (not orthostatic) should be screened for diabetes mellitus, connective tissue diseases, dysproteinemic conditions, hepatitis C, and human immunodeficiency virus (HIV).

Microscopic examination of urine. A careful microscopic analysis is considered to be the "poor man's renal biopsy." Cells and cellular casts are hallmarks of glomerular disease. When protein condenses in renal tubules, a cast of the internal shape of the tubule is created. Waxy or hyaline protein casts are always seen in patients with proteinuria but can also be seen in the urine of patients without glomerular disease and an otherwise normal urinalysis. RBC casts represent blood and protein derived from the glomerulus and are always indicative of glomerulonephritis. White blood cell casts or mixed cellular casts may also be present with glomerular disease.

Imaging studies. Radiocontrast agents cleared by glomerular filtration (e.g., diethylenetriamine pentaacetic acid) can be used to calculate GFR.

Ultrasonography. A renal ultrasonographic examination is very useful in defining renal size, identifying cysts, and screening for obstructive uropathy. Small dense "echogenic" kidneys on ultrasonography indicate a diffuse advanced stage of CKD. Exceptions to the typical inverse correlation between cortical thickness and CKD are diabetes, and infiltrative renal disease such as can occur with lymphoma, and amyloidosis, in which renal size may be increased.

Renal biopsy. A percutaneous renal biopsy should be performed only when the information will contribute to the treatment of the patient (i.e., alter therapy or provide critical prognostic information). Some treatable glomerular diseases, such as diabetes

mellitus, lupus, dysproteinemias, and antinuclear cytoplasmic antibody glomerulonephritis, can be diagnosed from serologic studies, which may then influence the decision on whether to biopsy a patient or not.. Common indications for renal biopsy are: (a) to establish a diagnosis in patients with idiopathic nephrotic syndrome or nonpostinfectious glomerulonephritis; (b) to establish the severity or prognosis of a CKD, such as that seen with lupus nephritis; or (c) to determine the etiology of acute renal failure that fails to resolve in a timely manner.

Percutaneous renal biopsy is done in some potential renal transplant recipients to determine the primary cause of CKD. Certain diseases such as membranoproliferative glomerulonephritis, focal glomerulosclerosis, IgA nephropathy, diabetic nephropathy, and oxalosis can recur in the transplanted kidney. It is important to consult an experienced renal pathologist for accurate interpretation of a renal biopsy. An open renal biopsy may be required in the severely obese, in noncooperative patients, and in patients with a solitary kidney who have evidence of renal disease.

Evaluation of the hypertensive patient for chronic kidney disease

Evaluation for CKD includes a history and physical examination seeking appropriate clues as to etiology (**Table C115.3**). Laboratory studies should always include a urinalysis, BUN, serum creatinine, electrolytes and serum albumin, spot urine A/C ratio, eGFR, and occasionally a 24-hour creatinine clearance, renal ultrasonography or renal biopsy (**Figure C115.2**).

Suggested Readings

American Diabetes Association. Diabetic nephropathy. *Diabetes Care* 2006;29:S83–S42.

Ginsberg JM, Chang BS, Matarese RA, et al. Use of single voided urine samples to estimate quantitative proteinuria. *N Engl J Med* 1983;309:1543–1546.

Jennette JC, Falk RJ. Glomerular clinicopathologic syndromes. In: Greenberg A, ed. *Primer on kidney disease*, 3rd ed. San Diego: Academic Press, 2001.

Levey AS, Greene T, Kusek J, et al. A simplified equation to predict glomerular filtration rate from serum creatinine [Abstract]. *J Am Soc Nephrol* 2000;11:155A.

Stevens LA, Levey AS. Chronic kidney disease in the elderly — how to assess risk. *N Engl J Med* 2005;352:2122–2124.

CHAPTER C116 ■ EVALUATION OF RENOVASCULAR DISEASE

STEPHEN C. TEXTOR, MD

KEY POINTS

- Renovascular disease can accelerate hypertension and limit perfusion of the kidney, worsening sodium retention and threatening its viability.
- Selection of diagnostic imaging modality depends on the specific objective: (a) identification or exclusion of main renal artery disease; (b) determining whether the entire renal mass is affected (bilateral, or solitary functioning kidney; (c) establishing severity, location, and suitability for revascularization; and (d) determining progression of disease.
- Noninvasive studies that focus mainly on imaging the renal vasculature [magnetic resonance (MR) angiography, computed tomographic (CT) angiography, or renal artery Doppler ultrasonography] are usually performed before angiography.
- Functional studies of renin release or lateralization of radionuclide (with or without blockade of the renin-angiotensin system) have limited predictive value.
- Full workup should only be contemplated when vascular intervention is feasible; whether the patient receives interventional or medical therapy depends on a number of factors, including the underlying risk factors, the disease type, and the characteristics of the lesion.

See also Chapters **A51** and **C168**

Renal arterial disease produces a broad spectrum of clinical manifestations. When the occlusive disease reaches a degree sufficient to reduce renal perfusion, activation of compensatory mechanisms (release of renin along with salt retention) can produce the syndrome of renovascular hypertension, whereas progression of atherosclerosis can lead to renal ischemia and loss of kidney function. Management of renovascular disease is currently debated and includes both medical and interventional approaches.

Renal artery stenosis versus renovascular hypertension

Renal artery stenosis is relatively common due to the widespread prevalence of atherosclerosis. Epidemiologic and imaging studies of the renal arteries indicate that some degree of atherosclerotic renal artery stenosis may be found in 20% to 45% of patients with disease of the coronary or peripheral vascular beds. Many renal artery stenotic lesions (<50% lumen occlusion) are of only minor hemodynamic significance. True renovascular hypertension refers to the syndrome of elevated arterial blood pressure (BP) produced by reduced renal perfusion, best defined by the degree

of BP reduction after successful renal revascularization. Arterial hypertension results from activation of multiple renal pressor mechanisms, including activation of the renin-angiotensin system and excessive salt and water retention; these compensations cause systemic arterial hypertension, which restores perfusion of the kidney.

Fibromuscular versus atherosclerotic disease

Fibromuscular disease of the renal arteries can appear at any age but has a marked predilection for young women. Atherosclerotic disease has become the predominant renal artery lesion in Western countries and increases in frequency with advancing age. Most atherosclerotic renovascular disease is superimposed on essential hypertension, which accounts in part for the low rate of true "cure" with successful renal revascularization. The effectiveness of recent antihypertensive therapy and constraints on the cost of diagnostic testing both contribute to the fact that many patients with renal artery stenosis and renovascular hypertension remain undetected. When BP can be controlled with a simple regimen and renal function remains stable, there is little impetus to pursue correctable causes of hypertension. As a result, renal artery stenosis is now frequently identified during angiography for other reasons, such as cardiac catheterization or evaluation of peripheral vascular disease.

Rationale for renovascular imaging

Concerns about progressive vascular occlusion, loss of kidney function, and episodes of pulmonary edema have become major stimuli for considering renovascular intervention. Hence, clinicians must consider what goals are achievable before undertaking diagnostic evaluation of the renal circulation. Often this centers on examining the role of renal artery lesions in producing a spectrum of manifestations (**Figure C116.1**). Studies to evaluate renovascular disease are typically directed toward one or more of the following: (a) establishing a causal role and hemodynamic significance related to generation of hypertension, with consideration of therapeutic intervention or (b) estimating the likelihood of benefit from renal revascularization by establishing that "critical" renal artery stenosis impairs the viability of the poststenotic kidney, which is at risk for progressive renal injury and "ischemic nephropathy." Advances in medical therapy have made "resistant hypertension" less important as a primary reason to evaluate renovascular disease.

Renovascular disease spectrum

Recognition that restoring kidney blood flow and pressures can lower arterial pressure has been a driving force behind the search for secondary hypertension. The degree of success in achieving that goal, however, depends strongly on the etiology of renovascular disease, and the duration of the hypertension. Among younger women, acute onset hypertension may be due to fibromuscular dysplasia, more often seen in the right renal artery; these individuals often respond to revascularization. Among older individuals with treatment resistant hypertension, atherosclerotic renovascular disease remains a relatively common secondary cause of hypertension.

Recent advances in imaging, medical therapy (especially agents capable of blocking the renin-angiotensin system), and endovascular techniques have combined to make this a controversial and rapidly changing clinical field. Curing hypertension in older individuals with atherosclerotic disease is uncommon, but intervention can reduce medication burden and improve BP control and is therefore a potential indication for intervention. Management of renovascular hypertension is further complicated by the fact that more elderly individuals than ever before develop symptoms referable to atherosclerotic renal vascular disease.

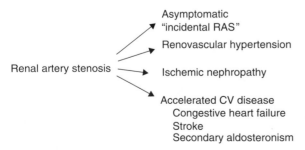

Figure C116.1 Issues in renovascular disease. RAS, renal artery stenosis; CV, cardiovascular.

Ischemic nephropathy

Natural history. Atherosclerotic renal artery stenosis is a progressive disorder. Prospective series suggest that progression to higher ultrasound velocities occurs in 31% of lesions overall and 49% of lesions, which are >60% occluded initially. Remarkably, few lesions (3%) progressed to total occlusion in this series. It must be emphasized that progression of the lesion does not always translate into clinical progression, with worsening hypertension or kidney function. Several series of "incidental" renal artery lesions followed without revascularization indicate that true clinical progression develops in 10% to 15% of individuals observed for 3 to 5 years. Specific characteristics that lead to progression are not known but likely include risk factors for atherogenesis, including cigarette smoking and dyslipidemia.

Role of comorbidities and global risk assessment. Rates of renal arterial disease progression are clinically important for several reasons. Because most renal artery lesions do not worsen rapidly, it is likely that many patients will die of other causes. Furthermore, for many patients, the hazards of vascular study and intervention (including complications of the procedure and restenosis) may outweigh the true clinical risk associated with renovascular disease. These features support a highly individualized approach before undertaking a diagnostic evaluation and committing to vascular repair. Remarkably, renal function and BP outcomes in reported series of patients subjected to either stenting or surgery do not differ greatly, whether the disease is bilateral or unilateral. However, the presence of bilateral disease is an independent predictor of cardiovascular (CV) mortality.

Predictors of response to intervention. Prediction of the response to revascularization remains a challenge. The most consistently useful predictor of benefit is a recent, major change in BP or renal function, which marks the acute development of a critical degree of arterial stenosis. Recent studies have tried to identify kidneys not likely to respond to restoration of blood flow.

Renal size. Presence of renal shrinkage (kidneys <8 cm in length) confers a negative prognosis.

Resistive index. Assessment of poststenotic renal blood flow and vascular resistance within the kidney (the "resistive index" obtained by Doppler ultrasonography) provides information about potential salvageability; a low resistive index improves the likelihood of a good response of BP or renal function response but findings are rarely absolute.

Kidney function. Assessment of kidney function and proteinuria is important. Serum creatinine levels >3 mg/dL indicate advanced renal insufficiency and predict low probability of recovery of renal function after either surgical or endovascular repair.

Proteinuria. The presence of proteinuria, particularly in subjects with diabetes, raises the possibility of other glomerular disease, which may not benefit from renal revascularization directly. However, it must be emphasized that renovascular lesions producing hypertension have been found associated with nephrotic range proteinuria (>3 g daily). This level of proteinuria can revert to normal after renal revascularization, angiotensin-converting enzyme (ACE) inhibition or nephrectomy. Hence, the presence of proteinuria itself must be considered nonspecific.

Laboratory diagnostic techniques

Plasma renin activity. Renal vein renin determinations illustrate the limitations of laboratory testing. Several studies indicate that lateralization of renal vein measurements provides strong positive predictive benefit (>90%) from renal revascularization regarding improved BP control. However, failure to find a lateralizing measurement is also commonly associated with clinical benefit (50%–60%). As a result, such measurements are of limited value in planning intervention.

Lateralizing studies. Many types of lateralization studies have been proposed to establish whether certain lesions impair blood flow or promote release of renin and to establish whether correction of the vascular lesion is likely to produce important improvement in either blood flow or renal function. Most of these studies, including radionuclide renography, measurement of bilateral renal vein renin levels, intravenous pyelography, and ureteral catheterization with split-renal function studies all assume that the "stenotic kidney" is being compared to a normal "contralateral" kidney. In reality, the contralateral kidney is often not normal due to parenchymal disease, to diffuse arterial disease, or to the absence of a contralateral kidney. Lateralizing tests may have value under specific circumstances such as identifying a "pressor" kidney before nephrectomy.

Renin-angiotensin-aldosterone system activation studies. Exaggerated activity of the renin-angiotensin-aldosterone system (RAAS) in renovascular hypertension is the premise underlying tests that measure responses of the RAAS to pharmacologic manipulation. These tests have the drawback of being sensitive to the effects of basal conditions [e.g., renal function, sodium intake, or drugs affecting renin release, including β-blockers, diuretics, sympatholytic agents, ACE inhibitors and angiotensin receptor blockers (ARBs)]. In clinical practice these have limited predictive value and are not used commonly.

Imaging studies

Renal artery lesions are commonly identified with the use of noninvasive imaging procedures. In many instances, these procedures are undertaken primarily to exclude either unilateral or bilateral renal artery disease.

Captopril renography. This test remains widely available and is usually applied to rule out high-grade renal artery disease. Administration of captopril (or other ACE inhibitors) amplifies the functional difference between kidneys by demonstrating accumulation of radionuclide (the fraction not removed by glomerular filtration) in the affected kidney. The renogram does not provide direct imaging of the renal vessels and must be considered an indirect assessment of renal blood supply.

When performed carefully in patients with near normal renal function, some series indicate that a normal captopril renogram excludes renal artery stenosis with high negative predictive value. Split-renal function measurements with renography indicate that recovery of function in the poststenotic kidney sometimes can be observed after renal revascularization. When renal function is poor (creatinine levels ≥ 2 mg/dL), the likelihood of false positive scans rises and it is less reliable.

Doppler ultrasonography. In most institutions, Doppler interrogation of the renal arteries is among the least expensive tests available. When carefully performed, Doppler studies can produce highly reliable estimates of renal artery flow velocity. A rise in velocity (to >200 cm/second) and/or higher than the aortic velocities (renal-aortic ratio ≥ 3.5) is considered predictive of >60% luminal narrowing. Studies of the flow velocity during diastole ("resistive index") suggest that high resistance is more likely to be associated with poor therapeutic responses of BP and renal function after renal revascularization, although this is not universally observed. Examination of the Doppler waveforms distal to the main renal artery segments within the kidney can establish disturbances in waveforms (designated "parvus and tardus") which indicate more proximal functional obstruction. Pressure gradients estimated by this technique can be used serially to track progression of a known stenotic lesion.

Drawbacks of ultrasonography include the fact that functional assessment of the kidney itself is limited, that it can be technically demanding and time consuming, and that some individuals are not technically suitable for study. Accessory renal arteries cannot be identified reliably by this method. Positive studies are nearly always confirmed at angiography but false-negative studies are common, particularly when body habitus makes location of the renal vessels difficult.

Computed tomographic angiography. Dynamic imaging using high-speed helical or multidetector computed tomography (CT) is now widely available for imaging both vascular and organ structure. These studies can provide measurements of parenchymal volume and perfusion with reliability, but do utilize significant iodinated contrast. This exposure poses a hazard in patients with renal insufficiency, particularly with diabetes. CT angiography has positive and negative predictive values comparable to magnetic resonance (MR) angiography and can more reliably detect small accessory vessels.

Gadolinium-contrast magnetic resonance angiography. MR imaging can visualize the main renal arteries and yield an approximate estimate of renal function by measuring clearance of the contrast agent. Predictive value for high-grade renal arterial lesions has been estimated above 90%. Although expensive, this method offers the most complete noninvasive imaging of the renal vasculature with a nonnephrotoxic agent. Recent reports of a rare fibrosing skin condition ("nephrogenic fibrosing dermopathy" now designated "nephrogenic systemic fibrosis") prompted concerns about excessive use of gadolinium in patients with advanced renal dysfunction. MR angiography is limited by offering best images of only the proximal renal artery segments and may miss distal lesions or accessory vessels.

Contrast arteriography. Conventional angiography remains the "gold standard" for evaluation and identification of renal artery lesions. It is now most commonly performed at the time of planned endovascular intervention with balloon angioplasty and/or stenting to restore vessel patency. Angiography may be performed at the time of imaging aorta and vessels for planned surgical procedures, which commonly involve both aortic and renal artery repair. The hazards of arteriography include atheroembolic disease and contrast nephrotoxicity, particularly in older subjects with preexisting renal insufficiency and/or diabetes.

Angiotensin-converting enzyme inhibitors and angiotensin receptor blockers in diagnosis of renovascular hypertension. Normal glomerular filtration depends on the efferent arteriolar actions of angiotensin II, particularly under conditions of reduced afferent BPs to the glomerulus. As a result, blocking the generation or actions of angiotensin II can reduce glomerular filtration pressure (see Chapter A51) and produce a hemodynamic change with "functional acute renal insufficiency." Widespread clinical use of agents that block the renin-angiotensin system has changed the presentation of renovascular disease because individuals with unsuspected renovascular disease are given these drugs. When renovascular disease is present, ACE inhibitor and ARBs tend to reduce glomerular filtration rate (usually by 30%–50% in unilateral disease). Corollaries to this observation are twofold: (a) the clinician must be attuned to the possibility of unsuspected renal artery disease when complications arise, such as when deteriorating renal function or "flash pulmonary edema" with circulatory congestion out of proportion to left ventricular systolic function; and (b) the clinician must consider the possibility of progressive atherosclerotic renal failure if stenotic lesions are not corrected.

Clinical decision-making

Clinicians managing patients with renovascular hypertension face a number of challenges. Decisions regarding the extent of diagnostic evaluation must be predicated upon a clear understanding from the outset of the implications of the results. In contemplating studies to identify renovascular hypertension, it is implicit that the *a priori* likelihood of both renovascular hypertension and the potential impact of vascular intervention are sufficient. At the same time, the clinician should consider whether the renal artery disease has the potential to adversely affect renal function and whether intervention should be undertaken for renal preservation (with intervention at the time of initial angiography). At present, there is little clear guidance from clinical trials and therefore individual decisions require astute clinical judgment. Prospective trials including the National Institutes of Health (NIH)-sponsored CORAL trial (Cardiovascular Outcomes in Renal Atherosclerotic Lesions) are now evaluating whether renal revascularization truly increases the benefits of optimized medical therapy. The CORAL study will be important to identify whether it is appropriate to intervene in "silent" renal artery stenosis. In particular, it has become common practice for cardiologists to perform renal artery stenting at the time of coronary artery intervention. This procedure should be discouraged because at present, there are no studies demonstrating improved mortality, renal function, or BP control.

Suggested Readings

Boudewijn G, Vasbinder C, Nelemans PJ, et al. Diagnostic tests for renal artery stenosis in patients suspected of having renovascular hypertension: a meta-analysis. *Ann Intern Med* 2001;135:401–411.

Caps MT, Perissinotto C, Zierler RE, et al. Prospective study of atherosclerotic disease progression in the renal artery. *Circulation* 1998;98:2866–2872.

Chabova V, Schirger A, Stanson AW, et al. Outcomes of atherosclerotic renal artery stenosis managed without revascularization. *Mayo Clin Proc* 2000;75:437–444.

Conlon PJ, Athirakul K, Kovalik E, et al. Survival in renal vascular disease. *J Am Soc Nephrol* 1998;9:252–256.

van Jaarsveld BC, Krijnen P, Derkx FHM, et al. The place of renal scintigraphy in the diagnosis of renal artery stenosis. *Arch Intern Med* 1997;157:1226–1234.

La Batide-Alanore A, Azizi M, Froissart M, et al. Split renal function outcome after renal angioplasty in patients with unilateral renal artery stenosis. *J Am Soc Nephrol* 2001;12:1235–1241.

Muray S, Martin M, Amoedo ML, et al. Rapid decline in renal function reflects reversibility and predicts the outcome after angioplasty in renal artery stenosis. *Am J Kidney Dis* 2002;39:60–66.

Radermacher J, Chavan A, Bleck J, et al. Use of Doppler ultrasonography to predict the outcome of therapy for renal-artery stenosis. *N Engl J Med* 2001;344:410–417.

Safian RD, Hanzel G. Treatment of renal artery stenosis. In: Creager MA, Loscalzo J, eds. *Vascular medicine: a companion to Braunwald's heart disease*. Philadelphia: WB Saunders, 2006:349–357.

Tan KT, van Beek EJ, Brown PW, et al. Magnetic resonance angiography for the diagnosis of renal artery stenosis: a meta-analysis. *Clin Radiol* 2002;57:617–624.

Textor SC. Pitfalls in imaging for renal artery stenosis. *Ann Intern Med* 2004;141:730–731.

Zeller T, Frank U, Muller C, et al. Predictors of improved renal function after percutaneous stent-supported angioplasty of severe atherosclerotic ostial renal artery stenosis. *Circulation* 2003;108:2244–2249.

CHAPTER C117 ▪ EVALUATION OF AORTOCAROTID BAROREFLEXES

ADDISON A. TAYLOR, MD, PhD AND NAVEED IQBAL, MD

KEY POINTS

- Hypertension leads to aortocarotid baroreceptor resetting, blunted orthostatic control of blood pressure (BP), and increased BP variability.
- Baroreflex failure with preganglionic disease (multiple systems atrophy) is associated with normal resting sympathetic nervous outflow but no response to postural stimulation; postganglionic disease (diabetes, amyloidosis) is associated with low sympathetic outflow in the supine position and with upright posture.
- Exaggerated baroreflex responses in the carotid sinus hypersensitivity (CSH) syndrome can cause severe hypertension alternating with hypotension, bradycardia, and syncope.
- Pathophysiologically based diagnoses of autonomic dysfunction in patients with hypertension or orthostatic hypotension and syncope can improve management.

See also Chapters A38, A56, and **C154**

The autonomic nervous system, through its sympathetic and parasympathetic divisions, modulates rapid adaptation of the cardiovascular system to changing conditions. This system is intimately involved in the maintenance of normal blood pressure (BP) during posture or temperature changes, metabolic alterations, or other environmental stresses. This precise regulation is achieved through a series of highly differentiated but closely integrated reflex arcs, including the aortocarotid (high-pressure) and cardiopulmonary (low-pressure) baroreflex arcs.

Applied pathophysiology

Components of baroreflex arcs. In its simplest form, the aortocarotid baroreflex arc consists of three basic components, as illustrated in **Figure C117.1.**

Sensory fibers. Sensory nerves arising from mechanoreceptor fibers in the heart and great arteries transmit afferent signals through the vagus and the glossopharyngeal cranial nerves and through the sympathetic nerves to the central nervous system (CNS). In the case of the low-pressure (cardiac) system, the sensed signal is volume-related cardiac stretch ("preload"); the aortocarotid system responds to pressure change and pulsatility ("afterload").

Internuncial neurons. Inhibitory internuncial neurons located in the nucleus tractus solitarius integrate signals from the afferent sensory nerves, which are combined with input from the hypothalamus and higher cortical centers to modulate the

activity of the rostral ventrolateral medulla, which controls efferent sympathetic flow.

Efferent fibers. Autonomic efferent arcs involve two neurons. The cell body of the first neuron in the sympathetic neuronal chain is located in the brain stem, and its axon terminates in the thoracic spinal sympathetic ganglion. The cell body of the second neuron in this chain is located in the sympathetic ganglion and terminates in an organ or vascular structure such as the myocardium or blood vessel wall. In contrast, the first neuron in the parasympathetic chain extends from the brain stem to the organ or vascular structure and synapses with a very short second neuron that is located entirely within that structure. Norepinephrine is the primary neurotransmitter released by the second neuron of the sympathetic chain, whereas acetylcholine is released by the second neuron of the parasympathetic chain.

Physiologic effects. The aortocarotid or arterial baroreflexes, also termed the *high-pressure baroreflexes,* derive their name from the anatomic location of their afferent fibers. The sensory nerve fibers from the carotid arteries and aortic arch that comprise the afferent limb of this baroreflex are coupled to mechanoreceptors in the wall of the arteries that are sensitive to changes in stretch or transmural pressure. Chemoreceptor cells sensitive to carbon dioxide and, to a lesser extent, oxygen are also present in this region.

Arterial baroreflexes. The aortocarotid baroreflex exhibits tonic activity under resting conditions. As illustrated by the black

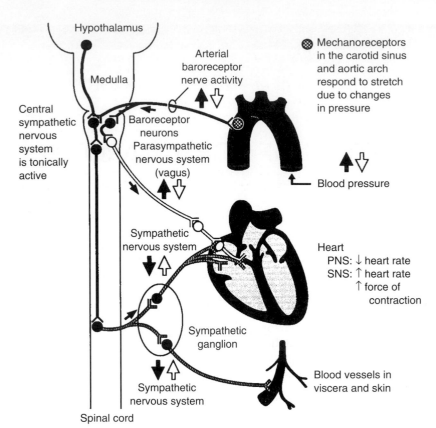

Figure C117.1 Schematic illustration of the essential components of the aortocarotid baroreflex arc. Autonomic neural responses to an increase in blood pressure (BP) are indicated by the *upward pointing black arrows* and autonomic neural responses to a decrease in BP by the *downward pointing white arrows*. PNS, parasympathetic nervous system; SNS, sympathetic nervous system.

arrows in **Figure C117.1**, a rise in BP increases aortocarotid baroreceptor nerve activity. This heightened baroreceptor nerve firing stimulates parasympathetic nerve activity, resulting in a reduction in heart rate and cardiac output, and reduces sympathetic nerve activity, causing vasodilation and decreased cardiac contractility. These compensatory hemodynamic changes tend to return the elevated BP toward its previous value. As illustrated by the white arrows in **Figure C117.1**, the opposite effects are produced by a reduction in BP.

Modulation of baroreflex function. Several factors modulate the cardiovascular response to baroreflex activation. These include origin and strength of the activating stimulus, the "set point" of the reflex, neuronal inputs from the hypothalamus and higher cortical centers, and input from brain stem centers that modulate other autonomic functions such as respiration or gastrointestinal motility. Conditions influencing the heart and conduit arteries and the embedded stretch receptors such as arteriosclerosis can also lead to impaired baroreflex control. The modulatory influence of neurohumoral and vasoactive substances (catecholamines, angiotensin, prostanoids, neuropeptides, etc.), and interactions of aortocarotid with cardiopulmonary baroreflex and chemoreflex arcs further modulate function of this complex system.

Assessment of baroreflex function

A variety of physiologic and pharmacologic maneuvers have been used to characterize the cardiovascular responses to autonomic reflex activation in healthy subjects and to evaluate the integrity of the autonomic cardiovascular reflexes in patients with specific cardiovascular diseases. Some of the maneuvers and their effects on baroreflexes are summarized in **Table C117.1**. Baroreceptor

sensitivity is the slope of the line relating the change in the R-R interval (reciprocal of the heart rate on electrocardiogram (ECG), representing cardiac sympathetic output) to the change in BP during the preceding two cardiac cycles (representing aortocarotid baroreflex input).

Bedside assessment. Although a quantitative assessment of baroreceptor sensitivity requires continuous monitoring of the ECG and beat-to-beat BP, a qualitative assessment of baroreflex arc integrity can be obtained at the bedside by measuring the change in heart rate from baseline during Valsalva's maneuver for 15 seconds. The heart rate typically increases 10 to 30 beats per minute by the end of a 15-second Valsalva maneuver in healthy individuals. Baroreceptor sensitivity has also been estimated by using parameters derived from spectral analysis of continuous indirect systolic BP recordings from finger arteries during spontaneous and synchronized breathing.

TABLE C117.1

PHYSIOLOGIC AND PHARMACOLOGIC MANEUVERS THAT MODULATE AUTONOMIC CARDIOVASCULAR REFLEXES IN HUMANS

Aortocarotid baroreflexes	
Activate	Deactivate
Neck pressure	Neck suction
Phenylephrine	Nitroglycerin
Angiotensin II	Amyl nitrite
Valsalva, phase IV	Nitroprusside

Laboratory assessment of autonomic function. BP and heart rate are the usual hemodynamic parameters monitored at the bedside to assess the effects of autonomic reflex activation. A more comprehensive evaluation is obtained if one or more of the following hemodynamic measurements are also included: cardiac output, cardiac contractility, venous capacitance, peripheral and central venous pressure, or limb (forearm or leg) blood flow. Direct measurements of peripheral muscle sympathetic nerve firing rates in the arm or leg using microneurographic techniques are basically limited to research applications that study regional differences in sympathetic neural activity. Power spectral analysis of heart rate variability or arterial pressure signals provides an indirect assessment of changes in autonomic function but there is controversy about which components of cardiovascular autonomic function are represented by low- versus high-frequency power spectra. Assessment of systemic and regional norepinephrine spillover rates, plasma norepinephrine and epinephrine concentrations, plasma renin activity, plasma angiotensin II concentrations, plasma arginine vasopressin, plasma atrial natriuretic peptide, and measurements of adrenergic receptor number or affinity on circulating leukocytes or platelets offer additional, although indirect, information about the neurohormonal consequences of autonomic reflex activation.

Tilt-testing and other maneuvers. Changes in arterial high-pressure baroreceptor activity can be induced by any physiologic or pharmacologic maneuver that produces an abrupt increase or decrease in BP (**Table C117.1**). For example, the transient hypotension that occurs with standing or passive tilt results in a reflex increase in heart rate, whereas the post-Valsalva increase in BP causes reflex slowing. Infusion of pressor substances (such as α-adrenergic agonists) increase BP and cause reflex slowing of the heart rate, whereas vasodilators (sodium nitroprusside or hydralazine) lower BP and augment sympathetic efferent nerve activity, heart rate, and cardiac contractility. The magnitude of the BP change in response to vasodilators and vasoconstrictors is inversely proportional to the degree of baroreceptor blunting. Maneuvers such as neck suction or neck pressure that alter the transmural pressure or stretch in the carotid sinus can also be used to activate or deactivate arterial baroreceptor reflexes (**Table C117.1**).

Age adjustment. Because baroreceptor sensitivity decreases with age, the baroreceptor response obtained in a patient with suspected autonomic abnormalities should be compared with the response obtained in healthy subjects of comparable age.

Impaired baroreflex function

Aortocarotid baroreflex abnormalities have been documented in a wide variety of clinical conditions in which autonomic neuronal control of BP is altered. Some of the more common conditions are summarized in **Table C117.2**. Optimal therapy in each of these conditions depends on the underlying pathophysiologic abnormality.

Symptoms. Conditions with impaired baroreflex function (most notably idiopathic orthostatic hypotension, multiple-system atrophy, and long-standing diabetes mellitus) are characterized by orthostatic lightheadedness, weakness, or syncope owing to interruption of the high-pressure baroreflex arc by the underlying disease. Palpitations and tachycardia may also occur, with or without accompanying BP change, as in the postural orthostatic tachycardia syndromes.

Laboratory abnormalities and therapeutic implications. Specific identification of the site of baroreflex dysfunction has therapeutic implications.

Preganglionic disease. When the disease affects primarily the preganglionic sympathetic nerves, as in multiple-system atrophy, supine values for plasma norepinephrine are normal and there is no increase with standing because the aortocarotid baroreflex arc is interrupted within the CNS. There is normal basal release of norepinephrine from the intact postganglionic nerve and sensitivity of vascular α-receptors to α-agonists is not altered. Orthostatic hypotension in patients with preganglionic disease often improves with a high-tyramine diet. Monoamine oxidase inhibitors can increase norepinephrine release from the normal postganglionic nerve and decrease its metabolism in the synaptic cleft in patients with preganglionic disease.

TABLE C117.2

SELECTED CLINICAL CONDITIONS ASSOCIATED WITH AUTONOMIC DYSFUNCTION

Cardiovascular conditions	Environmental	Primary/unknown
Hypertension	Microgravity (space)	Carotid sinus hypersensitivity
Congestive heart failure	Prolonged bed rest	Idiopathic orthostatic hypotension
Myocardial infarction	Genetic diseases	Baroreceptor failure
Mitral valve prolapse	Familial dysautonomia	Obstructive sleep apnea
Drugs/toxins	Dopamine β-hydroxylase deficiency	Neurocardiogenic syncope
α-Adrenergic agonists	Neoplastic disorders	Orthostatic tachycardia syndromes
β-Adrenergic agonists	Spinal meningiomas	Psychiatric diseases
Cocaine	Brain stem meningiomas	Panic disorder
Amphetamines	Systemic mastocytosis	Agoraphobia
Endotoxin shock	Neurologic diseases	Trauma
Certain snake venoms	Friedreich's ataxia	Spinal cord transection
Cigarette smoking	Guillain-Barré syndrome	
Endocrine/metabolic diseases	Parkinson's disease	
Diabetes mellitus	Central nervous system	
	demyelinating diseases	
Hyperthyroidism	Syringomyelia	
Fabry's disease	Multiple-system atrophy	
	Familial dysautonomia	

Postganglionic disease. Infiltrative or metabolic diseases affect primarily the postganglionic nerve, as in diabetes mellitus or amyloidosis, where peripheral autonomic function is markedly impaired. There is low supine resting plasma norepinephrine concentrations in these conditions and no increase with standing (a stimulus that usually results in an increase in plasma norepinephrine of 50% to 100% above the supine value). There is also adrenergic receptor upregulation, with increased sensitivity to α-adrenergic agonists (phenylephrine). Patients with diseases involving postganglionic nerves may respond to α-agonists such as phenylpropylamine, clonidine, and midodrine. Patients with hypotension, regardless of the site of baroreflex dysfunction, require fluid volume expansion with a high-salt diet, often combined with the mineralocorticoid hormone, fludrocortisone.

Refractory hypertension and orthostatic instability. Some conditions associated with baroreflex abnormalities have been treated by using implanted neural pacemakers to modify the baroreflex. Deep brain electrical stimulation of the subthalamic nucleus in patients with Parkinson's disease has been reported to improve their orthostatic instability, whereas electrical stimulation of the carotid sinus afferent nerves with an implantable pulse generator has been demonstrated to reduce BP in patients with drug resistant hypertension.

Carotid sinus hypersensitivity

Clinical findings. Carotid sinus hypersensitivity (CSH) is characterized by wide swings of BP, often in excess of 100 mm Hg, often with syncope or near-syncope. Symptoms may be produced by deformation of the carotid sinus by neck pressure, lateral rotation or hyperextension of the neck, or by wearing garments with tight-fitting collars that impinge on the carotid arteries. This condition has also been observed in patients when tumors of the neck impinge on the carotid artery or encircle the glossopharyngeal or vagus nerves and in patients with extensive scarring in the neck secondary to radical neck dissection or prior radiation. In most CSH patients, however, there is no obvious cause for the condition, although it tends to occur more frequently in the elderly. Diagnosis is established by demonstrating that massage of one carotid sinus for 5 to 10 seconds produces a fall of >50 mm Hg in the BP or a sinus pause of >3 seconds accompanied by near-syncopal or syncopal symptoms. There is some reluctance to perform carotid sinus massage in elderly patients; in this setting, pharmacologic maneuvers to raise and lower BP may be preferable.

Subtypes and therapeutic implications. Three different types of CSH have been noted and form the basis of the classification of this syndrome: (a) cardioinhibitory type (bradycardia only), (b) vasodepressor type (hypotension without bradycardia), and (c) mixed cardioinhibitory plus vasodepressor type.

Cardioinhibitory type. In patients who meet the criteria for cardioinhibitory carotid sinus syndrome, it is essential to repeat the carotid sinus massage (or pharmacologic study) after insertion of a temporary transvenous pacemaker to maintain the heart rate. This excludes the possibility of a vasodepressor component that was undetected during the initial evaluation. If no significant vasodepressor component is demonstrated during carotid sinus massage with cardiac pacing, a permanent cardiac pacemaker of the dual chamber type usually prevents further symptoms. In the newest pacemakers, a rate-drop algorithm is incorporated into the firmware that activates the pacemaker impulse in response to a predetermined level of reduction in heart rate.

Vasodepressor type. A patient who has a significant vasodepressor component should be managed medically with elastic support garments, α-agonists, and with fluid expansion in a manner similar to that described in the preceding text for orthostatic hypotension. Should these options fail, surgical interruption of the carotid sinus reflex by stripping the adventitia from the carotid artery or by transection of the glossopharyngeal nerve as it enters the brain can be considered; this procedure has been reported to prevent symptoms in a small series of patients.

Suggested Readings

Bannister R. *Autonomic failure: a textbook of clinical disorders of the autonomic nervous system*, 3rd ed. New York: Oxford University Press, 1992.

Baguet JP, Hammer L, Levy P, et al. Night-time and diastolic hypertension are common and underestimated conditions in newly diagnosed apnoeic patient. *J Hypertens* 2005;23:521–527.

Brignole M, Oddone D, Cogorno S, et al. Long-term outcome in symptomatic carotid sinus hypersensitivity. *Am Heart J* 1992;123:687–692.

Farquhar WB, Taylor JA, Darling SE, et al. Abnormal baroreflex responses in patients with idiopathic orthostatic intolerance. *Circulation* 2000;102:3086–3091.

Honzíková N, Nováalová Z, Závodná E, et al. Baroreflex sensitivity in children, adolescents, and young adults with essential and white-coat hypertension. *Klin Padiatr* 2006;218:237–242.

Jordan J, Biaggioni I. How to diagnose, how to treat: diagnosis and treatment of supine hypertension in autonomic failure patients with orthostatic hypotension. *J Clin Hypertens (Greenwich)* 2002;4:139–145.

Ketch T, Biaggioni I, Robertson R, et al. Four faces of baroreflex failure: hypertensive crisis, volatile hypertension, orthostatic tachycardia, and malignant vagotonia. *Circulation* 2002;105:2518–2523.

Parati G, Di Rienzo M, Mancia G. How to measure baroreflex sensitivity: from the cardiovascular laboratory to daily life. *J Hypertens* 2000;18:7–19.

Smit AA, Timmers HJ, Wieling W, et al. Long-term effects of carotid sinus denervation on arterial BP in humans. *Circulation* 2002;105:1329–1335.

Stemper B, Beric A, Welsch G. Deep brain stimulation improves orthostatic regulation of patients with Parkinson disease. *Neurology* 2006;67:1781–1785.

CHAPTER C118 ■ EVOLUTION OF AMERICAN, EUROPEAN, AND BRITISH HYPERTENSION GUIDELINES

HENRY R. BLACK, MD; BRYAN WILLIAMS, MD AND JOSEPH L. IZZO, Jr., MD

KEY POINTS

■ For a guideline to be widely followed, it must be realistic, clear, easy to use, and free of scientific, commercial, or governmental bias.
■ The scientific database used to formulate good guidelines includes a wide variety of information and expert opinion, not just randomized clinical trials (RCTs) or meta-analyses.
■ Any document that simply reviews current literature without providing a sophisticated interpretation does not provide necessary *guidance*.
■ A hypertension treatment guideline should focus on specific management guidance for hypertension and also provide guidance to reduce overall cardiovascular disease (CVD) risk, including cholesterol-lowering or aspirin therapy.
■ Worldwide guidelines are in agreement on almost all major issues regarding hypertension care.

See also Chapters B100, C103, **C105, C107,** and **C119**

Worldwide practice of medicine has continued to change since publication of the first randomized placebo-controlled clinical trial by the Medical Research Council of Great Britain in 1947 demonstrating that treatment of tuberculosis with streptomycin was superior to placebo. Since then innumerable randomized clinical trials (RCTs) have been conducted using various paradigms: placebo-controlled, active comparator, single-blind, double-blind, and open-label.

What are guidelines and what should they provide?

Essential characteristics. For a guideline to be widely followed, it must be realistic, clear, easy to use, and free of commercial, governmental, or scientific bias. Guidelines can be *focused* or *comprehensive* and provide more than just clinical advice to practitioners. They can be tools of social engineering and a way to translate science to public health. They should be able to be used by the widest possible variety of interested parties, including experts (real or imagined), generalists, patients, payers, policy makers, and journalists.

The "science-based" approach. Recent history is marked by the advent of a systematic approach to the study of disease known as *evidence-based* medicine. This pursuit has provided a platform for an ever-increasing number of guidelines to assist practitioners in managing patients more skillfully. Yet in fields

that are evolving rapidly, evidence from clinical trials is often dated. Furthermore, many trials provide conflicting information and, in the end, there cannot be a clinical trial to answer all possible clinical questions. Therefore, expert opinion is needed to make realistic assessments about the overall benefits and risks of existing therapies.

Guidelines should therefore be broadly "science based" but must also be innovative and represent best medical opinion. The information used to formulate a proper guideline must arise from all relevant scientific sources, not just RCTs or meta-analyses of these trials. Such sources of nonrandomized data include physiology, pathophysiology, epidemiology, outcomes research (registries and data bases), cohort studies, case–control studies, convenience samples, and clinical experience. Although a hierarchy of reliability of these information types has been widely adopted, all can be helpful to a greater or lesser degree. Any document that just reviews the current literature without providing a sophisticated expert interpretation is not very useful or reliable.

Responsibilities of hypertension guideline writers. No condition has been better studied using RCTs, than hypertension. Since 1967 when the first Veterans Administration Trial was published, thousands of investigators all around the world have designed and implemented hundreds of studies. But these trials, for the most part, address only one facet of the problem. An ideal guideline for hypertension should contain guidance on assessment and therapeutic intervention but must also address many other facets, including expert advice and guidance on defining hypertension and its variants, properly measuring blood pressure (BP), assessing and stratifying global risk, evaluating and managing diverse populations, using and interpreting new technologies and tests, and sustaining BP control over time.

Responsibilities of hypertension guideline users. It must always be remembered that guidelines simply provide *guidance,* not a set of immutable laws. An individual clinician's judgment about an individual patient must supercede the advice given by a committee that has not seen that individual patient and evaluated the individual's needs and priorities. He or she should understand what treatment goals are appropriate for which patient and how to deal with identifiable causes of hypertension and hypertensive emergencies. Most importantly, the guideline user must establish (and document) the priorities that are most important for that particular patient.

United States guidelines (1977–2003)

Several organizations have produced guidelines for hypertension in the United States but the periodic reports of the Joint National Committee on the Prevention (a term added in the 1990s), Detection, Evaluation, and Treatment of High Blood Pressure (JNC reports) are considered to be the most definitive. The JNC reports are the work of the National High Blood Pressure Education Program Coordinating Committee, a group of 41 organizations (both medical and lay). They have provided information on screening, how to measure BP, which tests to order, how to treat special populations (e.g., children, older persons, African Americans), and how to handle hypertensive emergencies. In all of the JNC reports, the foundation of therapy is therapeutic lifestyle modification. Important trends in the JNC reports are the continuing evolution of the BP classification system and the downward trend in treatment thresholds (**Figure C118.1**).

JNC 1–2. The JNC 1 (1976–77) classification system did not address systolic blood pressure (SBP), and drug therapy was only recommended for those with diastolic blood pressure (DBP) ≥105 mm Hg but therapy could be "considered" for those with DBP of 90 to 104 mm Hg. Thiazide diuretics were recommended as initial therapy. JNC 2 (1980) introduced the terms *mild, moderate,* and *severe* and classified hypertensive patients based strictly on DBP. This had the unfortunate consequence of implying that an individual with so-called mild hypertension (DBP 90–104 mm Hg) was not a significant risk. Accordingly, clinicians failed to appreciate that most hypertension-related target organ damage happens to patients with BPs in that range. JNC 2 offered the same treatment recommendations as JNC 1. These reports began the process of stepwise drug addition later called *stepped care.*

JNC 3–4. JNC 3 (1984) addressed SBP but only as "isolated systolic hypertension" (SBP ≥160 mm Hg) or as "borderline isolated systolic hypertension" (SBP 140–159 mm Hg) with a DBP <90 mm Hg, but did not suggest treating individuals with only SBP elevations. In that report β-blockers were added to the initial therapy recommendations and low doses rather than full or high dose of drugs were suggested as the appropriate way to start treatment. JNC 3 also pointed out for the first time those individuals with SBP levels <140 mm Hg who might be at some risk, calling them "high normal". Within the "stepped care" framework, JNC 4 (1988) added angiotensin-converting enzyme

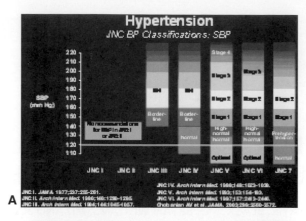

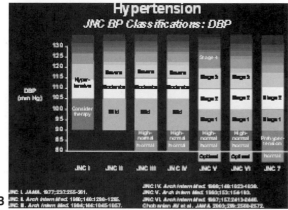

Figure C118.1 The evolution of blood pressure (BP) classification in the JNC reports. SBP, systolic blood pressure; DBP, diastolic blood pressure.

(ACE) inhibitors and calcium channel blockers (CCBs) as initial therapy options, despite the absence of RCTs.

JNC 5–6. The JNC 5 (1993) committee, writing as the "evidence-based" era became dominant, returned to recommending diuretics and β-blockers as "preferred" initial treatment. Although it was argued that these were the only classes of drugs shown to reduce morbidity or mortality in RCTs, the evidence for β-blocker benefits alone was inconsistent. More importantly, this report reclassified hypertensive patients using a new staging system; the terms mild, moderate and severe were dropped and for the first time, the role of a systolic hypertension was highlighted. JNC 6 (1997) dropped the term *preferred* antihypertensive drugs and suggested that any of seven classes of agents could be an appropriate initial treatment option. It reduced the number of BP stages from 4 to 3 and established the term *goal BP*. The standard goal was ≤140/90 mm Hg, but for high-risk patients with diabetes or chronic kidney disease (CKD), a lower target (≤130/85 mm Hg) was overwhelmingly recommended based on the notion that high-risk patients benefit the most from aggressive therapy. This assertion has since proved to be correct despite relatively thin evidence from clinical trials at the time. JNC 6 also introduced the term *compelling indication* to designate specific treatment for individuals who had particular comorbid conditions for which RCTs had demonstrated both BP-lowering and specific outcome benefits with selected antihypertensive drugs [e.g., ACE inhibitors for heart failure or diabetes mellitus (DM)]. In JNC 6, hypertensive patients with BP >160/100 mm Hg or with DM or CKD, drug treatment was recommended when lifestyle modification was started, but drugs were to be used only after 6 months of lifestyle modification in moderate-risk individuals or 12 months in those at lowest risk.

JNC 7. JNC 7 (2003), the most recent U.S. guideline and the first one published in a short ("express") and long (comprehensive) version, simplified the classification system by reducing the number of hypertension stages to 2. JNC 7 also introduced the term *prehypertension* to call attention to the BP-related risks in individuals with BP <140/90 mm Hg. JNC 7 presented a highly streamlined version of care in which risk-based care was dichotomized to those with or without target organ damage/diabetes (**Figure C118.2**). The importance of lifestyle modifications was heavily stressed and thiazide diuretics were recommended as initial treatment for "most" hypertensive patients, largely based on the results of the Antihypertensive Lipid Lowering Treatment to Prevent Heart Attack Trial (ALLHAT). ACE inhibitors, angiotensin receptor blockers (ARBs), CCBs, and β-blockers were all felt to be appropriate first-line treatment in certain patients, especially those with compelling indications. JNC 7 specifically recommended that all stage 2 hypertensive patients (SBP ≥160 mm Hg or DBP ≥100 mm Hg) be started on two-drug combinations, one of which should usually be a thiazide diuretic. The list of compelling indications was expanded to include heart failure, post–myocardial infarction, high coronary risk, and recurrent stroke. The goal BP for high-risk hypertensive patients was modified to ≤130/80 mm Hg to be in agreement with American Diabetes Association and National Kidney Foundation guidelines.

European and World Health Organization/International Society of Hypertension guidelines (2003–2007)

Several guidelines have emerged from Europe, where there has been a distinct emphasis toward characterizing the need for treatment on the basis of overall cardiovascular disease (CVD) risk.

Classifying overall risk level. The 2007 guideline from the European Society of Hypertension/European Society of Cardiology (ESH/ESC) for the treatment of hypertension classifies BP as similar to the World Health Organization/International Society of Hypertension (WHO/ISH) classification of BP (**Table C118.1**). However, the level of BP at which therapeutic intervention is recommended depends on the total CVD risk and the pattern of other comorbidities (**Table C118.2**), a theme common to the ESH/ESC and the WHO/ISH guidelines. At its most extreme, the 2007 ESH/ESC guideline recommends consideration of BP-lowering medication in people with "normal" BP (120–129/80–84 mm Hg) when there is clinical evidence of CKD or CVD. This is the most radical departure so far from the traditional concept of "normal" versus "abnormal" BP based on an arbitrary threshold, and is an attempt to view the relationship between BP and risk as a continuum, with the threshold for intervention defined by a person's CVD risk rather than by BP.

CVD risk is assumed to be sufficiently high to warrant intervention at lower BP thresholds when there is overt clinical evidence of CVD, cerebrovascular disease, or CKD. In addition,

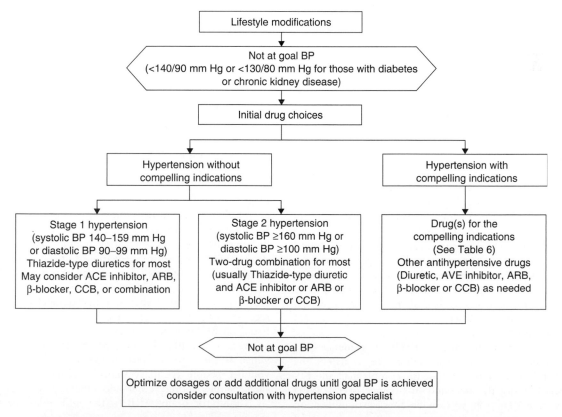

Figure C118.2 JNC 7 BP treatment algorithm. Risk stratification by blood pressure (BP) stage is matched by the level of therapeutic aggressiveness (choice of one or two drugs as initial therapy). Presence of "compelling indications" (heart failure, ischemic heart disease, diabetes, chronic kidney disease, or prior stroke) dictates type of drug chosen based on clinical trials.

TABLE C118.1

CLASSIFICATION OF BLOOD PRESSURE ACCORDING TO THE ESH/ESC GUIDELINE 2007

Category	Systolic (mm Hg)		Diastolic (mm Hg)
Optimal	<120	and	<80
Normal	120–129	and/or	80–84
High normal	130–139	and/or	85–89
Grade 1 hypertension	140–159	and/or	90–99
Grade 2 hypertension	160–179	and/or	100–109
Grade 3 hypertension	≥180	and/or	≥110
Isolated systolic hypertension	≥140	and	<90

Isolated systolic hypertension should be graded (1, 2, 3) according to systolic blood pressure values in the ranges indicated, provided that diastolic values are <90 mm Hg. Grades 1, 2, and 3 correspond to classification in mild, moderate, and severe hypertension, respectively. These terms have now been omitted to avoid confusion with quantification of total cardiovascular risk.

the presence of target organ damage (e.g., left ventricular hypertrophy, vascular structural change, albuminuria), or features of the metabolic syndrome prompts consideration of drug treatment at lower BP levels. Finally, those without overt disease or structural damage may also warrant intervention at lower levels of BP based on either aggregation of their number of conventional risk factors or more formal calculation of their CVD risk using the European Systematic Coronary Risk Evaluation (SCORE) chart. This chart is similar in concept to the Framingham risk charts but has been developed using mortality data from many countries to better reflect the CVD risk of European patients.

World Health Organization/International Society of Hypertension guidelines.
The most recent version of the WHO/ISH guidance was issued in 2003 as an update of its 1999 guideline. The WHO/ISH guidance is developed with a strong focus on the prevention and treatment of hypertension in the developing world. Like the European guidelines, the WHO/ISH report is also focused on BP management in the context of overall CVD risk and has used a simple way of calculating risk based on the number of risk factors and/or the presence of comorbidity or target organ damage. The greater the risk, the lower the BP threshold for intervention (Table C118.3).

Treatment targets.
The BP targets are specified for two broad groups: (i) uncomplicated hypertension and (ii) hypertension with higher CVD risk due to comorbidities. In general, the treatment target for uncomplicated hypertension is <140/90 mm Hg or <130/80 mm Hg for patients with diabetes, CVD, or CKD, although based on limited evidence.

Therapeutic interventions

Lifestyle changes. The WHO/ISH and ESH/ESC guidance both recognize the importance of lifestyle changes to (i) reduce the likelihood of developing hypertension, (ii) complement the BP-lowering effects of drug therapy, and (iii) reduce overall CVD risk. There is consistency in worldwide lifestyle modification recommendations: a strong endorsement to maintain an ideal body weight; undertake regular exercise; increase fruit and vegetable intake; limit sodium, total caloric, saturated fat, and

alcohol intake; and also to stop smoking. Lifestyle modifications are particularly important to the WHO/ISH because developing countries will soon contribute the greatest worldwide burden of hypertension-related deaths, many of which will be directly attributable to adopting a westernized lifestyle.

Specific drug choices. The ESH/ESC and the WHO/ISH guidelines both recognize that BP-lowering itself is the most important benefit from drug therapy. To aid drug therapy selection, both guidelines list contraindications to the major classes of BP-lowering drugs and list compelling and possible indications for the major classes of drugs. Mindful of the importance of cost of drugs in developing regions, the WHO/ISH guideline specifically endorses thiazide diuretics as initial therapy when there is no compelling indication for another major class of drug therapy, a recommendation similar to JNC 7 in the United States.

Combination drug therapies. All guidelines recognize that combinations of BP-lowering drugs are often required to achieve recommended BP goals, especially in those with high CVD risk or comorbidities, who are targeted to lower goals. The ESH/ESH guideline outlines a strategy for initial monotherapy (Figure C118.3) but also highlights the option of using low-dose combination therapy as initial treatment for those who have a very marked elevation of BP, high CVD risk, and a lower BP goal (<130/80 mm Hg). This strategy is similar to that recommended in JNC 7, although unlike JNC 7, the ESC/ESH guideline does not specify that the initial combination therapy should usually contain a thiazide diuretic; the WHO/ISH guideline does not contain specific guidance on combinations of drugs. Neither guideline contains recommendations or treatment algorithms for patients requiring more than two drugs to control BP.

United Kingdom perspectives: the National Institute for Clinical Excellence/British Hypertension Society guidelines.
In 2006, the British Hypertension Society (BHS) and the National Institute for Health and Clinical Excellence (NICE) joined forces to develop a guideline update on the management of hypertension. This guideline is different from the ESH/ESC and WHO/ISH guidance in that it focuses on hypertension management in primary care and uses a standardized and rigorous systematic review and cost-effectiveness analysis (consistent with NICE guidance in other therapeutic areas).

Initial therapy. The NICE/BHS guidance eliminated β-blockers as preferred initial therapy for hypertension and reserved their use for patients with specific indications (e.g., symptomatic angina or heart failure) or as a fourth-line add-on therapy. This decision was based on observations that β-blockers are less effective than other BP-lowering drugs in preventing major CVD events, especially stroke, and are therefore the least cost-effective treatment option. In addition, the BHS/NICE guideline also produced a simplified treatment algorithm (Figure C118.4) which recommended all older patients (aged 55 years or older) or blacks at any age initially receive a CCB ("C" drug) or thiazide-type diuretic ("D" drug), based on BP-lowering efficacy, outcomes, and cost-effectiveness analyses. NICE/BHS highlighted the absence of adequate data which is the basis of recommendations for initial therapy in younger people (younger than 55 years) and concluded that such people should commence therapy with an "A" drug: ACE inhibitor or an ARB (if the ACE inhibitor was not tolerated).

Additional antihypertensive therapy. The unique aspect of this guidance was the very prescriptive treatment algorithm for step 2

TABLE C118.2

ESH/ESC HYPERTENSION GUIDELINE 2007—BP THRESHOLDS FOR INTERVENTION ARE DEPENDENT CVD RISK AND CO-MORBID DISEASE

	Blood pressure (mm Hg)				
Other risk factors OD or disease	Normal SBP 120–129 mm Hg or DBP 80–84 mm Hg	High normal SBP 130–139 mm Hg or DBP 85–89 mm Hg	Grade 1 HT (SBP 140–159 mm Hg or DBP 90–99 mm Hg)	Grade 2 HT (SBP 160–179 mm Hg or DBP 100–109 mm Hg)	Grade 3 HT (SBP ≥ 180 mm Hg or DBP ≥ 110 mm Hg)
No other risk factors	No BP intervention	No BP intervention	Lifestyle changes for several months then drug treatment if BP uncontrolled	Lifestyle changes for several weeks then drug treatment if BP uncontrolled	Lifestyle changes + Immediate drug treatment
1–2 risk factors	Lifestyle changes	Lifestyle changes	Lifestyle changes for several weeks then drug treatment if BP uncontrolled	Lifestyle changes for several weeks then drug treatment if BP uncontrolled	Lifestyle changes + Immediate drug treatment
≥3 risk factors, MS or OD	Lifestyle changes	Lifestyle changes and consider drug treatment	Lifestyle changes + Drug treatment	Lifestyle changes + Drug treatment	Lifestyle changes + Immediate drug treatment
Diabetes	Lifestyle changes	Lifestyle changes + Drug treatment	Lifestyle changes + Drug treatment	Lifestyle changes + Drug treatment	Lifestyle changes + Immediate drug treatment
Established CV or renal disease	Lifestyle changes + Immediate drug treatment	Lifestyle changes + Immediate drug treatment	Lifestyle changes + Immediate drug treatment	Lifestyle changes + Immediate drug treatment	Lifestyle changes + Immediate drug treatment

OD, subclinical organ damage; SBP, systolic blood pressure; DBP, diastolic blood pressure; HT, hypertension; MS, metabolic syndrome; CV, cardiovascular.

(A + C or A + D), step 3 (A + C + D) and step 4 (addition of other agents, **Figure C118.4**). It is of interest that in this guideline "more diuretic" was the preferred option for people with drug-resistant hypertension before a fourth drug was added.

Treating total cardiovascular disease risk. Consistent with the shift toward characterizing patients on a global risk basis, the ESH/ESC guidelines and those in the United Kingdom (the Joint British Guidelines on Cardiovascular Disease Prevention) have provided explicit guidance on the need to consider concomitant risk-reduction strategies, especially in patients at higher risk. The importance of this multirisk factor intervention approach is that it aims to reduce risk, not just BP, and ensures that those at highest risk receive the most effective treatments to reduce that risk. This focus of multirisk factor intervention within a

TABLE C118.3

STRATIFICATION OF RISK ACCORDING TO WHO/ISH GUIDELINES

	Blood pressure (mm Hg)		
Other risk factors and disease history	Grade 1 (SBP 140–159 mm Hg or DBP 90–99 mm Hg)	Grade 2 (SBP 160–179 mm Hg or DBP 100–109 mm Hg)	Grade 3 (SBP ≥180 mm Hg or DBP ≥110 mm Hg)
No other risk factors	Low risk	Medium risk	High risk
1-2 risk factors	Medium risk	Medium risk	High risk
3 or more risk factors, or TOD, or ACC	High risk	High risk	High risk

SBP, systolic blood pressure; DBP, diastolic blood pressure; TOD, target organ damage; ACC, associated clinical conditions.

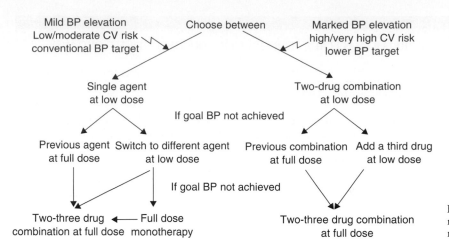

Figure C118.3 European Society of Hypertension/European Society of Cardiology (ESH/ESC) Guidance on monotherapy versus combination therapy strategies.

single guideline is an important difference between European and U.S. guidelines that have traditionally focused on individual risk factors. Accordingly, statin therapy should be considered in all hypertensive patients with overt CVD, type 2 DM, or a calculated CVD risk of $\geq$20%. In the absence of contraindications, low-dose aspirin is recommended for similar at-risk groups.

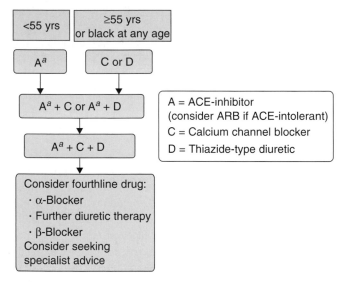

Figure C118.4 National Institute for Clinical Excellence/British Hypertension Society (NICE/BHS) Treatment Algorithm 2006. ARB, angiotensin receptor blocker; ACE, angiotensin-converting enzyme.

Suggested Readings

The ALLHAT Officers and Coordinators for the ALLHAT Collaborative Research Group. Major outcomes in high-risk randomized angiotensin-converting- enzyme inhibitor or calcium channel Blocker vs Diuretic. *JAMA* 2002;288:2981–2997.

Black HR. The paradigm has shifted to systolic blood pressure. *J Hum Hypertens* 2004;18:S3–S7.

British Cardiac Society, British Hypertension Society, Diabetes UK, HEART UK, Primary Care Cardiovascular Society, The Stroke Association. JBS 2: Joint British Societies' guidelines on prevention of cardiovasculardisease in clinical practice. *Heart* 2005;91(Suppl V):V1–V52.

Chobanian AV, Bakris GL, Black HR, et al. Joint National Committee on Prevention, Detection, Evaluation, and Treatment of High Blood Pressure. National Heart, Lung, and Blood Institute. National High Blood Pressure Education Program Coordinating Committee. Seventh report of the Joint National Committee on Prevention, Detection, Evaluation, and Treatment of High Blood Pressure. *Hypertension* 2003;42(6):1206–1252.

European Society of Hypertension (ESH)/European Society of Cardiology (ESC). 2007 Guidelines for the management of arterial hypertension. *Eur Heart J* 2007;12:1462–1536.

Joint National Committee on Prevention, Detection, Evaluation, and Treatment of High Blood Pressure. The sixth report of the Joint National Committee on Prevention, Detection, Evaluation, and Treatment of High Blood Pressure. *Arch Int Med* 1997;157:2413–2446.

National Institute for Clinical Excellence (NICE). *Clinical guideline 18 management of hypertension in adults in primary care 2004 and update 2006.* www.nice.org.uk/CG018 NICE guideline. 2006.

Prospective Studies Collaboration. Age-specific relevance of usual blood pressure to vascular mortality: a meta-analysis of individual data for one million adults in 61 prospective studies. *Lancet* 2002;360:1903–1913.

The Task Force for the Management of Arterial Hypertension of the European Society of Hypertension (ESC) and the European Society of Cardiology (ESH). 2007 Guidelines for the management of arterial hypertension. *Eur Heart J* 2007;28(12):1462–1536.

2003 World Health Organization (WHO)/International Society of Hypertension (ISH). Statement on management of hypertension. *J Hypertens* 2003;21:1983–1992.

CHAPTER C119 ■ OFFICE MANAGEMENT OF HYPERTENSION

JOSEPH L. IZZO, Jr., MD; HENRY R. BLACK, MD AND DOMENIC A. SICA, MD

KEY POINTS

- Demographic heterogeneity and the varying presence of associated disorders dictate a customized ("personalized") approach to hypertension management; each condition present must be managed independently yet within the context of the whole patient.
- All modifiable risk factors (weight, physical activity, smoking, hyperglycemia, hypercholesterolemia, and intake of alcohol, sodium, and potassium) must be managed aggressively in individuals with hypertension to optimally reduce morbidity and mortality.
- First-line antihypertensive drugs with proven outcome benefits are thiazide diuretics, angiotensin-converting enzyme (ACE) inhibitors, angiotensin receptor blockers (ARBs), and calcium channel blockers (CCB).
- Combinations of two first-line agents are usually needed to sustain systolic blood pressure (BP) reductions >20 mm Hg; primary two-drug combinations are: (a) thiazide diuretic with ACE inhibitor (or ARB) or (b) CCB with ACE inhibitor (or ARB).
- Disease-specific indications that influence drug choices include ischemic heart disease, heart failure, chronic kidney disease, cerebrovascular disease, or diabetes.
- Intermittent forms of hypertension, including white coat hypertension, do not always require antihypertensive drug therapy.

See also Chapters B89, B100, **C103, C104, C105, C106,** C114, **C118, C120, C122, C124,** and **C127**

Hypertension is by far the most important modifiable antecedent of adverse cardiovascular and renal events and remains the most common reason why adults see health practitioners. Systolic blood pressure (BP) is a more robust risk indicator and is therefore a more important therapeutic target than diastolic BP, especially in those older than 50 years. The risk of BP elevation is continuous; for each 20 mm Hg increase in systolic BP over the range of 115 to 185 mm Hg (or each 10 mm Hg increase in diastolic BP over the range of 75–115 mm Hg), the risk of ischemic heart disease (IHD) or stroke doubles.

The challenge of "customized" or "personalized" therapy

Managing hypertension is a complex process that blends focused BP control efforts with complementary strategies to manage variable patterns of coexisting conditions in what is an extremely heterogeneous population. Hypertension has different etiologies and presentations, from intermittent ("white coat") to highly complicated patterns that accompany cardiac, cerebrovascular, and renal diseases. At the same time, the presence of obesity and other risk factors also varies greatly and complicates treatment approaches. It is therefore logical to assume that every hypertensive individual should receive effective "customized" or "personalized" therapy. At the same time, it is a practical necessity to establish simple therapeutic guidelines for the management of any chronic disease. This creates a great degree of pressure on guideline writers and on clinicians, who have the substantial responsibility of synthesizing, interpreting, and prioritizing the huge amount of available information that can have a material effect on everyday medical practice (see Chapter C118).

Risk factor profiling and management

The strategic approach to hypertension begins with an assessment of global risk because therapeutic choices are based on the pattern of conditions present in the individual patient. Age, male gender, postmenopausal status, diabetes mellitus or insulin resistance, left ventricular hypertrophy (LVH), and dyslipidemia are independent factors that interact to increase cardiovascular disease (CVD) risk and amplify the impact of BP on CVD risk. The greater the number of cardiovascular risk factors, the greater the likelihood that any increase in BP >115/75 mm Hg will contribute to premature CVD and death.

Modifiable risk factors. In addition to BP, each patient should be assessed for the presence of modifiable risk factors (e.g., dyslipidemia, glucose intolerance, cigarette smoking, obesity, physical activity patterns, and intake of sodium, potassium, and alcohol). Although these conditions do not always directly affect the therapeutic approach to hypertension, their effective management is essential to global risk reduction (**Table C119.1**).

Target organ damage. Evaluation of hypertensive target organ damage is important (see Chapter C106) because the highest risk individuals are those with IHD, LVH, generalized atherosclerosis, heart failure (HF), cerebrovascular disease, renal damage, or retinopathy (**Table C119.2**). Most of these conditions have outcome studies that support the use of one or more specific antihypertensive drug classes as part of the antihypertensive therapy regimen.

White coat hypertension and exaggerated blood pressure variability. Even when BP is measured correctly (see Chapter C103), there are varying patterns of BP elevation in the medical setting and throughout everyday life. Nonsustained "white coat" hypertension (see Chapters B89, C105) carries with it much less risk than sustained hypertension but can be a challenge to accurate risk assessment and management decisions. Assessment of target organs is important because the presence of hypertensive organ damage rules out any "benign" aspect of the white coat syndrome and dictates the need for drug therapy. No study has yet demonstrated the benefit of pharmacologic therapy in the white coat syndrome but these individuals are

ideal candidates for aggressive lifestyle modification and careful follow-up. Unfortunately, stress-related BP increases (including the increments in BP measured in medical settings) usually do not respond well to standard antihypertensive drugs (including β-blockers). Preliminary data suggest that nontraditional methods such as device-guided deep-breathing or "yoga breathing" may favorably affect the white coat pattern.

Other forms of exaggerated BP variation, including an exaggerated morning BP surge or "masked hypertension" (BP elevations outside but not within the medical setting) increase cardiovascular risk and the need for drug therapy. Evening α-blocker therapy has been proposed as beneficial in blunting morning BP surges; masked hypertension should be approached as if the office BP is elevated by the same degree. Elderly individuals with baroreflex dysfunction exhibit marked BP variability that usually does not respond consistently to standard antihypertensive drugs. The goal of therapy is to blunt the variability to some degree but optimal BP control is unlikely; calcium channel blockers (CCBs) have the least negative effect on baroreflexes in these individuals.

Lifestyle modifications

In individuals with multiple risk factors, BP levels >130/80 mm Hg should be treated aggressively with all the tools available. Because "therapy" does not necessarily mean drugs, lifestyle modifications are indicated for all individuals, especially those that help bring BP, cholesterol, and glucose values into their optimal ranges (see Chapter C120 and **Table C119.1**). As a population goal, if everyone with a systolic BP >130 mm Hg followed lifestyle modification, complications of hypertension would be markedly diminished. Even if drug therapy is used, lifestyle modifications help optimize drug effects and minimize doses and numbers of agents needed. Weight control and physical activity are essential and should be addressed simultaneously. Body mass index should be 25 kg per m^2 or less and aerobic physical activity should be performed on at least three occasions per week of at least 30 minutes. Sodium intake should be <100 mEq per day (2.3 g of sodium) and potassium intake should be

---

TABLE C119.1

LIFESTYLE MODIFICATIONS[a]

Condition	Target	Initial therapy	Additional therapy
Obesity	<25 kg/m²	Weight reduction program	Weight loss drugs
Physical inactivity	Aerobic activity >90 min/wk	Aerobic exercise (self-directed)	Supervised program
Dysglycemia	Hemoglobin A_{1c} <6.5%	Weight loss Insulin sensitizers	Other oral agents Insulin
Dyslipidemia	LDL cholesterol <100 mg/dL	Weight loss Statins	Other agents
Cigarette smoking	Elimination	Smoking cessation program	Specific drugs
Excess alcohol intake	<2 oz alcohol/d	Counseling	—
Excess salt intake	<100 mEq sodium/d	Counseling	—
Inadequate potassium intake	>60 mEq/d	Counseling	—

[a]See text and Chapter C120.

TABLE C119.2

ASSESSMENT OF HYPERTENSIVE TARGET ORGAN DAMAGE[a]

Condition	Primary diagnostic clue	Confirmatory tests
Angina	History	ECG, echocardiography, angiography
Myocardial infarction		
Peripheral arterial disease	History	Ankle-brachial index, angiography
Left ventricular hypertrophy	ECG	Echocardiography
Heart failure	History and physical	Echocardiography
Stroke transient ischemic attack	History and physical	Carotid studies, cerebral imaging
Chronic kidney disease	Serum creatinine Microalbuminuria	Urinalysis, biopsy (rare)
Retinopathy	Funduscopic examination	Ophthalmology consult

ECG, electrocardiogram.
[a]See text and Chapter C107.

>60 mEq per day. Alcohol intake should be <2 oz per day and smoking should be eliminated.

General blood pressure target: <130/80 mm Hg

The general goal of BP management is to achieve sustained BP <130/80 mm Hg. This lower target ensures that most BP values will be below the JNC 7 threshold of <140/90. Lower BP targets have already been recommended for the most complicated cases: in JNC 7, BP<130/80 mm Hg was recommended for diabetes or chronic kidney disease. In 2007, the American Heart Association/American College of Cardiology (AHA/ACC) Scientific Statement on IHD suggested that the 130/80 mm Hg threshold should also be applied to anyone with a 10-year Framingham risk-equivalent >10%, known coronary artery disease, chronic angina, prior revascularization, peripheral arterial disease, or HF.

Stage 1 hypertension

Individuals with stage 1 hypertension (BP 140–159/90–99, an IHD risk >twofold over normotensive persons) should receive aggressive lifestyle management (**Table C119.1**). Generally they will also require antihypertensive drugs, alone or in combination.
First-line agents. Thiazides, angiotensin-converting enzyme (ACE) inhibitors, CCBs, and angiotensin receptor blockers (ARBs) have been proved to lower BP and to reduce morbidity from IHD, stroke, or HF. Accordingly, these drugs comprise first-line therapy for hypertension (**Table C119.3**) Combinations of two first-line agents are often needed to sustain systolic BP reductions >20 mm Hg; it is most effective to combine agents with complementary mechanisms of action, especially a vasodilator (i.e., a thiazide diuretic or CCB) with an agent that blocks the renin-angiotensin system (i.e., an ACE inhibitor or ARB).
Second-line agents. Second-line agents (adrenergic inhibitors, central agents, direct vasodilators; loop diuretics, aldosterone antagonists, renin inhibitors, and nitrates, **Tables C119.3 and C119.4**) may be useful to treat hypertension and one or more coexisting condition (e.g., β-blocker for migraine, night-time α-blocker for those with prostatism, or a significant early morning BP surge). At the same time, certain conditions common in hypertensive patients may diminish the attractiveness of other drugs (e.g., β-blockers in severe reversible airways disease or thiazide diuretics in recurrent gout.)

Generally these agents are best reserved for more difficult forms of hypertension.
Response heterogeneity and customized care. Although the average efficacy of certain drugs is different in various patient subgroups (e.g., less effectiveness of ACE inhibitors and ARBs in blacks), there is considerable interindividual variation in these response patterns. Nevertheless, certain trends have been consistently observed. In general, elderly individuals with wide pulse pressure (usually in the very elderly with isolated systolic hypertension) respond better to thiazide diuretics or CCBs than to drugs that block the renin-angiotensin or sympathetic nervous systems. The same general observation is true in blacks, but CCBs are also useful; some younger blacks also respond well to ACE inhibitors and ARBs. Patient profiling (e.g., cardiac output or plasma renin activity) has not proved beneficial in therapeutic decision making due to the wide variations within and between individuals under different physiologic and pathologic conditions. Clinicians can optimize therapy by comanaging hypertension and other conditions present in the individual patient. Many experts feel that thiazide diuretics are preferred in women because ACE inhibitors and ARBs are contraindicated in women of child-bearing potential and also because women are less tolerant of the ankle edema commonly caused by CCBs. Demographic trends in adverse effects can also affect drug choices; for example, ACE inhibitors are more likely to cause angioedema or cough in blacks.

Stage 2 hypertension

Individuals with stage 2 hypertension (BP >160/100 mm Hg; an IHD risk greater than fourfold over normotensive individuals) should receive aggressive lifestyle management and drugs to manage comorbidities (e.g., diabetes, dyslipidemia, end-organ damage). Initial use of standard two-drug antihypertensive therapy (**Tables C119.3 and C119.4**) is indicated for initial therapy, including fixed-dose combinations. Combinations of first-line agents with complementary mechanisms of action are preferred and should usually include a renin-angiotensin system blocker (ACE inhibitor or ARB) and a vasodilator (thiazide or

TABLE C119.3

SUBCLASSIFICATION OF ANTIHYPERTENSIVE DRUGS[a]

First-line agents	Second-line agents	Primary two-drug combinations	Primary three-drug combinations
Thiazide diuretics	β-Blockers	Thiazide + ACE inhibitor (or ARB)	Thiazide + CCB + ACE inhibitor (or ARB)
Calcium channel blockers	α-Blockers		
ACE inhibitors	Loop diuretics		
ARBs	Aldosterone antagonists		
	Direct vasodilators	CCB + ACE inhibitor (or ARB)	
	Renin inhibitors		
	Nitrates		

ACE, angiotensin-converting enzyme; ARB, angiotensin receptor blocker; CCB, calcium-channel blocker.
[a]First-line agents are those proved to reduce ischemic heart disease or stroke incidence. Second-line agents are useful in specific situations. Primary two-drug combinations utilize first-line drugs with complementary mechanisms of action.

CCB). BP control in stage 2 hypertension often requires three or more drugs; a recommended combination is thiazide diuretic + CCB + either ACE inhibitor or ARB. Second-line agents, especially aldosterone antagonists, loop diuretics, or adrenergic receptor blockers can be useful in situations where more than three medications are needed for BP control.

Disease-specific indications

The presence of any form of hypertension-related target organ damage warrants aggressive management to slow disease progression (**Table C119.4**). A comprehensive management plan must include vigorous lifestyle modification and disease-specific combinations of first-line antihypertensive drugs sufficient to control BP to <130/80 mm Hg; drugs to control cholesterol and blood sugar are commonly needed as well. Second-line antihypertensive drugs may also be needed to improve the natural history of hypertension-associated cardiovascular and renal diseases.

Ischemic heart disease and heart failure. The 2007 AHA/ACC guideline for BP management in IHD specifically recommends ACE inhibitors or ARBs for patients with all forms of the condition [angina, prior myocardial infarction (MI)] or revascularization, and HF). β-Blockers are recommended for angina, post-MI, HF, and certain arrhythmias; CCBs are alternative therapies for angina. Of note, in the Comparison of Amlodipine versus Enalapril to Limit Occurrences of Thrombosis (CAMELOT) study, individuals with BPs maintained below 120/80 mm Hg experienced regression of coronary atherosclerosis.

Stroke. Thiazide diuretics and CCBs have been associated with the lowest incidence rates of stroke in meta-analyses. There is no consistent agreement about BP targets in patients with known cerebrovascular disease but individuals in the Perindopril Protection against Recurrent Stroke Study (PROGRESS) who achieved consistent BP values <120/80 mm Hg had the lowest incidence of recurrent stroke or transient ischemic attack.

Chronic kidney disease and diabetes. Several professional societies, including the American Diabetes Association and the National Kidney Foundation/American Society of Nephrology have recommended use of combinations containing an ACE inhibitor or ARB to slow the progression of chronic kidney disease

to its end stage. Yet recent meta-analyses have questioned whether renal benefits are specific to renin-angiotensin-aldosterone system (RAAS) inhibitors or whether they are simply the result of superior BP control (<130/80 mm Hg). In individuals with marked albuminuria (>2,000 mg/day), even lower BP values may be beneficial and ACE inhibitors and ARBs may be of particular utility.

Resistant hypertension

Refractory hypertension exists when an appropriately dosed three-drug combination that includes a diuretic fails to control BP in an adherent patient. Perhaps the most common reason for true refractory hypertension is long-standing systolic hypertension in elderly people with severe arteriosclerosis. Workup for secondary forms of hypertension (especially sleep apnea, occult alcoholism, or hyperaldosteronism) or interfering drugs, [e.g., street drugs or nonsteroidal antiinflammatory drugs (NSAIDs)] may be warranted. Addition of a fourth or fifth drug may reduce BP to goal and referral to a hypertension specialist is often useful (see Chapter C106).

Other aspects of therapy

Patient education. An important part of chronic disease management is patient education. Hypertensive patients must act as partners with clinicians if sustained BP control is to be achieved. Patients should be aware of the consequences of poor BP control and should know the signs and symptoms of IHD and stroke. An educated patient is expected to be able to cite target BPs and should know the ranges of their home and office BP readings (see Chapter C114).

Achievable blood pressure control rates. The Healthy Persons 2000 and 2010 initiatives from the U.S. Department of Health and Human Services have set a goal BP attainment rate of 50% for the population. Current BP control rates are still <40% but appear to be increasing slowly. Several clinical trials suggest that target BP (using the definition <140/90 mm Hg) can be achieved in at least 70% of the population [e.g., ALLHAT, Controlled ONset Verapamil INvestigation of Cardiovascular Endpoints, (CONVINCE)] but higher control rates are expected in clinical trials because of selection of adherent participants, the organized framework of the trials; the use of reasonably

TABLE C119.4

MANAGEMENT OF HYPERTENSION[a]

| BP pattern (mm Hg) | Condition | Lifestyle modification | Initial treatment | | Additional therapy |
			First-line approach	Agents with potential problems	
Home BP <130/80 Office BP >140/90	"White coat" hypertension	Yes	Aggressive lifestyle modification	–	Nontraditional methods
Stage 1 HTN: Home or office BP >140–159/ 90–99	Elderly, ISH, Blacks	Yes	Specific first-line monotherapy[b] (Thiazide or CCB)	–	Primary two-drug combination[b]
	All others	Yes	Specific first-line monotherapy[b] (ACE inhibitor or ARB)	–	Primary three-drug combination[b] Intensify diuretic Rx; Add second-line agents
Stage 2 HTN: Home or office BP ≥160/100	All individuals	Yes	Primary two-drug combination[b] as initial therapy	–	Primary three-drug combination[b] Intensify diuretic Rx; Add second-line agent(s)
Disease-specific indication(s) and home or office BP >130/80	Ischemic heart disease	Yes	Specific drug(s) (β-blocker, CCB, ACE inhibitor or ARB)	Minoxidil, hydralazine	Primary two-drug combination[b] Add/intensify diuretic; Add second-line agents; Add nitrates
	Heart failure	Yes	1–3 drugs initially (ACE inhibitor or ARB ± β-blocker ± loop diuretic)	CCB, α-blocker	Add/intensify diuretic; Add aldosterone blocker Add inotrope
	Stroke/TIA	Yes	Specific first-line monotherapy[b] (Thiazide, CCB, or ARB)	β-Blocker, ACE inhibitor[b]	Primary two-drug combination[b] Add/intensify diuretic Add second-line agent(s)
	Chronic kidney disease	Yes	1–2 drugs initially (ACE inhibitor or ARB ± Thiazide or loop diuretic)	β-Blocker[c]	Add/intensify diuretic Add CCB Add α-blocker Other second-line agent(s)
	Diabetes	Yes	Specific first-line monotherapy[b] (ACE inhibitor or ARB)	β-Blocker[d]	Primary two-drug combination[b] Primary three-drug combination[b] Intensify diuretic Rx; Add alpha-blocker or other second-line agent(s)

First-line agents: thiazides, CCBs, ACE inhibitors, ARBs. Second-line agents: β-blockers, α-blockers, aldosterone blockers, loop diuretics, clonidine, minoxidil. ISH, isolated systolic hypertension; HTN, hypertension; TIA, transient ischemic attack; CCB, calcium channel blocker; ARB, angiotensin receptor blocker.
[a]See text and Tables C119.1–3.
[b]ACE inhibitors have been inconsistent in the primary or secondary prevention of stroke.
[c]β-Blockers may be less effective in reducing BP in volume-expanded states but are useful in the setting of ischemic heart disease, which is common in chronic kidney disease.
[d]β-Blockers there are needed for IHD managements but can cause weight gain and deterioration of glycemic control.

appropriate drugs and combinations, and the exclusion of patients with organ damage or very high BP levels. Nevertheless, improved BP control is clearly possible.

Barriers to blood pressure control. In the general population, at least 30% are not controlled due to the presence of white coat hypertension, isolated systolic hypertension in elderly people, clinical inertia and skepticism, and patient nonadherence (see Chapter C124). The barriers to long-term successful management of hypertension are formidable and must be addressed to achieve long-term adherence.

Health records deficiencies. Very few practitioners have access to electronic systems that allow adequate tracking of disease indicators (e.g., weight, BP, blood sugar), which must also be correlated with changes in therapy (e.g., antihypertensive drugs) over time. Only when graphic presentations of short-term and long-term BP trends are readily available can the optimal approach be taken (see Chapter C127).

System problems. Physician and provider attitudes are major determinants of overall control rates (See Chapter C124) but even when the caregivers are committed to reaching goal BP, a wide variety of other barriers, (e.g., limited patient contact time; inadequate reimbursement for services; and complex, competing, ever-changing managed-care formularies) act to reduce control rates. In general, the provider should be familiar with the local barriers and should work to minimize them.

Patient issues. The commitment of the patient to continue therapy remains critical. Several strategies are somewhat effective to improve adherence: fewer doses, fewer pills, fewer side effects, and matching the time of dosing to activities of daily living (e.g., morning teeth brushing or morning coffee) do work. Patients are more likely to take medication consistently if the dosage schedule is simple (once or, at most, twice per day). Fixed-dose combination drugs are also well received by patients.

Cost. Although the price of drugs would appear to be a major problem for adherence, most studies have shown that cost is usually not the rate-limiting problem. If, however, the patient cannot afford to buy the drug, then price becomes the most important factor. The clinician should not hesitate to ask about insurance status, the patient's drug plan, and whether he or she will be able to pay for the pills.

Suggested Readings

Chobanian AV, Bakris GL, Black HR, et al. Joint National Committee on Prevention DE, Treatment of High Blood Pressure. National Heart L, Blood I, National High Blood Pressure Education Program Coordinating C. Seventh report of the Joint National Committee on Prevention, Detection, Evaluation, and Treatment of High Blood Pressure. *Hypertension* 2003;42:1206–1252.

Cushman WC, Ford CE, Cutler JA, et al. Success and predictors of blood pressure control in diverse North American settings: the antihypertensive and lipid-lowering treatment to prevent heart attack trial (ALLHAT). *J Clin Hypertens* 2002;4:393–404.

Lewington S, Clarke R, Qizilbash N, et al. Age-specific relevance of usual blood pressure to vascular mortality: a meta-analysis of individual data for one million adults in 61 prospective studies. *Lancet* 2002;360:1903–1913.

Rosendorff C, Black HR, Cannon CP, et al. American Heart Association Council for High Blood Pressure R, American Heart Association Council on Clinical C, American Heart Association Council on E, Prevention. Treatment of hypertension in the prevention and management of ischemic heart disease: a scientific statement from the American Heart Association Council for High Blood Pressure Research and the Councils on Clinical Cardiology and Epidemiology and Prevention. *Circulation* 2007;115:2761–2788.

Singer GM, Izhar M, Black HR. Goal-oriented hypertension management: translating clinical trials to practice. *Hypertension* 2002;40:464–469.

Vasan RS, Larson MG, Leip EP, et al. Impact of high-normal blood pressure on the risk of cardiovascular disease. *N Engl J Med* 2001;345:1291–1297.

CHAPTER C120 ■ LIFESTYLE MODIFICATIONS

THEODORE A. KOTCHEN, MD AND JANE MORLEY KOTCHEN, MD, MPH

KEY POINTS

■ Cardiovascular disease (CVD) risk factors typically cluster within individuals; lifestyle modifications should address the overall risk of CVD.

■ Strategies to decrease CVD risk should include the following: prevention and treatment of obesity; appropriate amounts of aerobic physical activity; avoidance of diets high in sodium chloride, total fat, and/or cholesterol, meeting recommended dietary intakes for potassium, calcium, and magnesium, limiting alcohol consumption; and avoiding cigarette smoking.

■ Adoption of lifestyles targeted to reduce CVD risk has a favorable impact on CVD morbidity and mortality.

■ Successful strategies for implementing recommended lifestyle modifications remain a challenge.

See also Chapters B76, B90 to B96, **B98, C119,** C120, and C157

Risk factor clustering

Cardiovascular disease (CVD) risk factors tend to cluster within individuals. In the Framingham cohort at baseline, clustering of three or more risk factors occurred at twice the rate predicted by chance. Adolescents and adults with higher levels of blood pressure (BP) tend to have higher serum concentrations of total cholesterol, triglycerides, glucose, apolipoprotein B, and lower high-density lipoprotein (HDL) cholesterol values. Hypertensive individuals have an increased prevalence of dyslipidemia and glucose intolerance. Data from the National Health and Nutrition Examination Survey II (NHANES II) indicate that 40% of adults younger than 55 years with BPs >140/90 mm Hg have serum cholesterol concentrations >240 mg per dL, whereas cholesterol is elevated to this level in only 20% of normotensive age-matched control subjects. Likewise, of those individuals with blood cholesterol levels >240 mg per dL approximately 46% have BPs >140/90 mm Hg. This clustering of risk factors within individuals is in part heritable, and resistance to insulin-stimulated glucose uptake may be the common link between hypertension and dyslipidemia.

Epidemiologic observations, including data from the Framingham Study, clearly document the additive risk associated with an increasing number of risk factors. In hypertensive individuals, the metabolic syndrome (three or more of the following: hypertension, abdominal obesity, fasting blood glucose ≥110 mg/dL, fasting triglycerides ≥150 mg/dL, HDL cholesterol <50 mg/dL in women and <40 mg/dL in men) amplifies the cardiovascular risks associated with high BP. Hypertension and most of the other Framingham risk factors are strongly associated with obesity but in logistic regression models that predict CVD, obesity *per se* does not appear as a major, independent CVD risk factor.

Observations from autopsy studies document a strong relation between CVD risk factors and atherosclerosis in young people. The severity of asymptomatic coronary and aortic atherosclerosis is related to the number of premortem cardiovascular risk factors. Conversely, according to a recent report of cohort studies conducted in 366,599 young and middle-aged men and women, persons with a low CVD risk profile (serum cholesterol <200 mg/dL, BP <120/80 mm Hg, and no cigarette smoking) have a 72% to 85% lower mortality rate from CVD compared to those with one or more of these three risk factors. The recognition that CVD risk factors cluster within individuals dictates that any regimen for the prevention and treatment of hypertension should address overall CVD risk and not simply BP alone.

Impact of lifestyle interventions on blood pressure and other risk factors

BP is affected by body weight and diet composition. Table C120.1 lists specific dietary factors that may have an impact on both the prevalence of hypertension and level of BP.

Weight loss. Analysis of NHANES data suggests that the prevalence of hypertension in the United States is increasing,

---

TABLE C120.1

DIETARY FACTORS THAT MAY INFLUENCE BLOOD PRESSURE

Decrease blood pressure	Increase blood pressure
Potassium (2.7 g/d = 69 mEq/d)	Sodium chloride (8.3 g/d = 140 mEq/d)
Calcium (767 mg/d)	Alcohol (8.8 g/d)
Magnesium (283 mg/d)	Cholesterol (298 mg/d)
Protein (79 g/d)	Saturated fat (26.3 g/d)
	Carbohydrates (254 g/d)

Note: Numbers in parentheses refer to average daily consumption by U.S. adults, as determined from the Third National Health and Nutrition Examination Survey (NHANES III).

---

possibly as a consequence of the increasing prevalence of obesity and the aging of the population. Similarly, the prevalence of overweight and BP levels of children and adolescents have increased over the last decade. In short-term trials in both hypertensive and normotensive individuals, even modest weight loss (5%) can lead to a reduction in BP and an increase in insulin sensitivity. With a reduction in mean body weight of 9.2 kg, BP reductions of 6.3/3.1 mm Hg have been observed. Additional trials have documented that modest weight loss can prevent hypertension by approximately 20% among overweight, prehypertensive individuals and can facilitate medication step-down and drug withdrawal. Regular aerobic physical activity facilitates weight loss, decreases BP, and reduces the overall risk of CVD and all-cause mortality.

Alcohol. A meta-analysis of 15 randomized controlled trials reported that decreased consumption of alcohol in those with a moderate to large intake of alcohol similarly reduced BP by 3.3/2.0 mm Hg in hypertensive and nonhypertensive individuals.

Salt restriction. As reviewed in several meta-analyses, the lowering of BP by limiting sodium chloride (NaCl) intake to 75 to 125 mEq per day results in 4 to 6/2 to 4 mm Hg BP reductions in hypertensive individuals and lesser reductions in nonhypertensive individuals. Many of the trials included in these analyses were of short duration, and the full impact of NaCl reduction on BP may not have been realized, because this effect may increase over time if the dietary modification can be maintained. Moderate reduction of NaCl intake and weight loss, alone and in combination, have been shown to reduce BP and attenuate the development of hypertension in adults with prehypertension. In black hypertensive individuals, NaCl reduction from 170 to 85 mEq per day has been reported to reduce urine protein excretion as well as BP. In short-term trials, modest reduction in Na^+ intake (approximately 40%) also lowers BP in children and adolescents. The impact of reduction in NaCl intake on BP is enhanced when combined with increased dietary intakes of potassium (K^+) and calcium (Ca^{2+}), particularly in individuals consuming diets containing low amounts of these ions. Preliminary evidence suggests that variations of the angiotensinogen, α-adducin, and angiotensin-converting enzyme genes modify the BP responses to NaCl reduction and/or weight loss.

Dietary potassium. Results of two meta-analyses of clinical trials have shown that oral K^+ (60–120 mEq/day) lower both systolic and diastolic BP; the magnitude of the effect is greater in hypertensive individuals (4.4/2.5 mm Hg) than in nonhypertensive individuals (1.8/1.0 mm Hg) and increases with the duration of the trial. K^+ reduces BP to a greater extent in blacks than in whites. Ca^{2+} supplementation may result in a small but statistically significant reduction of systolic (1–2 mm Hg), but not diastolic BP. An increased Ca^{2+} intake has a greater impact on BP in individuals consuming Ca^{2+}-deficient diets but overall calcium supplementation has not reduced BP.

Dietary composition. Persons consuming vegetarian diets tend to have lower BPs than do nonvegetarians.

Dietary approaches to stop hypertension diet. The Dietary Approaches to Stop Hypertension (DASH) trial convincingly demonstrated that over an 8-week period, a diet high in fruits, vegetables, and low-fat dairy products lowered BP in individuals with BPs in the prehypertensive range or with the lower levels of stage 1 hypertension. Reduction of NaCl intake below 100 mEq per day augmented the effect of this diet on BP. Fruits and vegetables provide an enriched source of K^+, magnesium, fiber, and dairy products and are an important source of Ca^{2+}. Blacks are especially sensitive to the BP-lowering effects of a reduced NaCl intake, an increased K^+ intake, and the DASH diet. The DASH diet also lowers plasma concentration of homocysteine, another risk factor for coronary artery disease.

Multiple risk factor reduction. In a randomized, prospective clinical trial, the impact of a controlled meal plan that met the nutritional guidelines of the National Academy of Sciences was evaluated in men and women with essential hypertension, dyslipidemia, type 2 diabetes, or any combination of these diseases. Over a 10-week follow-up period, compared to participants consuming a self-selected diet, the intervention diet resulted in improvements in multiple risk factors, including hypertension, dyslipidemia, hyperinsulinemia, and excessive body weight.

Diabetes. The Diabetes Prevention Program Research Group conducted a large, randomized clinical trial involving U.S. adults who were at high risk for developing type 2 diabetes. Nondiabetic individuals with elevated fasting and postload plasma glucose concentrations were randomized to placebo, metformin, or a lifestyle modification program with the goals of at least a 7% reduction in body weight and 150 minutes of physical activity per week. Over an average follow-up of 2.8 years, the lifestyle intervention reduced the incidence of diabetes by 58%; metformin reduced diabetes incidence by only 31%. Similar beneficial results of diet and exercise on diabetes prevention have also been observed in other populations.

Impact of lifestyle interventions on overt cardiovascular disease

Observational evidence has consistently demonstrated a lower incidence of coronary heart disease (CHD) among groups with the highest intake of fruits, vegetables, and grains. An increased intake of fish oil may also reduce the risk of CHD and stroke.

Several prospective studies confirm these observations. In a cohort of 44,875 men aged between 40 and 75 years, a diet high in vegetables, fruit, legumes, whole grains, fish, and poultry and low in red meat, processed meat, high-fat dairy products, and refined grains reduced the risk of CHD over 8 years (relative risk, 0.70; $p < .0009$). Similarly, in a cohort of 42,254 women with a median follow-up or 5.6 years, participants reporting dietary patterns that included fruits, vegetables, whole grains, low-fat dairy products, and lean meats had a lower risk of all-cause mortality (relative risk, 0.69; $p < .001$), as well as a lower risk of mortality from cancer, CHD, and stroke.

Results of the Nurses' Health Study further document the beneficial impact of healthy lifestyles, including diet, on prevention of CHD. In that study, 84,129 middle-aged women were followed up over 14 years. The incidence of coronary events among those women who did not smoke, were not overweight, maintained a "healthful diet," exercised moderately to vigorously for half an hour a day, and consumed alcohol moderately was 80% lower than in the remainder of the population. Subjects were considered to consume a healthful diet if they scored in the highest 40% of the cohort on a composite measure based on a diet low in trans fat and glycemic load; high in cereal fiber, marine Omega-3 fatty acids, and folate; and with a high ratio of polyunsaturated to saturated fats.

Several prospective observational studies, including the Nurses' Health Study, have reported that low daily intakes of calcium, K^+, and magnesium are each associated with an increased risk of ischemic stroke in both men and women; diets rich in K^+, magnesium, and cereal fiber are associated with a reduced stroke risk.

Lifestyle recommendations for blood pressure control and cardiovascular health

Implementation of lifestyles that most favorably impact BP has implications for the prevention and treatment of hypertension and for population-based strategies to shift the overall distribution of risk downward. Even if lifestyle modification does not produce a sufficient reduction of BP to avoid drug therapy, the number of medications or dosages required for BP control may be reduced.

Obesity and physical activity. Physical activity or planned exercise should be an important component of any weight loss plan to prevent hypertension or reduce BP. It is likely that CVD mortality can best be reduced by motivating the large sedentary segment of the U.S. population to perform some level of physical activity on at least a weekly basis. Further reductions in mortality may be achieved by encouraging people who are occasionally physically active to become active on a more regular basis. Sedentary individuals with normal BP have a 20% to 30% increased risk of developing hypertension compared with their more active peers.

For most people, BP can be lowered with 30 minutes of moderately intense physical activity, such as a brisk walking, 6 to 7 days a week. In instances when less time is available, less frequent, more intense workouts are needed, such as running for 20 to 30 minutes 3 to 4 days a week. In either instance, if an exercise program is sufficiently well maintained, the long-term impact on BP can be substantial.

Salt intake. Any population-based guideline for an upper limit of dietary salt intake is arbitrary. Recommendations for reduction in salt intake should be both safe and palatable. For the general population, the American Heart Association recommends that the average daily consumption of salt in adults not exceed 6 g (approximately 1 tsp table salt). There is no evidence that lowering salt consumption to this level poses any health risk, and this recommendation is consistent with guidelines of a number of other agencies both in the United States and abroad. Lower salt intakes may be recommended for hypertensive individuals.

Potassium and other minerals. Adequate amounts of Ca^{2+}, K^+, and magnesium should be included within the overall diet. Except in patients who take a diuretic and may require a K^+ supplement, K^+ rich foods rather than supplements are the preferred source of K^+, for example, fruits and vegetables. Although Ca^{2+} supplementation is not recommended as a means of controlling BP, Ca^{2+} intake should be optimized to help prevent osteoporosis.

Alcohol. In aggregate, available evidence supports moderation of alcohol intake (among those who drink) as an effective approach to lower BP.

Stress. Emotional stress can raise BP acutely. Chronic exposure to environmental and occupational stress may also be associated with higher levels of BP. It has been suggested that psychosocial stress contributes to the increased prevalence of hypertension among inner-city blacks. However, controlled trials of relaxation therapies have not documented a consistent effect on BP. Currently, there is no compelling rationale for the use of relaxation therapies for the prevention or treatment of hypertension.

Dietary guidelines. Recommendations in the Seventh Report of the Joint National Committee on Prevention, Detection, Evaluation, and Treatment of High Blood Pressure (JNC 7) for

TABLE C120.2

LIFESTYLE MODIFICATIONS TO PREVENT AND MANAGE HYPERTENSION[a]

Modification	Recommendation	Approximate SBP reduction (range)
Weight reduction	Maintain normal body weight (body mass index 18.5–24.9 kg/m^2)	5–20 mm Hg/10 kg weight loss
Adopt DASH eating plan	Consume a diet rich in fruits, vegetables, and low-fat dairy products with a reduced content of saturated and total fat	8–14 mm Hg
Dietary sodium restriction	Reduce dietary sodium intake to no more than 100 mmol/d (2.4 g sodium or 6 g sodium chloride)	2–8 mm Hg
Physical activity	Engage in regular aerobic physical activity such as brisk walking (at least 30 min/d, most days of the week)	4–9 mm Hg
Moderation of alcohol consumption	Limit consumption to no more than two drinks (1 oz or 30 mL ethanol; e.g., 24 oz beer, 10 oz wine, or 2 oz 80-proof whiskey) per d in most men and to no more than one drink per d in women and lighter-weight persons	2–4 mm Hg

DASH, Dietary Approaches to Stop Hypertension.
[a]From U.S. Department of Health and Human Services. The Seventh Report of the Joint National Committee on Prevention, Detection, Evaluation, and Treatment of High Blood Pressure. NIH publication No. 03-5233, 2003.

lifestyle modifications to manage hypertension are presented in **Table C120.2.** These recommendations do not differ appreciably from the guidelines of the American Heart Association for the general population. More stringent guidelines may be recommended for high-risk individuals.

Antioxidants. Clinical trials have not identified any cardiovascular benefits of antioxidant administration and current guidelines do not recommend additional antioxidant or plant sterol supplementation beyond that in the diet for either the primary or secondary prevention of CVD. Fruits, vegetables, and whole grains are ordinarily rich in antioxidants, plant sterols, and fiber.

Prevention and implementation strategies

Potential risk factors for CVD can be identified in children and adolescents, for example, family history of CVD, obesity, and relatively high BP. For the primary prevention of CVD, it is important that healthy lifestyles be established at a young age. Recommendations should be comprehensive and address physical activity, nutrition, and smoking. Effective strategies will require a multifaceted approach for dealing with the population as a whole, targeted subgroups, and individuals with CVD risk factors and/or clinically evident CVD. Recommendations must also be practical if they are to be achieved, and dietary guidelines should be presented to the public in terms of overall diet and food choices. To facilitate change, different and culturally sensitive approaches may be targeted to special populations, such as children, the elderly, and minorities. Preliminary steps to the successful adoption of dietary change include assessment of the individual's readiness to make dietary change, current eating patterns and dietary intake, and the extent of family or social support. Development of strategies that are based on an understanding of the process of behavioral change may further assist in motivating people to make enduring lifestyle changes. It is also incumbent on the food industry to participate in this process by providing greater numbers of healthy food choices and by systematically reducing the NaCl content of processed foods. In the future, genetic studies may identify those individuals who are most likely to benefit from a specific lifestyle intervention.

Suggested Readings

American Heart Association. AHA Dietary Guidelines. Revision 2000: a statement for healthcare professionals from the Nutrition Committee of the American Heart Association. *Circulation* 2000;102:2284–2299.

Appel LJ, Brands MW, Daniels SR, et al. Dietary approaches to prevent and treat hypertension: a scientific statement from the American Heart Association. *Hypertension* 2006;47:296–398.

Appel LJ, Moore TJ, Obarzanek E, et al. A clinical trial of the effects of dietary patterns on blood pressure. *N Engl J Med* 1997;336:1117–1124.

Chobanian AV, Bakris GL, Black HR, et al. The seventh report of the Joint National Committee on Prevention, Detection, Evaluation, and Treatment of High Blood Pressure (JNC VII). *JAMA* 2003;289:2560–2572.

Diabetes Prevention Program Research Group. Reduction in the incidence of type 2 diabetes with lifestyle intervention or metformin. *N Engl J Med* 2002;346:393–403.

He FJ, MacGregor GA. Importance of salt in determining blood pressure in children: meta-analysis of controlled trials. *Hypertension* 2006;48:861–869.

Hu FB, Rimm EB, Stampfer MJ, et al. Prospective study of major dietary patterns and risk of coronary heart disease in men. *Am J Clin Nutr* 2000;72:912–921.

Kand TK, Schatzkin AM, Graubard BI, et al. A prospective study of diet quality and mortality in women. *JAMA* 2000;283:2109–2115.

Sacks FM, Svetkey LP, Vollmer WM, et al. Effects on blood pressure of reduced dietary sodium and the dietary approaches to stop hypertension (DASH) diet. *N Engl J Med* 2001;344:3–10.

Stampfer MJ, Hu FB, Manson JE, et al. Primary prevention of coronary heart disease in women through diet and lifestyle. *N Engl J Med* 2000;343:16–22.

Whelton PK, He J, Appel LJ, et al. Primary prevention of hypertension: clinical and public health advisory from the National High Blood Pressure Education Program. *JAMA* 2002;288:1882–1888.

CHAPTER C121 ■ EXERCISE THERAPY

DENISE G. SIMONS-MORTON, MD, PhD

KEY POINTS

- Moderate physical activity (150 minutes per week of brisk walking or similar activity, preferably 30 minutes a day on most days) is recommended for the vast majority of individuals with prehypertension and hypertension.
- Advice regarding increased physical activity should include a specific prescription of activity types and duration, behavioral counseling, and specific follow-up plans.
- Prior exercise stress testing is appropriate for individuals with one or more cardiovascular risk factors or with known cardiovascular symptoms or disease, and is suggested for persons with uncontrolled hypertension.

See also Chapters A41, **B91**, and **C163**

Physical activity is a key component of a healthy lifestyle. Low levels of physical activity contribute substantially to obesity, hypertension, dyslipidemia, diabetes, and premature cardiovascular disease (CVD). Increased physical activity, which is important for prevention and treatment of hypertension, is safe with appropriate screening and use of certain precautions.

Physical activity advice and counseling

Substantial scientific evidence supports prevention or treatment of hypertension with exercise. Aerobic activity (e.g., brisk walking, cycling, swimming) is recommended on a regular basis, preferably 5 or more days per week, for 30 minutes each day at moderate-intensity levels.

Physician endorsement. Physician advice to increase physical activity can be a strong motivator to patients; advice conveyed as a written prescription may enhance success. Behavioral research has found that provision of information alone is insufficient to achieve behavior change. Therefore, physician advice and prescription should be accompanied by education about general and specific aspects of recommended physical activity regimens as well as counseling.

Behavioral counseling and reinforcement. Physician advice followed by behavioral counseling provided by other members of the health care team is a reasonable and promising approach. Multiple contacts are needed to provide the necessary counseling for successful behavioral change. In conjunction with the team, patients should select an enjoyable activity, identify barriers and problem-solving tools to overcome them, set realistic goals, and ensure social support. Clinician feedback and positive reinforcement is also important. The ultimate goal is regular physical activity as a permanent lifestyle behavior; 30 minutes daily

of moderate-intensity activity should be considered a long-term (not a short-term) goal. Relapses to sedentary patterns should be considered temporary setbacks, not failures. Achievements should be reinforced, and short-term goals should be selected that are realistic. Follow-up visits should incorporate attention to physical activity, by the physician or by other medical staff, because behavioral intervention studies show that after follow-up intervention ceases, health behaviors begin to regress.

Activity intensity and monitoring. Intensity of activity can be determined in a variety of ways.

Heart rate. A traditional method is self-monitoring heart rate during exercise. Patients can be taught how to take a pulse (radial or carotid) or how to use a heart rate monitor. To identify the heart rate range corresponding to moderate-intensity aerobic activity (50%–69% of maximum heart rate), one can roughly estimate maximum heart rate by subtracting age from 220 and then multiplying by 50% and by 70%, respectively, to obtain the lower and upper values for the range. Therefore, for a 50-year old person, the target heart rate range for moderate-intensity exercise is from 85 to 120 beats per minute (bpm), calculated as follows:

$$\text{Lower limit: } (220 - 50) \times 0.50 = 85 \text{ bpm}$$
$$\text{Upper limit: } (220 - 50) \times 0.70 = 120 \text{ bpm}$$

An exercise heart rate anywhere within the heart rate range during activity is acceptable for achieving health benefits and improving fitness, but more intensive activity increases cardiorespiratory fitness to a greater degree. Individuals who are not used to physical activity should start at the lower end of the range, which will be more comfortable and safer. With increasing experience and fitness, heart rate values higher in the range can be targeted.

Perceived exertion scales. An alternative to heart rate monitoring is to achieve a relative perceived exertion of "moderate" or "equivalent to brisk walking." Perceived exertion or heart rate monitoring is preferred to providing an absolute pace in an exercise prescription, such as walking 4 miles per hour, because an individual's age and physical condition affect the actual and perceived intensity of the activity. The phrase *"brisk walking" or "walking as if you're in a hurry"* should adequately convey the picture of a moderate-intensity exercise to most patients. When an individual "breaks a sweat," it is likely that he/she has achieved at least a moderate-intensity activity.

Screening before exercise

Safety issues. Although some people with hypertension have greater blood pressure (BP) increases during exercise than people without hypertension, there is evidence that the benefits of exercise outweigh the transient risks. For safety and behavioral reasons, sedentary patients should start out slowly at a lower intensity and shorter duration of exercise than the ultimate goal. They could, for example, start with 10-minute walks 2 times a week and gradually increase over several weeks or months to 30 minutes of moderate-intensity activity 5 to 7 days a week.

Exercise-tolerance testing. People with CVD symptoms or known CVD need a medical history and examination and, if not contraindicated, an exercise test no matter what intensity of activity they wish to engage in; such patients may need to initiate exercise under medical supervision (**Table C121.1**). An exercise test, in addition to being diagnostic for ischemia and arrhythmias, can determine what intensity of exercise is safe (an intensity below which ischemia occurs) and whether exercise under supervision is necessary (if ischemia is seen, supervised exercise is recommended as well as appropriate treatment).

People with uncomplicated hypertension who are asymptomatic and wish to engage in moderate-intensity activity need no medical screening beyond routine evaluation. However, persons with BP ≥180/90 mm Hg may benefit from exercise tolerance testing (ETT) before starting an exercise program to assure BP does not rise to acutely dangerous levels during exercise as well as to evaluate propensity for ischemia and arrhythmias. For people with one or more CVD risk factor (hypertension, smoking, dyslipidemia, age older than 60 years, family history of early

heart disease) but no symptoms, screening may be appropriate before the individual undertakes a vigorous exercise program. An exercise test-derived maximum heart rate is useful in developing an individualized exercise prescription.

Contraindications to exercise. Absolute contraindications include acute ischemia, arrhythmias, and acute infections if marked by fever. Relative contraindications include valvular heart disease, advanced stages of heart failure (HF), ventricular aneurysm, certain electrolyte abnormalities (e.g., significant hypokalemia or hypocalcemia), some anemias, and certain chronic infectious diseases. Conditions such as diabetes, HF, and angina should be adequately controlled before beginning a vigorous exercise program.

Exercise and antihypertensive medications

Use of antihypertensive medication is not a contraindication to exercise participation, which should be encouraged in most patients with prehypertension or hypertension, whether taking antihypertensive drugs or not.

Enhancement of blood pressure lowering. Because of the BP-lowering effects of chronic aerobic exercise, individuals on antihypertensive medication who engage in a physical activity regimen may be able to achieve BP control on a lower level of medication, or possibly without medication, as long as the physical activity is continued regularly. In particular, exercise in conjunction with weight loss regimens is a particularly attractive adjunct to angiotensin-converting enzyme (ACE) inhibitor or angiotensin receptor blocker (ARB) therapy, which in turn do not intrinsically diminish exercise tolerance.

Other recommendations. Because β-blockers blunt the heart rate response to exercise, a perceived exertion of "moderate to very hard" or "equivalent to brisk walking" is a preferable recommendation to a target heart rate range. Persons on diuretics who exercise should pay particular attention to adequate hydration, particularly if they are also receiving ACE inhibitor or ARB therapy or if they exercise in hot climates and during the summer. Persons on antihypertensive agents should have extended cool-down periods at the end of an exercise session to reduce the likelihood of hypotensive episodes after abrupt cessation of activity.

TABLE C121.1

RECOMMENDATIONS FOR EXERCISE TESTING BEFORE EXERCISE PARTICIPATION

| Exercise intensity | No TOD or CVD, no risk factors, no symptoms, BP ≤180/110 mm Hg | No known TOD or CVD; 1 or more CVD risk factor | | Known TOD or CVD |
		No symptoms; BP ≤180/110 mm Hg	Symptoms or BP ≥180/110 mm Hg	
Moderate	Not necessary	Not necessary	Recommended	Recommended
Vigorous	Not necessary	May be beneficial	Recommended	Recommended

Target organ damage (TOD) and cardiovascular disease (CVD) include ischemic heart disease, heart failure, stroke, renal disease, neuropathy, or retinopathy; also includes diabetes as a "CVD equivalent".
CVD risk factors include hypertension, smoking, dyslipidemia, age older than 60 years, male gender or postmenopausal woman, family history of cardiovascular disease (in women <65 years or in men <55 years).
BP, blood pressure; TOD, target organ damage; CVD, cardiovascular disease.
(Adapted from American College of Sports Medicine. Position stand: exercise and hypertension. *Med Sci Sports Exerc* 2004;36(6):533–553.)

Suggested Readings

American College of Sports Medicine. Position stand: exercise and hypertension. *Med Sci Sports Exerc* 2004;36(6):533–553.

Fletcher GF, Blair SN, Blumenthal J, et al. Statement on exercise: benefits and recommendations for physical activity programs for all Americans: a statement for health professionals by the Committee on Exercise and Cardiac Rehabilitation of the Council on Clinical Cardiology, American Heart Association. *Circulation* 1992;86:340–344.

Marcus BH, Williams DM, Dubbert PM, et al. Physical activity intervention studies. What we know and what we need to know. A scientific statement from the American Heart Association Council on Nutrition, Physical Activity, and Metabolism (Subcommittee on Physical Activity); Council on Cardiovascular Disease in the Young, and the Interdisciplinary Working Group on quality of Care and Outcomes Research. *Circulation* 2006;114:2739–2752.

CHAPTER C122 ■ PATIENT EDUCATION

DANIEL W. JONES, MD

KEY POINTS

- Patient education requires large amounts of provider time but is an effective adjunct to hypertension management.
- Patient education is a continuous process involving a variety of health care workers.
- Resources for patient education are abundantly available, but quality varies.

See also Chapters C119, C123, and C124

Most experts and most clinicians consider patient education an integral part of hypertension patient management, but educational efforts are typically inconsistent.

Challenges to effective education

Hypertension is not obviously symptomatic and is often long lived in duration. Its treatment requires daily attention to lifestyle factors and medication for most patients. Patient education is a key element in promoting patient compliance. However, no other area of hypertension management is as challenging. Patient education requires large amounts of provider time and unfortunately is not reimbursable in most health systems. Some clinicians are unaware of the evidence for effectiveness of patient education in improving outcomes.

Benefits of education

A number of well-conducted studies clearly document the benefit of hypertension-related education. Morisky et al. evaluated three educational interventions: exit interviews, home visits, and group classes. After 5 years of follow-up, the intervention group had significantly better blood pressure control (79% controlled vs. 50% for a comparison group). Inconsistency is another problem. Because few studies have been done to guide the approach to patient education in hypertension, methods are often haphazard. Key patient education strategies have been previously outlined by Hill (**Table C122.1**).

Components of successful programs

The best providers plan for patient education just as they plan for any other component of disease-state management. Involvement of all members of the health care team improves effectiveness. In many settings, nurses and pharmacists provide much of the patient education; however, physician involvement is a necessary component. The simple mention of a concept by a physician (such as the need to lose weight) may improve the chances that educational efforts by other members of the team will be taken more seriously.

Educational materials. A crucial element in the success of any patient educational effort is the commitment of the provider to the educational process. It is impossible to draw the line between educating and motivating; good teachers are successful at both. Materials for use in patient education in blood pressure

---

TABLE C122.1

PATIENT EDUCATION STRATEGIES IN HYPERTENSION

Identify knowledge, attitudes, beliefs, and experience
Educate about condition and treatment
Tailor the regimen to the patient
Provide reinforcement
Promote social support
Collaborate with other professionals

TABLE C122.2

USEFUL WEB SITES FOR HYPERTENSION PATIENT EDUCATION

National High Blood Pressure Education Program (NHBPEP)
   http://www.nhlbi.nih.gov/about/nhbpep/index.htm
NHBPEP patient information
   http://www.nhlbi.nih.gov/health/publicheart/index.htm#hbp
NHBPEP your guide to lowering high blood pressure
   http://www.nhlbi.nih.gov/hbp/index.html
Dietary Approaches to Stop Hypertension (DASH) diet
   http://www.nhlbi.nih.gov/health/public/heart/hbp/dash/
      index.htm
American Heart Association
   http://www.americanheart.org
American Heart Association high blood pressure
   http://www.americanheart.org/presenter.jhtml?identifier=2114

avoiding the use of materials with poor objectivity. Two good sources of objective materials are the American Heart Association and the National High Blood Pressure Education Program of the National Heart, Lung, and Blood Institute. **Table C122.2** provides a list of web sites with patient information from each of these organizations. Printed materials in multiple languages aimed at various target groups are available, as well as materials in other educational formats, including video.

Suggested Readings

Green LW. Educational strategies to improve compliance with therapeutic and preventative regimens: the recent evidence. In: Haynes RB, Taylor DW, Sackett DL, eds. *Compliance in healthcare*. Baltimore: The Johns Hopkins University Press, 1979:157–173.

Grueninger UJ, Goldstein MG, Duffy PD. Patient education in hypertension: five essential steps. *J Hypertens* 1989;7:S93–S98.

Hill MN. Strategies for patient education. *Clin Exp Hypertens A* 1989;11:1187–1201.

Jones D, Basile J, Cushman W, et al. Managing hypertension in the south-eastern United States: applying the guidelines from the Sixth Report of the Joint National Committee on Prevention, Detection, Evaluation, and Treatment of High Blood Pressure. *Am J Med Sci* 1999;318:357–364.

Morisky DE, Levine DM, Green LW, et al. Five-year blood pressure control and mortality following health education for hypertension patients. *Am J Public Health* 1983;73:153 161.

management are plentiful. There are, however, several challenges to consider. Hypertension disproportionately affects the poor and the uneducated. Attention to use of materials suitable for a patient's learning level is crucial. Another major challenge is

---

CHAPTER C123 ■ ADHERENCE TO ANTIHYPERTENSIVE THERAPY

CHERYL R. DENNISON, ANP, PhD AND NANCY HOUSTON MILLER, RN

KEY POINTS

- Adherence (sometimes called concordance or compliance) is not an end in itself, but a means to improved care and outcomes.
- The extent to which patients are able to adhere to treatment recommendations is a major issue in blood pressure (BP) control and depends on many factors.
- Full benefits of antihypertensive therapy cannot be realized at current levels of adherence for most patients.
- Patients, providers, and health care organizations taking action can prevent, monitor, and address adherence problems by using effective strategies.

See also Chapters C106, **C119,** C122, C124, and C126

Despite available, effective treatment strategies, a large number of patients have uncontrolled blood pressure (BP) due to therapeutic nonadherence (not carrying out recommended medical or health advice), including failure to "persist" on medications. Typical adherence rates vary substantially in different populations and are much lower for lifestyle interventions and more for behaviorally demanding regimens. Nonadherence is an important, costly, and pervasive problem that contributes to relatively low rates of hypertension control worldwide, with unnecessarily high rates of complications such as stroke, coronary heart disease, heart failure, and end-stage renal disease. Nonadherence should be considered and monitored in patients who fail to reach goal BP, have "resistant" hypertension, or experience sudden loss of BP control.

Definition

Adherence is the extent to which the patient's behavior (in terms of taking medication, following a diet, modifying habits, or attending clinics) coincides with medical or health advice. Concordance and compliance are commonly used synonyms for adherence; some prefer "adherence" or "concordance" because they are nonjudgmental and reflective of a collaborative relationship, whereas "compliance" connotes a paternalistic provider–patient relationship.

More precise definitions vary according to the specificity of the recommended therapeutic behavior and the ability to measure the recommended behavior. For example, taking medication correctly at least 80% of the time is the most common practical definition of medication adherence. Not getting a prescription filled or refilled, taking the incorrect dose including taking too much medicine, taking a dose at the wrong time, forgetting to take a dose, or stopping a medication without the recommendation to do so, are other forms of nonadherence. Underdosing in different patterns, particularly 2- to 3-day drug holidays or omissions, is the most common form of medication nonadherence. In addition, missed appointments, continuation of unhealthy habits such as smoking tobacco, sedentary lifestyle, or a diet high in calories, fat, and sodium (Na^+) are prevalent, important forms of nonadherence to other aspects of the treatment regimen.

Measurement

A key challenge in managing nonadherence is the lack of accurate, practical, and affordable adherence measures in clinical practice. Methods to measure adherence to antihypertensive treatment are listed in **Table C123.1**.

Objective measures. Direct measures such as observation of drug levels in body fluids (e.g., blood, saliva, urine) are often impractical or unavailable and can be misleading. Indirect measures of adherence include prescription refills, electronic event monitoring, pill counts, clinical outcomes, self-report, and collateral report. Pharmacy records can be helpful in a health care system that includes integrated shared information. Evaluation of objective changes in BP, heart rate, or body weight may indicate adherence with recommendations; for example, a decrease in heart rate may indicate adherence with β-blocker therapy or increased physical activity. Lack of response to increments in treatment intensity and patients who fail to attend appointments are practical measures to assess adherence. Visit nonadherence and medication nonadherence often go together.

Self-reporting. Patient self-report of adherence is usually substantially overestimated because of the difficulty in recalling

---

TABLE C123.1

MEASURES OF ADHERENCE TO ANTIHYPERTENSIVE TREATMENT RECOMMENDATIONS

Self-report
  Use a nonthreatening approach: "Many people have difficulty taking all of their medications as prescribed. Have you missed any pills in the past week?" or "How many pills have you missed in the past week?"

Treatment response

Attendance at appointments

Hill-Bone High BP Compliance Scale[a]

How often do you	Response
1. Forget to take your HBP medicine?	1. All of the time
2. Decide NOT to take your HBP medicine?	2. Most of the time
3. Eat salty food?	3. Some of the time
4. Shake salt on your food before you eat it?	4. None of the time
5. Eat fast food?	
6. Make the next appointment before you leave the doctor's office?[b]	
7. Miss scheduled appointments?	
8. Forget to get prescriptions filled?	
9. Run out of HBP pills?	
10. Skip your HBP medicine before you go to the doctor?	
11. Miss taking your HBP pills when you feel better?	
12. Miss taking your HBP pills when you feel sick?	
13. Take someone else's HBP pills?	
14. Miss taking your HBP pills when you are careless?	

Pharmacy refills

Drug levels

Medication event monitors

HBP, high blood pressure.
[a]Scale and subscale scores are calculated by summing individual items.
Reducing sodium intake subscale: Items 3,4,5. Appointment keeping subscale: Items 6,7.
Medication taking subscale: Items 1,2, 8,9,10,11,12,13,14.
[b] Reverse code.

details of medication taking or attempting to please health care providers or avoid confrontation. Despite these problems, self-report remains an important aspect of adherence monitoring. The Hill-Bone High BP Compliance Scale is a brief tool to identify patients with various levels of adherence to medication taking, low Na^+ diet, and appointment keeping who would benefit from strategies to enhance adherence. This 14-item questionnaire can readily be completed by staff or patients while waiting to see a health care provider and has been shown to be predictive of BP control. In addition, the following simple validated question has been shown to predict 50% of those with low adherence to medications with a specificity of 87%: "Have you missed any pills in the past week?" Given the limitations with the existing methods of measuring adherence, the use of multiple methods is advised.

Factors associated with adherence

Although it is important for the patient to know the consequences of untreated hypertension and the benefits of therapy, such knowledge is not sufficient to assure adherence. Social, cultural, economic, and health care resource and access factors also influence adherence to the prescribed treatment regimen.

Positive factors. Seeing a health care provider regularly, having other health conditions, fear of complications of hypertension, a desire to control BP, and being on a medication regimen of lower complexity and cost are factors associated with higher rates of adherence. In addition, the frequency of BP monitoring at home and in the office is strongly associated with improved medication taking behavior and better BP control. Social support from family members and friends, employment, and health insurance also have been shown to be determinants of adherence and BP control.

Negative factors. The reasons for nonadherence are numerous. Problems with adherence are seen in patients of all ages, diseases, and severity of illness. Generally, adherence decreases over time particularly with long-term treatments. Level of education, knowledge about hypertension, socioeconomic status, and gender do not predict nonadherence. Nonhealthy behaviors, such as smoking, excessive alcohol intake, and sedentary lifestyle, are predictive of nonadherence. Moreover, nonadherence varies within and between recommended behaviors to control BP. Patients' actual and perceived barriers to BP control influence adherence behaviors.

Health care providers need to consider patients' beliefs, attitudes, perceptions, and prior experiences as well as their goals, values, and motivation. It is important to assess the reasons why patients do not follow advice. Factors in the social environment often create other priorities in daily life. Additional frequently cited reasons for not filling prescriptions or not taking medication as prescribed include a patient's belief that because their BP is now controlled, their hypertension is "cured", concern about side effects, not believing medication is beneficial, and cost.

Effective strategies to improve adherence

Successful BP control requires the initiation of appropriate therapies, achievement of the goal BP, and persistence of effective therapies over time. From a behavioral perspective, to achieve long-term BP control, patients must enter into and remain in care, make and maintain lifestyle changes, and for most, take medication as prescribed. Achieving and maintaining goal BP levels over time also requires continuous educational and behavioral strategies so that patients have the knowledge, skills, motivation, and resources to carry out treatment recommendations with minimal relapses. Successful adherence requires that patients know what steps to take and develop skills in problem identification and problem solving to address barriers as well as developing cues for memory enhancement. Strategies to help patients develop these skills needed to be adapted so that they are culturally salient and feasible for staff to implement.

Systematic studies. A recent review was conducted to determine the effectiveness of interventions to increase adherence to BP lowering medication in adults with essential hypertension in primary care with adherence to medication and BP control as outcomes but the number of randomized clinical trials (RCTs) in this area is limited. Simplifying dose regimens increased adherence in seven of nine studies, with a relative increase in adherence of 8% to 20%. Motivational strategies (including telephone-linked computer counseling, reminders, daily drug reminder charts, family member support, electronic medication aid cap, mail reminders and special unit-dose packaging) were successful in only 10 of 24 studies, with small increases in adherence (up to a maximum of 23%). Complex interventions (including worksite care through nurses; home visits, education, and special dosing devices, educational leaflets and newsletters, telephone and mailed reminders) involving more than one technique increased adherence in 8 of 18 studies (from 5% to 41%). Patient education alone seemed largely unsuccessful. Although more evidence is needed on the effect of various strategies through carefully designed RCTs, it is clear that the most effective approaches to improving medication adherence have been multifaceted, that is, targeting more than one factor with more than one intervention.

Multidisciplinary approach. A multidisciplinary team approach to hypertension care and control permits flexibility in matching patients' needs with the competencies of staff with different, yet complementary, skills and interests (see Chapter C126). Nonphysician health professionals, particularly nurses, pharmacists, and health educators have provided effective, safe, and well-received interventions that improve adherence and BP control. Nurse-supervised outreach workers, nurse case managers, and nurse practitioners, in collaboration with physicians and other health professionals have effectively improved outcomes. Studies within integrated health systems have demonstrated that when pharmacists, utilizing strategies to solve medication-related problems, are included as members of health care teams, BP control rates are increased and drug interactions, nonadherence, and costs reduced. Effective approaches designed to meet patient, provider, and organizational needs and minimize barriers to BP control have been delivered in nurse-managed clinics, work- and school-based programs, as well as pharmacy and community settings.

Health care provider actions to increase adherence

A combination of strategies is more likely to maximize long-term adherence by preventing, recognizing, and responding to adherence problems. There are evidence-based strategies for specific health care provider actions to improve adherence (**Table C123.2**).

Foster effective, communication with patients. In addition to patient education and skill building, effective communication and a trustful relationship between the patient and provider

HEALTH CARE PROVIDER ACTIONS TO INCREASE ADHERENCE WITH TREATMENT RECOMMENDATIONS

Foster effective communication with patients
- Provide clear, direct messages about importance of a behavior or therapy
- Provide verbal and written instruction, including rationale for treatments
- Develop skills in communication/counseling

Identify knowledge, attitudes, beliefs, and experiences
- Assess patient's understanding and acceptance of the diagnosis and expectations of being in care
- Discuss patient's concerns and clarify misunderstandings
- Elicit concerns and questions, provide opportunities for patient to state specific barriers to following advice

Educate patients about high blood pressure (BP) and treatment
- Inform patient of BP level
- Inform patient about recommended treatment and provide specific written information
- Emphasize need to continue treatment, that patient cannot tell if BP is elevated, and that BP control does not mean cure

Individualize the regimen
- Include patient in decision making
- Simplify regimen to once-daily dosing, if possible
- Incorporate treatment into patient's daily lifestyle
- Ask about behaviors to achieve BP control
- Agree with patient on realistic short-term goals for specific components of the medication and lifestyle modification plan
- Encourage discussion of diet and physical activity
- Encourage discussion of adverse drug effects and concerns
- Encourage self-monitoring with validated BP devices and diaries or logs for lifestyle behaviors
- Minimize cost of therapy; recognize financial issues and enlist local and national programs to assist in affording medications
- Indicate that adherence to the regimen will be a subject of discussion at the next visit
- Give positive feedback for behavioral and BP improvement
- Hold exit interviews to clarify regimen
- Schedule more frequent visits to counsel nonadherent patients
- Use telephone and mail contact to follow up patients who miss appointments
- Consider home visits
- Develop reminder systems to ensure identification and follow-up of nonadherent patients

Promote social support
- With patient permission, involve family or other social support in the treatment process
- Suggest common interest group activities (e.g., walking group) to enhance mutual support and motivation

Collaborate with other professionals
- Draw on complementary skills and knowledge of nurses, pharmacists, dietitians, optometrists, dentists, and physicians' assistants
- Refer patients for more intensive counseling

---

are of paramount importance in achieving sustained BP control. It is essential to provide clear, direct messages about the importance of adhering to the agreed-upon hypertension treatment plan. Because patients often receive multiple new messages during visits, it is important to provide verbal and written instructions so that the patient and family can review these separately from the encounter. Health professionals may need to further develop skills in effective communication and behavioral or motivational counseling to succeed in this area.

Identify knowledge, attitudes, beliefs, and experiences. Active participation by the patient as the decision maker and problem solver, with the health care provider functioning as advisor and guide, favors successful management of hypertension. This requires that patient's understanding and acceptance of the diagnosis and expectations of being in care are assessed, patient concerns addressed, and misunderstandings clarified.

Educate the patient about hypertension and treatment. Adequate knowledge of hypertension, consequences of

uncontrolled hypertension, and the treatment regimen is essential. In patient-centered care, patients are engaged in shared decision-making discussions to establish mutually agreed-upon BP goals. The patient always must be informed of BP values and pertinent test results and should "know their numbers." This provides an ideal opportunity to assess patient knowledge, educate, establish clear goals, and discuss progress toward goals. Patients must also be educated regarding the necessary self-monitoring skills (e.g., home BP monitoring).

Individualize the regimen. Successful education and counseling to promote adherence to the treatment regimen and BP control requires that health professionals individualize care to maximize the patient's motivation to remain in care, adhere to the lifestyle and medication regimens, and monitor progress toward goals. Efforts to individualize the regimen should focus on patient responses to the treatment regimen as well as self-care behaviors and skills necessary for hypertension control. The health care provider should work with the patient to mutually develop realistic, outcome-oriented goals and strategies for attaining the goals. Equally important, is frequent follow-up with the patient to assess progress toward goals and if necessary to revise strategies to improve the likelihood of attaining goals.

Simplifying the regimen with once (or at most twice) daily dosing significantly improves adherence. Incorporating the treatment regimen into the patient's daily lifestyle is required for long-term sustainability. The pairing of adherence behavior with daily habits (for example, linking pill-taking with events of daily living) avoids missed medication doses. Reminders by telephone, mail, or electronic aids enhance memory and appropriate behavior. Adherence packaging, such as blister packaging, help patients remember when to take their medication and notice if *they* have forgotten. One of the most successful strategies in many practices is the use of "pill boxes" with individual bins or multiple dose boxes for each day of the week.

Individualizing regimens also means helping individuals to modify lifestyle behaviors. This includes assessment of an individual's baseline behaviors, education about how to make the appropriate changes, counseling to develop strategies such as setting short-term goals and self-monitoring that will ensure the achievement and maintenance of the changes, constant follow-up with the patient to determine if adherence is a problem, working with patients to identify and resolve barriers to BP control, and reinforcement of progress toward the goal of change in behavior. A review of adherence in RCTs of cardiovascular disease prevention strategies identified the following successful approaches: signed agreements, behavioral skill training, self-monitoring, telephone/mail contact, spouse support, self-efficacy enhancement, contingency contracting, exercise prescriptions, external cognitive aids, persuasive communication, nurse-managed clinics, and work- or school-based programs.

Self-monitoring of BP at home or the worksite increases patient involvement and also provides much more frequent feedback on the basic relationship between adherence and BP levels than do physician office visits every 3 to 6 months. Self-monitoring of BP should be considered as a useful adherence-enhancing strategy especially when used in combination with other approaches such as patient reminders, counseling, and the use of nurse case managers.

Promote social support. With the patient's permission, the provider can educate family members or friends to participate in helping the patient with hypertension management. Family members can play a fundamental role providing daily reinforcement of the patient's efforts to achieve BP control. If the patient desires greater family participation, the patient should be encouraged to invite family members to attend and participate in clinic visits. In addition, some patients may benefit from small group activities, for example, clinic support groups or group visits, to enhance social support and motivation.

Collaborate with other professionals. Treatment should be planned in conjunction with the patient and other members of the multidisciplinary hypertension management team. The team may include health professionals from many disciplines and community health workers. Involving family, friends, community resources, and other health professionals can help patients to improve adherence and achieve and sustain BP control.

Multilevel approach to improve adherence

A multilevel approach is needed with patients, providers, and health care organizations taking action to increase adherence. The delivery of care needs to be organized to address potential and real problems with adherence at all levels simultaneously. It is important to work with individual patients to assure that they understand what is necessary to achieve treatment goals and that they participate in treatment decisions. Provider responsiveness to patient concerns as well as reinforcement and support are also necessary. Integrated systems approaches with continuous quality improvement enhance the training and practice of providers and patient outcomes.

Suggested Readings

Burke LE, Dunbar-Jacob JE, Hill MN. Compliance with cardiovascular disease prevention strategies: a review of the research. *Ann Behav Med* 1997;19:239–263.

Cappuccio FP, Kerry SM, Forbest L, et al. BP control by home monitoring: meta-analysis of randomised trial. *Br Med J* 2004;329:145.

Carter BL, Zillich AJ, Elliott WJ. How pharmacists can assist physicians with controlling BP. *J Clin Hypertens* 2003;5:31–37.

Haynes RB, Yao X, Degani A, et al. Interventions for enhancing medication adherence. *Cochrane Database Syst Rev* 2005;(4):CD000011.

Hill MN, Miller NM. Compliance enhancement: a call for multidisciplinary team approaches [Editorial]. *Circulation* 1996;93:4–6.

Kim MT, Hill MN, Bone LR, et al. Development and testing of the Hill-Bone compliance to high BP therapy scale. *Prog Cardiovasc Nurs* 2000;15:90–96.

Miller NM, Hill MN, Kotke T, et al. The multilevel compliance challenge: recommendations for a call to action. *Circulation* 1997;95:1085–1090.

Norby SM, Stroebel RJ, Canzanello VJ. Physician-nurse team approaches to improve BP control. *J Clin Hypertens* 2003;5:386–392.

Schroeder K, Fahey T, Ebrahim S. Interventions for improving adherence to treatment in patients with high BP in ambulatory settings. *Cochrane Database Syst Rev* 2004;(3):CD004804.

Svensson S, Kjellgren KI, Ahlner J, et al. Reasons for adherence with antihypertensive medication. *Int J Cardiol* 2000;76:157–163.

CHAPTER C124 ■ BARRIERS TO BLOOD PRESSURE CONTROL

DAVID J. HYMAN, MD AND VALORY N. PAVLIK, PhD

KEY POINTS

■ Most people with undiagnosed or uncontrolled hypertension see physicians regularly.
■ Most uncontrolled hypertension is caused by elevated systolic blood pressure (BP) but physicians have been unassertive in diagnosing and treating systolic hypertension, especially stage 1 (140–159 mm Hg).
■ Faulty BP measurement practices in physician offices contribute to poor hypertension control.
■ Lack of access to health care and patient nonadherence to treatment remain significant problems but do not totally account for the lack of BP control.

See also Chapters B96, B99, B102, **C123, C125, C126,** and **C127**

Hypertension control in the United States population

The Third National Health and Nutrition Examination Survey (NHANES III, 1988–1994) remains the most recent data analyzed for the role of health care utilization and blood pressure (BP) control. Hypertension control rates in the United States remain unacceptably low, with only approximately three-fourths of hypertensive individuals being aware of their condition, just over one-half of them are being treated, and slightly more than half of those treated are at BP goal, for a net control rate of 37%. Although this is a substantial improvement over the control rate in 1993 (27%), it is still far below our national goal of 50% by the Healthy People 2000 and 2010 initiatives (**Figure C124.1**).

Barriers to hypertension control can be classified into four groups: (1) unavailability of care, including lack of health insurance or the high cost of drugs, and systems issues; (2) physician-controlled decisions about the diagnosis and treatment of hypertension, or provider issues; (3) patient nonadherence to a prescribed drug regimen or follow-up schedule, or patient issues; and (4) societal impediments to a healthy lifestyle or behavioral issues.

Health care availability

NHANES III data show that most persons classified as having uncontrolled hypertension have health insurance and a usual source of medical care.
Care access. Persons who are "unaware" of having hypertension are of a mean age of 58 years; 90% of them have health insurance; approximately 80% have a usual source of health care; and 70% have seen a physician at least once within the last year,

with an average of more than three visits a year. More than 75% report having had a BP measurement within the last year. Persons who are aware of having hypertension but are untreated have demographic and health care access characteristics that are similar to those who are aware of their hypertension and are receiving

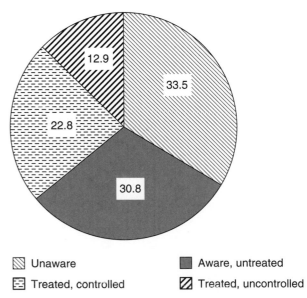

Figure C124.1 Hypertension control in the U.S. population (age adjusted), 2003–2004. (Reproduced with permission from Ong KL, Cheung BM, Man YB, et al. Prevalence, awareness, treatment, and control of hypertension among United States adults 1999–2004. *Hypertension* 2007;49(1):69–75.)

treatment. Persons being treated for hypertension, which is uncontrolled, are of average age of 65 years; approximately 95% have health insurance, a usual source of care, and have seen a physician at least once within the last year, with an average of six visits per year. The level of health care utilization among uncontrolled hypertensive individuals does not suggest that inaccessibility to health care services is the predominant reason for the lack of control.

Although it is important to recognize that lack of access to health care does not adequately explain the low levels of hypertension control in the United States, it is clear that hypertensive persons without health insurance or a source of primary care are at greater risk of having their BP being uncontrolled. Any change in the health care system that leaves more people uninsured or without a usual source of care would have an adverse impact on BP control levels. For example, Hispanic Americans with hypertension use health care the least and, therefore, have the lowest probability of being controlled. The fact that the vast majority of uncontrolled hypertensives who receive regular health care should not lessen the attention to other chronic health conditions that are present in the poorest and most vulnerable segments of the population.

Cost of care. Although the cost of drugs is a theoretical barrier to adequate hypertension control, diuretics, β-blockers, angiotensin-converting enzyme (ACE) inhibitors, and long-acting calcium channel blockers are now generic. Drugs in the first three classes can be obtained at a cost of $4 per month from at least one large national retailer. When drug costs do present a barrier to hypertension control for an individual, the cause is usually related to physician drug selection.

Physician-controlled barriers

Attitudes about systolic hypertension. Most (75%) of the undiagnosed, untreated, and treated but uncontrolled hypertension in the United States is systolic hypertension in persons whose diastolic BP is <90 mm Hg. **Table C124.1** reports the mean BP for different age groups and categories of hypertension control in the NHANES III survey sample. The average diastolic pressure exceeds 90 mm Hg only in the stratum of persons younger than 45 years (<20% of all hypertensive individuals).

In 2000, a clinical advisory was issued by the National High Blood Pressure Education Program recommending a "paradigm shift" in the criteria for diagnosis and treatment of hypertension. This paradigm shift related to systolic BP becoming the primary determinant of diagnosis and treatment decisions. This recommendation was restated in the JNC 7 report released in 2003. There is considerable evidence that uniform adoption of this recommendation would cause a major change in practice for United States physicians, and even more so for physicians in other countries. In a survey of self-reported physician behavior, many physicians admitted to not starting drug treatment for persistently elevated systolic BP if the diastolic BP was considered satisfactory. Moreover, many physicians acknowledged that they do not alter their therapeutic regimens in treated patients if systolic BP is elevated and the diastolic BP is at goal. Studies of physicians' actual practice have confirmed their self-reported behavior.

Physician inaction in the face of persistently elevated systolic BP has been documented through chart reviews in Veterans Affairs hospital clinics. In a large sample of practices in a major southwestern city, 25% of persons whose systolic BP was >140 mm Hg and whose diastolic BP <90 mm Hg were not even noted to be hypertensive. In treated hypertensive patients, diastolic BP persistently >90 mm Hg usually triggered intensification of treatment, whereas persistent systolic BP elevations did not. Oliveria et al. surveyed physicians about their reasoning during a specific patient encounter and reviewed the clinical records of that encounter. Physicians clearly did not act on persistently elevated systolic BPs and expressed explicit satisfaction with the less than optimal BP values achieved.

International studies of hypertension control also suggest that variation in individual physician treatment thresholds plays the dominant role in determining hypertension control rates. Despite the United States not having a national health insurance system, hypertension control in the country until recently was almost 70% better than in Canada, and approximately three to five times better than in England, Germany, Italy, Spain, or Sweden. It is unlikely that patient compliance or health care utilization explains these large differences.

The rate at which physicians adopt recommended changes in treatment practice is multifactorial and difficult to measure accurately. The concept of "clinical inertia" has been widely invoked to explain why physicians do not adopt certain

TABLE C124.1

BLOOD PRESSURE LEVELS IN UNCONTROLLED HYPERTENSIVES BY AGE[a]

Age-group	Hypertension present but subject unaware		Acknowledged, untreated hypertension		Treated, uncontrolled hypertension	
	Mean blood pressure (mm Hg)	SBP ≥140 mm Hg and DBP <90 mm Hg (%)	Mean blood pressure (mm Hg)	SBP ≥140 mm Hg and DBP <90 mm Hg (%)	Mean blood pressure (mm Hg)	SBP ≥140 mm Hg and DBP <90 mm Hg (%)
25–44 yr	138/91	51.9 ± 7.4	141/94	25.1 ± 7.9	147/95	29.1 ± 7.9
45–64 yr	148/86	69.4 ± 3.3	152/89	53.5 ± 4.8	150/87	66.1 ± 2.8
>65 yr	153/77	91.1 ± 1.1	160/81	81.5 ± 2.7	159/78	87.6 ± 1.3
All subjects	148/83	78.8 ± 2.0	151/88	59.1 ± 2.7	155/82	76.9 ± 1.5

DBP, diastolic blood pressure; SBP, systolic blood pressure.
[a]Plus-minus (±) values are mean ± standard error.
(From Hyman P. Characteristics of patients with uncontrolled hypertension in the United States. *N Engl J Med* 2001;345:479–486, with permission.)

"evidence-based" guidelines, but there has been very little discussion of the lack of randomized trials that demonstrate a benefit of treating a systolic BP in the 140 to 160 mm Hg range, or whether this lack of evidence contributes to physician inaction on this parameter. Professional organizations and regulatory agencies have used educational efforts and quality improvement and pay for performance programs to improve hypertension control rates, but the overall impact of these programs is unknown. An increase in control of treated hypertension in the elderly in the most recent national survey data may suggest a positive trend toward change and some managed care organizations now report the control rates in treated hypertensive patients of >60%.

Blood pressure measurement issues. Another factor that is controlled largely by physicians and is underappreciated as a barrier to hypertension control is inadequate BP measurement and follow-up practices. Most physicians appear to require a persistent BP reading over a specific threshold before intensifying medical treatment. Little is known about how physicians interpret a single office-based reading, consecutive readings in a single patient visit, or readings over a series of visits. Home BP monitoring by the patient is becoming more common but how it is used in physician decision making is not yet clear.

Actual BP measurement in office practice is often imprecise (see Chapter B102). Random errors in single BP measurements over time can mask a persistent BP elevation. In addition, there may be a systematic bias that could be very important to tighter control. Chart reviews from a large primary care clinic network show that physicians tend to selectively recheck BP values that are above the treatment goal but do not remeasure BPs in the normal range. Because of normal BP variation, repeat BP values may be lower and may delay treatment intensification.

Physicians also control the follow-up intervals, which are highly variable. If a physician's threshold for treating hypertension is a diastolic BP >90 mm Hg, for example, the number of persons who get treated could still be highly influenced by the follow-up strategy used. A physician who sees a patient with a diastolic BP of 92 mm Hg and reacts by advising the patient to return at weekly intervals and then initiates or intensifies BP treatment will better control hypertension than a physician who reacts to the same patient by simply saying, "Don't worry about it. We'll look at it again in 6 months."

Patient adherence (compliance)

Health professionals must beware of "shifting the blame" for uncontrolled hypertension to the patient. High treatment dropout rates motivated by drug side effects or other factors have been widely viewed as major obstacles to hypertension control. Although many studies showing a high dropout rate for *new*

patients with hypertension are well known, studies reporting that more than 95% of *established* hypertensive patients persist with treatment are not. Many physicians believe that drug side effects are a major contributor to lack of persistency of treatment but the basis for this claim is questionable, because most categories of antihypertensives used currently (including diuretics and β-blockers) have discontinuation rates in randomized double-blind trials that are similar to placebo.

Societal barriers to healthy lifestyle

Dietary patterns, such as high sodium intake, and lifestyle factors that lead to overweight are assumed to contribute to overall population prevalence, and lifestyle change has been the first line of treatment for hypertension since guidelines were first issued. However, with the proliferation of prepared and fast food, labor-saving devices, cars, and electronics, the prevalence of obesity in the United States has increased dramatically. In spite of this, an epidemiologic analysis showed that actual BP levels in the population actually fell over the period from 1960 to 1994, and the prevalence of hypertension in the United States has remained stable over the last 10 years. Societal factors, therefore, cannot be readily invoked as the limiting barrier to hypertension control in the United States.

Suggested Readings

Berlowitz D, Ash A, Hickey R, et al. Inadequate management of BP in a hypertensive population. *N Engl J Med* 1998;339:1957–1963.

Chobanian AV, Bakris GL, Black HR, et al. The seventh report of the Joint National Committee on Prevention, Detection, Evaluation, and Treatment of High BP: the JNC 7 report. *JAMA* 2003;289(19):2560–2572.

Franklin SS, Jacobs MJ, Wong ND, et al. Predominance of isolated systolic hypertension among middle-aged and elderly US hypertensives: analysis based on National Health and Nutrition Examination Survey (NHANES) III. *Hypertension* 2001;37(3):869–874.

Goff DC, Howard G, Russell GB, et al. Birth cohort evidence of population influences on BP in the United States, 1887–1994. *Ann Epidemiol* 2001;11(4):271–279.

Hyman D, Pavlik V. Self-reported hypertension treatment practices among primary care physicians. BP thresholds, drug choices, and the role of guidelines and evidence-based medicine. *Arch Intern Med* 2000;160:2281–2286.

Hyman D, Pavlik V, Vallbona C. Physician role in lack of awareness and control of hypertension. *Clin Hypertens* 2000;2:324–330.

Izzo JJ, Levy D, Black H. Clinical advisory statement. Importance of systolic BP in older Americans. *Hypertension* 2000;35:1021–1024.

Oliveria SA, Lapuerta P, McCarthy BD, et al. Physician-related barriers to the effective management of uncontrolled hypertension. *Arch Intern Med* 2002;162(4):413–420.

Ong KL, Cheung BM, Man YB, et al. Prevalence, awareness, treatment, and control of hypertension among United States adults 1999–2004. *Hypertension* 2007;49(1):69–75.

Pavlik VN, Hyman DJ, Vallbona C, et al. Selective physician BP remeasurement in the office setting may contribute to poor hypertension control. *Am J Hypertens* 2002;15(4 Pt 2):81A.

CHAPTER C125 ■ HYPERTENSION CONSULTATIONS

LAWRENCE R. KRAKOFF, MD

KEY POINTS

- The rationale for hypertension specialists arises from the complexity and diversity of healthcare systems and the overwhelming amounts of information in diverse medical specialties that relate to hypertension and its control.
- Hypertension specialists are familiar with complex diagnostic, evaluation, and treatment decisions needed in many patients with hypertension.
- Hypertension referrals are appropriate for establishing diagnoses (particularly for white coat hypertension or searching for identifiable causes of hypertension), or managing complex or refractory cases.
- Hypertension specialists have roles in planning health care protocols and systems, achieving better control rates, providing educational programs, quality assessment and systems improvements, and implementation of new guidelines and treatment paradigms.

See also Chapters **C119** and C124

The delivery of hypertension care

Health care system diversity and blood pressure control. Optimal management of the large fraction of the population with hypertension requires a complex and multicomponent health care system. The experience from clinical trials suggests that control of hypertension may be achieved in 50% to 60% of those enrolled. Yet, population surveys in the United States, report overall control of hypertension well below 40%. Control rates are even lower in other countries.

The diversity within the United States health care system is one reason for highly variable control rates. Most hypertensive patients are managed by primary care providers: internists, family practitioners, pediatricians, and nurse practitioners. There is also a wide variety of health care systems in noncentralized United States health care including the Veterans Administration Clinics, private practices, various group practices that are financed through varied mechanisms. Consultants advising primary care providers have different areas of expertise: Cardiologists, nephrologists, endocrinologists, clinical pharmacologists, and internists with special interests or training may be helpful resources.

Management of groups and populations. Recent trends indicate that hypertension control has become an even greater challenge for certain populations, especially older individuals. The lifetime risk of developing hypertension in suburban towns of the United States is now more than 85%. At the same time, the elderly population continues to grow. Individuals with

expert knowledge of cardiovascular epidemiology, prevention of hypertension, interpretation of relevant clinical trials, medical economics and population interventions will be of particular value to those responsible for providing and funding health care at the macro level. Educational interventions for groups of patients and providers, combined with mechanisms for feedback-alerts to providers are promising initiatives. National guidelines must be adapted to diverse local and community needs. Applying successful strategies from small trials to regional or national populations is being explored through the combination of expertise in hypertension in academic centers with networks recruiting local primary care providers. Hypertension experts may assist in finding strategies for overcoming barriers to optimal management through quality and process improvement. Experts may also participate in the development of care or surveillance systems outside of the offices and clinics that have been traditional sites of management. For example, management of hypertension at work-sites has become an attractive supplemental system that may be suitable for expansion. The growing use of home blood pressure (BP) recording with day-to-day management by nonphysician providers (e.g., nurse practitioners) supervised by hypertension consultants is a promising strategy for moving preventive medicine out of the clinic and into the home where the patient becomes, in effect, a provider of care. Some of the issues that require expertise for groups and populations are shown in **Table C125.1.**

PROBLEMS OF HYPERTENSION CARE IN POPULATIONS AND GROUPS THAT MAY REQUIRE "HYPERTENSION EXPERTS"

Problems	Skills or special knowledge required
Screening groups or populations	Methods of unbiased measurement, epidemiology, guidelines for classification of hypertension
Quality assessment for care	Knowledge of current guidelines, strategies for review, data management, interventions that may improve local practices
Interventions to improve control	Education of both patients and providers with strategies for feedback
New care systems	Knowledge of alternate strategies to conventional office-clinic based care, awareness of worksite, rural health care, special systems, home care strategies
Cost-effective care for systems with limited resources	Medical economics, cost-effective analysis, including pharmacy and formulary review, results of clinical trials

Guideline-based hypertension referrals

The current American guideline for hypertension management, JNC-7, offers a useful framework to describe how experts in clinical hypertension (consultants) might be effectively linked to management of patients with hypertension and their individualized special problems. Subjects are classified as normal, prehypertensive, or with stage 1 or stage 2 hypertension. High-risk subjects are classified as having "compelling indications" for therapy if they have diabetes or previous cardiac, cerebrovascular, or renal disease. There are also "special situations" identified by JNC-7 that may modify therapeutic recommendations, including pregnancy or prostate disease. Finally, there are "identifiable causes" for hypertension such as primary aldosteronism or sleep apnea syndrome.

Across the entire disease spectrum of individuals requiring surveillance or treatment, it is expected that primary care providers will manage the vast majority of cases with prehypertension and stage 1 hypertension (approximately 40% of the United States population). Many in this large group will have high risk profiles or identifiable causes of hypertension. Consultation with a hypertension expert will not often be needed. For this group, however, experts may play a different role in supervising and providing quality control for resources such as ambulatory BP recording or use of home BP measurement devices. In contrast, individual hypertension expert consultations will play a greater role in decisions for those with stage 2 hypertension, those with compelling indications, individuals who are refractory to treatment, or those with signs or symptoms consistent with an identifiable (secondary) form of hypertension.

Specific reasons for consultation

Common problems most appropriate for consultations by hypertension specialists are shown in **Table C125.2**.

PROBLEMS OF PATIENT CARE THAT MAY REQUIRE A "HYPERTENSION SPECIALIST" AND SOME OF THE SKILLS AND KNOWLEDGE BASE THAT WILL BE NEEDED TO DEAL WITH THESE PROBLEMS

Problems	Skills or special knowledge required
White coat or masked hypertension	Methods and interpretation of ambulatory blood pressures, home recordings
Refractory hypertension— apparent failure to respond to medications	Causes and management of complex drug regimens, awareness of issues related to out-of-clinic blood pressure assessment and compliance
Adverse reactions to antihypertensive medications	Clinical pharmacology: awareness of individual barriers to adherence including patient's perceptions, awareness of unusual drug reactions, specific management skills
Identifiable hypertension (renal diseases, adrenal or steroid abnormalities, sleep apnea syndrome, etc.)	Causes, diagnostic methods, specific management skills
High-risk conditions or complex conditions (carotid stenosis, peripheral artery disease, aortic aneurysm, other medical conditions requiring complex multidrug treatment)	Familiarity and experience in management of vascular, renal, and cardiac diseases, depression, panic disorder, chronic lung disease, sleep apnea, and rare disorders such as arteritis

White coat and masked hypertension. In the past, the diagnosis of white coat hypertension has been a problematic issue for all practitioners who care for younger healthy patients. Now that ambulatory BP monitoring has become widely available, reimbursable, and cost-effective, it can be ordered directly by primary practices without need for consultation. Similarly, as the role of home BP monitoring becomes more firmly established, the need for expert consultation for the diagnosis of white coat hypertension will diminish. Some individuals with normal office BP readings have consistently elevated home and nonoffice BP readings. This condition, currently termed *masked hypertension* needs special consideration for treatment with antihypertensive drugs, because no outcome trials are available for evidence-based guidance in their management.

Adverse drug effects, drug and food interactions. A common problem in the management of hypertension is adverse effects of medications. A specialist can be extremely useful in recommending alternate strategies for BP control. Rarely, pharmacogenetic differences in drug metabolism alter the effectiveness of certain regimens. Diet composition may need attention. For example, grapefruit can potentiate the antihypertensive action of felodipine and some other calcium-channel blockers.

Refractory hypertension. Refractory or resistant hypertension (failure to achieve adequate BP control with adequate doses of three or more antihypertensive drugs, one of which is a diuretic) will most likely remain the most frequent reason for consulting a hypertension expert. In these patients, there is need for a careful in-depth assessment to determine possible causes of the poor therapeutic response and to change the current therapeutic strategy. The consultant needs to be familiar with all the 'usual suspects' for refractory hypertension, including a false-positive diagnosis due to a prominent, white coat effect, poor adherence to treatment, inadequate doses of drugs, drug interactions, and many others. Systematic assessment of refractory hypertension by experts in clinics organized for this purpose appears to be effective in achieving higher rates of control.

Identifiable (secondary) forms of hypertension. Those problems related to identifiable hypertension listed in **Table C125.2** may require expertise from those with special competence or training, especially with regard to the planning and interpretation of the complex diagnostic tests that are sometimes employed.

High-risk and complicated hypertension. Management of those with compelling indications or special needs by specialists has already been mentioned. In addition, older patients with multiple risk factors or complex diseases (e.g., advanced atherosclerotic disease) often require specific expertise for assessment of aortic aneurysms, carotid and peripheral arteries and may be candidates for endovascular surgery. Some experience in geriatrics and psychiatry may assist in the management of patients with such disorders as dementia, panic disorder, or depression. Patients with advancing renal disease also present special challenges to the nephrologist-hypertension specialist and those with declining ventricular function challenge the cardiologist-hypertension specialist.

Hypertension specialist certification

With the advent of the American Society of Hypertension (ASH) Specialist Program, practitioners from many disciplines with particular expertise in clinical hypertension can be certified as specialists in hypertension. Qualifications include appropriate professional credentials and satisfactory completion of a qualifying examination. The European Hypertension Society has embarked on a similar pathway adapted to the variety of cultural and national patterns characteristic of the European community. Finding the appropriate relationship between a small number of experts with advanced skills in management of hypertension and the large number of primary care providers who detect and treat hypertension in the population at large will be a major challenge. The diverse health care systems and the resource limits within individual countries will be important determinants of how well BP can be controlled and how much that control can impact the increasing burden of preventable cardiovascular diseases.

Suggested Readings

Canzanello VJ, Jensen PL, Schwartz LL, et al. Improved blood pressure control with a physician-nurse team and home blood pressure measurement. *Mayo Clin Proc* 2005;80(1):31–36.

Chobanian AV, Bakris GL, Black HR, et al. The seventh report of the Joint National Committee on Prevention, Detection, Evaluation and Treatment of High Blood Pressure: The JNC 7 Report. *JAMA* 2003;289:2560–2572.

Egan BM, Lackland DT, Basile JN. American Society of Hypertension regional chapters: leveraging the impact of the clinical hypertension specialist in the local community. *Am J Hypertens* 2002;15(4 Pt 1):372–379.

Garg JP, Elliott WJ, Folker A, et al. Resistant hypertension revisited: a comparison of two university-based cohorts. *Am J Hypertens* 2005;18(5 Pt 1):619–626.

Krakoff LR. Systems for care of hypertension in the United States. *J Clin Hypertens* 2006;8(6):420–426.

Lloyd-Jones DM, Evans JC, Levy D. Hypertension in adults across the age spectrum: current outcomes and control in the community. *JAMA* 2005;294(4):466–472.

Oliveria SA, Lapuerta P, McCarthy BD, et al. Physician-related barriers to the effective management of uncontrolled hypertension. *Arch Intern Med* 2002;162:413–420.

Redon J, Campos C, Rodicio JL, et al. Prognostic value of ambulatory blood pressure monitoring in refractory hypertension: a prospective study. *Hypertension* 2001;31:712–718.

Roumie CL, Elasy TA, Greevy R, et al. Improving blood pressure control through provider education, provider alerts, and patient education: a cluster randomized trial. *Ann Intern Med* 2006;145(3):165–175.

Rudd P, Houston Miller N, Kaufman J, et al. Nurse management for hypertension. *Am J Hypertens* 2004;17:921–927.

CHAPTER C126 ■ NONPHYSICIAN PROVIDERS AND THE MANAGEMENT OF HYPERTENSION

BARRY L. CARTER, PharmD

KEY POINTS

- Clinical inertia, suboptimal treatment regimens, and poor patient adherence are frequent contributors to poor blood pressure (BP) control.
- Incorporating nonphysician providers (pharmacists, physician assistants, or nurses) into the management plan can greatly increase BP control rates.
- Health systems should explore strategies to develop and incorporate comprehensive care models for patients with hypertension.

See also Chapters C123 and **C124**

Barriers to blood pressure control

Many believe that poor blood pressure (BP) control is related to limited access to care, poor patient adherence, or an insufficient armamentarium of antihypertensive medications. Although these are important problems for some populations, it is becoming increasingly clear that these barriers to care are not nearly as problematic as were initially thought to be.

Physician attitudes are now recognized as major barriers to better BP control (see Chapter C124) through failure to intensify therapy despite frequent physician visits. The most common reasons for "resistant" hypertension referred to a hypertension center were drug-related causes (61%, including suboptimal regimens), patient nonadherence (13%), secondary hypertension (7%), or other (18%). Such studies suggest that clinical inertia and the use of suboptimal treatment regimens are the major causes of poor BP control.

There are many reasons why physicians might be willing to accept poor BP control in an individual patient including more urgent competing medical problems, BP close but not yet at goal although much closer than baseline, patient stressors the day of the clinic visit, or patient resistance to adding another medication. These issues can lead to complacency and thereby failure to achieve a goal BP.

Interventions to reduce clinical inertia

Many interventions have been tried to overcome the above-mentioned problems including patient education, provider reminders, provider education, as well as audit and feedback. These approaches, although generally effective, do not tend to be as productive as organizational and structural changes to the health care team. A literature synthesis for the Agency for Health Care Research and Quality (AHRQ) found that adding nonphysician members to assist with hypertension management is one of the most serviceable strategies. The Veterans Administration (VA)/Department of Defense (DoD) Hypertension guidelines state, "*If BP continues to be elevated, clinicians should consider…care management by a pharmacist in the follow-up and adjustment of medications to improve BP goal.*"

Hypertension management by pharmacists

Pharmacists working in a wide variety of settings have been able to assist physicians with hypertension management. In addition to traditional community pharmacies, clinical pharmacists have provided hypertension management within staff model managed care organizations, academic clinics, and Veterans Affairs Medical Centers (VAMCs). Each of these settings is circumstantially unique with differing infrastructures that impact how physicians might utilize pharmacists in hypertension management.

Physician–pharmacist collaborative models. Most hypertension management provided by pharmacists occurs in group practices and in close collaboration with physicians. Patients with hypertension were randomized to usual care (N = 99) or to a physician–pharmacist comanagement intervention group (N = 98) in an integrated health system in California. The pharmacists assessed patients every 2 to 4 weeks and then contacted the physician with recommendations based on an evidence-based algorithm. BP was reduced significantly more in the intervention group than in the usual care group ($p < .01$) at 6, 9, and 12 months (22 vs. 9, 25 vs. 10, and 22 vs. 11 mm Hg, respectively). Significantly more patients in the intervention group

(60%) achieved BP control than in the usual care group (43%, $p = .02$). In another study, patients with uncontrolled hypertension were randomized to a control (N = 46) or intervention (N = 49) group managed by a physician–pharmacist team and experienced better BP control (23 vs. 11 mm Hg, $p <.001$) than in the control group, with BP controlled in 55% of patients in the intervention versus 20% of the control group ($p <.001$). The physicians accepted 93% of the recommendations made by the pharmacist.

In a randomized, cluster-design controlled trial that included 24-hour ambulatory BP monitoring to confirm the efficacy of a physician–pharmacist collaborative intervention, over 9 months intervention, the office BP was significantly lower in the intervention group (124/75 mm Hg vs. 133/79 mm Hg, $p <.001$), 24-hour BP levels showed similar significant intervention effects [mean difference of 8.8 mm Hg for systolic blood pressure (SBP) and 4.6 mm Hg for diastolic blood pressure (DBP)]. Clinical pharmacists made 267 recommendations for change (2.6 per patient) and physicians accepted 256 (96%) of the recommendations (e.g., increase the existing drug dose in 34%, add a nondiuretic in 30%, or add a thiazide diuretic in 17%). Physicians in the control group changed medications only 100 times (1.28 per patient, $p <.001$ compared to the intervention group).

Community pharmacists.
Several studies have evaluated the ability of community pharmacists to assist physicians with hypertension management. Communication barriers can be a problem but these barriers can be overcome if the physician and pharmacist agree to collaborate and jointly establish policies and procedures. In other cases, the physician can either obtain permission for medical data to be shared or the pharmacist may visit the physician's office to review the patient's medical record.

The first study to evaluate pharmacist management of hypertension was actually conducted with a community pharmacist who evaluated patients with poor BP control, poor medication adherence, or adverse events. The pharmacist worked closely with two physicians in an urban health center, reviewed medical records in the physician's office, and made recommendations to the physicians. BP control deteriorated in the control group (163/93 vs. 166/101 mm Hg) but improved in the study group (157/99 vs. 146/90 mm Hg, between groups $p <.001$).

Carter et al. conducted a similar study within a private, rural medical practice that had a pharmacy housed in the building. Pharmacists reviewed medical records and made face-to-face recommendations to the physicians. SBP was significantly reduced in the intervention group (N = 25, 146 to 135 mm Hg, $p <.001$ for SBP) but not in the control group (N = 26, 147 to 142 mm Hg).

Management of hypertension by nurses
Nurses and, more recently, nurse practitioners have provided hypertension management for approximately 40 years in settings such as the VA, mobile clinics, home visits, work-based programs, and office or clinic settings. In systems with physician hypertension specialists, a team approach is often applied using nurses, dietitians, and nurse educators to care for patients. The nurse is often the primary caregiver for patients with hypertension, providing assessment of adverse reactions, evaluating medication adherence, and teaching patients to perform home BP monitoring.

Nurse specialists.
An early study randomized 457 hypertensive patients to a worksite-based nurse-run clinic or usual physician care outside the workplace. The nurses prescribed and adjusted drug therapy followed by a weekly chart review by physicians. After 6 months of follow-up, nurse-managed patients were more likely to adhere to the medication regimen (68% vs. 49%, $p <.005$) and to achieve goal BP (49% vs. 28%, $p <.001$).

Rudd et al. evaluated nurse case management of hypertension in a randomized controlled trial (76 managed by the primary physician, 74 received nurse-based care). Nurse case managers provided education regarding use of an automated BP device, strategies to improve medication adherence and identification of adverse drug events, and made medication dosage adjustments; new medication was started after physician consultation. The nurses conducted telephone interviews at 1 week and at 1, 2, and 4 months. SBP declined by 14.2 mm Hg in the intervention group compared to 5.7 mm Hg in the control group ($p <.01$). Medication adherence at 6 months was 81% in the intervention group and 69% in the control group ($p = .03$).

Nurse practitioners.
A large study evaluated primary care delivered by nurse practitioners compared to physicians in patients with any condition including hypertension. Patients were randomized to either a nurse practitioner (N = 806) or a physician (N = 510), both of whom had the same roles and responsibilities for prescribing medications, consulting, referring, or admitting patients. The primary outcome was a quality of life score, which was equivalent for the two groups. For the patients diagnosed with hypertension, BP was lower in the nurse practitioner group (137/82 mm Hg) than physician groups (139/95 mm Hg, $p = .28$ for SBP and $p = .04$ for DBP). Other studies have found that when nurse practitioners care for a wide variety of patients, BP control rates are similar to what is seen with physician-based care. In contrast, when the nurse model focuses on hypertension, BP control rates are often better than usual care.

Hypertension management with a nurse–pharmacist model
Most studies utilize either nurses or pharmacists for BP management. Whether a nurse, pharmacist, or both are employed often depends on which providers are available and the size and structure of the clinic or health system. Few studies describe true nurse–pharmacist models for hypertension management. A study conducted in the Madison VAMC evaluated the impact of a clinical pharmacist on physician prescribing, medication documentation, and patient compliance. The study included 75 control and 98 study group patients. At the end of the study, medication adherence was 72% in the intervention group and 20% in the control group ($p <.001$). BP was controlled in 69% of the intervention group and 29% of the control group ($p <.02$). Following this experience, the investigators evaluated whether the effect could be sustained after 4.75 years of follow-up. During this follow-up, a nurse clinician was included. The nurse and pharmacist had interchangeable roles and responsibilities. In the study group, 75% of patients were adherent to all medications compared to 20% in the control group ($p <.001$). BP was controlled in 90% of the intervention group compared to 20% in the control group ($p <.01$). The investigators concluded that the clinical pharmacist and a nurse clinician improved both medication compliance and BP control.

TABLE C126.1

STRATEGIES TO UTILIZE NONPHYSICIAN PROVIDERS

Barrier or problem	Actions by providers
Foster continuity, communication, and patient empowerment	
■ Insufficient time for education, counseling, and rapid follow-up	■ Use nurse (and/or pharmacist) case management to track patients and provide routine follow-up, especially when blood pressure (BP) is controlled with lifestyle and/or at goal
■ Insufficient follow-up between physician visits	■ Utilize community pharmacists to monitor BP between physician visits ■ Use telephone follow-up (nurse and/or pharmacist)
■ Patients lack of self-efficacy and do not understand their treatment	■ Establish BP goals and a plan. Include patients in decisions about prevention and treatment goals for BP ■ Use contracting strategies ■ Teach patients to use home monitoring
■ Poor lifestyle and medication adherence	■ Assess patient adherence at each visit ■ Anticipate barriers or occasional low adherence and discuss solutions ■ Nurse provides strategies to make behavioral change to improve lifestyle modification ■ Pharmacist assesses reasons for poor medication adherence and modifies regimen if necessary ■ Use self-report on adherence, pill counts, or electronic data ■ Contact community pharmacist to obtain refill history
■ Adverse reactions	■ Have a pharmacist assess and modify therapy when applicable
■ Missed appointments	■ Develop reminder systems to ensure identification and follow-up of patient status ■ Use telephone follow-up ■ Schedule evening/weekend office hours
Clinical inertia and suboptimal treatment regimens	
■ Therapy is not intensified even when BP is not controlled	■ Document the goal BP in the medical record ■ Assess the patient's progress toward goal BP at each visit ■ Benchmark BP control rates by provider or by clinic ■ Have a pharmacist assess any patient with poor BP control and adjust therapy
■ Suboptimal treatment regimens	■ Have a pharmacist assess any patient with poor BP control and adjust therapy ■ Add thiazide diuretic if not in regimen ■ Intensify medications and utilize combinations since most patients require two to three medications

Toward an integrated model

The keys to successfully implementing better BP care are role negotiation and frequent communication among the primary care physician, clinical pharmacist, nurse, and any other health care providers. In health systems where an interdisciplinary model has been implemented, BP control rates have been significantly improved.

Goal-orientated care. Regardless of which professionals are used for hypertension management, a goal-oriented approach is essential. All providers must take responsibility for achieving high

BP control rates in the system and for each patient. Achieving these goals may require a complete restructuring of care delivery. Providers must move from acute, crises-based care to a model of preventing and managing chronic conditions. Pharmacists, nurses, and other office personnel can help track patients, remind them of their upcoming office visit, and contact them when they do not show up for an appointment. **Table C126.1** provides some suggestions for utilization of nonphysician providers in the management of hypertension.

Efficiency and continuity.

Efficiency can be greatly improved by the use of telephone follow-up by the nurse to evaluate medication and diet adherence. If the clinic employs a pharmacist, he/she should assist the physician with designing a specific drug regimen that considers coexisting conditions and potential drug–drug interactions. The pharmacist should counsel patients about proper medication use, administration, storage, and potential adverse reactions. In addition, a nurse case manager, if available in a clinic, can provide continuity between physician visits, offer behavioral counseling to improve adherence to lifestyle modifications, and evaluate adverse reactions. Many clinics may not have a clinical pharmacist or nurse clinician/nurse practitioner but physicians can still solicit the support of selected community pharmacists to help with hypertension management. Despite increasing purchases of prescriptions by mail, the average patient visits their pharmacy at least monthly. Once a relationship and scope of practice has been negotiated, the pharmacist can assist with monitoring BP, assessing BP control, and monitoring for adverse reactions or drug interactions.

Patient education and accountability.

Pharmacists and nurses can help patients become more engaged in their management and teach them to perform home BP monitoring. The nurse can provide dietary and weight management counseling, adjust medications, and provide appropriate follow-up visits.

Suggested Readings

Alsuwaidan S, Malone DC, Billups SJ, et al. Characteristics of ambulatory care clinics and pharmacists in Veterans Affairs medical centers. IMPROVE investigators. Impact of managed pharmaceutical care on resource utilization and outcomes in Veterans Affairs medical centers. *Am J Health Syst Pharm* 1998;55:68–72.

Bond CA, Monson R. Sustained improvement in drug documentation, compliance, and disease control. A four-year analysis of an ambulatory care model. *Arch Intern Med* 1984;144:1159–1162.

Carter BL, Barnette DJ, Chrischilles E, et al. Evaluation of hypertensive patients after care provided by community pharmacists in a rural setting. *Pharmacotherapy* 1997;17:1274–1285.

Carter BL, Zillich AJ, Elliott WJ. How pharmacists can assist physicians with controlling BP. *J Clin Hypertens* 2003;5(1):31–37.

Rudd P, Miller NH, Kaufman J, et al. Nurse management for hypertension. A systems approach. *Am J Hypertens* 2004;17:921–927.

Schultz JF, Sheps SG. Management of patients with hypertension: a hypertension clinic model. *Mayo Clin Proc* 1994;69:997–999.

Shojania KG, McDonald KM, Wachter RM, et al. *Closing the quality gap: a critical analysis of quality improvement strategies, Volume 3-Hypertension Care.* AHRQ publication No. 04-0051-3, January 2005.

Veterans Administration, Department of Defense(VA/DoD). *VA/DoD Clinical practice guideline for diagnosis and management of hypertension in the primary care setting.* Department of Veterans Administration, Department of Defense, 2004. Revision July 2005.

Zillich AJ, Sutherland JM, Kumbera PA, et al. Hypertension outcomes through BP monitoring and evaluation by pharmacists (HOME study). *J Gen Intern Med* 2005;20:1091–1096.

CHAPTER C127 ■ HYPERTENSION RECORDKEEPING AND ELECTRONIC MANAGEMENT SYSTEMS

MARY K. GOLDSTEIN, MD, MS AND BRIAN B. HOFFMAN, MD

KEY POINTS

■ Flowsheets and tabular summaries of hypertension-related patient information improve care and facilitate treatment of hypertensive patients.
■ Graphic displays can communicate quantitative information and patterns rapidly and improve patient education.
■ Guideline-based decision support systems for each individual patient are being developed for use by clinicians at the time of medical decision making in outpatient clinics.

See also Chapters **C119,** C124, and C125

Rationale for improved recordkeeping systems

Despite comprehensive, evidence-based, national guidelines, clinical management of hypertension often falls short of adequate blood pressure (BP) control with optimal choices of drugs. To manage hypertension effectively over time, physicians and other health care professionals need rapid access to accurate medical record information about the patient's previous BPs and antihypertensive regimens. Such information can be difficult for the physician to extract from clinic charts unless they are structured to collect and display this specific information.

The increasing availability of electronic medical records offers an opportunity for improving the display of relevant clinical information. Electronic medical records, viewed at the time of clinic visits, can be used to present guideline-based recommendations about management of hypertension to physicians and other health care providers when medical decisions are actually being made.

Traditional data organization: a barrier to blood pressure control

Medical data in traditional clinical charts is often so extensive that it overwhelms the physician's capacity to synthesize and evaluate it in the time available for most clinic visits. Prioritization of information value also does not occur. In contrast, presentation of information in graphic format can vastly improve the recipient's perception of important disease and treatment patterns. An early example of the power of graphic display of information is the famous dot map of Dr. John Snow, the physician who, by plotting the location of each death, identified the Broad Street Water pump as the source of the cholera epidemic in London in 1854.

Improved information systems

Clinical information intended to help physicians provide care for hypertensive patients may most effectively take the form of flowsheets and summaries.

Flowsheets. Flowsheets and graphs have been used routinely in paper charts for outpatients in many clinical domains—for example, growth charts and immunization records for children, fundal height and other parameters in prenatal care, and hematologic and renal parameters together with drug doses in chemotherapy protocols. Flowsheets aimed at providing important information for the management of hypertension, on paper or in electronic format, should be prominently located in the medical record and should display details of BPs and doses of antihypertensive medications over a time frame relevant to the clinical setting. For example, intensive care unit flowsheets may show minute-to-minute changes in BP, whereas outpatient primary hypertension flowsheets typically show values over weeks, months, and sometimes years. Despite the fact that these are reasonably easy to maintain, hypertension flowsheets have not been widely used.

Electronic records. Periodic summaries from a paper chart aid in making necessary clinical decisions but are extremely labor intensive. In contrast, an electronic record lends itself readily to automating the rapid extraction and display of patient data important to a particular clinical domain. Patient summaries from electronic patient data may be presented in text format or, with

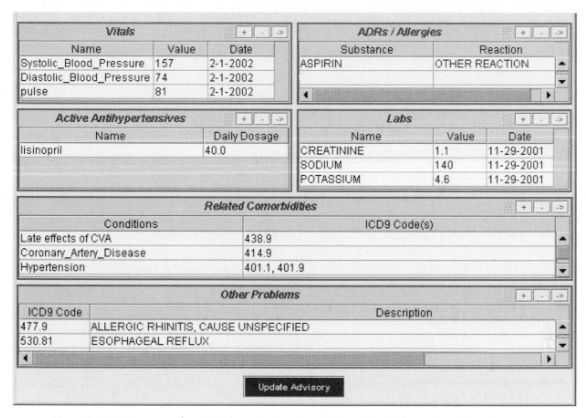

Figure C127.1 Summary of patient's hypertension-related information. Recent patient data relevant to treatment of hypertension are extracted from various locations in the electronic medical record and summarized in this window. Information content can be changed, using the + and − buttons. For example, new diagnoses can be added from a drop down menu, or present diagnoses can be deleted. Recommendations made by the program can be updated by clicking the Update Advisory button at the bottom of the screen. The recommendations of the program (for a different patient) are shown in **Figure C127.2.** CVA, cerebrovascular accident; ADR, adverse drug reactions.

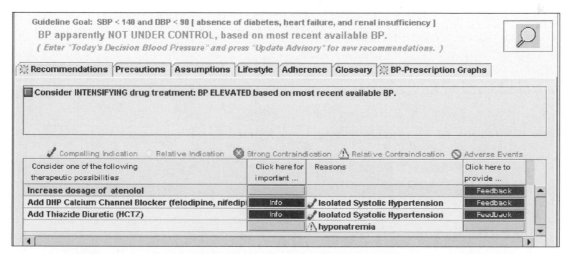

Figure C127.2 Display of guideline-based recommendations. The figure shows the mid-portion of a screen displayed in a pop-up window in the electronic medical record that includes goal BP (<140/90 mm Hg). Because this patient is above target, the information can be displayed in red letters. A series of tabs give options for the clinician to select options. The screen shows the Recommendations tab, which is the default display when the window pops up. Because the BP is not adequately controlled, the primary recommendation is to intensify drug treatment. The table shows recommended changes to drug treatment; recognizing that drug choices must be individualized and that guideline-based recommendations may not apply to each patient, clinicians are asked to consider the possibilities. The first column in the table shows the specific drug recommendations for this patient, including an increase in the dose of the current drug (atenolol) or the addition of a new drug. A variety of options are afforded in boxes that prompt the user to make choices derived from guidelines and prescription policies. BP, blood pressure; SBP, systolic blood pressure; DBP, diastolic blood pressure; DHP, dihydropyridine; HCTZ, hydrochlorothiazide.

the more recent wide availability of graphic user interfaces, in user-friendly visual displays.

Graphic displays. Many electronic medical record systems include graphing capabilities for display of single parameters. For example, the Computerized Patient Record System (CPRS) used nationally by the Department of Veterans Affairs (VA) in its hospitals and clinics includes a feature to display graphs of a single parameter in each instance for a time window selected by the user. This feature can be used to display every BP value entered into the patient's electronic record.

Summary of hypertension-related information. The electronic medical record can be organized to present a summary of the patient's relevant clinical information (**Figure C127.1**). The summary shows the most recent vital signs, known allergies or adverse reactions to drugs, the most recent relevant laboratory tests, a list of current antihypertensive medications, the diagnoses relevant to choice of antihypertensive medication, and other diagnoses.

Management decision support for hypertension management. The electronic medical record may be combined with hypertension guidelines to generate recommendations for management of each patient. A detailed description of the hypertension knowledge base for this program is beyond the scope of this chapter. These recommendations may be displayed visually. **Figure C127.2** shows one such display. In this case, the recommendations are shown with icons indicating the clinical significance of each recommendation (e.g., a compelling indication

per JNC 7). Additional information triggered by the patient data is available by clicking the Info button adjacent to the recommendation. The clinician can also provide feedback about the recommendation from a checklist of options by clicking the Feedback button.

Automated treatment for health evaluator and advisor-hypertension. The ability to display a graph of a patient's BPs over time is quite useful. It is also clinically advantageous to know what antihypertensive drugs, and at what doses, the patient was taking at the time these BP measurements were made. **Figure C127.3** shows a graphic display of BPs and antihypertensive drugs on the same time line. **Figures C127.1** to **C127.3** are from the Automated Treatment for Health Evaluator and Advisor-Hypertension (ATHENA-HTN), a hypertension advisory system built using EON technology for developing decision-support systems for guideline-based care. The graph shows the target BPs representing adequate control, individualized to take into account comorbidities such as diabetes. The dose of each antihypertensive drug is shown at the time the drug was introduced or changed. Gaps in availability of the drug—for example, due to the patient not refilling the prescription on time—suggest the need to ask the patient about barriers to medical refill or other potential medication adherence difficulties. A recent version of the VA's CPRS also includes functionality to permit graphing of different parameters on the same time line.

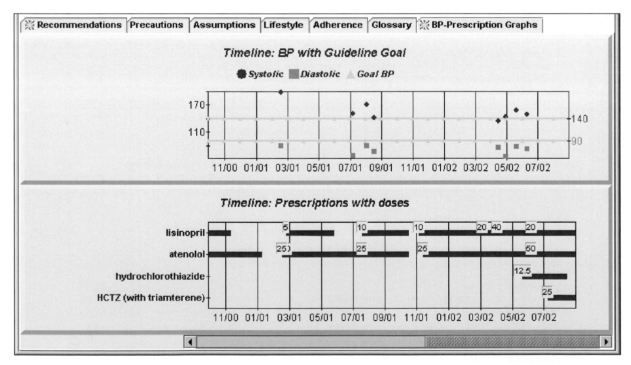

Figure C127.3 BPs and antihypertensive medications on the same timeline. This figure shows the BP-Prescription Graphs tab from a hypertension advisory program (Automated Treatment of Hypertension Evaluator and Advisor, ATHENA Decision-Support System). This tab also displays a time line with the patient's BP measurements (*top graph*) and antihypertensive drugs, including drug dose (*bottom graph*). The patient's goal BP (in this case 140/90 mm Hg) is shown as a gray line on the top graph so that it is readily apparent when the BP exceeds goal values. The drug display shows how many days of prescription drug the patient had available; gaps in the line are a clue to the possibility of the patient not refilling prescriptions in a timely manner. In this case, the patient's prescription for hydrochlorothiazide (HCTZ) was changed to a prescription for the combination of HCTZ/triamterene, with the newer prescription entered (appropriately) before the patient had run out of the previous one. BP, blood pressure.

Quality improvement and testing of records systems

Automation provides many opportunities to improve medical care and patient safety through alerts, reminders, and other such systems. Studies of accidents, particularly in the airline industry, have shown that the introduction of automated systems can also affect human problem solving in ways that can lead to unanticipated problems. Qualitative analysis of cognitive processes in medical work can inform design of more effective interfaces, for example, for computerized physician order-entry. New automated systems should be thoroughly tested in simulated clinical environments before they are deployed, and the systems should be monitored after implementation to detect and correct problems as they arise.

Health insurance portability and accountability act

The Health Insurance Portability and Accountability Act (HIPAA) of 1996, Public Law 104-191, specifies a number of regulations that include standard transaction and code sets and the national provider identifier, security standards, and a privacy rule that went into effect in April 2003. Physicians and health care systems should be aware of important security and privacy provisions of HIPAA.

Suggested Readings

Chan A, Martins S, Coleman R, et al. Post fielding surveillance of a guideline-based decision support system. In: Henriksen K, Battles JR, Marks ES, Lewin DI, eds. *Advances in patient safety: from research to implementation. Vol. 1. Research findings AHRQ publication number 05-0021-1.* Rockville: Agency for Healthcare Research and Quality, 2005:331–339.

Chobanian AV, Bakris GL, Black HR, et al. The Seventh Report of the Joint National Committee on Prevention, Detection, Evaluation, and Treatment of High BP: the JNC 7 report. *JAMA* 2003;289(19):2560–2572.

Goldstein MK, Coleman RW, Tu SW, et al. Translating research into practice: organizational issues in implementing automated decision support for hypertension in three medical centers. *J Am Med Inform Assoc* 2004;11(5):368–376

Goldstein MK, Hoffman BB, Coleman RW, et al. Patient safety in guideline-based decision support for hypertension management: ATHENA DSS. *J Am Med Inform Assoc* 2002;9(Suppl 6):S11–S16. Full text available through pubmedcentral:http://www.pubmedcentral.nih.gov/articlerender.fcgi?artid=419409.

Goldstein MK, Lavori P, Coleman R, et al. Improving adherence to guidelines for hypertension drug prescribing: cluster-randomized controlled trial of general versus patient-specific recommendations. *Am J Manag Care* 2005;11(11):677–685.

Johnson CD, Zeiger RF, Das AK, et al. *Task analysis of writing hospital admission orders: evidence of a problem-based approach. AMIA Annu Symp Proc* 2006:389–393.

McDonald CJ. Protocol-based computer reminders, the quality of care and the non-perfectibility of man. *N Engl J Med* 1976;295:1351–1355.

Shortliffe EH, Cimino JJ, Hannah KJ, Ball MJ, eds. *Biomedical informatics: computer applications in health care and biomedicine, Health informatics series,* 3rd ed. New York: Springer, 2006.

Tufts ER. *The visual display of quantitative information.* Cheshire: Graphics Press, 1983.

Walsh JME, McDonald K, Shojania KG, et al. *Quality improvement strategies for hypertension management: a systematic review. Med Care* 2006;44(7):646–657.

CHAPTER C128 ■ ANTIHYPERTENSIVE DRUGS: PHARMACOLOGIC PRINCIPLES AND DOSING EFFECTS

JOSEPH L. IZZO, Jr., MD AND DOMENIC A. SICA, MD

KEY POINTS

- Underdosing and inadequate titration of antihypertensive drugs contribute to our failure to get more hypertensive patients to goal blood pressure (BP).
- Dose–response effects exist for all classes of antihypertensive drugs but BP responses to dose titration are most apparent for sympatholytics, α-blockers, calcium antagonists, and diuretics.
- Maximal responses to angiotensin-converting enzyme (ACE) inhibitors and angiotensin receptor blockers (dose–response plateaus) vary across the population, with African Americans and older patients (often "low-renin" subgroups) demonstrating reduced maximal responses and less effect from dose titration.
- Dose–effect relationships are affected by genetic traits (e.g., salt-sensitivity) and environment-related conditions (e.g., dietary salt intake) as well as drug–drug interactions (e.g., ACE inhibitor effect is enhanced by diuretics or blunted by nonsteroidal antiinflammatory drugs).
- Combination drug therapy using agents with complementary mechanisms of action enhances population BP responses and reduces dose–response variability, making BP-lowering effects more predictable.

See also Chapters C119 and C129

Basic principles

Pharmacodynamics versus pharmacokinetics.
Pharmacokinetic properties are those related to absorption, distribution, and elimination of a drug. For most drugs and most patients, pharmacokinetic considerations are of minor importance in that they are already reflected in the approved dose ranges and dose intervals. Pharmacokinetic differences are most readily apparent in the use of certain drugs in subpopulations with impaired clearance. For example, a drug that is water soluble and principally eliminated by glomerular filtration often requires dosage adjustment in patients with renal impairment. From a practical point of view, it is the pharmacodynamic properties of a drug (i.e., characteristics that describe its biologic effects) that are of greatest interest clinically.

Efficacy and peak:trough effects.
Antihypertensive drugs are typically evaluated after single and multiple doses to determine the time course of their effects. From such studies, an area-under-the-curve (AUC) can be calculated for a drug and equated with a particular response. Because AUC is so cumbersome to obtain, peak and trough blood pressure (BP) effects are usually substituted. Peak-to-trough ratio by itself does not determine drug efficacy, however.

Establishing overall efficacy requires peak-to-peak and trough-to-trough comparisons of placebo to active drug. An antihypertensive drug is approved for once-daily use if its trough effect (24 hours after the last dose) is at least 50% of its peak effect. Clinically, trough BP readings, sometimes derived from ambulatory monitoring studies, are particularly useful in defining whether BP control has been effectively maintained throughout a dosing interval.

Dose–response relationships.
A fundamental concept in therapeutics is the log-linear dose–response curve (Hill-type curve), which is critical to an accurate understanding of the effects of a given drug (**Figure C128.1**). The effect of an adrenergic receptor antagonist is correlated with the logarithm of its concentration and, by extension, the logarithm of the dose. In the case of a true log-linear relationship, a tenfold increase in dose would be needed to double the effect (point A to B in **Figure C128.1**); doubling the dose would then be expected to increase the effect by the logarithm of 2 (approximately 0.3, i.e., from

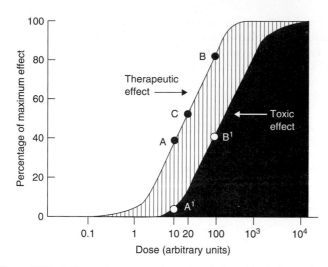

Figure C128.1 Theoretic therapeutic and toxic logarithmic-linear dose-response curves.

point A to C). If the relationship was log-linear, a fourfold dose increase would be needed to double the effect. In either case, it can be readily seen that small titration steps (increasing the existing dose by <100%) usually have relatively little incremental effect and delay goal achievement.

A corollary to the dose–response principle is that a drug exhibits a log–dose response for its toxic effects that is typically parallel and to the right of its therapeutic effect curve. Therefore, at any given clinical dose of an approved agent, the therapeutic effect is expected to be greater than the toxic effect (equivalent to moving from point B to B^1 in **Figure C128.1**). Decreasing the medication dose tends to decrease therapeutic and toxic effects but may result in a relatively greater decrease in toxicity (**Figure C128.1**, point A to A^1). The difference between the therapeutic and toxic effect curves is sometimes called the *therapeutic window* of a drug (cross-hatched area in Figure C128.1).

Factors affecting dose–response relationships

Population and within-individual pharmacodynamic differences. Dose–response relationships can be described in a number of ways. Population responses are often highly variable

and represent a wide range of individual responses that depend on genetic and environmental considerations that vary within and across individuals. For example, within an individual, environmentally driven characteristics such as sodium (Na^+) balance markedly affect responses to anti–renin-angiotensin drugs. Therefore, the shape and height of a dose–response curve varies within individuals and across the population depending on salt intake.

In a heterogeneous population, dose–response curves are more properly defined by their ranges than their mean values at any given dose (**Figure C128.2**). This is classically true for responses to either diuretics or renin-angiotensin system (RAS) blocking drugs, which have complementary biologic mechanisms. In a low-renin individual, the dose–response relationship to an ARB is relatively flat across all doses but the dose–response plateau can be raised by either salt depletion or concomitant diuretic use. In contrast, those in a high-renin state at the time of the drug intake have a vigorous response to an ARB. Thiazide diuretics (or calcium blockers), on the other hand, tend to be most effective in low-renin individuals. Combination of the two agents, because of their complementary mechanisms of action, shifts the dose–response relationship upward and to the left and also narrows the population (and perhaps within-individual) variability in response. Combinations are therefore more predictable and reliable than monotherapy.

Sympatholytics and dihydropyridines have relatively steep dose–response curves with somewhat less variation between individuals. A rough guide to the overall effectiveness of dose titration for antihypertensive drug classes is sympatholytics > calcium antagonists > diuretics > β-blockers = angiotensin-converting enzyme (ACE) inhibitors = ARBs.

Drug–drug interactions. In virtually all cases, addition of a diuretic to a preexisting drug regimen results in an enhanced response, typically reflected by (a) a leftward shift of the curve (less drug required to effect the same reduction in BP), (b) a greater peak (sometimes called *plateau*) response, or (c) a steepening of the response slope at its midpoint. In contrast, addition of a nonsteroidal antiinflammatory drug to a given antihypertensive regimen may have the opposite effect(s).

Pharmacogenetic differences. Race or ethnicity is a crude predictor of drug responses; black hypertensive individuals are generally less responsive to ACE inhibitors, ARBs, and direct renin inhibitors and more responsive to diuretics and calcium

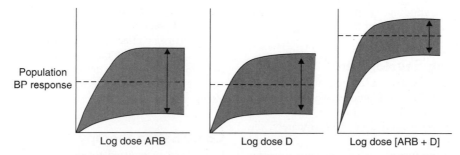

Figure C128.2 Combination of drugs with complementary mechanisms of action. There is wide population variation (*shaded areas, double arrows*) in blood pressure (BP) effects of either ARBs or diuretics (D) but the mean effect is similar (*dotted lines*). Because a lack of response to either agent tends to define a probable response to the other (by definition, the complementary mechanism of action), the combination of ARB and diuretic doubles the efficacy and simultaneously reduces population variation in responsiveness, making the combination more predictably effective in reducing BP.

antagonists. This response pattern is modified by Na$^+$ balance, however. An example of a true pharmacogenetic difference is the lower effectiveness of hydralazine in individuals who have inherited the rapid acetylator gene. As many as 70% of patients who respond inadequately to oral doses of 200 mg daily of hydralazine will be rapid acetylators. In these patients, the dose of the drug can be increased up to 400 mg daily, without risk of drug-induced lupus.

Pseudotolerance. Another major consideration in the pharmacodynamic dose–response relationship for an antihypertensive medication is the extent to which BP counterregulatory mechanisms are activated by BP lowering. Acute and chronic BP reductions often activate an interlinked series of mechanisms designed to restore BP. Reflex increases in cardiac output, peripheral vasoconstriction, and salt/water retention can result from baroreflex-mediated activation of the sympathetic nervous and RASs. These responses are most likely to occur when arterial dilator drugs (hydralazine, minoxidil, some calcium antagonists) or high-dose diuretics are used. Clinically, it can be difficult to gauge the extent to which counterregulatory systems are activated. A relatively reliable sign is an unexplained loss of previously established BP control. A clinically relevant increase in pulse rate (>10%) should prompt consideration of lowering the dose of the provoking agent or adding a β-blocker. Sodium retention, as a means by which BP control is lost, is easy to recognize if peripheral edema develops but sodium retention as a factor in loss of BP control can still occur without peripheral edema. If this is suspected, a diuretic can be started (or if one is already in use its dose can be increased) to effect a small weight loss.

Other physiologic adaptations. Some differences in responsiveness between acute and chronic dosing may occur as a result of metabolic changes or even changes in receptor density. True tachyphylaxis, in which enzyme induction increases drug metabolism, is generally not seen with antihypertensive drugs.

Duration of therapy. Very few long-term studies are available, but it appears that the full effects of some drugs may not be apparent until months or even years after therapy is begun. It has been speculated that favorable remodeling of the heart and blood vessels, a process that takes much longer than acute hemodynamic effects, can occur with certain agents. This view is consistent with the results of the Trial of the Prevention of Hypertension (TROPHY) study, where about 20% (2 mm Hg) of the effect of candesartan in prehypertension persisted 2 years after the drug was discontinued. Therefore, a dose–response relationship for an individual compound cannot be fully evaluated unless it is also considered as a function of time.

Impact of gaps in drug development

The drug approval process involves a complicated series of premarketing steps in which the manufacturer works with the United States Food and Drug Administration to demonstrate safety and efficacy of an experimental drug. Unfortunately, the rules for drug development have not been carefully scrutinized until relatively recently. In the process, it has become apparent that full dose ranges of approved agents have not been adequately investigated. This problem can influence the apparent risk-to-benefit ratio of a drug and affect prescribing habits.

Overdosing errors (lack of data on minimum therapeutic doses). Several antihypertensive medications were introduced at doses higher than those currently recommended, including thiazide diuretics, β-blockers, α-methyldopa, hydralazine,

and the ACE inhibitor captopril. In these cases, the failure to recognize the value of lower doses can be traced directly to a lack of data at the low end of the dose–response curves. A result of the administration of unnecessarily large doses of these medications is an impressive array of adverse effects, including proteinuria, dysgeusia, and leukopenia with captopril; sedation and depression with α-methyldopa; and a lupus-like syndrome associated with hydralazine. With thiazides, the use of lower doses, which are almost equally effective and are safer, was only determined by trial and error long after thiazides were approved for use.

Underdosing errors (lack of data on maximal therapeutic doses). Failure to explore the upper ranges of the dose–response relationship occurs commonly as well. There is a powerful reluctance of drug developers to push an investigational drug to its toxic limits for fear that development will be automatically terminated. In recent years, this problem has led to a consistent trend to underdose agents such as ARBs, which are yet to demonstrate toxic dose-dependent effects different from placebo.

Inadequate titration (failure to recognize dose-response effects). Characteristic dose–response relationships for many antihypertensive drugs have been artifactually masked during drug development and approval. This is because of the scientific inadequacy of typical end point–limited dose-titration trials. Such trials underrepresent the true "effective dose" (that meets a prespecified endpoint) and mix final results of lower and higher doses to determine overall efficacy. Because not all patients are tested at each dose (as would occur in a forced titration design), a false picture of the true dose–response relationship is created. The (heterogeneous) response to the lowest dose (including hyporesponders, normal responders, and hyperresponders) is relatively higher than the responses observed in subsequent dose titration steps that include predominantly individuals who are intrinsically more resistant to the drug. The result of this systematic selection bias is the appearance of an artifactually "flat" dose–response curve (i.e., a limited maximal effect or plateau). Such bias is amplified by the degree of heterogeneity of population responses (e.g., age- and race-dependent responses to ACE inhibitors and ARBs, which are erroneously believed to have essentially flat dose–response curves). Many of the pooled dosing studies on currently available ACE inhibitors and ARBs actually demonstrate an "inexplicable" reduction in BP effect at the highest tested dose—further evidence of the impact of dose-selection bias.

Inadequate 24-hour blood pressure control (inadequate trough doses). It is sometimes mistakenly assumed that the trough-to-peak effect ratio for a given drug is independent of dose. This is not the case, however, for many drugs, including ACE inhibitors, which tend to reach a plateau for peak effect at lower doses than those required to achieve a maximal trough effect.

Combination therapy

It has been recognized for decades that there is value to the use of drug combinations, not only to improve overall efficacy within and between individuals but also to reduce dose-dependent side effects.

Rationale. This notion was the foundation for the original triple-drug regimen of the 1970s (hydralazine, reserpine, and hydrochlorothiazide) and the stepped-care approach of the early Joint National Committee reports. Given the fact that multiple physiologic systems contribute to BP elevation and that most antihypertensive agents have a predominant (specific) mechanism of action related to one (or more) of these physiologic systems, it can be anticipated that multiple drugs will be needed to maintain BP control. Finally, it is generally recognized that "lower BP is better," yet most agents when used as monotherapy simply will not lower BP to optimal levels (ideally to ≤120/80 mm Hg, but at least to <140/90 mm Hg). Another feature of combination therapy that has received inadequate attention is the tendency for combinations, particularly those that use drugs with complementary mechanisms of action to reduce the population variation in responses, thereby increasing the predictability of response in diverse populations (**Figure C128.2**). The promptness of BP control is also improved, thereby reducing cardiovascular risk.

Fixed-dose combinations. Fixed-dose combination products were among the earliest effective oral antihypertensive agents, and many are still embraced by busy practitioners. Recent data demonstrate a rapid growth in the use of fixed-dose combinations because the efficacy and tolerability of these combinations are more acceptable now to both patients and practitioners. Given the relatively poor overall BP control rates, the potential to deliver simultaneously greater efficacy and safety, and the improved patient acceptance that they usually bring, fixed-dose products should be reconsidered for first-line therapy. Overall, combinations of a diuretic or calcium antagonist with an ACE inhibitor or ARB are very attractive two-drug combinations. The Avoiding Cardiovascular events through COMbination therapy in Patients Living with Systolic Hypertension (ACCOMPLISH) study will directly assess whether a diuretic or a calcium antagonist (or a calcium entry blocker) is the best drug to add to an ACE inhibitor.

Suggested Readings

Donnelly R, Elliott HL, Meredith PA. Concentration-effect analysis of antihypertensive drug response. Focus on calcium antagonists. *Clin Pharmacokinet* 1994;26:472–485.

Johnston GD. Dose-response relationships with antihypertensive drugs. *Pharmacol Ther* 1992;35:53–92.

Meredith PA, Elliot HL. Concentration-effect relationships and implications for trough-to-peak ratio. *Am J Hypertens* 1996;9:66S–70S.

Meredith PA, Reid JL. The use of pharmacodynamic and pharmacokinetic profiles in drug development for planning individual therapy. In: Laragh JH, Brenner BM, eds. *Hypertension: pathophysiology, diagnosis, and management*, 2nd ed. New York: Raven Press, 1995:2771–2783.

Sica DA. Rationale for fixed-dose combinations in the treatment of hypertension: the cycle repeats. *Drugs* 2002;62:443–462.

CHAPTER C129 ■ DRUG COMBINATIONS

ALAN H. GRADMAN, MD

KEY POINTS

- More than one drug is required to achieve goal blood pressure (BP) in the vast majority of hypertensive patients.
- Combining drugs that work by complementary pharmacologic mechanisms improves overall efficacy, speed of BP control, predictability, and tolerability.
- Fixed-drug combinations simplify treatment regimens and promote adherence.
- Most fixed-drug combinations include a diuretic or calcium channel blocker (CCB) with an angiotensin-converting enzyme (ACE) inhibitor, angiotensin receptor blocker (ARB), or β-blocker.

See also Chapters **C119** and C128

It is increasingly apparent that optimal strategies for sustained blood pressure (BP) control require the use of combinations of antihypertensive drugs.

Combination therapy in clinical trials

The major challenge in the contemporary treatment of hypertension is the prompt achievement and long-term maintenance of BP levels that are low enough to reduce the incidence of major cardiovascular (CV) endpoints. Controlled clinical trials, all of which are essentially combination drug trials, document that achieving the systolic and diastolic BP levels recommended by current guidelines is not possible with single agents; multidrug therapy has been necessary in approximately 75% of hypertensive individuals in these trials. In the Losartan Intervention for Endpoints (LIFE) trial in which treatment to goal (<140/90 mm

Hg) was aggressively pursued in >9,000 patients with left ventricular hypertrophy and an average baseline BP of 175/98 mm Hg, >90% required more than one antihypertensive agent. In Antihypertensive and Lipid-Lowering Treatment to Prevent Heart Attack Trial (ALLHAT), only 26% of subjects were at goal with a single agent. In patients with diabetes and renal insufficiency in whom BP targets are set lower (<130/80 mm Hg), more than three drugs were generally needed. In those with isolated systolic hypertension, achieving systolic BP levels <140 mm Hg necessitates the use of combination therapy in approximately two thirds of patients, and more than one third will require more than two drugs to reach goal.

Failure of single-drug regimens

Although considerable variation in individual response is observed in populations, most available drugs reduce diastolic BP by 4 to 8 mm Hg and systolic BP by 7 to 13 mm Hg when corrected for placebo effect. This magnitude of effect is insufficient to achieve goal BP in most hypertensive individuals. Furthermore a theoretical reduction in CV events by 50% would require a BP reduction of approximately 20/10 mm Hg based on worldwide observational studies.

There are several reasons for the therapeutic inadequacy of monotherapy. Reduction in BP by almost any pharmacologic approach activates counterregulatory mechanisms that oppose and thereby limit the action of the primary agent. Activation of "BP defense mechanisms" such as sympathetic nervous activation and renal salt and water retention counteract the effect of vasodilators. Concomitant conditions such as subclinical heart failure (HF), often unrecognized chronic kidney disease, or concurrent drug treatment (e.g., nonsteroidal anti-inflammatory agents) are other reasons for the limited ability of monotherapy to bring BP to goal.

Goals of combination therapy

The goals of combination drug therapy are to improve the long-term efficacy and tolerability of drug treatment, to facilitate the prompt achievement of target BP, and to increase predictability of responses in heterogeneous populations (see Chapter C128).
Efficacy. If the agents included in a combination additively reduce BP, BP goals will be met more often. Hypertension is typically a multifactorial problem and the exact pathophysiologic mechanisms operative in an individual patient are often obscure. Combining agents with complementary pharmacologic actions and targets can be expected to broaden the spectrum of response across a range of patient types, for example, those with high or low activity of the renin-angiotensin system. Particularly efficacious two-drug combinations include a thiazide diuretic (or calcium antagonist) together with an ACE inhibitor, angiotensin receptor blocker (ARB), or β-blocker .
Tolerability. Tolerability is improved if dose-dependent side effects (clinical or metabolic) are reduced by combining smaller doses of two drugs compared to using higher doses of individual agents. Most drugs exhibit parallel dose-response curves for their therapeutic and toxic effects (**Figure C128.1**). The degree to which these curves are separated constitutes the therapeutic index of the drug. If the curves are close together, increasing the BP response through dose titration leads to an increased frequency of side effects. Dose-dependent side effects are seen with all classes of antihypertensive agents except for angiotensin-converting enzyme (ACE) inhibitors and ARBs. Upward dose

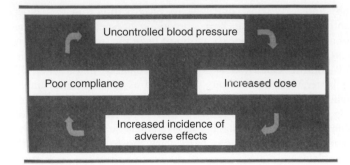

Figure C129.1 Potential consequences of monotherapy dose titration.

titration in an attempt to avoid the addition of a second agent is often a factor in the failure of monotherapy if side effects increase in the process (**Figure C129.1**). Appropriate combination therapy may also improve the tolerability of drugs included in the regimen if side effects associated with a particular drug are neutralized by the pharmacologic properties of a second agent. For example, the tendency for thiazides to cause hypokalemia is blunted by concomitant use of potassium-sparing diuretics, ACE inhibitors, or ARBs. Conversely, the combined use of drugs that may depress cardiac conduction, such as verapamil and β-blocker, should generally be avoided.
Prompt blood pressure control. Preventing CV complications necessitates timely control of elevated BP. Dose titration of individual agents is time consuming and often results in only modest additional BP reduction. In some cases, such as ACE inhibitors or ARBs, the dose–response curve is quite flat within individuals and titration is relatively ineffective. Early use of combination therapy reduces the need for multiple monotherapy titration steps and facilitates the more rapid attainment of target BP.
Predictability of response. Using drugs with complementary mechanisms of action increases the consistency of responses in heterogeneous populations. For example, a diuretic is somewhat more efficacious in a "low-renin" population (e.g., most older African Americans) and an ACE inhibitor is somewhat more efficacious in a "high-renin" population (e.g., obese young whites), the combination of diuretic and ACE inhibitor achieves equal BP control in both populations with less overall variability (see Chapter C128).

Fixed-dose combinations

Rationale. Traditional teaching has stressed avoidance of fixed-dose antihypertensive drug combinations based on the idea that maximum flexibility of dose titration should be maintained and that concomitant use of more than one medication makes it difficult to ascertain the cause of any side effect that may arise. There are certainly selected instances [e.g., patients with coronary artery disease (CAD) or HF, in whom the dose of β-blocker must be titrated to achieve a specific target heart rate] but in the vast majority of hypertensive patients, this consideration is of little importance. In contrast, the advantages of fixed-drug combinations are significant. The importance of partial or complete nonadherence to complicated multidose–multidrug regimens is an important factor in the failure of antihypertensive therapy; fixed-dose combinations simplify the therapeutic regimen and promote adherence. A consistent problem with fixed-dose products is cost, although generic competition eventually leads to lower prices. In some instances, costs to the patient may actually be less, based on the payment system being used. A final advantage derives from the fact that marketed fixed-drug combinations have been carefully studied and have received U.S. Food and Drug Administration (FDA) approval because they produce greater long-term BP reduction than monotherapy. Therefore, they constitute proven entities in comparison to randomly selected combinations of individual agents. A list of commonly used fixed-drug combinations is given in **Table C129.1**.

Clinical use. Fixed-dose combinations are most often used as the "second step" in patients who exhibit an inadequate response to the agent chosen initially. Low-dose combination therapy is an alternative strategy to the traditional approach of increasing the dose of the first drug until goal BP is reached or side effects supervene. Although the incremental reduction in BP is often not dissimilar, dose-dependent side effects are reduced, if not avoided, and the overall tolerability of treatment is improved.

Use of fixed-dose combinations is increasingly common as first-step therapy in hypertension. Recent developments make it now likely that many fixed-dose agents will receive indications for the initial treatment of hypertension. Several low-dose combinations, such as captopril and hydrochlorothiazide (HCTZ) and bisoprolol together with HCTZ have been approved by the FDA for this purpose. Fixed-dose combinations are most useful in patients with more severe hypertension in whom the likelihood is low that any single drug will achieve goal BP. JNC 7 recommended that combination drugs be used as first-line therapy in individuals with BP >20 mm Hg systolic or 10 mm Hg diastolic above goal. The initial use of a combination decreases the number of office visits and shortens the time period necessary to bring BP under control.

Importance of diuretics in combination therapy

There are many reasons to consider including a diuretic whenever combination therapy is required; these possibilities led the JNC 7 to recommend the use of thiazide diuretics *"alone or in combination for most"* hypertensives. Low-dose diuretics constitute an excellent therapeutic selection given their safety, efficacy, low cost, and proven ability to reduce clinical events. Unrecognized volume expansion is a common factor for the failure of monotherapy and the addition of a diuretic is frequently effective in countering this tendency. Diuretics offer additive BP-lowering effects when combined with many commonly used choices for initial therapy including ACE inhibitors, ARBs, and β-blockers. The combination of a diuretic and a calcium channel blocker (CCB) is less than additive in effect, perhaps because both increase renal sodium excretion (diuretic > CCB) and act as vasodilators (CCB > diuretic) in chronically lowering BP.

Specific combinations

Thiazides and potassium-sparing diuretics. Hypokalemia is an extremely important dose-related side effect of thiazide diuretics. Combining a thiazide with a potassium-sparing diuretic such as spironolactone, triamterene, or amiloride improves safety. Because of the greater incidence of hypokalemia and possible cardiac arrhythmias in susceptible subjects, HCTZ should be used at no more than 25 mg/day unless, perhaps, when combined with a potassium-sparing agent. The incremental reduction in BP from increasing the dose of HCTZ from 25 to 50 mg is minimal.

Thiazides with angiotensin-converting enzyme inhibitors or angiotensin receptor blockers. A large body of evidence supports the benefits of blocking the renin-angiotensin-aldosterone system (RAAS) on reducing clinical events, particularly in hypertensive patients with coexistent proteinuria, renal insufficiency, left ventricular hypertrophy, systolic dysfunction or established vascular or CAD. The combination of either an ACE inhibitor or an ARB with a low-dose diuretic is one of the most attractive approaches to contemporary combination therapy. The mechanisms of action of drugs included in these combinations are clearly complementary. Diuretics reduce intravascular volume, activating the RAAS. This results in vasoconstriction and a reduction in the magnitude of any observed BP reduction. In the presence of an ACE inhibitor or an ARB, activation of the RAAS is prevented, and the effects of combining these agents become additive. ACE inhibitor–thiazide and ARB-thiazide combinations are effective in black patients who, in general, demonstrate less BP reduction compared to whites when treated with ACE inhibitors or ARBs alone. Addition of an ACE inhibitor or ARB to a thiazide also tempers the degree to which serum potassium falls with diuretic therapy.

β-Blockers and thiazides. β-blockers are effective antihypertensive agents and are a preferred therapy in patients with ischemic heart disease. Their antihypertensive effects are mediated, in part, by suppression of renin release. Therefore, like the ACE inhibitors and ARBs, β-blockers attenuate the RAAS activation that accompanies the use of thiazide diuretics. Addition of diuretics also improves the effectiveness of β-blockers in blacks and others with low-renin forms of hypertension.

Calcium-channel blockers and angiotensin-converting enzyme inhibitors. CCBs are among the most potent antihypertensive agents and are an essential component of therapy in patients with very elevated BPs. When combined with ACE inhibitors, their BP-lowering effects are additive, and in the Anglo-Scandinavian Cardiac Outcomes Trial (ASCOT) was stopped prematurely because the combination of an ACE inhibitor and a CCB provided superior CV endpoint reduction compared to the combination of a β-blocker and a diuretic.

Addition of an ACE inhibitor significantly improves the tolerability profile of a CCB. ACE inhibitors can partially blunt the increases in heart rate that may accompany initiation of therapy with a dihydropyridine CCB and can neutralize (in part or completely) the edema occurring with a CCB, the most important dose-limiting side effect seen with these agents. In one study with felodipine, the incidence of edema was reduced from 10.8% to 4.1% by combining both classes of drugs. The cause for the edema produced by CCBs is believed to be arteriolar dilation without accompanying venular dilation, the result being an increased pressure gradient across capillary membranes in dependent portions of the body. Addition of an ACE inhibitor, by producing concurrent venodilation, reduces the pressure gradient and fluid transudation.

Calcium-channel blockers and angiotensin receptor blockers. Combinations of CCBs and ARBs have proved in clinical trials to be well tolerated and highly efficacious and promise to be useful additions to treatment choices for hypertension. There appears to be little difference in efficacy of ACE inhibitor–CCB combinations and ARB–CCB combinations but there may be a greater tendency for edema in the latter.

Calcium-channel blockers and β-blockers. This attractive combination is not available in the United States. β-Blockers lower BP by reducing cardiac output and renin release, whereas

TABLE C129.1

COMBINATION DRUGS FOR HYPERTENSION

Drug	Trade name
Thiazides and potassium-sparing diuretics	
Triamterene 37.5, 50.0, or 75.0 mg HCTZ 25 or 50 mg	Dyazide, Maxzide
Spironolactone 25 or 50 mg HCTZ 25 or 50 mg	Aldactazide
Amiloride 5 mg HCTZ 50 mg	Moduretic
ACE inhibitors and diuretics	
Benazepril 5, 10, or 20 HCTZ 6.25, 12.5 or 25 mg	Lotensin HCT
Captopril 25 or 50 mg HCTZ 15 or 25 mg	Capozide[a]
Enalapril 5 or 10 mg HCTZ 12.5 or 25 mg	Vaseretic
Lisinopril 10 or 20 mg HCTZ 12.5 or 25 mg	Prinzide, Zestoretic
ARBs and diuretics	
Candesartan 16 or 32 mg HCTZ 12.5 mg	Atacand HCT
Irbesartan 150 or 300 mg HCTZ 12.5 mg	Avalide
Losartan 50 or 100 mg HCTZ 12.5 or 25.0 mg	Hyzaar[a]
Telmisartan 40 or 80 mg HCTZ 12.5 mg	Micardis HCT
Valsartan 80, 160, or 320 mg HCTZ 12.5 mg or 25.0 mg	Diovan HCT
Olmesartan 20 or 40 mg HCTZ 12.5 or 25.0 mg	Benicar HCT
β-Blockers and diuretics	
Atenolol 50 or 100 mg Chlorthalidone 25 mg	Tenoretic
Bisoprolol 2.5, 5.0, or 10.0 mg HCTZ 6.5 mg	Ziac[a]
Metoprolol 50 or 100 mg HCTZ 25 or 50 mg	Lopressor HCT
Nadolol 40 or 60 mg Bendroflumethiazide 5 mg	Corzide
Propranolol 40 or 80 mg HCTZ 25 mg	Inderide
Propranolol (ER) 80, 120, 160 mg HCTZ 50 mg	Inderide LA
Timolol maleate, 10 mg/HCTZ, 25 mg	Timolide
CCBs and ACE inhibitors	
Amlodipine 2.5, 5.0, or 10.0 mg Benazepril 10, 20, or 40 mg	Lotrel
Felodipine (ER) 5 mg Enalapril 5 mg	Lexxel
Verapamil (ER) 180 or 240 mg Ttrandolapril 1, 2, or 4 mg	Tarka
CCBs and ARBs	
Amlodipine 5 or 10 mg Valsartan 160 or 320 mg	Exforge
Amlodipine 5 or 10 mg Olmesartan 20 or 40 mg	Azor

ACE, angiotensin-converting enzyme; ARBs, angiotensin receptor blockers; HCTZ, hydrochlorothiazide; CCBs, calcium channel blockers; ER, extended release.
[a]Approved by the U.S. Food and Drug Administration for initial therapy.
(Adapted from Joint National Committee on Prevention, Detection, Evaluation, and Treatment of High BP. The seventh report of the Joint National Committee on Prevention, Detection, Evaluation, and Treatment of High BP. *JAMA* 2003;289:2560–2572.)

dihydropyridine CCBs cause direct vasodilation. These complementary mechanisms results in fully additive BP reduction but addition of a thiazide diuretic is needed in some cases. A low-dose combination of felodipine extended release (ER) (2.5 mg) and metoprolol ER (25 mg) produced BP reduction comparable to maximum doses of each agent with an incidence of edema similar to placebo.

Angiotensin-converting enzyme inhibitors and angiotensin receptor blockers. ACE inhibitors and ARBs inhibit the RAAS by different pharmacologic mechanisms and their combination can result in additional BP reduction compared to monotherapy. A major problem with existing studies, however, is that submaximal doses of each agent have been combined. Even in the better studies, the combined effects are minimally additive compared to either agent combined with a diuretic or CCB, and this combination is generally not useful in managing difficult-to-control hypertension. Potential indications for ACE–ARB combinations are hypertension with proteinuric renal disease or HF due to systolic dysfunction. Clinical trials have yielded statistical benefits of the ACE–ARB combination in these conditions but it remains unclear whether the study designs allowed full optimization of doses of either component before combination.

Suggested Readings

Dahlof B, Sever PS, Poulter NR, et al. Prevention of cardiovascular events with an antihypertensive regimen of amlodipine adding perindopril as required versus atenolol adding bendroflumethiazide as required, in the Anglo-Scandinavian Cardiac Outcomes Trial-BP Lowering Arm (ASCOT-BPLA): a multicentre randomized controlled trial. *Lancet* 2005;366:895–906.

Fogari R, Zoppi A, Derosa G, et al. Effect of valsartan addition to amlodipine on ankle oedema and subcutaneous tissue pressure in hypertensive patients. *J Hum Hypertens* 2007;21(3):220–224.

Giles TD. Rationale for combination therapy as initial treatment for hypertension. *J Clin Hypertens* 2003;5(4 Suppl 3):4–11.

Gradman AH, Acevedo C. Evolving strategies for the use of combination therapy in hypertension. *Curr Hypertens Rep* 2002;4:343–349.

Gradman AH, Cutler NR, Davis PJ, et al Combined enalapril and felodipine extended release (ER) for systemic hypertension. *Am J Cardiol* 1997;79:431–435.

Kendall MJ. Approaches to meeting the criteria for fixed dose antihypertensive combinations. Focus on metoprolol. *Drugs* 1995;50:454–464.

Menard J, Bellet M. Calcium antagonists-ACE inhibitors combination therapy: objectives and methodology of clinical development. *J Cardiovasc Pharmacol* 1993;1:549–S54.

Neutel JM, Black HR, Weber MA. Combination therapy with diuretics: an evolution of understanding. *Am J Med* 1996;101:61S–70S.

Sica DA. Rationale for fixed-dose combinations in the treatment of hypertension: the cycle repeats. *Drugs* 2002;62:243–262.

Wolf G, Ritz E. Combination therapy with ACE inhibitors and angiotensin II receptor blockers to halt progression of chronic renal disease: pathophysiology and indications. *Kidney Int* 2005;67:799–812.

CHAPTER C130 ■ THIAZIDE AND LOOP DIURETICS

DOMENIC A. SICA, MD

KEY POINTS

- Thiazide diuretics are useful low-cost first-line agents in the treatment of systolic and diastolic hypertension that reduce cardiovascular (CV) morbidity and mortality.
- Benefits of thiazide diuretics are achieved at low doses [e.g., 12.5 mg to 25 mg of hydrochlorothiazide (HCTZ) or chlorthalidone daily].
- In combination with any other class of antihypertensive drugs, diuretics additively reduce blood pressure (BP).
- Mild biochemical abnormalities caused by low-dose diuretic therapy (hypokalemia, hyperglycemia, and hyperuricemia) are not associated with increased short-term mortality.
- Loop diuretics are not first-line therapy in hypertension and should be reserved for conditions with clinically significant fluid overload [e.g., renal failure, heart failure (HF), and fluid retention with vasodilator drugs, such as minoxidil].

See also Chapters **B100,** B102, C106, **C119,** and C166

Thiazide diuretics reduce extracellular fluid (ECF) volume, offset fluid retention caused by other drugs, and dilate peripheral arterioles on a long-term basis (**Table C130.1**). Loop diuretics are potent natriuretic agents that reduce both ECF volume and blood pressure (BP), particularly in conditions of reduced glomerular filtration, such as heart failure (HF) and renal failure.

THIAZIDES

Thiazide diuretics, initially used in the 1950s, were the first truly effective, well-tolerated, once-daily oral antihypertensive agents. Used alone or in combination with other antihypertensives, thiazides provide predictable and sustained antihypertensive effect in at least half of the hypertensive population, without serious side effects.

Mechanisms of action

The antihypertensive effect of thiazide and thiazide-like diuretics can be separated into acute, subacute, and chronic phases, corresponding roughly to 1 to 2 weeks, 4 to 8 weeks, and several months, respectively. Renal mechanisms are more prominent in the early phases, whereas vascular mechanisms predominate in the later phases.

Early renal (salt/water excretion) effects. Thiazide diuretics act by inhibiting the sodium $[Na^+]$/chloride $[Cl^-]$ reabsorption pump in the distal convoluted tubule, thereby increasing urinary excretion. In the acute phase, there is a variable, dose-dependent degree of ECF contraction but plasma volume returns to normal within several days. By increasing Na^+ availability at the distal tubule, thiazides lead to increased excretion of potassium (K^+) and magnesium. By a separate mechanism, thiazides decrease urinary calcium excretion; this feature distinguishes them from loop diuretics, which increase urinary calcium.

Chronic vascular (hemodynamic) effects. Early hemodynamic effects of thiazides include reduction in ECF volume, cardiac preload, and cardiac output. Chronically, however, as ECF and cardiac output return toward baseline, systemic vascular resistance decreases. In the "subacute" period between the acute and chronic phases, cardiac output and systemic resistance changes coexist but are in a transition state. The cellular mechanism for the relative vasodilation with thiazide-like diuretics remains unknown but is likely to involve alterations in vascular smooth muscle cell ion transport.

Outcome studies in hypertension

Early trials in diastolic hypertension. Diuretics were the foundation of an additive regimen used by the Veterans Administration (VA) Cooperative Study Group in the 1960s that convincingly proved the benefits of reducing BP. Both the first (diastolic ≥ 105 mm Hg) and second (diastolic, 90–104 mm Hg) VA trials demonstrated reduced cardiovascular (CV) morbidity and mortality with treatment. Subsequent trials over the next 2 decades followed the principle of "stepped-care" therapy (diuretic followed by adrenergic inhibitor, followed by vasodilator) first used in the VA studies. Beginning in the 1970s, this approach formed the basis for the seven reports of the Joint Committee on the Prevention, Detection, Evaluation, and Treatment of High Blood Pressure (JNC).

A meta-analysis of 18 trials and 48,220 patients has differentiated the effects of diuretics from β-blockers on health outcomes and found that low-dose diuretics are more effective than high-dose diuretics in the prevention of CV events. With low-dose diuretic therapy, stroke rates are reduced by 34%, coronary heart disease (CHD) by 28%, HF by 42%, total mortality by 10%, and CV mortality by 24%, all of which are statistically significant. High-dose diuretics also reduce strokes and HF.

Antihypertensive lipid-lowering heart attack trial study. The Antihypertensive Lipid-Lowering Treatment to Prevent Heart Attack (ALLHAT) Trial randomized >42,000 individuals with stage 1 or 2 hypertension to chlorthalidone, doxazosin, lisinopril, or amlodipine as initial treatment. Within 3 years, chlorthalidone proved to be superior to the α-blocker doxazosin with respect to the incidence of HF and this study arm was

stopped early for ethical reasons. At the end of the study in year 6, the remaining three arms were equivalent in their effect on the primary outcome [a composite of fatal CHD and nonfatal myocardial infarction (MI)]. Analysis of the secondary endpoints, however, demonstrated that chlorthalidone was superior to lisinopril at preventing stroke, likely related to superior BP control at the beginning of the study. Chlorthalidone was also superior to lisinopril and amlodipine in preventing HF within the first year but over the long term, both the angiotensin-converting enzyme (ACE) inhibitor and the diuretic reduced HF to a greater degree than amlodipine.

Isolated systolic hypertension. For the large majority of hypertensive patients, systolic BP is a better predictor of adverse outcomes than diastolic BP. The Systolic Hypertension in the Elderly Program (SHEP) in isolated systolic hypertension [(ISH), systolic BP ≥ 160, diastolic BP <90 mm Hg] studied the effects of chlorthalidone-based therapy compared to placebo on the incidence of stroke and other CV events over approximately 5 years. Chlorthalidone reduced the stroke rate by 36%, MI by 27%, HF by 54%, and overall CV morbidity by approximately 32%, all of which were highly statistically significant. In SHEP, the final achieved BP was 144/68, a reduction of 27/8 mm Hg from baseline (171/77 mm Hg) and 12/2 mm Hg lower than placebo.

Clinical use

Guidelines for the use of diuretics for the treatment of hypertension are provided in **Table C130.1**. Thiazide diuretics are among the most frequently prescribed antihypertensives. Hydrochlorothiazide (HCTZ) is the most commonly used agent, but chlorthalidone, metolazone, and numerous other thiazide-like diuretics provide similar antihypertensive effects.

Dosing. All thiazides can be given once daily, usually in the morning. It is now apparent that lower doses of thiazide diuretics than originally used are highly efficacious. In the elderly, a beginning dose of 12.5 mg and a maximum dose of 25 mg HCTZ (or its equivalent) are recommended. In the SHEP, 12.5 mg of chlorthalidone controlled >50% of patients for several years. In other groups of patients, it is rarely necessary or desirable to use ≥ 50 mg per day (or its equivalent) of a thiazide diuretic.

Efficacy: monotherapy versus combinations. The ability of diuretics to lower BP has been demonstrated in numerous clinical trials. As monotherapy, in low doses, diuretics control BP in approximately 50% of patients with stage 1 or early stage 2 hypertension. In combination with other drugs, diuretics can control up to 70% of patients. Diuretics can be successfully combined with β-blockers, ACE inhibitors, angiotensin receptor blockers (ARBs), centrally acting agents, renin inhibitors with roughly additive effects of the two individual components. In combination with calcium antagonists, the effects are incremental but not fully additive. In the VA monotherapy study, the combination of a diuretic with drugs from any other class provided the best antihypertensive effect as compared to combinations without a diuretic.

Population response patterns. Patient groups that exhibit a high degree of salt sensitivity (see Chapter B93), particularly the "low-renin groups" (e.g., blacks, the elderly, many diabetic patients), and those with relatively high cardiac output forms of hypertension (particularly obese individuals) respond particularly well to thiazide diuretic therapy. ISH is also usually responsive to thiazide therapy.

TABLE C130.1

DIURETIC DOSES AND CLINICAL USE

Drug	Trade name	Total daily doses (frequency)	Comments
Thiazide-type diuretics			
Chlorthalidone	Hygroton	12.5–50.0 (1)	More prolonged effect than hydrochlorothiazide
Hydrochlorothiazide	HydroDIURIL Microzide	12.5–50.0 (1)	
Indapamide	Lozol	1.25–5.0 (1)	
Metolazone	Zaroxylyn	2.5–10.0 (1)	Effective at glomerular filtration rate <40 mL, unlike other thiazide diuretics; very poor bioavailability
Metolazone	Mykrox	0.5–1.0 (1)	Improved bioavailability compared to metolazone (Zaroxylyn) results in lower dose being given
Loop diuretics			
Furosemide	Lasix	40–240 (2–3)	Shorter duration of action—multiple daily dosing to avoid rebound sodium retention
Bumetanide	Bumex	0.5–4.0 (2–3)	Same as furosemide
Torsemide	Demadex	5–100 (1–2)	Long duration of action
Ethacrynic acid	Edecrin	25–100 (2–3)	Only nonsulfonamide diuretic, ototoxicity

Dietary modifications. A low-sodium diet enhances the efficacy of diuretics and should be encouraged as an adjunctive measure. It is also generally recommended that hypertensive individuals should increase their daily intake of K^+, although it is unclear to what degree such an increase can fully overcome the kaliuretic effects of thiazides. Salt restriction can also have a modest but favorable effect on thiazide-induced kaliuresis.

Drug interactions. Beneficial interactions include a predictable, additive BP-lowering effect when thiazides are combined with other classes of antihypertensive agents. Adverse interactions include the blunting of thiazide effects by nonsteroidal antiinflammatory drugs and the potential to increase fatigue and lethargy, especially when combined with β-blockers. Thiazides also tend to exacerbate the hypokalemia induced by steroids or loop diuretics, although the latter interaction may be favorable in the treatment of hyperkalemia in HF, renal disease, or type IV renal tubular acidosis. Doses of lithium must usually be monitored closely in lithium-treated patients because thiazides can reduce lithium excretion.

Adverse effects

When diuretics were first introduced into clinical practice, high doses (up to 200 mg daily of HCTZ and chlorthalidone) were often used. With these doses came the potential for dangerous electrolyte changes; particularly hypokalemia. Many of these initial concerns are now less germane in that diuretics are now rather routinely given in much lower doses.

Volume depletion and hyponatremia. Severe volume depletion is uncommon with thiazide diuretics in ambulatory patients, particularly when low doses are used. Diuretic-related volume depletion becomes more pertinent when excessive fluid loss from other causes (e.g., vomiting, diarrhea, and malnutrition) has occurred and is more likely with loop diuretic therapy. Hyponatremia to dangerously low levels (<110 mEq/L) can occur in the setting of diuretic-induced volume contraction. This reaction is typically dose-dependent, more common in elderly women, and more apt to occur with thiazide than loop diuretics. Discontinuation of the diuretic, together with liberalization of

Na^+ intake and temporary restriction of water intake, corrects this abnormality. A diuretic can sometimes be restarted in such a patient; however, the dose should be reduced with careful monitoring for recurrence.

Hypokalemic alkalosis. Hypokalemia and "contraction alkalosis" may develop as a result of increased delivery of Na^+ and Cl^- to the distal nephron; together with increased levels of Na^+-retaining steroids, such as aldosterone, there is increased exchange of Na^+ for K^+ and hydrogen ions. Potassium loss occurs mostly in the first 3 to 7 days of diuretic therapy and thereafter tends to level off unless there is a particularly high Na^+ intake. Fewer than 10% of patients develop mild hypokalemia (serum K^+ values between 3–3.5 mmol/L with HCTZ doses in the order of 12.5–25 mg/day. The likelihood and the degree of hypokalemia can be further minimized by instituting a low Na^+/high K^+ diet. Other treatment strategies for diuretic-related hypokalemia include K^+ supplements or K^+ sparing diuretics.

A long-standing controversy persists about diuretic-induced hypokalemia and its potential association with ventricular arrhythmias and sudden cardiac death (SCD). Although a few studies in the early 1980s indicated a potential for arrhythmias in hypertensive subjects with diuretic-induced hypokalemia, many other studies, including ALLHAT, have been unable to substantiate the finding that small reductions in serum K^+ (<0.3 mmol/L) increase the risk of SCD. If hypokalemia does carry a cardiac risk, it is most likely in patients with myocardial ischemia, HF, or those being treated with digitalis preparations.

Lipids and glucose. Early trials suggested that thiazides modestly increase serum lipids, but in most of these studies, there was substantial long-term weight gain. In the ALLHAT study, minimally higher serum cholesterol was found in the chlorthalidone subgroup compared to either the lisinopril or amlodipine subgroups. Currently recommended doses of thiazides have a negligible effect on serum lipids.

Small changes in fasting glucose (~5 mg/dL) were seen with chlorthalidone in the ALLHAT study and the overall incidence of new-onset diabetes in the chlorthalidone group was 11.6% at the end of the study compared to approximately 8.1% with lisinopril and 9.8% with amlodipine, independent of serum K^+. The investigators argued that the absence of increased cardiovascular disease (CVD) endpoints after 4 to 6 years of chlorthalidone exonerates thiazides from any adverse role in promoting atherogenesis. Typically, however, diabetic CVD endpoints take approximately 2 decades to occur, so the significance of hyperglycemia induced by thiazides is not fully resolved.

Other complications. Thiazide-induced hyperuricemia relates to volume contraction and the competition of thiazides with uric acid for renal tubular secretion through the organic anion secretory pathway. In susceptible individuals, acute gouty arthritis may be precipitated with diuretic therapy, although it is not common. Lowering of serum magnesium (Mg^{2+}) with thiazides is fairly common, but the clinical significance of this finding is unclear; Mg^{2+} loss may increase the tendency toward hypokalemia and cardiac arrhythmias in patients with heart disease. In some hypokalemic patients, it is difficult to achieve normokalemia unless Mg^{2+} depletion is first treated. This, however, appears to be the case only at the extremes of Mg^{2+} depletion.

LOOP DIURETICS

Mechanisms of action

Tubular effects and hemodynamics. Loop diuretics (furosemide, ethacrynic acid, bumetanide, torsemide) act on membrane ion transport mechanisms in the thick ascending limb of the loop of Henle to prevent reabsorption of Cl^- and Na^+. These transporters are, to a degree, prostaglandin-sensitive; therefore, agents that interfere with prostaglandin synthesis (e.g., nonsteroidal antiinflammatory drugs) can blunt the tubular actions of loop diuretics. Loop diuretics are venodilators, accounting for their immediate preload-reducing effects in pulmonary edema. There is little arteriolar dilator effect of loop diuretics, so these agents are ineffective in reducing BP in the vast majority of individuals with hypertension.

Renal function and natriuresis

Normal renal function. When glomerular filtration rate is normal, a variety of mechanisms blunts the ability of loop agents to persistently reduce ECF volume or BP; in some cases, net volume expansion occurs as a result of stimulation of several reflex mechanisms. The initial diuresis (1–2 hours) with loop diuretics is typically followed by longer period of Na^+ retention that can result in neutral (or sometimes positive) Na^+ balance, even if the acute effect has been a significant initial natriuresis and diuresis. Mechanisms for this effect include altered intrarenal hemodynamics, tubular function, and stimulation of systemic "BP defense" mechanisms such as the renin-angiotensin and sympathetic nervous systems. Antinatriuresis is most commonly

seen with short-acting loop diuretics (furosemide), especially if given once daily.

Renal dysfunction. Loop diuretics provide consistent natriuresis and diuresis in patients with reduced glomerular filtration rates ($\leq$40–50 mL/minute) as may be seen with intrinsic renal disease or when renal blood flow is reduced in the advanced stages of HF. In these states, the renal and systemic antinatriuretic mechanisms are blunted. Loop diuretics also effectively reduce ECF volume and BP in hypertensive states marked by edema, as occurs in the nephrotic syndrome and with potent vasodilators such as minoxidil.

Practical pharmacology

Furosemide is relatively short-acting and may need to be used 2 to 3 times a day in some patients to achieve the desired effects. Torsemide has a prolonged duration of action (up to 24 hours) and may also exert weak direct vasodilator effects at nondiuretic doses. Torsemide is also distinctive among loop diuretics in that it is predictably well absorbed. In general, the adverse effects of loop diuretics are similar to those described for thiazide diuretics. Loop diuretics increase urinary calcium excretion and are not preferred agents in female patients with osteoporosis.

Suggested Readings

The Antihypertensive and Lipid-Lowering Treatment to Prevent Heart Attack Trial (ALLHAT). Major outcomes in high-risk patients randomized to angiotensin-converting enzyme inhibitor or calcium channel blocker versus diuretic. *JAMA* 2002;288:2981–2997.

Brater DC. Diuretic therapy. *N Engl J Med* 1998;339:387–395.

Freis ED. Critique of the clinical importance of diuretic-induced hypokalemia and elevated cholesterol level. *Arch Intern Med* 1989;149:2640–2648.

Kostis JB, Davis BR, Cutler J, et al. Prevention of heart failure by antihypertensive drug treatment in older persons with isolated systolic hypertension. *JAMA* 1997;278:212–216.

Kostis JB, Wilson AC, Freudenberger RS, et al. SHEP Collaborative Research Group. Long-term effect of diuretic-based therapy on fatal outcomes in subjects with isolated systolic hypertension with and without diabetes. *Am J Cardiol* 2005;95:29–35.

Moser M, Setaro JE. Antihypertensive drug therapy and regression of left ventricular hypertrophy: a review with a focus on diuretics. *Eur Heart J* 1991;12:1034–1039.

Psaty MB, Smith NL, Siscovick DS, et al. Health outcomes associated with antihypertensive therapies used as first line agents. *JAMA* 1997;277:739–745.

Sica DA. Diuretic-related side effects: development and treatment. *J Clin Hypertens (Greenwich)* 2004;6:532–540.

Turnbull F, Neal B, Algert C, et al. Blood Pressure Lowering Treatment Trialists' Collaboration. Effects of different blood pressure-lowering regimens on major cardiovascular events in individuals with and without diabetes mellitus: results of prospectively designed overviews of randomized trials. *Arch Intern Med* 2005;165:1410–1419.

Wu J, Kraja AT, Oberman A, et al. A summary of the effects of antihypertensive medications on measured blood pressure. *Am J Hypertens* 2005;18:935–942.

CHAPTER C131 ■ ALDOSTERONE BLOCKERS AND POTASSIUM-SPARING DIURETICS

MURRAY EPSTEIN, MD, FACP

KEY POINTS

- Aldosterone blockers provide effective antihypertensive treatment, especially in low-renin and salt-sensitive forms of hypertension.
- Newer, more selective aldosterone blockers (e.g., eplerenone) have fewer of the progestational and antiandrogenic effects than spironolactone, enhancing tolerability and potentially improving adherence to therapy.
- Aldosterone blockers provide an additional benefit in the treatment of heart failure when combined with angiotensin-converting enzyme (ACE) inhibitors, digoxin, and loop diuretics.
- Other potassium-sparing diuretics (amiloride or triamterene) are generally given for essential hypertension as a fixed-dose combination with hydrochlorothiazide (HCTZ).

See also Chapters A20 and **C167**

ALDOSTERONE BLOCKERS

Spironolactone, a nonselective aldosterone blocker, has been in clinical use for several decades. Owing to resurgent interest in aldosterone as a mediator of hypertension and cardiovascular disease, a selective aldosterone blocker (eplerenone) has been developed and is now in clinical use.

Rationale for aldosterone blockade

Hypertension. Aldosterone exerts multiple physiologic actions that raise blood pressure (BP), including mediation of increased extracellular fluid volume and promotion of vasoconstriction (Table C131.1). Aldosterone acts on mineralocorticoid receptors (MR) in epithelial cells in the distal tubule and collecting duct to promote sodium (Na^+) reabsorption and K^+ excretion.

Because aldosterone appears to constitute an important risk factor for cardiovascular disease, the use of aldosterone blockers, in addition to thiazides, angiotensin-converting enzyme (ACE) inhibitors, and angiotensin receptor blockers (ARBs) could provide additional benefit in the treatment of hypertensive end-organ damage. Thiazides increase aldosterone levels by reducing extracellular fluid volume; therefore the combination of thiazides and aldosterone antagonists has a rational basis. With drugs that block the formation or actions of angiotensin II (ACE inhibitors and ARBs), there is evidence that some patients may experience "aldosterone escape" during long-term treatment, in which aldosterone levels are initially suppressed but gradually return to baseline levels by mechanisms that remain to be fully elucidated. Spironolactone has additional renal effects: decreased urinary excretion of potassium (K^+), magnesium, and calcium.

Hypertensive end-organ damage. Pathophysiologic and outcome studies suggest another rationale for aldosterone blockade: prevention or reversal of cardiac target organ damage, especially fibrosis. In general, the endocrine/paracrine properties of aldosterone transduced through MR ("genomic effects") also affect function of the colon and exocrine (salivary and sweat) glands. In addition to the genomic effects of aldosterone, there are significant "nongenomic" effects in the heart, kidneys, and vasculature.

Heart failure. The renin-angiotensin-aldosterone system is markedly activated in heart failure and spironolactone and eplerenone have proved to be beneficial in reducing heart failure morbidity and mortality [Randomized Aldactone Evaluation Study (RALES) and Eplerenone Post-Acute Myocardial Infarction Heart Failure Efficacy and Survival Study (EPHESUS) trial, respectively] when added to standard therapy.

Vascular effects. In animal models, aldosterone blockade attenuates cardiac fibrosis in the damaged heart, reduces aortic fibrosis, and improves both large artery compliance as well as endothelial function. Clinical trials have shown that spironolactone reduces cardiac and vascular collagen turnover, improves reflex control (heart rate variability), reduces ventricular arrhythmias, improves endothelial function, and dilates blood vessels. In concert, these

PATHOPHYSIOLOGIC ACTIONS OF ALDOSTERONE THAT PROMOTE HYPERTENSION AND INCREASE CARDIOVASCULAR RISK

Sodium retention/volume expansion
Reduction in vascular compliance
Promotion of endothelial dysfunction
Upregulation of angiotensin II receptors
Potentiation of the pressor responses of angiotensin II
Increases in sodium influx in vascular smooth muscle cells
Fibrosis in the heart, kidneys, and vasculature
Activation of plasminogen-activator inhibitor-1
Stimulation of transforming growth factor β_1
Stimulation of reactive oxygen species
Hypertrophy of vascular smooth muscle cells and myocardial cells
Increase in blood lipid levels
Hypokalemia resulting in increased potential for cardiac arrhythmias, glucose intolerance, insulin resistance
Hypomagnesemia resulting in increased potential for cardiac arrhythmias

hemodynamic and humoral actions of aldosterone may translate into specific clinical benefits in hypertension and cardiovascular and renal diseases.

Proteinuria. Extensive preclinical and clinical evidence supports the efficacy of aldosterone blockers, when added to ACE inhibitors or ARBs, in attenuating proteinuria. These data suggest that aldosterone *per se* promotes renal injury; consequently add-on aldosterone blockade has the potential for attenuating renal injury.

Clinical use
Essential hypertension
Spironolactone. Spironolactone is indicated for treating hypertension and is particularly effective when given together with a thiazide-type diuretic. Similar to conventional thiazide-type or loop diuretics, aldosterone blockers provide effective antihypertensive treatment in most patients with low-renin forms of hypertension, particularly in blacks, the elderly, and many diabetic persons. Aldosterone blockers are also effective in the large subgroup of individuals with metabolic syndrome (obesity, hypertension, insulin resistance, dyslipidemia, accelerated

atherogenesis). Therefore, most hypertensive patients can be expected to have some level of response to aldosterone blockers.
Eplerenone. In developmental studies, the selective aldosterone blocker eplerenone safely and effectively lowered BP in patients with mild to moderate hypertension and diverse comorbidities, including left ventricular hypertrophy and diabetes mellitus. Eplerenone is indicated for hypertension and is equally effective in black and white patients. Eplerenone is effective and well tolerated when used alone or in combination with a variety of other agents, including ACE inhibitors, ARBs, calcium antagonists, and β-blockers.
Resistant hypertension. Aldosterone blockade has assumed an important role in the treatment of resistant hypertension, defined as failure to achieve goal BP despite treatment with full doses of three different antihypertensive agents, one of which is a diuretic. Several recent clinical studies indicate that aldosterone blockade provides significant incremental BP reduction when added to treatment regimens of patients with resistant hypertension. The dose range for spironolactone in these studies has typically been between 25 and 50 mg per day.
Hyperaldosteronism. Aldosterone blockers are effective in the therapy of various forms of hyperaldosteronism, including adrenal hyperplasia, adrenal adenoma, and glucocorticoid-remediable aldosteronism (GRA). Doses required in these conditions are often higher than those used in essential hypertension (Table C131.2).
Heart failure. In RALES, spironolactone was compared to placebo in its ability to reduce heart failure–related events. When given in addition to conventional therapy with ACE inhibitor, digoxin, and loop diuretic, spironolactone, 25 mg daily, reduced mortality and heart failure hospitalizations.

Applied pharmacology
Receptor pharmacology. Spironolactone is moderately more potent than eplerenone in competing for the mineralocorticoid receptor. Preclinical studies with eplerenone have demonstrated a >100-fold lower affinity for androgen and progesterone receptors than is the case for spironolactone and its active metabolite, canrenone.
Dosing. The recommended dosing range of spironolactone is 25 to 200 mg once or twice daily in mild to moderate hypertension, and that of eplerenone is a total dose of 50 to 100 mg given once or twice daily. Pharmacokinetic studies have not found any correlation between alterations in eplerenone disposition kinetics and degree of renal dysfunction. Spironolactone pharmacokinetics have not been examined in the setting of renal dysfunction.

DOSES OF ALDOSTERONE ANTAGONISTS IN VARIOUS CLINICAL CONDITIONS

Drug	Dosing frequency	Usual dose ranges (Total mg/d)		
		Essential hypertension	Hyperaldosteronism	Heart failure
Spironolactone (Aldactone)	q.d.–b.i.d.	25–200	50–200[a]	25–50
Eplerenone (Inspra)	q.d.–b.i.d.	50–100	—	—

[a]Similar doses may be effective in polycystic ovary syndrome, but the drug has not been approved specifically for that purpose.

Drug interactions. Favorable interactions include enhanced natriuresis and a potassium-sparing effect when aldosterone blockers are combined with loop or thiazide diuretics. Potentially unfavorable interactions include hyperkalemia when aldosterone antagonists are combined with ACE inhibitors or ARBs, particularly in patients who have renal insufficiency, diabetes mellitus, or hyporeninemic hypoaldosteronism (type IV renal tubular acidosis). Eplerenone should be used carefully with inhibitors of CYP3A4 activity (e.g., ketoconazole or verapamil) because its metabolism is CYP3A4 dependent.

Major adverse effects of mineralocorticoid receptor blockers

Sexual function. Although spironolactone is an effective antialdosterone agent, its use in patients is limited by its tendency to produce undesirable sexual side effects. At standard doses, impotence and gynecomastia are frequently noted in men, whereas premenopausal women may experience menstrual abnormalities. These adverse effects are due to the binding of spironolactone to progesterone and androgen receptors and represent a substantial reason for drug discontinuation. RALES reported a 10% incidence of gynecomastia or breast pain in its male subjects receiving 25 to 50 mg per day of spironolactone versus 1% on placebo ($p < .001$). The approval of the selective aldosterone blocker eplerenone provides a treatment with improved tolerability and reduced side effects. Consequently, eplerenone therapy should improve patient adherence with antialdosterone therapy compared to spironolactone.

Hyperkalemia. Particularly in the setting of reduced renal function (primarily chronic kidney disease and heart failure), potassium excretion is diminished. Another condition that predisposes to hyperkalemia is type IV renal tubular acidosis (hyporeninemic hypoaldosteronism) that is usually seen in long-standing diabetic patients. The obligatory tendency toward hyperkalemia in these conditions is further exacerbated by attenuation of aldosterone-dependent kaliuresis by MR blockade. In these conditions, careful monitoring of serum potassium, attention to dietary potassium restriction, and consideration for concomitant use of loop diuretics are important. Although untested formally, modest liberalization of sodium intake (to allow greater distal tubular sodium–potassium exchange) may also be useful.

OTHER POTASSIUM-SPARING DIURETICS

Other weaker diuretic compounds, such as amiloride and triamterene, can increase renal sodium excretion with relative potassium sparing. These agents tend to be relatively ineffective when used as monotherapy for hypertension but can be useful in combination with hydrochlorothiazide (HCTZ).

Amiloride

Mechanisms of action. Amiloride blocks epithelial sodium transport channels selectively. In the distal tubule, this action indirectly reduces aldosterone-sensitive sodium–potassium exchange and leads to increased urinary sodium excretion, with relative potassium sparing. Additional vasodilatory effects have been proposed. Comparing amiloride to MR antagonists, the former works at the basolateral membrane, whereas the latter works at the epithelial membrane and nuclear level.

Clinical use. In essential hypertension, amiloride is usually given as part of a fixed-dose combination with HCTZ. It is also sometimes used alone or in combination to treat GRA and other forms of hyperaldosteronism. Amiloride can be substituted for spironolactone when sexual side effects limit the use of the latter. Adverse effects with amiloride are usually mild and transient and typically include gastrointestinal discomfort or, occasionally, muscle cramps. Hyperkalemia can occur with amiloride particularly in patients with chronic kidney disease or in those receiving other compounds known to limit the renal excretion of potassium—such as ACE inhibitors, angiotensin receptor blockers, and nonsteroidal antiinflammatory drugs.

Triamterene

Triamterene also blocks epithelial sodium transport channels, although less avidly than amiloride. Used alone, triamterene has little effect on BP. Triamterene-thiazide combinations were extremely popular when it was believed that there was reduced potassium wasting when triamterene was added to thiazide (in doses of 50 mg daily or more). Because there is less potassium wasting with lower doses of thiazide (12.5–25 mg HCTZ), the use of triamterene combinations has waned. In clinical practice, gastrointestinal side effects sometimes limit its use. Triamterene is a weak folic acid antagonist, but megaloblastic anemia is rare. Triamterene is incompletely absorbed and can crystallize in the urine, potentially contributing to renal stone formation. Its use can be accompanied by an increase in serum concentrations or increased urinary uric acid excretion, requiring that it be used carefully, if at all, in patients with gout.

Suggested Readings

Calhoun DA. Use of aldosterone antagonists in resistant hypertension. *Prog Cardiovasc Dis* 2006;48:387–396.

Delyani JA. Mineralocorticoid receptor antagonists: the evolution of utility and pharmacology. *Kidney Int* 2000;57:1408–1411.

Epstein M. Aldosterone and the hypertensive kidney: its emerging role as a mediator of progressive renal dysfunction: a paradigm shift. *J Hypertens* 2001;19:829–842.

Epstein M. Aldosterone blockade: an emerging strategy for abrogating progressive renal disease. *Am J Med* 2006;119:912–919.

Epstein M, Williams GH, Weinberger M, et al. Selective aldosterone blockade with eplerenone reduces albuminuria in patients with type 2 diabetes. *Clin J Am Soc Nephrol* 2006;1:940–951.

Krum H, Nolly H, Workman D, et al. Efficacy of eplerenone added to renin-angiotensin blockade in hypertensive patients. *Hypertension* 2002;40:117–123.

Pitt B, Reichek N, Willenbrock R, et al. Effects of eplerenone, enalapril, and eplerenone/enalapril in patients with essential hypertension and left ventricular hypertrophy. The 4E-left ventricular hypertrophy study. *Circulation* 2003;108:1831–1838.

Pitt B, Zannad F, Remme WJ, et al. The effect of spironolactone on morbidity and mortality in patients with severe heart failure. *N Engl J Med* 1999;341:709–717.

Sica DA. Eplerenone: a new aldosterone receptor antagonist. Are the FDA's restrictions appropriate? *J Clin Hypertens (Greenwich)* 2002;4:441–445.

Weinberger MH, Roniker B, Krause SL, et al. Eplerenone, a selective aldosterone blocker, in mild-to-moderate hypertension. *Am J Hypertens* 2002;15:709–716.

CHAPTER C132 ▪ β-ADRENERGIC BLOCKERS

WILLIAM H. FRISHMAN, MD AND DOMENIC A. SICA, MD

KEY POINTS

- β-Blockers are appropriate for treatment of arterial hypertension, especially in patients who also have concomitant ischemic heart disease (IHD), heart failure (HF), or arrhythmias.
- β-Adrenergic blockers are highly heterogeneous with respect to various properties: degree of intrinsic sympathomimetic activity (ISA), membrane-stabilizing activity, $β_1$-selectivity, $α_1$-adrenergic blocking activity, solubilities and routes of systemic elimination, potencies, and duration of action.
- β-Adrenergic blockers reduce mortality and nonfatal reinfarction rates and improve clinical outcomes in patients with stable left ventricular dysfunction who are receiving conventional HF treatment.

See also Chapters A12, **B100,** and **C119**

β-Blockers are effective and safe and are widely used in the therapy for hypertension and other cardiovascular disorders.

Indications and outcome studies

Hypertension. The Seventh Report of the Joint National Committee on Prevention, Detection, Evaluation, and Treatment of High Blood Pressure (JNC 7) reiterated the recommendations of the previous JNC that β-adrenergic blockers are an appropriate first-line alternative in the treatment of hypertension. These recommendations were based on the reduction of morbidity and mortality in large clinical trials, but most of the benefit accrued to secondary cardiovascular protection (in established disease) rather than primary prevention of events. In the Antihypertensive and Lipid-Lowering Treatment to Prevent Heart Attack Trial (ALLHAT), β-blockers were used as second-line agents in combination with a diuretic, an angiotensin-converting enzyme (ACE) inhibitor, or a calcium channel blocker (CCB). Owing to the relative lack of evidence for primary prevention with β-blocker–based therapy, recent European guidelines suggest that these agents are best reserved for treatment of hypertensive patients with existing cardiovascular disease (CVD), especially those with ischemic heart disease (IHD), heart failure (HF), or certain arrhythmias. Of note, the apparent lack of effectiveness of β-adrenergic blockers in primary prevention has been attributed by some critics specifically to atenolol, the drug used most often worldwide. In that regard, almost all trials have employed atenolol once daily, a significant problem because the half-life of the drug is only 6 to 9 hours.

Angina pectoris. In the absence of contraindications, β-blockers are recommended as the initial therapy for long-term management of angina pectoris. In this regard, β-blockers provide similar clinical outcomes and fewer adverse events than CCBs

in randomized trials of patients who have stable angina. All β-blockers appear to be equally effective for relief of angina, probably due to a combination of heart rate control and blood pressure (BP) lowering. Combined therapy with nitrates and β-blockers may be more efficacious for the treatment of angina pectoris than the use of either drug alone. Combined therapy with β-blockers and CCBs may provide clinical benefit for patients with angina pectoris who remain symptomatic with either agent used alone.

Antiarrhythmic effects. The antiarrhythmic actions of β-blockers are considered to be a class effect but this categorization may be an oversimplification, especially for agents with intrinsic sympathomimetic activity (ISA) that may be less effective. β-Blockers alone and in combination with other antiarrhythmic drugs are important in the treatment of various cardiac arrhythmias, including ventricular tachyarrhythmias due to myocardial ischemia, mitral valve prolapse, and on occasion, atrial fibrillation. β-Blockers are also useful for treating symptomatic sinus tachycardia in patients with and without hypertension. Although β-blockers are not potent suppressors of premature ventricular contractions, they have been shown to reduce the incidence of sudden, presumably arrhythmic, death after myocardial infarction (MI).

Myocardial infarction. The 2001 American Heart Association and American College of Cardiology (AHA/ACC) guidelines for secondary prevention of MI recommend starting β-blockers in all post-MI patients and continuing therapy indefinitely. These recommendations are reiterated in JNC 7 and in the 2007 ACC/AHA guidelines for treatment of hypertension in IHD. The β-Blocker Heart Attack Trial (BHAT) using propranolol and the Norwegian Multicenter Study Group trial using timolol showed significant reductions in rates of mortality and/or reinfarction, but these studies did not include patients with symptomatic HF or those receiving contemporary HF therapies. Later trials, including the Survival and Ventricular Enlargement (SAVE) and the Acute Infarction Ramipril Efficacy (AIRE), showed that β-blockers provided an additional reduction in CVD mortality independent of ACE inhibitors. β-Blockers without ISA are the only agents conclusively shown to decrease the rate of sudden death, overall mortality, and recurrent MI in survivors of acute MI. Labetalol, the only β-blocker with significant α-blocking activity, has not been studied in the post-MI population. Carvedilol, which has weaker α-blocking activity than labetalol, reduced morbidity and mortality in the Carvedilol Postinfarct Survival Control in Left Ventricular Dysfunction (CAPRICORN) trial.

Heart failure. Two meta-analyses, each including more than 3,000 patients, evaluated HF trial results for numerous β-blockers including bisoprolol, bucindolol, carvediolol, metoprolol, and nebivolol. Both the meta-analyses showed a risk reduction for mortality, hospitalization for HF, and the combined endpoint of mortality and hospitalization. Several large trials have firmly established the benefits of β-blockers in HF, including the U.S. Carvedilol Program and three large mortality trials: the Metoprolol CR/XL Randomized Intevention Trial in Congestive Heart Failure (MERIT-HF), the Cardiac Insufficiency Bisoprolol Study II (CIBIS-II), and the Carvedilol Prospective Randomized Cumulative Survival (COPERNICUS) trial. In these studies demonstrating benefit, extended-release forms of the drugs were used or the shorter-acting agents were administered twice daily. There is currently not a single preferred β-blocker for the treatment of HF.

Antihypertensive mechanisms and pharmacokinetic differences

There is no consensus as to the mechanisms by which β-blocking drugs lower BP and it is likely that multiple modes of action (**Table C132.1**) are involved.

Drug differentiation

β-Adrenergic blocking drugs as a group have similar therapeutic effects despite their structural differences. Varied aromatic ring

TABLE C132.1

PROPOSED MECHANISMS TO EXPLAIN THE ANTIHYPERTENSIVE ACTIONS OF β-BLOCKERS

1. Reduction in heart rate and cardiac output
2. Central nervous system effect
3. Inhibition of renin release
4. Reduction in venous return and plasma volume
5. Reduction in peripheral vascular resistance (ISA drugs and α-, β-blockers)
6. Reduction in vasomotor tone
7. Improvement in vascular compliance
8. Resetting of baroreceptor levels
9. Effects on prejunctional β-receptors: reduction in norepinephrine release
10. Attenuation of pressor response to catecholamines with exercise and stress

(Modified from Frishman WH, Silverman R. Physiologic and metabolic effects. In: Frishman WH, ed. *Clinical Pharmacology of the β-Adrenoreceptor Blocking Drugs, 2nd ed.* Norwalk: Appleton-Century-Crofts, 1984:27–49.)

structures are the basis for variation in their pharmacokinetic differences, including completeness of gastrointestinal absorption, degree of first-pass hepatic metabolism, lipid solubility, protein binding, volume of distribution, penetration into the central nervous system, concentration in the myocardium, rate of hepatic biotransformation, pharmacologic activity of metabolites, and renal clearance. The relevance of these variations depends on the clinical conditions present in the individual being treated. In contrast to ACE inhibitors and angiotensin receptor blockers (ARBs), important differences in intrinsic chemical properties of β-adrenergic blocking drugs translate into significant clinical differences in effects (**Table C132.2**).

Solubility, elimination, and duration of effects. β-Blockers can be divided into two broad categories by their solubilities, which affect metabolism and elimination routes. Metabolism of β-blockers does not seem to be altered significantly by disease states and, in particular, by renal failure.

Lipid-soluble agents. Lipid-soluble agents are eliminated primarily by hepatic metabolism and tend to have relatively short plasma half-lives with wider variations in plasma concentrations. Propranolol and metoprolol are both lipid soluble, are almost completely absorbed by the small intestine, and are largely metabolized by the liver. They tend to have highly variable bioavailability and relatively short plasma half-lives. A lack of correlation between the duration of clinical pharmacologic effect and plasma half-life may explain why these drugs can be effective even when administered once or twice daily.

Water-soluble agents. Water-soluble agents (e.g., atenolol or nadolol) that are eliminated as intact molecules by the kidney tend to have longer half-lives and more stable plasma concentrations, potentially allowing once-daily administration. These agents are incompletely absorbed through the gut and are eliminated unchanged by the kidney. Differences do emerge when the durations of effect of individual β-blockers are compared (**Table C132.3**). Several β-blockers do not provide full 24-hour coverage (especially atenolol) and therefore often fail to adequately control BP for 24 hours or to be effective in blunting the early morning rise in BP. Dose titration is effective in some people, particularly in pulse-rate dependent forms of hypertension.

Extended-release formulations of carvedilol, metoprolol, and propranolol are available that allow effective, once-daily dosing of these drugs. There are also sustained and extended-release forms of propranolol indicated for nighttime dosing. Studies have shown that both long-acting propranolol and metoprolol provide much smoother daily plasma level curves than do comparable divided doses of conventional propranolol and metoprolol. Sublingual and nasal spray formulations that can provide immediate β-blockade are being tested in clinical trials. Ultra–short-acting β-blockers (esmolol) are available for use when a short duration of action is desired (e.g., in patients with questionable HF) or in the treatment of perioperative hypertension or supraventricular tachycardias. The short half-life (<15 minutes) relates to the rapid metabolism of the drug by blood and hepatic esterases.

β_1-Selectivity. Receptor selectivity has been used as a marketing theme for several β-blockers but the clinical relevance of this property is unclear. When used in very low doses (e.g., metoprolol 25 mg), β_1-selective blocking agents (atenolol, metoprolol, acebutolol, betaxolol, bisoprolol, and esmolol) inhibit cardiac β_1-receptors but have less influence on the β_2-receptors in bronchial and vascular smooth muscles (**Table C132.1**). In higher doses (e.g., metoprolol 50 mg/day or more), β_1-selective blocking agents also block β_2-receptors. Accordingly, β_1-selective agents

Part C: Clinical Management/Section IV: Antihypertensive Drugs

TABLE C132.2

PHARMACODYNAMIC PROPERTIES OF β-ADRENERGIC BLOCKING DRUGS USED IN HYPERTENSION

Drug	β_1-Blockade potency ratio (propranolol = 1.0)	Relative β_1-selectivity	Intrinsic sympathomimetic activity	Membrane-stabilizing activity
Acebutolol	0.3	+	+	+
Atenolol	1.0	++	0	0
Betaxolol	1.0	++	0	+
Bisoprolol[a]	10.0	++	0	0
Carteolol	10.0	0	+	0
Carvedilol[b]	10.0	0	0	++
Labetalol[c]	0.3	0	+	0
Metoprolol	1.0	++	0	0
Nadolol	1.0	0	0	0
Nebivolol[d]	10.0	++	0	0
Oxprenolol	0.5–1.0	0	+	+
Penbutolol	1.0	0	+	0
Pindolol	6.0	0	++	+
Propranolol	1.0	0	0	+
Sotalol	0.3	0	0	0
Timolol	0.6	0	0	0

+, modest effect; ++, strong effect; 0, no effect.
[a]Bisoprolol is also approved as a first-line antihypertensive therapy in combination with a very-low-dose diuretic.
[b]Carvedilol has peripheral vasodilating activity and additional α_1-adrenergic blocking activity.
[c]Labetalol has additional α_1-adrenergic blocking activity and direct vasodilatory activity (β_2-agonism); it is available for use in intravenous form for hypertensive emergencies.
[d]Nebivolol can augment vascular nitric oxide release.
(Adapted from Frishman WH. *Clinical Pharmacology of the β-Adrenoreceptor Blocking Drugs*, 2nd ed. Norwalk: Appleton-Century-Crofts, 1984.)

may be marginally safer than nonselective agents in patients with asthma or chronic obstructive pulmonary disease. A second theoretical advantage is that unlike nonselective β-blockers, β_1-selective blockers in low doses may not block the β_2-receptors that mediate dilatation of arterioles. This possibility remains unproven and β-blockers can be used in patients with peripheral vascular disease.

Intrinsic sympathomimetic activity or partial-agonist activity. Certain β-adrenergic receptor blockers (pindolol, acebutolol) are actually weak (partial) agonists that bind to β_1-adrenergic receptor sites, β_2-adrenergic receptor sites, or both. This combined action manifests itself as a neutral effect on heart rate when the sympathetic nervous system is not activated (e.g., supine rest) and as a blunted increase in heart rate when the sympathetic system is activated (e.g., exercise stress) (**Table C132.2**). In the treatment of patients with arrhythmias, angina pectoris of effort, or hypertension, drugs with mild-to-moderate ISA appear to be as efficacious as β-blockers lacking this property. β-Blocking agents with nonselective partial-agonist activity can reduce peripheral vascular resistance chronically and may also cause less depression of atrioventricular conduction. Marked tachycardia, tremor, and diaphoresis (epinephrine-like effects) can occur in patients with autonomic insufficiency who are given ISA drugs, but it is still debated whether the presence of ISA is clinically significant in routine clinical situations.

Combined α, β-adrenergic blocking activity. Labetalol, and to a much lesser extent carvedilol, are β-blockers that also antagonize α-adrenergic receptors. Like other β-blockers, they are useful in the treatment of hypertension and angina pectoris. However, unlike most β-blocking drugs, the additional α-adrenergic blocking actions lead to a reduction in peripheral vascular resistance that acts to maintain higher levels of cardiac output for a given level of BP. Clinically, the additional α-blockade may manifest itself as relative orthostatic intolerance, with an exaggerated postural decrease in BP.

Membrane-stabilizing activity. At concentrations well above therapeutic levels, certain β-blockers have a quinidine-like, local anesthetic membrane-stabilizing effect on the cardiac action potential that is potentially antiarrhythmic (**Table C132.2**). There is no evidence that MSA is responsible for any direct negative inotropic effect of the β-blockers on the usual dose range, but MSA may be responsible for myocardial depression in massive β-blocker intoxication.

Nitric oxide-releasing activity. Nebivolol, a β_1-selective blocker, has additional vasodilator actions related to an enhancement of nitric oxide activity. Whether this additional property in a β-blocker offers additional clinical benefits is yet to be determined.

Clinical usage

Blood pressure effects. Thirteen orally active β-adrenergic blockers are approved in the United States for the treatment of hypertension (**Tables C132.2 and C132.3**). In the usual prescribed dose, β-blockers have equivalent antihypertensive efficacy; however, a recent meta-analysis concluded that atenolol may have less protective effects on cardiovascular endpoints

TABLE C132.3

β-ADRENERGIC BLOCKING DRUGS: DOSES

Drug	Trade name	Usual range, mg (frequency/d)	Comment	Fixed-dose combination
Acebutolol	Sectral	200–800 (1)	β$_1$-selective, ISA	—
Atenolol	Tenormin	25–100 (1)	β$_1$-selective	Tenoretic
Betaxolol	Kerlone	10–20 (1)	β$_1$-selective	—
Bisoprolol	Zebeta	2.5–20.0 (1)	β$_1$-selective, indicated as first-step therapy as combination product	Ziac
Carteolol	Cartrol	2.5–10.0 (1)	—	—
Carvedilol	Coreg,	3.125–25.0 (1–2)	Combined α-, β-blocker, postural hypotension	—
	Coreg CR	10–80 (1)		
Labetalol	Normodyne, Trandate	100–400 (2)	Combined α,β-blocker, postural hypotension	—
Metoprolol	Lopressor, Toprol XL	25–200 (1,2)	β$_1$-selective, long-acting preparation available	—
Nadolol	Corgard	40–320 (1)	—	Corzide
Penbutolol	Levatol	10–20 (1)	—	—
Pindolol	Visken	5–15 (2)	ISA	—
Propranolol	Inderal, Inderal LA	10–240 (1–2)	Long-acting preparation available	Inderide
Timolol	Blocadren	20–60 (2)		Timolide

ISA, intrinsic sympathomimetic activity.

than other β-blockers. True dose equivalence among the various β-blockers has not been established. Uncommonly there is a paradoxical elevation of systolic pressure during β-blockade in persons with severe aortic arteriosclerosis, presumably due to the increased stroke volume caused by rate slowing in the setting of increased arterial stiffness. Escalating doses of β-blockers and combined α-, β-blockers can induce salt and water retention, making the addition of a diuretic necessary. Abrupt discontinuation of a β-blocker, particularly when administered in high doses, may be followed by tachycardia and angina in patients with coronary artery disease. Therefore, a step-wise reduction in dose is advised in all high-risk patients.

Response subgroups. There are few predictors of response to a β-blocker, but when hypertension is accompanied by a high pulse rate, the BP response is generally pronounced. β-Blockers are effective in hyperkinetic forms of hypertension as in individuals with a high "cardiac awareness profile" (somatic manifestations of anxiety, such as tremor, sweating, and tachycardia). There is a weak positive relationship between plasma renin activity and BP response to β-blockade. In small studies, individuals who responded to β-blockade also responded well to ACE inhibitor or ARB and less vigorously to diuretic or calcium antagonist. Certain patient subsets demonstrate lower response rates to β-blocker monotherapy, including those with low-renin hypertension and salt-sensitive individuals such as black hypertensive patients, but racial differences in the BP response to β-blockers are abolished by combination with a thiazide diuretic. Elderly and diabetic patients respond heterogeneously to β-blocker monotherapy.

Hypertensive urgencies and emergencies. In general, there is very little acute BP decrease when standard β-blockers are administered orally or parenterally. The notable exception to the rule is the combined α-, β-blocker labetalol, the only agent in the class indicated for parenteral management of hypertensive emergencies and for treatment of intraoperative and postoperative hypertension. Labetalol can also be used in its oral form to treat patients with hypertensive urgencies.

Other clinical uses. Orally active β-blockers are indicated for angina pectoris, hypertrophic cardiomyopathy, hyperdynamic

circulations, essential tremor, and migraine headaches and can be used with caution in pregnancy-associated hypertension. Some β-adrenergic blockers reduce the risk of mortality in survivors of acute MI and improve clinical outcomes in patients with HF. Although β-blockers reduce LV mass, they are generally less effective than other antihypertensives in this regard. Perioperative hypertension, which often has a hyperadrenergic component, may sometimes be effectively treated with β-blocker therapy. Whether these agents should be used "protectively" to reduce operative risk remains hotly debated, but their use in the preoperative period to protect high-risk patients undergoing noncardiac and cardiac surgery against myocardial ischemia has a theoretical rationale.

Combinations with other drugs. The antihypertensive effect of a β-blocker is fairly predictably enhanced by the simultaneous administration of a diuretic. Hydrochlorothiazide doses as low as 6.25 mg provide a substantial BP-lowering effect with a β-blocker and such additive effect has led to the approval of a combination of bisoprolol and hydrochlorothiazide as first-step therapy by the U.S. Food and Drug Administration. β-Blockers are also useful add-on therapy in the setting of vasodilator-related tachycardia, as may occur with hydralazine, minoxidil, and high-dose dihydropyridine CCBs.

Adverse effects and contraindications

Most β-adrenergic blockers, at least in the usual dose range, should not be used in patients with bronchospastic asthma, acutely decompensated HF, heart block (greater than first degree), or sick sinus syndrome. The drugs should be used with caution in insulin-dependent diabetes, because they may worsen glucose intolerance, mask the adrenergically driven symptoms of hypoglycemia, prolong recovery from hypoglycemia, or increase the magnitude of the hypertensive response to hypoglycemia. β-Blockers should not be discontinued abruptly in patients with known IHD. Long-acting dihydropyridines and nondihydropyridine agents are alternative drugs for relieving angina. Most β-blockers may increase plasma triglycerides and reduce high-density lipoprotein cholesterol levels. β-Blockers with ISA or α-blocking activity have little or no adverse effect on plasma lipids.

Combinations of diltiazem or verapamil with β-blockers may have additional depressant effects on the sinoatrial and atrioventricular nodes and may also promote negative inotropy. The addition of H_2-blocking agents to the combination of verapamil and β-blockers can also lead to myocardial depression. Combining a β-blocker and reserpine may result in marked bradycardia and syncope. Combination with phenylpropanolamine, pseudoephedrine, ephedrine, and epinephrine can cause significant elevations in BP due to unopposed α-receptor–induced vasoconstriction.

Suggested Readings

Abrams J, Frishman WH, Freedman J. Pharmacologic options for treatment of ischemic disease. In: Antman EM, ed. *Cardiovascular therapeutics*, 3rd ed. Philadelphia: Elsevier Science, 2007:77–120.

American College of Cardiology/American Heart Association. ACCAHA 2006 Guideline update on perioperative cardiovascular evaluation for noncardiac surgery: focused updated on perioperative beta blocker therapy. A report of the American College of Cardiology/American Heart Association Task Force on practice guidelines. *Circulation* 2006;113:2662–2674.

Bengtsson K, Melander O, Orho-Melander M, et al. Polymorphism in the β_1 adrenergic receptor gene and hypertension. *Circulation* 2001;104:187–190.

Devereux RB. Do antihypertensive drugs differ in their ability to regress left ventricular hypertrophy? *Circulation* 1997;95:1983–1985.

Frishman WH. Alpha and beta-adrenergic blocking drugs. In: Frishman WH, Sonnenblick EH, Sica D, eds. *Cardiovascular pharmacotherapeutics*, 2nd ed. New York: McGraw-Hill, 2002:67–97.

Frishman WH, Bryzinski BS, Coulson LR, et al. A multifactorial trial design to assess combination therapy in hypertension: treatment with bisoprolol and hydrochlorothiazide. *Arch Intern Med* 1994;154:1461–1468. [Published correction appears in 1995;155:709].

Frishman WH, Hainer JW, Sugg J. M-FACT Study Group. A factorial study of combination hypertension treatment with metoprolol succinate extended release and felodipine extended release. *Am J Hypertens* 2006;19:388–395.

Opie LH. Cardiovascular drug interactions. In: Frishman WH, Sonnenblick EH, Sica D, eds. *Cardiovascular pharmacotherapeutics*, 2nd ed. New York: McGraw-Hill, 2002:875–891.

Panjrath GS, Messerli FH. β-blockers for primary prevention in hypertension: era bygone? *Prog Cardiovasc Dis* 2006;49:76–87.

Reiter MJ. Cardiovascular drug class specificity: β-blockers. *Prog Cardiovasc Dis* 2004;47:11–33.

CHAPTER C133 ■ α-ADRENOCEPTOR ANTAGONISTS

JAMES L. POOL, MD

KEY POINTS

- Selective α_1-adrenoceptor antagonists lower blood pressure (BP) by blocking postsynaptic vasoconstrictor effects of norepinephrine.
- Hemodynamically, selective α_1-adrenoceptor inhibitors cause balanced arterial and venous dilation, with no increase in cardiac output, but tend to cause greater BP lowering in the upright compared to supine position.
- α_1-Adrenoceptor antagonists relieve lower urinary tract symptoms (LUTS) in patients with benign prostatic hyperplasia (BPH).
- α-Blockers are less effective than diuretics in reducing the incidence of heart failure.

See also Chapters A12 and C119

Several types of α-blocking drugs are used to treat hypertension and prostatism.

Selectivity of α-adrenoceptor antagonists

Clinically relevant α-adrenoceptor blockers can be classified according to their abilities to affect α_1 and α_2 receptor subtypes. In general, three subtypes exist: nonselective ($\alpha_1 + \alpha_2$) antagonists (phentolamine and phenoxybenzamine), selective presynaptic α_2-antagonists (yohimbine and rauwolscine), and selective postsynaptic α_1-antagonists (prazosin, terazosin, and doxazosin).

Selective α_1-antagonists. α_1-Receptors are predominantly located postsynaptically on vascular smooth muscle cells, where they mediate the vasoconstrictive action of norepinephrine (**Figure C133.1**). Prazosin, terazosin, and doxazosin are quinazoline compounds (**Table C133.1**) that are postsynaptic α_1-adrenoceptor antagonists approved for the treatment of hypertension. These drugs are highly selective for α_1-adrenoceptor subtypes (α_{1A}, α_{1B}, α_{1D}) and even when given in large doses, do not inhibit α_2-adrenoceptors, β-adrenoceptors, or the receptors for acetylcholine (muscarinic), dopamine, or 5-hydroxytryptamine.

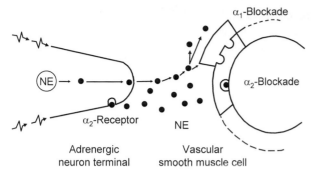

Figure C133.1 Mechanism of action of selective α₁-adrenoceptor blockade. NE, norepinephrine.

Nonselective α-antagonists. Nonselective agents are either competitive (phentolamine) or noncompetitive (phenoxybenzamine) with respect to receptor binding. Because α₂-adrenoceptors tonically inhibit neuronal norepinephrine release in the central nervous system (CNS) and periphery, nonspecific α-blockers (i.e., drugs with α₁ + α₂ antagonism) tend to increase sympathetic nervous outflow and neuronal norepinephrine release more than selective α₁-blockers. β-Adrenoceptor-mediated tachycardia and enhanced renin secretion occur with selective and nonselective agents. These properties help explain why nonselective α-blockers are not useful in the treatment of essential hypertension.

Selective α₂-antagonists. Selective blockade of presynaptic α₂-adrenoceptors with yohimbine increases blood pressure (BP) and heart rate; this agent is used occasionally in patients with autonomic insufficiency.

α-, β-adrenergic inhibitors. Labetalol, a nonselective β-blocker has demonstrable selective α₁-adrenoreceptor antagonist effects that are approximately 10% as potent as phentolamine. Carvedilol is another nonselective β-blocker with selective α₁-adrenoreceptor antagonist effects that are weaker than labetalol. Carvedilol, which is indicated for the treatment of heart failure and hypertension, acts predominantly as a β-blocker in clinical situations.

Diverse effects of α₁-receptors and antagonists

Blood pressure effects. Sympathetic overactivity in hypertension and accompanying excess stimulation of postsynaptic α₁-adrenoceptors is the core rationale for the use of selective α₁-adrenoceptor inhibitors as antihypertensive drugs. With these agents, the reduction in BP is achieved with little or no change in cardiac output because of balanced venous and arterial dilation. Favorable hemodynamic effects of selective α₁-inhibitors have also been demonstrated during exercise, when cardiac performance is better preserved with α₁-blockers than β-blockers.

Prostatism. α₁-Adrenoceptors regulate the degree of constriction of urinary tract sphincters. The sites of action of α₁-blockers when relieving lower urinary tract symptoms (LUTS) have not yet been established, but effects on prostatic and nonprostatic tissues are important. α₁-Adrenoceptors in the bladder, urethra, and vas deferens and in the CNS, ganglia and nerve terminals may all influence the clinical effects of α₁-blockers in LUTS.

Ventricular hypertrophy. Stimulation of cardiac α₁-adrenoceptors causes marked trophic effects, and regression of left ventricular hypertrophy has been reported with selective α₁-adrenoceptor inhibitors. Nevertheless, in clinical trials, α₁-blockers have not provided sustained morbidity or mortality benefit.

Heart failure: lack of effect. The Antihypertensive and Lipid-Lowering Treatment to Prevent Heart Attack Trial (ALLHAT) was completed with no significant difference in the primary endpoint [fatal congestive heart disease (CHD) and nonfatal myocardial infarction (MI)] among the four treatment groups—amlodipine, chlorthalidone, doxazosin, and lisinopril. However, the doxazosin arm (maximum dose 8 mg) was stopped prematurely because of (a) projected statistical futility to prove superiority to diuretic for the primary endpoint and (b) its lesser outcome benefit than chlorthalidone against secondary endpoints (25% higher incidence of combined cardiovascular disease and a twofold increased incidence of probable heart failure). Marginal positive results were found in retrospective analyses of the Valsartan Heart Failure Trial 2 (Val-HeFT2) study, in which α-blockade in combination with nitrates was beneficial in established heart failure.

Lipids. Although not specifically approved for dyslipidemia, selective α₁-adrenoceptor lowers total cholesterol by 2% to 3%, low-density lipoprotein (LDL) by 3% to 4%, and triglycerides by similar degrees while increasing high-density lipoprotein cholesterol. These effects are probably the result of several different mechanisms, including an increase in LDL cholesterol receptor number, a decrease in LDL cholesterol synthesis, stimulation of lipoprotein lipase activity, reduction of very low-density lipoprotein cholesterol synthesis and secretion, and a reduction in the absorption of dietary cholesterol. In addition, the 6-hydroxy and 7-hydroxy metabolites of doxazosin inhibit the oxidation of LDL cholesterol. The beneficial effects of α₁-blockers on lipids and glucose were observed in ALLHAT, although those who received doxazosin as initial therapy had more early cardiovascular events, especially heart failure. The rate of fatal and nonfatal MI (the primary endpoint) was not different in the doxazosin group.

Glucose tolerance. Another effect of selective α₁-inhibitors in hypertensive patients with insulin resistance, hyperglycemia, or noninsulin-dependent diabetes mellitus is an improvement in insulin sensitivity. There is usually a reduction in elevated serum insulin levels and a trend toward reduced fasting glucose levels. These "insulin sensitizing" effects are generally modest, however, and α₁-blockers are not specifically indicated for the treatment of hyperglycemic syndromes.

SELECTIVE α₁-ANTAGONISTS

Drug names	Dosing frequency	Starting dose (mg)[a]	Maintenance dose
Prazosin (Minipress)	b.i.d.–t.i.d.	1	5–10 mg twice daily
Doxazosin (Cardura)	q.d.–b.i.d.	1	4–16 mg once daily
Terazosin (Hytrin)	q.d.–b.i.d.	1	5–20 mg once daily

[a]A low starting dose is advised for these compounds to minimize the chance of postural hypotension or first-dose hypotension.

Treatment with selective α_1-blockers

Hypertension. Selective α_1-blockers (**Table C133.1**) have been shown to be effective antihypertensive agents, whether used as monotherapy or as part of a multidrug regimen. Age, race, and gender do not substantially influence BP responses to these agents. Approximately half of the essential hypertensive patients treated with α_1-blocker monotherapy achieve diastolic BPs <90 mm Hg, providing that adequate dosages are used. In large placebo-controlled studies, doxazosin or terazosin given once daily lowered BP by approximately 10/8 mm Hg in the standing position and by approximately 9/5 mm Hg in the supine position at 24 hours postdose.

Combination therapy. In general clinical practice, α_1-blockers have their widest application as a component of a multiple drug regimens for the treatment of stage 2 hypertension. They are useful adjuncts to achieve the lower BP targets needed (<130/80 mm Hg) in diabetes and chronic kidney disease (which often manifest increased sympathetic activity). Their effects are additive with angiotensin-converting enzyme (ACE) inhibitors, angiotensin receptor blockers, β-blockers, calcium channel blockers, diuretics, and direct-acting vasodilators. In the Anglo-Scandinavian Cardiac Outcomes Trial (ASCOT), subjects were assigned initially to either amlodipine 5 to 10 mg (N = 9,639), adding perindopril 4 to 8 mg as required to achieve <140/90 mm Hg, or to atenolol 50 to 100 mg (N = 9,618), adding bendroflumethiazide 1.5 to 2.5 mg as required. Long-acting doxazosin-gastrointestinal therapeutic system (GITS), a formulation not available in the United States, was added as a third-line agent to a total of 11,702 subjects on both regimens, with combined adjusted mean BP reductions of 11.4/6.4 mm Hg; 31% of randomized subjects reached the target BP after addition of doxazosin. For α_1-blockers to remain effective as monotherapy, they must usually be titrated to the high end of approved dose ranges (10–20 mg daily for prazosin or terazosin, 8–16 mg daily for doxazosin).

Diuretic therapy. Although less pronounced than with direct arterial vasodilators, α_1-blockers cause a degree of sodium and water retention in most patients. Concomitant use of a diuretic is almost always needed to sustain the antihypertensive effects of these drugs but also predisposes to a greater orthostatic BP decrease (lower upright than supine BP).

Pheochromocytoma and hypertensive crisis. Phentolamine, a parenteral drug, is used almost exclusively for emergent and urgent severe hypertension with excess catecholamine release. The oral, nonselective, and noncompetitive α-inhibitor phenoxybenzamine remains an important agent in the preoperative management of pheochromocytomas and cases of inoperable, metastatic pheochromocytoma.

Prostatism. α_1-Blockers, including alfuzosin and tamsulosin (which are not indicated for hypertension), are now widely used treatment for patients presenting with LUTS associated with benign prostatic hyperplasia (BPH) and bladder outlet obstruction.

Side effects

Selective α_1-antagonists are generally well tolerated with a shortlist of potential adverse effects including asthenia (2%), nasal congestion (2%), and dizziness (1%). The dizziness phenomenon with α_1-blockers is due in some cases to reduced cerebral blood flow and pressure in the upright position, especially when α_1-antagonists are used with diuretics (which further reduce cardiac preload). However, patients can experience dizziness without postural hypotension. There is also a significant "first-dose phenomenon" with severe hypotension after initial dosing, mostly with the short-acting α_1-blockers such as prazosin. The first-dose effect wanes rapidly, at least in part because of subsequent salt and water retention. Syncope is uncommon, occurring in <1% of patients when small doses (1 mg or less) are used initially but is also associated with addition of α_1-blockers to a multiple drug regimen (especially if a diuretic, β-blocker, or verapamil is being given). Individuals with alterations of urinary bladder function can develop incontinence with α_1-blocker-mediated relaxation of the bladder outlet. In placebo-controlled trials, small decreases in hemoglobin, white blood cell (WBC) count, total protein, and albumin levels have been attributed to hemodilution secondary to fluid retention.

Suggested Readings

ALLHAT Collaborative Research Group. Major cardiovascular events in hypertensive patients randomized to doxazosin vs. chlorthalidone: the antihypertensive and lipid-lowering treatment to prevent heart attack trial (ALLHAT). ALLHAT Collaborative Research Group. *JAMA* 2000;283:1967–1975.

Andersson KE. Alpha-adrenoceptors and benign prostatic hyperplasia: basic principles for treatment with alpha-adrenoceptor antagonists. *World J Urol* 2002;19:390–396.

Black HR, Keck M, Meredith P, et al. Controlled-release doxazosin as combination therapy in hypertension: the GATES study. *J Clin Hyp* 2006;8:159–166.

Cohn JN, Archibald DG, Ziesche S, et al. Effect of vasodilator therapy on mortality in chronic congestive heart failure. Results of a Veterans Administration Cooperative Study. *N Engl J Med* 1986;314:1547–1552.

Dahlof B, Sever PS, Poulter NR, et al. Prevention of cardiovascular events with an antihypertensive regimen of amlodipine adding perindopril as required versus atenolol adding bendroflumethiazide as required, in the Anglo-Scandinavian Cardiac Outcomes Trial-BP Lowering Arm (ASCOT-BPLA): a multicentre randomised controlled trial. *Lancet* 2005;366:895–906.

Frishman WH, Kotob F. Alpha-adrenergic blocking drugs in clinical medicine. *J Clin Pharmacol* 1999;39:7–16.

Guimaraes S, Moura D. Vascular adrenoceptors: an update. *Pharmacol Rev* 2001;53:319–356.

Kirby RS, Pool JL. Alpha-adrenoceptor blockade in the treatment of benign prostatic hyperplasia: past, present and future. *Br J Urol* 1997;80:521–532.

Roehrborn CG, Bartsch G, Kirby R, et al. Guidelines for the diagnosis and treatment of benign prostatic hyperplasia: a comparative, international overview. *Urology* 2001;58:642–650.

Sica DA, Pool JL. Current concepts of pharmacotherapy in hypertension—alpha-adrenergic blocking drugs: evolving role in clinical medicine. *J Clin Hypertens (Greenwich)* 2000;2:138–142.

Taylor AA, Pool JL. Clinical pharmacology of antihypertensive therapy. *Semin Nephrol* 2005;25:215–226.

CHAPTER C134 ■ CENTRAL AND PERIPHERAL SYMPATHOLYTICS

BARRY J. MATERSON, MD

KEY POINTS

- Central α_2-sympathetic agonists (methyldopa, guanabenz, guanfacine) reduce blood pressure (BP) by decreasing sympathetic nervous outflow, systemic vascular resistance, and heart rate.
- Clonidine is an agonist for both central α_2-adrenoceptors and I_1-imidazoline receptors; moxonidine and rilmenidine are predominantly I_1-receptor agonists with lesser α_2 effects.
- Central sympatholytics may be particularly useful in patients with concomitant anxiety, but major drawbacks include somnolence, dry mouth, rebound hypertension on withdrawal, and skin sensitivity reactions to transdermal delivery systems (clonidine).
- Peripheral sympatholytics (reserpine, guanethidine, guanadrel) deplete nerve terminal norepinephrine, decrease reflex peripheral arterial and venous constriction during upright posture, and predispose to orthostatic hypotension; sexual dysfunction and drug–drug interactions further limit their use.

See also Chapter A37

Drugs that reduce sympathetic neurotransmission were some of the earliest compounds used in hypertension. Despite their overall effectiveness in reducing blood pressure (BP), widespread clinical use remains limited by their high side effect profiles. All of the drugs of this class prescribed in the United States are available as generic preparations; ganglionic blocking agents are rarely used and are only available on a limited basis in the United States.

Central sympatholytics

Central sympatholytics (**Table C134.1**) directly reduce sympathetic outflow to the heart and blood vessels by their actions on brain stem sympathetic nervous control centers. They are particularly useful for patients who have hypertension with associated anxiety, especially that which is manifested by sympathetic overactivity. Central sympatholytics are often ineffective when used as single-drug therapy, in part due to salt and water retention; a thiazide-type diuretic is therefore a logical partner drug. Clonidine, the prototype of this class, was shown in the Veterans Affairs Cooperative Study to be somewhat more effective in whites than in blacks and is recognized as being more effective in older than in younger blacks.

Mechanisms of action

α_2-adrenoceptor stimulation. Stimulation of α_2-adrenoceptors in the rostral ventrolateral medulla (RVLM) nuclei in the brain stem inhibits sympathetic nervous outflow; subsequent reduction in peripheral sympathetic nerve activity causes a relative vasodilation, whereas reduced cardiac sympathetic nerve activity favors a decrease in heart rate. α-Methyldopa (which requires conversion to α-methylnorepinephrine), guanabenz, and guanfacine stimulate RVLM α_2-adrenoceptors but also inhibit noradrenergic nerves in the nucleus ceruleus, causing sedation; concomitant stimulation of α_2-receptors of the salivary glands causes dry mouth.

I_1-imidazoline receptor stimulation. Moxonidine and rilmenidine are relatively selective agonists for the I_1-imidazoline receptors of the RVLM and have less effect on the α_2-adrenoceptors. Nevertheless, they are not totally free from some sedation and dry mouth. Clonidine, the most widely used drug in this class, stimulates both the α_2-adrenoceptors and the I_1-imidazoline receptors. The physiologic effects of withdrawal of sympathetic nervous tone include parallel and balanced decreases in peripheral vascular resistance, heart rate, and systolic and diastolic BP.

Drug differentiation

Methyldopa. Methyldopa has a relatively slow onset of action and is primarily used to treat pregnancy-induced hypertension. Methyldopa is also a suitable alternative to clonidine in those patients in whom rebound hypertension or intolerable side effects occur. Treatment of hypertensive emergencies with intravenous methyldopa has been supplanted by more effective agents.

Hypersensitivity reactions, including hepatitis and Coombs-positive hemolytic anemia, have been seen with methyldopa but it is not necessary to stop methyldopa in patients who become Coombs positive but do not develop hemolytic anemia.

TABLE C134.1

CENTRAL SYMPATHOLYTICS: α_2-AGONISTS

Methyldopa	Aldomet	Oral: 125-, 250-, 500-mg tablets; oral suspension and parenteral (both 50 mg/mL); usual oral dose, 500–2,000 mg/d divided into two to four doses
Combinations	Aldoclor	Methyldopa + chlorothiazide
	Aldoril	Methyldopa + hydrochlorothiazide
Clonidine	Catapres	Oral: 0.1-, 0.2-, 0.3-mg tablets; usual dose, 0.2–0.6 mg in two doses
		Transdermal therapeutic system 1, 2, and 3 (containing 2.5, 5.0, and 7.5 mg, respectively); patch to be applied once weekly
Combination	Clorpres	Clonidine + chlorthalidone
Guanabenz	Wytensin	Oral: 4- and 8-mg tablets; usual dose, 8–32 mg/d in two doses
Guanfacine	Tenex	Oral: 1- and 2-mg tablets; usual dose, 1–2 mg at bedtime

Rare patients develop significant fever from methyldopa as well. Methyldopa and its metabolic products can interfere with some assays for catecholamines, which is less of a problem with the newer assays in use for catecholamine determination. Methyldopa can interfere with other therapeutic agents and its use with monoamine oxidase inhibitors is contraindicated due to the potential for hypertensive crisis.

Clonidine. Oral clonidine has a rapid onset of action (30–60 minutes) and is useful for managing hypertensive urgencies. An optional transdermal delivery system provides a constant dose of drug for 7 days, but takes 1 to 2 days to attain peak effect with BP effects lingering from 8 to 24 hours after the patch is removed. Best absorption from the patch occurs when it is placed on the chest or upper arm.

If high-dose clonidine (usually ≥ 1.0 mg, although sometimes lower) is used, sudden discontinuation can cause rebound hypertension with symptoms of excessive sympathetic discharge. Although much less common, rebound hypertension may also occur with the clonidine patch. Rebound hypertension may be accentuated if a β-blocker is used concomitantly. Skin hypersensitivity to the transdermal clonidine patch occurs in as many as 20% of patients.

Guanabenz. Guanabenz has limited clinical use but is somewhat similar to clonidine in its mechanisms and effects. It is somewhat longer acting and slightly less prone to rebound hypertension with sudden withdrawal. Efficacy can be less than clonidine in some patients but there is also less orthostatic hypotension.

Guanfacine. Guanfacine differs from the other members of this class in that its prolonged (24-hour) duration of action typically allows dosing to be once daily. Evening dosing is often recommended on the basis of the need for blunting the early morning surge in catecholamines and to utilize its mild sedative effects. As with other agents in this class, guanfacine works best when coadministered with a small dose of diuretic, which optimizes BP lowering with minimum central nervous system (CNS) adverse effects. Adverse effects increase significantly with doses >1 mg per day.

Imidazoline blockers. Moxonidine and rilmenidine are available in Europe, but not in the United States. Furthermore, the expectation that reduction of sympathetic outflow by use of moxonidine would benefit patients with heart failure was disproved in a clinical trial.

Adverse effects. Somnolence and dry mouth (40%) are the most common adverse drug reactions and the major reason central sympatholytics are discontinued. Other CNS depressants and ethanol enhance sedative effects. Dry mouth may be quite annoying to the patient, and decreased formation of saliva may increase the risk of dental caries and periodontal disease. Salivary substitutes may sometimes be needed in patients so affected.

Peripheral sympatholytics

Peripheral sympatholytics have a common mechanism of action that depletes norepinephrine at postganglionic sympathetic nerve endings. Reserpine has additional CNS mechanisms of action that other peripheral sympatholytics do not, so the adverse effects of all peripheral sympatholytics are not entirely comparable. Reserpine remains a widely used agent on a worldwide basis. Nevertheless, reserpine, guanethidine, and guanadrel have important and potentially dangerous interactions with other drugs that affect postganglionic catecholamine metabolism, and their use has decreased since the advent of more powerful and safer antihypertensive drugs. Guanadrel and guanethidine are only available on a limited basis.

Mechanisms of action. Drugs of this class work by entering sympathetic neurons through a catecholamine–hydrogen pump mechanism and displace norepinephrine from binding proteins in storage granules, exposing the catecholamine to oxidation. The result is intraneuronal norepinephrine depletion and reduced neurogenic vascular and cardiac tone. The ensuing reflex upregulation of peripheral adrenergic receptors in the catecholamine-depleted state leaves the individual predisposed to exaggerated pressor responses to endogenous and exogenous catecholamines and sympathomimetic agents. The ability to respond instantaneously to upright postural change with reflex peripheral vasoconstriction is also impaired, predisposing to orthostatic hypotension. In addition, reserpine depletes other tissue stores of catecholamines, including the heart, and reduces serotonin levels.

Drug differentiation. Reserpine is extremely long acting and can be an effective and very inexpensive antihypertensive agent in low doses (0.05 mg/day), especially when given with a diuretic. Most of its adverse effects occur with much higher dosage regimens. Guanethidine is difficult to titrate because of its wide therapeutic range, very long duration of action, and high rate of orthostatic symptoms. This compound is sufficiently potent that some cases of resistant hypertension can be resolved by the addition of as little as 10 mg of guanethidine. Guanadrel is shorter acting and easier to titrate than guanethidine and is observed to cause less diarrhea and orthostatic hypotension. Guanadrel is excreted renally and requires dosage adjustment in renally impaired patients. These drugs also typically cause dose-dependent salt and water retention, which attenuates their antihypertensive effect; therefore, diuretic add-on therapy is almost always necessary in their long-term use.

Adverse effects. Reserpine causes nasal stuffiness and has been associated with the development of depression. It can increase gastric acidity and the likelihood of acid-peptic disease and impact intestinal motility in such a way that ulcerative colitis may be worsened or biliary colic precipitated. Tricyclic antidepressants interfere with guanidine uptake by neurons and may decrease the hypotensive effect of guanethidine and guanadrel. If these drugs are added to monoamine oxidase inhibitors, a hypertensive crisis may be precipitated, so their use in Parkinson's disease is limited. Peripheral sympatholytics may also trigger a hypertensive crisis in the rare instance where an unrecognized pheochromocytoma is present. Frequent stools or diarrhea can be a problem with guanethidine, although less so with guanadrel. Retrograde ejaculation is another adverse reaction seen with these drugs.

Suggested Readings

Chobanian AV, Bakris GL, Black HR, et al. Seventh report of the Joint National Committee on Prevention, Detection, Evaluation, and Treatment of High BP. *Hypertension* 2003;42:1206–1252.

Cohn JN, Pfeffer MA, Rouleau J, et al. Adverse mortality effect of central sympathetic inhibition with sustained-release moxonidine in patients with heart failure (MOXCON). *Eur J Heart Fail* 2003;5:659–667.

Fenton C, Keating GM, Lyseng-Williamson KA. Moxonidine: a review of its use in essential hypertension. *Drugs* 2006;66:477–496.

Materson BJ. Combination therapy as the initial drug treatment for hypertension: when is it appropriate? *Am J Hypertens* 2001;14:293–295.

Materson BJ, Kessler WB, Alderman MH, et al. A multi-center, randomized, double-blind dose-response evaluation of step-2 guanfacine versus placebo in patients with mild-to-moderate hypertension. *Am J Cardiol* 1986;57:32E–37E.

Materson BJ, Reda DJ, Cushman WC, et al. Single-drug therapy for hypertension in men: a comparison of six antihypertensive drugs with placebo. *N Engl J Med* 1993;328:914–921.

Participating Veterans Administration Medical Centers. Low doses versus standard dose of reserpine: a randomized, double-blind, multi-clinic trial in patients taking chlorthalidone. *JAMA* 1982;248:2471–2477.

Veterans Administration Cooperative Study Group on Antihypertensive Agents. Multi-clinic controlled trial of bethanidine and guanethidine in severe hypertension. *Circulation* 1977;55:519–525.

CHAPTER C135 ◼ RENIN INHIBITORS

NORMAN K. HOLLENBERG, MD, PhD

KEY POINTS

- Inhibiting the action of renin blocks the renin-angiotensin-aldosterone system (RAAS) at its physiologic rate-limiting step.
- Renin inhibitors are effective, long-lasting antihypertensive agents with tolerability similar to other RAAS inhibitors.
- Ongoing clinical trials will prove whether this class of agents is effective in other cardiovascular or renal diseases.

See also Chapters **A13,** A16, A18, and C119

With the wide use of angiotensin-converting enzyme (ACE) inhibitors and angiotensin receptor blockers (ARBs), blockade of the renin-angiotensin-aldosterone system (RAAS) has come to play a central role in the management of hypertension. The newest RAAS blockers are part of the renin inhibitor class.

Comparing renin-angiotensin-aldosterone system blockers

Rationale for renin-angiotensin-aldosterone system blockade. Blockade of the RAAS results in a range of potential benefits, including favorable hemodynamic effects and prevention of angiotensin II (Ang II)-dependent generation of an array of potentially toxic factors, including proinflammatory cytokines, free oxygen radicals, and factors responsible for fibrosis at the tissue level (e.g., transforming growth factor β and plasminogen

activator inhibitor 1). Therefore, a reasonable goal is to render the RAAS system quiescent. During the last few years, attention has shifted from the question whether blocking the RAAS is useful in various patient populations to a new question: *How can we optimize blockade of the RAAS system?* Various studies have examined combinations of ACE inhibitor and ARB, very high-doses of ARBs, combinations of ACE inhibitor or ARB with a mineralocorticoid receptor antagonist, and most recently the utility of renin inhibition.

Rationale for renin inhibition. When the RAAS is blocked with an ACE inhibitor, the fall in Ang II within the kidney activates the short-feedback loop, causing a striking increase in the rate of formation and release of renin. This response, at least in part, offsets the useful actions of the ACE inhibitor or ARB.

It has been recognized for more than 50 years that a highly effective place to block the RAAS is at the interaction of renin with renin substrate [angiotensinogen (AGT)] because this is the physiologic rate-limiting step in the system. It is important to understand the concept of a "rate-limiting step;" although the idea of the lowest Km (the velocity an enzyme reaction) in a sequence can be difficult to conceptualize, the relationships become clearer if one looks at the actual concentrations of substrates and products in the renin cascade. The concentration of Ang I in the circulation is approximately double the concentration of Ang II. Therefore, there is a small gradient favoring conversion of Ang I to Ang II by ACE. In contrast, the concentration gradient between AGT and Ang I is almost 5,000:1. Clearly, if one wishes to most efficiently blunt the entire RAAS, an ideal location would be at the highest gradient in the cascade. The only class of agents that can render the RAAS fully quiescent is the renin inhibitor; the stoichiometry of a renin inhibitor is such that when adequate doses are given, there is sufficient renin inhibitor to block all renin that are present before therapy and those that are produced by the reactive (short feed-back loop) renin response.

Pharmacology

Early renin inhibitors were intravenous preparations that were capable of reducing angiotensin levels and blood pressure (BP) without any important adverse effects; these agents had relatively low potency, very poor oral bioavailability, a short duration of action, and a very high cost of synthesis. All these features made it unattractive to develop these compounds further. Aliskiren, an octanamide, is the first of a new class of nonpeptide, low-molecular weight, extremely active, transition-state renin inhibitors. These agents designed through molecular modeling are highly potent and very specific for human renin.

Pharmacokinetics. Aliskiren has very low bioavailability in the 2% to 3% range but is effective because of its considerable potency against human renin. After oral dosing, the plasma concentration of aliskiren peaks at 2 to 4 hours and exhibits a half-life in the range of 24 to 36 hours. Aliskiren modestly accumulates following daily administration. Ingestion of aliskiren with food reduces absorption but this effect is unlikely to be clinically meaningful. Aliskiren is not substantially cleared by the renal route; therefore, it does not require dosage adjustment on a pharmacokinetic basis when administered in the setting of renal failure.

Metabolism and drug interactions. On the basis of *in vitro* studies the CYP3A4 isozyme appears to be responsible for aliskiren metabolism, a finding that explains some of the drug–drug interactions with this compound: irbesartan decreases the maximum concentration [C_{max}] of aliskiren by 50%; when multiply dosed, coadministration of atorvastatin increases its C_{max} and area-under-the-curve (AUC) by 50%; aliskiren reduces the AUC and Cmax of furosemide by approximately 30% and 50%, respectively.

Pharmacodynamics

Animal models. The high specificity of aliskiren for primate renin has limited the studies that can be performed in animal models. Some studies have been performed in the sodium-depleted conscious marmosets, a primate model, where aliskiren reduced

BP strikingly for more than 24 hours without any effect on heart rate. There was the anticipated dose-related rise in active plasma renin concentration and suppression of plasma renin activity, indicative of renin inhibition. Despite the rise in plasma active renin, the concentrations of Ang I and Ang II remained very low, demonstrating effective RAAS blockade.

In double transgenic rats bearing the human renin and human AGT genes, it is possible to assess tissue injury with primate renin inhibitors. These rats, presumably as a by-product of their unusual renin state, develop severe hypertension and organ damage at a young age. Aliskiren, in this model, prolonged the survival with a fall in proteinuria as well as reduced tissue injury in the heart and kidney. Therefore, the preliminary data available from this model suggests that aliskiren has the potential to protect the heart and kidney from injury.

Clinical trials. There have been several BP trials in which aliskiren was compared either with placebo or an active control, including an ACE inhibitor, ARB, thiazide-type diuretic, and calcium channel blocker. Aliskiren proved to be as effective as the alternative agent and was very well tolerated in each of the studies. None of the clinical trials studied whether a specific patient population will show lesser or greater benefit beyond what might be derived from BP reduction alone. Ongoing studies are designed to address the efficacy of aliskiren in patients with diabetes mellitus, in those with proteinuria, in those with cardiovascular disease, and in the obese population. The current package label does not have this compound indicated in doses >300 mg.

Tolerability

Renin inhibitors, like other drugs that interfere with the RAAS system, are among the best-tolerated antihypertensives available. In the clinical studies to date, the most common adverse effect reported in aliskiren clinical trials is dose-related diarrhea, evident with daily doses of 600 mg. More complete RAAS blockade however, may bring about some problems such as effects on renal function or serum potassium concentration, especially in patients with diabetes mellitus, heart failure, or renal impairment.

Suggested Readings

Azizi M. Renin inhibition. *Curr Opin Nephrol Hypertens* 2006;15:505–510.
Azizi M, Web R, Nussberger J, et al. Renin inhibition with aliskiren: where are we now, and where are we going? *J Hypertens* 2006;24:243–256.
Cheng H, Harris RC. Potential side effects of renin inhibitors-mechanisms based on comparison with other renin-angiotensin blockers. *Expert Opin Drug Saf* 2006;5:631–641.
Fisher NDL, Hollenberg NK. Is there a future for renin inhibitors? *Expert Opin Investig Drugs* 2001;10:417–426.
Fisher NDL, Hollenberg NK. Renin inhibition: what are the therapeutic opportunities? *J Am Soc Nephrol* 2005;16:592–599.
Muller DN, Luft FC. Direct renin inhibition with aliskiren in hypertension and target organ damage. *Clin Am J Soc Nephrol* 2006;1:221–228.
O'Brien E. Aliskiren: a renin inhibitor offering a new approach for the treatment of hypertension. *Expert Opin Investig Drugs* 2006;15(10):1269–1277.
Staessen JA, Li Y, Richart T. Oral renin inhibitors. *Lancet* 2006;368:1449–1456.
Waldmeier FJ, Glaenzel U, Wirz B, et al. Absorption, distribution, metabolism and elimination of the direct renin inhibitor aliskiren in healthy volunteers. *Drug Metab Dispos* 2007;35(8):1418–1428.

CHAPTER C136 ■ ANGIOTENSIN-CONVERTING ENZYME INHIBITORS

DOMENIC A. SICA, MD

KEY POINTS

- All angiotensin-converting enzyme (ACE) inhibitors decrease production of angiotensin II, indirectly reduce sympathetic nervous system (SNS) activity, and increase bradykinin (BK) levels.
- Minor distinguishing features among ACE inhibitors include differing degrees of tissue binding and routes of elimination.
- ACE inhibitors slow the progression of target organ damage such as nephropathy (particularly with proteinuria), and heart failure (HF), while decreasing mortality in both the postmyocardial infarction and high-risk coronary artery disease patient.
- ACE inhibitor side effects include cough, angioedema, hyperkalemia, and a form of reversible functional renal insufficiency that derives from low renal perfusion pressure (HF and renal artery stenosis).

See also Chapters **A15,** A16, A18, **B100, C119,** C149, C151, C152, and C156

The pivotal role of angiotensin II (Ang II) in hypertension and end-organ disease derives not only from being a potent vasoconstrictor but also from activation of a wide range of neural, trophic, inflammatory, and procoagulant pathways. The utility of angiotensin-converting enzyme (ACE) inhibition is now well recognized and several ACE inhibitors are approved for various cardiac and renal conditions (**Table C136.1**).

Pharmacology

General. Ten ACE inhibitors are currently marketed in the United States (Tables **C136.1 and C136.2**). Although ACE inhibitors can be separated by differences in absorption, protein and tissue binding, half-life, and mode of disposition, all drugs in this class similarly reduce blood pressure (BP) at appropriate doses. With the exception of lisinopril and captopril, ACE inhibitors are prodrugs, which improves their absorption before hydrolysis to active diacids in the liver or intestine. ACE inhibitors structurally heterogeneous and are distinguished by having sulfhydryl (captopril), phosphinyl (fosinopril), or carboxyl (all other ACE inhibitors) side groups. ACE inhibitors localize (bind) to specific tissues in part related to their lipophilicity but whether greater tissue levels of lipophilic ACE inhibitors (e.g., quinapril or ramipril) offer any clinical benefit is unclear.

Class effect. Because there are few properties that definitively separate one ACE inhibitor from another, cost has become increasingly relevant. With no consensus definition of "class effect," it is unclear whether it is legitimate to switch from one compound in a class to another, especially when a higher-priced agent has been specifically studied in a disease state [e.g., heart failure (HF) or diabetic nephropathy]. Class effect seems to describe the pattern and degree of BP reduction with ACE inhibitors. For cardiovascular (CV) outcomes, however, equivalent doses have not been fully established for ACE inhibitors and substitution of one ACE inhibitor for another is at best done empirically.

Mechanisms of action

Neurohormonal effects. ACE is a pluripotent serine protease that catalyzes the conversion of angiotensin I (Ang I) to Ang II, while degrading bradykinin (BK) and other vasodilator peptides. ACE1 is identical to kininase II; therefore ACE inhibition also increases BK concentrations. An increase in BK stimulates the production of endothelium-derived relaxing factor (nitric oxide) and induces prostacyclin release, the result of which is vasodilation.

The degree of reduction in Ang II is an important but poorly defined factor in the chronic response to ACE inhibition. Long-term ACE inhibitor use has been associated in humans and animals with apparent "angiotensin-escape," (long-term return of plasma Ang II to pretreatment levels), ostensibly through generation of Ang II by non–ACE1-dependent pathways. Because of the negative feedback of Ang II on renin release, renin and Ang I concentrations increase during acute and chronic ACE inhibition, potentially providing additional substrate for ACE2 and other alternative pathway enzymes, such as chymases (see Chapter A16). The clinical relevance of these additional

TABLE C136.1

U.S. FOOD AND DRUG ADMINISTRATION–APPROVED INDICATIONS
FOR ANGIOTENSIN-CONVERTING ENZYME INHIBITORS

Drug	Hypertension	Heart failure	Diabetic nephropathy	High-risk cardiovascular disease
Captopril	●	● (Post-MI)[a]	●	
Benazepril	●			
Enalapril	●	●[b]		
Fosinopril	●	●		
Lisinopril	●	● (Post-MI)[a]		
Moexipril	●			
Perindopril	●			●[c]
Quinapril	●	●		
Ramipril	●	● (Post-MI)		●[c]
Trandolapril	●	● (Post-MI)		

MI, myocardial infarction.
[a]Captopril and lisinopril are indicated for heart failure treatment post–myocardial infarction and as adjunctive therapy for heart failure.
[b]Enalapril is indicated for high-risk individuals and for asymptomatic and symptomatic patients.
[c]On the basis of results of the Heart Outcomes Prevention Evaluation (HOPE) study and The European Trial on Reduction of Cardiac Events with Perindopril in Stable Coronary Artery Disease (EUROPA).

pathways is unclear, particularly because BP effects and beneficial outcomes with ACE inhibitors are so similar to those observed with angiotensin receptor blockers (ARBs).

Nonsteroidal anti-inflammatory drugs (NSAIDs) can blunt the BP-lowering effect of ACE inhibitors. Captopril may be more prone to an NSAID interaction because it directly stimulates prostaglandin synthesis. A portion of ACE inhibitor effect can be attributed to indirect reduction in sympathetic nervous system (SNS) activity. ACE inhibitors do not reduce resting plasma catecholamine concentrations but tend to blunt reflex sympathetic activation seen with volume depletion or vasodilating drugs.

Hemodynamic effects. ACE inhibition results in balanced reduction of cardiac preload (through their vasodilatory effects) and afterload (through direct and indirect arterial dilator effects). Because Ang II facilitates SNS activation, ACE inhibition tends to blunt stress-induced increases in catecholamines and heart rate. In hypertension, there is a modest reduction in systemic vascular resistance (SVR) without the reflex increase in cardiac output seen with arterial dilators. In HF, reductions in the very high SVR that characterize this syndrome allow partial normalization of reduced cardiac output, without increased myocardial oxygen consumption. The sympatholytic actions of ACE inhibitors may actually slow heart rate in HF, thereby increasing ventricular filling time and further improving contractile efficiency.

Hypertension

Blood pressure effects. BP responses to ACE inhibitors are comparable to that of most other drug classes, with response rates from 40% to 70% in stages 1 and 2 hypertension. On the basis of trials comparing trough:peak activity ratios with 24-hour ambulatory BP monitoring, several ACE inhibitors (fosinopril, lisinopril, perindopril, ramipril, and trandolapril) can be administered once daily.

Subgroups and response patterns. There is a limited relationship between plasma renin activity *per se* and the BP response to an ACE inhibitor. Certain patient subsets demonstrate lower response rates to ACE inhibitor monotherapy, including low-renin, salt-sensitive individuals (e.g., very elderly, diabetic, or black hypertensive persons). The low-renin state in elderly hypertensive patients is an exception in that it is not related to volume status. The elderly generally respond to ACE inhibitors, although reduced renal clearance sometimes leads to higher plasma concentrations. Black hypertensive patients are perceived as being less responsive to ACE inhibitors but this population is highly heterogeneous and includes many responders. Racial differences in BP response disappear when an ACE inhibitor is combined with a diuretic.

Dosing. If adequate doses of an ACE inhibitor are used, BP can be effectively lowered in many patients (**Table C136.2**) but the full ranges of ACE inhibitor doses have never been carefully studied. There is substantial variation between individuals and groups, as previously discussed. The dose–response curve for BP is steep at low doses and flat thereafter but not as flat as had been previously believed (see Chapter C128). Dose titration may help improve trough effects and prolong the duration of peak effect but has less impact on the peak effect itself. Duration of therapy also matters; recognition of the full BP response may require weeks or months. If a partial response to an ACE inhibitor occurs, therapy can be continued at a particular dose for a period of time. There is no evidence to support switching from an ACE inhibitor to an ARB if the former has failed. Of note, among antihypertensive compounds used to treat hypertension, the incidence of new-onset diabetes appears to be the lowest with ACE inhibitors and ARBs.

Combinations with other drugs

Diuretic or calcium antagonist. The antihypertensive effect of an ACE inhibitor is predictably enhanced by the coadministration of a diuretic or calcium antagonist. Fixed-dose combination products containing an ACE inhibitor and a diuretic capitalize on the rationale that sodium (Na^+) depletion activates the renin-angiotensin system (RAS) and thereby sensitizes the individual

TABLE C136.2

ANGIOTENSIN-CONVERTING ENZYME INHIBITORS: DOSAGE STRENGTHS AND TREATMENT GUIDELINES

Drug	Trade name	Usual total daily dose in hypertension (mg) (frequency/d)[a]	Usual total daily dose in heart failure (mg) (frequency/d)[a]	Comment	Fixed-dose combinations[b]
Benazepril	Lotensin	20–40 (1)	Not FDA approved for heart failure		Benazepril and hydrochloro-thiazide (Lotensin HCT)
Captopril	Capoten	75–300 (2–3)	18.75–150.00 (3)	Generically available	Captopril and hydrochloro-thiazide (Capozide[c])
Enalapril	Vasotec	5–40 (1–2)	5–40 (2)	Generic and intravenous	Enalapril and hydrochloro-thiazide (Vaseretic)
Fosinopril	Monopril	10–40 (1)	10–40 (1)	Renal and hepatic elimination	Fosinopril and hydrochloro-thiazide (Monopril-HCT)
Lisinopril	Prinivil, Zestril	10–40 (1)	5–20 (1)	Generically available	Lisinopril and hydrochlorothi-azide (Prinzide, Zestoretic)
Moexipril	Univasc	7.5–30.0 (1)	Not FDA approved for heart failure		Moexipril and hydrochloro-thiazide (Uniretic)
Perindopril	Aceon	4–16 (1)	Not FDA approved for heart failure	Indicated in high-risk vascular patients	
Quinapril	Accupril	20–80 (1)	10–40 (1–2)		Quinapril and hydrochloro-thiazide (Accuretic)
Ramipril	Altace	5–20 (1)	10 (2)	Indicated in high-risk vascular patients	
Trandolapril	Mavik	2–8 (1)	2–4 (1)	Renal and hepatic elimination	

FDA, U.S. Food and Drug Administration; HCT, hydrochlorothiazide.
[a]Lower doses are often recommended to initiate therapy. Higher doses are recommended for chronic therapy to provide full 24-hour coverage.
[b]Fixed-dose combinations in this class all contain a thiazide-type diuretic.
[c]Capozide is indicated for first-step treatment of hypertension.

to ACE inhibition. Diuretic doses as low as 6.25 mg of hydrochlorothiazide (HCT) can evoke this additive response, suggesting that even subtle alterations in Na$^+$ balance are sufficient to bolster the effect of ACE inhibitors. ACE inhibitors are also beneficially combined with calcium blockers, both in terms of increased efficacy and reduced edema.

Other combinations. Combining an ACE inhibitor and a β-blocker was at first considered useful because the β-blocker might blunt the hyperreninemia induced by an ACE inhibitor; however, in practice, only a marginal additional response occurs when these drug classes are combined. The combination of a peripheral α-antagonist and an ACE inhibitor will incrementally reduce BP but the combination of an ACE inhibitor and an ARB is not significantly better than either given alone at maximum doses.

Ischemic heart disease

The 2007 Scientific Statement of the American Heart Association and College of Cardiology on the treatment of hypertension in individuals with ischemic heart disease (IHD) recommends the use of ACE inhibitors for all forms of the syndrome, from high-risk individuals to those with known coronary artery disease (CAD) and HF (see Chapter C149).

Clinical trials. The Heart Outcomes Prevention Evaluation (HOPE) study comparing ramipril add-on (10 mg/day) to placebo in >9,500 high-risk patients was stopped early (after 4.5 years of treatment) because of a 22% reduction in relative risk of IHD endpoints in the ramipril group, with or without diuretic.

The individual components of the composite endpoint were also significantly reduced: 32% for stroke, 26% for CV death, and 20% for myocardial infarction (MI). The European Trial on Reduction of Cardiac Events with Perindopril in Stable Coronary Artery Disease (EUROPA) involved 12,218 patients with stable CAD randomized to ACE inhibitor (perindopril 8 mg/day) or placebo. After 4 years, perindopril reduced primary endpoint (CV disease, MI, or cardiac arrest) by 20% and the rate of fatal and nonfatal MI by 24%. The Prevention of Events with ACE Inhibition (PEACE) trial that added trandolapril (4 mg/day) to usual care in patients with stable CAD and preserved left ventricular function found no additional benefit of added ACE inhibition on CV death, MI, or coronary revascularization. In PEACE, however, subjects received highly effective background therapies (including aspirin and statins) and had very low event rates with or without ACE inhibition.

Clinical use. In HOPE, low-dose ACE inhibition (ramipril 2.5 mg/day) is ineffective in preventing CV events whereas higher doses (ramipril 10 mg) were beneficial. After MI, the patient must be first stabilized hemodynamically (i.e., without hypotension); a low dose of an oral ACE inhibitor should be initiated, generally within 24 hours of the event, particularly if the MI is anterior and associated with depressed left ventricular function with aggressive titration based on clinical status. Much of the positive hemodynamic effects and overall benefit of ACE inhibition are seen within the first month of therapy after an MI but do not appear to be related to a substantial decline in arrhythmia-related mortality.

Heart failure

Data from several placebo-controlled or open label trials have prompted a joint American College of Cardiology and American Heart Association task group to recommend ACE inhibitors as first-line agents in all stages of HF (see Chapter C151). ACE inhibitors improve exercise tolerance and symptomatology and substantially reduce the risk of death and hospitalization for HF. Statistically significant reductions in HF mortality have been observed with several ACE inhibitors including enalapril, captopril, ramipril, quinapril, trandolapril, and lisinopril.

Nephropathy. The collaborative study group of Lewis et al. and the Ramipril Efficacy In Nephropathy (REIN) study with ramipril demonstrated in diabetic patients and nondiabetic persons with renal involvement that ACE inhibitors effectively reduce both urine protein excretion and the rate of decline of renal function in excess of that expected with BP reduction alone. ACE inhibitors are of proven benefit in the setting of established insulin or noninsulin-dependent diabetic nephropathy, normotensive type 1 diabetes mellitus patients with microalbuminuria and a variety of nondiabetic renal diseases. Also, ACE inhibitors slow renal disease progression in blacks with hypertensive nephrosclerosis as demonstrated in the African-American Study of Kidney Disease (AASK).

Stroke. The Perindopril Protection against Recurrent Stroke Study (PROGRESS) reported that the *combination* of perindopril and indapamide reduced the recurrence of stroke in both normotensive and hypertensive patients; however, in this trial, stroke or CV disease reduction with perindopril alone was not significant, despite there being a several mm Hg reduction in BP. The absence of a stroke-protective effect with perindopril has been attributed to its marginally reducing BP and the low dose (2–4 mg) of perindopril used. The HOPE study, however, provided strong evidence that treatment with more appropriate doses of an ACE inhibitor (ramipril, 10 mg daily) substantially reduces the risk of stroke in high-risk cardiac patients. In contrast to these results is the Antihypertensive and Lipid Lowering Treatment to Prevent Heart Attack Trial (ALLHAT), which found that lisinopril-based treatment (without diuretic or calcium antagonist) was associated with a higher stroke rate in the entire study population (15%) and the black cohort (40%). These differences favoring diuretic over ACE inhibitor therapy relative to stroke, in part related to substantially inferior BP control with the latter and the failure of the study design to recapitulate standard medical practice. American Heart Association guidelines for the primary prevention of stroke recommend ramipril to prevent stroke in high-risk patients and in patients with diabetes and hypertension.

ACE inhibitors are effective antihypertensive agents and are particularly useful in hypertensive diabetic patients (with or without proteinuria) with a neutral, if not sometimes positive, effect on insulin resistance and hyperlipidemia. They are also useful in patients with isolated systolic hypertension or systolic-predominant forms of hypertension in that they improve vascular compliance. In patients with cerebrovascular disease, they preserve cerebral autoregulatory ability despite a reduction in BP. ACE inhibitors are not specific coronary vasodilators, but they do decrease myocardial oxygen consumption and thereby influence ischemia; therefore, they can be used effectively in patients with CAD.

Clinical usage

Nephropathy. ACE inhibitor regimens shown to slow the rate of chronic kidney disease (CKD) progression include captopril,

50 mg t.i.d.; enalapril, 20 mg per day; benazepril, 20 mg per day; and ramipril, 10 mg per day. It is presumed that renal failure increases the pharmacologic effect of these doses by reducing the renal clearance of the ACE inhibitor. Doses required to maximally reduce proteinuria may be greater than those needed to optimally lower BP.

Adverse effects

Renal function. A form of functional renal insufficiency has been observed with ACE inhibitors in patients with either a solitary kidney and high-grade renal artery stenosis or bilateral renal artery stenosis. This phenomenon occurs more commonly when conditions of dehydration, HF, and microvascular renal disease are superimposed on large vessel disease. The theme common to these conditions is one of reduced glomerular filtration pressures. When glomerular filtration pressures initially fall intrarenal production of Ang II increases, which supports glomerular filtration by efferent arteriolar constriction. The abrupt removal of Ang II, as occurs with ACE inhibitor therapy, relaxes efferent arterioles and thereby reduces glomerular pressure to a level too low to support filtration. Discontinuation of the ACE inhibitor or careful volume repletion usually corrects this problem.

Potassium. Hyperkalemia with ACE inhibitors generally arises only in predisposed patients with a reduced glomerular filtration rate or hypoaldosteronism (diabetics or HF patients with renal failure). Use of K+-sparing diuretics or K+ supplements increases the likelihood of hyperkalemia with an ACE inhibitor. Alternatively, ACE inhibitors minimize the fall in serum K+ produced by diuretics.

Cough. A dry, nonproductive cough can occur in patients treated with an ACE inhibitor. This is a *class effect* and has been attributed to increased levels of BK metabolites and other vasoactive peptides; therefore, once a cough has occurred with an ACE inhibitor switching to a different ACE inhibitor will not eliminate the cough. Typically, the cough disappears 1 to 2 weeks after discontinuation of the ACE inhibitor. ARBs can be considered in ACE inhibitor intolerant patients because this drug class does not have cough as an associated side effect.

Other. Angioneurotic edema is an unpredictable and potentially life-threatening complication of ACE inhibitor therapy, which fortunately is uncommon occurring in <1% of treated patients. It is approximately three times more common in blacks than in whites. Angioedema typically occurs shortly after beginning therapy with an ACE inhibitor, although it has also been seen years after beginning an ACE inhibitor. Angioneurotic edema has a distinctive pattern of involvement with severe swelling of the mouth, tongue, and upper airway and at its extreme can be life threatening. ACE inhibitors are contraindicated in pregnancy because they can also cause developmental defects if given in the second or third trimester of pregnancy but are not teratogenic *per se*.

Suggested Readings

Agodoa LY, Appel L, Bakris GL, et al. Effect of ramipril *versus* amlodipine on renal outcomes in hypertensive nephrosclerosis: a randomized controlled trial. *JAMA* 2001;285:2719–2728.

Casas JP, Chua W, Loukogeorgakis S, et al. Effect of inhibitors of the renin-angiotensin system and other antihypertensive drugs on renal outcomes: systematic review and meta-analysis. *Lancet* 2005;366:2026–2033.

Dzau VJ, Bernstein K, Celermajer D, et al. The relevance of tissue angiotensin-converting enzyme: manifestations in mechanistic and endpoint data. *Am J Cardiol* 2001;88:1L–20L.

Garg R, Yusuf S. Collaborative Group on ACE Inhibitor Trials. Overview of randomized trials of angiotensin-converting enzyme inhibitors on mortality and morbidity in patients with heart failure. *JAMA* 1995;273:1450–1456.

HFSA. Executive summary: HFSA 2006 comprehensive heart failure practice guideline. *J Card Fail* 2006;12:10–38.

Lewis EJ, Hunsicker LG, Bain RP, et al. The effect of angiotensin-converting enzyme inhibition on diabetic nephropathy. The Collaborative Study Group. *N Engl J Med* 1993;329:1456–1462.

Schoolwerth AC, Sica DA, Ballermann BJ, et al. Renal considerations in angiotensin converting enzyme inhibitor therapy: a statement for healthcare professionals from the Council on the Kidney in Cardiovascular Disease and the Council for High BP Research of the American Heart Association. *Circulation* 2001;104:1985–1991.

Schmieder RE, Hilgers KF, Schlaich MP, et al. Renin-angiotensin system and cardiovascular risk. *Lancet* 2007;369:1208–1219.

The SOLVD investigators. Effect of enalapril on survival in patients with reduced left ventricular ejection fractions and congestive heart failure. *N Engl J Med* 1991;325:293–302.

Yusuf S, Sleight P, Pogue J, et al. Effects of an angiotensin-converting enzyme inhibitor, ramipril, on cardiovascular events in high-risk patients. The Heart Outcomes Prevention Evaluation Study Investigators. *N Engl J Med* 2000;342:145–153.

CHAPTER C137 ■ ANGIOTENSIN RECEPTOR BLOCKERS

MICHAEL A. WEBER, MD

KEY POINTS

■ Angiotensin receptor blockers (ARBs) work primarily by selective blockade of AT_1 receptors; it remains unproved that agonist action of angiotensin II (Ang II) on unblocked vasodilatory AT_2 receptors enhances the antihypertensive and outcome effects of these agents.

■ ARBs are effective as monotherapy (especially in younger white subjects) but when combined with other antihypertensive agents (especially thiazide diuretics and calcium channel blockers) are effective in virtually all populations.

■ Positive outcome benefits with ARBs have been demonstrated in diabetic kidney disease, heart failure, ischemic heart disease, and stroke; this benefit pattern is similar to angiotensin-converting enzyme (ACE) inhibition.

■ ARBs reduce the incidence of atrial fibrillation and new-onset diabetes and favor regression of left ventricular hypertrophy.

See also Chapters **A17,** C119, C128, and C129

Angiotensin II receptor blockers (ARBs) are used primarily for the treatment of hypertension, although clinical trials have helped to define their use for such additional indications as heart failure, post–myocardial infarction, diabetic nephropathy, and stroke prevention. Because these drugs work by blocking the global effects of renin-angiotensin system activation, there was an early tendency to see them largely as better-tolerated alternatives to angiotensin-converting enzyme (ACE) inhibitors. It is now apparent that there are pharmacologic and clinical differences between these two classes.

Mechanisms of actions

Pharmacology. ARBs act by binding selectively to the angiotensin (Ang) AT_1 receptor. These nonpeptide oral agents can be either competitive (irbesartan, valsartan) or insurmountable (candesartan or the losartan metabolite Exp3174) receptor blockers. Some ARBs are prodrugs that depend on conversion to an active metabolite to produce most of their clinical effects. In the case of losartan and Exp3174, the parent compound also has some pharmacologic activity but because it is a much weaker agonist than its potent metabolite, its presence tends to diminish overall efficacy. Still, there is no evidence of meaningful clinical differences between drugs that work in their parent form and those that are prodrugs. ARBs have variable bioavailability, from 13% to 15% for eprosartan and candesartan to 60% to 80% for irbesartan. ARBs are generally administered once daily; minor pharmacokinetic differences exist among these agents but adequate doses of any of them produce reasonable 24-hour blood pressure (BP) control. There is also no evidence that any of the differing pharmacologic properties within the ARB class materially influence the outcome benefits if adequate doses are used.

Receptor subtypes. Four Ang II receptors have been described: AT$_1$, AT$_2$, AT$_3$, and AT$_4$ (see Chapter A17). So far, only the AT$_1$ and the AT$_2$ receptors have been well defined. The AT$_1$ receptor mediates most of the known physiologic actions of Ang II, including its hemodynamic and trophic effects. The AT$_2$ receptor is found primarily during fetal development and appears to mediate apoptosis and tissue remodeling/healing. Much of the time, AT$_2$ receptor expression is very low. Overall, the AT$_2$ receptor seems to have opposing or countervailing properties to the AT$_1$ receptor. Tissue culture studies have confirmed that AT$_1$ blockade reduces cell growth and that AT$_2$ blockade (with nonclinical experimental agents) increases cell growth. Simultaneous blockade of the AT$_1$ receptor and stimulation of the AT$_2$ receptor (the putative situation when an ARB is used) would, therefore, result in an enhanced antiproliferative effects. These interesting possibilities, which have yet to be fully defined in the clinical setting, are summarized in **Table C137.1**. It is possible that injurious stimuli such as high BP or other cardiovascular risk factors can evoke the expression of vascular AT$_2$ receptors, which would be expected to mediate vasodilation and inhibitory effects on cell growth. Recently, stimulation of AT$_2$ receptors has been shown to increase nitric oxide production and may even influence tissue kinin release.

Effects on renin-angiotensin-aldosterone system components. ARBs cause increases in plasma renin concentration, plasma renin activity, and circulating Ang I and Ang II concentrations, largely by inhibiting the negative feedback of Ang II on juxtaglomerular cells. The increased Ang II has no direct vasoconstrictive effect because the AT$_1$ receptor is blocked. Aldosterone levels tend to fall through AT$_1$ receptor blockade on adrenal zona glomerulosa cells, although this effect is surprisingly minimal.

Indications and outcome studies

Several clinical endpoint trials so far reported with ARBs indicate that they may provide outcomes benefits beyond their apparent clinically measured BP effects.

Hypertension

Losartan Intervention for Endpoint study. The Losartan Intervention for Endpoint (LIFE) study was a double-blind randomized trial in patients with left ventricular hypertrophy that compared 4,605 patients treated with losartan-based therapy to 4,588 patients on atenolol-based therapy. To achieve BP control, hydrochlorothiazide and other agents could be added to either drug. Despite virtually identical BP effects on brachial BPs (**Table C137.2**), losartan (compared to atenolol) reduced the primary composite endpoint (cardiovascular mortality, stroke, and myocardial infarction) by 13%, ($p = .021$), stroke by 25% ($p = .001$), new-onset diabetes by 25% ($p = .0001$), and permitted greater regression of left ventricular hypertrophy ($p = .001$). Those with diabetes at baseline (**Table C137.2**) had outcome benefits with losartan at least as great as the cohort as a whole. In the subgroup with isolated systolic hypertension, a marked beneficial effect of losartan was observed on the primary endpoint (25% reduction) and stroke (40% reduction) relative to atenolol. For reasons that are not clear, the losartan benefits in LIFE were not observed in the black study patients.

Valsartan Antihypertensive Long-Term Use Evaluation study. This valsartan-amlodipine comparison study in high-risk hypertensive patients was marred by design flaws affecting drug dosing that caused greater BP reduction in the amlodipine arm and a reduction in myocardial infarction in patients receiving this drug. However, when the two study arms were appropriately matched for BP, overall cardiac events, myocardial infarction, stroke, and mortality rates were similar but valsartan was associated with less heart failure and new-onset diabetes.

Diabetic nephropathy. The Reduction of Endpoints in NIDDM with the Angiotensin II Antagonist Losartan (RENAAL) study was a randomized double-blind placebo-controlled trial in hypertensive patients with diabetic nephropathy and albuminuria that compared the effects of losartan with conventional therapy (diuretics or β-blockers were primary agents; ACE inhibitors could not be used) in diabetic hypertensive patients with overt

---

TABLE C137.1

ANGIOTENSIN II RECEPTORS AND EFFECTS OF BLOCKADE

Vascular AT$_1$ receptors

  Constantly expressed
  Mediate vasoconstriction
  Mediate angiotensin II arterial wall growth effects

Vascular AT$_2$ receptors

  Expressed only after injury (sustained hypertension might provoke expression)
  Mediate vasodilation
  Mediate antiproliferative actions
  Activate other factors (e.g., nitric oxide, tissue kinins)

Potential double action of selective AT$_1$ blockers

  Directly block vasoconstrictor and growth actions of angiotensin II at AT$_1$ receptors
  Increase circulating angiotensin II levels
  Unblocked AT$_2$ receptors (if expressed), stimulated by increased angiotensin II activity, mediate vasodilation and growth inhibition
  Net effect: AT$_1$ blockade plus AT$_2$ stimulation

TABLE C137.2

LIFE STUDY[a]: ADJUSTED[b] HAZARD RATIOS (95% CONFIDENCE INTERVAL), LOSARTAN VERSUS ATENOLOL

	Whole study	Diabetic patients
Primary composite end point[c]	0.87 (0.77–0.98), $p = .021$	0.76 (0.58–0.98), $p = .031$
Cardiovascular mortality	0.89 (0.73–1.07), $p = .206$	0.63 (0.41–0.95), $p = .028$
Stroke	0.75 (0.63–0.88), $p = .001$	0.79 (0.55–1.14), $p = .204$
Myocardial infarction	1.07 (0.88–1.31), $p = .491$	0.83 (0.55–1.25), $p = .373$
New-onset diabetes	0.75 (0.63–0.88), $p = .001$	Not applicable

Total study: losartan (N = 4,605), atenolol (N = 4,588); diabetic patients: losartan (N = 586), atenolol (N = 609).
[a]Selected endpoints.
[b]For degree of left ventricular hypertrophy and Framingham risk score at baseline.
[c]Cardiovascular mortality, stroke, and myocardial infarction.

proteinuria (mean baseline albumin/creatinine ratio: 1,867 mg/g). Compared with conventional therapy over 3.5 years, losartan reduced the primary composite endpoint (doubling of serum creatinine, end-stage renal disease or death) by 16% ($p = .024$). Another study in diabetic nephropathy (baseline urinary albumin ~4 g/day), the Irbesartan type 2 Diabetic Nephropathy Trial (IDNT) compared irbesartan (150 or 300 mg daily) with conventional therapy and also with the calcium antagonist amlodipine (up to 10 mg daily) during a 3-year period. Despite similar brachial cuff BP reductions in the three groups, irbesartan reduced the primary composite endpoint (same as in RENAAL) by 20% ($p = .02$) compared with conventional treatment and by 23% ($p = .006$) compared with amlodipine.

Irbesartan MicroAlbuminuria-2 study. The Irbesartan Micro-Albuminuria 2 (IRMA 2) trial demonstrated that irbesartan 300 mg daily (but not 150 mg daily) was superior to conventional antihypertensive therapy during a 2-year period in preventing progression to overt nephropathy in type 2 diabetic hypertensive patients with microalbuminuria. Despite their clear renal protective effects, the three renal studies were not designed or powered to evaluate other cardiovascular endpoints.

Heart failure. Studies so far in heart failure have identified no meaningful differences between ARBs and ACE inhibitors on cardiovascular mortality and morbidity. In the Evaluation of Losartan in the Elderly (ELITE) Studies (I and II), outcome effects of losartan were not different from ACE inhibition in heart failure. The Valsartan Heart Failure Trial (ValHEFT) provided an indication for valsartan in the management of heart failure; the magnitude of benefit in those intolerant to ACE inhibitor was similar to that achieved with ACE inhibitors in general. The Candesartan in Heart Failure—Assessment of Mortality and Morbidity (CHARM) Alternative Study led to a heart failure indication for candesartan, again with benefits similar to those seen with ACE inhibitors.

Given that the doses employed in existing clinical trials were not always maximal, it remains unclear whether giving ARBs and ACE inhibitors in combination could confer additional benefits in heart failure. It appears most likely that the two drug types are best regarded as alternatives to each other. This conclusion is supported by the results of the Valsartan in Acute Myocardial Infarction (VALIANT) trial, conducted in patients with left ventricular systolic dysfunction following myocardial infarction, which showed similar effects of valsartan, captopril, and the combination valsartan–captopril on the primary mortality endpoint. In the CHARM-Preserved Study in patients with diastolic heart failure (preserved systolic function), there was a trend toward reduced heart failure hospitalizations with candesartan.

Atrial fibrillation. In the LIFE study, compared with β-blocker treatment, losartan reduced new-onset atrial fibrillation events by approximately one third. Moreover, in a study of patients whose atrial fibrillation was converted electrically or pharmacologically to sinus rhythm, irbesartan was significantly more effective than placebo in preventing recurrence of the arrhythmia.

Stroke. In addition to the LIFE study demonstrating stroke benefit of losartan, the Morbidity and Mortality After Stroke—Eprosartan versus Nitrendipine for Secondary Prevention (MOSES) trial demonstrated that eprosartan reduced recurrent stroke rates in hypertensive patients with a history of ischemic strokes to a greater degree than the dihydropyridine nitrendipine (previously demonstrated to confer primary stroke prevention in hypertension) despite equivalent effects on brachial cuff BP.

Clinical usage

Blood pressure effects. ARBs have antihypertensive efficacy comparable to other major antihypertensive drug classes. Some of the principal properties of these agents, together with information about dosing, are summarized in **Table C137.3**.

Dose–response effects are less pronounced with ARBs and the difference in BP-lowering efficacy between the usual starting doses and the maximum doses is often only 4 to 8 mm Hg, although there is considerable population heterogeneity in the peak dose–response (see chapter C127). As a practical matter, this property adds to the convenience of using these agents because for most of them there is at most a one-step titration regimen. The lack of dose-dependent side effects should encourage use of higher doses.

TABLE C137.3

AVAILABLE ANGIOTENSIN RECEPTOR BLOCKERS

Generic	Brand	Half-life (H)	Usual dose range[a] (mg)	Comments
Losartan	Cozaar; Hyzaar[b]	2	50–100	Active metabolite (E-3174), losartan is uricosuric, labeled indication in type 2 diabetic nephropathy
Valsartan	Diovan; Diovan HCT[b]	6	80–320	Labeled indication in congestive heart failure
Irbesartan	Avapro; Avalide[b]	11–15	150–300	Labeled indication in type 2 diabetic nephropathy
Eprosartan	Teveten	5–9	400–800	May have inhibitory effect on the sympathetic nervous system
Telmisartan	Micardis; Micardis HCT[b]	24	40–80	Dose-dependent bioavailability of 42%–58%, volume of distribution of 500 L
Candesartan cilexetil	Atacand; Atacand HCT	9–13	8–32	Active metabolite candesartan
Olmesartan medoxomil	Benicar	13	20–40	Active metabolite olmesartan

[a] Angiotensin receptor blockers are administered once daily although their effect may wane at the end of the dose interval occasionally requiring a second dose.
[b] Combination products containing hydrochlorothiazide.

Response variability. Some clinical trials have demonstrated differences in antihypertensive efficacy among these agents but it is important to recognize that such differences may be influenced partly by the populations chosen, dietary salt consumption, or selection of doses. ARBs appear to have equal BP effects in younger and older patients as well as in men and women. As with the ACE inhibitors, ARBs appear to have less monotherapeutic efficacy in black patients than in white. It is possible that this is an issue of dosing, for some of the early data with tasosartan (an effective ARB that was withdrawn because of a safety concern) suggested that black patients required doses approximately three times as high as white patients to achieve comparable BP responses. This is an important issue; as these drugs are used for a wider range of cardiovascular and diabetic disorders it is critical to ensure that their potential cardiovascular and renal protective effects are made available to all population groups. Racial differences in BP response are nonexistent when ARBs are combined with thiazide diuretics, an important factor in view of the growing routine use of two-drug fixed-dose combinations.

Combination with other drugs. Combinations of ARBs with diuretics are very efficacious, as are combinations with calcium channel blockers. Because of the difference in pharmacologic properties between the ACE inhibitors and ARBs, there has been interest in the possibility that they may provide effective combination therapy. Preliminary data have shown that reduction of proteinuria with combination treatment may be more effective than with either agent alone. Likewise, the ValHEFT and CHARM-Added studies also indicated that, under certain circumstances, combination therapy may be more effective than single-drug therapy, at least when usual clinical doses are employed. Results with BP have been mixed: early studies with losartan suggested that minimal additional BP-lowering effects were obtained when it was combined with an ACE inhibitor. When lisinopril was combined with irbesartan, the two drugs in usual clinical doses had similar antihypertensive effects, but their combination had a greater effect on BP than either alone. The current ONgoing Telmisartan Alone and in Combination with Ramipril Global Endpoint Trial (ONTARGET) clinical outcomes study in patients with previous histories or current evidence of disease factors that heighten cardiovascular risk is comparing ramipril with telmisartan and with the combination of the two

drugs. This trial will be reported in 2008 and could add important information about the indications for ARB therapy.

Adverse effects

One of the principal attributes of ARBs is the absence of dose-related symptomatic and metabolic adverse events. The incidence of side effects is not different from that in placebo-treated patients; in fact, the incidence of headache in clinical trials is usually higher with placebo than with ARBs. Cough is much less common than with ACE inhibitors but, like the ACE inhibitors, ARBs are contraindicated in pregnancy due to the potential for fetal abnormalities.

Suggested Readings

Brenner BM, Cooper ME, de Zeeuw D, et al. Effects of losartan on renal and cardiovascular outcomes in patients with type 2 diabetes and nephropathy. *N Engl J Med* 2001;345:861–869.

Cohn JN, Tognoni G, The Valsartan Heart Failure Trial Investigators. A randomized trial of the angiotensin-receptor blocker valsartan in chronic heart failure. *N Engl J Med* 2001;345:1667–1675.

Dahlof B, Devereux RB, Kjeldsen SE, et al. LIFE Study Group. Cardiovascular morbidity and mortality in the Losartan Intervention For End point reduction in hypertension Study (LIFE): a randomized trial against atenolol. *Lancet* 2002;359:995–1003.

Lewis EJ, Hunsicker LG, Clarke WR, et al. Renoprotective effect of the angiotensin-receptor antagonist irbesartan in patients with nephropathy due to type 2 diabetes. *N Engl J Med* 2001;345:51–60.

Parving HH, Lehnert H, Brochner-Mortensen J, et al. The effect of irbesartan on the development of diabetic nephropathy in patients with type 2 diabetes. *N Engl J Med* 2001;345:870–878.

Pitt B, Poole-Wilson PA, Segal R, et al. Effect of losartan compared with captopril on mortality in patients with symptomatic heart failure: randomized trial — the losartan heart failure survival study ELITE II. *Lancet* 2000;355:1582–1587.

Schrader J, Luders S, Kulschewski A, et al. MOSES Study Group. Morbidity and mortality after stroke, eprosartan compared with nitrendipine for secondary prevention: principal results of a prospective randomized controlled study (MOSES). *Stroke* 2005;36:1218–1226.

Wachtell K, Lehto M, Gerdts E, et al. Angiotensin II receptor blockade reduces new-onset atrial fibrillation and subsequent stroke compared to atenolol: the losartan intervention for end point reduction in hypertension (LIFE) study. *J Am Coll Cardiol* 2005;45(5):712–719.

Weber MA, Julius S, Kjeldsen SE, et al. BP dependent and independent effects of antihypertensive treatment on clinical events in the VALUE trial. *Lancet* 2004;363:2049–2051.

Yusuf S, Pfeffer MA, Swedberg K, et al. CHARM Investigators and Committees. Effects of candesartan in patients with chronic heart failure and preserved left-ventricular ejection fraction: the CHARM-Preserved Trial. *Lancet* 2003;362:777–781.

CHAPTER C138 ■ CALCIUM ANTAGONISTS

MATTHEW R. WEIR, MD

KEY POINTS

- Calcium antagonists (CAs) (sometimes called *calcium channel blockers*) are powerful arterial dilators that are effective as antihypertensive monotherapy and in combination with other agents; they are particularly useful in reducing the incidence of stroke.
- The antihypertensive properties of CAs remain robust in all forms of hypertension, in all races, and at any age; they are effective over a wide range of dietary salt intake, which makes them useful in patients who find it difficult to reduce dietary salt consumption.
- Cardiac effects differ among CAs; they are useful in angina, but their use in arrhythmias is complex. In contrast to dihydropyridine (DHP) CAs, nondihydropyridine CAs (verapamil and diltiazem) tend to slow heart rate.
- Monotherapy with DHP CAs may not provide optimal protection against heart failure (HF) or progressive renal disease, but combinations of CAs with other agents in these conditions are not contraindicated *per se* and may be useful; nondihydropyridine CAs reduce proteinuria.
- Common side effects of CAs are related to their arteriolar dilator properties, including edema, flushing, headache, and, sometimes, tachycardia.

See also Chapters **A8, A10,** and **B100**

Cellular calcium flux

Calcium (Ca^{2+}) plays a critical role in cellular communication, regulation, and function, and any manipulation of transmembrane Ca^{2+} flux affects a variety of cellular regulatory processes and functions (see Chapter A10). Normally, cells maintain a low resting intracellular concentration of Ca^{2+} in the face of large and inwardly directed concentration gradient ($\sim$10,000-fold). As Ca^{2+} enters the cell, it combines with Ca^{2+}-binding proteins to stimulate a number of second messenger systems and cellular responses, such as nerve excitation, cardiac and vascular smooth muscle contraction, and hormone secretion. Calcium channels can be differentiated into several subtypes, but the L-type channel is the one most directly associated with blood pressure (BP) control. L-channels have activator and antagonist binding sites that can be regulated (or altered experimentally) in disease states.

Calcium antagonists subtypes

Calcium antagonists (CAs, also called *calcium channel blockers*) belong to a structurally and pharmacologically diverse group of compounds that fit into three main subclasses: phenylalkylamines, benzothiazepines, and 1,4-dihydropyridines; the prototypes of these classes are verapamil, diltiazem, and nifedipine, respectively (**Table C138.1**). The pharmacologic mechanism of action common to these drugs is to decrease cellular Ca^{2+} entry through the L-type Ca^{2+} channel. CA subtypes are quantitatively and qualitatively distinct in that they have differential sensitivity and selectivity for binding the pharmacologic receptors along with the Ca^{2+} channel in various tissues. This differential selectivity of action has important implications for the use of these drugs in clinical medicine and explains why the CAs vary considerably in their effects on regional circulatory beds, sinus and atrioventricular nodal functions, and myocardial contractility. Therefore, the CAs have quite different clinical applications, contraindications, drug–drug interactions, and side effect profiles.

Actions

CAs have a very diverse profile of biologic activity owing to the ubiquitous presence of L-type calcium channels on excitable and transport tissues (**Table C138.1**).

Vasodilation. CAs uniformly reduce vascular resistance through L-channel blockade, which directly reduces intracellular Ca^{2+}. Experimental maximal vasodilatory responses are inversely related to the degree of activation of the renin-angiotensin system. At rest, CAs do not cause clinically discernible reflex-mediated sympathoneural activation but at higher doses or during periods of sympathetic excitation (stress or exercise), their sympathoexcitatory effects (increased plasma catecholamines and heart rate) are more apparent, especially with dihydropyridine (DHP) CAs. CAs are more effective vasodilators in constricted than in nonconstricted vascular beds and greater vasodepressor responses occur

TABLE C138.1

CALCIUM ANTAGONISTS: PHARMACOLOGY

Available compounds
    Phenylalkylamines: verapamil
    Benzothiazepines: diltiazem
    Dihydropyridines: nifedipine, amlodipine, felodipine,
       isradipine
Mode of action
    Decrease cellular calcium entry through the L-type
       channel
    Negative inotropic effect (nondihydropyridines)
    Reduction in total peripheral resistance
    Natriuresis
    Interference with angiotensin II, α_1- and α_2-mediated
       vasoconstriction
Indications for use
    All forms of hypertension
    Salt-sensitive hypertension
    Diastolic dysfunction (nondihydropyridines)
    Variant angina
    Cerebral vascular disease
    Cyclosporine hypertension
Contraindications/restrictions
    Heart block and heart failure (nondihydropyridines)
    Myocardial ischemia (short-acting dihydropyridines)
    Heart failure
        Prevention properties inferior to diuretic
        Interaction of verapamil or diltiazem with
           β-blockers
    Renal protection inferior to angiotensin-converting
       enzyme inhibitor
    Proteinuria reduction inferior to angiotensin-converting
       enzyme inhibitor (dihydropyridines)
Common side effects
    Tachycardia (dihydropyridines)
    Edema
    Flushing
    Headache
    Constipation (verapamil)

in patients with higher levels of BP. Although there are few head-to-head comparisons, it seems that there is little, if any, difference in BP-lowering potency between the various CAs, provided that sufficient doses of each drug are given.

Renal effects. CAs facilitate natriuresis by increasing renal blood flow, dilating afferent arterioles, and increasing glomerular filtration pressure. These hemodynamic events are marked by a diminished filtration fraction and reduced renal tubular sodium reabsorption. Non-DHP CAs (but not DHP CAs) diminish proteinuria, possibly by improving glomerular permselectivity to albumin but more likely by lowering renal perfusion pressure.

Cardiac effects. Cardiac contractility is largely unaffected by CAs, with the exception of patients who have systolic dysfunction heart failure (HF). CAs do not reduce exercise capacity in individuals with normal systolic function and have minimal blunting effect on stress-induced increases in systolic BP.

Dihydropyridine calcium antagonists. DHP CAs have little effect on resting heart rate when used chronically. Although they may cause reflex tachycardia early in the course of therapy or at very high doses, long-term studies show similar heart rates before and during therapy with usual clinical doses. Amlodipine and felodipine are relatively safe but not always beneficial in patients with systolic dysfunction but they may be used as part of a regimen that improves HF symptom control by lowering systolic BP and are safe. It has been suggested that CAs may be useful for the treatment of diastolic dysfunction, perhaps through direct effects on myocardial relaxation; benefits are more likely to occur with non-DHP CAs because of their greater heart rate–lowering potential.

Nondihydropyridine calcium antagonists. Non-DHP CA agents have more diverse cardiac effects. In the dose range used for the treatment of hypertension, non-DHP CAs usually have little effect on pulse rate. In some patients, however, pulse rates may be decreased by as much as 10% (by comparison, β-blockers usually lower heart rate by 15%–30%). Although verapamil has the greatest negative inotropic effect among the CAs, its ability to act as a coronary and systemic vasodilator usually counterbalances any adverse consequences of negative inotropism. Whereas diltiazem can reduce inoatrial and atrioventricular conduction rates, verapamil primarily affects atrioventricular nodal conduction. Consequently, both can be used in the treatment of acute or chronic supraventricular arrhythmias but verapamil is contraindicated in patients with preexcitation syndrome with rapid ventricular response because it may accentuate conduction through accessory pathways.

Pharmacology

Kinetics and dynamics. DHP CAs are reasonably well absorbed, but they tend to undergo extensive first-pass metabolism. In general, CA metabolites are inactive, with the possible exception of nifedipine; unlike other CAs, amlodipine does not have an extensive hepatic first-pass metabolism, which contributes to its more prolonged effect. Many of the CAs have been reformulated into sustained-release preparations, which allows for once-daily dosing. The pharmacokinetic properties of the two non-DHP CAs are somewhat similar (**Table C138.2**). The bioavailability of verapamil and diltiazem increases with chronic dosing, most likely secondary to saturable metabolism, which sufficiently increases the levels of verapamil or diltiazem to allow twice rather than three times daily dosing with immediate-release formulations (**Table C138.2**). Verapamil and diltiazem are also currently available in a variety of sustained-release formulations that allow once-daily dosing.

Several studies have demonstrated a consistent concentration–effect relationship for many of the CAs. This helps predict the effectiveness of long-term therapy from the first-dose response. In addition, the concentration–effect relationship illustrates the importance of pharmacokinetic differences between drugs and the influence of aging and disease on absolute drug effect. Withdrawal of CAs does not cause rebound hypertension, but rapid withdrawal may induce coronary artery spasm or angina pectoris, especially in patients with ischemic heart disease.

Alterations in effects. The pharmacokinetics of the CAs can be affected by many factors. In patients with renal insufficiency, the pharmacokinetics of these drugs are minimally changed. In hepatic disease states, diminished systemic clearance may necessitate dosage adjustments. Aging slows the metabolism of these drugs, presumably secondary to the accompanying decrease in hepatic blood flow, sometimes causing the need to use lower doses of CAs in the elderly. Grapefruit can alter the metabolism and activity of verapamil.

TABLE C138.2

CALCIUM ANTAGONISTS: DOSES

Drug	Trade name	Usual dose (frequency/d)	Comment	Fixed-dose combinations
Dihydropyridines				
Amlodipine	Norvasc	2.5–10.0 (1)	Very long acting	Amlodipine and benazepril (Lotrel)
Felodipine	Plendil	2.5–20.0 (1)	Plasma levels increased with grapefruit juice intake	Felodipine and enalapril (Lexxel)
Isradipine	DynaCirc, DynaCirc SR	2.5–5.0 (1–2)	Dose dependent increase in heart rate, similar to all Drugs in this class	
Nicardipine	Cardene-SR	30–60 (2)		
Nifedipine	Procardia XL, Adalat CC	30–120 (1–2)		
Nimodipine		60 (4–6)	Indicated for subarachnoid Bleed	
Nisoldipine	Sular	10–40 (1)		
Nondihydropyridines				
Diltiazem	Cardizem SR, Cardizem-CD or SR, Tiazac	120–360 (1)	Inhibits cytochrome CYP3A4	Diltiazem and enalapril
Verapamil	Calan, Calan-SR, Isoptin-SR, Covera-HS, Verelan-PM	120–360 (1)	Nocturnal dosing indicated for Covera-HS and Verelan-PM	Verapamil and trandolapril (Tarka)

Use in hypertension

Efficacy. Both DHP CAs and non-DHP CAs are effective alone and in combination with other agents in lowering BP. They are effective in isolated systolic hypertension (ISH), where nitrendipine lowered systolic BP by 10 mm Hg more than placebo in the Systolic Hypertension in Europe (SYST-Eur) trial and reduced all-cause cardiovascular (CV) morbidity and mortality by approximately 30%. The Hypertension Optimal Treatment (HOT) trial demonstrated that aggressive BP lowering to values below 140/90 mm Hg with a felodipine-based regimen was both safe and effective. In the Antihypertensive and Lipid-Lowering Treatment to Prevent Heart Attack Trial (ALLHAT), the systolic blood pressure (SBP) lowering with an amlodipine-based regimen was approximately 3 to 4 mm Hg more than that seen with lisinopril-based treatment and 1 to 2 mm Hg less than with a chlorthalidone-based regimen. The amlopidine-based regimen also reduced diastolic BP better than the other initial therapies, although the differences were modest.

CAs have been shown to be similarly effective and safe in their approved dosing range (**Table C138.3**), with monotherapy response rates in hypertension >50%. They work well in younger and older patients but are somewhat more effective than renin-angiotensin blocking drugs in black hypertensive patients. CA effectiveness is largely independent of salt intake or nonsteroidal antiinflammatory drug use, which makes them unique among antihypertensive drugs and are also effective in hypertension induced by cyclosporine or corticosteroids.

Drug combinations. The antihypertensive effect of CAs is generally additive with other antihypertensive drug classes, including thiazide diuretics. The addition of a DHP CA to a non-DHP CA can incrementally reduce BP. If CAs are to be combined with β-blockers, it is preferable to use a DHP CA to avoid atrioventricular block or a worsening of systolic function, which is a concern with diltiazem or verapamil.

CAs have been formulated in fixed-dose combinations with angiotensin-converting enzyme (ACE) inhibitors and angiotensin receptor blockers (ARBs) (see Chapter C129); four fixed-dose combinations are available, two combining ACE inhibitor with DHP CA (benazepril and amlodipine, enalapril and felodipine) and two combining ACE inhibitor with non-DHP CA (trandolapril and verapamil, enalapril and diltiazem). DHP CA combinations with ARBs are also available (amlodipine and valsartan, amlodipine and olmesartan).

Other beneficial effects of calcium antagonists

Stroke protection and cognitive function. Stroke-related morbidity and mortality in elderly patients with ISH was dramatically reduced (by ~40%) in the SYST-Eur and Systolic Hypertension in China (SYST-China) studies. In ALLHAT, the protection from stroke with amlodipine was equivalent to that seen with chlorthalidone and exceeded that observed with lisinopril. In SYST-Eur, a blunting of the age-related decline in cognitive function was also observed, perhaps due to the decline in BP or as a direct function of Ca^{2+} channel inhibition.

Angina and ischemic heart disease. CAs are approved and used for the treatment of classic, vasospastic, and unstable angina, especially in those who are unable to tolerate β-blockers. A working group representing the World Health Organization and the International Society of Hypertension has recently reviewed available data and concluded that beyond their BP-lowering effects, CAs have no independent beneficial or harmful effects on coronary heart disease (CHD) events, including fatal or nonfatal myocardial infarctions (MIs) and other deaths from CHD. ALLHAT demonstrated that the rates of coronary events and death were similar with amlodipine, chlorthalidone, and lisinopril-based regimens. In contrast, the Anglo-Scandanavian Cardiovascular Outcomes Trial (ASCOT) was terminated early for ethical reasons because CV event rates were lower with amlodipine-based therapy than with atenolol-based therapy. Verapamil has also been demonstrated to reduce reinfarction rate and post-MI morbidity and mortality when administered 1 to 2 weeks after an MI. Diltiazem has demonstrated benefit

TABLE C138.3

DRUG–DRUG INTERACTIONS WITH CALCIUM ANTAGONISTS

Calcium antagonist	Interacting drug	Result
Verapamil	Digoxin	↑ Digoxin levels by 50%–90%
Diltiazem	Digoxin	↑ Digoxin level by 40%
Verapamil	β-Blockers	↑ Atrioventricular nodal blockade, hypotension, bradycardia, asystole
Verapamil, diltiazem	Cyclosporine	↑ Cyclosporine levels by 30%–40%
	Cimetidine	↑ Verapamil and diltiazem levels by decreased metabolism
Verapamil	Rifampin/ phenytoin	↓ Verapamil levels by enzyme induction
Dihydropyridines	α-Blockers	Excessive hypotension
	Propanolol	Increased propanolol levels
	Cimetidine	Increased area under the curve and plasma levels of calcium antagonist
Nicardipine, amlodipine	Cyclosporine	↑ Cyclosporine levels (nicardipine 40%–50%, amlodipine 10%)

↑, increased; ↓, decreased.

in reducing the risk of reinfarction in patients with a non–Q wave MI.

In general, DHP CAs should not be given in the immediate post-MI period because their powerful vasodilatory effects can potentially reduce BP and thereby increase myocardial oxygen demand. In this regard, verapamil is probably the CA of choice in the post-MI patient, especially in those who are unable to tolerate β-blockers.

Arrhythmias. In the setting of arrhythmias or conduction disturbances, CA use can prove complicated. Non-DHPs can be useful in various supraventricular tachycardias, but they are usually contraindicated in the setting of heart block.

Heart failure. Amlodipine was found to be "neutral" (relatively safe but unhelpful) in patients with HF in the Prospective Randomized Amlodipine Survival Evaluation (PRAISE) trial. In ALLHAT, amlodipine was decidedly inferior to chlorthalidone in preventing HF regardless of gender, age, race, or glycemic status.

CAs should not generally be used in people with significant HF risk. In those with overt HF, CAs should only be considered for use if severe hypertension is present and proves difficult to control with non-CA agents.

Progressive renal disease and proteinuria
Dihydropyridine calcium antagonists. Careful review of clinical trial data in patients with renal disease indicates that monotherapy with DHP CAs may not slow progression of renal disease as well as ACE inhibitors or ARBs. The African-American Study of Kidney disease (AASK) in nephrosclerosis compared combination therapy based on amlodipine to combinations based on ramipril or metoprolol. Individuals with a urinary protein:creatinine ratio >0.22 (corresponding to proteinuria excretion >300 mg/day) or renal impairment (baseline glomerular filtration rate <40 mL/minute) experienced a worsening of proteinuria and an accelerated rate of decline in renal function if randomized amlodipine compared to ramipril. In contrast,

during the second phase of the Appropriate Blood Pressure Control in Diabetes (ABCD) study in relatively healthy diabetic patients with normal renal function, there was no difference between ACE inhibitor (lisinopril) and the DHP CA nisoldipine with respect to protection against renal deterioration or worsening of proteinuria. Therefore, it would be premature to conclude that DHP CAs should not be used in patients with renal disease, especially because the combination of an ACE inhibitor and a CA has not been tested adequately, and lower BP by itself is known to be protective.

Nondihydropyridine calcium antagonists. Data for non-DHP CAs are somewhat different; small studies with these agents have found that they reduce proteinuria to a degree similar to that observed with ACE inhibitors; however, long-term renal outcome studies with non-DHP CAs have not been completed. In a large Italian trial in diabetes, the addition of verapamil to benazapril caused no further reduction in protein excretion rate.

Raynaud's phenomenon, cerebral vasospasm, and migraine headache. Peripheral vasospastic conditions can be improved with CAs, both DHP and non-DHP.

Adverse effects

Safety issues. Review of available observational studies does not support claims of an adverse effect of CAs on cancer or bleeding risk. In ALLHAT, there were no differences among chlorthalidone, amlodipine, and lisinopril with respect to bleeding episodes or cancer rates; in fact cancer was higher in those whose initial therapy was lisinopril. There was a higher rate of suicide and unintentional injury with amlodipine, which is probably a chance finding.

Side effects. DHP CAs are generally well tolerated but have common dose-dependent side effects that may limit tolerability and are related to their actions as arteriolar dilators: headache, flushing, tachycardia, and peripheral edema. The peripheral edema seen with CAs is not caused by net salt and water retention but rather to greater arteriolar than venous dilation and an increase in lower extremity transcapillary pressure gradients. This phenomenon is dose dependent and is linked to prolonged upright or sitting posture; pedal edema is less common with non-DHP CAs. ACE inhibitors (and perhaps ARBs) are more effective than diuretics in treating the edema, probably because of their relative abilities to lower tissue hydrostatic pressures through balanced arterial and venous dilation. CAs are not associated with abnormalities in electrolyte, carbohydrate, or lipid metabolism.

Drug–drug interactions. Drug–drug interactions are not uncommon with CAs (**Table C138.3**). For example, verapamil and diltiazem decrease cyclosporin metabolism by inhibition of its CYP3A4-mediated metabolism and in so doing reduce the amount of drug needed to be taken to maintain therapeutic drug levels.

Suggested Readings

Ad Hoc Subcommittee of the Liaison Committee of the World Health Organization and the International Society of Hypertension. Effects of calcium antagonists on the risks of coronary heart disease, cancer and bleeding. *J Hypertens* 1997;15:105–115.

Agodoa LY, Appel L, Bakris GL, et al. African-American Study of the Kidney Disease and Hypertension (AASK) Study Group. Effect of ramipril *vs* amlodipine on renal outcomes in hypertensive nephrosclerosis: a randomized controlled trial. *JAMA* 2001;6:2774–2776.

Elliott HL, Meredith PA. Pharmacokinetics of calcium antagonists: implications for therapy. In: Epstein M, ed. *Calcium antagonists in clinical medicine*, 3rd ed. Philadelphia: Hanley & Belfus, 1997:69–92.

Epstein M. Calcium antagonists in the management of hypertension. In: Epstein M, ed. *Calcium antagonists in clinical medicine*, 3rd ed. Philadelphia: Hanley & Belfus, 2002:293–314.

Hansen JE Treatment with verapamil after an acute myocardial infarction: review of the Danish studies on verapamil in myocardial infarction (DAVIT I and II). *Drugs* 1991;42:43–53.

Lewis FJ, Hunsicker LG, Clarke WR, et al. Renoprotective effect of the angiotensin-receptor antagonist irbesartan in patients with nephropathy due to type 2 diabetes. *N Engl J Med* 2001;345:851–860.

Materson BJ, Reda DJ, Cushman WC, et al. Single drug therapy for hypertension in men: a comparison of six antihypertensive agents with placebo. The Department of Veterans Affairs Cooperative Study Group on Antihypertensive Agents. *N Engl J Med* 1993;328:914–921.

Piepho RW, Culbertson VL, Rhodes RS. Drug interactions with the calcium-entry blockers. *Circulation* 1987;9:181–194.

Saunders E, Weir MR, Kong BW, et al. A comparison of the efficacy and safety of a β-blocker, a calcium channel blocker, and a converting enzyme inhibitor in hypertensive blacks. *Arch Intern Med* 1990;150:1707–1713.

Schrier RW, Estacio RO, Esler A, et al. Effects of aggressive blood pressure control in normotensive type 2 diabetic patients on albuminuria, retinopathy and strokes. *Kidney Int* 2002;61:1086–1097.

CHAPTER C139 ■ DIRECT ARTERIAL DILATORS

C. VENKATA S. RAM, MD, FACC, MACP AND ANDREW FENVES, MD, FACP

KEY POINTS

- "Pseudotolerance" to the effects of direct arterial dilators (reflex increases in sympathetic nervous and renin-angiotensin activity and accompanying salt and water retention) limits effectiveness of arterial dilators as monotherapy.
- "Triple therapy" (vasodilator + adrenergic inhibitor + diuretic) is necessary with arterial dilator drugs to limit side effects and counteract pseudotolerance mechanisms.
- Hydralazine use is limited mainly to pregnancy and hospitalized patients, although hydralazine-nitrate combinations are sometimes used in heart failure; minoxidil is generally limited to use in refractory hypertension or renal failure.
- Vasodilators are not generally appropriate in high-risk cardiac patients.
- Metabolism of hydralazine, which is used to treat hypertension in pregnancy, is genetically determined.

See also Chapters C119 and C147

By definition, arterial dilator drugs directly relax vascular smooth muscle cells. The mechanisms of action of the main arteriolar dilators used in clinical practice now, hydralazine and minoxidil, are not fully known but ultimately involve a change in the balance between the vasoconstrictive influences of cytosolic calcium and the vasodilatory influences of cyclic guanosine monophosphate.

Clinical aspects of use of these drugs are summarized in **Table C139.1**.

Pseudotolerance

Mechanisms. Arterial dilators are initially effective in lowering blood pressure (BP) but over time, their effects tend to wane.

TABLE C139.1

CLINICAL USE OF DIRECT VASODILATORS

| Drug (brand name) | Oral dosing | | | Comments |
	Initial dose (mg)	Dosing frequency	Total maintenance dose (mg/d)	
Hydralazine (Apresoline)	25	b.i.d.–t.i.d.	100–300	Mainly used in pregnancy Usually part of triple therapy with diuretic and adrenergic inhibitor Substitute for ACE inhibitors in ACE inhibitor–intolerant heart failure Reversible lupus-like side effects
Minoxidil (Loniten)	2.5–5	q.d.–b.i.d.	10–40	Only for severe refractory hypertension Must be used with diuretic and adrenergic inhibitor or ACE inhibitor Causes hypertrichosis

This pattern is called *pseudotolerance* because it does not generally represent a loss of direct drug effect but rather the response of the major "BP defense" mechanisms: the sympathetic nervous system (SNS), the renin-angiotensin-aldosterone system (RAAS), and renal salt and water retention. The first step in the pseudotolerance response is probably baroreceptor-mediated sympathetic activation, resulting in tachycardia, an increase in cardiac output, and heightened myocardial oxygen demand. Subsequent RAAS activation and renal salt and water retention work in a counterproductive manner to maintain the increase in cardiac output through increased cardiac preload and stroke volume despite the fact that resting heart rate returns toward normal. These features make it risky to use vasodilator monotherapy in patients with known or possible coronary artery disease (CAD).

Implications for therapy. Blocking pseudotolerance mechanisms forms the rationale for the addition of antiadrenergic drugs (β-blockers or sympatholytic agents) and diuretics to arterial dilators to comprise "standard triple therapy." Many of the unpleasant side effects of arterial dilators (e.g., flushing, headache, and palpitations) can also be overcome by adding antiadrenergic agents and diuretics (**Figure C139.1**). When used in this manner, vasodilators can be helpful in the long-term management of otherwise difficult to treat hypertension.

Hydralazine

Hydralazine, a classic direct arteriolar dilator, was introduced in the early 1950s for the treatment of hypertension. Although hydralazine reduces BP, pseudotolerance and immunologic problems limit its use.

Pharmacokinetics and metabolism. After oral administration, 90% of hydralazine is absorbed from the gastrointestinal tract. The plasma half-life of hydralazine is only 4 hours, but its clinical action lasts from 8 to 12 hours after oral dosing. An oral dose of 75 to 100 mg is equipotent to 10 to 25 mg given parenterally. Very little of the unchanged drug appears in the urine and the extensive metabolism largely depends on the genetically determined amount of N-acetyltransferase in the individual. "Slow" acetylators have higher plasma concentrations after a given dose of hydralazine and greater drug-induced toxicities than fast acetylators (each approximately half of the U.S. population).

Clinical use. Hydralazine is used most commonly as a parenteral agent in hypertensive emergencies, most notably pregnancy-associated hypertension. Although an effect on BP may be seen in a few minutes, the maximum effect occurs between 15 and 75 minutes after administration. The usual parenteral dose is 20 to 40 mg, which may be repeated every 2 to 4 hours as necessary.

Hydralazine is used infrequently in essential hypertension as part of a multiple-drug regimen and is given twice daily despite its relatively short half-life. Usually, it is added as the third or fourth agent to patients unresponsive to various combinations of diuretics, β-blockers, calcium channel blockers, and RAAS blocking agents. When a β-blocker is contraindicated, other antiadrenergic drugs, usually central α-agonists, are appropriate alternative choices to facilitate pulse rate reduction. The oral dose requirements to achieve the therapeutic goal are somewhat unpredictable but therapy is often initiated with doses of 10 to 25 mg twice daily, which can be increased at weekly intervals to a top-end dose of 100 to 200 mg twice daily.

Hydralazine–nitrate combinations. The combination of nitrate and hydralazine lowers BP but now has a specific indication for the treatment of heart failure in blacks. The

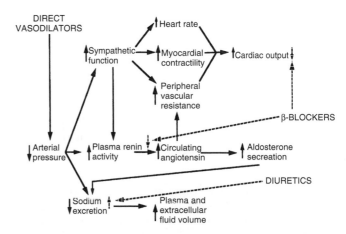

Figure C139.1 Hemodynamic consequences of direct vasodilators and the influence of concomitant therapy with a diuretic and β-blocker. Effects of concomitant therapy are shown by *dashed arrows.*

current formulation is a fixed-dose combination product (BiDil) of isosorbide dinitrate 20 mg and hydralazine 75.5 mg that is given as one or two tablets three times daily.

Side effects and toxicity. Hydralazine causes numerous bothersome and sometimes serious side effects. The total daily dose is limited to 200 to 300 mg because higher doses pose a risk of inducing a lupus-like syndrome; fast acetylators may receive higher doses without appreciable toxicity. Some patients develop nausea and vomiting and, occasionally, peripheral neuropathy. Fluid retention can cause not only edema but also pseudotolerance to the vasodepressor effect of hydralazine, an effect that can be overcome by diuretic therapy, dietary restriction of salt intake, or both. Hydralazine-induced lupus usually presents with arthralgias and may be accompanied by malaise, weight loss, skin rash, splenomegaly, as well as pleural and pericardial effusion. Hydralazine-induced lupus appears between 6 and 24 months after the therapy is begun, occurs mainly in slow acetylators, and is more common in women. The syndrome is reversible after discontinuation of therapy, and full recovery occurs within weeks. In contrast to systemic lupus erythematosus, hydralazine-induced lupus is associated with antibodies directed against single-stranded DNA (surprisingly with very high titers) rather than against the native double-stranded DNA. Antibodies to histones are also frequently present. Patients with hydralazine-induced lupus rarely develop glomerulonephritis.

Minoxidil

Minoxidil is a more potent vasodilator than hydralazine but is similar in its overall hemodynamic actions. Its mechanisms of action may involve stimulation of certain potassium channels that act to limit calcium entry into cells. Although minoxidil is extremely effective as a vasodilator, its adverse effects limit its use in clinical practice to hypertensive patients who are refractory to all other drugs.

Pharmacokinetics and metabolism. Minoxidil is completely and rapidly absorbed from the gastrointestinal tract. In patients with advanced renal failure, the absorption of the drug is delayed. It is predominantly metabolized in the liver. The elimination half-life of minoxidil varies from 3 to 4 hours, although the duration of action may be much more prolonged lasting as long as 12 to 72 hours.

Clinical use. Minoxidil is frequently necessary in patients with renal insufficiency and is effective regardless of the severity or etiology of hypertension and the status of renal function. Before minoxidil became available, bilateral nephrectomy was the only therapeutic option in patients with uncontrolled hypertension and renal damage. After an initial decrease in glomerular filtration rate (GFR), prolonged minoxidil therapy can stabilize or improve renal function. Sustained BP control with minoxidil has occasionally resulted in the discontinuation of dialysis in patients with an acute or chronic component of hypertensive nephrosclerosis. The improvement in GFR is primarily due to

effective BP control rather than a specific renoprotective effect of minoxidil.

Minoxidil should always be administered as part of "triple therapy" with an adrenergic inhibitor and a potent diuretic, usually of the loop-active variety, with doses of the latter two drugs adjusted as needed to control minoxidil-induced tachycardia and edema formation. A combination of a loop-active diuretic and a thiazide-type diuretic may be necessary to treat refractory edema. In the event of contraindications to a β-blocker, a central sympatholytic drug or a rate-reducing calcium channel blocker can be substituted. The usual starting dose of minoxidil is from 2.5 to 5 mg daily. Doses are then titrated to 10 to 40 mg given once or twice daily. A few patients, particularly those with advanced renal failure, may require doses above 40 mg daily to achieve the necessary therapeutic effect.

Side effects. Fluid retention and symptoms of reflex activation of sympathetic activity are almost uniform. On electrocardiogram (ECG), ST-segment depression and T-wave changes are sometimes seen in patients receiving minoxidil; whether this observation represents cardiac ischemia or is a manifestation of left ventricular hypertrophy is unclear. Pericardial effusion, including tamponade, has also been reported in patients receiving minoxidil therapy. The true incidence of this side effect is not known because many patients receiving minoxidil are already predisposed to develop fluid retention as a result of cardiac or renal dysfunction. Elevated pulmonary artery pressures have been documented in patients receiving chronic minoxidil therapy, an effect less likely to occur in patients receiving β-blockers concurrently. Hypertrichosis occurs in most patients treated with minoxidil. Such excessive hair growth is particularly evident on the forehead and face, neck, shoulders, arms, and legs and limits it use in women. The specific mechanism for minoxidil-induced hair growth is not known, but it is probably related to increased blood flow to the hair follicles. Hypertrichosis can be treated with depilatory agents. In those instances where hair growth is unacceptable, minoxidil may need to be discontinued with the excess hair disappearing within a few weeks.

Suggested Readings

Campese VM. Minoxidil: a review of its pharmacological properties and therapeutic use. *Drugs* 1981;22:257–278.

Handler RP, Federman JS. Hydralazine-induced lupus. *N Y State J Med* 1982; 82:1288.

Koch-Weser J. Medical intelligence drug therapy. *N Engl J Med* 1976;295:320–323.

Lundeen TE, Dolan DR, Ram CV. Pericardial effusion associated with minoxidil therapy. *Postgrad Med* 1981;70:98–100.

Mitchell HC, Pettinger WA. Renal function in long-term minoxidil treated patients. *J Cardiovasc Pharmacol* 1980;2:S163–S172.

Ram CV. Clinical considerations in combined drug therapy of hypertension. *Pract Cardiol* 1984;10:83–105.

Sica DA. Minoxidil: an underused vasodilator for resistant or severe hypertension. *J Clin Hypertens (Greenwich)* 2004;6:283–287.

Zacest R, Gilmore E, Koch-Weser J. Treatment of essential hypertension with combined vasodilation and beta-adrenergic blockade. *N Engl J Med* 1972; 286:617–622.

CHAPTER C140 ■ NITRATES, DOPAMINE AGONISTS, POTASSIUM CHANNEL OPENERS, AND SEROTONIN-RELATED AGENTS

ALEXANDER M. M. SHEPHERD, MD, PhD

KEY POINTS

- Nitrates can be used to lower blood pressure (BP) in urgent or emergent situations; they are limited in use by tolerance and tend to lower central systolic BP more than peripheral systolic BP.
- Parenteral dopamine (DA) agonists (fenoldopam) are useful in urgent or emergent situations, particularly in hypertension with renal insufficiency.
- Potassium channel openers and serotonin antagonists have low efficacy as monotherapy and have frequent side effects.
- Imidazolines are being investigated for use in human hypertension.

See also Chapters **A12, A24, A25, C139,** and C147

Nitrates

Organic nitrates have been used for many years orally, transdermally, and parenterally in the therapy of hypertension and angina pectoris.

Mechanisms of action. Nitrates require enzymatic hydrolysis to release the freely diffusible gas nitric oxide (NO), which vasodilates by stimulating the formation of cyclic guanosine monophosphate (cGMP) in vascular smooth muscle cells (see Chapter A21). Hemodynamically, these agents cause balance preload and afterload reduction but also commonly cause tachycardia. Nitrates are especially effective in dilating the coronary and cerebral circulations, leading simultaneously to their powerful actions to reduce myocardial ischemia and cause a vascular type of headache. Nitrates tend to also reduce aortic systolic BP to a greater degree than brachial systolic BP (see Chapter C112) due to their actions to reduce pressure wave reflection and central systolic pressure augmentation. One small study suggests that nitrates are particularly useful when combined with other agents in the treatment of isolated systolic hypertension.

Nitrate tolerance. A major limitation to the use of nitrates as antihypertensive drugs is the rapid development of nitrate tolerance during chronic dosing. The basis for this tolerance is not entirely understood but may occur because of upregulation of the cGMP-dependent kinase type 1β (GLK1β) and downregulation of the GLK1α. GLK1β is less effective in stimulating large-conductance Ca^{2+}-dependent potassium channels, resulting in progressively less relaxation of vascular smooth muscle and

less clinical effect. Nitrate tolerance is especially prevalent with timed-release preparations or with the required multiple daily doses of isosorbide dinitrate (ISDN) or mononitrate. One mechanism to combat nitrate tolerance is a "drug holiday"; in treating angina, instead of giving the drug every 8 hours, a dose is omitted to permit resensitization of vascular smooth muscle. This practice has the obvious drawback of leaving the individual without effective therapy for several hours, significantly lessening the value of these agents in the treatment of hypertension. Furthermore, the need for multiple daily doses makes nitrates relatively unattractive as chronic antihypertensive agents.

Nitroglycerin and sodium nitroprusside. These agents are given predominantly for the urgent or emergent treatment of hypertension or angina pectoris. Nitroglycerin (NTG) is preferred for acute myocardial ischemia or dissecting aortic aneurysm. Nitroprusside (NTP) is more potent in reducing BP as it acts more selectively in reducing afterload. Their actions are very short-lived and they usually require careful BP monitoring. Transdermal nitrates, either in a paste or patch form, are used most commonly in ischemic heart disease but can also impact the BP.

Hydralazine-nitrate combinations. A fixed-combination product of hydralazine and ISDN, has been found to be effective in treating congestive heart failure in African Americans. Presumably, the basis for this efficacy is the arterial and venous dilation caused by ISDN and the further reduction in afterload caused by hydralazine. It has also been suggested that the nitrate portion of this combination increases NO bioavailability whereas hydralazine decreases nitrate tolerance. Although this combination is currently untested in hypertension it would be expected to lower BP.

Dopamine agonists

Several decades of research have resulted in the synthesis of molecules with greater selectivity for dopamine (DA) receptors than DA, which also activates β-adrenergic and α-adrenergic receptors in a dose-dependent manner. Because the vasculature has a high density of vasodilatory dopaminergic receptors, DA and related agonists can lower BP at relatively low doses.

Fenoldopam. The first highly selective dopaminergic agonist to reach the market is fenoldopam mesylate, which stimulates DA_1 receptors. It is approved for the acute in-hospital management (for up to 48 hours) of severe hypertension. It has limited oral bioavailability and a very short elimination half-life (5–9 minutes), restricting its use to hypertensive emergencies. Fenoldopam is administered by constant intravenous infusion, beginning with a dose of 0.1 μg/kg/minute. Doses are increased by 0.05 to 0.10 μg/kg/minute every 10 to 20 minutes as necessary up to 1.5 μg/kg/minute.

Renal effects. Fenoldopam potently dilates a number of vascular beds, especially the renal circulation, in a dose-dependent manner and acutely improves glomerular filtration and urinary flow rates and is natriuretic and kaliuretic. Several studies of fenoldopam have shown that it is as effective as sodium NTP; in addition it does not have toxic metabolic byproducts (thiocyanate is a metabolite of sodium NTP). Fenoldopam is also useful for the intraoperative control of BP and possibly for its salutary effect on renal blood flow. The latter may be of particular importance in the at-risk renal patient receiving contrast media. BP monitoring during fenoldopam administration can be less rigorous than that required for sodium NTP, permitting its use in less intensive medical settings.

Drug interactions. Fenoldopam has expected interactions with other drugs that affect the dopaminergic system, including monoamine oxidase inhibitors, metoclopramide, bromocriptine, most antipsychotics, and tricyclic antidepressants. The beneficial effects of natriuresis with fenoldopam may be partially offset by activation of the renin-angiotensin axis. Fenoldopam should be used cautiously with β-blockers because inhibition of the reflex sympathetic response can result in unexpected hypotension. Fenoldopam increases intraocular pressure slightly but this does not preclude its use in most patients.

DA_2 agonists. Selective peripheral DA_2 agonists could be useful in the chronic therapy of hypertension because they would be expected to reduce sympathetic nervous outflow. Unfortunately, currently available drugs such as bromocriptine also cross the blood–brain barrier and cause unacceptable side effects. Other DA agonists (quinpirole, carmoxirole, and ropinirole) can stimulate the pituitary gland and the chemoreceptor trigger zone in the area postrema, which lie outside the blood–brain barrier, resulting in inhibition of prolactin release, nausea, and vomiting. Further research may produce DA_2 agonists with acceptable side effect profiles and improved bioavailability.

Potassium channel openers

The large number of subtypes of K^+ channels in cell lines presents both a challenge and a therapeutic opportunity. K^+ channel openers increase intracellular K^+ and cause cell membrane hyperpolarization, which in turn causes vascular relaxation by preventing the opening of voltage-activated calcium (Ca^{2+}) channels. Several organ systems are affected by K^+ channel openers, including the cardiovascular, respiratory, reproductive, genitourinary, gastrointestinal, muscular, and central nervous systems, as well as the skin and eye.

Compounds that directly "open" adenosine triphosphate-sensitive K^+ channels include cromakalim (and its negative enantiomer levcromakalim), aprikalim, pinacidil, minoxidil, diazoxide, KR-30450, BRL-34915, and nicorandil; all are potent vasodilators in humans. Because it contains a nitrate moiety, nicorandil also induces vascular muscle relaxation by activation of guanylyl cyclase in addition to its primary effect on K^+ channels. Its dual action results in increased coronary artery blood flow and decreased cardiac work because of afterload reduction. Nicorandil may precondition the myocardium to future ischemic insults by selectively activating mitochondrial adenosine-dependent potassium (K_{ATP}) channels, thereby promoting myocardial capillary and arteriolar growth. If this proves to be clinically relevant, nicorandil and its future "dual-action" congeners may be a significant advance in the therapy of hypertension and ischemic heart disease.

Serotonin-related agents

Serotonin has diverse cardiophysiologic effects through its actions on the different serotonin receptor subtypes that mediate its biologic actions. The vasoconstrictive effects of serotonin are mediated by 5-hydroxytryptamine type 2 ($5\text{-}HT_2$) serotonergic receptors, which also enhance the vasoconstrictive effects of angiotensin II and norepinephrine. Selective $5\text{-}HT_{2B}$ blockers (SB204741 and SB200646) are peripheral vasodilators.

Several molecules that affect peripheral or central serotonin metabolism have been studied in humans, including ketanserin, which is thought to lower BP principally by $α_1$-adrenergic blockade without cardiac stimulation, as well as flesinoxan, urapidil, and 5-methylurapidil. Ketanserin has been studied in preeclampsia but it lacks antihypertensive efficacy in a substantial proportion of these patients, even at high doses. Urapidil stimulates $5\text{-}HT_{1a}$ receptors centrally and also acts as a peripheral postsynaptic $α_1$-receptor antagonist.

Beneficial effects on platelet function and fibrinolysis may account for improved outcomes in long-term trials [Prevention of Atherosclerotic Complications with Ketanserin (PACK) and Prognosis of Ischemic Risk in Atheromatous Patients under Mediatensyl (PRIHAM), with urapidil]. In addition, there may be beneficial effects on lipid profiles or insulin resistance with urapidil. Unfortunately, $5\text{-}HT_2$ serotonergic blockers may prolong the QT_c interval, particularly in hypokalemic patients, which may pose a potential risk in patients treated with these drugs.

Imidazolines

Imidazolines, compounds with five-member rings containing two nitrogens (e.g., moxonidine and rilmenidine), are chemically related to clonidine, which also interacts with imidazoline (I_1)-receptors. In humans, these compounds decrease BP by reducing sympathetic nervous output and cause a balanced decrease in venous and arterial constriction without changing heart rate or cardiac output. Moxonidine and rilmenidine have approximately equal to 30-fold greater affinity for the imidazoline receptor compared with $α_2$ receptors, which decreases the likelihood of central nervous system side effects (especially sedation and dry mouth) and potentially improves tolerability. Moxonidine use is associated with adverse outcomes in heart failure.

Suggested Readings

Barbato JC. Nicorandil; the drug that keeps on giving. *Hypertension* 2005;46:647–648.

Dooley M, Goa KL. Urapidil. A reappraisal of its use in the management of hypertension. *Drugs* 1998;56:929–955.

Frishman WH, Hotchkiss H. Selective and nonselective dopamine receptor agonists: an innovative approach to cardiovascular disease treatment. *Am Heart J* 1996;132:861–870.

Goldberg ME, Cantillo J, Nemiroff MS, et al. Fenoldopam infusion for the treatment of postoperative hypertension. *J Clin Anesth* 1993;5:386–391.

Messerli F. Moxonidine: a new and versatile antihypertensive. *J Cardiovasc Pharmacol* 2000;35:553–556.

Murphy MB, Murray C, Shorten GD. Fenoldopam: a selective peripheral dopamine-receptor agonist for the treatment of severe hypertension. *N Engl J Med* 2001;345:1548–1557.

Stokes GS, Bune AJ, Huon N, et al. Long-term effectiveness of extended-release nitrate for the treatment of systolic hypertension. *Hypertension* 2005;45:380–384.

Taylor AL, Ziesche S, Yancy C, et al. African-American Heart Failure Trial Investigators. Combination of isosorbide dinitrate and hydralazine in blacks with heart failure. *N Engl J Med* 2004;351:2049–2057.

Ziegler D, Haxhiu MA, Kaan EC, et al. Pharmacology of moxonidine, an I1-imidazoline receptor agonist. *J Cardiovasc Pharmacol* 1996;27:S26–S37.

CHAPTER C141 ■ VASOPRESSIN INHIBITORS

HARALAMBOS GAVRAS, MD, FRCP AND IRENE GAVRAS, MD

KEY POINTS

■ There are two types of arginine vasopressin (AVP) receptors: V_1 (vasoconstrictor) and V_2 (aquaretic) receptors.

■ V_2 receptor antagonists ("vaptans") reduce urine osmolality, increase urinary volume and free water excretion, but do not change urinary sodium excretion.

■ The dual V_1 and V_2 antagonist conivaptan is recommended for short-term IV use in hypervolemic and euvolemic hyponatremia.

■ Oral vaptans may be of use in euvolemic and hypervolemic forms of hyponatremia, and in edematous states [e.g., heart failure (HF), cirrhosis, nephrotic syndrome, and possibly polycystic kidney disease] but have no clear role in the treatment of hypertension.

See also Chapters **A22, A39,** and **A60**

Applied pathophysiology

Antidiuretic hormone [(arginine vasopressin, (AVP)] has mainly two actions: (1) organ-specific vasoconstriction mediated through V_{1a} receptors on vascular smooth muscle cells and (2) antidiuresis exerted through V_2 receptors in renal vascular endothelium and basolateral membranes of renal collecting tubular cells. The hydro-osmotic "aquaretic" effect involves activation of aquaporin-2 (AQP-2) water channels, resulting in excretion of water but not electrolytes. Other possible actions include a V_{1B} receptor-mediated stimulation of adrenocorticotropin release, platelet aggregation, and inhibition of sympathetic neuronal function. The V_1-mediated effect of AVP is one of the three major systemic vasopressor mechanisms [the other two being the renin-angiotensin system (RAS) and the sympathetic nervous system (SNS)], that can contribute to elevated peripheral vascular resistance in heart failure (HF) and possibly some forms of hypertension. The V_2-mediated effect is responsible for the abnormal intravascular fluid volume expansion with dilutional hyponatremia, characteristic of the syndrome of inappropriate antidiuretic hormone secretion (SIADH), as well as the compensatory extracellular volume expansion accompanying a variety of edematous states, including HF, nephrotic syndromes, and cirrhosis. Inhibition of AVP by blocking its receptors with selective V_1 or V_2 receptor antagonists, or possibly with dual V_1V_2 antagonists could be clinically useful.

Hemodynamic effects of arginine vasopressin

Hypertension. Experimental animal studies using V_1 inhibition demonstrated that salt-induced hypertension was partly AVP dependent and partly SNS dependent and was characterized by peripheral vasoconstriction with diminished (not expanded) intravascular fluid volume, the opposite of the pattern seen in SIADH (dilutional hyponatremia and intravascular fluid volume expansion but no hypertension or peripheral edema). In humans, the contribution of AVP to blood pressure (BP) maintenance appears to be minimal under usual physiologic conditions with normal or mildly elevated BP levels. In contrast, in patients with severe resistant hypertension, although V_1 inhibition alone causes a small decrease in BP, when it is added to preexisting SNS-RAS blockade, a much larger decrease in BP is observed, although the magnitude of the depressor effect is not related to pretreatment AVP levels. AVP becomes more important hemodynamically in cases of dehydration, hypovolemia, or orthostatic intolerance due to autonomic insufficiency.

Heart failure. Neurohormonal activation involving three major vasopressor systems (the RAS, the SNS, and AVP) is an important pathogenic mechanism as well as a prognostic indicator of poor outcome in HF. The role of AVP in HF is least well defined, partly due to limited availability of effective AVP receptor antagonists. AVP peptide analogs with dual V_1V_2 blocking capacity were tested in experimental animals with HF and were found to produce initially a brisk aquaretic response that was subsequently diminished, suggesting tachyphylaxis. However, the effect could be partially sustained if the antagonist was administered on alternating days rather than daily. Unfortunately, in humans such compounds turned out to act more as agonists than antagonists of the V_2 receptor. In patients with HF, V_1 inhibition causes hemodynamic improvement with a fall in peripheral resistance and increase in cardiac output in 30% of patients, especially those with elevated AVP levels at baseline.

Vasopressin antagonists

Species specificity has been a major obstacle to the successful development of AVP antagonists, as many peptide and nonpeptide compounds that were found to be active antagonists in animals, turned out to be either inactive or even act as partial agonists in humans. This is the main reason for the delay in development of clinically useful AVP antagonists until recently. There is still no selective V_1 antagonist being developed for clinical use, although a number of nonpeptide selective V_2 or dual V_1V_2 antagonists have become available for human use in recent years and constitute a new class of drugs: the "vaptans."

Vaptans. Four nonpeptide AVP antagonists are currently in various stages of clinical development for the treatment of hyponatremia. Conivaptan (Vaprisol) is a dual V_1V_2 antagonist that recently obtained U.S. Food and Drug Administration (FDA) approval and is now marketed for IV use only. Three others, lixivaptan, tolvaptan, and satavaptan are selective V_2 antagonists suitable for oral administration but are still not commercially available.

Conivaptan. Conivaptan is indicated for both euvolemic and hypervolemic forms of dilutional hyponatremia associated with hypothyroidism, renal dysfunction, and various malignancies. Especially at risk are elderly patients in critical care and postsurgical units, in whom neurologic symptoms such as confusion and altered mental status may go undiagnosed. Notably, the SIADH can also be triggered by a number of commonly used medications, such as antidepressants and other psychotropic agents, in which cases it is usually underdiagnosed due to its vague and insidious symptomatology. Conivaptan is recommended at the dose of 20 to 40 mg per day IV for up to 4 days, with close monitoring of serum Na^+ levels. It is not being developed for longitudinal oral use because of potential drug interactions with compounds, whose metabolism involves the CYP3A4 isozyme, which is strongly inhibited by conivaptan.

Tolvaptan. In the Acute and Chronic Therapeutic Impact of a Vasopressin (ACTIV) antagonist in congestive heart failure (CHF) (ACTIV in CHF), there was improvement in low serum Na^+ levels, increased urinary Na^+ excretion and weight loss at 60 days but no significant improvement in signs and symptoms of congestion with 30 to 90 mg daily of tolvaptan compared to placebo. However, a meta-analysis suggested a tendency to reduced mortality with active treatment in the higher-risk patients. This finding prompted the initiation of two additional trials: a larger multicenter outcome trial (EVEREST) found that tolvaptan at 30 mg per day had no effect on long-term morbidity or mortality from HF; the Multicenter Evaluation of Tolvaptan Effect on Remodeling (METEOR) trial found no beneficial or adverse effect on left ventricular remodeling after 1 year of tolvaptan (30 mg/day) in a well-treated cohort of HF patients with an ejection fraction <30%. A meta-analysis combined the results from two studies in of hyponatremia [including chronic HF, cirrhosis, SIADH or other causes—the Study of Ascending Levels of Tolvaptan in Hyponatremia (SALT)-1 and SALT-2 studies] and found that a 30-day course of tolvaptan increased serum Na^+ concentrations, along with physical and mental well-being. Mild side-effects (e.g., thirst, dizziness, and hypotension) were seen and hyponatremia recurred within a few days of discontinuation of therapy.

Other vaptans. Lixivaptan has been studied in a number of small clinical trials involving patients with SIADH, cirrhosis or HF, for up to 7 days. As with tolvaptan, there was a significant dose-related increase in serum Na^+ concentration and urine volume starting at the dose of 50 mg daily. The published experience with satavaptan is limited; however, it has been studied at 5 and 10 mg doses in patients with SIADH; both doses effectively increased free water clearance and normalized serum Na^+ values. In an open-label extension of these studies, some patients have been successfully treated with no evidence of drug escape.

Adverse effects. Vaptans are generally well-tolerated, despite some dizziness, hypotension, and commonly, increased thirst. Volume depletion and a decline in glomerular filtration rate occasionally occur in vaptan-treated patients. Volume depletion is dose dependent and a function not only of drug half-life but also of fluid intake. Prolonged severe hyponatremia and overly rapid correction of hyponatremia may result in permanent neurologic damage but there have been no reports of demyelination. The potential for interaction with compounds that undergo CYP3A4 metabolism exists because vaptans variably inhibit the CYP3A4 isozyme; monitoring may be necessary if these compounds become available for long-term oral use.

Suggested Readings

Adrogué HJ, Madias NE. Hyponatremia. *N Engl J Med* 2000;342:1581–1589.

Creager MA, Faxon DP, Cutler SS, et al. Contribution of vasopressin to vasoconstriction in patients with congestive heart failure: comparison with the renin-angiotensin system and the sympathetic nervous system. *J Am Coll Cardiol* 1986;7:758–765.

Gavras H. Pressor systems in hypertension and congestive heart failure: role of vasopressin. *Hypertension* 1990;16:587–593.

Gavras H, Gavras I. Salt-induced hypertension: the interactive role of vasopressin and of the sympathetic nervous system. *J Hypertens* 1989;7:601–606.

Gheorghiade M, Gattis WA, O'Connor CM, et al. Effects of tolvaptan, a vasopressin antagonist, in patients hospitalized with worsening heart failure: a randomized controlled trial. *JAMA* 2004;291:1963–1971.

Goldsmith SR, Gheorghiade M. Vasopressin antagonism in heart failure. *J Am Coll Cardiol* 2005;46:1785–1791.

Greenberg A, Verbalis JG. Vasopressin receptor antagonists. *Kidney Int* 2006;69: 2124–2130.

Ribeiro A, Mulinari R, Gavras I, et al. Sequential elimination of pressor mechanisms in severe hypertension in humans. *Hypertension* 1986;8(Suppl I):I–169– I–173.

Schrier RW, Gross P, Gheorghiade M, et al. Tolvaptan, a selective oral vasopressin V$_2$-receptor antagonist for hyponatremia. *N Engl J Med* 2006;355:2099– 2112.

Siragy HM. Hyponatremia, fluid-electrolyte disorders, and the syndrome of inappropriate antidiuretic hormone secretion: diagnosis and treatment options. *Endocr Pract* 2006;12:446–457.

CHAPTER C142 ■ ENDOTHELIN ANTAGONISTS

WILLIAM J. ELLIOTT, MD, PhD

KEY POINTS

- Endothelin (ET) and its two major receptors (ET$_A$ and ET$_B$) are involved in many pathologic processes, including systemic and pulmonary hypertension and cerebral vasoconstriction.
- Bosentan, a relatively nonselective ET antagonist, has been approved for pulmonary hypertension; it does lower systemic blood pressure (BP) at high doses but has significant toxicity.
- Darusentan, a more selective ET$_A$ receptor antagonist being developed for resistant hypertension, may have a better side effect profile and greater systemic BP effects.
- Development of ET antagonists continues for systemic and pulmonary hypertension, heart failure (HF), cerebral vasospasm, kidney disease, and prostate cancer; hepatotoxicity has been a major hurdle.

See also Chapter **A21**

Since 1988, when the endothelin (ET) system was discovered, more than 19,000 publications and 2,500 review articles have described its physiology and pharmacology. Antagonists selective for the ET$_A$ receptor and others less selective (i.e., those that also block the ET$_B$ receptors) are under development (**Table C142.1**). These compounds offer benefit in humans or in animal models of many human diseases, including hypertension (both systemic and pulmonary), heart failure (HF), diabetic nephropathy and albuminuria, vascular and cardiac remodeling, cerebral vasospasm, erectile dysfunction, prostate cancer, glioma, and malignant melanoma.

The first two selective ET antagonists were peptides, which limited their study in humans. BQ-123 (~818-fold more selective for the ET$_A$ receptor) and BQ-788 (~1,083 times more selective for the ET$_B$ receptor) are used mostly in laboratory and mechanistic studies because they must be administered intravenously. Selectivity of an ET antagonist for these receptor subtypes may be important because activation of ET$_B$ receptors leads to vasodilation and release of nitric oxide in humans, whereas activation of ET$_A$ receptors produces vasoconstriction, smooth muscle cell hyperplasia, and hypertrophy.

Nonselective antagonists

Bosentan

Essential hypertension. The first pivotal study of bosentan in mild-moderate hypertension, studied a dose range of 100 to 2,000 mg per day. After 4 weeks of treatment, bosentan at doses ≥ 500 mg per day, was effective in lowering both seated systolic and diastolic blood pressure (BP) at trough in both office and ambulatory measurements. There were no significant differences across the groups in heart rate, plasma norepinephrine or creatinine concentrations, plasma renin activity, or angiotensin II levels, but higher levels of both ET-1 and big ET were seen in some of the groups given bosentan. Symptomatic adverse effects were common at higher doses (43% of those given 2,000 mg/day, vs. 37% for placebo vs. 34% for the comparator, enalapril); a first-dose effect typical of vasodilators (headache, flushing) and more chronically, pedal edema were seen. There were also mild, transient elevations of one or more liver function tests in 5%.

Pulmonary hypertension. Subsequent studies showed an effective dose-dependent lowering of pulmonary arterial pressure and bosentan has now received marketing approval (Tracleer) but is extremely expensive (>$2,000 per month). Oral therapy is

ENDOTHELIN ANTAGONISTS AND THEIR POTENTIAL USES

Agent	Selectivity for ET_A/ET_B receptor	Potential primary use
Bosentan	~20	Pulmonary hypertension
Tezosentan	~30	Not effective in heart failure
Enrasentan	~110	Not effective in heart failure
Darusentan	~130	Resistant hypertension
Ambrisentan	~260	Pulmonary hypertension
Avosentan	50–600	Type 2 diabetic nephropathy
Clazosentan	~1,000	Cerebral vasospasm
Atrasentan	~1,860	Prostate cancer
Sitaxsentan	~6,500	Pulmonary hypertension
TBC-3711	~100,000	Resistant hypertension
Edonentan	~80,000	Heart failure (perhaps)

initiated at a dose of 62.5 mg twice daily, and increased to 125 mg twice daily after 4 weeks. Monthly liver function and pregnancy tests, as well as quarterly blood counts, are required during follow-up.

Adverse effects. Drug–drug interactions have been reported for bosentan, which is a mild inducer of CYP2C9 and CYP3A4, and as such its concurrent use with simvastatin, cyclosporine, or warfarin will reduce the levels of these compounds. Alternatively, the levels of bosentan increase when coadministered with ketoconazole or cyclosporine.

Tezosentan. This nonselective ET antagonist has a short elimination half-life when administered intravenously. At least five small safety studies in patients with acutely decompensated HF yielded rather equivocal results, but two larger and identically-designed studies of morbidity and mortality (Value of Endothelin Receptor Inhibition with Tezosentan in Acute Heart Failure Studies, VERITAS-1 and 2) were stopped prematurely due to a low probability of showing a significant beneficial effect after either 1 or 7 days.

Enrasentan. This drug binds to both the ET_A and ET_B receptors but is more selective than bosentan. On the basis of positive results in animal models of hypertension and HF, it was compared to placebo in the Enrasentan Cooperative Randomized Evaluation (ENCOR) trial, involving 419 patients with New York Heart Association (NYHA) class II-III HF who were also given "standard therapy." The results showed a trend in favor of placebo, with approximately a threefold increase in risk of HF hospitalization for those randomized to enrasentan.

Selective endothelin-A receptor antagonists

Darusentan. Darusentan is more selective for the ET_A receptor than bosentan and has been tested in doses of 10 to 100 mg per day in hypertension. After 6 weeks of treatment, there was a dose-dependent decrease in both systolic and diastolic BP and no change in heart rate, but headache (13.5%), flushing (9.4%), and peripheral edema (7.3%) were seen in those who received the 100 mg per day dose. In 115 subjects with "resistant hypertension" titrated doses of 10 to 300 mg were tested. After 10 weeks of darusentan, the placebo-corrected change in seated office BP was $-11.6 \pm 3.3/-5.8 \pm 2.3$ mm Hg ($p = .02/.004$); ambulatory BPs

were also lower. There were no serious adverse events, but pedal edema occurred in 17.3% of the darusentan-treated subjects. These results led to the design and recruitment for an even larger trial of darusentan in resistant hypertension. Darusentan had previously shown no significant improvement in either left ventricular systolic volume or outcomes compared to placebo in 642 patients with HF in the Endothelin-A Receptor Antagonist Trial in Heart Failure (EARTH) trial.

Ambrisentan. This weakly selective ET_A receptor antagonist has a relatively long serum elimination half-life (9–16 hours), which makes once-daily dosing possible. It is approved (as Letairis) for the treatment of pulmonary hypertension. There have been no liver function test abnormalities observed, but, like bosentan, it is not recommended for patients with moderate or severe hepatic impairment and pregnancy tests and monitoring of liver function tests are required monthly. Because ambrisentan is metabolized by CYP3A4, and CYP2C19, coadministration with cyclosporine, ketoconazole-like, or omeprazole-like drugs should be done only with caution.

Avosentan. This compound is only weakly selective for the ET_A receptor and could be reclassified as a nonselective antagonist. A major developmental area for avosentan had been in the area of diabetic nephropathy but a study against placebo in 2,364 type 2 diabetic patients with nephropathy was terminated early by the sponsoring company because of safety concerns.

Clazosentan. Clazosentan is a much more selective antagonist that prevents cerebral vasoconstriction in animal models and may have beneficial effects in hypertension and renal dysfunction. It is currently being tested as an intravenous therapy for preventing delayed cerebral vasospasm in patients with subarachnoid hemorrhage, where it appears to effectively reduce cerebral vasospasm but does not improve outcomes.

Atrasentan. This orally available selective ET_A receptor antagonist is being tested in hormone-refractory metastatic prostate cancer because of the recognition that ET is involved in the regulation of apoptosis and angiogenesis in this disease. A recent meta-analysis of data from 1,002 patients treated with atrasentan (10 mg/day orally) in phase II and phase III trials showed that atrasentan significantly prolonged the disease progression and onset of bone pain.

Sitaxsentan. This selective ET_A receptor antagonist has >90% oral bioavailability and a 10-hour serum elimination half-life. It has been studied in pulmonary hypertension in a number of clinical trials that have involved >1,000 patients. Because sitaxsentan inhibits the metabolism of warfarin, a dose adjustment is needed when it is coadministered with sitaxsentan.

TBC-3711. The experimental compound TBC-3711 is a selective ET_A receptor antagonist being developed for resistant hypertension. It has oral bioavailability of >80% and a 6- to 7-hour serum elimination half-life.

Edonentan. The most selective ET_A receptor to be tested in animal models of HF and pulmonary hypertension is edonentan. It replaced an earlier analog because of its higher selectivity, but has not yet been given to humans.

Future developments

Many other ET receptor antagonists are currently in development, with the hope that they will avoid the hepatotoxicity and drug–drug interactions seen with bosentan. It is unlikely that any ET receptor antagonist will avoid the anemia (thought to be dilutional because of concomitant weight gain and peripheral edema), vasodilator-type symptomatic adverse effects, and, most importantly, the teratogenicity and fetal mortality seen in animal studies that resulted in a "black-box warning" in the product information for both bosentan and ambrisentan.

Suggested Readings

Anand I, McMurray J, Cohn JN, et al. Long-term effects of darusentan on left-ventricular remodelling and clinical outcomes in the Endothelin-A Receptor Antagonist Trial in Heart Failure (EARTH): Randomised, double-blind, placebo-controlled trial. *Lancet* 2004;364:347–354.

Battistini B, Berthiaume N, Kelland NF, et al. Profile of past and current clinical trials involving endothelin receptor antagonists: The novel "-sentan" class of drug. *Exp Biol Med* 2006;231:653–695.

Black HR, El Shahawy M, Weiss RJ, et al. Darusentan: antihypertensive effect in patients with resistant systolic hypertension [Abstract]. *J Am Coll Cardiol* 2006;47:299A.

DORADO. *DORADO—Fixed doses of darusentan as compared to placebo in resistant hypertension*. Available on the Internet at http://www.clinicaltrials.gov/ct/show/NCT00330369. Accessed 21 JUN 2007.

Krum H, Viskoper RJ, Lacourcière Y, et al. Bosentan Hypertension Investigators. The effect of an endothelin-receptor antagonist, bosentan, on blood pressure in patients with essential hypertension. *N Engl J Med* 1998;338:784–790.

Liu C, Chen J. Endothelin receptor antagonists for pulmonary arterial hypertension. *Cochrane Database Syst Rev* 2006;3:CD004434.

Nakov R, Pfarr E, Eberle S, et al. HEAT Investigators. Darusentan: an effective endothelin. A receptor antagonist for treatment of hypertension. *Am J Hypertens* 2002;15:583–589.

Vatter H, Seifert V. Ambrisentan, a non-peptide endothelin receptor antagonist. *Cardiovasc Drug Rev* 2006;24:63–76.

CHAPTER C143 ■ ANTIHYPERTENSIVE EFFECTS OF NONANTIHYPERTENSIVE DRUGS

ROSS D. FELDMAN, MD

KEY POINTS

- Thiazolidinediones (glitazones) and statins have small blood pressure (BP)-lowering effects.
- Aspirin, only when taken at bedtime, lowers BP.
- Selective phosphodiesterase-5 inhibitors (sildenafil and related compounds) can lower BP but they interact with nitrates or other vasoactive drugs and may cause severe hypotension.

See also Chapters A30, A32, A64, C158, and C159

The history of pharmacology is replete with drugs that are ultimately used for indications quite disparate from their originally approved uses such as β-adrenoceptor antagonists for heart failure (HF). Several currently available classes of drugs approved for non–blood pressure (BP)-related indications may also lower BP, although the U.S. Food and Drug Administration (FDA) has not approved the medications for hypertension.

Among the drugs to be considered are those effective in reducing other risk factors that commonly impact the development or consequences of atherosclerotic disease, but whose antihypertensive effects are not widely appreciated, especially thiazolidinediones, statins, and aspirin. Notably, there is also a range of drugs that may improve BP control "secondarily" such as rimonabant, the endocannabinoid-1 receptor antagonist effective in the treatment of obesity. A direct effect of this agent on BP is possible but the weight loss itself would be expected to lower BP.

Thiazolidinediones

Atherosclerotic risk factors cluster with an incidence more frequent than that predicted by chance. The so-called metabolic syndrome (insulin resistance syndrome) is characterized by obesity, hypertension, dyslipidemia, and insulin resistance, the last of which may be the common basis for the vascular and lipid abnormalities evident in these patients. On the basis of the premise that insulin resistance might be the "final common pathway" linking the components of the metabolic syndrome, the antihypertensive effects of drugs that improve insulin resistance have been studied. Foremost are the thiazolidinediones, also known as *glitazones* or *insulin-sensitizers*. Several members of this family, including troglitazone (now removed from the market) and rosiglitazone have been shown to reduce BP, although quite modestly. In the recent Diabetes REduction Assessment with ramipril and rosiglitazone Medication (DREAM) study, BP in normotensive patients was 2/1 mm Hg lower with rosiglitazone treatment.

The mechanism underlying the BP-lowering effect of glitazones remains unclear but may relate to reducing sympathetic nervous system activity or on endothelial function, which is abnormal in diabetes. Endothelial dysfunction has been attributed to a range of mechanisms, including impaired fatty acid metabolism, persistent hyperinsulinemia, and chronic hyperglycemia. Several glitazones, including pioglitazone and rosiglitazone, have been shown to improve flow-mediated vasodilation in subjects with insulin resistance. It is also possible that the antihypertensive effects of these compounds are related to their regulation of peroxisome proliferator–activated receptors (PPAR). The effect is probably not related to insulin *per se* (a vasodilator) because BP reduction does not occur with agents that either increase insulin secretion (sulfonylureas) or improve insulin action (metformin).

Regardless of the mechanism of the antihypertensive effects of glitazones, recent concerns about their neutral to potentially detrimental effects on cardiovascular endpoints make it unlikely these drugs will ever be utilized primarily for their BP-lowering effects.

Statins

Antihypertensive effects have been demonstrated with statin therapy in hypertensive but not normotensive subjects, with BP-lowering effects as high as 5 to 10 mm Hg in stage 1 hypertensive patients. This effect can be missed in short-term studies because it is not always evident until 2 to 3 months of therapy. The delayed effect is consistent with the concept that the BP reduction is related to a change in vascular structure and is not due to reduced lipid levels *per se*. It is unclear whether the antihypertensive effects of statins are class specific or whether similar effects occur with other drugs that lower cholesterol. Pravastatin and simvastatin are agents reported to reverse endothelial dysfunction and vascular compliance in hypercholesterolemic subjects. Statins reduce vascular free-radical release, decrease vascular smooth muscle cell migration and proliferation, and have direct antiinflammatory effects but the impact of these changes on hypertension remains to be established.

Aspirin

Several studies have documented the antihypertensive effects of low-dose acetylsalicylic acid (ASA) taken at bedtime (−7/−5 mm Hg in hypertensive patients) but not with a morning dosing regimen. The time-dependent effects of aspirin may represent antioxidant effects in parallel with the chronobiology of the generation of reactive oxygen species. This effect of aspirin is unlikely to be shared by other cyclooxygenase inhibitors, which tend to raise BP.

Selective phosphodiesterase inhibitors

Selective inhibitors of phosphodiesterases (PDEs), especially PDE-5 and others important in the metabolism of cyclic guanosine monophosphate (cGMP), may be useful in lowering BP but none of these compounds currently have an indication for hypertension. PDE-5 inhibitors increase cGMP concentrations in vascular smooth muscle, the predominant mechanism by which endothelial cells modulate vasodilatation after nitric oxide synthase activation. In contrast, organic nitrates act as nitric oxide donors that relax vascular smooth muscle but because they rapidly desensitize guanylyl cyclase, their hypotensive effects are rapidly attenuated during chronic therapy. Sildenafil is currently indicated in the treatment of pulmonary hypertension.

The breakdown of cGMP is regulated by several subfamilies of PDEs, including types 3, 4, and 5. There is increasing evidence that inhibitors of these PDEs, particularly the PDE-5 inhibitor sildenafil, have a significant antihypertensive effect. In the largest controlled study to date, sildenafil treatment was associated with a small but significant reduction in BP (4/4 mm Hg) in normotensive subjects, without a change in either resting or exercise-related heart rate. Limitations in the duration of action of sildenafil as well as variability in its bioavailability make it unlikely that sildenafil will ever be approved as an antihypertensive drug but other agents with a longer duration of action may prove useful. Marked vasodilation is seen when sildenafil is used in combination with nitrates or α-blockers in patients and severe hypotension has occurred. As a result, sildenafil should not be used in individuals who require these agents.

Suggested Readings

Arruda-Olson AM, Mahoney DW, Nehra A, et al. Cardiovascular effects of sildenafil during exercise in men with known or probable coronary artery disease: a randomized crossover trial. *JAMA* 2002;287:719–725.

Bellosta S, Bernini F, Ferri N, et al. Direct vascular effects of HMG-CoA reductase inhibitors. *Atherosclerosis* 1998;137:5101–5109.

Borghi C, Veronesi M, Prandin MG, et al. Statins and BP regulation. *Curr Hypertens Rep* 2001;3:281–288.

Curioni C, André C. Rimonabant for overweight or obesity. *Cochrane Database Syst Rev* 2006; Issue (4):CD006162.

Egan BM, Greene EL, Goodfriend TL. Nonesterified fatty acids in BP control and cardiovascular complications. *Curr Hypertens Rep* 2001;3:107–116.

Esposito K, Ciotola M, Carleo D, et al. Effect of rosiglitazone on endothelial function and inflammatory markers in patients with the metabolic syndrome. *Diabetes Care* 2006;29(5):1071–1076.

Hermida RC, Ayala DE, Calvo C, et al. Differing administration time-dependent effects of aspirin on BP in dipper and non-dipper hypertensives. *Hypertension* 2005;46(4):1060–1068. [Epub 2005 Aug 8.]

Gerstein HC, Yusuf S, Bosch J, et al. DREAM (Diabetes REduction Assessment with ramipril and rosiglitazone Medication) Trial Investigators. Effect of rosiglitazone on the frequency of diabetes in patients with impaired glucose tolerance or impaired fasting glucose: a randomised controlled trial. *Lancet* 2006;368:1096–1105.

Nissen SE, Wolski K. Effect of rosiglitazone on the risk of myocardial infarction and death from cardiovascular causes. *N Engl J Med* 2007;356:072761.

Ogihara T, Rakugi H, Ikegami H, et al. Enhancement of insulin sensitivity by troglitazone lowers BP in diabetic hypertensives. *Am J Hypertens* 1995;8:316–320.

Sung BH, Izzo JL Jr, Dandona P, et al. Vasodilatory effects of troglitazone improve BP at rest and during mental stress in type 2 diabetes mellitus. *Hypertension* 1999;34:83–88.

CHAPTER C144 ■ BLOOD PRESSURE–RAISING EFFECTS OF ANTI-INFLAMMATORY DRUGS, ANGIOGENESIS INHIBITORS, AND CHOLESTEROL-ESTER-TRANSFER PROTEIN INHIBITORS

RAYMOND R. TOWNSEND, MD

KEY POINTS

- Usage of nonsteroidal anti-inflammatory drugs (NSAIDs) and cyclooxygenase-2 inhibitors (COXIBs) increase blood pressure (BP) in normotensive and hypertensive people.
- Reductions in sodium excretion and vasodilatory prostaglandins are thought to be mechanisms for increased BP with these agents.
- NSAIDs and COXIBs inhibitors can reduce antihypertensive drug effects but less so with calcium antagonists compared to other classes of agents.
- Angiogenesis inhibitors and cholesteryl-ester-transfer protein (CETP) inhibitors can increase BP but mechanism(s) for these effects remain to be determined.

See also Chapters A15, A25, A26, **A28, A30,** A49, **C106,** and C166

Nonsteroidal anti-inflammatory drugs (NSAIDs) and selective cyclooxygenase-2 inhibitors (COXIBs) are frequently prescribed to treat fever, and both acute and chronic pain conditions. These circumstances are common in hypertensive patients, so primary blood pressure (BP) effects or interactions of NSAID/COXIB drugs with antihypertensive drugs are important.

NONSTEROIDAL ANTI-INFLAMMATORY DRUGS AND CYCLOOXYGENASE-2 INHIBITORS

Mechanisms of blood pressure–raising effects

The principal pharmacologic effect associated with either NSAID or COXIB usage is blockade of prostaglandin production. The cyclooxygenase-1 (COX-1) enzyme, largely responsible for gastric cytoprotection, is spared by COXIBs but not by NSAIDs. The COX-2 enzyme is the source of much of the circulating and kidney-derived prostaglandin E$_2$ (PGE$_2$) and prostacyclin (PGI$_2$). Although COX-2 was originally believed to be expressed mostly during inflammation, recent investigations show that it is also expressed physiologically and that its inhibition blunts the BP-lowering effect of certain antihypertensive medications, especially angiotensin-converting enzyme (ACE) inhibitors. Blockade of the COX-2 enzyme by both NSAIDs and COXIBs is thought

to be the principal mechanism by which BP increases. At least two separate pathways have been proposed by which prostaglandins modulate BP (**Figure C144.1**).

Blockade of prostaglandin-induced vasodilation. PGE$_2$ and PGI$_2$ are direct vasodilators that bind to prostaglandin receptors on vascular smooth muscle cell membranes, where they directly produce vasodilation and counteract vasoconstriction caused by humoral factors such as angiotensin-II or catecholamines. Both NSAIDs and COXIBs decrease the production

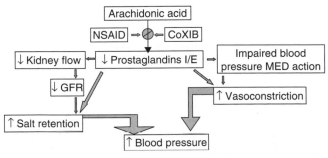

Figure C144.1 Diagram showing main mechanisms by which nonsteroidal anti-inflammatory drug (NSAID) and cyclooxygenase-2 (COXIB) therapies influence blood pressure. MED, medication; GFR, glomerular filtration rate.

of vasodilatory prostaglandins, thereby resulting in vaso-constriction.

Kidney effects. The natriuretic actions of prostaglandins also contribute to their systemic hemodynamic effects. Renal prostaglandin production occurs principally in the medulla, where prostaglandins (mainly PGE_2) promote sodium (Na^+) loss through their actions on cells in the loop of Henle. Blockade of natriuresis with NSAIDs or COXIBs results in Na^+ and water retention, weight gain, edema, and frequently an increase in BP. Additionally, renal prostaglandin production occurs in the glomerular circulation where it is important in maintaining glomerular blood flow and glomerular filtration. Because prostaglandins are vasodilatory, prostaglandin production blockade by NSAIDs or COXIBs can decrease renal blood flow and glomerular filtration, thereby activating intrarenal Na^+-retaining mechanisms. These actions of prostaglandins are clinically more important in situations such as heart failure (HF) and chronic kidney disease (CKD), in which there is greater dependence on prostaglandins to maintain maximal glomerular blood flow and filtration. Infrequently, in older patients on thiazide diuretics, the combined renal effects of NSAIDs can result in disproportionate water (over Na^+) retention due to loss of the natural antagonism of vasopressin, with development of hyponatremia, sometimes severe.

Blood pressure modulation by prostaglandins in disease states. Prostaglandins act more as modulators of BP regulation than primary mediators of vascular tone in health. As a result, the effects of prostaglandin blockade are more evident when challenges to BP control are present (e.g., reduced renal function, aging, diabetes, or salt loading), with a stronger tendency to increased BP. Volume depletion, impaired kidney function, or HF typically result in renal vasoconstriction. Blockade of prostaglandins can further compromise an already diminished glomerular filtration rate (GFR) and exacerbate Na^+ retention.

Blood pressure-raising effects of nonsteroidal anti-inflammatory drugs and cyclooxygenase-2 inhibitors

Obtaining precise estimates of the effect on NSAID and COXIB therapy on BP in humans is hampered by the heterogeneity of the agents and the conflicting results in published studies.

Hypertensives versus normotensives. NSAIDs and COXIBs have BP-increasing effects that tend to be greater in hypertensive patients than in normotensive persons, usually in the range of 2 to 6 mm Hg (**Table C144.1**). The BP increases appear to be dose-related for both NSAIDs and COXIBs and predominantly affect systolic BP, perhaps because NSAID use is highest in older individuals with systolic hypertension.

Inter-individual variability. Although the NSAID data in **Table C144.1** are reported as changes in "mean BP," the systolic BP that increases during NSAID or COXIB therapy have significant interindividual variability. Many patients have no change in BP, whereas others may have as much as a ≥ 20 mm Hg increase in systolic BP. The latter patients are more likely to be older, have some degree of reduced renal function, are more salt sensitive, and generally have higher systolic BPs before exposure to the NSAID. The usage of NSAIDs or COXIBs in these populations therefore justifies close monitoring for BP consequences. Older patients taking NSAIDs are also more

TABLE C144.1

HYPERTENSIVE EFFECTS BY CLASS AND AGENT AND BLOOD PRESSURE STATUS

	Hypertensives	Normotensives
NSAIDs (pooled)	3.6–5.4	1.0–1.1
Indomethacin	4.8–6.0	1.0
Naproxen	3.1–6.1	ND
Piroxicam	2.9–6.2	ND
Sulindac	(−)1.6–2.2	(−)1.6
Aspirin	(−)1.8–1.0	0.6
COXIBs		
Rofecoxib	2.6–4.7	3.4
Celecoxib	(−)0.4	4.3
Etoricoxib	1.3–3.2[a]	
Lumiracoxib	0.4[a]	

Data for nonsteroidal anti-inflammatory drugs are changes in mean arterial pressure in mm Hg; data for cyclooxygenase-2 inhibitors are systolic blood pressure changes in mm Hg.
NSAIDS, nonsteroidal anti-inflammatory drugs; COXIBs, cyclooxygenase-2 inhibitors; ND, no data; (−), negative value.
[a]Hypertensive and normotensive combined, systolic blood pressure reported.

likely to initiate antihypertensive drug therapy. All classes of antihypertensive drug therapy, with the exception of the calcium antagonists, appear to have their antihypertensive effectiveness reduced by NSAIDs and COXIBs.

Nonsteroidal anti-inflammatory drugs. Metaanalyses have evaluated the degree of BP elevation associated with NSAID use and serve as the basis for the data in **Table C144.1**. However, metaanalyses are less robust than a well designed and properly powered clinical trial but available trial data are limited to younger, often healthy (as opposed to having arthritis) individuals treated over short periods (often 4–6 weeks). Therefore, existing data are not robust.

There appears to be variability in the hypertensive effects within the classes of NSAIDs. Aspirin in doses up to 1.5 g daily has no appreciable BP effect. Sulindac also demonstrates little prohypertensive effect, perhaps related to a peculiarity in renal metabolism in which the drug is selectively inactivated within the kidney. Indomethacin has the most extensive documentation prohypertensive effects followed by piroxicam.

Cyclooxygenase-2 inhibitors. COXIB effects on renal hemodynamics are similar to those of the NSAIDs. Several large trials of COXIB therapy, which typically enrolled subjects with and without hypertension, show that systolic BP can increase up to 4 mm Hg from baseline on average. More patients experienced either an increase of systolic BP of >20 mm Hg or a final systolic BP >140 mm Hg with rofecoxib compared with other COXIBs. Rofecoxib was removed from the market in September 2004 because of a small but definite increase in heart attack frequency. Similarly, valdecoxib was also withdrawn from the market approximately 6 months later in 2005 for safety reasons. As with NSAIDs, treatment with calcium antagonist therapy seems protective against BP increases with COXIBs. The newer COXIBs (lumiracoxib and etoricoxib) may have less BP-increasing effects.

Renovascular hypertension

A circumstance in which NSAIDs can *lower* BP is renovascular hypertension. Renin release in the presence of a renal artery stenosis is importantly influenced by PGI_2. Blockade of the COX-2 enzyme (which generates PGI_2) or absence of the PGI receptor (IP in a genetic model) reduces BP in renovascular hypertension.

ANGIOGENESIS INHIBITORS

This class of cancer chemotherapeutic agents is relatively new and little is known about why they raise BP. Because this class reduces blood vessel growth, vascular rarefaction (loss of vessel bed) is one mechanism by which they may increase BP. The agent bevacizumab inhibits the action of vascular endothelial growth factor (VEGF). The actions of VEGF include stimulation of nitric oxide (NO) generation; loss of this NO generation could contribute to an increase in BP with angiogenesis inhibitors. In a study of the oral Raf kinase inhibitor and VEGF receptor antagonist sorafenib (BAY 493006) where BP (not tumor response) was the primary endpoint, systolic BP increased by >10 mm Hg after 3 weeks of treatment in 75% of the patients, with or without underlying hypertension, and persisted for up to 3 months. The recovery time for BP to return to baseline values with angiogenesis inhibitor discontinuation is not known.

CHOLESTEROL-ESTER-TRANSFER PROTEIN INHIBITORS

This class of agents works through inhibition of the cholesteryl-ester-transfer protein (CETP), which promotes the relocation of cholesterol from high-density lipoprotein (HDL) to apolipoprotein B (apoB)-containing lipoproteins, including low-density lipoprotein (LDL). Blockade of CETP therefore increases HDL-cholesterol. At least one agent in development in this class (torcetrapib) demonstrated a 4- to 5-mm Hg average increase in systolic BP in some studies, with some patients experiencing substantially greater increases in BP. These changes and an adverse cardiovascular event profile truncated clinical development. The mechanism of this effect remains speculative at this time and it is not known whether future agents in this class will have the same effect on BP.

Suggested Readings

Curtis SP, Ng J, Yu Q, et al. Renal effects of etoricoxib and comparator nonsteroidal anti-inflammatory drugs in controlled clinical trials. *Clin Ther* 2004;26:70–83.

Fitzgerald GA. The choreography of cyclooxygenases in the kidney. *J Clin Invest* 2002;110:33–34.

Imanishi M, Kawamura M, Akabane S, et al. Aspirin lowers blood pressure in patients with renovascular hypertension. *Hypertension* 1989;14:461–468.

Johnson AG, Nguyen TV, Day RO. Do nonsteroidal anti-inflammatory drugs affect blood pressure? A metaanalysis. *Ann Intern Med* 1994;121:289–300.

Krum H, Aw TJ, Liew D, et al. Blood pressure effects of COX-2 inhibitors. *J Cardiovasc Pharmacol* 2006;47(Suppl 1):S43–S48.

Matchaba P, Gitton X, Krammer G, et al. Cardiovascular safety of lumiracoxib: a meta-analysis of all randomized controlled trials > or =1 week and up to 1 year in duration of patients with osteoarthritis and rheumatoid arthritis. *Clin Ther* 2005;27:1196–1214.

Pope JE, Anderson JJ, Felson DT. A metaanalysis of the effects of nonsteroidal anti-inflammatory drugs on blood pressure. *Arch Intern Med* 1993;153:477–484.

Schwartz JI, Vandormael K, Malice MP, et al. Comparison of rofecoxib, celecoxib, and naproxen on renal function in elderly subjects receiving a normal-salt diet. *Clin Pharmacol Ther* 2002;72:50–61.

Veronese ML, Mosenkis A, Flaherty KT, et al. Mechanisms of hypertension associated with BAY 43-9006. *J Clin Oncol* 2006;24:1363–1369.

Wilson SL, Poulter NR. The effect of non-steroidal anti-inflammatory drugs and other commonly used non-narcotic analgesics on blood pressure level in adults. *J Hypertens* 2006;24:1457–1469.

SECTION V ■ MANAGING HYPERTENSION IN SPECIAL POPULATIONS

CHAPTER C145 ■ TREATMENT OF PREHYPERTENSION

HENRY R. BLACK, MD AND JOSEPH L. IZZO, Jr., MD

KEY POINTS

- The term *prehypertension* first appeared in the 7th report of the Joint National Committee (JNC 7) to describe the "intermediate" blood pressure (BP) values (120–139/80–89 mm Hg) between true normotension (<120/80 mm Hg) and traditional hypertension (>140/90 mm Hg).
- Cardiovascular disease (CVD) and stroke risks in prehypertension are roughly double those of normotension.
- Prehypertension management centers around lifestyle modifications (weight control, increased physical activity, reduction of dietary sodium and alcohol), which have been shown to lower BP modestly in clinical studies.
- The Trial of Prevention of Hypertension (TROPHY) demonstrated that angiotensin receptor blockade effectively lowers BP and subsequent incidence of hypertension in prehypertensives; studies are needed to determine if prehypertensive persons with increased risk from prediabetes, hypercholesterolemia, or microalbuminuria benefit from drug therapy.

See also Chapters B90, **B92,** C105, **C119,** and **C120**

Prehypertension is the term used to describe intermediate blood pressure (BP) values between "true normotension" (<120/80 mm Hg) and "traditional hypertension" (≥140/90 mm Hg) in the fraction (almost one fourth) of the U.S. population at increased risk for cardiovascular (CV) disease. In the Framingham studies, the 12-year risk of ischemic heart disease in individuals with systolic BP in the 130 to 139 mm Hg range was roughly twice that of those whose values remained <120 mm Hg. These trends are virtually identical to the estimates obtained from worldwide experience in almost 1 million adults that included systolic BPs from 115 to 185 mm Hg: each 20 mm Hg increase in systolic BP (or 10 mm Hg diastolic BP) doubled the risk of a fatal heart attack or stroke over the next 12 years. Current debate centers on how to prevent the onset of hypertension and reduce morbidity and mortality in a cost-effective manner in prehypertensives.

Definition and rationale of prehypertension

The seventh report of the Joint National Committee on the Prevention, Detection, Evaluation and Treatment of High Blood Pressure (JNC 7) coined the term *prehypertension* (BP 120–139/80–89 mm Hg). The reason to draw attention to this category included the appreciable morbidity and mortality attributable to the continuous relationship between BP and CV disease risk, even when BP is not markedly elevated. Age is closely related to BP; systolic BP increases at a rate of approximately 0.5 mm Hg per year on average, although with wide variation. Those with the lowest BP

values at any age have proportionally lower systolic BP values in later life, whereas the opposite is true for those in the highest BP values. Therefore, those with the highest systolic BP values exhibit "premature hypertension." For those who maintain a normal BP in their middle years (age 55–65), the "lifetime burden" of becoming hypertensive (systolic BP in excess of 140 mm Hg) still exceeds 90%.

Although the relationships among age, systolic BP, and global CV disease risk are continuous, practical issues dictate that individual categories assist patient and clinicians in decision making. Prehypertension can only be applied if there are no major comorbidities; by definition, an individual cannot be "prehypertensive" if he/she has target organ complications of hypertension (ischemic heart disease, heart failure, kidney disease, or prior stroke) or is under current treatment for hypertension.

Clinical trials in prehypertension
Lifestyle modification
Trials of hypertension prevention. The Trials of Hypertension Prevention (TOHP), phase 2 showed that modest weight loss (by 4.3–4.5 kg, with or without sodium restriction to 80 mmol/day) reduced BP by 4.0/2.8 mm Hg at 6 months in overweight (110%–165% of desirable body weight) prehypertensive persons (diastolic BP of 83–89 mm Hg with systolic BP <140 mm Hg) compared to usual care. At 36 months, however, the reduction in BP was only 1.1/0.6 mm Hg and at 48 months, the incidence of

hypertension (BP ≥140/90 mm Hg or the use of antihypertensive drugs) was actually less in each active intervention group than with usual care [relative risk (RR) 0.78–0.82]. Those subjects who maintained the 6-month weight loss (≥4.5 kg) for the next 30 months had sustained BP reductions and were 65% less likely to become hypertensive. Overall likelihood of becoming hypertensive in the intervention group was 42% lower at 6 months, 22% lower 0.78 at 18 months, and only 19% at 36 months than the control group. After 7 years of follow-up in 181 of the more than 2,800 participants, the incidence of hypertension was 18.9% in the weight loss group and 40.5% in the combined group. This study has just published one of the first long-term observational follow-up studies with 10- to 15-year data from 2,415 of the participants. The risk of having a CV event was lowered by a statistically significant 25% in the intervention group after appropriate adjustments.

DASH Trial. The Dietary Approaches to Stop Hypertension (DASH) study enrolled 459 (133 hypertensive, 326 prehypertensive) adults with systolic BP <160 mm Hg and diastolic BP 80–95 mm Hg. Sodium intake and body weight were maintained at constant levels. The best results were seen in those who were fed a diet high in fruits, vegetables, and dairy products and low in saturated and total fat: approximately 5.5/3 mm Hg in hypertensive persons and approximately 3.5/2.1 mm Hg in prehypertensive persons (p <.001 and <.004). In a second study, reduced sodium intake (65 vs. 100 vs. 142 mmol/day in a crossover design of 1 month each) was combined with the basic DASH regimen in 412 individuals; reducing sodium intake from 142 to 65 mmol/day reduced systolic BP by 7.1 mm Hg in the prehypertension cohort compared to the DASH diet alone. Of note, the DASH diet is particularly effective in older individuals.

PREMIER Trial. The PREMIER trial has further addressed the success of a lifestyle modification regimen to prevent BP increases in the prehypertensive population. This study compared a comprehensive behavioral intervention using conventional recommendations, a similar intervention plus the DASH diet, and advice only in 810 individuals with stage 1 hypertension (37%) or prehypertension (63%). At 6 months, systolic BP was reduced by 4.3 mm Hg (p <.001) in the hypertensive persons receiving the DASH diet compared to 2.1 mm Hg lower in the advice-only group; 35% had normal BPs in the comprehensive intervention group compared to 19% who received advice only. At 18 months, 24% still had nonhypertensive BPs in the intervention group.

Angiotensin receptor blocker therapy

TROPHY Study. The Trial of Prevention of Hypertension (TROPHY) tested the concept of whether treatment of prehypertension with angiotensin receptor blocker (ARB) could change the age-related progression to sustained hypertension. The group studied included predominantly overweight [body mass index (BMI) ≥30 kg] whites with office BPs averaging 134/85 mm Hg. The final study design included lifestyle counseling for all, with a parallel-arm comparison between placebo (administered for 4 years) and ARB (candesartan 16 mg daily for 2 years, followed by placebo for 2 years). The principal dependent variable was cumulative incidence of new hypertension (BP ≥140/90 mm Hg) at 2 and 4 years. The study was positive; those who received ARB had significantly less hypertension at 2 years (−66%). What was mildly surprising is that the benefit of ARB appeared to persist at 4 years, where the treatment group still experienced 16% less hypertension than the placebo group. Also mildly surprising was the degree of immediate BP response to ARB (~10 mm Hg within the first month) and the rapidity of

disappearance of the effect (increase of ~8 mm Hg within 1 month of ARB cessation). The residual difference between groups (~2 mm Hg) has been interpreted as possible evidence of favorable resetting of BP control mechanisms or remodeling of the vasculature. What is clear is that the BP in prehypertension is tonically dependent on ongoing activation of the renin-angiotensin system.

Other studies. Skov et al. studied ARB therapy in 110 offspring of hypertensive parents, aged 29 to 30, with baseline BP 129/79 mm Hg. Candesartan 16 mg/day for 12 months was given in parallel with placebo; as in TROPHY, both groups received an additional 2 years of placebo therapy. After 1 year of active treatment, 24-hour mean ambulatory BP was 3.9/3.4 mm Hg lower than baseline in the ARB-treated group whereas BP rose minimally (0.3/0.6 mm Hg) in the placebo group. Six months after stopping candesartan, BPs rose to identical levels as the placebo group. Active therapy caused greater regression of left ventricular mass (−9.4 g/m^2 vs. −3.3 g/m^2, p = .02) and also reduced renal vascular resistance. Adverse reactions were negligible and similar in both groups. This study provides evidence of favorable effects of ARBs on BP and target organ function in very healthy individuals.

Treatment recommendations

Existing guidelines: lifestyle modifications. First and foremost is adherence to the prescient recommendations of JNC 7 that anyone with BP values >120/80 mm Hg should sustain an optimal lifestyle by practicing weight control, maintaining adequate physical activity and modest dietary salt restriction, and avoiding tobacco and excessive alcohol consumption. These recommendations now have a strong rationale based on clinical trials [TOHP, DASH, PREMIER]. Lifestyle modifications are important at all ages. A 2006 Scientific Statement from the American Heart Association reviewed the evidence that dietary approaches can prevent the development of sustained hypertension in those with prehypertension.

Drug therapy. A more politically charged question is whether prehypertension should be treated with drugs. Current cynicism, inertia, and high costs of health care continue to mitigate against drug treatment of prehypertension. It is extremely difficult to perform meaningful cost–benefit analyses in prehypertension because the model assumptions tend to drive results in low risk populations.

A compelling case for drug therapy can be made for those prehypertensive persons with coexisting glucose intolerance, hyperlipidemia, or microalbuminuria. Any of these conditions roughly doubles cardiovascular disease (CVD) risk, which is equivalent to the risk of traditional hypertension (BP >140/90 mm Hg). Results of TROPHY are encouraging and strongly suggest that the best current choice is probably the ARB class (at least in the overweight white population) due to their proven BP benefits and extremely benign adverse effect profile. The hypothesis that early ARB therapy may prevent the onset of microalbuminuria and diabetic kidney disease is currently being tested in the Randomised Olmesartan And Diabetes MicroAlbuminuria Prevention Study (ROADMAP) trial. The only significant concern is that women of childbearing potential should not take ARBs due to possible fetal abnormalities. Whether adequate BP reduction in prehypertension would occur with ARB therapy in blacks or other demographic groups is unknown; it is possible that low-dose calcium channel blocker (CCB) or diuretic therapy would be more appropriate for some people.

Suggested Readings

Appel LJ, Champagne CM, Harsha DW, et al. PREMIER Collaborative Res Group. Effects of comprehensive lifestyle modification on blood pressure control: main results of the PREMIER clinical trial. *JAMA* 2003;289:2083–2093.

Appel LJ, Moore TJ, Obarzanek E, et al. DASH Collaborative Research Group. The effect of dietary patterns on blood pressure: results from the DASH clinical trial. *N Engl J Med* 1997;336:1117–1124.

Chobanian AV, Bakris GL, Black HR, et al. The seventh report of the Joint National Committee on Prevention, Detection, Evaluation, and Treatment of High Blood Pressure—JNC 7 Express. *JAMA* 2003;289:2560–2572.

Cook NR, Cutler JA, Obarzanek E, et al. Long term effects of dietary sodium reduction on cardiovascular disease outcomes: observational follow-up of the trials of hypertension prevention (TOHP). *Br Med J* 2007;334:885–888,

Elmer PJ, Obarzanek E, Vollmer WM, et al. PREMIER Collaborative Res Group. *Ann Intern Med* 2006;144:485–495.

Julius S, Nesbitt SD, Egan BM, et al. Trial of preventing hypertension study I. Feasibility of treating prehypertension with an angiotensin-receptor blocker. *N Engl J Med* 2006;354:1685–1697.

Sacks FM, Svetkey LP, Vollmer WM, et al. DASH-Sodium Collaborative Resserch Group. *N Engl J Med* 2001;344:3–10.

Skov K, Eiskjær H, Hansen HE, et al. Treatment of young subjects at high familial risk of future hypertension with an angiotensin-receptor blocker. *Hypertension* 2007;50:89–95.

The Trials of Hypertension Prevention Collaborative Research Group. Effects of weight loss and sodium reduction intervention on blood pressure and hypertension incidence in overweight people with high-normal blood pressure. The Trials of Hypertension Prevention, phase II. *Arch Intern Med* 1997;157:657–667.

CHAPTER C146 ■ TREATMENT OF THE ELDERLY HYPERTENSIVE: SYSTOLIC HYPERTENSION

JAN N. BASILE, MD

KEY POINTS

- Hypertension affects up to 75% of individuals 60 years and older, the most rapidly growing segment of our population.
- cardiovascular (CV) risk in the elderly is related to increased systolic blood pressure (BP) and pulse pressure and to decreased diastolic blood pressure (DBP); systolic blood pressure (SBP) reduction is the major target for improving outcomes in the elderly patient.
- Hypertension therapy in older individuals should include lifestyle modification, especially weight loss and sodium restriction, which may decrease the need for antihypertensive medication.
- If low-medication doses are initially used, significant attention must be paid to subsequent titration; combination therapy is usually required for optimal BP control.

See also Chapters **A45,** B76, B92, B93, **C103,** C105, and C149

The *elderly*, defined as individuals 60 years or older, represent the most rapidly growing segment of our population that is projected to double over the next 25 years. Hypertension [blood pressure (BP) ≥140/90 mm Hg] confers a three- to four-fold increased risk for cardiovascular disease (CVD) in older individuals; for every 20 mm Hg increase of systolic blood pressure (SBP) >115 mm Hg, mortality from ischemic heart disease and stroke doubles in all age-groups older than 40 years. Recent recommendations emphasize that SBP should be the primary target in the management of elderly patients with hypertension. Unfortunately, at most 20% of elderly hypertensive persons have BPs controlled to values <140/90 mm Hg.

Age and blood pressure patterns
Isolated systolic hypertension. Isolated systolic hypertension [ISH, SBP ≥140 mm Hg and diastolic blood pressure (DBP)

<90 mm Hg] represents the most common form of hypertension in the elderly. Its prevalence increases with age; two-thirds of individuals 60 years and older and three-fourths of those older than 75 years have ISH. SBP is the most appropriate parameter for risk stratification in the elderly. In an analysis of the Framingham Heart Study, knowledge of SBP alone allowed correct classification of the stage of hypertension in 99% of adults older than 60 years, whereas DBP alone resulted in only 66% of patients being correctly classified.

Blood pressure patterns and risk. Increases in DBP or SBP are directly associated with increased CVD risk in younger populations but in those older than 60 years , increased SBP and *decreased* DBP mark increased risk. Accordingly, in the elderly, the pulse pressure (SBP–DBP) is a stronger predictor of CVD risk than is increased SBP or decreased DBP individually. To date there has not been a clinical trial that has shown that reducing pulse pressure reduces risk, so lower SBP continues to be the primary goal for decreasing cardiovascular (CV) risk in the elderly patient with hypertension.

Pathophysiology

An age-related increase in aortic stiffness explains most of the frequent development of ISH in the elderly. DBP elevation caused by constriction of smaller arterioles also contributes to SBP elevation but it is primarily the loss of distensibility of the larger arteries, especially the aorta that is the hallmark of the condition. Elevated systolic pressure increases left ventricular (LV) work and therein the risk of developing LV hypertrophy, whereas decreased DBP can potentially compromise forward blood flow in diastole, especially in the coronary arteries.

Clinical evaluation

All hypertensive persons should be systematically evaluated, irrespective of age, using standard criteria (see Chapter C105).

Office blood pressure evaluation. A few caveats apply to BP measurement in the elderly because BP is more variable in the older patient and BP measurement techniques can pose special problems. Care should be taken to allow the patient to become accommodated to the measurement setting. Sitting BPs require feet on the floor and back supported in a chair (see Chapter C103). Orthostatic BP decreases that exceed 20/10 mm Hg signal increased CVD risk and potential medication intolerance. Therefore, BP should also be measured in the supine and standing positions in all elderly patients. Rarely, peripheral arteries may become calcified leading to a measured BP value considerably in excess of actual intra-arterial pressure ("pseudohypertension"). Pseudohypertension should be suspected when medication causes hypotensive symptoms in elderly patients with normal or elevated BP when measured or in those with persistently high BP without evidence of target organ damage.

Home blood pressure monitoring. If home BP values are monitored, there is often an exaggerated BP variation in general, including exaggerated diurnal variation, with extremely high first-morning readings followed by much lower values throughout the day. The elderly are also more likely to develop post-prandial hypotension, particularly after a large meal.

Secondary hypertension. Most elderly patients do not have a reversible form of hypertension (**Table C146.1**). Among reversible causes of hypertension in the elderly, renovascular disease is not uncommon and often goes unrecognized in the elderly hypertensive. If BP is controlled and renal function remains normal, there is little benefit from its detection, however, because other comorbidities are more likely to cause death. In addition, renovascular repair with surgery or stenting does not often cure the hypertension; it merely reduces the average number of medications required for BP control by about one.

Evidence-based benefits of therapy in the elderly

Lifestyle modification. Weight loss is of particular value in reducing systolic BP in the elderly (see Chapter B92) and may reduce or even eliminate the need for pharmacologic therapy. Reduced sodium intake is recommended because most older hypertensive persons are salt sensitive (see Chapter B93). The Trial of Non-pharmacologic Interventions in the Elderly (TONE) showed that restricting salt intake to 80 mmol (2 g) per day modestly reduced SBP and DBP during the 30-month trial; 40% of those treated with

a low-salt diet were able to discontinue medication. The combination of weight loss and salt restriction reduced BP more than either strategy by itself; the need for antihypertensive therapy was eliminated in almost half the participants. The elderly should also be encouraged to avoid excessive alcohol intake and remain as physically active as is feasible.

Treatment of isolated systolic hypertension. There is no longer any doubt that controlling SBP in the older patient reduces the CVD and renal complications of hypertension. Several large, prospective placebo-controlled systolic/diastolic hypertension trials conducted over the last 3 decades found a reduction in CV morbidity and mortality when DBP was lowered to <90 mm Hg (**Table C146.2**). Other randomized, placebo-controlled trials have shown significant benefit from drug treatment in elderly patients with ISH (**Table C146.3**).

The systolic hypertension in the elderly program study. The Systolic Hypertension in the Elderly Program (SHEP) achieved a favorable reduction in stroke and CVD events using a diuretic-based strategy [with or without a β-blocker (**Table C146.2**)]. In those with stage 2 ISH (SBP ≥160 mm Hg and DBP <90 mm Hg), effective treatment reduced stroke, heart failure, coronary events,

---

TABLE C146.1

INDICATIONS TO EVALUATE FOR SECONDARY HYPERTENSION IN THE OLDER PATIENT

New onset stage 2 hypertension
Unprovoked hypokalemia or refractory hypokalemia while on diuretic therapy
Hypertension refractory to a three-drug regimen, one of which is a thiazide
Symptoms suggestive of pheochromocytoma
Continued creatinine rise on appropriate antihypertensive therapy

---

TABLE C146.2

PERCENTAGE EVENT REDUCTION IN CLINICAL TRIALS IN OLDER HYPERTENSIVE PATIENTS

	Stroke	Coronary artery disease	Congestive heart failure	All cardiovascular disease
Systolic/diastolic				
Australian	33	18	—	31
EWPHE	36	20	22	29[a]
STOP	47[a]	13[b]	51[a]	40[a]
MRC	25[a]	19	—	17[a]
HDFP	44[a]	15[a]	—	16[a]
Isolated systolic				
SHEP	33[a]	27[a]	55[a]	32[a]
Syst-EUR	42[a]	30	29	31[a]
Syst-China	38[a]	27	—	25[a]

EWPHE, European Working Party on High BP in the Elderly; STOP, Swedish Trial in Old Patients; MRC, Medical Research Council; HDFP, Hypertension Detection and Follow-Up Program; SHEP, Systolic Hypertension in the Elderly Program; Syst-EUR, European Trial on Isolated Systolic Hypertension in the Elderly; Syst-China, Systolic Hypertension in China.
[a]Statistically significant.
[b]Myocardial infarction only.

TABLE C146.3

MAJOR CLINICAL TRIALS SHOWING BENEFIT OF TREATING ISOLATED SYSTOLIC HYPERTENSION

	SHEP (N = 4,736)	SYST-EUR (N = 4,695)	SYST-CHINA (N = 2,394)
Baseline BP, SBP/DBP (mm Hg)	160–219/<90	160–219/<95	160–219/<95
BP reduction, SBP/DPB (mm Hg)	27/9	23/7	20/5
Drug therapy	Chlorthalidone	Nitrendipine	Nitrendipine
	Atenolol	Enalapril/Hydrochlorothiazide	Captopril/Hydrochlorothiazide
Outcomes (% ↓)			
Stroke	33	42	38
Coronary artery disease	27	30	27
Congestive heart failure	55	29	—
All cardiovascular disease	32	31	25

↓, decrease; DBP, diastolic blood pressure; SBP, systolic blood pressure; SHEP, Systolic Hypertension in the Elderly Program; Syst-EUR, European Trial on Isolated Systolic Hypertension in the Elderly; Syst-China, Systolic Hypertension in China.
(From Jamerson K, Giles T, Sica D, et al. Inhibiting both RAS and SNS for high blood pressure control: myths and facts. *J Clin Hypertens* 2000;2:331–338, with permission.)

and mortality by approximately one third. Benefit occurred when SBP was reduced by at least 12 mm Hg more than placebo (and to a level ~25 mm Hg below the entry SBP).

The European trial on isolated systolic hypertension in the elderly study. The European Trial on Isolated Systolic Hypertension in the Elderly (Syst-EUR) compared placebo to a moderately long-acting dihydropyridine (DHP) calcium channel blocker (CCB), nitrendipine in individuals with baseline SBP >160 and DBP <95 mm Hg. BP reductions and CVD benefits similar to SHEP were seen. A meta-analysis of eight placebo-controlled trials in the elderly by Staessen et al. (including a total of 15,693 patients followed up for 4 years) found active treatment reduced coronary events by 23%, strokes by 30%, CV deaths by 18%, and total deaths by 13%, with the benefit particularly high in those older than 70 years.

Other studies. Benefit occurs in those older than 80 years but limited data are available for those 85 years or older. The Hypertension in the Very Elderly Trial (HYVET) pilot study enrolled more than 1,200 patients at least 80 years of age with systolic/diastolic hypertension and found a trend toward increased mortality but reduction in stroke compared to placebo with just 1 year of therapy. The main HYVET trial should provide more definitive information on these trends. In the Hypertension Optimal Treatment (HOT) trial in 19,000 subjects with hypertension, one third of whom were older than 65 years; the lowest incidence of CV events occurred in those with a mean SBP of 139 mm Hg, with no additional benefit or risk from lowering BP further.

Drug treatment recommendations

Stage 1 ISH affects 25% of the elderly population, so clinicians should strive to treat these individuals to the goals advised in JNC 7.

Treatment goals. Although none of the trials achieved an average SBP of <140 mm Hg, the Seventh Report of the Joint National Committee on Prevention, Detection, Evaluation, and Treatment of High BP (JNC 7) and a recent consensus statement recommend the minimum goal for therapy to be SBP <140 mm Hg and DBP <90 mm Hg, unless the patient has diabetes mellitus, chronic kidney disease, or coronary artery disease, where

the goal is <130 mm Hg for SBP and <80 mm Hg for DBP. Data to support these recommendations included natural history studies and limited interventional data. Although the vascular risk of stage 1 ISH (SBP 140–159 mm Hg/DBP <90 mm Hg) is well established, it should be recognized that no trial has been completed in stage 1 ISH and no study has tested how low the SBP target should be in ISH.

Initial drug choice. Although JNC 7 does not recommend a preferred initial therapy in older patients with ISH, it does recommend thiazide diuretics for most individuals with hypertension. Other consensus groups recommend diuretics or calcium antagonists as first-line therapy in those with ISH based on placebo-controlled outcome trials. Several trials in the elderly have suggested that the initial agent chosen is less important than the level of BP reduction achieved. However, there are major shortcomings in the assumptions and designs of these studies; accordingly, the question of superiority of one antihypertensive class over another in elderly patients with ISH still remains to be answered. Although all classes of antihypertensive agents can lower SBP and DBP in the elderly, most outcome trials showing a reduction in vascular morbidity and mortality used diuretics and, when necessary, added a β-blocker. β-Blocker therapy is no longer recommended as monotherapy in the elderly unless prescribed for ischemic heart disease, post–myocardial infarction (MI), or heart failure with reduced ejection fraction. A recent British hypertension treatment guideline suggested that β-blockers have limited to no clinical benefit in uncomplicated hypertension and as such are now viewed as third-or fourth-line agents in those older than 55 years of age.

Combination therapy. Most elderly patients require two or more drugs to achieve the recommended SBP goal of <140 mm Hg. In all antihypertensive drug trials, second- and third-line agents were added to achieve better BP control; therefore, hypertension trials should be viewed as combination drug trials. In the SHEP and the Syst-EUR trials, 40% to 50% of participants required at least two drugs (**Table C146.3**) to achieve a SBP mean of approximately 145 mm Hg, whereas DBP was <80 mm Hg. In routine practice, if the SBP goal is achieved, the DBP goal is almost always reached as well. According to recent guidelines, initiating therapy with two drugs, either separately or as a fixed-dose combination, should be considered in patients whose SBP goal is at least 20 mm Hg above the desired goal of <140 mm Hg or lower for those with diabetes, chronic renal disease, and coronary artery disease. The use of fixed-dose combination therapy may have particular benefit in the elderly, who are often on many concomitant medications for other comorbidities. In addition to increasing the likelihood of attaining BP goals, fixed-dose combination therapy may allow lower doses of the component agents to be used, reducing the dose-dependent side effects often seen with higher dose monotherapy, while providing the simplicity and convenience of multiple BP-lowering medications in one tablet and reduce the overall pill burden.

Underdosing problems. Many physicians believe that the usual dose of the initial agent in older hypertensive persons should be half of that used in younger hypertensive persons based on the fear of excessive BP responses due to slowed renal or hepatic metabolism. Unfortunately, this practice often leads to underdosing and reduced BP control rates. Although it may be prudent to titrate more slowly, a schedule of 4-week visits is reasonable. If not used initially, a thiazide diuretic should be included in most regimens to enhance the efficacy of other BP-lowering agents.

Potassium maintenance. Serum potassium should be kept normal especially in diuretic-treated elderly hypertensives. A recent retrospective analysis of SHEP found that 7% of the participants on the long-acting diuretic chlorthalidone developed hypokalemia (serum potassium <3.5 mEq/L) by the 1-year visit. Those individuals who developed hypokalemia had an event rate similar to those in the placebo group, whereas those with levels >3.5 mEq per L had significantly fewer CV events, suggesting that serum potassium should be kept above 3.5 mEq/L. Interestingly only 11% of those whose initial treatment was chlorthalidone in the Antihypertensive and Lipid Lowering Trial to reduce Heart Attack (ALLHAT) needed potassium supplementation.

Fears of excessive blood pressure lowering. The J-curve hypothesis states that lowering DBP below a certain critical value increases the risk of CV death in those with underlying CVD. This issue has been extensively debated. In that regard, a retrospective analysis of the SHEP trial has suggested that the few patients whose DBP was lowered to <55 mm Hg experienced no benefit in outcome when compared to the placebo group. It has been discussed in detail in the recent American Heart Association/American College of Cardiology Consensus statement on the treatment of hypertension in individuals with ischemic heart disease (see Chapter C149). That document suggests that the J-curve is most likely explained by noncardiac factors yet it recommends caution in lowering DBP to values <60 mm Hg.

Suggested Readings

Benetos A, Thomas F, Bean K, et al. Prognostic value of systolic and diastolic BP in treated hypertensive men. *Arch Intern Med* 2002;162:577–581.

Bulpitt C, Beckett N, Cooke J, et al. Hypertension in the Very Elderly Trial Working Group. Results of the pilot study for the hypertension in the very elderly trial. *J Hypertens* 2003;21:2409–2417.

Franklin SS, Khan SA, Wong ND, et al. Is pulse pressure useful in predicting risk for coronary heart disease? The Framingham Heart Study. *Circulation* 1999;100:354–360.

Hansson L. How far should we lower BP in the elderly. *Cardiovasc Drugs Ther* 2001;15:275–279.

Hansson L, Lindholm LH, Ekbom T. STOP-Hypertension-2 study group. Randomized trial of old and new antihypertensive drugs in elderly patients: cardiovascular mortality and morbidity in the Swedish Trial in Old Patients with Hypertension-2 (STOP-2) study. *Lancet* 1999;354:1751–1756.

Izzo J, Levy D, Black HR. Clinical advisory statement. Importance of systolic BP in older Americans. *Hypertension* 2000;35:1021–1024.

SHEP Cooperative Research Group. Prevention of stroke by antihypertensive drug treatment in older persons with isolated systolic hypertension. *JAMA* 1991;265:3255–3264.

Somes G, Pahor M, Shorr RI, et al. The role of diastolic BP when treating isolated systolic hypertension. *Arch Intern Med* 1999;159:2004–2009.

Staessen JA, Fagard R, Thijs L, et al. Morbidity and mortality in the placebo controlled European trial on isolated systolic hypertension (Syst-Eur) in the elderly. *Lancet* 1997;350:757–764.

Staessen JA, Gasowski J, Wang JC, et al. Risk of untreated and treated isolated systolic hypertension in the elderly: meta-analysis of outcome trials. *Lancet* 2000;355:865–872.

CHAPTER C147 ■ TREATMENT OF HYPERTENSIVE URGENCIES AND EMERGENCIES

DONALD G. VIDT, MD

KEY POINTS

- A patient presenting with severe hypertension [usually blood pressure (BP) >180/110 mm Hg] must be triaged and treated according to the nature and severity of the symptoms and associated comorbidities.
- Markedly elevated BP by itself, in the absence of symptoms or target organ damage, does not automatically require emergency therapy; oral agents and follow-up care within a few days are indicated.
- Hypertensive urgencies are severe BP elevations (BP >180/110 mm Hg) that are not immediately life threatening but are associated with either symptoms (e.g., severe headache) or moderate target organ damage (e.g., elevated serum creatinine); treatment with oral agents and follow-up within 24 to 72 hours are indicated.
- Hypertensive emergencies exist when BP is very high (often >220/140 mm Hg) and acute target organ damage is present (e.g., heart failure, acute myocardial infarction, aortic aneurysm, hypertensive encephalopathy, or hemorrhagic stroke); hospitalization (usually in an intensive care unit), close BP monitoring, and parenteral therapy are indicated.
- Discharging a patient from an emergency room (ER) or outpatient setting without a confirmed follow-up appointment is a missed opportunity to improve BP control or to pursue appropriate diagnostic studies for secondary hypertension.

See also Chapters C106, C119, C143, C159, and C170

Most emergency department patients with severely elevated blood pressure (BP) do not receive the evaluation, treatment modifications, or discharge instructions consistent with current guidelines. Two recent studies evaluated the emergency department management of patients with severe hypertension: fewer than 10% received all recommended studies, serum chemistries were performed in 70% to 73%, an electrocardiography in 53% to 70%, a chest x-ray in 24% to 46%, urinalysis in 43% to 44%, and funduscopic examination in <36%. Also of concern was the observation in both studies that although follow-up care was often recommended, it was infrequently scheduled in writing.

Triaging severe hypertension

Triage and management decisions in a patient who presents acutely with severely elevated BP (usually >180/110 mm Hg in adults) depend more on the nature and severity of the comorbidities than on the BP itself. Broadly speaking, individuals with severe elevations of BP can be divided into three broad categories that can overlap: (a) BP >180/110 mm Hg without symptoms or acute signs of organ damage, (b) hypertensive urgencies, with BP >180/110 mm Hg and symptoms or modest organ damage, or (c) hypertensive emergencies, often with BP >220/140 mm Hg, associated with life-threatening organ dysfunction.

The clinician faced with acute management decisions in a patient with severe hypertension must usually decide how to triage the patient and treat the BP before the workup is complete. The algorithm in **Table C147.1** provides a framework for identification of true hypertensive emergencies and guides management decisions, especially the decision to use oral medications or admit the patient for parenteral therapy.

A thorough but expeditiously performed history and physical evaluation with selected laboratory studies can help in assessing the immediate clinical status of the patient, provide clues to any underlying etiology of the hypertension, assess the degree of target organ involvement, and help select the most appropriate pharmacologic therapy. Initial laboratory studies should include a urinalysis with sediment examination, an electrocardiogram, a hemogram, and a complete chemistry profile. A computed tomographic scan of the head should be considered in the comatose patient or when the clinical examination suggests cerebrovascular ischemia or hemorrhage. Cardiac studies are dictated by the presenting syndrome.

Treatment of severe hypertension

The most important aspect of management of severe hypertension (BP >180/110 mm Hg) is the recognition that immediate

TABLE C147.1

ALGORITHM FOR TRIAGE AND MANAGEMENT

	Severe hypertension	Hypertensive urgency	Hypertensive emergency
BP	>180/110 mm Hg	>180/110 mm Hg	Often >220/140 mm Hg
Symptoms	Often asymptomatic Headache Anxiety	Severe headache Shortness of breath Edema	Prolonged chest pain/unstable angina Severe shortness of breath Motor impairment/neurologic deficit Altered mental status Uncontrollable bleeding
Workup results	No target organ damage/clinical cardiovascular disease	Target organ damage/clinical cardiovascular disease may be present	Pulmonary edema/heart failure Acute MI Cerebrovascular accident Encephalopathy Renal insufficiency Preeclampsia Renal failure Aneurysm
Acute management	Initiate/resume medication(s) Increase dosage of inadequate agent Observe for 1–3 h	Lower BP with oral or parenteral agents as underlying conditions warrant Adjust current therapy Observe for 3–6 h	Order baseline laboratories Initiate intravenous line Monitor vital signs May initiate disease-appropriate parenteral therapy in the emergency room
Plan	Arrange follow-up >72 h If no prior evaluation, schedule appointment	Arrange follow-up evaluation (24–72 h)	Immediate admission to intensive care unit Treat to appropriate goal BP Additional diagnostic studies as warranted

BP, blood pressure; MI, myocardial infarction.
(Adapted from Vidt DG. Emergency room management of hypertensive urgencies and emergencies. *J Clin Hypertens (Greenwich)* 2001;3:158–164.)

normalization of the BP is not necessary. Acute pain, emotional distress, or abrupt withdrawal of prior therapy (especially oral clonidine) can cause transient BP elevations. If it is known that the hypertension is sustained, it is usually appropriate to prescribe a two-drug therapy as recommended by JNC 7 for stage 2 hypertension (BP >160/100 mm Hg). An effort should be made to identify individuals at risk for secondary hypertension (e.g., those with renal or adrenal causes of hypertension, drug-induced hypertension), which are much more common in patients with severe hypertension syndromes. It is also important to counsel the patient on the importance of long-term BP control and to schedule follow-up within 1 week or less.

Hypertensive urgencies

The term *hypertensive urgency* implies the need for immediate intervention; it must be applied cautiously because precipitous BP reduction may present more immediate danger than having severe hypertension (**Table C147.2**). This lesson was learned from studying the adverse cardiac ischemic consequences caused by the formerly common emergency room (ER) practice of using oral nifedipine for virtually any patient who presented with marked BP elevation. This category is somewhat nebulous but includes symptoms such as severe headache or shortness of breath, evidence of non–life-threatening target organ damage such as elevated serum creatinine, T-wave changes on electrocardiogram (ECG), or microangiopathic changes in the peripheral blood smear.

Therapy. Agents that reliably cause an immediate fall in BP include central sympatholytics (clonidine 0.1–0.2 mg), labetalol (200–400 mg), and amlodipine (2.5–5 mg). Responses

to angiotensin-converting enzyme (ACE) inhibitors are more variable. For many patients with urgent hypertension without symptoms of major target organ dysfunction, initiation of therapy with two oral agents is appropriate to lower BP to an intermediate target over 24 to 72 hours as noted for severe hypertension. Be aware that aggressive dosing of oral agents may necessitate a longer period of observation in the ER to minimize the risk of significant hypotension following discharge. Appropriate follow-up within 3 days of the incident should be scheduled and written instructions provided to the patient.

Hypertensive emergencies

Almost all hypertensive emergencies (**Table C147.3**) are caused or exacerbated by intense systemic vasoconstriction, often with profound (but masked) blood volume reduction. The goal of therapy is to reduce vasoconstriction while maintaining adequate perfusion of target organs. The heart, brain, and kidneys have autoregulatory mechanisms that protect them from acute ischemia when BP is abruptly reduced and these mechanisms normally operate over a wide range of BPs. The lower limit of autoregulation in hypertensive patients is shifted upward, however, so that precipitous BP lowering to very low levels can theoretically lead to circulatory collapse in the brain, heart, or kidney. In reality, with judicious, gradual BP-lowering, hypoperfusion is rarely seen and autoregulatory mechanisms reset to more normal levels.

Immediate treatment goals. Therapy is often initiated before the results of laboratory studies are available; additional diagnostic studies may be undertaken in situations in which

TABLE C147.2

HYPERTENSIVE URGENCIES (NOT ACUTELY LIFE-THREATENING; MORE SEVERE FORMS MAY BE HYPERTENSIVE EMERGENCIES)

Extensive body burns
Acute glomerulonephritis with severe hypertension
Scleroderma crisis
Acute systemic vasculitis with severe hypertension
Surgery-related hypertension
    BP >180/110 mm Hg in patients requiring immediate surgery
    Postoperative hypertension[a]
    Severe hypertension after kidney transplantation
Severe epistaxis
Drug-related hypertension
    Rebound hypertension after sudden withdrawal of
        antihypertensive agents (most cases)
    Monoamine oxidase inhibitor interactions (food or drug)
Episodic/severe hypertension associated with chronic spinal cord
    injury
Autonomic hyperreflexia syndrome (baroreflex dysfunction)

the cause of the hypertension or the etiology of stroke remains in doubt. Aggressive treatment is appropriate but initial therapy aimed at partial reduction of BP is probably safer for most patients with a hypertensive emergency; achievement of normotensive BP levels is not indicated. The general goal of initial therapy is to reduce mean arterial BP by no more than 25% within 2 hours or to a BP in the range of 160/100 mm Hg (a mean arterial pressure ~120 mm Hg).

Specific syndromes. Specific therapies are indicated by the types of organ damage present.

Heart failure and acute myocardial infarction. In patients with an acute aortic dissection or acute heart failure, an immediate reduction of BP to lower levels may be indicated to maintain adequate pump function. A recent scientific statement from the American College of Cardiology and American Heart Association recommended that patients with ischemic heart disease should be

TABLE C147.3

LIFE-THREATENING HYPERTENSIVE EMERGENCIES (MILDER FORMS MAY BE HYPERTENSIVE URGENCIES, SEE TABLE C147.2)

Hypertensive encephalopathy
Acute cerebrovascular disease
    Intracerebral hemorrhage
    Subarachnoid hemorrhage
    Acute atherothrombotic brain infarction
Acute left ventricular failure with pulmonary edema
Acute myocardial infarction or unstable angina
Acute aortic dissection
Eclampsia or severe hypertension during pregnancy
Catecholamine excess states
    Pheochromocytoma crisis
    Overdose with sympathomimetics or drugs with similar
        action (phencyclidine, cocaine, phenylpropanolamine)
    Severe drug withdrawal states
Head trauma
Postcoronary artery bypass hypertension
Uncontrollable postoperative bleeding

aggressively managed to achieve a target BP of <130/80 mm Hg within several days, although the speed of the initial BP reduction is dependent on the clinical conditions present. Adequate BP reduction is mandated for any patient receiving thrombolytic therapy (see Chapter C149).

Acute stroke. In patients with an acute cerebrovascular accident, the benefits of marked reduction of BP are still debated but it is likely that pathogenetic differences in stroke mechanisms (e.g., thrombotic vs. hemorrhagic) may call for different approaches. In the case of hemorrhagic stroke, an argument can be made for more aggressive BP reduction, although initially to intermediate values such as 160/100 mm Hg. In ischemic stroke, concerns persist that acute BP reductions may compromise perfusion to the ischemic penumbra, the at-risk zone adjacent to the infarct. Of note, there is as yet no systematic evidence that this fear is justified. To be prudent, however, BP reductions in most stroke patients should be accomplished over a period of hours, with careful attention paid to any changes in neurologic status. As with acute myocardial infarction (MI), patients who are candidates for thrombolysis require more fastidious BP control to minimize hemorrhagic consequences or extension of the stroke (see Chapter C153).

Hypertensive encephalopathy. Hypertensive encephalopathy is a potentially lethal complication of severe hypertension that occurs when an increase in BP exceeds the autoregulatory ability of the brain to maintain constant cerebral perfusion. The resulting disruption of the blood–brain barrier causes diffuse cerebral edema and neurologic dysfunction. The presence of papilledema is the *sine qua non* of hypertensive encephalopathy, which should be suspected when there is a significant elevation of BP accompanied by other neurologic signs and symptoms. This is a diagnosis of exclusion and requires that stroke, intracranial hemorrhage, seizure disorder, mental disorder, mass lesions, vasculitis, and encephalitis be ruled out. When hypertensive encephalopathy is suspected, BP should be promptly lowered with nitroprusside or labetalol with careful monitoring in an intensive care facility with frequent neurologic assessments. BP reduction is often associated with dramatic improvement in cerebral function; subsequent deterioration in neurologic function however, requires reevaluation and consideration of other possible diagnoses.

Specific drugs. In keeping with the vasoconstrictive nature of hypertensive emergencies, the parenteral drugs that are safest and most effective are listed in **Table C147.4**. Of the available choices, parenteral labetalol is particularly attractive because it does not require intraarterial BP monitoring, tends to protect the heart, and counteracts the marked sympathetic overactivity and tachycardia that often accompany a hypertensive emergency. Sodium nitroprusside is particularly attractive in hypertensive encephalopathy because it can be precisely controlled, has a rapid onset of action and short half-life, and because it has minimal adverse effects on cerebral or coronary blood flow. Intravenous nicardipine has been used successfully in the management of hypertensive encephalopathy. Other choices depend on the individual patient characteristics and the goals of immediate therapy; fenoldopam may be useful when renal insufficiency is present.

With the exception of pulmonary edema or marked fluid overload, diuretics are not indicated for initial therapy in hypertensive emergencies (owing to the volume contraction that usually accompanies the condition). Loop-diuretics in particular are not recommended for the routine treatment of hypertensive urgencies or emergencies in the absence of fluid overload because they can cause additional reflex vasoconstriction

TABLE C147.4

DRUGS USEFUL FOR HYPERTENSIVE EMERGENCIES

Agent	Dose	Onset/duration of action (after discontinuation)	Precautions
PARENTERAL VASODILATORS			
Sodium nitroprusside	0.25–10.00 µg/kg/min as i.v. infusion[a]; maximal dose for 10 min only	Immediate/2–3 min after infusion	Nausea, vomiting, muscle twitching; with prolonged use, may cause thiocyanate intoxication, methemoglobinemia acidosis, cyanide poisoning; bags, bottles, and delivery sets must be light resistant
Glyceryl trinitrate	5–100 µg as i.v. infusion[a]	2–5 min/5–10 min	Headache, tachycardia, vomiting, flushing, methemoglobinemia; requires special delivery systems due to the drug's binding to polyvinyl chloride tubing
Nicardipine	5–15 mg/h i.v. infusion	1–5 min/15–30 min, but may exceed 12 h after prolonged infusion	Tachycardia, nausea, vomiting, headache, increased intracranial pressure, possible protracted hypotension after prolonged infusions
Verapamil	5–10 mg i.v.; can follow with infusion of 3–25 mg/h	1–5 min/30–60 min	Heart block (first-, second-, and third-degree), especially with concomitant digitalis or β-blockers; bradycardia
Fenoldopam	0.1–0.3 mg/kg/min i.v. infusion	<5 min/30 min	Headache, tachycardia, flushing, local phlebitis
Hydralazine	10–20 mg as i.v. bolus or 10–40 mg i.m.; repeat every 4–6 h	10 min i.v./>1 h (i.v.), 20–30 min i.m./4–6 h i.m.	Tachycardia, headache, vomiting, aggravation of angina pectoris
Enalaprilat	0.625–1.250 mg every 6 h i.v.	15–60 min/12–24 h	Renal failure in patients with bilateral artery stenosis, hypotension
PARENTERAL ADRENERGIC INHIBITORS			
Labetalol	10–80 mg as i.v. bolus every 10 min; up to 2 mg/min as i.v. infusion	5–10 min/2–6 h	Bronchoconstriction, heart block, orthostatic hypotension
Esmolol	500 µg/kg bolus injection i.v. or 25–100 µg/kg/min by infusion May repeat bolus after 5 min or increase infusion rate to 300 µg/kg/min	1–5 min/15–30 min	First-degree heart block, congestive heart failure, asthma
Phentolamine	5–15 mg as i.v. bolus	1–2 min/10–30 min	Tachycardia, orthostatic hypotension

[a]Requires a special delivery system.

in the renin-angiotensin-aldosterone and sympathetic nervous systems. "Standard" β-blockers (i.e., those without the α-blocking property of labetalol) are generally ineffective in lowering BP in hypertensive emergencies, presumably because they have no vasodilator capacity. Parenteral esmolol may be indicated if myocardial ischemia, tachycardia, or other catecholamine-sensitive arrhythmias are present.

Follow-up care

Regardless of the type of hypertensive emergency or the antihypertensive agent used to control BP, the objective should be to start an oral regimen as soon as the patient can tolerate it, thereby allowing earlier tapering and discontinuation of parenteral agents, and hospital discharge. Switching abruptly from intravenous to oral therapy may result in a precipitous rise in BP if appropriate agents are not chosen, so patients should be monitored carefully during this period. If clinically stable and appropriate follow-up care can be arranged, even those patients who needed emergent or urgent treatment can safely be discharged on oral medications with a follow-up visit within 24 to 72 hours in the outpatient setting. To discharge a patient from an ER or outpatient setting without a confirmed follow-up appointment is a missed opportunity to get that patient back into treatment—optimal control of BP should be a management priority.

Suggested Readings

Bender SR, Fong MW, Heitz S, et al. Characteristics and management of patients presenting to the emergency department with hypertensive urgency. *J Clin Hypertens (Greenwich)* 2006;8:12–18.

Elliott WJ. Clinical features in the management of selected hypertensive emergencies. *Prog Cardiovasc Dis* 2006;48:316–325. [Review].

Gales MA. Oral antihypertensives for hypertensive urgencies. *Ann Pharmacother* 1994;28:352–358.

Grossman E, Messerli FH, Grodzicki T, et al. Should a moratorium be placed on sublingual nifedipine capsules given for hypertensive emergencies and pseudoemergencies? *JAMA* 1996;276:1328–1331.

Hix JK, Vidt DG. Hypertensive emergencies and urgencies: uncontrolled severe hypertension. In: Battegay EJ, Lip GYH, Bakris GL, eds. *Hypertension—principles and practice*. Boca Raton: Taylor & Francis, 2005:651–669.

Karras DJ, Kruus LK, Clenki JJ, et al. Evaluation and treatment of patients with severely elevated BP in academic emergency departments: a multicenter study. *Ann Emerg Med* 2006;47:230–236.

Vaughan CJ, Delanty N. Hypertensive emergencies. *Lancet* 2000;356:411–417.

Vidt DG. Emergency room management of hypertensive urgencies and emergencies. *J Clin Hypertens (Greenwich)* 2001;3:158–164.

Vidt DG. Hypertension curriculum review. Hypertensive crises: emergencies and urgencies. *J Clin Hypertens* 2004;6(9):520–525.

CHAPTER C148 ■ TREATMENT OF HYPERTENSION IN MINORITIES

MAHBOOB RAHMAN, MD, MS AND JACKSON T. WRIGHT, Jr., MD, PhD

KEY POINTS

- In the black population, monotherapy with renin-angiotensin system (RAS) blockers [angiotensin-converting enzyme (ACE) inhibitors, angiotensin receptor blockers, (ARBs) or β-blockers] is somewhat less effective in lowering blood pressure (BP) than monotherapy with diuretic or calcium blocker, but there is wide variation in response to all antihypertensive drug classes in all populations.
- The combination of a diuretic [or calcium channel blocker (CCB)] with an RAS blocker is equally effective in all racial subgroups studied.
- ACE inhibitors and ARBs appear to be less effective than thiazide-type diuretics or calcium blockers in preventing cardiovascular (CV) complications of hypertension in blacks, although either drug is recommended for any hypertensive patient with heart failure (HF) or chronic kidney disease,
- Few data are available on efficacy of different drugs in non-black minorities but greater rates of ACE inhibitor side effects occur in some minorities: angioedema and cough in blacks, cough and flushing in Asians.
- Drug cost and social issues may need to be considered more often in low-income minority groups.

See also Chapters **B84, B85, B86, B87,** and **B88**

Hypertension and hypertensive target organ damage are both more prevalent and severe in certain minority populations, especially blacks, and clinicians should therefore be especially vigilant in the evaluation and treatment of these populations. Differences in epidemiology, severity, and response to antihypertensive drug classes between population subgroups are also influenced by cultural and social factors, along with access to health care. To date, however, consistently reproducible genetic differences have not been established for any of these parameters. Furthermore, racial and ethnic differences are qualitative rather than quantitative. Therefore, although characteristics of hypertension differ slightly among racial and ethnic groups, the presentation and management of hypertension in minority populations is for the most part similar to that of the rest of the population.

Epidemiologic overview

The United States is an increasingly diverse nation of individuals from various racial and ethnic origins. In 2000, the U.S. Census Bureau reported population percentages of whites, 75.1%; blacks, 12.9%; Mexican American, 7.3%; other Hispanics, 6.5%, Asian and Pacific Islanders, 4.5%; and Native Americans, 1.5%. In the last decade, the country has experienced a marked increase in minority populations and immigrants, and this trend is expected to continue. As immigrant populations acculturate, their risks for cardiovascular (CV) disease change. Because of the greater prevalence and severity of hypertension in African Americans (and until recently, the smaller size of other minority groups in the United States), more data on hypertension are available in African Americans compared to other racial-ethnic groups. Data from the third National Health and Nutrition Survey (NHANES 1999–2002) indicate that there remains significant racial/ethnic variability in the prevalence, awareness, treatment, and control of hypertension in the United States.

Blacks. The prevalence of hypertension in African Americans is higher than in whites and Mexican Americans (**Table C148.1**). Hypertension-related mortality remains five to seven times higher in the African-American community and left ventricular hypertrophy (LVH), coronary heart disease (CHD), and stroke are two to four times higher in African Americans than in whites; moreover, CHD typically develops several years earlier. Differences in obesity and lifestyle factors in young adults contribute to the higher baseline blood pressure (BP) and greater BP increase over time in blacks relative to whites. In blacks, the excess prevalence of obesity, diabetes mellitus (DM), and LVH add to the risk of end-organ complications—a risk already substantially increased based on the severity of the underlying hypertension. These circumstances make the need for aggressive BP control even more critical

Hispanic Americans. Age-adjusted BP levels in Hispanic populations generally parallel those of the racial group to which they belong. BP is generally the same or lower than that of non-Hispanic whites, despite the high prevalence of obesity and type 2 DM. Mexican Americans in general have lower hypertension prevalence and severity than do non-Hispanic whites. Mexican Americans have lower hypertension control rates; despite this, they have similar rates of CHD as do whites. Conversely, they have higher rates of end-stage renal disease (ESRD) primarily due to their having increased rates of obesity and diabetes. Low socioeconomic status compounded by language barriers may affect preventive and primary health care in this sector of the population.

Asians and Pacific Islanders. Native Hawaiians appear to be at greater risk for coronary artery disease (CAD), and the group as a whole has poorer health outcomes and lower life expectancy than other groups in Hawaii, due, at least in part, to their increased prevalence of obesity and DM. Although NHANES II reported that 27% of all U.S. adults 20 to 59 years of age were overweight in 1985, a study of residents of Hawaiian Homestead lands on the largely rural island of Molokai found that 65% of these native Hawaiians (20–59 years of age) were overweight. The South Asian countries of India, Pakistan, Bangladesh, Sri Lanka, and Nepal make up one fourth of the world's population; South Asians have the highest rates of CAD of any ethnic group studied but recent data suggest that this can be largely explained by higher levels of traditional risk factors at younger ages. The age-adjusted prevalence of myocardial infarction or angina was approximately three times higher in South Asian men compared to the Framingham Offspring Study (7.2% vs. 2.5%) but was similar in women (0.3% vs. 1%).

Native Americans. Although the data are extremely limited, the prevalence of hypertension in Native Americans is probably similar to that in the general population. As in other populations, hypertension incidence is associated with obesity, age, and DM prevalence.

Clinical trials comparing drug therapies in minorities

There are few studies specifically designed to evaluate racial and ethnic differences in antihypertensive drug response. Clinically significant ethnic and racial differences in treatment response have not been reported for most population subgroups. However, while a great deal of population variability in response exists, angiotensin-converting enzyme (ACE) inhibitors, angiotensin receptor blockers (ARBs), and β-blockers are consistently less effective in lowering BP in black hypertensives compared to thiazide diuretics and calcium channel blockers (CCBs). The only trial specifically designed to examine the effect of various antihypertensive agents in black compared to white patients, the Antihypertensive and Lipid-Lowering Treatment to Prevent Heart Attack Trial (ALLHAT) showed treatment based on an ACE inhibitor (or an α-blocker) was associated with poorer BP control than treatment based on a thiazide diuretic, with a greater risk of CV events, especially stroke and heart failure (HF). CCBs show similar BP reduction and CV protection compared to diuretics in black hypertensive patients but a substantially higher rate of HF. Outcome studies comparing ARBs with other agents have included few blacks but also suggest less CV protection in black patients. ACE inhibitors (and presumably ARBs) are more effective than β-blockers and dihydropyridine CCBs in preventing progression of renal disease in multiple populations, including black patients with hypertension and chronic kidney disease.

TABLE C148.1

HYPERTENSION IN MINORITIES

Race/ethnicity	Hypertension prevalence	Awareness	Under current treatment	Controlled hypertension
Total	28.6	63.4	45.3	29.3
White non-Hispanic	27.4	62.9	48.6	29.8
Black, non-Hispanic	40.5	70.3	55.4	29.8
Mexican American	25.1	49.8	34.9	17.3

All values are reported as %.
Adapted from *MMWR* 2005;54(1):7–9

Management

Evaluation. The evaluation of hypertension in minorities is similar regardless of subgroup. In all, evaluation is directed at assessing the severity and presence of other risk factors, target organ damage, and likelihood of secondary hypertension. The higher frequency of early onset, severe, resistant essential hypertension makes the identification of secondary hypertension more challenging in black hypertensive patients. Sleep disordered breathing also occurs more commonly in blacks and in the Asian population, and this racial difference is greatest at early ages. Therefore, evaluation for sleep disordered breathing and other secondary causes of hypertension should be considerations based on the nature of the clinical presentation.

Lifestyle modification. Lifestyle modification deserves special attention in minority populations. The increasing problem of obesity in these populations makes it mandatory to emphasize caloric restriction and exercise as part of the treatment plan for hypertension. Reduction of sodium intake should also be strongly emphasized in minority populations. In addition, the Dietary Approaches to Stop Hypertension (DASH) trials clearly demonstrated the BP-lowering efficacy of diets high in fruits, vegetables, grains, and low-fat dairy products, and reduces BP even in the absence of weight reduction. Reduced sodium intake as a complement to the DASH diet reduces BP further. It is noteworthy that blacks showed the greatest BP reduction with this diet, which was as effective as most pharmacologic monotherapies. It has been speculated that increased potassium content of the DASH diet is an important aspect of its beneficial effects.

Monotherapy. There are no compelling data to suggest that the treatment of minorities should differ substantively from the population as a whole. On the basis of the ALLHAT results, diuretics are considered by many practitioners as "preferred" initial therapy in black hypertensives. β-Blockers, ACE inhibitors, and CCBs also reduce CV event rates and are reasonable alternatives in those unable to take diuretics in most populations. However, ALLHAT suggested both greater BP reduction and CV event reduction with CCBs in black hypertensive patients than with ACE inhibitors or α-blockers, and in other studies, CCBs were more effective in lowering BP than β-blockers. Although data are limited, there is no indication of differences in BP efficacy of specific drugs in other population subgroups.

Need for combination therapy. BP control can be enhanced by combining agents from different classes rather than simply increasing monotherapy doses. In research studies and in clinical practice, diuretics are commonly used in combination with other classes of agents to achieve BP goals. Interracial BP response differences for ACE inhibitors, ARBs, or β-blockers are all but eliminated when any of these agents is combined with a thiazide-type diuretic or a CCB. Furthermore, the fact that most hypertensives require more than one antihypertensive agent to reach their BP goal diminishes the relevance of the debate over which of several agents should be prescribed as initial therapy.

Medication side effects. The incidence of side effects with ACE inhibitors appears to be higher in blacks than in the general population. In particular, cough and especially angioedema occur at roughly two to three times the rates seen in whites. On the basis of anecdotal experience, cough and flushing are also prominent in Asians receiving ACE inhibitors. The reasons for these racial differences are not yet known, but different patterns of bradykinin breakdown are suspected.

Cost and other issues. The cost of drugs may also represent a significant hurdle and the lower income levels of many minority populations can influence the likelihood of long-term adherence to therapy. It is fortunate that in addition to noteworthy effects on BP lowering and reduction in clinical endpoints, thiazide-type diuretics are very inexpensive, usually costing pennies per day. Increased availability of generic ACE inhibitors and CCBs, as well as β-blockers and centrally acting agents, will increase the number of affordable options for most patients. Many pharmaceutical firms offer special programs to aid economically disadvantaged patients, which can also be exploited. Other social and cultural issues may also affect an individual's willingness to accept lifestyle changes or take medications. Health care providers should be familiar with these issues and be prepared to work with individuals to overcome such barriers to therapy.

Suggested Readings

The ALLHAT Officers and Coordinators for the ALLHAT Collaborative Research Group. Major cardiovascular events in hypertensive patients randomized to doxazosin vs chlorthalidone. *JAMA* 2000;283:1967–1975.

Enas EA, Garg A, Davidson MA, et al. Coronary heart disease and its risk factors in the first generation immigrant Asian Indians to the USA. *Indian Heart J* 1996;48:343–353.

Hajjar I, Kotchen TA. Trends in prevalence, awareness, treatment, and control of hypertension in the United States, 1988–2000. *JAMA* 2003;290(2):199–206.

Hyman DJ, Pavlik VN. Characteristics of patients with uncontrolled hypertension in the United States. *N Engl J Med* 2001;345:479–486.

Joshi P, Islam S, Pais P, et al. Risk factors for early myocardial infarction in South Asians compared with individuals in other countries. *JAMA* 2007;297:286–294.

Julius S, Alderman MH, Beevers G, et al. Cardiovascular risk reduction in hypertensive Black patients with left ventricular hypertrophy: The LIFE Study. *J Am Coll Cardiol* 2004;43:1047–1055.

Oparil S, Wright JT Jr. Ethnicity and BP. *J Clin Hypertens (Greenwich)* 2005;7(6):357–364.

Wright JT Jr, Agodoa L, Contreras G, et al. Successful BP control in the African American study of kidney disease and hypertension. *Arch Intern Med* 2002;162:1636–1643.

Wright JT Jr, Bakris G, Greene T, et al. AASK Study Group. Effect of BP lowering and antihypertensive drug class on progression of hypertensive kidney disease: results from the AASK trial. *JAMA* 2002;288:2421–2467.

Wright JT Jr, Dunn JK, Cutler JA, et al. Outcomes in hypertensive black and non-black patients treated with chlorthalidone, amlodipine, and lisinopril. *JAMA* 2005;293(13):1595–1608.

CHAPTER C149 ■ TREATMENT OF HYPERTENSIVE PATIENTS WITH ISCHEMIC HEART DISEASE

CLIVE ROSENDORFF, MD, PhD, FRCP

KEY POINTS

■ Goal blood pressure (BP) is <130/80 mm Hg for patients at high risk for, or with existing ischemic heart disease (IHD); the degree of BP lowering is the major determinant of cardiovascular risk reduction.
■ Recommended first-line choices for BP control in high-risk patients include angiotensin-converting enzyme (ACE) inhibitors, angiotensin receptor blockers (ARBs), thiazide diuretics, or calcium antagonists (CAs); addition of a second drug is often necessary to achieve target BP.
■ Recommended first-line choice for BP control in stable angina is a β-blocker, or if contraindicated, a long-acting CA; ACE inhibitors and thiazide diuretics also improve outcomes.
■ In patients hospitalized with an acute coronary syndrome, hypertension should be treated with a β-blocker; alternative choices in the absence of ventricular dysfunction include substitution of verapamil or diltiazem or addition of a long-acting dihydropyridine.

See also Chapters A65, **B77**, C109, C110, and **C119**

Ischemic heart disease [IHD, also referred to as *coronary artery disease* (CAD)] limits myocardial perfusion and therefore oxygen supply. Systolic hypertension increases myocardial oxygen demand because of the increased output impedance to left ventricular (LV) ejection, and is a common cause of LV hypertrophy. The combination of decreased oxygen supply and increased oxygen demand explains why hypertensive patients are more likely than normotensive people to have a myocardial infarction (MI) or other major coronary event, and are at higher risk of dying after an acute MI.

Blood pressure components and ischemic heart disease

Diastolic blood pressure and the J-curve. Many studies have shown that there is a continuous relationship between diastolic blood pressure (DBP) and the risk of a coronary event: the lower the DBP, the lower the risk. However, there has been concern that coronary blood flow could be impaired and IHD risk could increase if the DBP (the coronary filling pressure) goes below the lower limit of coronary autoregulation, thereby producing a J-shaped curve. The concern is heightened in IHD patients with hypertension and LV hypertrophy, who may have an altered autoregulatory threshold, increased afterload, and intrinsically greater myocardial oxygen demand due to the LV hypertrophy. Yet there are no reliable clinical data about what the autoregulatory threshold may be. The Hypertension Optimal Treatment (HOT) trial, designed to investigate this issue, did find a very small upswing in major cardiovascular events (MI and

cardiovascular mortality, but not stroke or renal failure) at DBP levels below 70 mm Hg. This apparent myocardial susceptibility to low diastolic perfusion pressures is consistent with the notion that stroke morbidity and mortality is best correlated with systolic blood pressure (SBP), whereas the best predictor of coronary events may be pulse pressure.

Systolic blood pressure. Pulse pressure is usually greatest in isolated systolic hypertension (ISH), where DBP is often below 70 mm Hg before or during treatment. In the elderly with ISH (and low DBP), no J-shaped curve has been described. In fact, the three outcome trials in the elderly with ISH [Systolic Hypertension in the Elderly Program (SHEP), Systolic Hypertension in Europe (SYST-Eur), and Systolic Hypertension in China (SYST-China)] together showed decreases of 25% in MI including sudden death in the active treatment group compared with those who received placebo. These studies also demonstrate the value of SBP reduction in reducing IHD events. Diabetic patients benefited significantly from aggressive BP lowering in the HOT trial.

Goals of antihypertensive therapy

Target blood pressure. There is very good epidemiologic evidence from the Prospective Studies Collaboration, based on their meta-analysis of almost 1 million adults from 61 prospective studies that IHD risk is continuous over the range of 115/75 to 185/115 mm Hg, and that each 20/10 mm Hg increment doubles IHD risk. Despite this continuity, practical matters dictate that target BP values should be established. Taken together, there are ample data to support the recommendation

TABLE C149.1

SUMMARY OF THE MAIN RECOMMENDATIONS

	General CAD prevention	High CAD risk[a]	Stable angina	UA/NSTEMI	STEMI
BP target (mm Hg)	<140/90	<130/80	<130/80	<130/80	<130/80
Lifestyle modification[b]	Yes	Yes	Yes	Yes	Yes
Specific drug indications	Any effective antihypertensive drug or combination[c]	ACE I *or* ARB *or* CCB *or* thiazide diuretic *or* combination	β-Blocker *and* ACE I (or ARB)	β-Blocker (if patient is hemodynamically stable) *and* ACE I (or ARB[d])	β-Blocker (if patient is hemodynamically stable) *and* ACE I (or ARB[d])
Comments	If SBP ≥160 mm Hg or DBP ≥100 mm Hg, then start with two drugs		If β-blocker contraindicated, or if side effects, can substitute diltiazem or verapamil (but not if bradycardia or LVD) Can add dihydropyridine CCB (not diltiazem or verapamil) to β-blocker A thiazide diuretic can be added for BP control		

CAD, coronary artery disease; UA, unstable angina; NSTEMI, non–ST-elevation myocardial infarction; STEMI, ST-segment elevation myocardial infarction; ACE-I, angiotension-converting enzyme inhibitor; ARB, angiotensin receptor blocker, CCB, calcium-channel blocker; LVD, left ventricular dysfunction; BP, blood pressure.
[a]Diabetes, chronic kidney disease, known CAD or CAD equivalent (carotid artery disease, peripheral arterial disease, abdominal aortic aneurism), or 10-year Framingham risk score of ≥10% .
[b]Weight loss if appropriate, healthy diet (including sodium restriction), exercise, smoking cessation, alcohol moderation.
[c]Evidence supports ACE inhibitor (or ARB), CCB, or thiazide diuretic as first line therapy.
[d]If anterior MI, if hypertension persists, if LV dysfunction or HF, or if the patient has diabetes.

to lower BP to <130/80 mm Hg in any patient at high risk for developing cardiovascular disease (**Table C149.1**). High risk may be defined as the presence of a "coronary risk equivalent" (diabetes, prior IHD event, chronic kidney disease, carotid artery disease, peripheral arterial disease, abdominal aortic aneurysm, or a 10-year Framingham risk score of ≥10%).

Speed of blood pressure lowering. No studies have addressed prospectively the appropriate speed of BP lowering in patients with established occlusive IHD. General opinion remains that BP should be lowered cautiously, maintaining DBP above 60 mm Hg if the patient has diabetes or is older than 60 years. In older hypertensive individuals with wide pulse pressures, lowering SBP may cause very low DBP values (<60 mm Hg). This should alert the clinician to assess carefully any untoward signs or symptoms, especially those compatible with myocardial ischemia. In the very old (those older than 80 years), antihypertensive therapy is effective in decreasing the frequency of strokes, but similar evidence for reducing IHD events is less certain.

Prevention of ischemic heart disease with antihypertensive drugs

Lifestyle modifications remain important in the prevention and therapy of IHD but drug therapy is also proven to further reduce morbidity and mortality (**Tables C149.1 and C149.2**). In general, angiotensin-converting enzyme (ACE) inhibitors, angiotensin receptor blockers, calcium antagonists, or thiazide diuretics or their combination are preferred as first-line drugs for the treatment of hypertension in patients at high risk for IHD.

Diuretics and β-blockers. Early clinical trials [Hypertension Detection and Follow-Up Program (HDFP), Medical Research Council (MRC), SHEP, Swedish Trial in Old Patients with Hypertension (STOP), and MRC-elderly] used diuretics, sympathetic blocking agents, and β-blockers to investigate the value of primary prevention. These studies showed a significant benefit

of treatment for reducing stroke morbidity and mortality in all age-groups, whereas reduction in IHD events was less impressive. In SHEP, the benefit of diuretic or β-blocker therapy on MI (25% reduction) was not as great as it was for stroke (36% reduction). Many explanations have been advanced for the dissociation between stroke and IHD outcomes, including the potential arrhythmogenic effects of diuretic-induced hypokalemia.

Antihypertensive and lipid-lowering treatment to prevent heart attack trial (ALLHAT). This very large trial in high-risk hypertensive patients showed no significant difference between chlorthalidone, lisinopril, and amlodipine in preventing the combined primary endpoint of nonfatal MI plus coronary heart disease (CHD) death, combined CHD (primary endpoint, coronary revascularization, or hospitalized angina), or all-cause mortality. There was superiority of a diuretic (chlorthalidone) over the ACE inhibitor lisinopril in preventing stroke, and over the α-blocker doxazosin, the calcium antagonist (CA) amlodipine, and lisinopril in preventing heart failure (HF) but BP control was not equal in all treatment arms. The results of ALLHAT were interpreted by the authors to recommend thiazide diuretics as first-line therapy for hypertensive patients unless there was a contraindication to using them. A more conservative position is that of the Joint National Committee (JNC 7) that diuretics are appropriate therapy for most individuals, alone or in combination; JNC 7 did not identify any class of drugs as "first line."

Calcium antagonists. Trials of CAs for the primary prevention of cardiovascular complications of hypertension [SYST-Eur, SYST-China, Prospective Randomized Evaluation of the Vascular Effects of Norvasc Trial (PREVENT), Multicenter Isradipine Diuretic Atherosclerosis Study (MIDAS), Nordic Diltiazem Study (NORDIL), and Intervention as a Goal in Hypertension Treatment (INSIGHT)] tended to show a significant degree of prevention of stroke, compared to placebo, diuretic, β-blocker alone, or combined therapy. The absolute risk reduction in IHD deaths and nonfatal coronary events was less impressive, with

TABLE C149.2

KEY CLINICAL TRIALS OF ANTIHYPERTENSIVE DRUGS IN THE PREVENTION OF IHD

Trial/study acronym	Report	Duration (yrs)	Treatment	Patients	Mean age	Total coronary events/ 1,000 patients/yr	
						Active	Control/reference
DIURETICS OR β-BLOCKERS vs. PLACEBO							
HDFP	1979	5	Diuretics (± reserpine/ methyldopa ± hydralazine ± guanethidine) vs. referred care	10,940	51	6	7
MRC	1985	5	Bendrofluazide or propanolol vs. placebo	17,354	51	5	4
SHEP	1991	4.5	Chlorthalidone (± atenolol) vs. placebo	4,736	72	15[a]	20
STOP	1992	2	3 β-blockers + HCTZ vs. placebo	1,627	76	17[a]	25
MRC-Elderly	1992	5.8	Atenolol or HCTZ + amiloride vs. placebo	4,396	70	7(diuretic)[a] 12(β-blocker)	13
CALCIUM CHANNEL BLOCKERS vs. PLACEBO							
Syst-Eur	1997	2	Nitrendipine(± enalapril ± HCTZ) vs. placebo	4,695	70	34[a]	44
Syst-China	1998	2	Nitrendipine (± captopril ± HCTZ) vs. placebo	2,394	67	5	7
PREVENT	2000	3	Amlodipine vs. placebo	825	57	21[a]	25
CAMELOT	2004	2	Amlodipine vs. placebo	1,318	57	14	19
ACE INHIBITORS vs. PLACEBO							
HOPE	2000	5	Ramipril vs. placebo	9,297	67	93[a]	104
EUROPA	2003	4	Perindopril vs. placebo	13,655	60	19[a]	24
PEACE	2004	5	Trandolapril vs. placebo	8,920	64	17	18
CAMELOT	2004	2	Enalapril vs. placebo	1,328	58	13	19
CALCIUM CHANNEL BLOCKERS vs. OTHER AGENTS							
MIDAS	1996	3	Isradipine vs. HCTZ	883	59	14	8
NORDIL	2000	5	Diltiazem (± ACE I ± diuretic or α-blocker) vs. diuretic + β-blocker (± ACE-I or α-blocker)	10,881	60	6	7
INSIGHT	2000	4	Nifedipine (± atenolol or enalapril) vs. HCTZ + amiloride (± atenolol or enalapril)	6,321	65	16	17
ALLHAT	2000	4.9	Amlodipine (+ atenolol, clonidine, reserpine, hydralazine) vs. chlorthalidone (+ atenolol etc.)	24,303	67	19	19
INVEST	2003	2	Verapamil SR (+ trandolapril + HCTZ) vs. atenolol (+ trandolapril + HCTZ)	22,576	67	30	30
CONVINCE	2003	3	Verapamil (± other) vs. atenolol or HCTZ	8,241	66	12	12
ASCOT–BPLA	2005	5.5	Amlodipine (± perindopril) vs. atenolol (± bendroflumethiazide)	19,257	63	14[a]	16
ACE INHIBITORS vs. OTHER AGENTS							
UKPDS	1998	9	Captopril (± furosemide ± nifedipine ± methyldopa ± prazosin) vs. atenolol (± furosemide ± nifedipine ± methyldopa ± prazosin)	758	56	26	23
CAPP	1999	6	Captopril vs. β-blockers (± diuretics)	10,985	53	13	13

TABLE C149.2

(CONTINUED)

Trial/study acronym	Report	Duration (yr)	Treatment	Patients	Mean age	Total coronary events/ 1,000 patients/yr	
						Active	Control/reference
STOP-2	1999	6	ACE-I vs. calcium antagonists or diuretic and/or β-blocker	6,614	76	13	14(diuretic/ β-blocker) 17(calcium antagonist)
ABCD	1998	5	Enalapril (± metoprolol ± HCTZ) vs. nisoldipine (± metoprolol ± HCTZ)	470	58	4[a]	21
ALLHAT	2002	4.9	Lisinopril vs. amlodipine vs. chlorthalidone	23,056	67	19	19
ANBP -2	2003	4.1	Enalapril (+ others) vs. HCTZ (+ others)	6,083	72	14	16
ANGIOTENSIN RECEPTOR BLOCKERS vs. OTHER AGENTS							
LIFE	2002	4.8	Losartan vs. atenolol	9,193	67	16	15
VALUE	2004	4.2	Valsartan (+ HCTZ + others) vs. amlodipine (+ HCTZ + others)	15,245	67	11.4	9.6
VALIANT	2006	3	Valsartan vs. captopril	9,818	5	144	147

[a]$p < 0.05$.

IHD, ischemic heart disease; HDFP, Hypertension Detection and Follow-Up Program; MRC, Medical Research Council; SHEP, Systolic Hypertension in the Elderly Program; STOP, Swedish Trial in Old Patients with Hypertension; PREVENT, Prospective Randomized Evaluation of the Vascular Effects of Norvasc Trial; CAMELOT, Comparision of Amlodipine vs. Enalapril to Limit Occurrences of Thrombosis; HOPE, Heart Outcomes Prevention Evaluation; EUROPA, events with Perindopril in stable coronary Artery disease; PEACE, Prevention of Events with Angiotensin-Converting Enzyme Inhibition; MIDAS, Multicenter Isradipine Diuretic Atherosclerosis Study; NORDIL, Nordic Diltiazem Study; INSIGHT, Intervention as a Goal in Hypertension Treatment; ALLHAT, Antihypertensive and Lipid-Lowering Treatment to Prevent Heart Attack Trial; INVEST, International Verapamil–Trandolapril Study; CONVINCE, Controlled Onset Verapamil Investigation of Cardiovascular Endpoints; ASCOT-BPLA, Anglo-Scandinavian Cardiac Outcomes Trial–Blood Pressure Lowering Arm; UKPDS, U.K. Prospective Diabetes Study; CAPP, Captopril Prevention Project; ABCD, Appropriate Blood Pressure Control in Diabetes; ANBP, Australian National Antihypertensive Trial; LIFE, Losartan Intervention for Endpoint; VALUE, Valsartan Long-term Use Evaluation; VALIANT, Valsartan in Acute Myocardial Infarction Trial; HCTZ, hydrochlorothiazide; ACE-I, angiotensin-converting enzyme inhibitor.

the exception of the SYST-Eur study. In SYST-Eur, however, the reference drug was placebo; a significant number of patients in the active treatment group received an add-on agent, including enalapril, which may have influenced the results. A meta-analysis of CAs as first-line antihypertensive treatment (Pahor, et al.) suggested that CAs were inferior to angiotensin-converting enzyme (ACE) inhibitors, with a greater risk for MI (26%), HF (25%), and major cardiovascular events (10%), although they were as effective as ACE inhibitors in the reduction of all-cause mortality and stroke. More recently the Anglo-Scandinavian Cardiac Outcomes Trial–Blood Pressure Lowering Arm (ASCOT–BPLA) showed that a regimen based on amlodipine (with addition of ACE inhibitor if needed) had fewer coronary events than an atenolol-based regimen (to which a thiazide could be added).

Angiotensin-converting enzyme inhibitors. Trials of ACE inhibitors [U.K. Prospective Diabetes Study (UKPDS) and Captopril Prevention Project (CAPPP)] showed significant benefit of BP lowering on overall cardiovascular morbidity and mortality, especially stroke, but did not demonstrate a clear-cut benefit of ACE inhibitors over conventional therapy (diuretics, β-blockers, or both) for the prevention of acute coronary events. However, in STOP-2, ACE inhibitors were significantly better than CAs and also better than conventional therapy (diuretics, β-blockers, or both) in reducing MI but the low power of the study precluded reaching statistical significance. All of these studies suffer from significant design flaws.

In more recent trials of ACE inhibitors in patients with established IHD or high risk for IHD, the benefits of ACE inhibitors were clear. In the Heart Outcomes Prevention Evaluation (HOPE), after 5 years, the relative risk for cardiovascular death in the ramipril-treated group was 0.74; for MI, 0.80; for revascularization procedures, 0.85; for cardiac arrest, 0.63; and for HF, 0.77 (all highly significant vs. the placebo-treated group). The results applied equally to hypertensive and nonhypertensive patients, and to patients with known IHD and those without coronary vascular disease. Substudies of HOPE revealed that ACE inhibition reduced progression of atherosclerosis and improved myocardial remodeling. Although originally billed as a study demonstrating results not explained by BP reduction, subgroup analysis demonstrated a substantial BP effect (>10 mm Hg) on 24-hour ambulatory BP. In the EURopean trial On reduction of cardiac events with Perindopril in stable coronary Artery disease (EUROPA), perindopril therapy was associated with a 20% relative risk reduction in the primary composite endpoint of cardiovascular death, MI, or cardiac arrest compared to placebo therapy. These relatively recent studies have served to reinforce the general idea, based on many trials, that ACE inhibition is protective in high-risk patients with and without LV dysfunction.

Angiotensin receptor blockers. The use of angiotensin receptor blockers (ARBs) for the treatment of hypertension in patients with IHD has a solid foundation in animal studies and surrogate endpoint studies in humans. The Losartan Intervention for Endpoint (LIFE) study showed that losartan prevents more strokes and cardiovascular deaths than atenolol, but there were no significant differences in the rate of MI or hospital admissions for angina in this study. Protection by ARBs against cardiovascular events was similar to that produced by a CA in the Valsartan Long-term Use Evaluation (VALUE) trial, and similar to ACE inhibition in the Valsartan in Acute Myocardial Infarction Trial (VALIANT).

Treatment of hypertension in patients with stable angina

Nonpharmacologic and risk-factor management. The treatment of patients with symptomatic IHD is directed toward preventing MI and death and toward reducing the symptoms of angina and the occurrence of ischemia (**Table C149.1**). Treatment of risk factors include, in addition to BP control, smoking cessation, tight glycemic control, exercise training, lipid lowering, and weight reduction in obese patients. There is compelling evidence for the use of antiplatelet agents, aspirin if not contraindicated, otherwise clopidogrel.

Pharmacologic therapy.

β-blockers. The mainstay of therapy remains β-blockers, which reduce anginal symptoms, improve mortality, and lower BP; these drugs remain as first-line therapy in hypertensive patients with IHD and stable angina. β-Blockers reduce cardiac output and BP by slowing heart rate, which reduces myocardial oxygen demand. The slowing of heart rate prolongs diastolic perfusion time of the coronary arteries, thereby enhancing myocardial perfusion and improving ventricular mechanics. In addition, BP can also be reduced by blockade of β-adrenoreceptors on the cells of the renal juxtaglomerular apparatus, the major source of circulating renin; this mechanism variably contributes to BP reduction.

Diabetes is not a contraindication to the use of β-blockers, although the patient should be made aware that the hyperadrenergic symptoms of hypoglycemia may be masked. In hypertensive LV failure, β-blockers (especially carvedilol, metoprolol, and bisoprolol) may be used as a component of the antifailure therapy, but should be started at a very low dose and titrated up very slowly.

Other agents. When there are contraindications to the use of β-blockers, such as asthma or chronic obstructive airways disease with a significant bronchospastic component, severe peripheral vascular disease, or severe bradyarrhythmias such as a high degree of atrioventricular block or the sick sinus syndrome, CAs, either long-acting dihydropyridine agents (such as amlodipine, felodipine, or a long-acting formulation of nifedipine) or nondihydropyridine drugs such as verapamil or diltiazem, are appropriate therapy for angina and hypertension.

One controlled study [Total Ischemic Burden European Trial (TIBET)] comparing β-blockers with CAs has reported equal efficacy in controlling stable angina, but most studies have shown β-blockers to be superior [Angina Prognosis Study in Stockholm (APSIS), Total Ischemic Burden Bisoprolol Study (TIBBS)]. Combining a β-blocker with an appropriate CA enhances antianginal efficacy. Because of the increased risk of severe bradycardia or heart block if β-blockers are used together with verapamil or diltiazem, long-acting dihydropyridine CAs are preferred for combination therapy. Mainly on the basis of the HOPE and EUROPA data, a good case can be made for the inclusion of an ACE inhibitor in the treatment regimen, and, from ALLHAT, for a thiazide diuretic. Other important therapies are short- or long-acting nitrates, and antiplatelet and lipid-lowering agents.

Treatment of hypertension in patients with acute coronary syndromes

Unstable angina and non–ST segment elevation myocardial infarction. Hospitalization, usually in a coronary care unit, is indicated for: (a) patients with unstable angina (rest angina, new onset angina, increasing frequency and intensity of previously stable angina, or angina within 6 weeks of MI, but with normal cardiac markers of ischemia) or (b) with non–ST segment elevation MI [non–ST elevation myocardial infarction (NSTEMI), elevated markers of myocardial injury, such as troponin I or T, or the MB isoenzyme of creatine kinase, but without ST segment elevation (Table C149.1)].

General care. Anti-ischemic therapy includes bed rest, continuous electrocardiogram monitoring, intravenous nitroglycerin, supplemental oxygen, morphine sulfate, and a β-blocker or alternatively, a nondihydropyridine CA (verapamil or diltiazem) in the absence of contraindications and severe LV dysfunction. An ACE inhibitor should be added in patients with anterior MI, diabetes, uncontrolled hypertension, or LV systolic dysfunction Diuretic therapy is often necessary for long-term BP control, especially if a state of volume overload is present.

Anticoagulation. Because of the increased risk of hemorrhagic stroke in patients with uncontrolled hypertension who are given antiplatelet or anticoagulant therapy, hypertension should be treated aggressively. Antiplatelet therapy with aspirin or clopidogrel and anticoagulant therapy with intravenous unfractionated heparin subcutaneous low-molecular-weight heparin or a direct thrombin inhibitor, is standard therapy. A platelet glycoprotein IIb/IIIa receptor antagonist (e.g., intravenous abciximab, eptifibatide or tirofiban) can be added in patients with continuing ischemia or other high-risk features, and in patients in whom a percutaneous coronary intervention is planned.

Other measures. Lipid-lowering therapy is needed for patients whose low-density lipoprotein cholesterol is >100 mg/dL, or whose high-density lipoprotein cholesterol is <40 mg/dL. High risk patients with LV systolic dysfunction, left main IHD, or severe three-vessel disease, or two-vessel disease with severe proximal left anterior descending coronary artery involvement should be considered for coronary artery bypass grafting; lesser degrees of IHD should be evaluated for percutaneous coronary intervention on an individual basis. Follow-up BP should be controlled with a goal BP of <130/80 mm Hg.

ST-segment elevation myocardial infarction

General care. The management of ST-segment elevation myocardial infarction (STEMI) is similar to that for unstable angina and NSTEMI, except that arrhythmia control and primary percutaneous transluminal angioplasty and stenting, or thrombolytic therapy, become more important.

Antihypertensive drugs. In the absence of contraindications, all patients with STEMI, whether they are hypertensive or not, should receive a β-blocker and ACE inhibitor. If the patient is hemodynamically stable (no hypotension, cardiogenic shock or HF) intravenous therapy with a short-acting β_1-selective β-blocker should be started as soon as possible, followed by an oral β-blocker within the first 2 days. Many randomized clinical trials have shown a significant morbidity and mortality benefit of ACE inhibitors started early in the course of acute STEMI, particularly with anterior MI, persistent hypertension, left ventricular dysfunction (LVD), or diabetes. CAs do not reduce mortality rates in the setting of acute MI and should not be used except when β-blockers are contraindicated or inadequately controlling angina or supraventricular tachycardia, or when adjunct therapy for BP control is necessary. Nondihydropyridine CAs, such as diltiazem and verapamil, should not be used in patients with bradyarrhythmias or impaired LV function and should be used with caution if β-blockers are also being given.

Suggested Readings

Antman EM, Anbe DT, Armstrong PW, et al. ACC/AHA Guidelines for the management of patients with ST-elevation acute myocardial infarction – executive summary. *Circulation* 2004;110:588–636.

Anderson JL, Adams CD, Antman EH, et al. Acc/AHA 2007 Guidelines for the Management of Patients with unstable Angina/non–ST elevation myocardial infarction—Executive summary. *J Am Coll Cardiol* 2007;50:652–2756.

Gibbons RJ, Abrams J, Chatterjee K, et al. ACC/AHA 2002 Guideline update for the management of patients with chronic stable angina—summary article. *Circulation* 2003;107:149–158.

Rosendorff C. Ischemic heart disease in hypertension. In: Braunwald E, Black HR, Elliott WJ, eds. *Hypertension: a companion text to Braunwald's heart disease.* Philadelphia: WB Saunders, 2007:327–339.

Rosendorff C, Black HR, Cannon CP, et al. AHA scientific statement: the treatment of hypertension in the prevention and management of ischemic heart disease. *Circulation* 2007;115:2761–2788.

CHAPTER C150 ■ MANAGEMENT OF HYPERTENSIVE PATIENTS WITH LEFT VENTRICULAR HYPERTROPHY AND DIASTOLIC DYSFUNCTION

RICHARD B. DEVEREUX, MD

KEY POINTS

- Left ventricular hypertrophy (LVH) is an independent risk factor that doubles the risk of cardiovascular (CV) events and deaths.
- There are four basic patterns of left ventricular dysfunction with LVH: low midwall shortening (MWS) with a normal or minimally reduced ejection fraction (EF); impaired diastolic filling with reduced late-diastolic compliance (i.e., restrictive physiology); reduced EF; or combinations of impaired relaxation and compliance.
- Optimal management of LVH depends on accurately delineating the pattern of left ventricular dysfunction, relating the symptom complex to the underlying disorder, and matching the treatment to the pattern observed.
- Regression of LVH improves CV function and prognosis.

See also Chapters **A58, A59,** A60, A73, **B78,** C149, and C151.

Left ventricular hypertrophy (LVH) is a direct consequence of hypertension that functions as an independent factor for cardiovascular (CV) disease events. Effective antihypertensive therapy reduces LVH, improves cardiac function, and reduces risk.

Prognostic and therapeutic implications of left ventricular hypertrophy and abnormal left ventricular geometry

Individuals with echocardiographic or electrocardiographic (ECG) evidence of LVH are more than twice as likely to experience CV events and death (**Figure C150.1**) (see Chapter B78) in a variety of population-based samples, including blacks, whites, women, men, and patients with or without coronary artery disease (CAD). A

genetic component also exists for LVH (see Chapter A73). The attributable risk of LVH for all-cause mortality is even greater than that of single- or multi-vessel CAD or low left ventricular ejection fraction (LVEF). In addition, concentric LVH, characterized by a high relative wall thickness, is associated with a further increment in the rate of CV events. Finally, an increasing number of studies using echocardiography or ECG have identified associations between LVH regression and a lowered event rate, suggesting that LVH regression should be a treatment goal in hypertension.

Assessment of left ventricular hypertrophy
Echocardiography. Echocardiography provides a sensitive and widely available tool for evaluating LV structure and

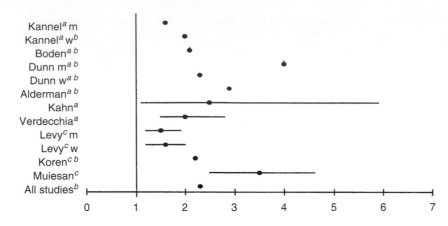

Figure C150.1 Mean risk ratios (*solid circles*) and, when available, 95% confidence interval (*horizontal lines*) of baseline left ventricular hypertrophy (LVH) for subsequent cardiovascular morbidity in available studies. m, in men; w, in women. [a]electrocardiographic LVH; [b]p <.05; [c]echocardiographic LVH. (From Vakili BA, Okin PM, Devereux RB. Prognostic significance of left ventricular hypertrophy. *Am Heart J* 2001;141:334–341, with permission.)

function. Primary LV measurements of septal and posterior wall thickness and of LV internal dimension by methods recommended by the American Society of Echocardiography M-mode or two-dimensional (2D) allow calculation of LV mass using a formula validated by necropsy (r = 0.92, N = 52), with good reproducibility in a large series of hypertensive adults (intraclass correlation coefficient = 0.93). The relative wall thickness (ratio of LV wall thickness to chamber radius) provides a useful measure of LV concentricity.

High ejection fraction paradox. Echocardiograms or nuclear angiograms show a high LVEF in 15% to 20% of patients with stage 1 hypertension despite increased afterload. Part of this apparent paradox is due to a technical artifact caused by the fact that EF has been traditionally measured at the endocardium, whereas the average myocardial fiber is located at the midpoint of the wall. LV wall thickening raises EF for any level of midwall shortening (MWS). Therefore, myocardial contractility is assessed more accurately by expressing MWS as a percentage of the value predicted for circumferential end-systolic stress at the level of the LV midwall. Stress-corrected MWS is subnormal in approximately 20% of patients with stage 1 or stage 2 hypertension and is above the upper limit of normal in only 2% or fewer of hypertensive patients.

Monitoring left ventricular hypertrophy as a surrogate endpoint. If regression of LVH is to be used as a surrogate endpoint in the treatment of hypertensive patients, the methods of monitoring LV mass need to be reliable with little regression to the mean. The reliability of echocardiographically determined LV size and wall thicknesses and LV mass and geometry, as expressed by relative wall thickness, was assessed in a sample of hypertensive patients with LVH recruited into the Prospective Randomized Enalapril Study Evaluating Regression of Ventricular Enlargement (PRESERVE) trial (N = 183). Readings by a blinded highly experienced reader of two echocardiograms performed approximately 6 weeks apart showed that there was a close relationship between LV mass on the first and second echocardiograms (intraclass correlation coefficient = 0.93, p <.001), with no evidence of regression to the mean, except at the highest level of LV mass.

Clinical studies of left ventricular hypertrophy regression

Meta-analyses. A meta-analysis of LVH regression considered 80 double-blind, randomized, parallel-group controlled clinical studies published through 2002 that included 17 placebo arms

(N = 346) and 146 active treatment arms (N = 3,767). There were 24 studies (N = 730) with diuretics, 30 (N = 608) with β-blockers, 44 (N = 1,113) with calcium antagonists (CAs), and 39 (N = 1,068) with angiotensin-converting enzyme (ACE) inhibitors; mean duration of treatment was 29 weeks. Several factors other than treatment influenced the degree of LVH regression. In analyses that adjusted for treatment duration and change in diastolic blood pressure (BP), there was a significant difference (p = .004) among medication classes: LV mass index decreased by 13% with angiotensin II receptor blockers [angiotensin receptor blockers (ARBs), 95% CI, 8,18%], by 11% with CAs (95% CI, 9,13%), by 10% with ACE inhibitors (95% CI, 8,12%), by 8% with diuretics (95% CI, 5,10%), and by 6% with β-blockers (95% CI, 3,8%). In pair-wise comparisons, ARBs, CAs, and ACE inhibitors were more effective at reducing LV mass than β-blockers (all p < .05).

Direct comparisons. Other studies have revealed a greater reduction of 24-hour BP in diuretic-treated patients but greater LV mass reduction with ACE inhibition. The PRESERVE trial compared the effects of once-daily enalapril and slow-release nifedipine. More than 70% of patients had effective BP control, and both medications reduced LV mass index substantially (by 15–17 g/m^2) at 6 and 12 months; decreased relative wall thickness suggested favorable LV remodeling. The Losartan Intervention for Endpoint Reduction in Hypertension (LIFE) trial studied composite endpoint reduction [stroke, myocardial infarction (MI), CV death] in 9,193 individuals with LVH in a randomized, double-blind, parallel-group design comparing the effects of losartan versus atenolol. Cornell voltage-duration product and the Sokolow-Lyon voltage combination were reduced significantly more (both p <.001) by losartan than atenolol therapy despite equivalent BP lowering. In the large (N = 960) echocardiographic substudy of LIFE, prevention of increased stroke volume during antihypertensive therapy potentiated the LVH regression at any given degree of BP reduction. Furthermore, the degree of LVH regression was proportional to the degree of improvement in LV systolic and diastolic function. In the LIFE study, echocardiographic and ECG assessment of LVH at baseline and annually during the study provided the opportunity to assess the relation of LVH regression to prognosis, with control for in-treatment BP, randomized antihypertensive medication, and a spectrum of CV risk factors and diseases. These analyses showed that treatment reduced the rate of CV events and all-cause mortality associated with absence versus presence of LVH (detected by either method), with estimated benefits as high as 50%.

Assessment of diastolic function

Pathophysiology. LV diastolic function can be defined by the relation between LV filling rates and filling pressures. Because noninvasive methods do not provide intracardiac pressure measurements, LV diastolic filling is analyzed in two phases. Early diastolic filling is predominately influenced by active myocardial relaxation together with the left atrium:LV pressure gradient. Late-diastolic filling is reduced by increasing passive stiffness of the LV (usually due to fibrosis), higher LV relative wall thickness, or a reduced left atrium:LV pressure gradient.

Mitral flow analysis. Measurements needed to produce a simple classification of the patterns of LV diastolic filling are based on Doppler analysis of mitral valve flow patterns. Critical measurements include (a) the peak early diastolic and atrial-phase filling velocities (E and A); (b) time required for E velocity to reach 0 ("deceleration time"); and (c) the interval between LV ejection for one heart beat and the beginning of transmitral blood flow for the next beat ("isovolumic relaxation time"). In middle-aged to elderly adults, E/A <0.8 is subnormal and a ratio higher than 1.5 is supranormal, suggesting the presence of impaired relaxation or "restrictive cardiomyopathy" due to increased LV stiffness. The deceleration time is normally 150 to 250 milliseconds, with longer values suggesting impaired relaxation and shorter ones seen with restrictive physiology. Isovolumic relaxation times ≥105 milliseconds are prolonged in middle and older age. Impaired relaxation can be diagnosed confidently by the combination of low E/A, long isovolumic relaxation time, and long deceleration time. Restrictive filling can be diagnosed by the combination of a short deceleration time and an isovolumic relaxation time, with E/A >1.5.

Tissue Doppler. The newer method of tissue Doppler imaging identifies impaired LV relaxation by the rate of deceleration of the mitral valve annulus; abnormal E' velocity is <8 cm per second. LV diastolic pressure is elevated when the ratio of the E wave of transmitral blood flow to the tissue Doppler E' exceeds 15.

Spectrum of left ventricular dysfunction in hypertension and left ventricular hypertrophy

LV dysfunction in hypertensive patients occurs as part of a complex spectrum that includes reduced contractility, LV geometric adaptation, abnormalities of LV diastolic filling, and dilated cardiomyopathy. Optimal management requires an orderly approach that delineates and relates the pattern of LV dysfunction to the symptoms and the selected therapy.

Left ventricular filling patterns in hypertension. In population-based samples of individuals with stage 1 or 2 hypertension, 30% to 50% have evidence of impaired LV relaxation, 3% show signs of restrictive LV filling, and 40% to 60% have normal transmitral flow patterns of LV filling. In hypertensive patients with the highest BPs, approximately two-thirds have abnormal relaxation, 4% have evidence of restrictive filling, one eighth show a "pseudonormal" filling pattern (combining features of impaired relaxation and restrictive filling); only approximately one sixth have normal filling.

Left ventricular dysfunction. In hypertension, the spectrum of LV dysfunction includes reduced EF, reduced myocardial contractility with preserved EF, impaired early diastolic LV relaxation, restrictive LV passive filling in late diastole, and various combinations of these abnormalities. Patterns of LV dysfunction are influenced by age, level of BP, and concomitant diseases. Reduced LVEF is relatively rare in uncomplicated asymptomatic patients with stage 1 hypertension without diabetes or renal failure (<2%). Mildly elevated EF may be seen in as many as 15% of such patients (high EF paradox). In the biracial, population-based sample of hypertensive adults in the Hypertension Genetic Epidemiology Network Blood Pressure Study (HyperGEN), which did not exclude symptomatic individuals, 10% had mildly reduced EF (40%–54%), and 3% had LVEF <40%. Among the patients with the highest levels of BP in the LIFE cohort, approximately 20% had an LVEF ≤54%.

Predictors of heart failure. In echocardiographic surveys, approximately 5% of hypertensive patients have mildly decreased LVEF, and 1% have severely reduced EF (<40%) without overt HF. HF occurs in fewer than 1% of hypertensive patients with normal EF, 5% with mild LV systolic dysfunction, and >25% with EF <40%. Similarly, HF occurs in approximately 2% of those with normal mitral E/A ratios, 5% with low E/A and in 25% with high E/A ratios. Subtle symptoms are probably more common than overt HF, including avoidance of previously routine activities and reduced performance on objective exercise tests.

Left ventricular dysfunction and future cardiovascular events. In a >10-year follow-up of initially asymptomatic hypertensive patients, low stress-corrected LV-MWS predicted CV events and CV death, whereas low EF was too infrequent to be a significant predictor. Despite a normal EF (≥55% cutoff, there may be subnormal MWS when the LV wall thickness is increased (>1.1 cm or >1.3 cm, respectively. CV death rates are increased in individuals at the extremes of low or high E/A ratios, independent of LVEF.

Management of left ventricular dysfunction

Correct management of LV dysfunction depends on matching the profile of the abnormality to the treatment.

Impaired diastolic function with normal (or increased) systolic function. No available treatment directly improves LV diastolic filling as its exclusive primary action. Because of the strong associations between poorly controlled hypertension and abnormal LV geometry (concentric or eccentric hypertrophy or concentric remodeling), the goals of treatment should be to optimize BP control and to normalize LV geometry. There are no guideline-specified BP targets for diastolic dysfunction but a reasonable target is BP <130/80 mm Hg as is recommended for individuals with CAD. With respect to individual drug choices, available clinical final data favor ARBs, ACE inhibitors, and long-acting CAs in that order. In a patient with dyspnea or other features of HF (often an elderly female with long-standing isolated systolic hypertension), echocardiogram may reveal a small LV chamber size associated with high EF, poor relaxation, and the formation of systolic intracavitary gradients within the LV. In these patients, slowing the heart rate with β-blockers, verapamil, or diltiazem may be beneficial. Diuretics or marked sodium-restriction, as often leads to volume depletion, may exacerbate this condition. Restrictive filling is usually associated with myocardial fibrosis; aldosterone antagonists, which may ameliorate cardiac fibrosis, may have a role in treating this condition but must be studied further to allow specific recommendations regarding their use.

Hypertension with low left ventricular midwall function. Low LV-MWS is strongly associated with LV hypertrophy and high relative wall thickness. Therapy should be aimed primarily at reversing LVH; ACE inhibitors, ARBs, CAs, diuretics, and β-blockers all have documented benefit, in descending order.

Hypertension with mild left ventricular systolic dysfunction. The syndrome of low LVEF is defined by an EF <55% by echocardiography (or <50% by nuclear angiogram or cardiac catheterization). LV diastolic filling pattern is then assessed by Doppler mitral inflow patterns or nuclear angiography. If BP is not controlled, a slightly reduced LVEF is most likely due to increased afterload. The treating physician should select an appropriate antihypertensive medication and then reevaluate LV function when BP is controlled. If arterial pressure is only minimally elevated or in the high normal range and LVEF is reduced, medications known to benefit patients with severe LV systolic dysfunction should be used, including ACE inhibitors, ARBs, β-blockers, or spironolactone. It is highly probable but as yet unproven that lower BP targets (130/80 mm Hg or lower) should be sought, as in patients with ischemic heart disease, diabetes, or chronic kidney disease.

Impaired systolic and diastolic function. Virtually all cases of significant LV systolic dysfunction also have corresponding diastolic dysfunction. Reduced systolic function is usually due to CAD or cardiomyopathy, which may occur in approximately 1% of hypertensive patients without overt HF. In this setting, it is appropriate to use ARBs, ACE inhibitors, β-blockers, hydralazine–nitrate combinations, or spironolactone. However, the prognosis is still poor in patients with evidence of restrictive LV filling. Investigation of agents to treat myocardial fibrosis or impaired relaxation directly is in its early phases.

Suggested Readings

Bella JN, Palmieri V, Liu JE, et al. Mitral E/A ratio as a predictor of mortality in middle-aged and elderly adults: the Strong Heart study. *Circulation* 2002;105:1928–1933.

Devereux RB, Bella JN, Palmieri V, et al. Prevalence and correlates of left ventricular systolic dysfunction in a bi-racial sample of hypertensive adults: the HyperGEN study. *Hypertension* 2001;38:417–423.

Devereux RB, Palmieri V, Sharpe N, et al. Effects of once-daily angiotensin converting enzyme inhibition and calcium channel blockade-based antihypertensive treatment regimens on left ventricular hypertrophy and diastolic filling in hypertension: the PRESERVE trial. *Circulation* 2001;104:1248–1254.

Devereux RB, Roman MJ, Paranicas M, et al. A population-based assessment of left ventricular systolic dysfunction in middle-aged and older adults: the strong heart study. *Am Heart J* 2001;141:439–446.

Devereux RB, Wachtell K, Gerdts E, et al. Prognostic significance of left ventricular mass change during treatment of hypertension. The LIFE study. *JAMA* 2004;292:2350–2356.

Gandhi SK, Powers JC, Nomeir AM, et al. The pathogenesis of acute pulmonary edema associated with hypertension. *N Engl J Med* 2001;344:17–22.

Okin PM, Devereux RB, Jern S, et al. The LIFE Study Investigators. Regression of electrocardiographic left ventricular hypertrophy during antihypertensive treatment and the prediction of major cardiovascular events: the LIFE study. *JAMA* 2004;292:2343–2349.

Roman MJ, Alderman MH, Pickering TG, et al. Differential effects of angiotensin converting enzyme inhibition and diuretic therapy on reductions in ambulatory blood pressure, left ventricular mass, and vascular hypertrophy. *Am J Hypertens* 1998;11:387–396.

Vakili BA, Okin PM, Devereux RB. Prognostic significance of left ventricular hypertrophy. *Am Heart J* 2001;141:334–341.

Wachtell K, Bella JN, Rokkedal J, et al. Change in diastolic left ventricular filling after one year of antihypertensive treatment: the LIFE trial. *Circulation* 2002;105:1071–1076.

CHAPTER C151 ■ TREATMENT OF HYPERTENSIVE PATIENTS WITH LEFT VENTRICULAR SYSTOLIC DYSFUNCTION

JOHN B. KOSTIS, MD

KEY POINTS

- Left ventricular systolic dysfunction and heart failure (HF) are common complications of aging and hypertension, in part because of increased survival after myocardial infarction (MI).
- HF can be staged according to the recommendations of the American College of Cardiology/American Heart Association (ACC/AHA) Consensus Statement: stage A (at risk), stage B (asymptomatic left ventricular dysfunction), stage C (symptomatic HF), and stage D (end-stage disease).
- Control of hypertension and fastidious management of cholesterol and other risk factors for coronary artery disease (CAD) are essential for the prevention and treatment of HF. In high-risk individuals, blood pressure (BP) should be <130/80; in patients with overt HF, BP should be reduced to the lowest tolerable levels.
- Additional therapeutic recommendations include angiotensin-converting enzyme (ACE) inhibitors for stages A through D, β-blockers as well as aldosterone receptor antagonists for stages B through D, and digitalis/diuretics for stages C through D HF.
- Optimal management of patients with late stage C and stage D HF requires organized HF clinics.

See also Chapters A58, A59, A60, B78, C109, C110, and **C111**

Demographic trends in heart failure

In the last several decades, age-adjusted mortality from cardiovascular (CV) disease has decreased by approximately 50% in men and women and in different racial subsets. Fatality from acute myocardial infarction (MI) has also decreased with the advent of thrombolytic therapy, percutaneous interventions, and adjunctive pharmacologic therapy. These factors, as well as the relatively poor control of hypertension in the community and the aging of the general population, have resulted in an increased incidence of left ventricular (LV) systolic dysfunction and heart failure (HF). The prognosis of hypertensive HF patients is poor because of the high rate of morbid and mortal events imposed by systolic LV dysfunction and the frequently coexisting coronary artery disease (CAD). Better blood pressure (BP) control and use of renin-angiotensin blocking drugs, β-blockers, and aldosterone receptor antagonists have greatly improved survival.

Definition and prognosis

The Heart Failure Society of America (HFSA) 2006 guideline offers the following definition of HF: HF is a syndrome caused by cardiac dysfunction, generally resulting from myocardial muscle dysfunction or loss, and characterized by LV dilation or hypertrophy. Whether the dysfunction is primarily systolic or diastolic or mixed, it leads to neurohormonal and circulatory abnormalities, usually resulting in characteristic symptoms such as fluid retention, shortness of breath, and fatigue, especially on exertion. In the absence of appropriate therapeutic intervention, HF is usually progressive at the levels of cardiac function and clinical symptoms. The severity of clinical symptoms may vary substantially during the course of the disease process and may not correlate with changes in underlying cardiac function. Although HF is progressive and often fatal, patients can be stabilized, and myocardial dysfunction and remodeling may improve, either spontaneously or as a consequence of therapy. In physiologic terms, HF is a syndrome characterized by elevated cardiac filling pressure or inadequate peripheral oxygen delivery, at rest or during stress, caused by cardiac dysfunction.

Heart Failure Society of America Evaluation guidelines

HFSA Guidelines recommend the following items for the evaluation for patients with a new diagnosis of HF: (a) assess clinical severity of HF by history and physical examination, (b) assess cardiac structure and function, (c) determine the etiology of HF, (d) evaluate for CAD and myocardial ischemia, (e) evaluate the risk of life-threatening arrhythmia, (f) identify any exacerbating factors for HF, (g) identify comorbidities that influence therapy, and (h) identify barriers to adherence and compliance.

New York Heart Association Functional Classification

The New York Heart Association (NYHA) Functional Classification is widely used in HF management and is recommended by the HFSA:

Class I   No limitation of physical activity. Ordinary physical activity does not cause undue fatigue, palpitation or dyspnea.

Class II   Slight limitation of physical activity. Comfortable at rest, but ordinary physical activity results in fatigue, palpitations, or dyspnea.

Class III   IIIA: Marked limitation of physical activity. Comfortable at rest, but less than ordinary activity causes fatigue, palpitation, or dyspnea.
IIIB: Marked limitation of physical activity. Comfortable at rest, but minimal exertion causes fatigue, palpitation, or dyspnea.

Class IV   Unable to carry on any physical activity without discomfort. Symptoms of cardiac insufficiency present at rest. If any physical activity is undertaken, discomfort is increased.

Pathogenesis of left ventricular systolic dysfunction

LV dysfunction and systolic HF in most people are the result of two overlapping but distinct pathways: hypertension and CAD.

Hypertension and aging. Uncontrolled hypertension and aging interact to exacerbate the development of HF, especially in the presence of obesity or diabetes, which further contribute to increased LV mass, LV wall thickness, and abnormal diastolic LV filling patterns. Impaired LV filling may cause the syndrome of HF with preserved ejection fraction (EF) ("diastolic HF or diastolic dysfunction") with symptoms due to high pulmonary venous pressure and decreased cardiac output. In addition, LV hypertrophy due to systolic overload imposed by hypertension is associated with changes in gene expression. Impairment of systolic function is initially compensated for by increased LV thickness, but ultimately, LV remodeling associated with neurohormonal activation, increased wall tension, apoptosis, myocyte loss, fibrosis, chamber dilatation, and depressed systolic function leads to HF.

Coronary artery disease. The second pathway that commonly leads from hypertension to HF is LV systolic dysfunction after acute MI. MI leads to reduced cardiac output, neurohormonal activation, and remodeling, resulting in LV dilatation, elevated filling pressure, systolic dysfunction, and systolic HF. Other causes unrelated to hypertension include dilated cardiomyopathy of viral, alcoholic, toxic, or other etiologies. Regardless of the cause of LV dysfunction, uncontrolled hypertension further increases the LV wall tension and LV work due to systolic overload.

Diagnosis

Overt HF is usually recognized by its congestive symptoms, but early LV systolic dysfunction may be difficult to diagnose because it can be relatively asymptomatic. Typical signs are often absent or masked in many older people. Echocardiography should be performed in virtually all patients to establish the levels of systolic and diastolic function. On occasion, nuclear studies may also be helpful. Measurement of brain natriuretic peptide (BNP) has been used as an indicator of ventricular function but the reliability of this marker is reduced by pulmonary and renal diseases and diastolic dysfunction.

Prevention of heart failure in hypertension

Prevention of HF is a major objective of antihypertensive therapy and fastidious control of BP should be maintained by vigorous antihypertensive therapy. Controlling hypertension prevents LV hypertrophy and acute MI, both of which reduce the incidence of HF. Achieving the latter goal requires attention to the total risk profile of the patient and includes interventions aimed at encouraging physical activity, control of diabetes, avoidance of smoking and overweight, control of dyslipidemia, and use of aspirin by high-risk patients.

Blood pressure targets. According to the HFSA 2006 Guidelines, target BP in patients with hypertension and HF is <130/80 mm Hg. According to JNC 7 and the 2007 American College of Cardiology/American Heart Association (ACC/AHA) statement on the treatment of hypertension in ischemic heart disease, a target BP <140/90 mm Hg can be used for individuals with low CAD risk and no overt disease, whereas anyone with a coronary heart disease equivalent should have BPs controlled to <130/80 mm Hg.

Choice of drugs. Substantial BP lowering may require treatment with several drugs, including an angiotensin-converting enzyme (ACE) inhibitor or an angiotensin receptor blocker (ARB), a diuretic, and often a β-blocker or calcium channel blocker (CCB). Spironolactone may also be of use. Virtually all available clinical trials have used drug combinations. In the Losartan Intervention for Endpoint Reduction in Hypertension Study (LIFE) in patients with hypertension and LV hypertrophy, losartan and atenolol achieved similar peripheral BP reductions, but losartan was superior in causing regression of LV hypertrophy and decreasing clinical morbid and mortal events. In the LIFE study, a very small percentage of subjects (11%–12%) were treated with only one drug. In the Antihypertensive and Lipid-Lowering Treatment to Prevent Heart Attack Trial (ALLHAT) study, a diuretic, a CCB, an ACE inhibitor, and a peripheral α-blocker were compared to a diuretic with respect to CV outcomes. In this trial, the risk for HF was lower with chlorthalidone compared to the other agents. In the Anglo-Scandinavian Cardiac Outcomes Trial (ASCOT), amlodipine-based therapy (with perindopril as a step 2 drug) was superior in reducing central systolic BP and overall CV events compared to atenolol (with a diuretic as a step 2 drug). The addition of a statin at a fixed dose, with no titration to a goal, further decreased CV risk.

Treatment of systolic dysfunction

Goals of therapy. The treatment of patients with hypertension and LV systolic dysfunction, with or without overt HF, should alleviate symptoms, prevent hospitalization, slow or reverse progressive LV remodeling, and decrease mortality.

Blood pressure targets. Effective treatment of HF often lowers BP to values below currently recommended targets, although the lowest "reasonable" BP for HF is the subject of debate. Systolic BP values <100 mm Hg have been commonly observed in clinical trials that demonstrated increased survival. There are no specific threshold BP levels as long as there is no functional impairment. Some patients, especially those with intervening large MIs, develop marked LV dilatation, severe LV dysfunction, and low systolic BP (below 100 mm Hg). β-Blockers and ACE inhibitors and often digitalis should still be given to these patients, while carefully titrating diuretics. When symptomatic hypotension limits the ability to titrate β-blockers and ACE inhibitors or ARBs, a lower dose of both drugs rather than a high dose of one is often necessary. In stage D HF, hypotension rather than hypertension is associated with a worse prognosis.

Heart failure treatment guidelines. Current recommendations for therapy are based on the ACC/AHA staging system (Table C151.1).

Stage A ("at risk"). Therapy includes control of systolic and diastolic hypertension; treatment of lipid abnormalities; avoidance of behaviors that may increase the risk of HF (e.g., smoking, alcohol consumption, and illicit drug use); ACE inhibition in patients with atherosclerotic disease, diabetes mellitus, or hypertension and associated CV risk factors; control of ventricular rate in patients with supraventricular tachyarrhythmias; and treatment of thyroid disorders.

Stage B ("asymptomatic"). Therapy includes ACE inhibition and β-blockade in patients with a history of MI, regardless of EF; in those with a reduced EF, whether or not they have experienced an MI ; and in patients with a recent MI, regardless of EF.

Stage C ("symptomatic"). Therapy includes (unless contraindicated) digitalis, diuretics in patients with fluid retention, ACE inhibition, β-adrenergic blockade in all stable patients, aldosterone blockade in patients with recent MI or current NYHA class III/IV, withdrawal of drugs known to adversely affect the clinical status of HF patients (e.g., nonsteroidal antiinflammatory drugs, most antiarrhythmic drugs, and most CCBs) and exercise training of ambulatory patients. An ARB may be used in patients who do not tolerate ACE inhibitors because of cough or angioedema.

Stage D ("end-stage"). In addition to measures listed for patients in stages A, B, and C, the therapy of stage D ("end-stage") HF includes identification and control of fluid retention, potential evaluation for heart transplantation, referral to an HF management program, intravenous infusions of a positive inotropic agent, valve repair or replacement for severe secondary mitral regurgitation, mechanical assist devices, or hospice care.

Specific drugs

Angiotensin-converting enzyme inhibitors. The recommendation that ACE inhibitors should be used in patients with hypertension and all stages of LV systolic dysfunction is supported by *post hoc* analyses of the hypertensive subsets of large controlled clinical trials, including the Studies of Left Ventricular Dysfunction (SOLVD) with enalapril, the Acute Infarction Ramipril Efficacy Study (AIRE) and the Trandolapril Cardiac Event Study (TRACE). The Heart Outcomes Protection Evaluation (HOPE) with ramipril demonstrated a decreased occurrence of HF among high-risk patients (including those with hypertension).

TABLE C151.1

STAGES IN THE EVOLUTION OF HEART FAILURE (HF) AND RECOMMENDED THERAPY BY STAGE

	Stage A	Stage B	Stage C	Stage D
Classification	At high risk for HF without structural heart disease or symptoms of HF	Structural heart disease without symptoms of HF	Structural heart disease with prior or current symptoms of HF	Refractory HF requiring specialized interventions

Characteristics	Patients with
	  Hypertension
	  Coronary artery disease
	  Diabetes mellitus
	Or
	Patients
	  Using cardiotoxins
	  With family history of cardiomyopathy
		Patients with
		  Previous myocardial infarction
		  Left ventricular systolic dysfunction
		  Asymptomatic valvular disease
			Patients with
			  Known structural heart disease
			  Shortness of breath
			  Fatigue or reduced exercise tolerance
				Patients with marked symptoms at rest despite maximal medical therapy
				Patients recurrently hospitalized or those who cannot be safely discharged from the hospital without specialized interventions

Therapy	Treat hypertension
	Smoking cessation
	Treat lipid disorders
	Regular exercise
	Discourage alcohol intake and illicit drug use
	ACE inhibition (appropriate patients)
		All measures under stage A
		ACE inhibitors (in appropriate patients)
		β-Blockers (in appropriate patients)
			All measures under stage A
			Drugs for routine use:
			  Diuretics
			  ACE inhibitors
			  β-Blockers
			  Digitalis
			  Dietary salt restriction
				All measures under stages A, B, and C
				Mechanical assist devices
				Heart transplantation
				Continuous palliative (not intermittent) i.v. inotrope infusions
				Hospice care

ACE, angiotensin-converting enzyme.
(Adapted from Hunt SA, Baker DW, Chin MH, et al. ACC/AHA guidelines for the evaluation and management of chronic heart failure in the adult: executive summary. A report of the American College of Cardiology/American Heart Association Task Force on Practice Guidelines (Committee to revise the 1995 Guidelines for the Evaluation and Management of Heart Failure). *J Am Coll Cardiol* 2001;38:2101–2112.)

Angiotensin receptor blockers. ARBs should be given to HF patients who do not tolerate ACE inhibitors. ARBs have been shown to be superior to placebo in the Candesartan in Heart Failure Assessment of Reduction in Morbidity and Mortality (CHARM)-Alternative Trial, Reduction of Endpoints in NIDDM with the Angiotensin II Antagonist Losartan (RENAAL) and the Valsartan Heart Failure Trial (ValHEFT). ARB therapy was superior to CCBs in the Irbesartan Diabetic Nephropathy Trial (IDNT) and the Valsartan Antihypertensive Long-term Use Evaluation (VALUE) trial. Significant differences between ACE inhibitors and ARBs have not been observed in the few trials where a direct comparison was made [Losartan Heart Failure Survival Study (ELITE II), Optimal Trial in Myocardial Infarction with the Angiotensin II Antagonist Losartan (OPTIMAAL) and Valsartan In Acute Myocardial Infarction (VALIANT) trial].

β-Blockers. β-Blocker therapy reduces mortality in patients with hypertension, HF, and CAD. β-Blockers exert beneficial effects in HF by reducing heart rate, controlling BP, controlling supraventricular and ventricular arrhythmias (if present), and exerting antiischemic effects. In a meta-analysis of controlled trials using carvedilol or bisoprolol, β-blocker use was associated with a 30% reduction in mortality and a 40% reduction in hospitalizations in patients with class II and III HF. β-Blockers have reduced cardiac mortality and morbidity in patients with CAD in the majority of over 40 clinical trials.

The use of β-blockers is associated with adverse metabolic effects, including raised triglycerides, lowered high-density lipoprotein cholesterol, and glucose intolerance. However, given their demonstrated benefit in hypertension, HF, and CAD, β-blockers generally should not be withheld for fear of adverse effects. In patients with mild or moderate reversible airway disease, low doses of a cardioselective β-blocker do not usually produce clinically significant adverse respiratory effects, but physicians should be aware of the potential for metabolic and bronchoconstrictive adverse effects and take appropriate measures to counteract them.

Diuretics. Diuretic therapy is an essential adjunct to β-blocker and ACE inhibitor therapy to decrease congestive symptoms and signs of HF (pulmonary congestion, hepatomegaly, and edema). In early LV dysfunction, hydrochlorothiazide can be used, but as cardiac or renal function deteriorates, loop diuretics become increasingly necessary.

Aldosterone antagonists. The addition of aldosterone antagonists can decrease mortality in HF patients already receiving ACE inhibitors or β-blockers [The Randomized Aldosterone Evaluation Study (RALES) with spironolactone]; and in survivors of acute MI [Eplerenone Post–Acute Myocardial Infarction Heart Failure Efficacy and Survival Study (EPHESUS)].

Other treatments

Patients with acute decompensated HF require hospitalization in the presence of hypotension, worsening renal function, altered mentation, dyspnea at rest, rapid atrial fibrillation, or acute coronary syndromes. Routine use of hemodynamic monitoring is not recommended. Intravenous vasodilators and intravenous inotropes may be considered when filling pressures are elevated.

Arrythmia management. Electrophysiologic testing is not routinely recommended unless there is history of syncope or symptomatic ventricular tachyarrhythmia. Biventricular pacing should be considered in patients with a wide QRS and severe LV systolic dysfunction who have moderate to severe HF despite optimal medical therapy. Prophylactic implantable cardioverter-defibrillator (ICD) placement should be considered in patients with left ventricular ejection fraction (LVEF) <30% as well as in patients undergoing implantation of a biventricular pacing device for resynchronization therapy. ICD implantation is also recommended for survivors of cardiac arrest from ventricular tachyarrhythmia without evidence of acute MI or occurring >48 hours after the onset of MI in the absence of a recurrent ischemic event.

Surgical procedures. Surgical approaches in highly selected patients may include myocardial revascularization, insertion of assist devices, and cardiac transplantation. Evaluation for heart transplantation is recommended in patients with severe HF, debilitating refractory angina, or ventricular arrhythmia that cannot be controlled by other means. Isolated mitral valve repair or replacement for severe mitral regurgitation in the presence of severe systolic dysfunction is not recommended. Permanent mechanical assistance may be considered in highly selected patients. Partial left ventricular systolic resection (Batista procedure) is not recommended for nonischemic cardiomyopathy.

Disease management and support programs

Management programs should include comprehensive education and counseling individualized to patient needs. These needs are best met by organized HF clinics whose programs include promotion of self care, including self-adjustment of diuretic therapy in appropriate patents (or with family member/caregiver assistance); emphasis on behavioral strategies to increase adherence; vigilant follow-up after hospital discharge or after periods of instability; optimization of medical therapy, and increased access to providers; early attention to signs and symptoms of fluid overload, assistance with social and financial concerns. Control of hyperlipidemia, usually requiring statins, and immunization for influenza and pneumococcal pneumonia are useful. Prevention and control of diabetes and its complications are important.

Suggested Readings

American College of Cardiology/American Heart Association Task Force on Performance Measures. ACC/AHA clinical performance measures for adults with chronic heart failure. A report of the American College of Cardiology/American Heart Association Task Force on Performance Measures (Writing Committee to Develop Heart Failure Clinical performance Measures). *J Am Coll Cardiol* 2005;46(6):1144–1178.

Cook JR, Glick HA, Gerth W, et al. The cost and cardioprotective effects of enalapril in hypertensive patients with left ventricular dysfunction. *Am J Hypertens* 1998;11:1433–1441.

Fortuno MA, Ravassa S, Fortuno A, et al. Cardiomyocyte apoptotic cell death in arterial hypertension: mechanisms and potential management. *Hypertension* 2001;38:1406–1412.

Frohlich ED. Fibrosis and ischemia: the real risks in hypertensive heart disease. *Am J Hypertens* 2001;14:194S–199S.

Furberg CD, Psaty BM, Pahor M, et al. Clinical implications of recent findings from the antihypertensive and lipid-lowering treatment to prevent heart attack trial (ALLHAT) and other studies of hypertension. *Ann Intern Med* 2001;135:1074–1078.

Garg R, Yusuf S. Overview of randomized trials of angiotensin-converting enzyme inhibitors on mortality and morbidity in patients with heart failure. Collaborative group on ACE inhibitor trials. *JAMA* 1995;273:1450–1456.

Heart Failure Society of America. Executive summary: HFSA 2006 Comprehensive heart failure practice guideline. *J Card Fail* 2006;12(1):10–38.

Kostis JB. The effect of enalapril on mortal and morbid events in patients with hypertension and left ventricular dysfunction. *Am J Hypertens* 1995;8:909–914.

Kostis JB, Davis BR, Cutler J, et al. SHEP Cooperative Research Group. Prevention of heart failure by antihypertensive drug treatment in older persons with isolated systolic hypertension. *JAMA* 1997;278:212–216.

Rosendorff C, Black HR, Cannon CP, et al. Treatment of hypertension in the prevention and management of ischemic heart disease. A scientific statement from the American Heart Association council for high blood pressure research and the councils on clinical cardiology and epidemiology and prevention. *Circulation* 2007;115:2761–2788.

CHAPTER C152 ■ TREATMENT OF HYPERTENSIVE PATIENTS WITH PERIPHERAL ARTERIAL DISEASE

JEFFREY W. OLIN, DO

KEY POINTS

■ Lifestyle modification (weight loss, smoking cessation, exercise) should be part of the management of peripheral arterial disease (PAD); a structured walking program significantly increases the pain-free and maximum walking distance in patients with intermittent claudication.

■ Patients with PAD should be treated as if they have coronary artery disease (CAD), with optimized medical management of hyperlipidemia, hypertension, and hyperglycemia along with antiplatelet drugs.

■ Vigorous blood pressure (BP) lowering is important in all patients with PAD, especially diabetic patients; angiotensin-converting enzyme (ACE) inhibitor may be the antihypertensive agent of choice in patients with PAD.

■ β-Adrenergic blocker therapy does not worsen intermittent claudication in most subjects with PAD.

See also Chapters A65, **B81, C113, C120,** and **C149**

It is estimated that 2% to 5% of all patients with hypertension have symptoms suggestive of intermittent claudication (IC) at presentation; an ankle-brachial index (ABI) of ≤0.9 [indicating peripheral arterial disease (PAD)] was present in 25.5% of 1,537 participants in the Systolic Hypertension in the Elderly Program (SHEP). In addition, 50% to 92% of patients with PAD have high blood pressure (BP). The Seventh Report of the Joint National Committee on Prevention, Detection, Evaluation, and Treatment of High Blood Pressure (JNC 7) included PAD as a coronary heart disease (CHD) equivalent. Treating hypertension in all patients (including those with PAD) reduces the risk of myocardial infarction (MI), stroke, heart failure (HF), and death. There are limited available data on whether treatment of hypertension *per se* prevents the development of claudication or alters the natural history of PAD. Any class of antihypertensive medication may be used to treat the hypertension seen in these patients. The Treatment of Mild Hypertension Study (TOMHS) did show, however, that drug treatment in combination with lifestyle modification was superior to nutritional–hygienic treatment alone in preventing the development of IC and PAD over an average follow-up period of 4.4 years.

Recognition of peripheral arterial disease

Patients with PAD may present with the symptom complex of IC: discomfort, aching, cramping, pain, tightness, tiredness or heaviness in the buttocks, hip girdle, thighs, or calf muscles brought on by exercise and relieved by rest. There are three clinical features in patients with IC:

■ The discomfort is reproducible with a consistent level of exercise from day to day.
■ The discomfort completely resolves within 2 to 5 minutes after exercise has been stopped unless the patient has walked to the point of severe leg pain.
■ The discomfort occurs again at approximately the same distance once walking has been resumed.

For detailed description of evaluation, see Chapter C113.

Lifestyle modifications

JNC 7 endorsed lifestyle modifications as important adjunctive therapy in patients with PAD.

Exercise therapy. A structured walking program significantly increases pain-free and maximum walking distances in patients with IC. In 26 trials of exercise conditioning summarized by Hiatt and Regensteiner, claudication pain improved an average of 134% (range, 44%–290%) and peak walking time increased an average of 96% (range, 25%–183%). Studies using validated disease-specific questionnaires have shown that exercise in PAD improves quality of life. In addition, a regular walking program can lower BP, and triglycerides, raise high-density lipoprotein cholesterol, reduce glucose intolerance and insulin resistance, and most importantly, improve survival.

TABLE C152.1

CLAUDICATION WALKING PROGRAM

Patients who have intermittent claudication can benefit from a
regular walking program. Studies have shown that regular
exercise, particularly walking, can improve your symptoms of
leg pain

Follow these steps:

- Perform warm up and cooldown periods of 5–10 min each.
  This includes stretching of the legs, calves, and upper body.
  Begin walking slowly, and gradually build up your pace
- Walk for approximately 30 sec after you begin to experience
  leg discomfort or tiredness. Then stop completely and stand
  until the discomfort goes away. Walk at a pace so that you
  have to stop at approximately two blocks. Then begin
  walking again. Repeat this for 45 min at least 5 d a wk
- If you can walk more than four blocks, increase your
  walking pace so that you get discomfort at two blocks. In
  other words, if your legs usually start to hurt after walking
  four blocks, walk faster so that you feel the pain or
  discomfort after two blocks
- This walking program needs to be done at least five times a
  wk for 45 min in order to be maximally effective
- Do not force yourself to walk with pain. Stop 30 sec after the
  discomfort or tiredness starts

The period of walking should be 45 minutes long including
periods of rest (**Table C152.1**). During the exercise sessions,
the patient should walk until a mild or moderate level of pain
or discomfort is reached, followed by a rest period until the
discomfort abates. After the pain is gone, the patient should
resume walking until a moderate level of claudication pain
is reached, again followed by another rest period. Although
exercise is clearly effective, it has several limitations. Best
results are achieved in a supervised setting similar to cardiac
rehabilitation and require a motivated patient but lack of coverage
of a supervised program by most insurance companies has
limited its widespread use. The beneficial effects of walking
disappear quickly once the patient stops walking on a regular
basis.

Smoking cessation. Discontinuing cigarette smoking may be
the single most important factor that determines whether PAD
progresses and discontinuation of smoking may have a favorable
effect on walking tolerance. It is therefore important to encourage
and provide patients with the means to discontinue smoking.

Special considerations

A summary of treatment recommendations for patients with PAD
is provided in **Table C152.2**.

***Coronary artery disease in patients with peripheral
arterial disease.*** Resting ABI is an important predictor of
cardiovascular (CV) mortality in patients with PAD, which is
approximately 30% at 5 years, 50% at 10 years, and 75% at
15 years. Most deaths due to MI or stroke; the relative risk of
dying of any CV disease in patients with PAD is six to seven
times that of a control population. One study in patients with
diabetes mellitus (DM) suggested that intensively treating BP in
patients with PAD can have an overall favorable effect on the CV
event rate (**Figure C152.1**). Therefore patients with PAD should

TABLE C152.2

MEDICAL THERAPY OF PERIPHERAL ARTERIAL DISEASE

Stop smoking

Achieve ideal body weight

Walking exercise program (see Table C152.1)

Achieve goal blood pressure. [Use ACE (or angiotensin II receptor
blocker) as agent of first choice]

If hypertension is not present, consider ACE inhibitor for
cardiovascular protection

Control lipids (goal low-density lipoprotein <100 mg/dL). In high
risk consider LDL <70 mg/dL

Control diabetes

Administer antiplatelet therapy (clopidogrel or aspirin)

Consider use of cilostazol for symptoms of claudication if exercise
alone is ineffective

ACE, angiotensin-converting enzyme; LDL, low-density lipoprotein.

be treated as though they have coronary artery disease (CAD),
including the use of antiplatelet therapy.

Lipid-lowering therapy. Most patients with PAD have
abnormal blood lipids, including increased serum triglycerides,
increased total and low-density lipoprotein (LDL) cholesterol,
or decreased high-density lipoprotein cholesterol. In addition
to lifestyle modification (restriction of dietary fat, weight loss,
exercise), most patients should be on a statin to lower the
LDL cholesterol to <100 mg/dL and there are some studies
suggesting that further lowering to 70 mg/dL may be beneficial;
however goal LDL cholesterol levels this low have not been
specifically studied as to their impact on PAD and PAD-related
events. Statins are a very effective class of cholesterol-lowering
drugs that have been shown to decrease coronary event rates,
allow for regression of atherosclerosis, and help to normalize
endothelial function. Several reports have demonstrated improved
walking distance or leg functioning with statin use in patients with
PAD.

Glucose intolerance and diabetes mellitus. In individuals
with PAD who are also overweight coexisting glucose intolerance
or insulin resistance calls for increased exercise and weight
reduction. Approximately 35% to 40% of patients with PAD have
DM. Aggressive management of DM is indicated. Angiotensin-
converting enzyme (ACE) inhibitors or angiotensin receptor
blockers (ARBs) are the drugs of choice in patients with PAD, DM,
and hypertension. If hyperkalemia or worsening renal dysfunction
limits the use of these drug classes, other forms of antihypertensive
therapy can be used.

Although it is important to lower BP to goal levels in all
patients, it is especially so in patients with diabetes and PAD.
The Appropriate Blood Pressure Control in Diabetes (ABCD)
Trial randomized 480 normotensive (diastolic BP 80–89 mm
Hg) diabetic patients to a 2×2 factorial study with moderate or
intensive BP reduction, either with ACE inhibitor (enalapril) or
calcium blocker (nisoldipine). Mean BP at follow-up was lower
in the intensively treated group (128/75 mm Hg) compared to the
placebo group (138/81 mm Hg, p <.0001). After a follow-up of
5 years, the CV event rate was 13.6% in the intensively treated
group and 39% in the moderately treated group (p = .046), with
a marked inverse relationship between ABI and CV events in

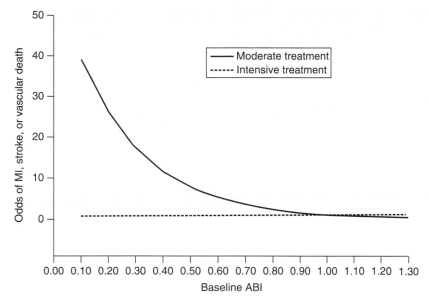

Figure C152.1 Relationship between ankle-brachial index (ABI) and cardiovascular events after adjusting for age, sex, duration of diabetes mellitus, systolic blood pressure, smoking status, total cholesterol level, history of myocardial infarction (MI) or stroke, neurologic stage, and adjusted Cornell voltage. Odds are calculated using moderate treatment and a baseline ABI of 1 as a reference. Patients randomized to moderate treatment (placebo; *solid line*) had an inverse relationship between ABI and events ($p = .009$). Patients intensively treated with nisoldipine or enalapril (*dotted line*) had no relationship between ABI and events, thereby demonstrating the protective effects of blood pressure treatment. MI, myocardial infarction. (From Mehler PS, Coll JR, Estacio RO, et al. Intensive blood pressure control reduces the risk of cardiovascular events in patients with peripheral arterial disease and type 2 diabetes. *Circulation* 2003;107:753–756, with permission.)

the moderately treated group compared to the intensively treated group ($p = .009$) (**Figure C152.1**). Although the findings in Fig. C152.1 are striking, the number of patients was small; a similar larger study is needed in patients with DM and PAD.

Antihypertensive drugs and peripheral arterial disease

JNC 7 confined its remarks to treating hypertension in patients with PAD to one sentence. "Any class of antihypertensive drugs can be used in most patients with peripheral arterial disease." Despite the high prevalence of PAD in older patients (>age 70 or those >50 with a history of smoking or DM) and the fact that most patients with PAD have hypertension, there is very little written about the most effective way to treat these patients. Direct-acting vasodilators, calcium channel blockers (CCBs), α_1-blockers, ACE inhibitors, and ARBs are all effective arteriolar vasodilators, but they do not dilate atherosclerotic vessels and, therefore, cannot be expected to improve symptoms of claudication. In general, antihypertensive drugs have no measurable effect on walking distance or calf blood flow.

β-*Blockers.* The commonly held belief that β-blocking agents should be avoided in PAD was challenged in a carefully performed meta-analysis of 11 randomized controlled trials by Radack and Deck, who concluded that β-adrenergic blocker therapy does not worsen intermittent claudication. Ten of 11 studies in this meta-analysis showed that pain-free and maximal treadmill walking distances were not decreased by atenolol, labetalol, or pindolol.

As a general rule, β-blockers should not be considered a first line agent in the treatment of hypertension in patients with PAD but if there is a clear indication for β-blocker use (HF, post-MI, angina pectoris, or arrhythmias), a β-blocker can and should be used. Patients with vasospastic diseases (e.g., Raynaud's phenomenon, chronic pernio) and hypertension should generally not receive β-blockers, because the frequency and degree of vasospasm may increase with the use of these drugs. Under these circumstances, CCBs and α-blockers may lower the BP while decreasing the severity and frequency of vasospasm.

Angiotensin-converting enzyme inhibitors. Although ACE inhibitors can effectively lower BP in many patients with PAD, most studies have shown that they do not significantly improve walking distance. Renal function should be followed closely in patients with PAD who are on ACE inhibitors because the prevalence of atherosclerotic renal artery stenosis (RAS) occurs in approximately 40% of patients with PAD or abdominal aortic aneurysm; high-grade bilateral RAS occurs in 10% to 15% of these patients.

ACE inhibitors may lower CV events. In the Heart Outcomes Prevention Evaluation Study (HOPE), of the 9,297 patients entered, 4,051 patients (44%) had PAD (ABI <0.9). In the entire group, the primary end point (MI, stroke, CV death) occurred in 17.7% of patients randomized to placebo and 14.1% of patients randomized to ramipril, a relative risk reduction of 22%. The primary endpoint occurred in 22% of patients with PAD who received placebo compared to 14.3% of patients without PAD receiving placebo (an ~50% increase in relative risk). Despite initial reports that ramipril benefits in HOPE effects were "independent of BP" (non-standardized clinic BP differences between ramipril and placebo were 3/2 mm Hg at year 2 and 3/1 mm Hg at year 5), an important 24-hour ambulatory BP substudy in a small subset of patients with PAD revealed a 24-hour BP reduction of 10/4 mm Hg with ramipril, enough of a change to explain all of the CV benefits attributed to ACE inhibition in this study.

Abdominal aortic aneurysms

Fastidious BP control to the lowest appropriate (asymptomatic levels is the cornerstone of nonsurgical management of abdominal aortic aneurysms. Although the data is limited and there are no large randomized trials, animal and human data suggest that β-blockers may slow the rate of aneurysmal expansion. Therefore, in the patient with an abdominal aortic aneurysm, β-blocker therapy is the antihypertensive treatment of choice if there are no contraindications to its use. Surgical resection or endovascular exclusion (aortic stent graft) of an abdominal aortic aneurysm should be considered for all symptomatic patients and in the asymptomatic patient with an aneurysm ≥5.5 cm or in patients in whom the rate of aneurysmal expansion exceeds the expected rate of approximately 0.4 cm per year.

Suggested Readings

Caprie Steering Committee. A randomized blinded trial of clopidogrel versus aspirin for patients at risk of ischaemic events (CAPRIE). *Lancet* 1996;348:1329–1339.

Clement DL. European Society of Hypertension Scientific Newsletter: control of hypertension in patients with peripheral artery disease. *J Hypertens* 2006;24:2477–2478.

Criqui MH, Langer RD, Fronek A, et al. Mortality over a period of 10 years in patients with peripheral arterial disease. *N Engl J Med* 1992;326:381–386.

Gardner AW, Poehlman ET. Exercise rehabilitation programs for the treatment of claudication pain. A meta-analysis. *JAMA* 1995;274:975–980.

Hiatt WR. Medical treatment of peripheral arterial disease and claudication. *N Engl J Med* 2001;344:1608–1621.

Hirsch AT, Haskal ZJ, Hertzer NR, et al. ACC/AHA 2005 Practice Guidelines for the management of patients with peripheral arterial disease (lower extremity, renal, mesenteric, and abdominal aortic): a collaborative report from the American Association for Vascular Surgery/Society for Vascular Surgery, Society for Cardiovascular Angiography and Interventions, Society for Vascular Medicine and Biology, Society of Interventional Radiology, and the ACC/AHA Task Force on Practice Guidelines (Writing Committee to Develop Guidelines for the Management of Patients With Peripheral Arterial Disease). *J Am Coll Cardiol* 2006;47:1239–1312.

Norgren L, Hiatt WR, Dormandy JA, et al. TASC II working group. Inter-society consensus for the management of peripheral arterial disease (TASC II). *Eur J Vasc Endovasc Surg* 2007;33(Suppl 1):S1–S75.

Olin JW. Hypertension in peripheral arterial disease. *Vasc Med* 2005;10:241–246.

Radack K, Deck C. Beta-adrenergic blocker therapy does not worsen intermittent claudication in subjects with peripheral arterial disease: a meta-analysis of randomized controlled trials. *Arch Intern Med* 1991;151:1769–1776.

Svensson P, de Faire U, Sleight P, et al. Comparative effects of ramipril on ambulatory and office blood pressures: a HOPE substudy. *Hypertension* 2001;38:E28–E32.

CHAPTER C153 ■ TREATMENT OF HYPERTENSIVE PATIENTS WITH CEREBROVASCULAR DISEASE

ROBERT D. BROWN, Jr., MD, MPH

KEY POINTS

- Specific blood pressure (BP) targets have not yet been identified in patients with acute cerebrovascular events, but precipitous decline in BP after ischemic stroke may increase infarct size.
- In acute ischemic stroke, moderate BP elevation can usually be managed conservatively, but BP must be more tightly controlled if thrombolytic therapy is used.
- In intracerebral and subarachnoid hemorrhage (SAH), hypertension should be treated if it is of moderate to marked severity.
- For secondary prevention, people with a transient ischemic attack (TIA) or cerebral infarction benefit from reduction in BP; those able to achieve BP values <120/80 mm Hg have the fewest recurrent events.

See also Chapters **A66,** A67, A68, **B79,** and **C114**

Hypertension is an important risk factor for transient ischemic attack (TIA), cerebral infarction, intracerebral hemorrhage (ICH), and subarachnoid hemorrhage (SAH), and is also commonly noted in conjunction with asymptomatic cerebrovascular occlusive disease. Optimal blood pressure (BP) treatment thresholds in people with cerebrovascular disease have not been established. It is commonly accepted that BP treatment goals are different based on the nature of the cerebrovascular ischemic symptoms, the cause of the ischemic event, presence of intracerebral ICH or SAH, and the timing after the event.

Acute cerebral ischemia and infarction

Hypertension after cerebral infarction is quite common. The causes of the elevated BP include pain, undiagnosed or undertreated preexisting hypertension, anxiety or agitation, reaction to artificial ventilation, physiologic response to hypoxia, or increased intracranial pressure (ICP).

Acute management considerations. In the setting of cerebral infarction, cerebral blood flow is more directly dependent on systemic BP because of impaired autoregulation in the area of the infarct. In theory, insufficient BP may lead to reduced perfusion in the peri-infarct area and increased infarct size. Management is currently based on anecdotal experience, findings from animal studies, knowledge of intracranial vascular autoregulation, and clinical experience because there are no large trials defining optimal BP management after cerebral infarction. Most neurologists believe it is prudent to allow BP to remain elevated immediately after an acute ischemic stroke (with occasional exception), realizing that in most patients, BP will decline spontaneously with time. Therefore, it is recommended that if thrombolysis is not utilized, elevated BP after cerebral infarction should be left untreated unless the systolic BP is >220 mm Hg or the mean BP is >120 mm Hg. There is no evidence that the risk of hemorrhagic transformation, occurrence of brain edema, early recurrent stroke, or other deleterious outcomes is increased with a conservative approach. Particularly in persons with a history of hypertension, more aggressive management of acutely elevated BP is more likely to increase infarct size, resulting in a poorer outcome.

Blood pressure goals. Antihypertensive drugs are often withheld unless the estimated mean arterial pressure (MAP) is >120 mm Hg, systolic BP >220 mm Hg or diastolic BP >120 mm Hg (**Table C153.1**). If these criteria for treatment are met, an initial BP goal would be to reduce BP by 15% during the first 24 hours. If less severe hypertension (systolic BP 185–220 mm Hg; diastolic BP 110–120 mm Hg; mean BP 110–120 mm Hg) is associated with hemorrhagic transformation, hypertensive encephalopathy, acute myocardial infarction, acute renal failure, acute pulmonary edema, or dissection of the thoracic aorta,

parenteral drug therapy should be initiated and BP titrated to lower levels.

Influence of thrombolytic therapy. In the National Institute of Neurological Disorders and Stroke intravenous tissue plasminogen activator (t-PA) stroke study, patients were excluded from receiving intravenous t-PA for acute ischemic stroke if the BP was >185 mm Hg systolic or ≥110 mm Hg diastolic or if ongoing aggressive management was needed to meet these criteria. If intravenous t-PA is used, the goal BP should be <185 mm Hg systolic and <110 mm Hg diastolic (**Table C153.1**). In addition, if more than two doses of labetalol or other ongoing aggressive maneuvers are necessary to bring BP to <185 mm Hg systolic or <110 mm Hg diastolic, thrombolysis should be used with extreme caution.

Choice of agents. The best agent to use in the setting of acute ischemic stroke is not clear. Aggressive management with agents such as intravenous sodium nitroprusside or intravenous nicardipine is typically not needed unless diastolic BP is >140 mm Hg (**Table C153.1**). Parenteral agents that are easily titrated with immediate-onset, minimal effect on cerebral blood flow and a low likelihood of causing precipitous decline in BP should be initiated (e.g., intravenous labetalol or low-dose intravenous enalapril). The response to intravenous enalapril, however, can be unpredictable and sometimes reduces BP excessively.

Chronic management after cerebral infarction

After a cerebral infarct has occurred, aggressive long-term management of hypertension is a key factor in secondary

---

TABLE C153.1

HYPERTENSION MANAGEMENT IN ACUTE CEREBROVASCULAR DISORDERS

BP level (mm Hg)	Management
Cerebral Infarction, not a Candidate for Thrombolysis	
Diastolic BP >140	Sodium nitroprusside, i.v., 0.5–1 µg/kg/min
Systolic BP >220 or diastolic BP 121–140; mean BP >120	Labetalol, 10 mg i.v. over 1–2 min, repeat or double every 10–20 min, up to 300 mg. Alternate: enalaprilat, 1 mg over 5 min, then 1–5 mg every 6 h
Systolic BP 185–220 or diastolic BP 105–120	No acute treatment, unless hemorrhagic transformation, hypertensive encephalopathy, acute myocardial infarction, acute renal failure from accelerated hypertension, acute pulmonary edema, or aortic dissection
	Treat factors that may contribute to increased BP, including pain, agitation, headache, bladder distension, and hypoxia
Systolic BP <185 or diastolic BP <105	No acute treatment
Cerebral Infarction, Candidate for Thrombolysis	
Systolic BP >185 or diastolic BP >110, before treatment	Labetalol, 10 mg i.v. over 1–2 min, repeat or double every 10–20 min, up to 300 mg
Intracerebral Hemorrhage	
Systolic BP >230 or diastolic BP >140	Sodium nitroprusside, i.v., 0.5–1 µg/kg/min.
Mean BP >130 mm Hg, systolic BP 180–230 or diastolic BP >105–140	Labetalol, 10 mg i.v. over 1–2 min, repeat or double every 10–20 min, up to 300 mg. Alternate: enalaprilat, 1 mg over 5 min, then 1–5 mg every 6 h.
Mean BP <130, systolic BP <180 or diastolic <105	No acute treatment
Subarachnoid Hemorrhage	
Diastolic BP >140	Sodium nitroprusside, i.v.
Mean BP >130 and diastolic BP <140	Labetalol or enalaprilat, i.v., as noted for cerebral infarction and intracerebral hemorrhage
Mean BP <130	No acute treatment
BP, blood pressure.	

prevention. Both systolic and diastolic BP control are important and isolated systolic hypertension should not be ignored. The beneficial effects of BP reduction in this setting include reduced risk of a second cerebrovascular event, myocardial infarction and cardiovascular mortality. Long-term hypertension management can be implemented within a few days of cerebral infarction.

History of untreated or treated hypertension. If there is a history of untreated hypertension, antihypertensive medications may be initiated 12 hours after the ischemic stroke if the initial BP is >220/120 mm Hg or 24 hours after the ischemic stroke if the initial BP is <220/120 mm Hg. For previously treated patients with initial BP >220/120 mm Hg (or mean pressure >120 mm Hg), usual dosing of all antihypertensive medications may be resumed on the first day after ischemic stroke. For those with entry BPs <220/120 mm Hg (or a MAP <120 mm Hg), usual antihypertensive medications can be resumed at half doses 24 hours after stroke; if the BP decline is not marked, full medication doses may be used. Patients with a history of hypertension can be treated to standard BP control targets (<140/90 mm Hg in general or <130/80 mm Hg for patients with diabetes, chronic kidney disease, or ischemic heart disease).

No history of hypertension. For those without a history of hypertension, if the BP is >140/90 but <220/120 mm Hg (or MAP <120 mm Hg), the decision regarding antihypertensive management should be made within the first several days of the ischemic stroke. Those with higher BP (>220/120 mm Hg or MAP >120 mm Hg) will have been treated acutely as outlined in the preceding text and chronic antihypertensive management may be initiated after baseline BP is clarified, 24 to 48 hours after stroke onset.

Long-term blood pressure targets. Patients who have had a TIA or cerebral infarction may benefit from a slight reduction in BP levels even if BPs are <140/90 mm Hg and there is no history of hypertension. In the Perindopril Protection against Recurrent Stroke Study (PROGRESS), patients receiving combination antihypertensive therapy experienced a mean reduction of BP of 9/4 mm Hg and had the greatest reduction in the risk of recurrent events.

Choice of agents. The specific medication selected is likely not as important as the overall reduction in BP. Prevention of recurrent stroke, other cardiovascular events, and cognitive decline are important goals of antihypertensive treatment. The ability to prevent stroke has been demonstrated for several classes of drugs including diuretics in the Systolic Hypertension in the Elderly Program (SHEP), calcium antagonists in the Systolic Hypertension in Europe and Hypertension Optimal Treatment trials, angiotensin-converting enzyme (ACE) inhibitors in the Heart Outcomes Prevention Evaluation (HOPE), angiotensin receptor blockers in the Losartan Intervention for Endpoint Reduction in Hypertension Trial (LIFE) and the Acute Candesartan Cilexetil Evaluation in Stroke Survivors (ACCESS) study. Recurrent stroke rates were reduced by a combination of perindopril and indapamide in the PROGRESS study but the effect of ACE inhibitor alone was neutral.

Other considerations. Aspirin is common therapy following a stroke and may sometimes attenuate the effect of certain antihypertensive medication classes. Lipid lowering is indicated in many stroke patients in that stroke recurrence is lessened in patients so treated, a process which occurs independent of the degree of cholesterol reduction. In addition to medical management, lifestyle changes should be implemented including weight loss, increased physical activity, reduction in sodium intake, and smoking cessation.

Intracerebral hemorrhage

BP elevation is common after intracerebral hemorrhage but it is unclear whether aggressive BP management lessens the chance of increasing hemorrhage size or recurrence or leads to other deleterious outcomes, such as diffuse cerebral ischemia or periinfarct zonal ischemia. In consideration of this delicate balance, for persons with spontaneous intracerebral hemorrhage, antihypertensive medications are typically initiated acutely if MAP is >130 mm Hg or the systolic and diastolic BP are >180 or >105 mm Hg, respectively. The initial management goal should not be to rapidly achieve normotension. If there is no evidence of increased ICP, then the BP goal would be a MAP of 110 mm Hg or BP of 160/90 mm Hg. If there is suggestion that the ICP is elevated, then the ICP should be monitored and the cerebral perfusion pressure (MAP–ICP) should be kept >60 mm Hg. Patients with a history of hypertension should be managed with particular care and the goal levels may not be quite as strict. Given that increased ICP is more common in intracerebral hemorrhage than in cerebral infarction, a higher BP may be necessary to maintain a stable cerebral perfusion pressure for the former. The antihypertensive agents recommended under these circumstances are similar to those used for cerebral infarction (**Table C153.1**).

Subarachnoid hemorrhage

The management of hypertension with SAH is controversial. Studies have not consistently defined a higher rate of rebleeding or death in persons with increased systolic BP. Among those with persistently elevated BP (MAP >130 mm Hg), very careful reduction with labetalol or nitroprusside is reasonable (**Table C153.1**). Should any evidence of clinical deterioration or vasospasm occur, antihypertensive therapy should be halted and fluid resuscitation begun.

Suggested Readings

Adams HP Jr, Adams RJ, Brott T, et al. Guidelines for the early management of patients with ischemic stroke: a scientific statement from the Stroke Council of the American Stroke Association. *Stroke* 2003;34(4):1056–1083.

Bosch J, Yusuf S, Pogue J, et al. The HOPE Investigators. Use of ramipril in preventing stroke: double blind randomised trial. *BMJ* 2002;324:1–5.

Broderick J, Adams HP Jr, Barsan W, et al. Guidelines for the management of spontaneous intracerebral hemorrhage: a scientific statement from the Stroke Council of the American Stroke Association. *Stroke* 1999;30:905–915.

Chobanian AV, Bakris GL, Black HR, et al. The seventh report of the Joint National Committee on Prevention, Detection, Evaluation, and Treatment of High BP: the JNC 7 report. *JAMA* 2003;289(19):2560–2572.

Mayberg MR, Batjer HH, Dacey R, et al. Guidelines for the management of aneurysmal subarachnoid hemorrhage: a statement for healthcare professionals from a special writing group of the Stroke Council, American Heart Association. *Circulation* 1994;90:2592–2605.

The National Institute of Neurological Disorders and Stroke rt-PA Stroke Study Group. Tissue plasminogen activator for acute ischemic stroke. *N Engl J Med* 1995;333:1581–1587.

PROGRESS Collaborative Group. Randomised trial of a perindopril-based blood-pressure-lowering regimen among 6105 individuals with previous stroke or transient ischaemic attack. *Lancet* 2001;358:1033–1041.

Powers WJ. Acute hypertension after stroke: the scientific basis for treatment decisions. *Neurology* 1994;43:461–467.

The Stroke Prevention by Aggressive Reduction in Cholesterol Levels (SPARCL) Investigators. High-dose atorvastatin after stroke or transient ischemic attack. *N Engl J Med* 2006;355:549–559.

Wijdicks EF, Vermeulen M, Murray GD, et al. The effects of treating hypertension following aneurysmal subarachnoid hemorrhage. *Clin Neurol Neurosurg* 1990;92:111–117.

CHAPTER C154 ■ TREATMENT OF ORTHOSTATIC DISORDERS AND BAROREFLEX FAILURE

DAVID ROBERTSON, MD

KEY POINTS

■ Postural tachycardia syndrome (POTS) is characterized by a large increase in heart rate with little change in blood pressure (BP) on standing; there are many causes but limited treatment strategies.

■ Autonomic failure is characterized by severe supine hypertension and marked upright hypotension, often with syncope, that is accentuated by hypovolemia or exercise; treatment is directed toward symptom relief and restoring functional capacities for daily life.

■ Acute baroreflex failure is characterized by episodic severe hypertension, tachycardia, headache, and sweating, sometimes followed by hypotension; hypertensive crises may follow minor emotional or physical stimulation; treatment is directed toward reducing BP and excess sympathetic or vagal activity.

See also Chapters A38 and **C110**

Disorders of autonomic cardiovascular regulation commonly present with extreme variation of heart rate or blood pressure (BP) and are often associated with assumption of the upright posture. Autonomic disorders may be considered in three categories: (a) mild dysautonomias, in which tachycardia may be present but orthostatic hypotension is usually absent; (b) severe dysautonomias (autonomic failure), rare conditions in which there is always orthostatic hypotension, often with other neurologic problems; and (c) baroreflex failure, in which exaggerated BP and heart rate variation is exacerbated by emotional or physical stress rather than postural change.

Postural tachycardia syndrome

The mild dysautonomias include neurally mediated syncope, in which there are episodic decreases in BP or heart rate, associated with fainting, almost always in the upright posture. The other major mild dysautonomia is postural tachycardia syndrome (POTS). POTS has the clinical hallmark of rapid heart rate on standing without orthostatic hypotension; it is not a single disease, but rather a syndrome.

Pathogenesis. The pathophysiologic bases underlying POTS can encompass structural, endocrinologic, renal, immune, toxic, and neuropathic processes (**Figure C154.1**). Among the structural entities, examples include absent venous valves and varicose veins. Volume deficits may be of two types: persistent hypovolemia (Bartter's syndrome and Gitelman's syndrome) or orthostatic hypovolemia resulting from excessive transudation of fluid from the vascular compartment into the interstitial fluid compartment during upright posture. Autoimmune mechanisms may be important

in some cases of POTS. Recently, an antibody against the α_3 subunit of the N_N-nicotinic receptor on autonomic ganglia has been detected in approximately 15% of a subgroup of patients with autonomic disorders, including POTS. Neuropathic POTS is usually due to a partial dysautonomia.

Rarely a genetic syndrome of norepinephrine transporter (NET) dysfunction gives rise to POTS. Patients with NET dysfunction complain of palpitations and orthostatic tachycardia, dizziness and lightheadedness on standing, occasional fainting, reduced exercise capacity, and fatigue. The NET is a unique gene product that subserves "reuptake" functions at the level of noradrenergic synapses (uptake-1). NET is likely to be of particular importance in terminating adrenoreceptor activation in the heart, where synapses are narrow and NET is responsible for removal of 90% of the norepinephrine in the synapse.

Diagnostic criteria. POTS is characterized by four major criteria: (a) symptoms of sympathetic activation with upright posture, (b) orthostatic increase in heart rate $\geq$30 beats per minute, (c) normal orthostatic BP maintenance (BP drop $\leq$20/10 mm Hg), (d) high plasma norepinephrine during standing ($\geq$600 pg per mL). POTS represents the "final common pathway" for dozens of genetic and acquired autonomic and cardiovascular entities (**Table C154.1**).

There remain many uncertainties about POTS, including its prevalence; we do not understand where the normal spectrum ends and where POTS begins. POTS and deconditioning share many of the clinical features and their separation can prove challenging. Most patients with POTS reduce their levels of physical activity and therefore present with both POTS and

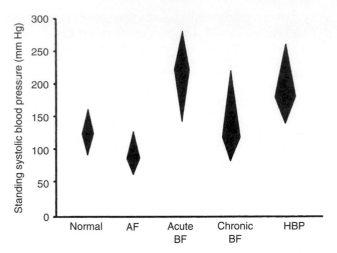

Figure C154.1 Representative standing systolic blood pressures (BPs) recorded in in-patients and healthy subjects. The widest point of each *diamond* depicts the most common standing systolic pressure seen in typical patients, whereas the height depicts the range of pressures seen throughout the day. Patients with autonomic failure (AF) have the lowest standing pressure. In the acute phase of baroreflex failure (acute BF), usually days to weeks immediately after acute bilateral damage to the cranial nerves IX and X, extremely high pressures are similar to essential hypertension (HBP). After several months (chronic BF), the standing systolic pressure is usually near normal, but greater variability is still seen. (From Robertson D, Biaggioni I, Burnstock G, Low PA, eds. *Primer on the autonomic nervous system.* San Diego: Academic Press, 2004, with permission.)

deconditioning. Finally, we know very little about the long-term outcomes of POTS.

Treatment. Fortunately, we are acquiring an armamentarium of treatment strategies, which may result in improvement in symptoms in individual patients. These strategies include (a) orthostatic "exercise," (b) increased salt and water ingestion, (c) sodium-retaining steroid (fludrocortisones), (d) low-dose β-blockade, (e) low-dose α_2 agonist (clonidine), and (f) low-dose α_1 agonist (midodrine). Responses to these strategies are quite variable in their magnitude and duration, however, and it is often wise to consider referral of POTS patients to physicians with substantial clinical experience.

Autonomic failure

Pathogenesis. Multiple system atrophy (Shy-Drager syndrome) is a severe dysautonomia in which central control of autonomic function is impaired. The accompanying neurodegenerative

TABLE C154.1

POSTURAL TACHYCARDIA SYNDROME: MANY NAMES

Effort syndrome
Hyperdynamic β-adrenergic state
Idiopathic hypovolemia
Irritable heart
Mitral valve prolapse syndrome
Neurocirculatory asthenia
Orthostatic intolerance
Soldier's heart
Vasoregulatory asthenia

symptoms include cerebellar, extrapyramidal, and sometimes pyramidal abnormalities. Other severe dysautonomias include infiltrative autonomic neuropathy due to diabetes mellitus or amyloidosis. In the latter disorders, the primary problem is damage to the peripheral autonomic nerves. Finally, there are neurodegenerative disorders such as "pure autonomic failure," Parkinson's disease with autonomic failure, and genetic disorders such as dopamine β-hydroxylase deficiency, in which congenital absence of norepinephrine causes profound orthostatic hypotension (**Figure C154.2**). Usually a supine and upright BP, heart rate, and plasma catecholamines suffice to diagnose severe dysautonomias. A fat pad biopsy can confirm amyloidosis.

Treatment. The purpose of therapeutic interventions in patients with autonomic failure is to increase functional capacity rather than to achieve any particular level of BP. Drug treatment of orthostatic hypotension can be beneficial for selected patients. On the whole, however, severely affected patients are often extremely difficult to manage. The aim is for patients to have a 3-minute standing time, which usually enables them to go about daily activities. Factors such as prior ingestion of food and drugs as well as the rate of ventilation should be taken into account when assessing the patient's standing time or BP.

Importance of volume maintenance. Maximizing circulating blood volume is extremely important in treating orthostatic hypotension in autonomic failure. In addition to the absence of BP counterregulation by the sympathetic nervous system, relative and absolute volume depletion is present. There is often a reduction in central blood volume and many patients have a reduced total blood volume, low-normal values of central venous pressure, right atrial pressure, and pulmonary wedge pressure, even in the supine position. Liver blood flow is reduced considerably by upright posture, and blood-flow dependent drug metabolism may therefore be altered.

Patients with autonomic failure cannot adequately conserve sodium during low-salt intake. This may be due to decreased

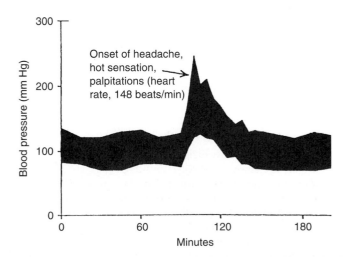

Figure C154.2 Blood pressure (BP) monitoring in a 43-year-old man approximately 2 weeks after surgical removal of a carotid body tumor. While BP was being monitored, the patient's right hand was immersed in ice water for 60 seconds. The BP immediately rose and continued to rise for several minutes after discontinuation of the cold stimulus. Symptoms appeared during this time and then resolved as BP and heart rate returned to normal during the following 30 minutes. On some occasions, the patient had spontaneous paroxysms of similar magnitude. (From Robertson D, Hollister AS, Biaggioni I, et al. The diagnosis and treatment of baroreflex failure. *N Engl J Med* 1993;329:1449–1455, with permission.)

renal nerve activity and perhaps to enhanced dopamine actions. In addition, renin responses to a low-salt diet and upright posture are reduced or absent in autonomic failure. Elevated supine pressure probably also contributes to the failure of the kidney to conserve salt and water through pressure-diuresis, especially overnight; relative hypovolemia and orthostatic hypotension may be worse in the morning and improve during the day. Salt intake should be liberalized in all patients except in those few with coexisting heart failure. Slight pedal edema is well tolerated and a welcome sign of higher intravascular volume as well as increased interstitial hydrostatic pressure. Fludrocortisone is also commonly used.

Elastic support garments. Waist-high, custom-fitted elastic support stockings that exert graded pressure on the lower body and increase interstitial hydrostatic pressure give some symptomatic relief; support stockings are not of much use unless they reach the waist. An abdominal binder in association with elastic stockings is even more useful and often better tolerated. Abdominal binders augment venous return from the splanchnic bed, a major source of venous pooling. However, patients must be cautioned not to wear these stockings when supine or at night, because the increased central blood volume can contribute to a marked increase in supine BP. Antigravity and shock suits have been used in the past with some success, but are awkward and bring undue attention to the patient's problems.

Activities. Patients should avoid activities that involve straining or lifting heavy objects because acute increases in abdominal or intrathoracic pressure compromise venous return and can precipitate hypotension. Coughing and straining at stool or with voiding may particularly bring on hypotension. Working with one's arms above shoulder level (e.g., shaving) can lower pressure dramatically. Ambulation or shifting weight from leg to leg as opposed to standing motionless takes advantage of muscular pumping on the veins. A slightly stooped walking posture may be helpful. Squatting and standing with the legs in a "scissor" position are valuable emergency methods of increasing venous return, particularly when presyncopal symptoms occur. Patients may sit with their legs over the side of the bed before standing. This minimizes hemodynamic stress, because assumption of the upright posture is broken down into two movements: (a) assumption of the seated posture and (b) standing from the seated posture.

Food intake. The effect of food and water on BP in chronic orthostatic hypotension can be important. In healthy subjects, there is a slight tachycardia with little or no fall in BP after eating. However, patients with autonomic failure, similar to the elderly or those taking sympatholytic agents, may exhibit large postprandial falls in BP due to exaggerated splanchnic vasodilation. Even a modest amount of food may cause problems, especially if the sugar content is high.

Exercise. A graded program of isotonic exercise such as walking is sometimes beneficial. More vigorous exercise such as jogging is rarely tolerated because post–exercise decreases in BP can be severe. Swimming is usually well tolerated because in water, orthostatic hypotension is attenuated. Climbing stairs is a common hypotensive stimulus.

Drug therapy. Various drugs can be considered in treating autonomic failure and orthostatic hypotension of diverse causes, but none are more useful than fludrocortisone and midodrine.

Fludrocortisone. Fludrocortisone (Florinef) has been the pharmacologic cornerstone in the treatment of autonomic failure for 50 years. Although some patients respond to 0.1 mg daily, 0.1 mg twice daily is usually more effective, with some patients needing 0.1 mg three times a day. Weight gain commonly occurs with fludrocortisone therapy and should be targeted at 3 to 8 lb. Fludrocortisone should generally be avoided in patients who by physical examination or history are on the verge of heart failure. The drug is begun at a dose of 0.1 mg once daily and titrated higher at 1- to 2-week intervals depending on the therapeutic response. Standing time, weight, supine BP, the presence or absence of rales and a gallop rhythm, and plasma-potassium and magnesium concentrations should be monitored. Many patients develop a reduction in potassium or magnesium concentration in plasma after 2 to 4 weeks of an adequate dosage of fludrocortisone, which may range from mild to severe; potassium replacement is occasionally necessary. Only a minority of patients require replacement of magnesium, which may best occur with slow-release preparations of magnesium chloride. A twice-daily dosage regimen with magnesium supplements minimizes diarrhea.

Midodrine. Midodrine is an α_1 agonist prodrug that raises BP through direct vasoconstriction. The dosage ranges from 5 mg daily (2.5 mg on awakening and again at noon) to dosages as high as 10 mg three times a day. The most common limitation in the treatment of orthostatic hypotension is development of unacceptable levels of supine hypertension, which is present in most patients, especially those receiving fludrocortisones, but may occur even in the absence of any treatment. Avoiding midodrine use after 5 PM reduces nocturnal (supine) hypertension.

Management of supine hypertension. It is often necessary to accept relatively high levels of supine BP to keep the individual functionally mobile, although one must always try to avoid very high supine BP values (>200 mm Hg systolic). Most patients can maintain supine BPs in the 140 to 180/90 to 100 mm Hg range. Supine hypertension can be minimized by placing the head of the bed on blocks to approximately 5 to 15 degrees. In addition to attenuating nocturnal diuresis, this reduces the notable worsening of symptoms in the morning. Head-up tilt at night may also minimize nocturnal shifts of interstitial fluid from the legs into the circulation. Ingesting a sweet at bedtime, together with a short-acting antihypertensive drug (e.g., hydralazine, nitrate, clonidine, and nifedipine) can attenuate nocturnal hypertension.

Baroreflex failure

Baroreflex failure is the most dramatic of autonomic disorders (**Figures C154.1** and **C154.2**).

Pathogenesis and presentation. Sudden loss of baroreflex innervation causes acute baroreflex failure, with severe hypertension and tachycardia in the supine and upright postures. BPs as high as 300/160 mm Hg occur, often accompanied by subjective sensations of warmth, flushing, palpitations, severe headache, and diaphoresis that are commonly mistaken for pheochromocytoma. After a few days, the sustained hypertensive phase gives rise to the more chronic labile BP phase. The hallmark of this phase is hypertension and tachycardia alternating with periods of hypotension, with or without bradycardia. The pressor crises tend to be preceded by minor emotional or physical perturbations, which usually last <1 hour, and include heat and flushing sensations. Patients sometimes exhibit emotional volatility but it is not always clear whether these features are result of the pressor crisis or the cause of it. Late in the disorder, the hypotensive phase may gradually become more pronounced and the hypertensive crises more attenuated. Etiologies of baroreflex failure include trauma, neck irradiation, and familial paraganglioma syndrome.

Diagnosis. Common findings are supranormal pressor responses to handgrip, cold pressor, and especially mental arithmetic testing. Perhaps the most helpful agent in diagnosing baroreflex failure is a low (0.1 mg) dose of clonidine; which often lowers BP by 30 to 70 mm Hg in a patient with baroreflex failure. Between crises, plasma norepinephrine levels are usually normal but during attacks, plasma norepinephrine may rise to values of 1,000 to 2,000 pg per mL (similar to values observed in myocardial infarction, severe heart failure, or some pheochromocytomas). Over time, the pressor crises in baroreflex failure tend to become attenuated, whereas worsening more commonly occurs in pheochromocytoma, an important point in differentiating these conditions. Urinary norepinephrine levels in baroreflex failure are usually at the upper border or slightly above normal range. Rarely, selective baroreflex failure (Jordan syndrome) occurs, in which parasympathetic efferent nerves to the heart are preserved, and marked bradycardia or asystole may arise from the "malignant vagotonia."

Therapy. The treatment of baroreflex failure is often very difficult. The initial sustained hypertension phase requires hospitalization in an intensive care unit and control with nitroprusside and sympatholytic agents. In the first 2 or 3 days, apneic spells can occur, especially if narcotics are employed, so continuous monitoring is necessary. Once the chronic labile phase is reached, oral or transdermal clonidine is usually effective, but high doses (0.6 to 1.8 mg daily in divided doses) are sometimes required, which may exacerbate hypotension and sedation.

Recognition of the relationship between emotional upset and pressor crises is important. In some cases, spontaneous biofeedback treatment may reduce the number and severity of attacks. Over long periods of time, most patients may be graduated from clonidine to propranolol or benzodiazepine with continued adequate control. In the rare patient with Jordan syndrome, the additional problem of episodic malignant vagotonia may require placement of a pacemaker to prevent cardiac arrest, after which long-term management of hypertension by guanethidine and attenuation of hypotension by fludrocortisone may be required. Unfortunately, guanethidine is no longer on the American market, but can be obtained abroad.

Suggested Readings

Heusser K, Tank J, Luft FC, et al. Baroreflex failure. *Hypertension* 2005;45(5):834–839.

Jacob G, Raj SR, Ketch T, et al. Postural pseudoanemia: posture-dependent change in hematocrit. *Mayo Clin Proc* 2005;80(5):611–614.

Jacob G, Shannon JR, Costa F, et al. Neuropathic postural tachycardia syndrome. *N Engl J Med* 2000;343:1008–1014.

Jordan J, Shannon JR, Black B, et al. Malignant vagotonia due to selective baroreflex failure. *Hypertension* 1997;30:1072–1077.

Ketch T, Biaggioni I, Robertson RM, et al. Four faces of baroreflex failure. Hypertensive crisis, volatile hypertension, orthostatic tachycardia, and malignant vagotonia. *Circulation* 2002;105:2517–2522.

Robertson D, Biaggioni I, Burnstock G, et al. eds. *Primer on the autonomic nervous system*. San Diego: Academic Press, 2004.

Robertson D, Hollister AS, Biaggioni I, et al. The diagnosis and therapy of baroreflex failure. *N Engl J Med* 1993;329:1449–1455.

Shannon JR, Flattem NL, Jordan J, et al. Orthostatic intolerance and tachycardia associated with norepinephrine-transporter deficiency. *N Engl J Med* 2000;342:541–549.

Shibao C, Gamboa A, Diedrich A, et al. Management of hypertension in the setting of autonomic failure: a pathophysiological approach. *Hypertension* 2005;45(4):469–476.

Timmers HJ, Wieling W, Karemaker JM, et al. Denervation of carotid baro- and chemoreceptors in humans. *J Physiol* 2003;553(Pt 1):3–11.

CHAPTER C155 ■ SEXUAL DYSFUNCTION AND HYPERTENSION

L. MICHAEL PRISANT, MD, FAHA, FACC, FACP

KEY POINTS

■ The prevalence of sexual dysfunction increases with age and concomitant cardiac disease, hypertension, obesity, reduced physical activity, diabetes mellitus, or tobacco use.

■ High-dose diuretics and drugs affecting sympathetic neurotransmission commonly cause sexual dysfunction.

■ Switching antihypertensive drugs, weight reduction, and phosphodiesterase-5 inhibitors can improve sexual dysfunction.

■ Phosphodiesterase-5 inhibitors should not be used in patients with unstable cardiac conditions; they interact with nitrates, α_1-blockers and perhaps other vasoactive drugs to cause hypotension that is sometimes severe.

See also Chapters **C105** and **C119**

Sexual dysfunction is a potential problem in the management of hypertensive patients in several ways. Sexual dysfunction is a marker of atherosclerosis, impairs quality of life, and is associated with nonadherence to treatment.

Risk factors for sexual dysfunction

Epidemiologic studies. The National Health and Social Life Survey recently questioned 1,749 women and 1,410 men between the ages of 18 to 59 years and found sexual dysfunction to be more common in women (43%) than men (31%). In the Massachusetts Male Aging Study (MMAS), a random survey of noninstitutionalized men between 40 and 70 years of age, the incidence of erectile dysfunction (ED) was 25.9 cases per 1,000 man-years. Overall, 9.6% of subjects experienced complete ED, whereas 48% of men had no ED. In addition to a sexual activity survey, blood pressure (BP), height, weight, sociodemographic data, health status survey, medications, psychological tests (dominance, anger, and depression), lipids and sex steroid hormones were measured. There was a direct relationship of ED with increasing age. Complete ED was more common with certain diseases, including treated heart disease (39%), treated diabetes mellitus (28%), untreated peptic ulcer (18%), treated hypertension (15%), untreated arthritis (15%), and untreated allergy (12%). Medications associated with complete ED in the MMAS included vasodilators (36%), cardiac drugs (28%), hypoglycemic agents (26%), and antihypertensive drugs (14%). The use of tobacco was associated with a two- to threefold increase in the rate of ED, independent of clinical condition

or concomitant drug use; among subjects using antihypertensive drugs, the rate of complete impotence among nonsmokers was 7.5% compared to 21% among smokers.

Hypertension and antihypertensive drugs. When compared to untreated normotensive patients, untreated hypertensive patients have a higher rate of ED. It is a common belief that antihypertensive drugs cause ED, but short-term exposure to various hypertensive medicines over a 6- to 14-week period was not associated with an increased rate of self-reported ED study in an analysis comparing several drugs (**Figure C155.1**). One of the best prospective studies to examine sexual dysfunction in men and women was the Treatment of Mild Hypertension Study (TOMHS). In this 4-year, double-blind, randomized, controlled trial of 902 men and women with stage 1 diastolic hypertension, all subjects were treated with lifestyle changes and then randomized to treatment with placebo; acebutolol, 400 mg/day; amlodipine, 5 mg/day; chlorthalidone, 15 mg/day; doxazosin, 2 mg/day; or enalapril, 5 mg/day. If the BP remained elevated, the dose of the medication was doubled. If the BP remained elevated, then chlorthalidone (15–30 mg/day) in the nondiuretic groups or enalapril (2.5–5 mg/day) in the diuretic group was added. The rate of sexual dysfunction in TOMHS was 14.4% in men and 4.9% in women. Of the 233 patients on no antihypertensive drugs at baseline, the rate of ED was 9.9%, compared to 17.6% among the 324 patients who were already receiving antihypertensive medications. The rate of ED increased progressively from 7.5% for the age-group 45 to 49 years to 18% for the group 60 years or older. Baseline ED was significantly related to systolic BP, ranging from 8.1% in subjects with systolic BP <130 mm Hg

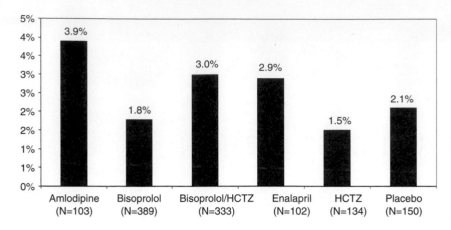

Figure C155.1 Prevalence of short-term self-reported erectile dysfunction. There was no significant difference among the groups receiving therapy for 6 to 14 weeks in a meta-analysis of studies. HCTZ, hydrochlorothiazide. (Modified from Prisant LM, Weir MR, Frishman WH, et al. Self-reported sexual dysfunction in men and women treated with bisoprolol, hydrochlorothiazide, enalapril, amlodipine, placebo, or bisoprolol/hydrochlorothiazide. *J Clin Hypertens (Greenwich)* 1999;1:22.)

to 20.9% in subjects with systolic BP ≥160 mm Hg. Through 24 months, the rate of ED was highest among subjects treated with chlorthalidone (17.1% vs. 8.1% with placebo, $p = .025$) and was lowest in subjects receiving doxazosin (5.6%, similar to placebo, $p = .60$). From 24 to 48 months, there was very little worsening of ED in subjects treated with chlorthalidone (17.1%–18.3%) but subjects receiving placebo had increased ED (8.1%–16.7%). At 48 months, there was no difference among the various antihypertensive treatment groups (**Figure C155.2**).

Management

Antihypertensive drugs. It is important to gather information about sexual function before starting antihypertensive drug therapy because all antihypertensive drugs can be associated with this side effect, as can hypertension itself. TOMHS is consistent

with other studies that suggest that diuretics may be associated with more sexual dysfunction than some other agents. In contrast to common belief, β-blockers were not associated with a higher rate of ED in TOMHS than other antihypertensive drugs but acebutolol was the β-blocker used in TOMHS (a partial agonist compound that may differ from atenolol or propranolol). Other studies show that the rate of ED is generally higher in men receiving multiple antihypertensive drugs. There are fewer data for women. As with men, there is a higher likelihood of sexual dysfunction with spironolactone, reserpine, and peripheral and central sympatholytics. Switching to alternative antihypertensive agents, such as angiotensin-converting enzyme (ACE) inhibitors, angiotensin II receptor blockers, or α_1-blockers may lessen if not eliminate the problem. Weight reduction has been shown to improve sexual function in men and women treated with

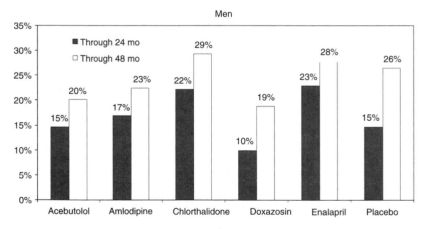

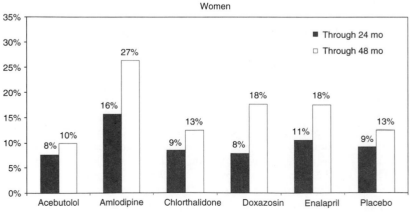

Figure C155.2 Incidence of reported decrease in sexual frequency through 24 and 48 months by gender and treatment group. Through 24 months, the rate of ED was highest among male subjects treated with chlorthalidone and was lowest in subjects receiving doxazosin. At 48 months, there was no difference among the various antihypertensive treatment groups. (Adapted from Grimm RH Jr, Grandits GA, Prineas RJ, et al. Long-term effects on sexual function of five antihypertensive drugs and nutritional hygienic treatment in hypertensive men and women. Treatment of Mild Hypertension Study (TOMHS). *Hypertension* 1997;29:8–14.)

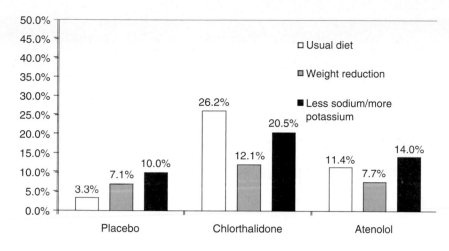

Figure C155.3 Worsening of erectile dysfunction at 6 months by drug and nonpharmacologic intervention. Chlorthalidone was associated with more erectile dysfunction than placebo or atenolol. Weight reduction reduced these effects of chlorthalidone. (Modified from Wassertheil-Smoller S, Oberman A, Blaufox MD, et al. The Trial of Antihypertensive Interventions and Management (TAIM) Study. Final results with regard to blood pressure, cardiovascular risk, and quality of life. *Am J Hypertens* 1992;5:37–44.)

chlorthalidone (**Figure C155.3**). Smoking cessation is advised for anyone with ED.

Phosphodiesterase-5 (PDE5) inhibitors. Sildenafil, vardenafil, and tadalafil are approved drugs for ED and are effective in hypertensive men. These selective drugs increase cyclic guanosine monophosphate in the corpus cavernosum, relax the helicine arteries, and allow blood to fill the lacunar spaces of the corpus cavernosum. For women, attention to foreplay, arousal, and lubrication can be helpful when hypertension-related sexual dysfunction is present. The limited data on sildenafil use in women would suggest limited, if any, benefit.

Blood pressure effects. PDE5 inhibitors reduce BP in normotensive individuals: sildenafil 100 mg, $-3.7/-3.6$ mm Hg; vardenafil 20 mg, $-7.5/-8$ mm Hg; and tadalafil 20 mg, $-1.6/-0.8$ mm Hg. Greater declines in BP may be observed in hypertensive (treated or untreated) patients. Compared to placebo, the maximum decrease in BP from 0 to 4 hours after 100 mg of sildenafil in amlodipine-treated hypertensives was $-8/-7$ mm Hg supine and $-10/-8$ mm Hg standing. The higher the baseline systolic or diastolic BP, the greater the ensuing decline in BP. Vardenafil 20 mg resulted in a $-6/-5$ mm Hg decrease in BP when coadministered with slow-release nifedipine 30 to 60 mg daily. Tadalafil 10 to 20 mg decreased BP maximally $-8/-4$ mm Hg in individual studies with various classes of antihypertensive drugs.

Hypotension. Caution is necessary when combining α_1-blockers and PDE5 inhibitors. Doxazosin 4 mg and sildenafil 25 mg reduced supine BP an additional $-7/-7$ mm Hg. Simultaneous administration of terazosin 10 mg and vardenafil 10 to 20 mg reduced standing systolic BP -14 to -23 mm Hg. Simultaneous administration of doxazosin 8 mg and terazosin 20 mg reduced BP $-9.8/-5.3$ mm Hg. PDE5 inhibitors must not be used in a patient taking nitrates. The clinician must be certain before prescribing a PDE5 inhibitor or a nitrate that the patient is not taking the other medication.

Contraindications and other side effects. A recent heart attack or stroke, obstructive hypertrophic cardiomyopathy, moderate-to-severe aortic stenosis, malignant arrhythmias, accelerated or malignant hypertension, unstable or refractory angina, uncompensated heart failure, and concomitant use of nitrates in any form precludes the safe use of PDE5 inhibitors. Side effects of PDE5 inhibitors include occasional headaches, facial flushing, dysuria, nasal stuffiness, esophageal reflux, lightheadedness, and color vision disturbances. Rare cases of nonarteritic anterior ischemic optic neuropathy have been reported with PDE5 inhibitors but the causal relationship has not been proved.

Suggested Readings

Duncan L, Bateman DN. Sexual function in women. Do antihypertensive drugs have an impact? *Drug Saf* 1993;8:225–234.

Feldman HA, Goldstein I, Hatzichristou DG, et al. Impotence and its medical and psychosocial correlates: results of the Massachusetts male aging study. *J Urol* 1994;151:54–61.

Grimm RH Jr, Grandits GA, Prineas RJ, et al. Long-term effects on sexual function of five antihypertensive drugs and nutritional hygienic treatment in hypertensive men and women. Treatment of Mild Hypertension Study (TOMHS). *Hypertension* 1997;29:8–14.

Johannes CB, Araujo AB, Feldman HA, et al. Incidence of erectile dysfunction in men 40 to 69 years old: longitudinal results from the Massachusetts male aging study. *J Urol* 2000;163:460–463.

Kostis JB, Jackson G, Rosen R, et al. Sexual dysfunction and cardiac risk (the Second Princeton Consensus Conference). *Am J Cardiol* 2005;96:313–321.

Laumann EO, Paik A, Rosen RC. Sexual dysfunction in the United States: prevalence and predictors. *JAMA* 1999;281:537–544.

Prisant LM. Phosphodiesterase-5 inhibitors and their hemodynamic effects. *Curr Hypertens Rep* 2006;8:345–351.

Prisant LM, Carr AA, Bottini PB, et al. Sexual dysfunction with antihypertensive drugs. *Arch Intern Med* 1994;154:730–736.

Prisant LM, Loebl DH, Waller JL. Arterial elasticity and erectile dysfunction in men. *J Clin Hypertens (Greenwich)* 2006;8(11):768–774.

Prisant LM, Weir MR, Frishman WH, et al. Self-reported sexual dysfunction in men and women treated with bisoprolol, hydrochlorothiazide, enalapril, amlodipine, placebo, or bisoprolol/hydrochlorothiazide. *J Clin Hypertens (Greenwich)* 1999;1:22–26.

CHAPTER C156 ▪ TREATMENT OF HYPERTENSION WITH CHRONIC RENAL INSUFFICIENCY OR ALBUMINURIA

ATUL R. CHUGH, MD AND GEORGE L. BAKRIS, MD

KEY POINTS

- ▪ Blood pressure (BP) control is the most important aspect of the prevention and treatment of advancing chronic kidney disease (CKD), regardless of etiology; BP should be maintained at ≤130/80 mm Hg or lower if tolerated, although evidence is limited for this recommendation.
- ▪ Three or more appropriately dosed antihypertensive medications are often necessary to achieve this goal; an angiotensin-converting enzyme (ACE) inhibitor or an angiotensin receptor blocker (ARB) should be included in the antihypertensive regimen and uptitrated to maximal recommended doses unless hyperkalemia (serum K ≥6 mEq/L) develops.
- ▪ Dietary recommendations must include potassium restriction for more advanced cases of CKD (stages 4 and 5)
- ▪ An increase in serum creatinine (Cr) of 30% in individuals with baseline creatinine <3 mg/dL, age older than 65 years [or a corresponding decrease in estimated glomerular filtration rate (eGFR)] within 4 months of therapy with an ACE inhibitor or ARB correlates with long-term preservation of renal function.
- ▪ Antihypertensive treatment should ideally reduce albuminuria by >30% after 6 months because this reduces the risk of dialysis by 46% to 72% at 5 years.

See also Chapters A42, **A50, A69, B80, B100, C115,** and **C119**

Chronic kidney disease (CKD) is defined as kidney damage present for at least 3 months with confirmation by biopsy or an estimated glomerular filtration rate (eGFR) <60 mL/minute (stage 3 CKD, see Chapter C115) or the presence of albuminuria. Approximately 11% of the U.S. population has CKD with projections indicating a doubling of its prevalence in the near-term future. As noted, most patients with CKD are either at stage 2 or 3. Diabetes is often listed as the leading cause of end-stage renal disease (ESRD), with hypertension second but this system underrepresents the role of hypertension in ESRD because there is little or no progression of CKD in diabetic patients in the absence of hypertension. Together, hypertension and diabetes account for >75% of patients with ESRD. More than 80% of patients with CKD have hypertension and the most common medical cause for refractory or difficult-to-treat hypertension is CKD.

Impaired glomerular filtration rate

eGFRs are calculated by major laboratories and many web sites including www.kidney.org/professionals/KDOQI/gfr_calculator .cfm have an on-line calculator for use. **Tables C115.1** and **C156.1** display the National Kidney Foundation (NKF) stages,

criteria, and prevalence of CKD in the United States. The ranges of values of serum creatinine (Cr) that correspond to these levels of glomerular filtration rate (GFR) are noted in **Table C156.1**.

Albuminuria

Definition and screening. Microalbuminuria (30–300 mg/day in a 24-hour collection or 20–200 mg/g creatinine on spot urine) is an independent marker for cardiovascular disease (CVD) and ESRD risk (**Figure C156.1**). Prediction of CKD progression is well established in diabetic patients with micro- and macroalbuminuria (>300 mg/day). The 2007 American Diabetes Association (ADA)-NKF guidelines has recommended screening for microalbuminuria in those at increased risk for renal or cardiovascular (CV) diseases. If proteinuria or microalbuminuria is present, further diagnostic testing is warranted and aggressive risk factor modification is recommended.

Benefits of treatment. Several large clinical trials show that reduction of macroalbuminuria by >30% within 6 months of starting treatment conferred a decreased risk of CKD progression and CV risk. As a result, recent guidelines now recommend repeated measurement of proteinuria (macroalbuminuria) at

TABLE C156.1

U. S. CHRONIC KIDNEY DISEASE (CKD) STAGE, ESTIMATED GLOMELULAR FILTRATION RATE (EGFR), PREVALENCE, AND SERUM CREATININE RANGES[a]

CKD stage		Demographics		Typical serum creatinine ranges (mL/min) in youth and old age for each stage of CKD	
Stage	eGFR (mL/min)	N (1,000s)	% of population	Age 21	Age 75
1	>90	10,259	5.8	0.8–1.0	0.7–0.9
2	60–89	21,794	12.3	1.1–2.0	1.0–1.5
3	30–59	5,910	3.3	2.1–3.5	1.6–2.2
4	15–29	363	0.2	3.6–7.5	2.3–3.5
5	<15 or dialysis	300	0.15	>7.6	>3.5

[a]Serum creatinine values are proportional to muscle-mass and are therefore substantially higher in men than women and in younger than older people. (Coresh J, Astor BC, Greene T, et al. Prevalence of chronic kidney disease and decreased kidney function in the adult U.S. population: Third National Health and Nutrition Examination Survey. *Am J Kidney Dis* 2003;41(1):1–12.)

6- and 12-month intervals with a focus on reducing the levels of protein excretion in concert with blood pressure (BP).

Sodium restriction. It should not be assumed that lowering BP *per se* with a renin-angiotensin-aldosterone system (RAAS) blocker would automatically lower proteinuria, as sodium (Na$^+$) intake is a key variable that will influence the degree to which urine protein excretion is reduced. Everyone with proteinuria needs to be counseled on dietary sodium restriction and generally should not consume more than 2 to 3 g per day of Na$^+$. Studies where diuretics were given as a surrogate for reduced Na$^+$ intake did not fully restore the maximal antiproteinuric effects of a RAAS blocker.

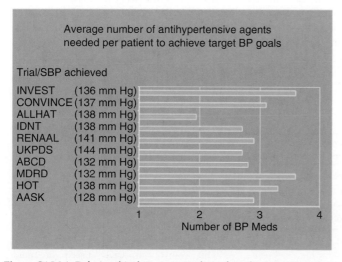

Figure C156.1 Relationship between number of antihypertensive agents and achievement of goal BP in randomized clinical trials that evaluated two different levels of BP. Data are from the low BP goal. BP, blood pressure; SBP, systolic BP; INVEST, INternational VErapamil SR-Trandolapril study; CONVINCE, Controlled Onset Verapamil Investigation of Cardiovascular Endpoints; ALLHAT, Antihypertensive and Lipid- Lowering Treatment to Prevent Heart Attack; IDNT, Irbesartan Diabetic Nephropathy Trial; RENAAL, Reduction of Endpoints in NIDDM with the Angiotensin II Antagonist Losartan; UKPDS, United Kingdom Prospective Diabetes Study; ABCD, Appropriate Blood Pressure Control in Diabetes; MDRD, Modification of Diet in Renal Disease; HOT, Hypertension Optimal Treatment; AASK, African-American Study of Kidney Disease and Hypertension; Meds, medications.

Lower blood pressure. Recent meta-analyses of more than 1,800 nondiabetic hypertensives with proteinuria support the idea that BP values should be as low as is practical in CKD patients. Lower risk of progression to ESRD was found in patients with >1 g proteinuria when systolic BP values were in the 120 to 130 mm Hg range. In a *post hoc* analysis of the Modification of Diet in Renal Disease (MDRD) trial, a low mean arterial BP of <92 mm Hg (compared to a range of 102–107 mm Hg) reduced the rate of progression to ESRD after 12 years, with a trend noted after 6 years.

Specific treatment strategies

BP reduction, regardless of the class of agents used, slows the age-related progression of CKD.

Current blood pressure targets. The Seventh Report of the Joint National Committee on Prevention, Detection, Evaluation, and Treatment of High BP (JNC 7), along with many other guidelines, state that the BP goal for those with CKD should be <130/80 mm Hg or lower based on data from retrospective analysis of multiple trials. For those with no albuminuria or microalbuminuria, a systolic BP <140 mm Hg is probably sufficient to provide a degree of renal protection. Renoprotection is a phenomenon that has been attributed uniquely to RAAS blockade, largely based on animal studies suggesting a disproportionally favorable effect of angiotensin-converting enzyme (ACE) inhibitors on intrarenal pressure. A recent meta-analysis, however, suggests that BP lowering itself may be the common denominator in renoprotection, irrespective of the class of agents used in the absence of proteinuria >300 mg/day (see Chapter B100).

Nonpharmacologic therapy. Patient education regarding diet and exercise must be stressed in the CKD patient with hypertension. More specifically, reduction in dietary Na$^+$ intake may reduce BP and albuminuria significantly. Patients with CKD differ substantially from patients with normal renal function in their ability to tolerate increased dietary K$^+$, so the Dietary Approaches to Stop Hypertension (DASH) diet (rich in fruits and vegetables) can only be applied safely in those with early stage 3 CKD with (GFR >50 mL/minute). Hyperkalemia is often worsened by concomitant salt restriction in the CKD patient.

Need for multiple drugs. A review of clinical trials shows that patients with CKD of any etiology required an average of 3.2 different antihypertensive medications per day to achieve target BPs (**Figure C156.1**). Use of fixed-dose combination antihypertensive medications [e.g., an ACE inhibitor combined with either a diuretic or a calcium channel blocker (CCB)] helps reduce pill burden and copayment costs. Such combinations can usually be used once daily, which may improve individual patient medication adherence and overall BP control, and ultimately lead to more consistent and cost-effective population control of hypertension.

Dialysis patients. The BP goal in people on dialysis is still under study but it is believed that BP goals in people on dialysis be <130/80 mm Hg. Volume status is important in achieving better BP control and patient adherence to a limited volume intake between dialysis sessions and strict attention to "target weight" are necessary. These patients also have a very high frequency of BP nondipping at night, a pattern that may respond to more vigorous dialysis. In some patients, however, vigorous ultrafiltration is associated with severe symptoms of fatigue, lethargy, nausea, and muscle cramping. Such individuals should be considered for more intensive antihypertensive drug management, including nocturnal drug dosing, particularly with α-blockers, which may help control daytime BPs as well as restore more normal circadian rhythms. Calcium antagonists and β-blockers may also be helpful.

A suggested approach to achieve blood pressure goals. On the basis of JNC 7 guidelines, patients with CKD and a level of blood pressure index (BPI) >20/10 mm Hg above goal (i.e., systolic BP ≥150 or diastolic BP ≥90 mm Hg) should be started on two antihypertensive agents simultaneously. A systematic approach is presented in **Figure C156.2**. Generally, all patients with CKD should be started on an ACE inhibitor or an angiotensin receptor blocker (ARB), with a goal of reaching a final BP of 130/80 mm Hg or lower. Doses of these drugs used in CKD trials are generally higher than those observed in clinical practice and the highest appropriate dose of each agent should be considered in all patients to best comply with available clinical trial evidence. Diuretic therapy is almost always necessary and calcium antagonists can be added as third-line therapy as needed. α-Blocking drugs are also useful in many patients, as are thiazide-loop diuretic combinations, especially when dosed more than once daily. Patients with symptomatic heart failure (HF) or coronary artery disease, which is relatively common in CKD, may also require β-blockers.

Specific antihypertensive drugs

Renin-angiotensin-aldosterone system blockers. A regimen that blocks the RAAS is widely recommended as the cornerstone of treatment.

Progression of renal disease. Although all antihypertensive agents that reduce BP slow CKD progression, no regimen is more efficacious than one containing a RAAS blocker. Trials examining the progression rate of both advanced diabetic and nondiabetic nephropathy in patients randomized to either an ACE inhibitor or an ARB have generally demonstrated significant decreases in disease progression.

Use in advanced chronic kidney disease. RAAS blockade–induced rises in serum Cr are well documented but levels at which treatment should be curtailed are not well defined. Some authorities recommend stopping treatment with ACE inhibitors or ARBs if serum Cr increases by >50% above baseline within the first 4 months of therapy (baseline creatinine ≤3 mg/dL). However, a 30% increase in serum Cr occurring within the first 4 months of ACE inhibitor or ARB therapy also predicts long-term preservation of renal function. After serum Cr reaches approximately 5 mg/dL, there is no evidence that continuation of ACE inhibitors or ARBs confers any additional benefit in lowering BP or slowing ESRD progression. Chronic volume depletion or bilateral renal artery stenosis should also be considered if >30% rise in serum Cr is seen. If serum K^+ remains <6 mEq/L during a period of serum Cr change, stabilization is usually seen and later increases in K^+ are not usually problematic.

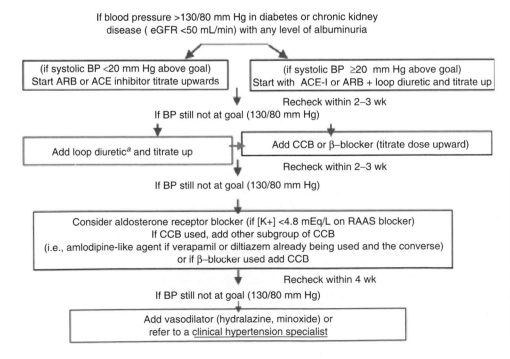

Figure C156.2 A suggested paradigm for BP control in CKD based on guideline recommendations and clinical trial paradigms showing favorable outcomes on CKD progression. BP, blood pressure; CKD, chronic kidney disease; eGFR, estimated glomerular filtration rate; ARB, angiotensin receptor blocker; ACE-I, angiotensin-converting enzyme inhibitor; CCB, calcium-channel blocker; RAAS, renin-angiotensin-aldosterone system. (From Khosla N, Bakris GL. Lessons learned from recent hypertension trials about kidney disease. *J Clin Hypertens* 2006;1:229–235, with permission.)
*a*Given twice daily.

Angiotensin-converting enzyme inhibitor combinations.
ACE inhibitor–diuretic combinations are useful as initial therapy to achieve the BP goal of <130/80 mm Hg. The use of a diuretic potentiates the BP-lowering effects of ACE inhibitors and this combination is particularly useful in blacks and the elderly. CCBs are useful second-line agents that demonstrate an additive BP-reducing capability in combination with first-line therapy. A reduction in CV events has also been noted with an ACE inhibitor/CCB combination. The combination of a nondihydropyridine (DHP) and DHP–calcium antagonist (CA) allows consistent BP reduction, probably in part because the non-DHP–CA can increase the half-life of the DHP–CA by CYP3A4 inhibition and reduced drug metabolism.

Calcium channel blockers.
In hypertension trials in people without CKD, CCBs consistently reduce the risk of stroke and myocardial infarction, which are 10 to 100 times more prevalent than ESRD. The effects of CCBs on CKD, however, appear to depend on the stage of CKD.

Early stages of chronic kidney disease. In the Appropriate Blood Pressure Control in Diabetes (ABCD) Study, nitrendipine equaled enalapril in its ability to prevent proteinuria or increased serum Cr in Stage 1–2 CKD. In those with Stage 1–2 nonproteinuric CKD, CCBs effectively prevent or slow CKD progression as demonstrated in a subpopulation of blacks with hypertensive nephrosclerosis without proteinuria [African-American Study of Kidney Disease and Hypertension (AASK)]; the rate of renal functional deterioration in the amlodipine arm was not significantly different than the ramipril arm.

Advanced chronic kidney disease. In two separate trials of advanced CKD, DHP CCB-based therapy failed to significantly slow CKD progression and favored an increase in albuminuria. Whether these potentially adverse effects of DHP–CCBs in advanced CKD patients can be attenuated by RAAS blockers is debated. In the Reduction of Endpoints in NIDDM with the Angiotensin II Antagonist Losartan (RENAAL) trial, CKD progression slowed in similar manner in individuals who received losartan with or without DHP–CCBs. Therefore, it appears that CCBs may be used as needed for BP control in CKD patients. Non-DHP–CCBs such as diltiazem or verapamil may have more favorable effects than DHPs on urine protein excretion in short-term studies but their long-term effects on CKD progression have not been studied.

Diuretics.
Thiazide diuretics (i.e., hydrochlorothiazide, chlorthalidone) improve the chances of achieving target BP goals. These agents have additive BP-reducing effects, with common side effects such as hypokalemia lessened by the concomitant use of an ACE inhibitor, ARB or an aldosterone receptor antagonist. CV events have been shown to decrease with RAAS blocker/diuretic combinations. However, the choice of diuretic in the CKD patient with hypertension should be guided by the GFR. In those with a GFR <50 mL/minute, a loop diuretic administered at least twice daily is typically required for an optimal BP-lowering effect to occur. However, chlorthalidone is much longer acting than hydrochlorothiazide and works somewhat better when GFR is below 60 mL/minute, albeit with a lesser potency than a loop diuretic. In patients with low-normal to normal K^+ levels, the use of a K^+-sparing diuretic can be considered in the early stages of CKD. However, eplerenone in combination with ACE inhibition was studied in hypertensive patients with proteinuria with similar reductions in urine protein excretion similar to what has been seen with an ACE inhibitor/ARB combination.

Other agents.
Given that activation of the sympathetic nervous system invariably accompanies CKD, long acting α-blockers (or α-β–blockers) can be helpful as third or fourth-line therapy for patients with CKD or prostatic hypertrophy. β-Blockers are also reasonable alternatives in CKD patients if coronary disease or HF is present. Centrally acting agents such as clonidine are alternative third- or fourth-line drugs but they should generally not be used with β-blockers because of the potential for exacerbation of rebound hypertension and because of potential adverse outcomes of the combination in HF.

Suggested Readings

American Diabetes Association. American Diabetes Association: clinical practice recommendations. *Diabetes Care* 2007;30:Sl–S56.

Am J Kidney Dis. KDOQI Clinical practice guidelines and clinical practice recommendations for diabetes and chronic kidney disease. 2007;49 (2 Suppl 2): S12–154.

Bakris GL, Fonseca V, Katholi RE, et al. GEMINI Investigators. Differential effects of beta-blockers on albuminuria in patients with type 2 diabetes. *Hypertension* 2005;46(6):1309–1315.

Bakris GL, Weir MR, Secic M, et al. Differential effects of calcium antagonist subclasses on markers of nephropathy progression. *Kidney Int* 2004;65(6):1991–2002.

Bakris GL, Weir MR, Shanifar S, et al. Effects of BP level on progression of diabetic nephropathy: results from the RENAAL study. *Arch Intern Med* 2003;163(13):1555–1565.

Coresh J, Astor BC, Greene T, et al. Prevalence of chronic kidney disease and decreased kidney function in the adult US population: Third National Health and Nutrition Examination Survey. *Am J Kidney Dis* 2003;41(1):1–12.

K/DOQI clinical practice guidelines on hypertension and antihypertensive agents in chronic kidney disease. *Am J Kidney Dis* 2004;43:S1–290.

Khosla N, Bakris GL. Lessons learned from recent hypertension trials about kidney disease. *Clin J Am Soc Nephrol* 2006;1:229–235.

Rahman M, Pressel S, Davis BR, et al. Renal outcomes in high-risk hypertensive patients treated with an angiotensin-converting enzyme inhibitor or a calcium channel blocker vs a diuretic: a report from the antihypertensive and lipid-lowering treatment to prevent heart attack trial (ALLHAT). *Arch Intern Med* 2005;165 (8):936–946.

Sarafidis PA, Khosla N, Bakris GL. Antihypertensive therapy in the presence of proteinuria. *Am J Kidney Dis* 2007;49(1):12–26.

Wright JT, Bakris G, Greene T, et al. Effect of BP lowering and antihypertensive drug class on progression of hypertensive kidney disease: results from the AASK trial. *JAMA* 2002;288:2421–2431.

CHAPTER C157 ■ TREATMENT OF THE OBESE HYPERTENSIVE PATIENT

XAVIER PI-SUNYER, MD, MPH

KEY POINTS

- Obesity [body mass index (BMI)] and central fat distribution (waist measurement) correlate with high blood pressure (BP).
- Changes in diet and activity usually improve control of BP.
- Pharmacotherapy for weight loss in obese hypertensive patients could include sibutramine (which may increase BP), orlistat (which causes steatorrhea), or possibly rimonabant.
- Higher doses of antihypertensive medications and drug combinations may be needed in obese hypertensive patients.

See also Chapters **A34,** A35, A36, **A46,** A47, **B92,** C158, and C159

The relationship between obesity and blood pressure (BP) has been reported in a large number of cross-sectional and longitudinal population-based studies. In the Framingham study, for every 10% increase in relative weight, systolic BP increased by 6.5 mm Hg. Because the clinical consequences of hypertension are more likely to occur in obese than lean individuals, it is disquieting that so many obese patients are not treated more aggressively for hypertension.

Blood pressure measurement

The measurement of BP in an obese patient can be difficult. To obtain accurate readings, the compression cuff must be large enough; a cuff that is too small often gives a falsely high reading. Obese arms with a severe taper are especially problematic. Often, thigh cuffs are required; the cuff bladder should be wide enough to cover at least three-fourth of the circumference and approximately two-thirds of the length of the upper arm. The patient should sit in a quiet room for 5 minutes before the measurement and two or more readings should be taken with initial verification in the contralateral arm.

Assessment of fat burden

Total fat burden and body fat distribution are important distinctions.

Body mass index. The total fat burden is best assessed in a simple and economical manner by calculating the body mass index (BMI) of an individual:

$$BMI = weight \ (kg)/height^2(m)$$
$$= [weight \ (lb)/height^2(in.)] \times 703$$

BMI correlates relatively well with total body fat except in very muscular individuals. Central or upper body obesity has more specifically been associated with increased BP in many population-based studies. "Overweight" is currently defined as a BMI of 25 to 29.9 kg/m^2 and obesity as a BMI >30 kg/m^2.

Waist to hip ratio. Central (visceral) obesity is best documented by measuring waist circumference; values >102 cm in males and >88 cm in women are abnormal according to the National Institutes of Health and the World Health Organization. A waist to hip ratio has also been used as a measure of obesity; ratios >1.0 in men and >0.85 in women are considered abnormal. Some authorities feel that simply measuring waist circumference is adequate to assess risk and estimate central obesity, with little additional benefit of measuring the waist to hip ratio.

Weight loss therapy

Weight loss therapy is recommended for every overweight or obese patient with hypertension.

Public health issues. Although culturally sensitive programs need to be initiated for specific population groups, it is important to note that all geographic racial and cultural subgroups in the United States manifest increasing cardiovascular risk with increasing weight. There is no reason to believe that all groups do not profit equally from weight loss and risk factor reduction. Older individuals, in general, take on similar or greater risks for morbidity with increasing weight than do younger subjects.

Therapeutic goals. The initial goal of weight loss therapy, to reduce body weight by 10% to 15% from baseline, has been shown to improve BP and a number of comorbid conditions. This amount of weight loss has been found to be practical and can often be maintained with behavioral treatment or pharmacotherapy. Optimal weight loss tends to occur over a time frame of 6 months, with a reasonable and sustainable rate of loss of 1 to 2 lb (0.45–0.90 kg) per week.

General evaluation. When beginning to work with an obese patient, a careful preliminary assessment must be made that includes discussion of the patient's usual diet, food preferences, and eating habits (time, place, and person). A careful history of previous weight loss attempts and why such attempts may have failed (or only partially succeeded) and physical activity habits should be documented. The prospective weight loser must be realistic about how much weight will be shed. Many patients lose motivation if they are unable to achieve ideal body weight in a short period of time. The provider should educate the patient that a 10% to 15% weight loss, will take time if the patient is to remain healthy and be able to sustain the weight loss; instruction on the cardiovascular consequences of obesity is also important.

Psychosocial evaluation. Losing weight is a difficult process and a patient needs to be appropriately motivated to sustain the process. It is important not to try to embark on such an arduous program unless the patient truly wants to lose weight and is motivated to do so. A readiness assessment needs to be made, noting psychological attitudes toward weight loss, capacity to increase physical activity, ability to understand nutritional guidelines, and self-control skills. Also, the environmental ambience and social support structure of the patient should be considered; joint weight loss programs undertaken with spouses or "significant others" should be considered, especially if the patient is not the primary preparer of food.

Behavior modification. Behavior modification is important if the weight loss is to be sustained. Behavior modification is not an arcane art; it can be used by any primary care provider interested in identifying simple ways to break old habits and develop new ones. In many cases, behavioral modification can be effectively performed by allied health professionals in conjunction with physician reinforcement.

Behavior modification emphasizes gradual, permanent changes in eating and exercise habits. There are five major areas in which altering behavior helps weight loss: (a) changing eating habits, (b) increasing physical activity, (c) altering attitudes, (d) developing support systems, and (e) acquiring education about nutrition. The primary focus is on self-control to achieve a gradual change in habits through incorporation of an individual's food preferences into dietary planning. The provider must be supportive and not demand perfection because there will be lapses along the way. The program for weight loss and weight maintenance must be adaptable to meet the needs of a diversity of patients. Therefore, there is no standardized set of rules to optimize weight reduction in a given patient.

Dietary changes. The strategies for weight loss include a hypocaloric diet and behavior modification strategies to maintain these lifestyle changes over the long term. The hypocaloric diet may be a low-fat diet, but what is most important is an overall decrease in calories. The nutritional plan must be individualized. It should take into consideration food preferences, availability, and taste, as well as cultural preferences and socioeconomic factors. In addition, attention needs to be paid to other concurrent dietary considerations required for comorbid conditions (e.g., hypertension and the potential need to restrict sodium or increase potassium, or hypercholesterolemia and the need to reduce the intake of saturated fats).

The nutritional plan must be a long-term one that emphasizes the need to reduce calories for weight loss and then weight maintenance. The typical U.S. diet consists of 14% protein, 40% fat, and 46% carbohydrate, of which 28% is complex carbohydrates and 18% is sugar. The best plan is to educate the patient with regard to high- and low-calorie-dense foods. High-fat foods should be reduced, and heavy intake of sugar should be discouraged. Portion sizes should be reduced and fiber intake should be increased. The DASH (Dietary Approaches to Stop Hypertension) diet, in conjunction with a decrease in dietary sodium, has been reported to be successful in hypertensive patients. This diet is rich in fruits and vegetables, low in saturated and total fat, and rich in low-fat dairy foods. Alcohol should be eliminated or drastically curtailed. The aim is for a 500 to 1,000 kcal deficit per day for the weight loss phase and then a decreased calorie intake of approximately 30 kcal per kg for weight maintenance. All these suggestions fit well with the Recommended Dietary Guidelines and the food pyramid promulgated by the U.S. Departments of Agriculture and of Health and Human Services. In some individuals, it may be more helpful to use a lower-calorie diet of approximately 800 kcal for a period of 12 to 24 weeks, and this is often done with liquid formulas.

Physical activity. Obese persons are extraordinarily sedentary. Physical activity is a crucial component for a weight loss and maintenance program. Exercise is important in obese hypertensive patients because it can have a direct effect in improving BP control and insulin sensitivity as well as on weight loss and its maintenance. Exercise increases energy expenditure, and what an obese patient needs is not only a decrease in caloric intake but also an increase in energy expenditure. Physical activity may take many forms, depending on the interests and capabilities of the patient. The important parts of an exercise program are intensity, duration, and frequency. A patient should be advised to start slowly and for short periods, but to exercise at least 5 times a week from the beginning. The plan should be to begin with low-intensity aerobic exercise (walking is probably best) and gradually work toward more intensive activity (e.g., jogging, swimming, biking, tennis). Activity should be done 5 to 7 days per week for approximately 30 minutes per day overall but may be divided into shorter segments if necessary. The exercise prescription should be individualized to the lifestyle of the individual. If social interaction and spousal or family support can be built into the exercise, the exercise program is more likely to be sustained. Enlisting outside resources such as swimming pools, health clubs, and gyms can be very helpful.

Maintenance of weight loss. After successful weight loss, the likelihood of weight loss maintenance is enhanced by a program consisting of periodic dietary counseling and regular physical activity that should be continued indefinitely. This needs to include continued contact with the physician and other providers to ensure a persistence of the new lifestyle changes that have been instrumental in the loss of weight.

Weight loss drugs. In patients with a BMI >27 kg/m², if a 6-month trial of diet, exercise, and behavior therapy has not proven successful, pharmacotherapy can be tried. Currently, there are three weight loss drugs that have clinical promise. Studies of all antiobesity drugs are notable for their high attrition rates and lack of data on major obesity-related morbidity and mortality.

Sibutramine. Sibutramine (Meridia) is a serotonin and norepinephrine reuptake inhibitor that reduces food intake by enhancing satiety. It is typically given in a dose range of 10 to 15 mg once daily. In randomized clinical trials for up to 2 years, a loss of approximately 10 to 15 lb (4.5–6.8 kg) was seen. Sibutramine can increase BP and heart rate; if these effects are significant, withdrawal of the drug may be necessary. The drug is contraindicated in patients with coronary artery disease and should be used sparingly (if at all) in patients with poorly controlled hypertension. Milder side effects include dry mouth, constipation, insomnia, dizziness, and nausea. Data on its safety and efficacy are only available for 2 years of continuous use.

Orlistat. Orlistat (Xenical) is an inhibitor of intestinal lipase that impairs fat transport by the gut, thereby decreasing absorption of the most calorie-dense foods. It is generally given in a dose of 120-mg three times daily with meals. This drug causes steatorrhea as part of its action, with soft and more frequent stools. It has approximately the same effectiveness as sibutramine over a 1-year period, with 55% of orlistat-treated patients losing more than 5% of their body weight and 25% losing more than 10% of their body weight (compared to 33% and 15%, respectively, achieving the same mean weight loss in the placebo-treated group). This drug has undergone 2-year clinical trials with no significant adverse side effects except for a small reduction of fat-soluble vitamins. To prevent possible deficiencies of fat-soluble vitamins, a daily multivitamin is recommended with its use. Currently, (in 2007) orlistat at a 60-mg dose has been approved for use without a prescription.

Rimonabant. Rimonabant is the first of the endocannabinoid receptor antagonists. Weight loss induced by rimonabant is similar to sibutramine. Improvements in high-density lipoprotein (HDL) cholesterol and triglyceride concentrations and reductions in BP have been reported. Rimonabant has been studied in more than 6,600 volunteers in a dose range of 5 to 20 mg once daily; 20 mg is most effective. In a 2-year study (RIO-North America), subjects who had been on active drug for a year, were rerandomized to continued rimonabant or placebo for an additional year; those on placebo therapy regained most of the weight (approximately 8% of body weight) they had lost, whereas the rimonabant groups had sustained weight loss. Patient drop-out rates for psychiatric disorders (predominantly depression) in rimonabant trials have been 6% to 7% but patients with significant mental illness were excluded from rimonabant trials. Rimonabant was approved for weight loss by the European Agency for the Evaluation of Medicinal Products and is under active review by the U.S. Food and Drug Administration.

Surgery. For the high-risk obese (BMI >40 kg/m^2 or BMI >35 kg/m^2 with significant comorbidities or adverse health conditions), obesity surgery is an appropriate, even life-saving option. Any procedure should be performed by an interested and experienced surgeon and the medical center should have a multidisciplinary team approach to allow the necessary long-term follow-up care. Types of procedures vary among institutions and operator skill and familiarity with a particular technique is an important factor in any potential surgical recommendation.

Blood pressure management

BP control often remains a significant problem in obese patients because not all patients experience a return to normal BP values even if they lose weight. For these obese hypertensive patients, effective antihypertensive drug therapy needs to be instituted or maintained. The general principles of management for obese patients are not different from that of nonobese patients but there are a few caveats.

Diuretics such as hydrochlorothiazide may be required in higher doses to have an adequate effect but they also tend to increase blood glucose levels and lower potassium levels at these higher doses. Because of these issues, it is often preferable to use somewhat lower doses of diuretics in combination with ACE inhibitors or angiotensin receptor blockers. β-Blockers may be effective at high doses in obese patients, but they may also induce worsening of insulin resistance and glucose intolerance and may cause fatigue and reduced exercise tolerance. α-Adrenergic receptor blocking agents may increase insulin sensitivity and are theoretically attractive in obese hypertensive patients, but these agents do not protect as well against heart failure (which is common in obesity) as other antihypertensive drugs. ACE inhibitors and angiotensin receptor blockers are useful in obese patients, improving insulin sensitivity, reversing left ventricular hypertrophy, and protecting the kidneys. Calcium antagonists tend to lower BP at the expense of dependent edema, which can be lessened or eliminated by combining the calcium antagonist with an ACE inhibitor or an angiotensin receptor blocker. Increased physical activity also combats edema in obese patients.

Suggested Readings

Carroll JF, Kyser CK. Exercise training in obesity lowers BP independent of weight change. *Med Sci Sports Exerc* 2002;34:596–601.

Chobanian AV, Bakris GL, Black HR, et al. Seventh report of the Joint National Committee on Prevention, Detection, Evaluation, and Treatment of High BP, National Heart, Lung, and Blood Institute, National High BP Education Program Coordinating Committee. *Hypertension* 2003;42:1206–1252.

National Heart, Lung, and Blood Institute. Clinical guidelines on the identification, evaluation, and treatment of overweight and obesity in adults—the evidence report. *Obes Res* 1998;6:515–2095.

Padwal RS, Majumdar SR. Drug treatments for obesity: orlistat, sibutramine, and rimonabant. *Lancet* 2007;369:71–77.

Pischon T, Sharma AM. Recent developments in the treatment of obesity-related hypertension. *Curr Opin Nephrol Hypertens* 2002;11:497–502.

Pi-Sunyer FX. A review of long-term studies evaluating the efficacy of weight loss in ameliorating disorders associated with obesity. *Clin Ther* 1996;18:1006–1035.

Sacks FM, Svetkey LP, Vollmer WM, et al. Effects on BP of reduced dietary sodium and the Dietary Approaches to Stop Hypertension (DASH) diet. *N Engl J Med* 2001;344:3–10.

Schotte DE, Stunkard AJ. The effects of weight reduction on BP in 301 obese patients. *Arch Intern Med* 1990;150:1701–1704.

CHAPTER C158 ■ TREATMENT OF HYPERTENSIVE PATIENTS WITH ABNORMAL BLOOD GLUCOSE

GUIDO LASTRA, MD; SAMY I. McFARLANE, MD, MPH AND JAMES R. SOWERS, MD

KEY POINTS

- Dysglycemia (elevated fasting blood glucose) increases cardiovascular disease (CVD) risk at levels above 100 mg/dL.
- Treatment goals for CVD risk factors in diabetics are blood pressure (BP) <130/80 mm Hg, low-density lipoprotein (LDL) cholesterol <70 mg/dL, and hemoglobin A1c <6.5%, respectively.
- The Steno-2 study showed that comprehensive, aggressive hygienic, and pharmacologic management reduced macrovascular (coronary disease or stroke) and microvascular (retinal or renal disease) events by approximately 50% compared to usual care.
- Combination drug therapy is necessary in the management of hypertension (HTN), hyperglycemia, and dyslipidemia in diabetic patients.

See also Chapters A34, **A47,** A63, **B90,** B92, and **B100**

Risk factor interactions

Cardiovascular disease (CVD) risk factors, [e.g., hypertension (HTN), impaired glucose homeostasis, atherogenic dyslipidemia, obesity, and albuminuria] frequently coexist and interact.

Hypertension and hyperglycemic syndromes. The clustering of major CVD risk factors, collectively known as the *cardiometabolic syndrome* (CMS), significantly increases the risk of CVD and type 2 diabetes mellitus (DM2). A single final common pathophysiologic abnormality that explains all aspects of the CMS seems improbable but the statistical association of the components of the CMS suggests multiple overlapping disease mechanisms. CVD is the major cause of premature death in patients with DM2, and HTN plays a key role in the development of both chronic kidney disease (CKD) and CVD. HTN also markedly increases the risk for CVD in patients with DM2. In the Multiple Risk Factor Intervention Trial, HTN, hypercholesterolemia, and tobacco abuse had a more severe effect on CVD in diabetic patients compared to nondiabetic persons.

Obesity and insulin resistance. Obesity and resistance to the physiologic actions of insulin play a major role in the pathophysiology of DM2 and diastolic HTN. Roughly half of all hypertensive patients are obese and insulin resistant, and the prevalence of HTN in patients with DM2 is up to three times greater than in age- and sex-matched patients with diabetes. There is a significant association between insulin resistance indices and BP in white Europeans, independent of other factors, including age, gender, or obesity. Indeed, a reduction of 30% in insulin sensitivity predicts future increases in diastolic BP; the influence of insulin resistance on BP is stronger than the effect of increasing age or obesity.

Angiotensin and oxidative stress. Systemic and local renin-angiotensin-aldosterone systems (RAAS) are activated in the setting of obesity and CMS. Adipose tissue, particularly the visceral-type, expresses all components of the renin-angiotensin system (RAS) (see Chapter A34). In addition to the well-established effects of the RAS on aldosterone secretion and renal tubular reabsorption of sodium (Na^+), tissue RAS overactivity contributes to insulin resistance through stimulation of angiotensin II (Ang II) type 1 receptors and increased production of reactive oxygen species (ROS) in adipocytes, skeletal muscle, and CV tissue (see Chapter A63). In turn, increased oxidative stress induces a shift toward endothelial dysfunction and atherogenesis, which add to the effects of fatty acids and adipokines. Therapeutic blockade of the RAS abrogates exaggerated production of ROS and corrects insulin resistance in experimental models.

Blood pressure issues in cardiometabolic syndrome and diabetes mellitus 2

Importance of blood pressure control. Tight BP control is the most important means of reducing CVD risk in CMS and DM2. Treatment is challenging because patients with DM2 require multiple medications to control BP, blood glucose, and cholesterol. Data from the United Kingdom Prospective Diabetes Study (UKPDS) demonstrated a 45% reduction in relative risk of fatal or nonfatal stroke with tighter BP control [mean BP achieved in the "tight" control group was 10/5 mm Hg lower (to 144/82 mm Hg) than the group randomized to "less tight" control]. The incidence of CVD in diabetic participants in the Hypertension Optimal Treatment study was reduced by roughly 50% in the group randomized to a goal diastolic BP <80 mm Hg (achieved diastolic BP 81 mm Hg) compared to those whose goal was <90 mm Hg (achieved diastolic BP 85 mm Hg). Similar trends have been observed for systolic HTN control with nitrendipine in patients older than 60 years in the Systolic Hypertension in Europe trial, in whom stroke rates in diabetics were reduced. CVD-related findings were also consistent with results from the Systolic Hypertension in the Elderly Program study, in which patients with DM2 derived additional reductions in CVD event rates when compared to the nondiabetic participants. The worldwide BP goal is now <130/80 mm Hg, as articulated by the American Diabetes Association (ADA) and the Seventh Joint National Committee for the Prevention, Detection, Evaluation, and Treatment of High Blood Pressure (JNC 7). Data from the Antihypertensive and Lipid-Lowering Treatment to Prevent Heart Attack Trial (ALLHAT) trial support current recommendations from the ADA and JNC 7 in patients with DM2.

Salt sensitivity and volume. Increased sensitivity to dietary Na^+ is greater in hypertensive patients with DM2, obesity, renal insufficiency, or low-renin status and in blacks and the elderly. Weight reduction and moderate salt restriction have been shown in clinical trials to reduce BP in both type 1 and 2 diabetic patients with HTN.

Loss of nocturnal decline of blood pressure. In patients with DM2, there is a loss of the normal nocturnal drop in BP and heart rate by 24-hour ambulatory monitoring ("nondipping"), which conveys excessive risk for stroke and myocardial infarction (MI). Microalbuminuria and increased left ventricular mass are also associated with nondipping in diabetic patients.

Orthostatic hypotension. In patients with diabetes and autonomic dysfunction, excessive venous pooling can cause immediate or delayed orthostatic hypotension, potentially compromising cerebral blood flow and leading to intermittent lightheadedness, fatigue, unsteady gait, and syncope. Orthostatic hypotension is itself a risk factor. All diabetic patients should have their BP periodically measured in the sitting and standing positions at each visit; a supine BP should also be measured at regular intervals. The increased propensity for orthostatic hypotension in patients with diabetes renders α-adrenergic receptor blockers less desirable agents for these patients. In addition, doses of all antihypertensive agents must be titrated more carefully in patients with diabetes particularly when orthostatic HTN exists. Hypotension and syncope may be a more serious problem in these patients than their HTN.

Essentials of therapy

Therapeutic lifestyle changes. The cornerstone of management of HTN and hyperglycemia is the early establishment of therapeutic lifestyle changes (TLC) to maintain optimal weight, BP, cholesterol, and glucose. Reduction in calories, refined carbohydrates, Na^+ and saturated fat intake, as well as increased nonsoluble fiber and potassium, leads to weight loss, improved glycemic control and increased insulin sensitivity. Increased regular aerobic physical activity reduces BP and improves control of dyslipidemia. In the Finnish Diabetes Prevention Program (DPP),

TLC was proved useful in the prevention of new-onset DM2 in subjects with impaired glucose tolerance.

Dietary intervention in diabetes. The primary goals of nutritional intervention in patients with diabetes are (a) to attain and maintain optimal body weight and (b) to use a low-fat, high-fiber, low-sodium diet to promote BP and lipid lowering. The ADA suggests an increase in carbohydrate or monounsaturated fat to compensate for the reduction in saturated fat in fatty meats, butter, eggs, and so on. However, replacement of saturated fat with complex carbohydrates may cause postprandial hyperglycemia in diabetic patients that can be ameliorated by smaller feedings and increased fiber intake. Overall, a weight reduction, "Heart Smart" diet is appropriate for all diabetic patients due to their intrinsic risk for CVD.

Comprehensive therapy. Patients with diabetes must receive comprehensive instruction in all aspects of therapeutic lifestyle modification. A model for comprehensive care is the protocol developed for the Steno-2 study, which compared state-of-the-art comprehensive diabetic care to usual community care and found superior outcomes using a "center approach" (an experienced multidisciplinary team of physicians and other professionals) and aggressive targets for diabetes (hemoglobin A1c <6.5%), total cholesterol (<175 mg/dL) and BP (<130/80 mm Hg), adjusted downward from higher targets at the beginning of the study as guidelines changed. Patients receiving intensive therapy had a 53% lower risk of combined CV and cerebrovascular disease endpoints [95% confidence interval (CI) 27%–74%], along with lower rates of nephropathy (by 61%, 95% CI 13%–87%), retinopathy (by 55%, 95% CI 14%–79%), and autonomic neuropathy (by 63%, 95% CI 21%–92%).

Blood pressure control. Foremost in the comprehensive approach needed for patients with the CMS and DM2 are weight control and aggressive treatment of HTN to BP values <130/80 mm Hg. Interruption of the RAS is considered to be another cornerstone of pharmacologic therapy to reduce macrovascular (atherosclerotic) and microvascular (ocular and renal) complications (see **Table C158.1**), although it remains unclear whether the beneficial effects of anti-RAS therapy are attributable simply to better systemic and microcirculatory BP control (see Chapter B100) or to direct reduction in the "toxic" effects of angiotensin II.

Antihypertensive drugs

Combination antihypertensive therapy. Achieving a BP goal of ≤130/80 in patients with diabetes and HTN almost always requires two or more antihypertensive medications; in one study of 1,372 patients with HTN and diabetes, the average number of medications required for a mean population goal BP of 130/85 mm Hg was 3.1; stated another way, more than half of the subjects did not reach target BP on three drugs. This number of medications is consistent with the findings from a number of large outcomes trials.

Angiotensin-converting enzyme inhibitors. Angiotensin-converting enzyme (ACE) inhibitors lower BP in the patient with HTN and diabetes but often require the addition of a diuretic to maximize their BP-lowering effect. ACE inhibitors decrease the morbidity and mortality that accompanies systolic forms of heart failure (HF), attenuate albuminuria and renal disease progression, and reduce CV risk (**Table 158.1**). These

TABLE C158.1

BENEFITS OF RENIN-ANGIOTENSIN SYSTEM BLOCKERS IN PREVENTING CARDIOVASCULAR EVENTS IN DIABETES

Trial	Study population	Mean duration (yr)	RAS blockade strategy	Primary outcome	Relative risk
CAPPP (1999)	Hypertensive patients	6.1	ACE inhibitor	Composite of myocardial infarction, stroke, and other cardiovascular deaths	0.79 (0.67–0.94)
HOPE (2000)	Vascular disease or diabetes + one other cardiovascular risk factor + low ejection fraction or heart failure	5	ACE inhibitor	Composite of myocardial infarction, stroke, and other cardiovascular deaths	0.66 (0.51–0.85)
DREAM (2006)	No cardiovascular disease	3	ACE inhibitor	Development of diabetes or death	0.91 (0.81–1.03) Non-significant
ALLHAT (2003)	Hypertension and at least one other CHD risk factor	4.9	ACE inhibitor	Combined fatal CHD or nonfatal myocardial infarction	0.70 (0.56–0.86)
CHARM (2003)	Heart failure	3.2	ARB	All-cause mortality	0.78 (0.64–0.96)
VALUE (2004)	Hypertensive patients at high cardiovascular risk	4.2	ARB	Composite of cardiac mortality and morbidity	0.77 (0.69–0.86)

RAS, renin-angiotensin system; CAPPP, Captopril Prevention Project; ACE, angiotensin-converting enzyme; HOPE, Heart Outcomes Prevention Evaluation; DREAM, Diabetes REduction Assessment with rampiril and rosiglitazone Medication; ALLHAT, Antihypertensive and Lipid-Lowering Treatment to Prevent Heart Attack Trial; CHD, coronary heart disease; CHARM, Candesartan in Heart Failure—Assessment of Mortality and Morbidity; ARB, angiotensin receptor blocker; VALUE, Valsartan Antihypertensive Long-term Use Evaluation.

benefits have been shown in randomized controlled trials such as the Captopril Prevention Project and the Microalbuminuria Cardiovascular and Renal Outcome–Heart Outcomes Prevention Evaluation (MICRO–HOPE) study. In the main study, ramipril diminished the self-reported new-onset diabetes rate; in both the main HOPE study and MICRO–HOPE (patients with diabetes and proteinuria), ACE inhibitor treatment was associated with a significant reduction in the risk of the combined CVD and microvascular endpoints.

Angiotensin receptor blockers. Three major studies—the Reduction of Endpoints in NIDDM with the Angiotensin II Antagonist Losartan Study (RENAAL), the Irbesartan Microalbuminuria Type 2 Diabetes in Hypertensive Patients Study, and the Irbesartan in Diabetic Nephropathy Trial—have shown that angiotensin receptor blockers (ARBs) are effective in reducing BP and the progression of renal disease in hypertensive patients with DM2. ARBs are considered to be an acceptable initial therapy alternative to ACE inhibitors in patients with DM2 and proteinuria, HF, systolic dysfunction, post–myocardial infarction, and mild renal insufficiency. In that regard, the RENAAL study documented reduction in the initial hospitalization rate for HF. In the Losartan Intervention for Endpoint (LIFE) trial, losartan was statistically significantly superior to atenolol in diabetic patients with HTN and left ventricular hypertrophy, reducing fatal and nonfatal strokes by 25%, and new onset of diabetes by 25% compared to atenolol.

Diuretics. Low-dose diuretics are effective antihypertensive agents in patients with or without diabetes. The adverse metabolic effects observed with large diuretic doses [e.g., 50–200 mg of hydrochlorothiazide (HCTZ)] have been observed much less so with low-doses (12.5–25 mg HCTZ). Diuretics are often required for good BP control in diabetic patients, many of whom are salt sensitive. The use of thiazide diuretics in diabetic patients is particularly well supported by ALLHAT, where approximately 15,000 of the 42,000 patients were diabetic at the outset of the trial.

Calcium channel blockers. Monotherapy with nondihydropyridine calcium channel blockers (CCBs) (e.g., verapamil or diltiazem) may have more beneficial effects on proteinuria than dihydropyridines (e.g., nifedipine or amlodipine) but when CCBs are combined with ACE inhibitors or ARBs as first-line treatments and good BP control is achieved, there is likely to be little difference among CCBs on renal endpoints. CCBs are especially useful in elderly patients with isolated systolic HTN and are as effective as thiazide diuretics in preventing major coronary events and strokes in diabetic patients with HTN. Dihydropyridine CCB therapy, however, may not protect as well against HF as thiazide-type diuretics.

β-Blockers. β-Blockers can be used in patients with diabetes but not as first-line agents according to many experts. Hypertensive patients receiving β-blockers (generally in conjunction with thiazide-type diuretics) have a higher risk of new-onset diabetes than those on no medication or other antihypertensive medications. Nevertheless, in the UKPDS study, atenolol was at least as effective as the ACE inhibitor captopril in reducing microvascular complications of diabetes, stroke, and death related to diabetes.

Suggested Readings

Coccheri S. Approaches to prevention of cardiovascular complications and events in diabetes mellitus. *Drugs* 2007;67:997–1026.
Gaede P, Vedel P, Larsen N, et al. Multifactorial intervention and cardiovascular disease in patients with type 2 diabetes. *N Engl J Med* 2003;348(5):383–393.

Heart Outcomes Prevention Evaluation Study Investigators. Effects of ramipril on cardiovascular and microvascular outcomes in people with diabetes mellitus: results of the HOPE study and MICRO-HOPE substudy. *Lancet* 2000;355:253–259.

Lewis EJ. Treating hypertension in the patient with overt diabetic nephropathy. *Semin Nephrol* 2007;27:182–194.

Lindholm LH, Ibsen H, Dahlof B, et al. LIFE Study Group. Cardiovascular morbidity and mortality in patients with diabetes in the Losartan Intervention For Endpoint reduction in hypertension study (LIFE): a randomised trial against atenolol. *Lancet* 2002;359:1004–1010.

Manrique C, Lastra G, Sowers JR. Hypertension and the cardiometabolic syndrome. *J Clin Hypertens* 2005;7:471–476.

Sowers JR. Obesity as a cardiovascular risk factor. *Am J Med* 2003;115(Suppl 8A):37S–41S.

Sowers JR. Insulin resistance and hypertension. *Am J Physiol Heart Circ Physiol* 2004;286:H1597–H1602.

Sowers JR, Haffner S. Treatment of cardiovascular and renal risk factors in the diabetic hypertensive. *Hypertension* 2002;40:781–788.

CHAPTER C159 ■ DYSLIPIDEMIA MANAGEMENT IN HYPERTENSIVES

PETER P. TOTH, MD, PhD

KEY POINTS

■ Hypertensive patients commonly have dyslipidemia, a widely prevalent, modifiable risk factor for coronary artery disease (CAD); usually serum low-density lipoprotein cholesterol (LDL-C) [and non–high-density lipoprotein cholesterol (HDL-C)] are elevated or serum HDL-C is low.

■ A complete fasting lipoprotein profile (total cholesterol, HDL-C, LDL-C, and triglycerides) should be performed on anyone undergoing screening for dyslipidemia; secondary causes of dyslipidemia should be considered in all cases.

■ The treatment of dyslipidemia is associated with reduced risk for cardiovascular morbidity and mortality; serum levels of LDL-C and non–HDL-C should be treated to risk-stratified goal levels. HDL-C level should be raised when it is low.

■ Primary and secondary prevention begins with lifestyle modification in all patients with dyslipidemia; medications (statins, fibrates, niacin, ezetimibe, bile acid–binding resins, fish oil) should be used as specified by national guidelines if lifestyle modifications fail.

See also Chapters **B76, B77, B92,** and **C120**

Pathophysiology

The dyslipidemias are a heterogeneous group of highly prevalent metabolic disorders whose etiologies are strongly influenced by genetic, dietary, and lifestyle factors. Abnormalities in lipid metabolism are quite varied and are attributable to: (a) a large number of polymorphisms in cholesterol and lipid biosynthetic enzymes and cell-surface receptors; (b) the mass and composition of ingested sterols and lipids; (c) the capacity for gastrointestinal (GI) absorption and intracellular mobilization of lipids and cholesterol; and (d) metabolic background, including insulin resistance, alcoholism, nephrotic syndrome, and thyroid dysfunction.

Cardiovascular disease risk

Dyslipidemia is highly correlated with increased risk for atherosclerotic disease and its clinical sequelae, including myocardial infarction (MI), cerebrovascular accident, intermittent claudication, need for lower limb amputation, renal arterial stenosis, and sudden death. Dyslipidemia is an important risk factor for cardiovascular disease (CVD) in both men and women and in all demographic, racial, and ethnic groups yet studied.

It is well-known from multiple prospective epidemiologic studies that risk factors cluster. Approximately two-thirds of all patients presenting with the diagnosis of hypertension will also have dyslipidemia. Given this high incidence of dyslipidemia in hypertensive patients, it is important that they be screened for dyslipidemia and, if it is found, be treated so as to ensure optimal reduction of risk for developing CVD and CVD-related events. In the Anglo-Scandinavian Cardiac Outcomes Trial, it was clearly demonstrated that treating dyslipidemia in hypertensive patients provides significant CVD risk reduction. Subgroup analyses from numerous other placebo-controlled, prospective intervention trials have substantiated this finding.

Dyslipidemia screening

A complete fasting (12–14 hours) lipoprotein profile should be performed on patients screened for dyslipidemia. A lipid profile should provide a quantitative estimate of serum triglycerides, total cholesterol, low-density lipoprotein cholesterol (LDL-C), and high-density lipoprotein cholesterol (HDL-C). Non–HDL-C is defined as the difference between total cholesterol and HDL-C, and represents the total atherogenic lipoprotein burden in serum [LDL-C, lipoprotein(a), and very low-density lipoprotein cholesterol (VLDL-C)]. LDL, VLDL, and Lp(a) particles are atherogenic because they are the delivery vehicles for cholesterol and lipid into the subendothelial space of arteries and promote foam cell, fatty streak, and atheromatous plaque formation. HDL particles are antiatherogenic. The HDLs drive reverse cholesterol transport, a process by which excess lipid from macrophage foam cells and atheromatous plaque is extracted and delivered back to the liver for elimination through the GI tract. The HDLs also exert multiple antioxidative, antithrombotic, and antiinflammatory effects along arterial walls that are widely assumed to be atheroprotective.

Management guidelines

The National Cholesterol Education Program Adult Treatment Panel III (NCEP ATPIII) has promulgated guidelines for dyslipidemia management in a rigorous and evidence-based manner.

Risk stratification. Specific LDL-C and non–HDL-C targets are specified by the stratification of patient risk. Initial risk stratification is performed by counting the number of risk factors a patient has. CVD risk factors include cigarette smoking, age >45 in men and >55 in women, HDL <40 mg per dL, hypertension [blood pressure (BP) >140/90 mm Hg or use of antihypertensive agents], family history of premature coronary artery disease (CAD; CAD in male first-degree relatives of age <55 years; CAD in female first-degree relatives of age <65 years), and age (men ≥45 years, women ≥55 years). A HDL ≥60 mg per dL is a protective factor and allows for the subtraction of one point from the total risk factor burden. If the patient has 0 to 1 risk factors, he/she is categorized as low risk (10-year Framingham risk <5%). However, if the patient has two or more risk factors, then it is recommended that a full Framingham risk score be calculated so as to differentiate moderate (<10%, 10-year risk), moderately high (10%–20%, 10-year risk), and high risk (>20%, 10-year risk) patients. An electronic version of a Framingham risk calculator for men and women can be downloaded at http://hp2010.nhlbihin.net/atpiii/riskcalc.htm.

Patients are also characterized by high risk if they have CAD (defined as a history of MI, stable/unstable angina, revascularization with coronary artery bypass grafting or percutaneous angioplasty) or a CAD risk equivalent [defined as diabetes mellitus, peripheral vascular disease, significant carotid artery disease (transient ischemic attack or stroke from carotid origin or >50% obstructive atheromatous plaque in a carotid artery), and abdominal aortic aneurysm]. In an addendum to ATPIII, the NCEP introduced the category of very high risk. Examples of very high risk patients include those with a history of an acute coronary syndrome (ACS) or those with CAD who are diabetic, smoke, or have multiple inadequately controlled risk factors.

Metabolic syndrome. The metabolic syndrome is a manifestation of insulin resistance and is defined by the presence of three or more of the following features: (1) *abdominal obesity* (men, waist >40 inches, women, waist >35 inches); (2) *triglycerides*

≥150 mg per dL; (3) *HDL-C*, in men <40 mg per dL, in women <50 mg per dL; (4) *BP* ≥130/85 mm Hg; and (5) *fasting glucose* ≥100 mg per dL. In patients with the metabolic syndrome, there is a very high prevalence of concomitant hypertension and mixed dyslipidemia. The metabolic syndrome is not a CAD risk equivalent. However, because these patients by definition have ≥2 risk factors, they should all have a 10-year Framingham risk score calculated in order to determine their specific LDL-C and non–HDL-C goals. All risk factors which comprise the metabolic syndrome in an individual patient should be managed aggressively.

Treatment goals. The NCEP has defined an optimal LDL-C for all patients as <100 mg per dL. It has also defined risk-stratified targets for LDL-C and non–HDL-C (**Table C159.1**). Until the guidelines are formally changed, LDL-C goals of <100 mg per dL and <70 mg per dL are *therapeutic options* for patients with moderately high and very high risk, respectively. The primary target of dyslipidemia management is LDL-C goal attainment. The secondary goal of lipid management is to attain non–HDL-C goals, particularly if baseline triglycerides are >200 mg per dL. The non–HDL-C goal is simply the LDL-C goal plus 30 mg per dL. If HDL-C is <40 mg per dL, it is recommended that effort be made to raise HDL-C through intensive therapeutic lifestyle modification and pharmacologic intervention, as needed. The NCEP has not defined risk-stratified goals for HDL-C. Consistent with guidelines issued by the American Diabetes Association, in hypertensive patients who are diabetic, HDL-C should be increased to >40 mg per dL in men and to >50 mg per dL in women.

A simple rule of the thumb for lipid management is that when it comes to LDL-C, lower is better; in contrast, when it comes to HDL-C, higher is better. Torcetrapib is a cholesterol ester transfer protein inhibitor capable of raising HDL-C up to 70% in clinical trials. Recent studies showed that torcetrapib actually increased risk for cardiovascular events and had no effect on rates of atheromatous plaque progression. Unfortunately, in addition to raising serum levels of HDL-C and inducing further reductions in LDL-C, torcetrapib also increased BP significantly and may have exerted direct vasculotoxicity. Consequently, studies with this agent are not believed to have negated the importance of therapeutic HDL elevation.

Although most health care providers know that a patient with CAD or a CAD risk equivalent should be treated to an LDL-C <100 mg per dL, studies have demonstrated that only 18% to 25% of these patients achieve this target. It is strongly recommended that hypertensive patients with dyslipidemia be treated to their risk-stratified lipoprotein targets.

Therapeutic lifestyle change

Therapeutic lifestyle change (TLC) is a critical part of managing all patients at risk for CVD. Patients who smoke should be unequivocally encouraged to stop and this advice should be repeated at every visit. Smoking induces endothelial cell dysfunction, increases the oxidation of LDL thereby rendering it more atherogenic, and promotes the catabolism of serum HDL. The daily intake of dietary cholesterol should be <200 mg and the percentage of saturated fat in the diet should be <7%. Total fat intake should be in the range of 25% to 35% of total caloric intake. The caloric distribution of other nutrients should consist of: 20% monounsaturated fat, 10% polyunsaturated fat, 50% to 60% carbohydrate, and 15%

TABLE C159.1

LOW-DENSITY LIPOPROTEIN (LDL) CHOLESTEROL GOALS AND THRESHOLDS FOR INITIATING LIFESTYLE CHANGE
AND PHARMACOLOGIC INTERVENTION

Risk category [a,b]	LDL goal	LDL level at which to initiate TLC	LDL level at which to consider drug therapy
CHD or CHD risk equivalents (10-year risk >20%)	<100 mg/dL (optional goal <70)[c]	≥100 mg/dL All patients regardless of LDL	≥130 mg/dL (100–129 mg/dL: drug optional) ≥100 mg/d[d] (<100 mg/dL: drug optional)
2+ Risk factors (10-year risk 10%–20%)	<130 mg/dL (optional goal <100)	≥130 mg/dL All patients regardless of LDL	≥130 mg/dL (>100 mg/dL: drug optional[d])
2+ Risk factors (10-year risk ≤10%)	<130 mg/dL	≥130 mg/dL	≥160 mg/dL
0–1 Risk factor[c]	<160 mg/dL	≥160 mg/dL	≥190 mg/dL (160–189 mg/dL: LDL-lowering drug optional)

LDL, low-density lipoprotein; TLC, therapeutic lifestyle change; CHD, coronary heart disease.
[a]CHD risk equivalents include diabetes mellitus, peripheral vascular disease, carotid artery disease (CAD), abdominal aortic aneurysm, and a 10-year Framingham risk >20%.
[b]Risk factors included in Framingham risk evaluation are age, systolic blood pressure, total cholesterol, HDL-C, and smoking status.
[c]The optional goal of <70 mg per dL is particularly targeted at patients who are at "very high" risk, that is, patients with a recent acute coronary syndrome and patients with CAD and poorly controlled risk factors (diabetes, cigarette smoking, multiple components of the metabolic syndrome).
(Adapted from Grundy SM, Cleeman JI, Merz CN, et al. Implications of recent clinical trials for the National Cholesterol Education Program Adult Treatment Panel III guidelines. *Circulation* 2004;110(2):227–239.)

protein. Patients should be encouraged to increase their intake of mono- and polyunsaturated fat and to decrease the intake of saturated and trans fat because these dietary modifications reduce serum levels of LDL-C. A consultation with a dietitian improves compliance and the probability of success. Viscous fiber and plant stanol supplements decrease GI cholesterol absorption. Patients should exercise for 20 to 30 minutes daily. Exercise promotes weight loss and reduces visceral adiposity and insulin resistance. Reductions in insulin resistance are associated with reduced serum triglycerides and increased HDL-C. Emphasis must be placed on lifelong adherence to TLC as therapeutic success most frequently decreases as a function of time.

TLC is crucial to the management of patients with the metabolic syndrome. Hypertriglyceridemia is quite common in these patients. If triglycerides remain elevated (200–499 mg/dL) after the NCEP LDL-C target is achieved, then the patient should be treated with a triglyceride-lowering drug (e.g., a fibrate or niacin). If triglycerides exceed 500 mg per dL, the patient should be treated with triglyceride-lowering medication and a very low fat diet (≤15% of total daily calories) in order to reduce risk for CVD *and* pancreatitis. In patients with severe hypertriglyceridemia, lipoprotein lipase deficiencies are frequently present and triglycerides can be >1,000 mg per dL. In addition to the aforementioned therapies, these patients may benefit from adjuvant therapy with orlistat, a drug that reduces fat absorption from the GI tract.

Antilipidemic medications
Statins
Actions. Statins are reversible, competitive inhibitors of the rate-limiting step of cholesterol biosynthesis, 3-hydroxy-3-methylglutaryl coenzyme A (HMG-CoA) reductase. The statins (atorvastatin, fluvastatin, lovastatin, pravastatin, rosuvastatin, and simvastatin) are the most potent drugs available for reducing

serum LDL-C. In addition to inhibiting cholesterol biosynthesis, the statins increase the systemic clearance of atherogenic lipoproteins by upregulating surface expression of the LDL receptor on hepatocytes. These drugs also decrease hepatic VLDL secretion, thereby reducing serum levels of triglycerides, and also increase serum HDL-C.

Clinical use. The magnitude of LDL-C reduction is dose and compound dependent, with pravastatin (up to 34%) and rosuvastatin (up to 63%) having the lowest and highest capacities, respectively. Each doubling of a statin's dose provides an additional 6% reduction in serum LDL-C.

Statins have substantially impacted modern cardiovascular care. In numerous large-scale, placebo-controlled clinical trials performed in both primary and secondary prevention cohorts, the statins significantly decrease rates of atheromatous plaque progression, MI, stroke, stable and unstable angina, and coronary and all-cause mortality. Statins reduce event rates in men and women, hypertensive patients, diabetic patients, smokers, and patients older than 70 years.

Patients on statin therapy should be counseled about the potential for hepatotoxicity, myalgia, and myopathy (including rhabdomyolysis). The mechanism of transaminase elevations with statin therapy does not preclude their safe use in patients with fatty liver disease. Statin-related myopathy may be compound-specific. It typically resolves shortly after discontinuation of the medication although it may linger for week to months in the occasional patient. There are also a number of other side effects purported to occur with statin therapy, including changes in memory and thinking, sleep abnormalities, mood change, and peripheral neuropathy among others. In the instance where such side effects arise medication discontinuation with the intent of determining whether symptom resolution occurs is the prudent course of action. The statins should not be used in women who are pregnant, contemplating a pregnancy, or lactating.

Fibrates

Actions. Fibrates activate lipoprotein lipase (an enzyme that hydrolyzes triglycerides in VLDL and chylomicrons) by decreasing the expression of apoprotein CIII (an inhibitor of this enzyme) and increasing levels of apoprotein CII (an activator of lipoprotein lipase). In addition to stimulating hepatic secretion of HDL, the fibrates reduce HDL catabolism through hepatic lipase, an enzyme that breaks down HDL particles that are enriched with triglycerides. Fibrates decrease serum triglycerides by 25% to 50% and increase HDL-C by approximately 10%.

Clinical use. Fibrates are well suited to the treatment of patients with high triglycerides and low HDL-C (frequently characteristic of patients with the metabolic syndrome and type 2 diabetes mellitus). Three studies (the Helsinki Heart Study, Veterans Affairs High-Density Lipoprotein Intervention Trial, and the Bezafibrate Infarction Prevention Study) have shown significant cardiovascular event reductions using fibrate therapy in such patients. Fibrates have not yet been shown to reduce risk for mortality. In the Fenofibrate Intervention and Event Lowering Trial, fenofibrate therapy in diabetic patients was associated with significant reductions in risk for nonfatal MI, need for coronary revascularization, hospitalization for angina pectoris, laser photocoagulation for retinopathy, and need for lower extremity amputations.

The use of statin and fibrate combination therapy has increased in parallel with the rising incidence of complex dyslipidemias. Gemfibrozil inhibits the glucuronidation of statins, which prolongs their functional availability. This can elevate the risk for hepatotoxicity and myopathy/rhabdomyolysis. When considering statin/fibrate combination therapy, fenofibrate is a safer choice as it does not block the glucuronidation of statins. When serum triglycerides do not normalize during treatment with a low fat diet and a fibrate, additional intervention with orlistat or high dose fish oil can be considered. Fish oil capsules containing ω-3 (eicosapentaenoic acid) and ω-6 (docosahexaenoic acid) fatty acids lower serum triglyceride levels and raise HDL-C in a dose-dependent manner.

Fibrate therapy is associated with a low risk of myopathy and mild elevations in serum transaminases and can increase the risk for cholelithiasis. Fibrate use is occasionally accompanied by an increase in serum creatinine values of unknown etiology.

Niacin

Actions. Niacin beneficially impacts lipoprotein metabolism by raising HDL by reducing HDL particle uptake and catabolism by hepatocytes. Niacin also decreases hepatic VLDL and triglyceride secretion by (a) decreasing the release of fatty acids from adipose tissue into the liver by inhibiting lipase activity and (b) reducing triglyceride formation within hepatocytes by inhibiting diacylglycerol acyltransferase. Niacin therapy is associated with decreased LDL-C because of reduced VLDL availability and increased catabolism of apoB100.

Clinical use. Niacin used as either monotherapy or in combination with a statin has been shown to reduce risk for MI, stroke, and rates of atheromatous plaque progression. Niacin therapy can be challenging to initiate and maintain due to its side-effect profile, most commonly prostaglandin-mediated cutaneous flushing. The frequency and severity of flushing can be reduced by taking a 325-mg tablet of aspirin 1 hour before taking niacin. Limiting fat intake for 2 to 3 hours before niacin ingestion also reduces flushing as fat is a source of arachidonic acid, the substrate for cyclooxygenase. Niaspan is a sustained-release formulation of niacin associated with less flushing. Other side effects include transient disturbances in glycemic control, pruritus, acanthosis nigricans, and increased serum levels of uric acid.

Ezetimibe

Actions. Dietary and biliary cholesterol is absorbed across the surface of jejunal enterocytes. Ezetimibe (Zetia) is a cholesterol absorption inhibitor. Ezetimibe inhibits a sterol transporter in enterocytes identified as Niemann-Pick C1 Like-1 protein, which translocates both cholesterol and phytosterols.

Clinical use. The mean LDL-C reduction with ezetimibe is 20%, but up to 24% of patients experience a reduction of >25%. Ezetimibe increases HDL-C by up to 4% and decreases triglycerides by up to 8%. Ezetimibe does not reduce the absorption of steroid hormones (ethinyl estradiol, progesterone), bile acids, or fat-soluble vitamins (A, D, E, or α- and β-carotenes). The incidence of liver toxicity with ezetimibe is nearly equivalent with placebo and there is no evidence of elevated risk for myopathy. Ezetimibe can also be safely used in combination with other statins and reduces the need for statin titration. Ezetimibe provides additive changes in lipoprotein levels to that observed with statin therapy.

Bile acid–binding resins

Actions. Bile acid sequestrants (BAS) are oral anion exchange resins that electrostatically bind bile acids in the GI tract and prevent them from being reabsorbed along the terminal ileum into the enterohepatic circulation. The BAS decrease serum LDL-C by increasing (a) the catabolism of cholesterol through 7-α-hydroxylase, the rate-limiting enzyme for the conversion of cholesterol into bile acids, and (b) the expression of LDL receptors on the surface of hepatocytes which promotes the clearance of apoB100-containing lipoproteins from plasma.

Clinical use. At maximum doses, the BAS increase HDL-C by 3% to 5% and decrease serum LDL-C by 15% to 30%. The BAS should be used in combination with a statin whenever possible because these drugs increase hepatic HMG-CoA reductase activity and cholesterol biosynthesis, potentially negating the therapeutic efficacy of the BAS over time. Although occasionally useful, these agents are poorly tolerated and rarely necessary.

Suggested Readings

Armani A, Toth PP. Colesevelam hydrochloride in the management of dyslipidemia. *Expert Rev Cardiovasc Ther* 2006;4(3):283–291.

Davidson M, Toth PP. Statins, fibrates, and niacin in the management of dyslipidemias. *Prog Cardiovasc Dis* 2004;47:73–104.

Expert Panel on Detection, Evaluation, and Treatment of High Blood Cholesterol in Adults. Executive summary of the third report of the National Cholesterol Education Program (NCEP) Expert Panel on Detection, Evaluation, and Treatment of High Blood Cholesterol in Adults (Adult Treatment Panel III). *JAMA* 2001;285:2486–2497.

Grundy SM, Cleeman JI, Merz CN, et al. Implications of recent clinical trials for the National Cholesterol Education Program Adult Treatment Panel III guidelines. *Circulation* 2004;110(2):227–239.

Heart Protection Study Collaborative Group. MRC/BHF Heart Protection Study of cholesterol lowering with simvastatin in 20,536 high-risk individuals: a randomised placebo-controlled trial. *Lancet* 2002;360:7–22.

Sever PS, Dahlöf B, Poulter NR, et al. ASCOT Investigators. Prevention of coronary and stroke events with atorvastatin in hypertensive patients who have average or lower-than-average cholesterol concentrations, in the Anglo-Scandinavian Cardiac Outcomes Trial—Lipid Lowering Arm (ASCOT-LLA): a multicentre randomised controlled trial. *Lancet* 2003;361:1149–1158.

Toth PP. Clinician update: HDL and cardiovascular risk. *Circulation* 2004;109: 1809–1812.

Toth PP. Low-density lipoprotein reduction in high risk patients: how low do you go? *Curr Atheroscler Rep* 2004;6:348–352.

Toth PP, Davidson MH. Cholesterol absorption blockade with ezetimibe. *Curr Drug Targets* 2005;5(6):455–462.

CHAPTER C160 ■ TREATMENT OF PREGNANT HYPERTENSIVE PATIENTS

SANDRA J. TALER, MD

KEY POINTS

- Hypertensive disorders have a high rate of recurrence (20%–50%) in subsequent pregnancies; most women with chronic hypertension in pregnancy have stage 1 hypertension and are candidates for nondrug (lifestyle modification) therapy.
- Preeclampsia occurs in 25% of women with chronic hypertension.
- There is no evidence that pharmacologic treatment leads to improved neonatal outcomes; meta-analyses suggest that all antihypertensive medications can retard intrauterine growth.
- Angiotensin-converting enzyme (ACE) inhibitors, angiotensin receptor blockers (ARBs), and direct renin inhibitors should be avoided in pregnancy at all stages, including conception.

See also Chapters **A54** and **B82**

The key to management of hypertension in pregnancy is to differentiate preeclampsia, a pregnancy-specific syndrome of exaggerated vasoconstriction and reduced organ perfusion, from preexisting chronic hypertension. Hypertension during pregnancy is classified into one of five categories (**Table C160.1**).

Prepregnancy assessment and counseling

Assessment of hypertension. Ideally, women with hypertension should be evaluated before conception to define the severity of their hypertension and plan for potential lifestyle changes. If systolic blood pressure (SBP) is ≥180 mm Hg or diastolic blood pressure (DBP) is ≥110 mm Hg, or if treatment requires multiple antihypertensive agents, the woman should be evaluated for potentially reversible causes. Although evaluation for secondary causes can usually be deferred until after delivery, all hypertensive women should be screened for pheochromocytoma at the time of discovery of the hypertension owing to the high associated morbidity and mortality of this condition if not diagnosed antepartum. Home blood pressure (BP) monitoring is a useful adjunct to close medical supervision. In hypertensive women planning to become pregnant, some practitioners change to antihypertensive medications known to be relatively safe during pregnancy, such as β-blockers, α-methyldopa or hydralazine.

Assessment of target organs. Women with a history of hypertension over several years should be evaluated for target organ damage (TOD), including left ventricular hypertrophy (LVH), retinopathy, and renal disease. If these conditions are present, women should be advised that pregnancy might worsen disease severity. Women with chronic hypertension may be at higher risk for adverse neonatal outcomes independent of the development of preeclampsia if proteinuria is present early in pregnancy. The risks of fetal loss and acceleration of maternal renal disease increase at serum creatinine levels >1.4 mg per dL at conception, although it may be difficult to separate the effects of pregnancy from progression of the underlying renal disease. Preeclampsia is significantly more common in women with chronic hypertension, with an incidence of approximately 25%. Risk factors for superimposed preeclampsia include renal insufficiency, a history of hypertension for 4 years or longer, and hypertension in a prior pregnancy.

Lifestyle counseling. Chronic hypertension before pregnancy requires planning for lifestyle changes. Hypertensive women are advised to restrict aerobic exercise during pregnancy based on theoretic concerns that inadequate placental blood flow may increase the risk of preeclampsia. Weight reduction is not recommended during pregnancy, even in obese women. Sodium restriction is recommended only for those women who have been successfully treated by this approach before pregnancy. As in all pregnancies, the use of alcohol and tobacco is strongly discouraged.

Renin-angiotensin blocking drugs

Use of angiotensin-converting enzyme (ACE) inhibitors or angiotensin receptor blockers (ARBs) during the second and third trimesters of pregnancy has been linked to oligohydramnios, fetal abnormalities (intrauterine growth retardation, hypocalvaria, renal dysplasia, anuria, and renal failure), and death. A recent epidemiologic study found first trimester exposure to ACE inhibitors

CLASSIFICATION OF HYPERTENSION IN PREGNANCY

Diagnosis	Criteria
Chronic hypertension	BP ≥140 mm Hg systolic or 90 mm Hg diastolic before pregnancy or before 20-wk gestation
	Persists >12 wk postpartum
Preeclampsia	BP ≥140 mm Hg systolic or 90 mm Hg diastolic with proteinuria (>300 mg/24 h or 200 mg/g creatinine) after 20-wk gestation
	Can progress to eclampsia (seizures)
	More common in nulliparous women, multiple gestation, women with hypertension for ≥4 yr, family history of preeclampsia, hypertension in previous pregnancy, renal disease
Chronic hypertension with superimposed preeclampsia	New onset proteinuria after 20 wk in a woman with hypertension
	In a woman with hypertension and proteinuria before 20 wk gestation:
	Sudden two- to threefold increase in proteinuria
	Sudden increase in blood pressure (BP)
	Thrombocytopenia
	Elevated aspartate aminotransferase or alanine aminotransferase
Gestational hypertension	Hypertension without proteinuria occurring after 20 wk gestation
	Temporary diagnosis
	May represent preproteinuric phase of preeclampsia or recurrence of chronic hypertension abated in midpregnancy
	May evolve to preeclampsia
	If severe, may result in higher rates of premature delivery and growth retardation than mild preeclampsia
Transient hypertension	Retrospective diagnosis
	BP normal by 12 wk postpartum
	May recur in subsequent pregnancies
	Predictive of future essential hypertension

was associated with a 2.7-fold higher risk of major congenital malformations of the cardiac and central nervous system, compared to other antihypertensive agents or untreated hypertension. These data support avoidance of all renin-angiotensin system blocking medications, including direct renin inhibitors, during all stages of pregnancy, including at conception. Women of childbearing age must be cautioned regarding the risks of early exposure and should be converted to treatment with other antihypertensive agents when planning for pregnancy.

Treatment of stage 1 (chronic) hypertension during pregnancy

Nondrug therapy. Most women with chronic hypertension in pregnancy have stage 1 hypertension (SBP of 140 to 159 and/or, DBP of 90 to 99 mm Hg) and are at low risk for cardiovascular complications during pregnancy. These women are candidates for nondrug therapy because there is no evidence that pharmacologic treatment leads to improved neonatal outcomes. Because BP

usually falls during the first half of pregnancy, hypertension may be relatively easy to control with few, if any, medications.

Drug therapy. The benefit of continued administration of antihypertensive drugs to pregnant women with chronic hypertension continues to be an area of debate. Some centers manage chronic hypertensive patients by stopping antihypertensive medications while maintaining close observation. For women with evidence of TOD and for those on multiple agents, medications may be tapered on the basis of BP readings but should be continued, if needed, to control BP. There is evidence from several studies that antihypertensive medications prevent BP from increasing to very high levels during pregnancy. Treatment should be reinstituted once BP reaches levels of 150 to 160 mm Hg systolic or 100 to 110 mm Hg diastolic.

Fetal safety concerns. The primary goal of treating chronic hypertension is to reduce maternal risk, but the agents selected must be safe for the fetus. α-Methyldopa is preferred by many as first-line therapy on the basis of reports of stable uteroplacental blood flow and fetal hemodynamics and follow-up studies up to 7.5 years showing no long-term adverse effects on development of children exposed to α-methyldopa *in utero*. Other treatment options are listed in **Table C160.2**. On the basis of a meta-analysis of 45 randomized controlled trials of treatment of pregnant women with mean arterial pressures (MAP) of 107 to 129 mm Hg, there are still concerns regarding the safety of any drug treatment. In this analysis of trials using α-methyldopa, β-blockers, thiazide diuretics, hydralazine, calcium channel blockers, and clonidine, there was a direct linear relationship between the treatment-induced fall in MAP and the proportion of small-for-gestational-age infants. The type of hypertension, category of antihypertensive

TREATMENT OF CHRONIC HYPERTENSION IN PREGNANCY

Agent	Comments
α-Methyldopa	Preferred on the basis of long-term follow-up studies supporting safety
	Dose range 250–500 mg, two to four times daily
Labetalol	Increasingly preferred to methyldopa owing to reduced side effects
	Dose range 100–200 mg two to four times daily
β-Blockers	Reports of intrauterine growth retardation (atenolol), generally safe
Clonidine	Limited data
Calcium antagonists	Limited data, no increase in major teratogenicity with exposure
	Nifedipine dosing 30–90 mg daily
	Amlodipine dosing 2.5–10 mg daily
Diuretics	Not first-line agents, probably safe
ACE inhibitors, angiotensin II receptor antagonists, renin inhibitors	Contraindicated, reported congenital malformations, fetopathy, and death

ACE, angiotensin-converting enzyme.

agent, and duration of therapy appeared not to explain this relationship. A subsequent expanded meta-analysis strengthened this association. Over the range of reported treatment-induced BP differences, a 10-mm Hg fall in MAP was associated with a 176-g decrease in birth weight.

Treatment of stage 2 (chronic) hypertension

There are few placebo-controlled trials evaluating the treatment of stage 2 hypertension in pregnancy. A recent Cochrane analysis concluded that there was insufficient data on which to determine the superiority of one agent over another. Until better evidence is available, the clinician's experience and familiarity with a specific drug should determine the choice of therapy, among those agents classified as being safe. Early reports of experience with severe chronic hypertension in the first trimester describe fetal loss rates of 50% and significant maternal mortality, with most of the poor outcomes occurring in those pregnancies complicated by superimposed preeclampsia.

Other considerations

Influence of renal disease. Women with progressive renal diseases should be encouraged to complete their childbearing while renal function is relatively well preserved. Among women with serum creatinine levels <1.4 mg per dL, fetal survival is only moderately reduced and the underlying disease does not generally worsen during pregnancy. A decrease in birth weight correlates directly with rising maternal serum creatinine concentration. In pregnant women with moderate or severe renal insufficiency, hypertension may accelerate the underlying renal disease and markedly reduce fetal survival. As renal failure progresses, the hypertension acquires an element of volume overload and may require sodium restriction, use of diuretics, or dialysis. Chronic dialysis during pregnancy is associated with significant maternal morbidity and fetal loss and conception should be discouraged. Renal transplant recipients are advised to wait 1.5 to 2 years after successful transplantation and to pursue pregnancy only if renal function is stable with serum creatinine values of 2 mg per dL or less. Rates of prematurity are high in transplant recipients; therefore all pregnancies in transplant recipients are considered to be high risk.

Treating hypertension during lactation. Breast-feeding can usually be done safely with certain limits on antihypertensive drug choices. In mildly hypertensive mothers who wish to breast-feed for a few months, medication may be withheld with close monitoring of BP. After nursing has stopped, antihypertensive therapy can be reinstituted. For patients with more severe BP elevation on a single antihypertensive agent, the clinician may consider reducing the dosage while closely monitoring mother and infant. The available data regarding excretion of antihypertensive agents in human breast milk suggest that all studied agents are excreted into human breast milk, although there are differences in the milk-to-plasma ratio related to lipid solubility and extent of ionization of the drug at physiologic pH. No short-term adverse effects have been reported from exposure to α-methyldopa or hydralazine. Propanolol and labetalol are preferred if a β-blocker is indicated. Diuretics may reduce milk volume and thereby suppress lactation. ACE inhibitors, ARBs (and probably renin inhibitors) should be avoided because of concerns of adverse neonatal renal effects. Given the scarcity of data, breast-fed infants of mothers taking antihypertensive agents should be closely monitored for potential adverse effects.

Preeclampsia

Historically, efforts to prevent and treat preeclampsia were limited by lack of knowledge of its underlying cause. Recent studies implicate an imbalance between circulating antiangiogenic and proangiogenic factors in the pathogenesis of this syndrome. Preeclampsia is also recognized as a state of reduced placental/fetal perfusion and subsequent extensive dysfunction of the maternal vascular endothelium (see Chapter A54).

Prevention. Prevention has focused on identification of women at higher risk, followed by close clinical and laboratory monitoring aimed at early recognition of the disease and institution of intensive monitoring or delivery when indicated. Despite the encouraging results of early small trials, none of the large multicenter trials of aspirin has demonstrated any benefit compared with placebo. The prevailing opinion is that women without risk factors do not benefit from treatment, but selective treatment for certain women at high risk (specifically women with the antiphospholipid antibody syndrome) may be reasonable. Randomized trials of calcium supplementation have demonstrated reductions in incidence of preeclampsia in high-risk women with low calcium intake. For low-risk women in the United States, there is no evidence of benefit with calcium-enriched diets. It was originally believed that antioxidant vitamin administration might reduce the risk of preeclampsia; however, trials using the antioxidant vitamins C (1,000 mg/day) and E (400 IU) in nulliparous women appear not to reduce the risk of preeclampsia.

General management principles. Treatment for preeclampsia consists of hospitalization for bed rest, control of BP, administration of magnesium sulfate for seizure prophylaxis when signs of impending eclampsia are present, and timely delivery. Therapy is palliative and does not alter the underlying pathophysiology of the disease; at best, it may slow progression of the condition and provide time for fetal maturation. Delivery is always the appropriate therapy for the mother but may compromise a fetus of <32-weeks gestation. For a preterm fetus with no evidence of fetal compromise in a woman with mild disease, valuable time may be gained by postponing delivery. Antihypertensive therapy should be prescribed only for maternal safety; it does not improve perinatal outcomes and may adversely affect uteroplacental blood flow.

It is unusual for preeclampsia to remit spontaneously, and, in most cases, the disease worsens. Regardless of gestational age, delivery should be strongly considered when there are signs of fetal distress, or intrauterine growth retardation, or signs of maternal risk including severe hypertension, hemolysis, elevated liver enzymes, and low platelet count (termed the *HELLP syndrome*), deteriorating renal function, visual disturbance, headache, or epigastric pain. Vaginal delivery is preferable to cesarean delivery to avoid the added stress of surgery. Close BP monitoring should continue after delivery because hypertension and preeclampsia may persist or even present postpartum.

Blood pressure management. As many women with preeclampsia were previously normotensive with BPs in the range of 100 to 110/70 mm Hg, acute elevations to what might be deemed otherwise minimal and not particularly worrisome (i.e., 150/100 mm Hg) may cause significant symptomatology and require immediate treatment. Severe hypertension, defined as SBP ≥170 mm Hg and/or DBP ≥110 mm Hg, should be treated promptly. Whatever the level of BP elevation when therapy is started, it should be reduced gradually so as to avoid hypotension.

Selection of antihypertensive agents and route of administration depends on anticipated timing of delivery. If it is likely to be

TABLE C160.3

TREATMENT OF ACUTE SEVERE HYPERTENSION IN PREECLAMPSIA

Drug	Dosage
Hydralazine	5 mg intravenous bolus, then 10 mg every 20–30 min to a maximum of 25 mg, repeat in several hours as necessary
Labetalol (second line)	20 mg intravenous bolus, then 40 mg 10 min later, 80 mg every 10 min for two additional doses to a maximum of 220 mg

more than 48 hours until delivery, oral α-methyldopa is preferred owing to its safety record and extensive experience. Oral labetalol is an alternative choice, with other β-blockers and calcium channel blockers being acceptable alternatives based on limited data. If delivery is imminent, parenteral agents such as hydralazine or labetalol are practical and effective (**Table C160.3**). Antihypertensives are administered before induction for persistent diastolic levels of 105 to 110 mm Hg or higher, aiming for levels of 95 to 105 mm Hg.

Recurrence of hypertension

Hypertensive disorders have a high rate of recurrence (20% to 50%) in subsequent pregnancies whether classified as gestational hypertension, preeclampsia, or preeclampsia superimposed on chronic hypertension. Risk factors for recurrence include early onset of hypertension in the first pregnancy, a history of chronic hypertension, persistent hypertension beyond 5 weeks postpartum, and high baseline BP early in pregnancy. Remote hypertension is more common after gestational hypertension. New data suggest that women with preeclampsia also have a greater tendency to develop hypertension than those who have had normotensive pregnancies.

Suggested Readings

Buchbinder A, Sibai B, Caritis S, et al. Adverse perinatal outcomes are significantly higher in severe gestational hypertension than in mild preeclampsia. *Am J Obstet Gynecol* 2002;186:66–71.

Cooper WO, Hernandez-Diaz S, Arbogast PG, et al. Major congenital malformations after first-trimester exposure to ACE inhibitors. *N Eng J Med* 2006;354:2443–2451.

Duley L. Drugs for treatment of very high BP during pregnancy. *Cochrane Database Syst Rev* 2006;3:CD001449.

National High BP Education Program Working Group on High BP in Pregnancy. Report of the National High BP Education Program Working Group on high BP in pregnancy. *Am J Obstet Gynecol* 2000;183:S1–S22.

Sibai BM. Chronic hypertension in pregnancy. *Obstet Gynecol* 2002;100:369–377.

Von Dadelszen P, Magee LA. Fall in mean arterial pressure and fetal growth restriction in pregnancy hypertension: an updated metaregression analysis. *J Obstet Gynaecol Can* 2002;24:941–945.

Von Dadelszen P, Magee LA. Antihypertensive medications in management of gestational hypertension-preeclampsia. *Clin Obstet Gynecol* 2005;2:441–459.

Von Dadelszen P, Ornstein MP, Bull SB, et al. Fall in mean arterial pressure and fetal growth restriction in pregnancy hypertension: a meta-analysis. *Lancet* 2000;355:87–92.

CHAPTER C161 ■ TREATMENT OF HYPERTENSIVE CHILDREN AND ADOLESCENTS

BONITA FALKNER, MD

KEY POINTS

■ Children and adolescents with hypertension, diabetes, or chronic kidney disease benefit from treatment to lower blood pressure (BP) to <90th percentile for age.
■ Evaluation for underlying cause, comorbidity, and target organ damage provide information to guide BP treatment decisions in children and adolescents.
■ Lifestyle changes benefit children with prehypertension and hypertension.
■ Pharmacologic treatment should be tailored to each child's circumstances.

See also Chapters **B83** and C163

Definition of hypertension in children

Hypertension in childhood and adolescence is defined as systolic or diastolic blood pressure (BP) at or above the 95th percentile for age, sex, and height. Childhood prehypertension is defined as a systolic or diastolic BP between the >90th and 95th percentile. For adolescents, a BP ≥120/80 mm Hg but <the 95th percentile) represents prehypertension. Tables that provide BP values for the 90th, 95th, and 99th percentile by sex, age, and height can be obtained from www.nhlbi.nih.gov/guidelines/hypertension/child_tbl.htm.

Goals of evaluation and therapy

The challenge clinically is to identify, evaluate, and treat those children who will benefit from interventions to lower BP. Children with levels of BP that are extremely elevated (>5 mm Hg above the 99th percentile) require careful evaluation for correctable forms of hypertension. These children benefit from treatment to lower BP irrespective of its cause. Children who have renal disease or diabetes should receive treatment to bring BP below the 90th percentile for renal protection. No data are available on the benefits of interventions to lower BP in the prehypertension range in children who do not have diabetes or renal disease but evidence now indicates that these children will continue to have higher BP levels throughout life and will progress to clinical hypertension at an early age. It is therefore appropriate to implement lifestyle modification strategies for childhood prehypertension.

Evaluation

Additional clinical information can be helpful in guiding decisions about drug therapy. A basic evaluation including an assessment of renal function and renal anatomy (renal ultrasound) should be performed. Many children with minimal elevations of BP for age are also overweight or obese; those with BP elevation (>90th percentile) should be evaluated for metabolic risk factors including glucose and lipid parameters and should be asked about symptoms of sleep apnea. Assessment for evidence of target organ damage is recommended including an echocardiogram to detect left ventricular hypertrophy. Another study that can provide useful information for management decisions is 24-hour ambulatory blood pressure monitoring (ABPM). As with adults, this procedure can provide information on levels and variability of BP. Echocardiogram and ABPM values should be reported and interpreted using the pediatric reference data.

Nonpharmacologic therapy in children and adolescents

Nonpharmacologic therapies for BP control are recommended for children with minimal elevations of BP or prehypertension. Children who have significant hypertension or those with uncorrectable conditions such as chronic kidney disease (CKD) will probably not respond to lifestyle modification alone, although these interventions often allow better BP control with lower doses of drugs. Weight reduction, dietary modification, and physical exercise regimens are difficult to effect in the young, but they do provide enduring benefits with minimal risk.

Weight reduction. Childhood obesity has become a major health problem that requires substantial public health efforts. Overweight children and adolescents with high BP should be strongly encouraged to lose excess weight and should be provided the education and support necessary to be successful in such efforts. The recently developed childhood growth grids

TABLE C161.1

DRUGS FOR TREATMENT OF CHRONIC HYPERTENSION IN CHILDREN

Class	Drug	Dose[b]	Dosing Interval	Evidence[c]	FDA labeling[d]	Comments[ed]
Angiotensin-converting enzyme (ACE) inhibitor	Benazepril	Initial: 0.2 mg/kg/d up to 10 mg/d Maximum: 0.6 mg/kg/d up to 40 mg/d	q.d.	RCT	Yes	1. All ACE inhibitors are contraindicated in pregnancy—females of childbearing age should use reliable contraception
	Captopril	Initial. 0.3–0.5 mg/kg/dose Maximum: 6 mg/kg/d	t.i.d.	RCT, CS	No	2. Check serum potassium and creatinine periodically to monitor for hyperkalemia and azotemia
	Enalapril	Initial: 0.08 mg/kg/d up to 5 mg/d Maximum: 0.6 mg/kg/d up to 40 mg/d	q.d.–b.i.d.	RCT	Yes	3. Cough and angioedema are reportedly less common with newer members of this class than with captopril
	Fosinopril	Children >50 kg Initial: 5–10 mg/d Maximum: 40 mg/d	q.d.	RCT	Yes	4. Benazepril, enalapril, and lisinopril labels contain information on the preparation of a suspension; captopril may also be compounded into a suspension
	Lisinopril	Initial: 0.07 mg/kg/d up to 5 mg/d Maximum: 0.6 mg/kg/d up to 40 mg/d	q.d.	RCT	Yes	5. FDA approval for ACE inhibitors with pediatric labeling is limited to children ≥6 yr of age and to children with creatinine clearance ≥30 mL/min/1.73 m²
	Quinapril	Initial: 5–10 mg/d Maximum: 80 mg/d	q.d.	RCT, EO	No	
Angiotensin receptor blocker	Irbesartan	6–12 yrs: 75–150 mg/d >13 yr: 150–300 mg/d	q.d.	CS	Yes	1. All ARBs are contraindicated in pregnancy—females of childbearing age should use reliable contraception
	Losartan	Initial: 0.7 mg/kg/d up to 50 mg/d Maximum: 1.4 mg/kg/d up to 100 mg/d	q.d.	RCT	Yes	2. Check serum potassium, creatinine periodically to monitor for hyperkalemia and azotemia
						3. Losartan label contains information on the preparation of a suspension
						4. FDA approval for ARBs is limited to children ≥6 yr of age and to children with creatinine clearance ≥30 mL/min/1.73 m²
α- And β-blocker	Labetalol	Initial: 1–3 mg/kg/d Maximum: 10–12 mg/kg/d up to 1,200 mg/d	b.i.d.	CS, EO	No	1. Asthma and overt heart failure are contraindications 2. Heart rate is dose-limiting 3. May impair athletic performance 4. Should be used cautiously in insulin-dependent diabetic patients
β-Blocker	Atenolol	Initial: 0.5–1 mg/kg/d Maximum: 2 mg/kg/d up to 100 mg/d	q.d.–b.i.d.	CS	No	1. Noncardioselective agents (propranolol) are contraindicated in asthma and heart failure
	Bisoprolol/ HCTZ	Initial: 2.5/6.25 mg/d Maximum: 10/6.25 mg/d	q.d.	RCT	No	2. Heart rate is dose-limiting 3. May impair athletic performance
	Metoprolol	Initial: 1–2 mg/kg/d Maximum: 6 mg/kg/d up to 200 mg/d	b.i.d.	CS	No	4. Should be used cautiously in insulin-dependent diabetic patients
	Propranolol	Initial: 1–2 mg/kg/d Maximum: 4 mg/kg/d up to 640 mg/d	b.i.d.–t.i.d.	RCT, EO	Yes	5. A sustained-release formulation of propranolol is available that is dosed once-daily

(continued)

TABLE C161.1

(CONTINUED)

Class	Drug	Dose[b]	Dosing Interval	Evidence[c]	FDA labeling[d]	Comments[ed]
Calcium channel blocker	Amlodipine	Children 6–17 yrs: 2.5–5 mg once daily	q.d.	RCT	Yes	1. Amlodipine and isradipine can be compounded into stable extemporaneous suspensions
	Felodipine	Initial: 2.5 mg/d Maximum: 10 mg/d	q.d.	RCT, EO	No	2. Felodipine and extended-release nifedipine tablets must be swallowed whole
	Isradipine	Initial: 0.15–0.2 mg/kg/d Maximum: 0.8 mg/kg/d up to 20 mg/d	t.i.d.–q.i.d.	CS, EO	No	3. Isradipine is available in both immediate-release and sustained-release formulations; sustained release form is dosed q.d. or b.i.d.
	Extended-release nifedipine	Initial: 0.25–0.5 mg/kg/d Maximum: 3 mg/kg/d up to 120 mg/d	q.d.–b.i.d.	CS, EO	No	4. May cause tachycardia
Central α-agonist	Clonidine	Children ≥12 yrs: Initial: 0.2 mg/d Maximum: 2.4 mg/d	b.i.d.	EO	Yes	1. May cause dry mouth and/or sedation 2. Transdermal preparation also available 3. Sudden cessation of therapy can lead to severe rebound hypertension
Diuretic	HCTZ	Initial: 1 mg/kg/d Maximum: 3 mg/kg/d up to 50 mg/d	q.d.	EO	Yes	1. All patients treated with diuretics should have electrolytes monitored shortly after initiating therapy and periodically thereafter
	Chlorthalidone	Initial: 0.3 mg/kg/d Maximum: 2 mg/kg/d up to 50 mg/d	q.d.	EO	No	2. Useful as add-on therapy in patients being treated with drugs from other drug classes
	Furosemide	Initial: 0.5–2.0 mg/kg/dose Maximum: 6 mg/kg/d	q.d.–b.i.d.	EO	No	3. Potassium-sparing diuretics (spironolactone, triamterene, amiloride) may cause severe hyperkalemia, especially if given with ACE inhibitor or ARB
	Spironolactone	Initial: 1 mg/kg/d Maximum: 3.3 mg/kg/d up to 100 mg/d	q.d.–b.i.d.	EO	No	4. Furosemide is labeled only for treatment of edema but may be useful as add-on therapy in children with resistant hypertension, particularly in children with renal disease
	Triamterene	Initial: 1–2 mg/kg/d Maximum: 3–4 mg/kg/d up to 300 mg/d	b.i.d.	EO	No	5. Chlorthalidone may precipitate azotemia in patients with renal diseases and should be used with caution in those with severe renal impairment
	Amiloride	Initial: 0.4–0.625 mg/kg/d Maximum: 20 mg/d	q.d.	EO	No	
Peripheral α-antagonist	Doxazosin	Initial: 1 mg/d Maximum: 4 mg/d	q.d.	EO	No	May cause hypotension and syncope, especially after first dose
	Prazosin	Initial: 0.05–0.1 mg/kg/d Maximum: 0.5 mg/kg/d	t.i.d.	EO	No	
	Terazosin	Initial: 1 mg/d Maximum: 20 mg/d	q.d.	EO	No	

TABLE C161.1

(CONTINUED)

Class	Drug	Dose[b]	Dosing Interval	Evidence[c]	FDA labeling[d]	Comments[ed]
Vasodilator	Hydralazine	Initial: 0.75 mg/kg/d Maximum: 7.5 mg/kg/d up to 200 mg/d	q.i.d.	EO	Yes	1. Tachycardia and fluid retention are common side effects 2. Hydralazine can cause a lupus-like syndrome in slow acetylators 3. Prolonged use of minoxidil can cause hypertrichosis 4. Minoxidil is usually reserved for patients with hypertension resistant to multiple drugs
	Minoxidil	Children <12 yr: Initial: 0.2 mg/kg/d Maximum: 50 mg/d Children ≥12 yr: Initial: 5 mg/d Maximum: 100 mg/d	q.d.–t.i.d.	CS, EO	Yes	

FDA, U.S. Food and Drug Administration; ACE, angiotensin-converting enzyme; ARB, angiotensin receptor blocker; b.i.d, twice-daily; HCTZ, hydrochlorothiazide; q.d., once-daily; q.i.d., four times daily; t.i.d., three times daily.
[a]Includes drugs with prior pediatric experience or recently completed clinical trials.
[b]The maximum recommended adult dose should not be exceeded in routine clinical practice.
[c]Level of evidence upon which dosing recommendations are based (CS, case series; EO, expert opinion; RCT, randomized controlled trial)
[d]FDA-approved pediatric labeling information is available. Recommended doses for agents with FDA-approved pediatric labels are the doses contained in the approved labels. Even when pediatric labeling information is not available, the FDA-approved label should be consulted for additional safety information.
[e]Comments apply to all members of each drug class except where otherwise stated.

(www.cdc.gov/growthcharts) for body mass index (BMI) are helpful in identifying the degree of excess weight and providing feedback to the child and family.

Diet modification. The contribution of sodium (Na^+) intake to elevations in BP in the young is less clear than it is in adults. Because the intake of Na^+ in Westernized societies is excessive, moderate Na^+ restriction is appropriate and seemingly without adverse nutritional consequences. Reduction in Na^+ intake to 2,500 mg per day or less is recommended for all hypertensive children and adolescents. This reasonable goal can be achieved by reducing the intake of processed foods, eliminating foods with obvious salt added (pretzels and "chips") and limiting the intake of table salt. The Dietary Approach to Stop Hypertension (DASH) study detected a beneficial effect on BP in adults of a diet that increased intake of a combination of dietary nutrients. A comparable study is yet to be conducted in children or adolescents. In view of the progressive dietary reduction in fresh fruits and vegetables and increasing intake of processed foods among the young, it is prudent and likely beneficial to encourage diet modifications that replace processed foods with fresh fruits and vegetables and low-fat dairy products that also increase dietary intake of potassium, calcium, vitamins, and other micronutrients. A reasonable approach is the "five a day" (five servings a day of fruits or vegetables).

Exercise. Secular reductions in physical activity have resulted in a more sedentary lifestyle among children and adolescents. Aerobic exercise decreases BP in hypertensive adolescents and is generally recommended for enhancing weight loss and improving cardiovascular fitness. At the other end of the spectrum, weight lifting and excessive muscle mass raises BP and should be discouraged. Physical activities and sports that emphasize aerobic exercise should be encouraged for children and adolescents. Sports participation does not impose a significant risk in hypertensive athletes. However, before sports participation a hypertensive child or adolescent should be evaluated medically and for those who require pharmacologic therapy, BP should be adequately controlled.

Other measures. In addition to the above lifestyle changes, use of tobacco, alcohol, and street drugs should be strongly discouraged. Adolescent boys with high BP who are active in competitive athletics or body-building activities should be cautioned against the use of anabolic steroids due to the potential adverse effects of these substances on BP.

Pharmacologic therapy in children and adolescents

Pharmacologic therapy for hypertension in the young is challenging for pediatricians because there are limited clinical trial data on the efficacy, safety, and dose responses for many antihypertensive drugs in children. In addition, the tablet strengths available make precise dose adjustments for small children difficult. The goal of pharmacotherapy is to restore the BP level to normal (below the 90th percentile) and in so doing lessen the risk of target organ damage.

Individualized therapy. When pharmacologic therapy is used, treatment should be individualized to achieve BP control efficiently with one or a combination of drugs at the lowest effective doses. Treatment should generally be initiated with a single antihypertensive agent with dose titration if needed. If BP control is not achieved, a second drug is added. Alternatively, if the first drug has no or insufficient effect following titration to the maximum recommended dose, or if the drug is not tolerated, then a different class of drug can be substituted. This approach differs from what has been suggested by JNC 7 wherein two drugs from different classes are advocated in those individuals whose BP is >20/10 mm Hg above target.

Specific drug choices. Thiazide diuretics, which are commonly used as a first choice drug in adults, are generally not used as the first step in antihypertensive therapy for pediatric patients, except in cases of overt fluid overload. Adrenergic blocking agents are effective for BP control but these agents can produce fatigue and compromise physical performance. Pharmacokinetic

TABLE C161.2

DRUGS FOR TREATMENT OF HYPERTENSIVE EMERGENCIES IN CHILDREN

Drug	Class	Dose[b]	Route	Comments
MOST USEFUL[a]				
Esmolol	β-Blocker	100–500 µg/kg/min	i.v. infusion	Very short-acting—constant infusion preferred; may cause profound bradycardia; produced modest reductions in BP in a pediatric clinical trial
Hydralazine	Vasodilator	0.2–0.6 mg/kg/dose	i.v., i.m.	Should be given every 4 hr when given as an i.v. bolus; recommended dose is lower than FDA label
Labetalol	α- And β-blocker	bolus: 0.2–1.0 mg/kg/dose up to 40 mg/dose infusion: 0.25–3.0 mg/kg/hr	i.v. bolus or infusion	Asthma and overt heart failure are relative contraindications
Nicardipine	Calcium channel blocker	1–3 µg/kg/min	i.v. infusion	May cause reflex tachycardia
Sodium nitroprusside	Vasodilator	0.53–10 µg/kg/min	i.v. infusion	Monitor cyanide levels with prolonged (>72 hr) use or in renal failure; or coadminister with sodium thiosulfate
OCCASIONALLY USEFUL[c]				
Clonidine	Central α-agonist	0.05–0.1 mg/dose, may be repeated up to 0.8 mg total dose	p.o.	Side effects include dry mouth and sedation
Enalaprilat	ACE inhibitor	0.05–0.1mg/kg/dose up to 1.25 mg/dose	i.v. bolus	May cause prolonged hypotension and acute renal failure, especially in neonates
Fenoldopam	Dopamine receptor agonist	0.2–0.8 µg/kg/min	i.v. infusion	Produced modest reductions in BP in a pediatric clinical trial in patients up to 12 yr
Isradipine	Calcium channel blocker	0.05–0.1 mg/kg/dose	p.o.	Stable suspension can be compounded.
Minoxidil	Vasodilator	0.1–0.2 mg/kg/dose	p.o.	Most potent oral vasodilator; long-acting

ACE, angiotensin-converting enzyme; i.m., intramuscular; i.v., intravenous; p.o., oral.
[a]Useful for hypertensive emergencies and some hypertensive urgencies.
[b]All dosing recommendations are based upon expert opinion or case series data except as otherwise noted.
[c]Useful for hypertensive urgencies and some hypertensive emergencies.

and pharmacodynamic response data in children are emerging for newer classes of antihypertensive drugs, including calcium channel blockers (CCBs), angiotensin-converting enzyme (ACE) inhibitors, and angiotensin receptor blockers (ARBs). Each can be used once daily. These drugs are effective and well tolerated in children and appear to have a good safety margin but ACE inhibitors and ARBs should be used with caution in sexually active adolescent girls because of the potential for fetal developmental defects from these drugs. The currently available information on the antihypertensive drugs used in children and adolescents is summarized in **Table C161.1.**

Hypertensive emergencies. Children who are symptomatic and have stage 2 hypertension, may require hospital admission for treatment and close monitoring of vital signs and neurologic status. The focus of treatment is to lower the BP as well as to identify the cause of the severe hypertension. Although acute elevations of BP associated with symptoms of target organ damage must be treated promptly to prevent serious complications, rapid decreases in BP should be avoided. The goal should be to decrease the BP to a safe level within a few hours, followed by a more gradual decrease to treatment goal. The treatment of hypertensive emergencies in children has traditionally relied on the use of parenteral drugs. **Table C161.2.** provides the doses of drugs used to treat hypertensive emergencies in children.

Summary

Treatment of hypertension in children and adolescents, both pharmacologic and lifestyle modification, should be tailored for each patient. The availability of the newer classes of drugs has extended the range of choices in medications to treat both chronic hypertension and hypertensive emergencies. These medications, especially those that have an extended duration of action, can provide the advantage of minimal side effects and improved compliance.

Suggested Readings

Bonilla-Felix M, Portman RJ, Falkner B. Systemic hypertension. In: Burg FD, Ingelfinger JR, Polin RA, et al. eds. *Gellis and Kagan's current pediatric therapy*, 17th ed. Philadelphia: WB Saunders, 2002:556–563.

Daniels SR, Kimball TR, Morrison JA, et al. Indexing left ventricular mass to account for differences in body size in children and adolescents without cardiovascular disease. *Am J Cardiol* 1995;76:699–701.

National High BP Education Program Working Group. The fourth report on the diagnosis, Evaluation, and Treatment of High BP in Children and Adolescents. *Pediatrics* 2004;114:555–576.

Sacks FM, Svetkey LP, Vollmer WM, et al. The DASH-Sodium Collaborative Research Group. Effects on BP of reduced dietary sodium and the dietary approaches to stop hypertension (DASH) diet. *N Engl J Med* 2001;344:3–10.

Soergel M, Kirschstein M, Busch C, et al. Oscillometric twenty-four hour ambulatory BP values in healthy children and adolescents: a multicenter trial including 1141 subjects. *J Pediatr* 1997;130:178–184.

CHAPTER C162 ■ MANAGEMENT OF HYPERTENSION AND PSYCHIATRIC DISORDERS

STEVEN L. DUBOVSKY, MD

KEY POINTS

■ In view of the frequent coincidence of hypertension and psychiatric disorders, especially of mood and anxiety, clinicians treating hypertension should be able to assess patients rapidly for concurrent psychiatric illnesses.

■ When treating hypertension in a psychiatric patient, the effects of any psychiatric medications on blood pressure (BP) should be considered.

■ If the psychiatric disorder is inadequately treated, factors specific to the disorder may be interfering with treatment adherence.

■ More severe psychiatric illnesses should be treated by a psychiatrist; a close collaboration between the psychiatrist and the clinician treating BP is often beneficial.

See also Chapters C106, C119, and C123

Psychiatric patients are more likely to have hypertension, and hypertensive patients are more likely to have comorbid psychiatric illnesses. As many as 48% of Americans have one or more lifetime affective episodes (disturbances of mood, either unipolar or bipolar), so clinicians who treat hypertension will inevitably encounter patients with psychiatric illnesses. In addition, an increasing number of psychiatric medications affect appetite and body weight and may interfere with the desired effects of antihypertensive drugs.

Interactions between hypertension and psychiatric disorders

Several factors are of interest in understanding the high coincidence of mood and anxiety disorders with hypertension and the interacting effects of their respective treatments.

Epidemiology. In a study of more than 20,000 seriously mentally ill patients in Ohio, hypertension (22%) and obesity (24%) were the most common medical comorbidities seen. Danish investigators compared more than 25,000 patients with bipolar disorder with 114,000 controls and found that patients with bipolar disorder were 1.27 times more likely to have hypertension. Hypertensive patients are also significantly more likely than the general population to have panic disorder or generalized anxiety disorder; hypertensive patients are prone to react to everyday challenges with anxiety and to have an increased risk of an anxiety disorder (22%). Clinically significant depression is also common and depressed hypertensive patients are more likely to be alcoholic and nonadherent to treatment.

Shared disease mechanisms. Hypertension and mood disorders (especially bipolar mood disorders) are both associated with hyperactive cellular calcium signaling, and elevations of platelet intracellular calcium ion concentrations have been reported both in essential hypertension and bipolar disorder. In anxiety disorders and depression, chronic overactivity of the sympathetic nervous system (SNS), diet, lifestyle, and obesity are important contributing factors.

Blood pressure effects of psychiatric drugs. Hypertension is a common side effect of a number of psychiatric medications, especially those that increase noradrenergic neurotransmission (e.g., reuptake inhibitors such as desipramine) or dopamine (DA) (e.g., bupropion, venlafaxine, and stimulants). Venlafaxine, especially at higher doses, can cause severe elevations in blood pressure (BP) and hypertensive crises. Monoamine oxidase inhibitors (MAOIs), phenelzine, isocarboxazid, tranylcypromine, selegeline, which are used to treat refractory and bipolar depression and some anxiety disorders, interact with tyramine-containing foods such as cheese to cause severe hypertension.

Psychiatric effects of antihypertensive drugs. The clinician must be aware of the psychiatric side effects of antihypertensive medications. Depression can be caused by reserpine, methyldopa, and less so by α-adrenergic blocking agents or nifedipine. Propranolol has traditionally been thought to induce depression regularly but abnormal dreams, sedation, and sexual dysfunction are more common than depression with this agent. β-Adrenergic blocking agents can also occasionally cause mania or confusion.

Substance abuse. Cocaine and alcohol abuse are common in depression and can lead to major problems in BP control. Substance abuse should be considered in any patient with refractory hypertension.

Psychiatric comorbidities and therapeutic adherence.
Approximately 50% of hypertensive patients discontinue their antihypertensives, often because of adverse effects. In a study of 233 patients who experienced multiple nonspecific adverse effects to several different medications (especially weakness, dizziness, fatigue or generally feeling ill) diastolic BP was higher and there was an increased prevalence of generalized anxiety, panic attacks, and depression. Such patients tend to be hypervigilant for anything that seems strange, dangerous or negative, perhaps leading them to focus excessively on side effects to which other patients might not pay attention. In general, patients with chronic mental disorders are less compliant with all forms of medical treatment.

There are many specific reasons why patients with chronic mental illnesses have difficulty adhering to treatment. Psychotic patients may be suspicious of the medication or the physician. Anxious patients tend to interpret minor side effects in a catastrophic manner and frequently question their safety in the physician's hands. Depressed patients may feel that they do not deserve to be well or may even covertly be attempting to commit suicide. Some patients who have been emotionally deprived and whose only caretaking is in the form of a doctor–patient relationship may hang on to that relationship by remaining ill and needing more appointments. Some people who feel chronically powerless and frustrated achieve a sense of power by defeating the physician's attempts to make them well. Addressing these issues is often necessary if the patient is to benefit from treatment for any medical condition, requiring close collaboration between the internist and the psychiatrist.

Diagnostic issues

In view of the high likelihood that hypertensive patients will have comorbid anxiety, mood disorders, or substance abuse, all patients should be screened for these conditions. Screening for anxiety disorders (**Table C162.1**), unipolar depression, and bipolar disease involves careful questioning and an understanding of the response to past treatment efforts with anxiolytics,

TABLE C162.1

PHYSICAL SYMPTOMS COMMONLY EXPERIENCED BY ANXIOUS PATIENTS

Shortness of breath
Light headedness
Paresthesias
Difficulty concentrating
Insomnia
Aches and pains
Jaw clenching
Back pain
Multiple somatic complaints
Choking
Chest pain
Tremor
Sweating
Palpitations
Feeling easily fatigued

antidepressants, and mood-stabilizing agents but in most cases, a few simple questions may be all that is required.

Effects of psychotropic medications
Some medications commonly used to treat psychiatric disorders can also be useful in hypertension, whereas others should be avoided.

Anxiolytics
Benzodiazepines. Acute anxiety is usually treated with benzodiazepines, which act on the γ-aminobutyric acid (GABA) receptor complex organized around the chloride ion channel. Occupation of benzodiazepine receptors increases affinity of GABA receptors for their agonist, increasing chloride influx and hyperpolarizing neurons in limbic and arousal centers. Reduction of activity in the locus ceruleus reduces activation of the SNS and tends to limit adrenal epinephrine release, both of which can impact favorably the heart rate (HR) and BP. Benzodiazepines have additive sedative effects with other sedating medications and may also have additive BP-lowering effects with antihypertensives in certain patients.

Abrupt discontinuation of benzodiazepines results in discontinuation syndromes, which are milder with a later onset but more prolonged with longer-acting preparations and more rapid and intense but of shorter duration with short-acting preparations. Benzodiazepine withdrawal results in sympathetic rebound, confusion, myoclonus, seizures, and elevated BP and pulse. However, more prolonged and attenuated forms of withdrawal associated with discontinuation of longer half-life benzodiazepines (e.g., chlordiazepoxide or diazepam) can result in sustained low level increases in BP.

Buspirone. Buspirone, a serotonin 5HT1A receptor partial agonist, is frequently administered for milder forms of chronic anxiety. Buspirone has a slow onset of action and does not cause sedation, psychomotor impairment, dependence, or withdrawal. It is preferred for patients who cannot tolerate these side effects (e.g., professional drivers, patients with pulmonary disease) and for patients with a history of substance abuse. Because of its serotonergic action, buspirone can have dangerous interactions with MAOIs.

Antidepressants. Several classes of antidepressants are available (**Table C162.2**). With the exception of bupropion, all of these medications are effective for anxiety and depression. Regardless of their structure, most of these medications block reuptake of serotonin, norepininephrine, or DA, thereby increasing intrasynaptic availability of these neurotransmitters in both the central and peripheral nervous system. Drugs that enhance DA activity can also elevate BP but this effect is highly variable.

Tricyclic antidepressants. Noradrenergic reuptake inhibitors (e.g., desipramine) can cause tachycardia, elevated BP, sweating, and tremor. Tricyclic antidepressants (TCAs) also interfere with the action of antihypertensives that must be taken up into presynaptic sympathetic neurons to work (e.g., guanethidine or reserpine). Anticholinergic side effects of the TCAs such as tachycardia, dry mouth, blurred vision, urinary retention, and constipation are most marked with tertiary amines such as amitriptyline, imipramine, trimipramine, and doxepin and lower with secondary amines such as desipramine and nortriptyline. Postsynaptic α_1 blockade results in BP lowering with all TCAs, but highly noradrenergic TCAs (desipramine) can elevate BP. All of the TCAs have the potential to increase appetite and weight.

Selective serotonin reuptake inhibitors. Medications that increase serotonergic activity (e.g., serotonin reuptake inhibitors) do

TABLE C162.2

ANTIDEPRESSANTS

Drug	Neurotransmitter action	Usual dose (mg)	Blood pressure effects	Comments
Tricyclic antidepressants (TCA)				
Imipramine	5HT, NE uptake inhibition	150–300	Postural hypotension	Adjusted by blood level
Desipramine	NE uptake inhibition	150–300	Increased BP	Therapeutic window
Amitriptyline	5HT, NE uptake inhibition	150–300	Postural hypotension	Anticholinergic
Nortriptyline	NE uptake inhibition	75–150	Increased pulse and BP	Therapeutic window
Doxepin	NE uptake inhibition; H1 blockade	150–300	Postural hypotension	Useful as antihistamine and for peptic ulcer
Trimipramine	NE, 5HT uptake inhibition	150–300		As for doxepin
Maprotiline	NE uptake inhibition	150–225		Tetracyclic structure; seizures at doses >225 mg/d
Amoxapine	NE uptake inhibition, D2 blockade	150–300	Increased BP or postural hypotension	Neuroleptic effect can cause extrapyramidal side effects; seizures at high doses
Clomipramine	5HT, NE uptake inhibition	150–250	Postural hypotension	Only TCA effective for OCD
Serotonin reuptake inhibitors				
Fluoxetine	5HT uptake inhibition	10–40	Negligible	Half-life 3 d
Paroxetine		10–50		Anticholinergic; causes weight gain; not for use in children
Sertraline		50–200		Minimal P450 effects
Fluvoxamine		150–300		Only SSRI requires divided dosing
Citalopram		20–40		No P450 interactions
Escitalopram		10–20		S-enantiomer of citalopram with similar effects
Third-generation antidepressants				
Trazodone	5HT2, α₁ antagonism	50–600	Hypotension	Can cause priapism at any dose; requires divided dosing as antidepressant
Nefazodone	5HT2 antagonism, 5HT uptake inhibition	200–600	Hypotension	Can improve sleep structure; rare cases of severe/fatal hepatotoxicity reported
Bupropion	NE, DA uptake inhibition	150–450	Mild hypertension	No sexual or cardiac effects; seizure risk at doses >450 mg
Serotonin norepinephrine reuptake inhibitors (SNRIs)				
Venlafaxine	5HT, NE, DA uptake inhibition	75–375	Severe hypertension possible at higher doses	Useful for severe and treatment-resistant depression; divided dose necessary at higher doses of XR formulation
Duloxetine	5HT, NE uptake inhibition	60–120	Mild hypertension possible	b.i.d. dosing
Monoamine oxidase inhibitors				
Phenelzine	Inhibition of intraneural metabolism of 5HT, NE, DA	30–90	Hypotension; hypertension with dietary interactions	Anticholinergic; causes weight gain
Isocarboxazid	As for phenelzine	20–60	As for phenelzine	Less sedation and weight gain than phenelzine
Tranylcypromine	As for phenelzine; metabolite releases DA	30–90	Less hypotension than phenelzine; spontaneous hypertension possible	More activating; amphetamine-like actions
Selegiline	As for tranylcypromine	20–50	No hypotension; no dietary interactions at doses ≤10 mg	Minimal antidepressant effect at doses <20 mg; patch available but benefit may not justify cost

b.i.d., twice daily; 5HT, serotonin; NE, norepinephrine; HR, heart rate; BP, blood pressure; H1, histamine 1 receptor; D2, dopamine 2 receptor; 5HT2, serotonin-2 receptor; SSRI, selective serotonin reuptake inhibitor; OCD, obsessive compulsive disorder; DA, dopamine; XR, extended release.

not typically increase BP and are more likely to cause headaches, gastrointestinal hypermotility, sedation, and sexual dysfunction; selective serotonin reuptake inhibitors (SSRIs) can also have noradrenergic side effects such as tachycardia and sweating. Medications in this class differ in their elimination half-lives and in their capacity to inhibit CYP450 enzymes. For example, fluoxetine and paroxetine are potent inhibitors of CYP2D6, which metabolizes metoprolol and propranolol. Trazodone is primarily an antagonist of serotonin 5HT2 receptors. Concomitant blockade of α_1 adrenergic receptors can cause priapism that is not dose related or hypotension. Nefazodone combines SSRI and 5HT2 antagonist properties and has negligible effects on BP. Norepinephrine (NE) and, to some extent, DA reuptake inhibition by bupropion conveys the potential to increase BP. Venlafaxine, which is particularly useful for treatment-resistant depression, inhibits serotonin reuptake at doses <75 mg. As the dose increases, norepinephrine reuptake and then DA reuptake are also inhibited. The latter effect produces a risk of a significant increase in BP in some patients and should not be given to hypertensive patients. Duloxetine inhibits reuptake of serotonin and norepinephrine, but not DA, at all doses, resulting in a lower risk of hypertension. Mirtazepine antagonizes serotonin 5HT2 and 5HT3 receptors as well as presynaptic norepinephrine α_2 receptors, which increases norepinephrine release, with the potential to elevate BP. Venlafaxine, bupropion, and mirtazepine are therefore not initial choices for hypertensive patients with depression.

Monoamine oxidase inhibitors. Despite their potential to cause dangerous hypertensive reactions when combined with tyramine-containing foods and some dopaminergic agents, MAOIs have a primary hypotensive effect, especially phenelzine and isocarboxazid. Additive hypotensive effects with medications used to treat hypertension are more common than are hypertensive reactions with these compounds.

Mood stabilizers. Diverse medication classes have mood-stabilizing effects, including lithium, some anticonvulsants (valproate, carbamazepine, oxcarbazepine, possibly levetiracetam), and calcium channel blockers (CCBs). Lithium slows the rate of depolarization of the sinus node and slows conduction through the AV node, which can reduce HR with only a minimal impact on BP. Carbamazepine can occasionally slow HR and lower BP, especially in older women. Carbamazepine is a potent inducer of CYP 3A4, whereas valproate can displace a number of medications from binding proteins.

Antipsychotics. Two broad categories of antipsychotic medications are available: neuroleptics and "atypical" agents. Representative members of each group are illustrated in **Table C162.3**.

Neuroleptics. The "typical" neuroleptic antipsychotic drugs have more neurologic side effects than the newer "atypical" or "second generation" antipsychotics. Low potency neuroleptics (e.g., chlorpromazine, thioridazine), which are administered in higher doses, are less likely to cause parkinsonism, akathisia, and other acute extrapyramidal syndromes but they have more anticholinergic and hypotensive side effects (as a result of α-adrenergic blockade) and cause more weight gain, similar to the TCAs. High-potency neuroleptics induce more severe acute extrapyramidal side effects but they are associated with less hypotension and fewer anticholinergic side effects.

Atypical agents. The atypical antipsychotics comprise a diverse group of compounds that seem to have a lower incidence of acute extrapyramidal side effects and fewer anticholinergic side effects than the neuroleptics. Aripiprazole and ziprasidone do not have significant cardiovascular (CV) side effects, whereas hypotension

TABLE C162.3

SOME ANTIPSYCHOTIC DRUGS

Drug	Cardiac/blood pressure effects
Low potency neuroleptics	
Chlorpromazine	Weight gain, hypotension, heart block
Thioridazine	Weight gain, hypotension, anticholinergic effects, sudden cardiac death
High-potency neuroleptics	
Haloperidol	Torsades de pointe
Fluphenazine	Hypotension
Atypical antipsychotics	
Risperidone	Prolactinemia, hypotension
Olanzapine	Weight gain, diabetes, sedation
Quetiapine	Sedation, weight gain
Ziprasidone	Agitation
Aripiprazole	Affect blunting
Clozapine	Sedation, hypotension, weight gain, diabetes, cardiomyopathy

may occasionally occur with risperidone and more commonly with olanzapine, quetiapine, or clozapine. Of greatest concern for BP control is the tendency of olanzapine or clozapine to cause weight gain, diabetes mellitus, or hyperlipidemia. Body weight, blood sugar, and BP should be monitored periodically in all patients taking atypical antipsychotics other than ziprasidone and aripiprazole, as well as the low potency neuroleptics.

Stimulants. Stimulants [e.g., methylphenidate, dextroamphetamine, and mixed amphetamine salts (Adderall)] are well-established treatments for attention deficit disorder and are also used to treat narcolepsy and some cases of depression. All of these medications elevate BP as a result of a direct action on DA receptors or release of DA from presynaptic sympathetic neurons. Atomoxetine is a noradrenergic tricyclic with a capacity to elevate BP and interfere with antihypertensive agents that must be taken up into presynaptic neurons. Stimulants can also displace other medications from binding proteins, elevating free drug levels.

Psychiatric effects of antihypertensive drugs

A number of medications, the primary use of which is to treat hypertension, also have psychiatric applications (**Table C162.4**).

β-Adrenergic blockers. The β-adrenergic blocker pindolol was initially reported to augment antidepressants but this effect has not been confirmed. Propranolol continues to be an effective treatment for performance anxiety when given in a single dose and is used regularly as a treatment for akathisia induced by antipsychotic drugs. As in other settings, the benefit of propranolol can be limited by sedation.

Clonidine. Clonidine is used routinely for hyperactivity in children with attention deficit hyperactivity disorder (ADHD) and may reduce hypertension caused by stimulants coadministered to treat inattention. Clonidine is effective but the risks (sedation, cognitive impairment, and aggravation of depression) often outweigh the benefits, especially because clonidine-induced rebound hypertension may be exacerbated by stimulants.

Calcium channel blockers. Verapamil has been shown to be superior to placebo and similar to lithium in the treatment of mania, and in some studies it has been useful as maintenance treatment. Verapamil is not only a consideration in hypertensive

TABLE C162.4

ANTIHYPERTENSIVES USED TO TREAT ANXIETY

Medication	Disorder/ symptoms	Comments
Captopril	Depression	Usually well tolerated
Pindolol	Depression	Not confirmed in controlled trials
Propranolol	Performance anxiety, akathisia	Sedation and sexual side effects
Clonidine	Hyperactivity in ADHD	Cognitive dysfunction, sedation, and rebound hypertension can be problems
Prazosin	Nightmares in PTSD	Dosing limited by daytime sedation
Verapamil	Bipolar disorder	Especially in pregnant patients needing pharmacotherapy; immediate release form often necessary

ADHD, attention deficit hyperactivity disorder; PTSD, post-traumatic stress disorder

patients with bipolar disorder, but is also useful in patients with cognitive dysfunction because it lacks the cognition-suppressing side effects of other mood stabilizers. Sustained release preparations are not as reliably effective for this indication as are immediate release forms of verapamil. Nimodipine has also been found to be useful in bipolar disorder.

α-Blockers. Prazosin has recently been shown to reduce nightmares and arousal in response to trauma-specific cues, and to improve sleep in post-traumatic stress disorder.

Angiotensin-converting enzyme inhibitors. Captopril has been noted in case series to improve mood in depressed hypertensive patients.

Suggested Readings

Barger SD, Sydeman SJ. Does generalized anxiety disorder predict coronary heart disease risk factors independently of major depressive disorder? *J Affect Disord* 2005;88:87–91.

Baune BT, Adrian I, Arolt V, et al. Associations between major depression, bipolar disorders, dysthymia and cardiovascular diseases in the general adult population. *Psychother Psychosom* 2006;75:319–326.

Bosworth HB, Bartash RM, Olsen MK, et al. The association of psychosocial factors and depression with hypertension among older adults. *Int J Geriatr Psychiatry* 2003;18:1142–1148.

Davies SJC, Jackson PR, Ramsay LE, et al. Drug intolerance due to nonspecific adverse effects related to psychiatric morbidity in hypertensive patients. *Arch Intern Med* 2003;163:592–600.

Dubovsky SL. Calcium antagonists in manic-depressive illness. *Neuropsychobiology* 1993;27(3):184–192.

Gump BB, Matthews KA, Eberly LE, et al. Depressive symptoms and mortality in men: results from the Multiple Risk Factor Intervention Trial. *Stroke* 2005;36:98–102.

Johannessen L, Strudsholm U, Foldager L, et al. Increased risk of hypertension in patients with bipolar disorder and patients with anxiety compared to background population and patients with schizophrenia. *J Affect Disord* 2006;95:13–17.

Khurana RN, Baudendistel TE. Hypertensive crisis associated with venlafaxine. *Am J Med* 2003;115:676–677.

Kim MT, Han HR, Hill MN, et al. Depression, substance use, adherence behaviors, and blood pressure in urban hypertensive black men. *Ann Behav Med* 2003;26:24–31.

Miller BJ, Paschall CB, Svendsen DP. Mortality and medical comorbidity among patients with serious mental illness. *Psychiatr Serv* 2006;57:1482–1487.

CHAPTER C163 ■ HYPERTENSION IN ATHLETES

JOHN J. LEDDY, MD, FACSM

KEY POINTS

■ Elevated blood pressure (BP) is one of the most common abnormalities found during the preparticipation physical evaluation of athletes and hypertension (HTN) is the most common cardiovascular (CV) disease encountered in the athletic population.

■ Athletes often have the "white coat effect"; additional BP recordings outside the office should be obtained and compared to office readings.

■ The 36th Bethesda Conference classified sports according to varying physiologic demands and provided specific recommendations for the evaluation, treatment, and sport participation of athletes with HTN; sports governing bodies also proscribe the use of certain medications.

■ Angiotensin-converting enzyme (ACE) inhibitors and other vasodilators are generally the medications of choice for active and athletic patients.

See also Chapters B91, C103, C112, and C121

Blood pressure patterns in athletes and physically active people

Sustained hypertension. Hypertension (HTN) in adults older than 18 years is defined as blood pressure (BP) elevations ≥140/90 mm Hg on at least two separate occasions; in children and adolescents as average systolic or diastolic BP ≥ the 95th percentile for gender, age, and height. HTN prevalence in the physically active is approximately 50% lower than in the general population, but the risk of HTN is increased in some athletes and physically active patients, including blacks, the elderly, the obese, and those with diabetes or renal disease. Wheelchair athletes with spinal cord injuries may also have severe BP elevations because of loss of autonomic control of BP. Almost 80% of adolescents with BP >142/92 mm Hg during a preparticipation physical evaluation (PPE) will eventually develop chronically elevated BP; therefore, BP should be closely monitored in all athletes and physically active patients.

White coat hypertension. It is critical to avoid a cavalier diagnosis of HTN because athletes often have the "white coat effect" (marked home–office BP difference). In a study of 410 athletes (aged 16.4 ± 2.6 years), 18 hypertensive patients (4.4%) were detected and evaluated with a 24-hour ambulatory blood pressure monitoring (ABPM). Sixteen of these had "white coat hypertension" (normal 24-hour average, daytime and nocturnal BP). Therefore, out-of-office BP recordings should be obtained in anyone with elevated office readings, either with home self-recorders or automatic ambulatory monitors.

Isolated systolic hypertension. Many conditioned athletes (particularly young men) have "athlete's heart" with very high resting stroke volume and cardiac output with low systemic vascular resistance and heart rate. Pulse pressure and systolic BP are high in these individuals, very often in the range of prehypertension and occasionally in the range of stage 1 HTN.

Spurious systolic hypertension. Another hemodynamic anomaly leading to high systolic BP and wide pulse pressure is the syndrome of "spurious systolic hypertension (SSH)," where amplification of the systolic pulse wave within the vasculature can lead to "hypertensive" BP values in the arm despite low or normal central systolic BP (see Chapter C112). This condition was discovered through the use of radial tonometry. Using a definition for SSH as a brachial systolic BP >140 with a central systolic BP <125 mm Hg, Hulsen et al. found 57 cases among young men and three cases among young women among the 750 participants in the Atherosclerosis Risk in Young Adults Study. 20-year Framingham risk scores in the SSH group were intermediate between normotensive and hypertensive patients but not significantly different from normotensive persons. Therefore, any risk increment attributable to SSH appears to be minimal at best but the natural history of the condition requires further study.

Evaluation

History. The athlete should be questioned about family history of HTN and premature cardiovascular (CV) disease and any symptoms of exertional chest pain, unusual dyspnea, or declining performance. Behavioral history is also important, including intake of sodium and saturated fats (e.g., in processed and "fast" foods), the use of alcohol, drugs (specifically, stimulants taken before competitions, or cocaine), tobacco, human growth hormone, or anabolic steroids. Alcohol consumption is frequent in scholastic athletes, the use of which in the evening can cause elevated morning BP readings. Athletes may be taking other substances or over-the-counter medications that can increase BP, including nonsteroidal anti-inflammatory drugs (NSAIDs), caffeine, diet pills, decongestants, herbs, and dietary supplements (especially those purported to increase energy or control weight), which often contain "natural" stimulants such as guanara, ma huang, and ephedra. Female athletes should be questioned about oral contraceptives because approximately 5% of all women who take them develop HTN over a 5-year period.

Physical examination. Standard BP measurement techniques should be rigorously employed (see Chapter C103). Particular attention should be paid to the measurement conditions (sitting quietly for 5 minutes with the back supported in a chair, feet on the floor, and the arm supported at the level of the heart), cuff size (large adult size for mid-arm circumference >33 cm and a child's cuff for mid-arm circumference <23 cm) and inflation technique (at least 20 mm greater than the disappearance of the radial pulse to avoid the "auscultatory gap"). If the arm BP is elevated, take the measurement in one leg (particularly in patients younger than 30 years). Initially, take pressures in both arms; if the BPs differ, use the arm with the higher BP. A full examination and standard screening should be performed (see Chapter C105). Secondary HTN probably has roughly the same prevalence in athletes as it does in the age-adjusted general population.

Echocardiogram. Any athlete with sustained BP elevation is recommended to have an echocardiogram. Left ventricular hypertrophy (LVH) beyond the "athlete's heart" should limit participation until the BP is normalized. This may be a problem for highly trained athletes because the distinction between the physiologic hypertrophy of "athlete's heart" and the pathologic hypertrophy of hypertensive heart disease is often unclear. Athletic LVH tends to be eccentric and associated with large chamber sizes and normal diastolic function whereas hypertensive LVH tends to be concentric and may be associated with diastolic dysfunction. In particular, intensive weight training and power lifting tend to cause concentric LVH, whereas aerobic activities tend to cause eccentric hypertrophy. Hypertensive athletes with ambiguous findings on echocardiography require cardiology consultation and may need to undergo a brief period of deconditioning (to look for partial regression of left ventricle wall thickness) or have genetic testing to evaluate for the possibility of familial hypertrophic cardiomyopathy.

Participation recommendations for athletes with hypertension

Task Force Five of the 36th Bethesda Conference provides recommendations for athletes with CV or structural abnormalities to prevent sudden cardiac death or disease progression (**Table C163.1**).

Because different sports place different physiologic demands on the athlete, sports are categorized into two general types: dynamic (producing a volume load on the LV) and static (producing a pressure load on the LV). Sports are further classified according to level of intensity: low, medium, and high, and also as to whether there is a contact/collision component (**Figure C163.1**). Physicians can use **Figure C163.1** as a guide to help to determine whether it is reasonably safe to recommend participation in competitive

TABLE C163.1

SUMMARY OF RECOMMENDATIONS OF THE 36TH BETHESDA CONFERENCE FOR HYPERTENSION (HTN) IN ATHLETES

1. Before training for competitive athletics, full assessment of blood pressure (BP) is needed. If office BP high (≥140/90 mm Hg), home BP of 24-h ambulatory BP should be measured to exclude "white coat" HTN. Those with pre-HTN (120/80 mm Hg up to 139/89 mm Hg) should be encouraged to modify lifestyle but should not be restricted from physical activity. Those with sustained HTN should have echocardiography. Left ventricular hypertrophy (LVH) beyond that seen with "athletes' heart" should limit participation until BP is normalized by appropriate drug therapy.
2. The presence of stage 1 HTN in the absence of target organ damage including LVH or concomitant heart disease should not limit the eligibility for any competitive sport. Once training is begun, the hypertensive athlete should have BP remeasured every 2–4 mo (or more frequently, if indicated) to monitor the impact of exercise.
3. Athletes with stage 2 HTN, even without evidence of LVH or other target organ damage should be restricted, particularly from high static sports (classes IIIA–IIIC), until hypertension is controlled by lifestyle modification or drug therapy.
4. All drugs being taken must be registered with appropriate governing bodies to obtain a therapeutic exemption.
5. When HTN coexists with another cardiovascular (CV) disease, eligibility for participation in competitive athletics is usually based on the type and severity of the associated condition.

(From Kaplan NM, Gidding SS, Pickering TG, et al. Task Force 5: systemic hypertension. *J Am Coll Cardiol* 2005;45:1346–1348, with permission.)

sports for athletes with HTN or to suggest activities suitable for cross-training to keep athletes active and aerobically conditioned during workup or treatment.

Many physical activities involve both static and dynamic components. For example, distance running has low static and high dynamic demands, water skiing has principally high static and low dynamic demands, and rowing has both high static and dynamic demands. Therefore, sports can be classified (**Figure C163.1**) as IIIC (high static, high dynamic), IIB (moderate static, moderate dynamic), IA (low static, low dynamic), and so on. For example, an athlete with stage II HTN that contraindicates sports associated with high pressure loads on the LV would be advised to avoid sports classified as IIIA, IIIB, and IIIC but may be able to participate in a IA sport until evaluation is complete and the BP is under control. Such decisions must be individualized. Physicians must also be aware that many athletes now use heavy resistance weight training (high static and low dynamic demand) for increasing strength and power in sports that do not include heavy static demands during competition (e.g., tennis, basketball). It may be possible to modify the training regimen to reduce the CV demands to an acceptable level.

Treatment of the hypertensive athlete

Untreated HTN in athletes may be accompanied by some limitation in exercise performance.

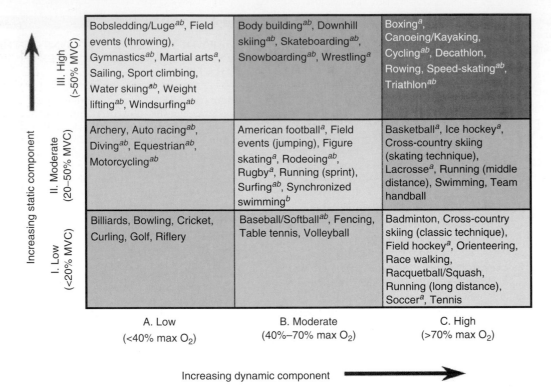

Increasing static component

III. High (>50% MVC)

II. Moderate (20–50% MVC)

I. Low (<20% MVC)

A. Low (<40% max O₂)

B. Moderate (40%–70% max O₂)

C. High (>70% max O₂)

Increasing dynamic component

Figure C163.1 Classification of sports. This classification is based on peak static and dynamic components achieved during competition. It should be noted, however, that higher values may be reached during training. The increasing dynamic component is defined in terms of the estimated percent of maximal oxygen uptake (max O_2) achieved and results in an increasing cardiac output. The increasing static component is related to the estimated percent of maximal voluntary contraction (MVC) reached and results in an increasing blood pressure (BP) load. The lowest total cardiovascular (CV) demands (cardiac output and BP) are in box 1A and the highest in box IIIC. Boxes IIA and IB depict low moderate, boxes IIIA, IIB and IC depict moderate, and boxes IIIB, and IIC depict high moderate total CV demands, respectively. [a]Danger of bodily collision; [b]Increased risk if syncope occurs. (Reprinted from Mitchell JH, Haskell W, Snell P, et al. Task Force 8: classification of sports. *J Am Coll Cardiol* 2005;45:1364–1367, with permission.)

Lifestyle modification. Although healthy lifestyle behaviors may not eliminate the need for antihypertensive drug therapy, they may reduce the amount of medication needed. Dietary and lifestyle changes include decreasing sodium intake (especially for African-American patients, the elderly and those with diabetes); increasing potassium intake (especially important in endurance athletes, who may be hypokalemic); losing weight; decreasing alcohol consumption; avoiding tobacco in any form, drugs of abuse (especially sympathomimetics such as cocaine or ephedra), androgens, anabolic steroids, growth hormone, and NSAIDs; applying relaxation techniques; and, for athletes in static sports, performing regular aerobic exercise.

Medication choices. The most common medications used for the treatment of HTN in athletes are the vasodilators. Angiotensin-converting enzyme (ACE) inhibitors are a good choice because they have no major effects on energy metabolism and cause no impairment of maximum oxygen uptake. The major side effect is a dry, nonproductive cough and rarely angioedema, which is approximately three- to five-fold more common in African Americans than whites or Asians. Because there have been anecdotal reports of postural hypotension after intense exercise in patients taking ACE inhibitors, an adequate cool-down period is recommended. Their effectiveness may be improved by adding a thiazide in a low dosage, especially in African Americans. The potassium-sparing effect of ACE inhibitors may

be increased when these agents are taken concomitantly with NSAIDs. Angiotensin-II receptor blockers (ARBs) produce similar effects as ACE inhibitors; however, they do not cause a dry cough. Patients of childbearing age should use some form of contraception if they are taking an ACE inhibitor, an ARB or a renin inhibitor (RI). ARBs, RIs and the calcium channel blockers are reasonable alternatives for athletes intolerant of ACE inhibitors. Thiazide diuretics are useful as second-line therapy in salt-sensitive athletes and physically active patients with HTN. They should be given in a low dosage and, in some patients, combined with a potassium-sparing agent. Thiazides are a good choice in patients who exercise only casually, in physically active elderly patients, and in African-American patients. Possible side effects include hypovolemia, orthostatic hypotension, and urinary loss of potassium and magnesium. These side effects can lead to muscle cramps, arrhythmias, and rhabdomyolysis in patients who are exercising intensely or competing in warm weather. β-Blockers are a poor choice for athletes because they limit exercise capacity.

Banned substances. Physicians and athletes need to be aware that the World Anti-Doping Agency, the U.S. Olympic Committee, and the National Collegiate Athletic Association have banned the use of some antihypertensive medications. Sports regulatory bodies have banned the use of all diuretics, so thiazides cannot be used by elite athletes who require random drug testing. β-Blockers are banned for archery and shooting sports.

Suggested Readings

Chick TW, Halperin AK, Gacek EM. The effect of antihypertensive medications on exercise performance: a review. *Med Sci Sports Exerc* 1988;20:447–454.

Hulsen HT, Nijdam ME, Bos WJ, et al. Spurious systolic hypertension in young adults: prevalence of high brachial systolic blood pressure and low central pressure and its determinants. *J Hypertens* 2006;24:1027–1032.

Kaplan NM, Gidding SS, Pickering TG, et al. Task Force 5: systemic hypertension. *J Am Coll Cardiol* 2005;45:1346–1348.

Kouidi E, Fahadidou-Tsiliroglou A, Tassoulas E, et al. White coat hypertension detected during screening of male adolescent athletes. *Am J Hypertens* 1999;12:223–226.

Mahmud A, Feely J. Spurious systolic hypertension of youth: fit young men with elastic arteries. *Am J Hypertens* 2003;16:229–232.

Mitchell JH, Haskell W, Snell P, et al. Task Force 8: classification of sports. *J Am Coll Cardiol* 2005;45:1364–1367.

National High Blood Pressure Education Working Group on High Blood Pressure in Children and Adolescents. The fourth report on the diagnosis, evaluation, and treatment of high blood pressure in children and adolescents. *Pediatrics* 2004;114: 555–576.

Niedfeldt MW. Managing hypertension in athletes and physically active patients. *Am Fam Physician* 2002;66:445–452.

O'Connor FG, Meyering CD, Patel R, et al. Hypertension, athletes, and the sports physician: implications of JNC VII, the fourth report, and the 36th Bethesda conference guidelines. *Curr Sports Med Rep* 2007;6:80–84.

World Anti-Doping Agency. *The World Anti-Doping Code. The 2007 Prohibited List. International Standard*, 2007. Accessed 6/12/07. http://www.usantidoping .org/files/active/athletes/2007%20Prohibited%20List.pdf.

CHAPTER C164 ■ PERIOPERATIVE MANAGEMENT OF HYPERTENSION

JOHN D. BISOGNANO, MD, PhD AND MICHAEL W. FONG, MD

KEY POINTS

■ Patients with preexisting hypertension have greater blood pressure (BP) lability and likelihood of electrocardiographic changes during anesthesia but it has not been clearly established that modest elevations of BP increase cardiovascular (CV) morbidity and mortality in the perioperative period.

■ BP elevations >180/110 mm Hg during surgery warrant therapy with intravenous agents.

■ Continuing home BP medications until surgery and reestablishing a good regimen postoperatively are key strategies to preventing perioperative hypertension and its potential complications.

See also Chapter C146

Perioperative hypertension is an elevation of blood pressure (BP) in the pre-, intra-, or postoperative period that most commonly occurs in patients with preexisting hypertension and is thought to confer an increased risk for adverse cardiovascular (CV) events. Treatment guidelines for chronic hypertension management in the clinic setting are clear but there is no current consensus on the level of BP elevation in the perioperative period that warrants treatment. Moreover, existing perceptions about risk are based on observational studies, with little or no prospective randomized evidence to support them. The incidence of the problem has also not been well described, in part, because of an absence of uniform definitional criteria for what constitutes perioperative hypertension.

Pathophysiology

Blood pressure regulatory systems. BP elevations are sustained by the sympathetic nervous system (SNS), renin-angiotensin system (RAS), and possibly vasopressin, all of which increase the concentration of intracellular free calcium and degree of constriction of vascular smooth muscle cells. Anesthesia predominantly interferes with the SNS, and differences among initial responses to anesthetic agents and their subsequent withdrawal are mainly related to their effects on the SNS (**Table C164.1**). Decreased sympathetic tone during anesthesia results in a relative decrease in cardiac preload and afterload and reduced release of renin. Under these circumstances endogenous vasopressin assumes a greater homeostatic role facilitating BP regulation through binding to V_1 receptors.

Effect of intubation. Stimulation of the larynx by endotracheal intubation causes a subcortical reflex response that results in sympathetic activation, with increased heart rate (HR) and mean arterial BP. Anesthetic agents are given before intubation to minimize this response but intubation can increase BP acutely by as much as 25 mm Hg. Advanced age and preexisting hypertension exacerbate this phenomenon. HR increases almost invariably with intubation but BP response depends on the type of laryngoscope and tube used; the MacIntosh laryngoscope results in a significant

TABLE C164.1

ANESTHETICS AND OTHER AGENTS

Agent	Effect	Duration
Narcotics		
Alfentanil (Alfenta)	Blunts the sympathetic response	10–15 min
Fentanyl (Sublimaze)		30–45 min
Sufentanil (Sufenta)		60 min
Meperidine (Demerol)		2–3 h
Morphine sulfate		2–4 h
Sedative/Hypnotics		
Etomidate (Amidate)	BP unchanged	3–10 min
Propofol (Diprivan)	Decreases BP	5–10 min
Methohexital (Brevital)	Decreases BP	5–10 min
Thiopental (Pentothal)	BP unchanged	5–15 min
Ketamine (Ketalar)	BP unchanged	5–15 min
Muscle relaxants		
Depolarizing		
Succinylcholine (Anectine)	BP unchanged	4–6 min
Nondepolarizing		
Mivacurium (Mivacron)	Unchanged or decreased BP	5–15 min
Rocuronium (Zemuron)	BP unchanged	30–60 min
Vecuronium (Norcuron)	BP unchanged	30–60 min
Atracurium (Tracrium)	Decreases BP	30–60 min
Cistracurium (Nimbex)	BP unchanged	30–60 min
Pancuronium (Pavulon)	Increases BP	45–60 min
Maintenance agents		
Inhalation		
Sevoflurane (Ultane)	Activate the sympathetic nervous system	4–14 min
Desflurane (Suprane)		5–16 min
Isoflurane (Forane)		7–10 min
Intravenous	Decreases BP	
Propofol (Diprivan)	BP unchanged	5–10 min
Ketamine (Ketalar)	Decreases BP	5–15 min
Narcotic agents	Decreases BP	As in the preceding text
Benzodiazepines		Variable
Emergence/Reversal agents		
Anticholinesterase		
Edrophonium	BP unchanged	60–70 min
Neostigmine	BP unchanged	60–80 min
Anticholinergics		
Atropine	BP unchanged	60–90 min
Glycopyrrolate	BP unchanged	2–4 h

BP, blood pressure.

increase in BP but the Trachlight lightwand and laryngeal mask airway Fastrach do not raise BP.

Anesthetic agents. With the use of *inhaled* agents during the maintenance period of anesthesia, sympathetic activation can still occur raising the BP by 20 to 30 mm Hg and the HR by 15 to 20 beats per minute in normotensive patients. The response in patients with preexisting hypertension tends to be much more robust, with BP elevations as great as 90 mm Hg and increases in HR up to 40 beats per minute. In contrast, *intravenous* anesthesia is more commonly associated with inhibition of the SNS and loss of baroreceptor reflex control, which cause the mean arterial BP to fall as anesthesia progresses. Patients with preexisting hypertension tend to have a greater degree of BP lability, and significant drops in BP can occur with the potential for precipitating cerebral or myocardial ischemia.

Perioperative risk

Perioperative hypertension (diastolic BPs >110 mm Hg) is thought to be associated with an increased risk for adverse outcomes [CV death, myocardial infarction, cerebrovascular accident, heart failure (HF), and life-threatening arrhythmias] but there are few convincing data to corroborate any impact of lesser BP elevations. Minor complications such as tachycardia, bradycardia, and hypotension are relatively common in hypertensive patients during the perioperative period. The hypothesis that CV risk can be reduced by postponing surgery to control hypertension has also never been studied prospectively in a randomized manner. In general, studies attempting to assess if admission arterial pressure correlates with perioperative risk have been substantially underpowered and have not looked at BP as a continuous variable.

A meta-analysis of observational studies was recently performed in an attempt to answer the question of whether the diagnosis of hypertension itself results in a greater perioperative risk. Although the odds ratio in this meta-analysis was statistically significant, the effect was small, likely due in part to the low perioperative event rate and the heterogeneity between the groups. ***Systolic hypertension.*** The risk of systolic hypertension is also not clear, although one study demonstrated that patients with systolic BP >200 mm Hg during carotid endarterectomy were at greater risk of neurologic deficits. In a prospective study examining patients undergoing elective cardiac surgery, isolated systolic hypertension conferred a small but statistically significant increase in the risk of perioperative morbidity compared to the general population. Also, if systolic BP is >180 mm Hg, electrocardiogram (ECG) abnormalities are more frequent, BP lability during surgery is increased, and there is a trend toward myocardial ischemia in the postoperative period. ***Target organ damage.*** There does appear to be a trend toward increased risk for adverse outcomes in those with elevated BPs and evidence of target organ damage at the time of admission. As in the broader population, overall increases in CV events have not been definitively established, however, due to their low incidence and the relatively small sample sizes in existing studies.

Therapy

Current guidelines. The 2002 American College of Cardiology/American Heart Association (ACC/AHA) guideline for the management of preoperative hypertension lists uncontrolled hypertension as a minor risk factor for perioperative myocardial infarction, HF, or death. This guideline does advocate treating JNC-6 stage 3 hypertension (systolic BP >180 mm Hg or diastolic BP >110 mm Hg) before surgery. Ideally, this is accomplished by establishing an adequate oral antihypertensive regimen and controlling BP over several days to weeks. If surgery is urgently needed, control of BP can be achieved over minutes to hours with the administration of intravenous agents, especially labetalol. ***Specific drugs.*** The importance of maintaining antihypertensive regimens before surgery is worth noting. The discontinuation of a stable outpatient regimen has the potential to lead to uncontrolled hypertension preoperatively, especially if there is cessation of sympatholytic drugs (clonidine or rarely, β-blockers). **Angiotensin-converting enzyme inhibitors and angiotensin receptor blockers.** There has been much debate in the literature over the use of angiotensin-converting enzyme (ACE) inhibitors and angiotensin receptor blockers (ARBs) in the perioperative period due in part to their potential central vagotonic effects. These agents alone or in combination have been associated with moderate hypotension and bradycardia, particularly when discontinued <10 hours before surgery. At least one prospective randomized trial has shown these effects to be more pronounced with ARBs and a few experts have recommended discontinuing ACE inhibitors or ARBs at least 24 hours before surgery. There is mixed evidence that prophylaxis with glycopyrrolate, a muscarinic anticholinergic agent, can attenuate these effects.

Diuretics. Careful attention must be paid to the potassium level in patients on diuretics. In addition to increasing the risk for arrhythmias and postoperative ileus, hypokalemia may potentiate the effects of depolarizing and nondepolarizing muscle relaxants.

Calcium channel blockers. In one observational study in older patients with hip fractures, the use of calcium channel blockers (CCBs) was associated with an increased risk for perioperative blood transfusion, presumably due to inhibition of platelet aggregation. Although the finding is interesting, the study looked at a very specific population and the results have not been confirmed by a randomized trial.

β-Blockers. β-Blockers have been shown to reduce perioperative CV complications in high-risk patients in randomized-controlled trials, and should be used whenever possible in this population. Use of these agents in low-risk populations is probably unnecessary and may actually increase the risk of adverse outcomes.

Intraoperative hypertension

Several factors should be taken into consideration when deciding whether to intervene for intraoperative hypertension. Traditional concerns about microcirculatory damage (e.g., retinopathy) in the setting of a hypertensive emergency may be less relevant in the intraoperative setting but at the same time, elevated systolic BP during surgery may increase bleeding or adversely affect cardiac afterload, especially in patients with compromised myocardial function or during cardiopulmonary bypass.

Blood pressure levels. Although no clear guidelines exist for when to treat intraoperative hypertension, there does not seem to be a higher incidence of adverse outcomes with systolic BPs <180 mm Hg. For systolic BP values >180 mm Hg, there are even fewer data but treatment is generally favored. Observational data suggests that increases in BP >20% above baseline in patients with preexisting hypertension or diabetes increases perioperative complications. Therefore, invasive arterial monitoring during major surgery is warranted, and a 20% deviation may be used as a starting point at which to consider therapy in those patients.

Specific drugs. Measures commonly used to control hypertension during this period include deepening of sedation, the use of vasodilators such as nitroglycerin or nitroprusside, or a combination of the two. Suppressing cardiac SNS activity with β-blockers, particularly following activation by inhaled maintenance agents, can also be useful. β-Blockers have been shown

TABLE C164.2

USEFUL INTRAVENOUS ANTIHYPERTENSIVE AGENTS

ACE inhibitors
Enalaprilat
β-Blockers
Esmolol
Labetalol (α/β)
Metoprolol
Propranolol
Calcium channel blockers
Nicardipine
Diltiazem
Diuretics
Bumetanide
Furosemide
Torsemide
Vasodilators
Hydralazine

ACE, angiotensin-converting enzyme.

to reduce perioperative CV complications in high-risk patients in randomized-controlled trials, and should be used whenever possible in this population.

Postoperative hypertension

Immediate postoperative period. As patients emerge from surgery, anticholinesterase or anticholinergic agents are frequently given to reverse the neuromuscular blockade used during anesthesia. Although atropine and glycopyrrolate are known to cause tachycardia, they generally do not cause a substantial increase in BP. Postanesthesia BP elevation is frequently caused by sympathetic activation due to patient anxiety and pain on awakening, along with withdrawal from continuous-infusion narcotics. Invasive arterial monitoring should be continued until it is evident that the patient is stable.

Thresholds at which to start therapy have not been defined, but BP >180 mm Hg systolic or >110 mm Hg diastolic should serve as a rough starting point for initiating treatment in the early postoperative period. Intravenous agents of any class can be used during the immediate postoperative period (**Table C164.2**); however, agents with a slightly longer duration of action may be preferable so that it may be easier to return the patient to an oral regimen. Because of the large volume shifts that occur during surgery, administration of blood, saline, or loop diuretics may be necessary depending on the individual's needs. Adequate pain control with intravenous or oral analgesic agents is also particularly important, and should not go unattended.

Late postoperative period. In the late postoperative period, the goal should be to reestablish the prior outpatient regimen. Postoperative arrhythmias (e.g., atrial fibrillation) may necessitate preferred use of β-blockers or rate-reducing CCBs.

Suggested Readings

Charlson ME, MacKenzie CR, Gold JP, et al. What patterns identify patients at risk for postoperative complications? *Ann Surg* 1990;212:567–580.

Colson P, Ryckwaert F, Coriat P. Renin angiotensin system antagonists and anesthesia. *Anesth Analg* 1999;89:1143–1155.

Comfere T, Sprung J, Kumar MM, et al. Angiotensin system inhibitors in a general surgical population. *Anesth Analg* 2005;100:636–644.

Eagle KM, Berger PB, Calkins H, et al. ACC/AHA guideline update for perioperative cardiovascular evaluation for noncardiac surgery—executive summary. *Circulation* 2002;105:1257.

Forrest JB, Rehder K, Calahan MK, et al. Multicenter study of general anesthesia. III. Predictors of severe perioperative adverse outcomes. *Anesthesiology* 1992;76:3–15.

Howell SJ, Sear JW, Foex P. Hypertension, hypertensive heart disease and perioperative cardiac risk. *Br J Anaesth* 2004;92(4):570–583.

Kihara S, Brimacombe J, Yaguchi Y, et al. Hemodynamic responses among three tracheal intubation devices in normotensive and hypertensive patients. *Anesth Analg* 2003;96:890–895.

Laslett L. Hypertension: preoperative assessment and perioperative management. *West J Med* 1995;162:215–219.

Prys-Roberts C, Meloche R. Management of anesthesia in patients with hypertension or ischemic heart disease. *Int Anesthesiol Clin* 1980;18:181.

Vuylsteke A, Feneck RO, Jolin-Mellgard A, et al. Perioperative BP control: a prospective survey of patient management in cardiac surgery. *J Cardiothorac Vasc Anesth* 2000;14(3):269–273.

SECTION VI ■ MANAGEMENT OF SECONDARY HYPERTENSION

CHAPTER C165 ■ MANAGEMENT OF SLEEP APNEA

VIREND K. SOMERS, MD, PhD AND SEAN M. CAPLES, DO

KEY POINTS

■ Obstructive sleep apnea (OSA) syndrome is widely prevalent in the general population and is especially frequent in patients who are obese or hypertensive.

■ Repetitive nocturnal hypoxemia results in acute neurohumoral activation and increased blood pressure (BP), which may carry over into the daytime.

■ Effective treatment of OSA not only attenuates the acute neurohumoral and pressor responses, but may also result in sustained reduction in daytime sympathetic activity and lower daytime BPs in hypertensive patients.

■ Principal treatment options include positional therapy, continuous positive airway pressure (CPAP), oral appliances, and weight loss.

See also Chapters A46, **A55,** and C106

Patients with obstructive sleep apnea (OSA) are often, but not always, obese. The disease process is characterized by repetitive nocturnal obstructive events secondary to upper airway collapse. The exact pathophysiology underlying the predisposition to airway collapse is not well understood but may relate to a number of factors including accumulation of adipose tissue, craniofacial characteristics, abnormal upper airway tone, and dysfunctional neural mechanisms regulating airway patency.

Hypertension in obstructive sleep apnea

Repetitive nocturnal desaturation episodes can be quite profound, reaching levels of oxygen saturation <50%. Hypoxemia, together with CO_2 retention, excites the peripheral and central chemoreflexes, causing sympathetic activation, vasoconstriction, and marked increases in blood pressure (BP). The hypoxemic and other metabolic stresses secondary to repetitive nocturnal OSA may also induce production of humoral substances with significant pressor and trophic consequences, including release of catecholamines, endothelin, and cytokines. The pressor effects of endothelin, for example, may persist for a number of hours.

Over the long term, the arousals from sleep and the neural, humoral, and metabolic responses to repetitive nocturnal hypoxemia may result in severe daytime somnolence, cognitive impairment, increased daytime BPs, and predisposition to ventricular dysfunction and heart failure.

Diagnosis and quantitation

There are no uniform criteria for evaluation and treatment for OSA. Formal diagnostic testing is not always necessary to institute innocuous therapy (i.e., positional manipulations) or behavioral modifications that may improve nighttime sleep. On the other hand, patients with some degree of risk based on this evaluation should undergo further workup. Simple overnight oximetry does have a role, particularly when interpreted by an experienced clinician. However, a "normal" appearing overnight oximetry does not rule out clinically significant OSA and should not preclude full polysomnographic (PSG) study in a patient at risk.

Clinical presentation. The decision to undertake a diagnostic evaluation is based on evidence of clinical impairment (daytime somnolence, impaired driving) in the setting of a compatible history (loud snoring, witnessed apneas) or physical examination (tonsillar enlargement, retrognathia), or both. The presence of coexistent cardiovascular disease or an associated risk factor often heightens clinical suspicion.

Obesity and sleep apnea. OSA is frequently associated with obesity, and a large percentage of patients with the syndrome are overweight. The impact of weight gain on OSA severity may be related to cervical fat deposition, intrapharyngeal adipose tissue accumulation, and effects of truncal obesity on lung volumes. Weight loss, whether from medical or dietary intervention or from bariatric surgery, has consistently been shown to improve disordered breathing during sleep. The response of OSA to weight loss varies from person to person, but even modest reductions (10% of body weight) have been shown to be of benefit. Moreover, weight loss is beneficial for overall health, particularly in those patients who have associated hypertension and other cardiovascular disease. Bariatric surgery, a potentially effective treatment for morbid obesity, also results in marked attenuation of sleep apnea severity.

Polysomnography. Diagnosis is based on clinical suspicion followed by confirmation using PSG monitoring of the electroencephalogram, eye movements, muscle tone, abdominal and chest movement, airflow, oxygen saturation, and, occasionally, intrathoracic pressure monitoring. The quantification of apneas and hypopneas detected during an overnight polysomnogram is referred to as the *apnea-hypopnea index* (AHI). An AHI <5 events per hour is seen in healthy adults. *Mild OSA* has been defined as an AHI from 5 to 20, *moderate* from 20 to 40, and *severe* as >40, although the shortcomings of the AHI should be noted. For example, this metric fails to quantify the degree of oxyhemoglobin desaturation, a potentially important variable in the setting of cardiovascular disease. Although significant OSA may be found in 2% to 4% of the adult population, the prevalence of the disorder is increased in patients with hypertension, of whom 30% to 40% may have OSA. The prevalence of OSA may be even higher in patients with resistant hypertension, particularly if they are obese.

Treatment of obstructive sleep apnea

Mild OSA may be treated with conservative measures with the option of more aggressive, and potentially invasive, therapies later if initial treatment fails. On the other hand, moderate to severe OSA requires more aggressive therapy at the outset, with behavioral modifications as an adjunct therapy.

Continuous positive airway pressure. Continuous positive airway pressure (CPAP) is the established gold-standard treatment for patients with moderate to severe disease. CPAP involves delivery of positive pressure through a nasal mask, thereby acting as a pneumatic splint to prevent collapse of the pharyngeal airway during sleep. It is often titrated with the guidance of PSG monitoring, although autotitrating devices have been increasingly used in lieu of in-laboratory titration. CPAP provides a number of advantages as the primary form of treatment; it is noninvasive, safe, effective, and rapidly and easily applied. Patients with daytime sleepiness consequent upon OSA respond best to CPAP therapy, even in those with a mildly abnormal AHI. Coexistent cardiovascular disease or increased cardiovascular risk may lower the threshold for treatment

Adverse effects of CPAP are few but often relate to nasal congestion or mask interface problems, both of which are

often readily addressed. As with any medical therapy, patient compliance is variable and ranges from 40% to 80%. Recent advances in positive pressure airway therapy include autotitrating units that adjust the pressure applied from minute to minute, based on measurement of dynamic obstruction throughout the night. Bilevel positive airway pressure (BiPAP) may be useful in patients with abnormal daytime ventilation who also have nocturnal sleep apnea, such as those with neuromuscular disease.

Positioning during sleep. Many patients have worsening of sleep apnea in the supine position when gravity causes the tongue and other soft tissue to fall back against the posterior pharyngeal wall, thereby predisposing to airway collapse. Manipulation of body position improves the rate of disordered breathing events during sleep. This may involve sleeping on one's side and, occasionally, head and trunk elevation to 30 degrees from horizontal, which affords the airway greater stability against early closure. Other maneuvers aimed at avoiding the supine position and maintaining the lateral recumbent position may be used, such as body-length pillows along the dorsal surface of the body. Placement of tennis balls within a pocket sewn into the back of a T-shirt worn at night provides a deterrent to the supine position. Over time, the patient should become conditioned to sleeping in the lateral recumbent position but positional therapy alone may effectively treat some patients or may be used as part of a multifaceted approach to nonpositional disordered breathing.

Oral appliances. The use of oral appliances in OSA, derived primarily from case series, is based on their ability to hold the tongue forward or to primarily reposition the mandible and tongue anteriorly. These appliances are molded to the shape of the mouth and teeth; because they have the potential to worsen airway obstruction, they should be fitted by a dentist or surgeon specialized in this field. These devices have been known to aggravate temporomandibular joint dysfunction, although newer "adjustable" appliances allow for titration of the mandibular position over time. Devices may be useful as an adjunct to weight loss and positional therapy in patients with mild OSA but a trial of CPAP should be considered before using an intraoral device due to the proven efficacy of CPAP. In patients with moderate or severe disease, intraoral devices should be reserved for those who do not tolerate or who refuse CPAP or surgical therapy.

Surgical procedures. Several surgical procedures have been developed to allow sustained weight loss or to alleviate upper airway obstruction and improve airflow in patients with OSA.

Bariatric surgery. Surgical induction of weight loss, such as with bariatric surgery, can markedly reduce OSA. Although not specifically indicated for OSA therapy, bariatric surgery is appropriate for many patients with OSA, who often have body mass indices >150% of normal.

Oropharyngeal surgery. Surgery may be the preferable treatment option for patients with a specific underlying identifiable oropharyngeal abnormality that is causing mild to moderate OSA. Examples include persistent tonsillar enlargement, nasal turbinate hypertrophy unresponsive to medical management, and nasal septal deviation. This may be especially attractive in young patients as well as older patients with few comorbidities.

Surgery is sometimes performed on patients without strictly defined anatomic lesions, with variable results. A common technique is uvulopalatopharyngoplasty, aimed at reducing obstruction at the oropharyngeal or retropalatal region. This entails excision of the uvula, tonsillar tissue, and portions of the soft palate. Because preoperative assessment is not highly specific for oropharyngeal forms of airway obstruction, only a minority of

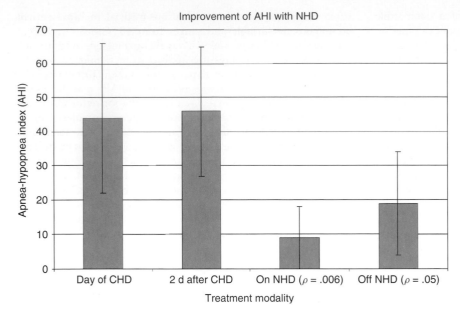

Improvement of AHI with NHD

Figure C165.1 Significant reduction in the apnea-hypopnea index (AHI) with the use of nocturnal hemodialysis (NHD), as compared to limited benefits from conventional hemodialysis (CHD). Study participants underwent 6 to 15 months of daily nocturnal hemodialysis, which caused a significant reduction in their AHI ($p = .006$). Also, on a night without NHD, participants still demonstrated a significant decrease in their AHI ($p = .05$). (Adapted from Hanly PJ, Pierratos A. Improvement of sleep apnea in patients with chronic renal failure who undergo nocturnal hemodialysis. *N Engl J Med* 2001;344:102–107.)

patients have long-term correction of OSA with these procedures. It is important to obtain follow-up PSGs to assess responses and the potential need for adjunctive CPAP therapy.

Tracheostomy. Tracheostomy was the first successful therapy for sleep apnea and is the only reliably effective surgical procedure to treat OSA. However, because of the associated morbidity, it should be reserved for those cases that are refractory to other measures or for patients with clinical urgency, such as severe hypoxemia or cardiac arrhythmias.

Drug therapy. Drugs that promote healthy weight loss are theoretically beneficial for patients with OSA. Other pharmacologic approaches have been largely unrewarding: sex hormone supplementation, respiratory stimulants, agents that act on brain stem neurotransmitters controlling the upper airway dilator muscles, and serotonin agonists and antagonists.

Sleep apnea in hemodialysis and pacemaker patients.

Interest in sleep-related clinical syndromes is accelerating and novel approaches to treatment of OSA are being described. In patients with OSA and end-stage renal failure, marked improvement in AHI occurred in patients treated with intensive nighttime hemodialysis (**Figure C165.1**). A small case series suggesting the value of nocturnal atrial overpacing in patients

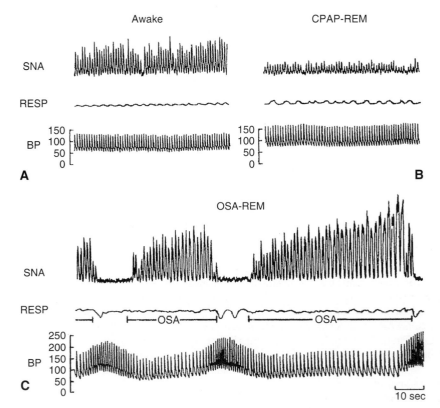

Figure C165.2 Recordings of sympathetic nerve activity (SNA), respiration (RESP), and intraarterial blood pressure (BP) in the same subject when awake (**A**), with obstructive sleep apnea (OSA) during rapid eye movement (REM) sleep (**C**), and with elimination of OSA by continuous positive airway pressure (CPAP) therapy during REM sleep (**B**). SNA is high during wakefulness, and increases further with OSA during REM. BP increases from 130/65 mm Hg when awake to 240/110 mm Hg at the end of apnea. Overall, nocturnal BP is increased. Elimination of apnea by CPAP (**B**) results in decreased sympathetic traffic and prevents BP surges during REM sleep. (From Somers VK, Dyken ME, Clary MP, et al. Sympathetic neural mechanisms in obstructive sleep apnea. *J Clin Invest* 1995;96:1897–1904, with permission.)

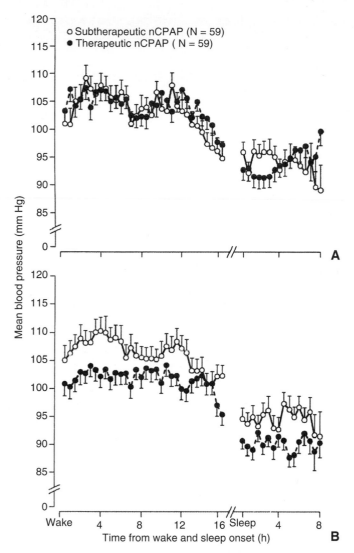

CPAP are proportional to the reduction in BP. In a normotensive individual, severe sleep apnea can result in elevation of nocturnal BPs to levels as high as 240/110 mm Hg. Because hypertension in OSA is associated with a potentiated chemoreflex response to hypoxemia, adrenergic and pressor responses to equivalent levels of hypoxemia seem to be more marked in hypertensive individuals. Therefore, BP responses to CPAP may be enhanced in hypertensive individuals with severe nocturnal apneas.

Chronic effects. It is not clear why recurrent nocturnal apneas should elicit responses that carry over into daytime wakefulness. High levels of sympathetic activity are evident in sleep apnea patients even when awake and in the absence of apneas.

Normotensive patients. In normotensive otherwise-healthy patients with OSA who are on no medications, treatment of sleep apnea results in a gradual decrease in tonic resting daytime sympathetic drive. This reduction in sympathetic activity becomes evident only after 1 month of treatment but is not accompanied by any substantial reduction in BP or heart rate. The absence of a significant BP reduction after chronic treatment of normotensive patients with sleep apnea has been consistent across a number of studies. Therefore, although CPAP treatment lowers nocturnal BP, daytime BPs in the longer term are less affected in normotensive individuals.

Hypertensive patients. Effects on BP appear to be clearer in hypertensive patients. As with normotensive patients, treatment with CPAP in a hypertensive patient acutely decreases the nighttime BP but also results in a significant reduction in daytime BP measurements (**Figure C165.3**). There are emerging data suggesting that patients with hypertension resistant to combination therapy should be evaluated for OSA, regardless of whether they are overweight or obese. If the apnea can be treated successfully, BP may decrease and the number and dosages of medications may be reduced.

Heart failure. In some patients with heart failure who also have OSA, treatment of sleep apnea may significantly reduce the BP and ameliorate heart failure symptoms in individuals with systolic or diastolic ventricular dysfunction.

Figure C165.3 Randomized trial comparing men with sleep apnea who were treated with therapeutic versus subtherapeutic CPAP (1 cm H_2O) over a 1-month period. Mean ambulatory blood pressure (BP) profile before (**A**) and after (**B**) treatment. Benefit was seen during sleep and wakefulness. Patients with severe apnea showed a better response, as did those on antihypertensive medications. nCPAP, nasal continuous positive airway pressure. (From Pepperell JC, Ramdassingh-Dow S, Crosthwaite N, et al. Ambulatory BP after therapeutic and subtherapeutic nasal continuous positive airway pressure for obstructive sleep apnea: a randomized parallel trial. Lancet 2002;359(9302):204–210, with permission.)

with OSA was not reproduced in a number of subsequent trials.

Benefits of treatment

Acute effects. Effective treatment and prevention of the repetitive nocturnal desaturation have immediate effects on the humoral and reflex responses to hypoxemia and hypercapnia (**Figure C165.2**). Specifically, administration of CPAP results in a marked reduction in sympathetic traffic and prevents the repetitive surges in BP that are evident at the end of the apneic events. Furthermore, several hours of treatment with CPAP induces a fall in other pressor and trophic substances such as endothelin and erythropoietin; endothelin changes after acute treatment with

Suggested Readings

Cleator IGM, Birmingham CL, Kovacevic S, et al. Long-term effect of ileogastrostomy surgery for morbid obesity on diabetes mellitus and sleep apnea. *Obes Surg* 2006;16:1337–1341.

Faccenda IF, Mackay TW, Boon NA, et al. Randomized placebo-controlled trial of continuous positive airway pressure on BP in the sleep apnea-hypopnea syndrome. *Am J Respir Crit Care Med* 2001;163:344–348.

Gangwisch JE, Heymsfield SB, Boden-Albala B. Short sleep duration as a risk factor for hypertension. Analyses of the First National Health and Nutrition Examination Survey. *Hypertension* 2006;47:833–839.

Haas DC, Foster GL, Neito FJ, et al. Age-dependent associations between sleep-disordered breathing and hypertension. Importance of discriminating between systolic/diastolic hypertension and isolated systolic hypertension in the Sleep Heart Health Study. *Circulation* 2005;111:614–621.

Hanly PJ, Pierratos A. Improvement of sleep apnea in patients with chronic renal failure who undergo nocturnal hemodialysis. *N Engl J Med* 2001;344:102–107.

Narkiewicz K, Kato M, Phillips BG, et al. Nocturnal continuous positive airway pressure decreases daytime sympathetic traffic in obstructive sleep apnea. *Circulation* 1999;100:2332–2335.

Pepperell JCT, Ramdassingh-Dow S, Crosthwaite N, et al. Ambulatory BP after therapeutic and subtherapeutic nasal continuous positive airway pressure for obstructive sleep apnea, a randomised parallel trial. *Lancet* 2002;359:204–210.

Peppard PE, Young T, Palta M, et al. Prospective study of the association between sleep-disordered breathing and hypertension. *N Engl J Med* 2000;342:1378–1384.

Somers VK, Dyken ME, Clary MP, et al. Sympathetic neural mechanisms in obstructive sleep apnea. *J Clin Invest* 1995;96:1897–1904.

Unterberg C, Luthje L, Szych J. Atrial overdrive pacing compared to CPAP in patients with obstructive sleep apnoea syndrome. *Eur Heart J* 2005;26:2568–2575.

CHAPTER C166 ■ MANAGEMENT OF DRUG-INDUCED AND IATROGENIC HYPERTENSION

EHUD GROSSMAN, MD; FRANZ H. MESSERLI, MD, FACC AND DOMENIC A. SICA, MD

KEY POINTS

■ A variety of therapeutic agents and chemical substances induce transient or sustained hypertension or counteract the effects of antihypertensive therapy.

■ Careful evaluation of a patient's drug regimen may identify chemically induced hypertension or preclude the need for antihypertensive therapy.

■ When drug- or chemically induced hypertension is identified, discontinuation of the causative agent is preferred but specific antihypertensive therapies or dose adjustments may be needed if continued use of the offending agent is necessary.

See also Chapters C105, C106, C143, C144, and C166

Hypertension related to drugs and other chemical substances represents a modifiable source of secondary hypertension that can obviate the need for unnecessary and costly evaluations or potentially dangerous drug interactions (**Table C166.1**). Withdrawal of the offending agent is often possible but specific therapies are sometimes necessary.

Steroids

Corticosteroids. Hypertension occurs in at least 20% of patients treated with synthetic corticosteroids in dose-dependent fashion; oral cortisol at doses of 80 to 200 mg per day can increase systolic blood pressure (BP) as much as 15 mm Hg within 24 hours. Glucocorticoid-induced hypertension occurs more often in elderly patients and in patients with a positive family history of essential hypertension. Mineralocorticoids (e.g., 9-α fluoroprednisolone and 9-α fluorocortisol), and other compounds such as licorice and carbenoxolone that inhibit 11-β hydroxysteroid dehydrogenase enzyme increase exchangeable sodium (Na^+) and blood volume, induce hypokalemia with metabolic alkalosis, and suppress plasma renin and angiotensin II. Skin ointments, antihemorrhoidal preparations, ophthalmic drops, asthma inhalers, and nasal allergy sprays may contain substances with significant mineralocorticoid activity (particularly 9-α fluoroprednisolone) and some contain sympathomimetic amines. Inhibition of enzymatic degradation of steroids by ketoconazole can lead to mineralocorticoid-related hypertension. Discontinuation of steroids or ketoconazole is needed if BP is to be lowered without pharmacologic therapy. If steroid treatment cannot be interrupted, diuretics or calcium antagonists may be used; adjunctive therapy with sympatholytic drugs is sometimes necessary.

Sex hormones. Oral contraceptives induce hypertension in approximately 5% of users of high-dose compounds that contain at least 50 μg of estrogen and 1 to 4 mg of progestin; small increases in BP have been reported in users of low-dose estrogen formulations. Women with a history of high BP during pregnancy, those with a family history of hypertension, cigarette smokers, obese women, blacks, diabetic patients, and those with renal disease may experience small BP increases with oral contraceptives; occasionally, severe hypertension occurs. Postmenopausal oral estrogen replacement therapy (ERT), with or without progestins, often increases systolic BP by 1 to 2 mm Hg but rarely causes severe hypertension. ERT use has been associated with increased cardiovascular (CV) morbidity and mortality and is no longer recommended unless severe menopausal symptoms are present. Men receiving estrogen for the treatment of prostatic cancer may also exhibit an increase in BP. Danazol, a semisynthetic androgen used in the treatment of endometriosis and hereditary angioedema has been reported to induce hypertension and fluid retention.

Nonsteroidal anti-inflammatory drugs

Nonsteroidal antiinflammatory drugs (NSAIDs) can induce an increase in BP by as much as 5 mm Hg (mean BP) and interfere with antihypertensive treatment (see Chapter C144). NSAID users also have a 40% increased risk of hypertension compared with nonusers. Elderly patients, those with pre-existing hypertension, salt sensitivity, renal failure, or renovascular hypertension are at a higher risk of developing severe hypertension with NSAIDs. NSAIDs may interact with some antihypertensive agents such as diuretics, β-blockers, and angiotensin-converting enzyme (ACE)

MANAGEMENT OF DRUG-INDUCED HYPERTENSION

Substance	Management	Comments
Steroids		
Glucocorticoids	Discontinue; if not possible, start diuretics	Monitor potassium
Mineralocorticoids	Discontinue; if not possible, start diuretics	Monitor potassium
Sex hormones		
Nonsteroidal anti-inflammatory drugs	Calcium antagonists	Assess the risk of an increase in BP against the expected benefit; among cyclooxygenase-2 inhibitors, celecoxib affects BP less than rofecoxib
Drugs affecting the sympathetic nervous system		
Ophthalmic solutions	Initial therapy, α-blockers or α-,β-blockers	Avoid β-blockers
Antiemetic agents		Transient increase in HR
Yohimbine hydrochloride	Discontinue	Avoid in hypertensive patients and in those treated with tricyclic antidepressants
Glucagon (only in patients with pheochromocytoma)	Initial therapy, intravenous phentolamine, oral phenoxybenzamine, or α_1-blockers	
Cocaine	Initial therapy, α-blockers, nitroglycerin, and verapamil	Most patients do not require treatment
Anorexics	Discontinue treatment	
Nasal decongestant	Initial therapy, α-, β-blockers	
Cough medications	Discontinue treatment	
Sibutramine	Discontinue sibutramine or modify antihypertensive therapy	In obese hypertensive patients, the BP reduction achieved by weight loss negates the potential increase related to the drug
Clozapine	Discontinue; if not possible, start α-blockers or nifedipine	
Bromocriptine		Avoid use for suppression of lactation
Disulfiram	Avoid alcohol intake	
Antidepressants		
Monoamine oxidase inhibitors	Initial therapy, α-blockers	
Tricyclic antidepressants	Initial therapy, α-blockers	
Serotonin agonist	Initial therapy, α-blockers	
Anesthetics and narcotics		Anesthetics and narcotics
Ketamine hydrochloride	Initial therapy, clonidine or α-blockers	Ketamine hydrochloride
Desflurane	Initial therapy, α-blockers or α-, β-blockers	Desflurane
Naloxone	Initial therapy, α-blockers	Naloxone
Sevoflurane	Clonidine or combination of diltiazem and nicardipine	Sevoflurane
Miscellaneous		
Cyclosporine	Discontinue or switch to tacrolimus; if not possible, start calcium antagonists; other drugs are also effective	Calcium antagonists may increase cyclosporine blood levels; multidrug therapy may be necessary
Tacrolimus	Discontinue; if not possible, start calcium antagonists	
	Other drugs are also effective	
Recombinant human erythropoietin	Lower the dose; if unsuccessful, start calcium antagonists or α-blockers; diuretics and angiotensin-converting enzyme inhibitors may be less effective	Dialysis with conventional antihypertensive treatment may be effective; phlebotomy may rapidly lower BP
Alcohol	Moderate alcohol intake or cessation	

inhibitors but typically do not interfere with the actions of calcium channel blockers and possibly central sympatholytic drugs, the antihypertensive efficacy of which is apparently unrelated to prostaglandin production. Individual NSAIDs vary considerably in their effect on BP; indomethacin, naproxen, and piroxicam are typically associated with the greatest increases in BP. Among selective NSAIDs, rofecoxib is more likely than celecoxib to raise systolic BP but a recent meta-analysis has shown that selective cyclooxygenase-2 (COX-2) inhibitors increase BP more than nonselective agents. Low-dose aspirin has no major effect on BP control in hypertensive patients (see Chapter C143). It is prudent to balance the risk of an increase in BP against the expected benefit of treatment with an NSAID; if their use is warranted, calcium antagonists and increased diuretic doses may be needed to control BP.

Dietary substances

Alcohol. Excessive alcohol use, either acute or chronic, has clearly been shown to raise BP and can induce resistance to antihypertensive therapy. The dose-dependent BP effects of alcohol are independent of obesity, Na^+ and K^+ intake, or cigarette smoking. Abstinence or at least moderation of alcohol intake to no more than 1 to 2 oz of alcohol daily is the best approach. In some cases, BP control is extremely difficult unless there is complete abstinence from alcohol. Failure on the part of a patient to divulge their level of alcohol intake should always be a consideration in the patient with resistant hypertension.

Caffeine. Caffeine acutely and transiently increases BP but chronic hypertension is unusual because of rapid tolerance to its pressor effects. BP effects of caffeine are more pronounced in men, in those with a positive family history and in African-American subjects. Strategies for reducing or eliminating caffeine intake should be considered in persistently hypertensive subjects.

Dietary supplements. Herbal products have the potential to increase BP and to interfere with antihypertensive treatment. Much of this evidence is anecdotal but some reports have shown that dietary supplements containing ephedra alkaloids can increase BP; these have been banned for sale in the United States since 2004.

Drugs affecting sympathetic neurotransmission

Sympathomimetic amines. Phenylephrine (Neo-Synephrine) administration in an ophthalmic or intranasal solution has been reported in isolated cases to increase BP and dipivalyl adrenaline, a prodrug used topically in the management of chronic simple glaucoma, can reversibly increase BP. The addition of sympathomimetic agents to β-blockers can also increase BP, presumably because of unopposed α-adrenergic vasoconstriction.

Cocaine. Acute cocaine use can cause a massive increase in sympathetic nervous traffic and circulating catecholamines as a result of facilitated catecholamine release and blockade of neuronal norepinephrine reuptake. Clinically, there is acute tachycardia and marked BP increase but not chronic hypertension unless an insidious form of cocaine-induced renal failure is also present. Most patients with cocaine-related hypertension do not require antihypertensive drug therapy, but if treatment is necessary, α-adrenergic receptor antagonists or combined α-, β-blockers are logical choices. Nitroglycerin and verapamil have also been used to treat cocaine-induced hypertension and coronary arterial vasoconstriction and should be considered if cocaine intoxication is complicated by myocardial ischemia.

Antidepressants. Monoamine oxidase inhibitors (MAOIs) can induce severe hypertension if patients consume large quantities of foods containing tyramine (e.g., some cheese varieties). Tranylcypromine is the most hazardous of these compounds, whereas moclobemide and brofaromine seem to be the least likely to raise BP. α-Adrenergic receptor blockers and α/β-blockers seem appropriate for initial treatment. Tricyclic antidepressants increase BP, mainly in patients with panic disorders. Buspirone and other serotonin receptor type 1α agonists have also been reported to increase BP, especially in those also on MAOI. Venlafaxine has a dose-dependent effect on BP that may become clinically significant at high doses. Episodes of severe hypertension have been described in patients treated with other antidepressant agents such as fluoxetine, fluoxetine plus selegiline, and thioridazine. Carbamazepine used for bipolar depression and seizures may also induce hypertension although this is a very uncommon phenomenon. Selegiline, a type B MAOI mainly used for Parkinson's disease may also increase BP when it is coadministered with other anti-Parkinson agents or dopamine. Clozapine may also raise BP

by both sympathetic nervous system (SNS) activation and weight gain, and α-adrenergic receptor antagonists are the treatment of choice (see Chapter C162).

Antiobesity drugs. Sibutramine, a novel serotonin and noradrenaline reuptake inhibitor, is an antiobesity drug that may increase heart rate and BP. In obese hypertensive patients, the BP reduction achieved by weight loss may effectively counterbalance the potential BP increase related to the drug. In a recent combined analysis of two placebo-controlled trials sibutramine treatment did not elicit a critical increase in BP even in hypertensive patients. Nevertheless, obese patients being treated with sibutramine should be monitored periodically for changes in BP. If sibutramine-related hypertension occurs, a combination of ACE inhibitor with a diuretic or calcium channel blocker is effective.

Other agents. Bromocriptine is commonly used for prolactin inhibition and suppression of puerperal lactation. Although bromocriptine most commonly has a sympatholytic hypotensive effect, severe hypertension with subsequent stroke has been reported in the postpartum period. The α_2-antagonist yohimbine is essentially the opposite of clonidine and commonly raises BP; it should be avoided in hypertensive patients or those treated with tricyclic antidepressants. Antiemetic agents such as metoclopramide, alizapride, and prochlorperazine increase BP transiently in patients treated with cisplatin. Glucagon may induce severe hypertension in patients with pheochromocytoma. Acute BP increases under any of these situations is best treated by withdrawal of the offending agent; if needed, a variety of oral or parenteral agents, including α-blockers (phentolamine, phenoxybenzamine, or doxazosin) or the α/β-blocker labetalol, can be useful to lower BP immediately.

Anesthetics and narcotics

Ketamine hydrochloride, desflurane, and sevoflurane have been reported to severely increase BP by stimulating the SNS. Treatment with sympatholytic agents such as α-blockers, α,β-blockers, or clonidine usually lowers BP in patients so treated. The simultaneous use of vasoconstrictors (e.g., felypressin) with topical cocaine can result in severe hypertension. A hypertensive response to naloxone (opiate antagonist), especially during attempted reversal of narcotic-induced anesthesia in hypertensive patients, has also been reported. The opioid antagonist naloxone can acutely reverse the antihypertensive effects of clonidine and thereby cause an acute hypertensive urgency/emergency.

Anti–human immunodeficiency virus treatment

Highly active antiretroviral therapy (HAART) can increase systolic BP. The tendency to cause insulin resistance with this regimen is somewhat less than with the first generation of protease inhibitors. The reaction to HAART is more pronounced in the elderly and in those with higher baseline systolic BP, higher baseline cholesterol levels, and low baseline CD4 cell count. BP should be periodically measured and treated as necessary in HIV-infected patients on HAART.

Immunosuppressives and antineoplastic agents

Calcineurin inhibitors (cyclosporin and tacrolimus) may increase BP in patients with organ transplants, autoimmune diseases, or dermatologic disorders. The risk of hypertension with these agents is unrelated to sex or race, but is dose related, increases with age of the patient, and is exacerbated by preexisting hypertension or renal failure. BP usually falls after the withdrawal of cyclosporine but may not remit completely. Calcium channel blockers are useful agents but multidrug therapy is usually necessary. Tacrolimus produces less hypertension than cyclosporine and should be considered as an option in patients with cyclosporine-induced hypertension (see Chapter C171). Hypertensive reactions associated with paclitaxel and angiogenesis inhibitors (e.g., bevacizumab) occur in a dose-dependent manner.

Recombinant human erythropoietin

Recombinant human erythropoietin (r-HuEPO) increases BP in a dose-related manner and leads to hypertension in 20% to 30% of patients with kidney failure who receive it. Hypertension develops variably, from as early as 2 weeks to several months after initiating r-HuEPO. Part of the mechanisms may be related to increased blood viscosity; gradual subcutaneous dose titration reduces the rate of rise of hematocrit and blunts the onset of hypertension. When HuEPO-related hypertension occurs, diuretic therapy or increased dialytic ultrafiltration is usually needed to improve volume control but on occasion, multiple drugs may be required. If these measures are unsuccessful, the dose of r-HuEPO should be lowered or therapy should be held for several weeks.

Heavy metals

Epidemiologic studies have confirmed the high incidence of hypertension among patients exposed to lead, even at low levels (<40 μg/dL, see Chapter B95). Blood lead level has been positively associated with both systolic and diastolic hypertension,

especially in postmenopausal women, and lead exposure appears to predate many cases of pregnancy-related hypertension. Some reports suggest that arsenic or cadmium exposure may also induce hypertension in humans. Chelation is not a therapy usually recommended. Specific therapies have not been tested in this variant of hypertension.

Suggested Readings

Brem AS. Insights into glucocorticoid-associated hypertension. *Am J Kidney Dis* 2001;37:1–10.

Clyburn EB, DiPette DJ. Hypertension induced by drugs and other substances. *Semin Nephrol* 1995;15:72–86.

Grossman E, Messerli FH. High blood pressure. A side effect of drugs, poisons, and food. *Arch Intern Med* 1995;155:450–460.

Haller CA, Benowitz NL. Adverse cardiovascular and central nervous system events associated with dietary supplements containing ephedra alkaloids. *N Engl J Med* 2000;343(25):1833–1838.

Jordan J, Scholze J, Matiba B, et al. Influence of Sibutramine on blood pressure: evidence from placebo-controlled trials. *Int J Obes Relat Metab Disord* 2005;29(5):509–516.

Noordzij M, Uiterwaal CS, Arends LR, et al. Blood pressure response to chronic intake of coffee and caffeine: a meta-analysis of randomized controlled trials. *J Hypertens* 2005;23(5):921–928.

Palacios R, Santos J, Garcia A, et al. Impact of highly active antiretroviral therapy on blood pressure in HIV-infected patients. A prospective study in a cohort of naive patients. *HIV Med* 2006;7:10–15.

Richard CL, Jurgens TM. Effects of natural health products on blood pressure. *Ann Pharmacother* 2005;39(4):712–720.

Sowers JR, White WB, Pitt B, et al. The effects of cyclooxygenase-2 inhibitors and nonsteroidal anti-inflammatory therapy on 24-hour blood pressure in patients with hypertension, osteoarthritis, and type 2 diabetes mellitus. *Arch Intern Med* 2005;165(2):161–168.

Yoshita K, Miura K, Morikawa Y, et al. Relationship of alcohol consumption to 7-year blood pressure change in Japanese men. *J Hypertens* 2005;23(8):1485–1490.

CHAPTER C167 ■ MANAGEMENT OF HYPERALDOSTERONISM AND HYPERCORTISOLISM

DAVID A. CALHOUN, MD

KEY POINTS

- Hypokalemia is a late and variable manifestation of primary aldosteronism (PA); early in the disease, normokalemic hypertension is most common.
- There are no universally agreed-upon criteria for the diagnosis of PA.
- Reported prevalence rates of PA vary widely but are generally proportional to blood pressure (BP) (<1%–2% in mild hypertension to >20% in resistant hypertension).
- Morning plasma aldosterone:renin activity ratio is the most common screening test; confirmation of PA requires 24-hour urinary aldosterone collection after salt loading.
- Most patients with Cushing's syndrome or hypercortisolism develop hypertension.

See also Chapters A19, **A20**, A72, and **C131**

PRIMARY ALDOSTERONISM

Primary aldosteronism (PA) is most often caused by bilateral nodular hyperplasia; discrete aldosterone producing adenoma (APA) is very uncommon. Differentiation of subtype is clinically relevant because unilateral APAs can be surgically cured, whereas nodular hyperplasia is recurrent and is treated with medications.

Prevalence

PA, first described by Jerome Conn in 1955, has been considered to be an uncommon cause of hypertension, with an estimated prevalence of <1% in general hypertensive populations. Prevalence rates are dependent on the sensitivity and specificity of the analyses used, however, and techniques vary widely among laboratories. Several reports now suggest that PA is more common than thought. Chilean investigators screened more than 700 hypertensive patients for PA and found an overall prevalence of 6.7%.

The prevalence of PA appears to be proportional to the level of blood pressure (BP) at presentation. PA is uncommon (<2%) in patients with stage 1 hypertension but has a prevalence of 8% in stage 2 hypertension (≥160/100 mm Hg) and 13% in patients with BP ≥180/110 mm Hg; other studies in patients with resistant hypertension suggest a prevalence rate of as much as 20% (**Figure C167.1**). In these studies, the large majority of patients with PA were not hypokalemic at the time of diagnosis, suggesting that hypokalemia is a late manifestation of PA. Earlier diagnosis is due in part to increasing awareness of the disease and the widespread availability of more standardized assays for plasma aldosterone

and plasma renin activity (PRA), and in some cases, changes in diagnostic criteria.

Evaluation

Screening. PA must be distinguished from normal reactive hyperaldosteronism caused by volume depletion, often due to diuretic therapy. Screening for PA is generally recommended in (a) patients with hypokalemia (serum K^+ <3.5 mEq/L), (b) patients with resistant hypertension, (c) patients with a history of BP >180/110 mm Hg, or (d) patients with an adrenal mass. The most common screening test for PA is the plasma aldosterone:PRA ratio aldosterone renin **ratio** (ARR). This technique is highly sensitive but has a high false-positive rate, generally because PRA, the denominator, can be very low (in some laboratories <0.1 ng/mL/hour). Accordingly, some laboratories use a minimum PRA of <0.5 ng/mL/hour. The screening cutoff value for ARR varies; values >20 to 30 are considered suspicious; some experts also require a minimum plasma aldosterone >12 ng per dL.

Patient preparation. Hormonal testing is usually performed in the early morning in freely ambulatory patients. Hypokalemia should be corrected for at least 4 weeks before measurement of plasma aldosterone because low serum potassium (K^+) levels suppress aldosterone release. Aldosterone antagonists (spironolactone, eplerenone) can falsely increase plasma aldosterone levels and must be withdrawn for 4 weeks before testing is undertaken. Potassium-sparing diuretics (e.g., amiloride or triamterene) can stimulate aldosterone through increased serum K^+ and should also be withdrawn whenever possible. Nevertheless, for practical reasons, ARR is most often measured with patients remaining

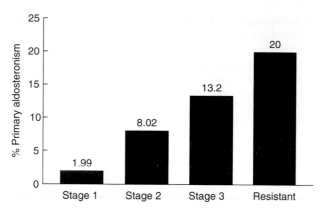

Figure C167.1 Prevalence of primary aldosteronism according to severity of hypertension (JNC 6 stage 1 140–159/90–99, stage 2 160–179/100–109, stage 3 ≥180/≥110 mm Hg; resistant, >140/90 mm Hg on three or more antihypertensive medications). JNC, Joint National Committee on Prevention, Detection, Evaluation, and Treatment of High Blood Pressure. (Reprinted with permission from Calhoun DA. Resistant hypertension. In: Oparil S, Weber MA, eds. *Hypertension: a companion to Brenner and Rector's the kidney.* Philadelphia: WB Saunders, 2005:620.)

on therapy. A high ARR observed during angiotensin-converting enzyme (ACE) inhibitor, angiotensin receptor blocker (ARB), or diuretic use is even more suspicious for aldosterone excess because these medications tend to lower ARR by raising PRA and lowering aldosterone.

Confirmatory tests. Because of the high false-positive rate of ARR screening testing, PA must be confirmed by aldosterone

suppression testing in all cases. In some cases it may be appropriate to omit the ARR and proceed directly to suppression testing.

Dietary salt loading. Dietary salt loading as an outpatient is the simplest and most practical option for suppression testing. Patients ingest a normal diet with additional salt (4–6 g/day for 3–4 days in tablet form, as 1 tsp table salt added to food each day, or as supplements including soups and bouillon). After salt loading, a 24-hour urine is collected for aldosterone, creatinine, and sodium. The cutoff values vary between laboratories; a 24-hour urinary aldosterone >12 to 14 μg per 24 hours is considered definitive for PA as long as the Na excretion rate exceeds 200 mEq per 24 hours. In patients who habitually ingest >200 mEq Na per day, additional salt loading is not needed to interpret plasma or urinary aldosterone levels (**Figure C167.2**). Dietary salt loading is generally safe and well tolerated but modest elevations in BP occasionally occur.

Fludrocortisone suppression testing (FST). Fludrocortisone (0.1 mg 4 times daily for 4 days) has been combined with a high salt diet (≥12 g daily) in some centers, although both the frequency and dose of fludrocortisone are very high. The fludrocortisone suppression testing (FST) with high doses of fludrocortisone carries a risk of a significant hypertension and hypokalemia and is not recommended for individuals with chronic kidney disease (CKD), advanced age, or heart failure. Failure to suppress the morning upright plasma aldosterone level to <6 ng per dL is considered a positive indicator of PA.

Intravenous salt loading. Intravenous infusion of 2 L of normal saline over 4 hours is normally expected to suppress plasma aldosterone to <10 ng per dL. Saline infusion testing should

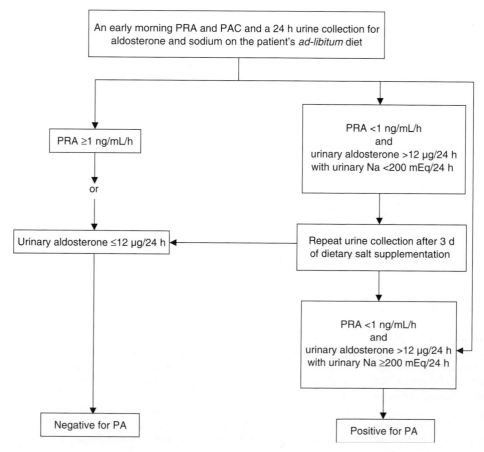

Figure C167.2 Flow chart for the diagnostic evaluation for primary aldosteronism (PA). PRA, plasma renin activity; PAC, plasma aldosterone concentration; Na, sodium. (Adapted Nishizaka MK, Pratt-Ubunama M, Zaman MA, et al. Validity of plasma aldosterone-to-renin activity ratio in African-American and white subjects with resistant hypertension. *Am J Hypertens* 2005;8:805–812.)

be done in the morning because the normal diurnal rhythm for aldosterone includes a decrease during the afternoon.

Captopril suppression testing. The captopril suppression test is the least well-validated alternative test. PRA and aldosterone are measured before and 2 hours after oral administration of captopril 25 mg; the test is considered positive if plasma aldosterone cannot be suppressed below 15 ng per dL. Patients should be withdrawn from ACE inhibitors or ARBs for 2 to 4 weeks before testing.

Imaging studies. Patients confirmed with PA should also have adrenal imaging for possible APA. Computed tomography (CT) imaging using thin-cut (2–3 mm) sections of the adrenals is widely available but has relatively poor sensitivity and specificity. The concordance between CT imaging and adrenal vein sampling (AVS) is only approximately 40% and if CT scanning alone is used to guide therapy, inappropriate treatment (medical vs. surgical) may occur in up to half the patients. CT imaging, however, is still justified as part of the evaluation for PA in order to (a) visually localize tumors before AVS, (b) to identify particularly large tumors (>3–4 cm) that may warrant resection because of increased risk of cancer, and (c) visualize the local anatomy before AVS or adrenalectomy, including potentially localizing the origin of the adrenal veins.

Adrenal vein sampling. Patients with biochemical and anatomic evidence suggestive of APA should have AVS because those with a confirmed APA or unilateral hyperplasia (a rare form of PA) will potentially benefit from adrenalectomy if there is lateralization of aldosterone secretion. An experienced radiologist is essential to obtain samples for aldosterone and cortisol (the latter as a control for nonspecific adrenal steroid release). AVS is a technically difficult procedure, particularly in the right adrenal vein. The procedure is best performed after withdrawal of medications that may affect aldosterone secretion (e.g., spironolactone, eplerenone, other potassium-sparing diuretics, ACE inhibitors, or ARBs).

Treatment

The decision between medical and surgical treatment for PA can be difficult. Medical therapy for bilateral hyperplasia or bilateral adenoma is recommended. Although surgery is considered the treatment of choice for APA in many centers, medical therapy is also a realistic option, in part because APAs very rarely undergo malignant degeneration and postprocedural hypertension is common.

Adrenalectomy. An APA is suggested by more severe hypertension, a history of hypokalemia, higher plasma or urinary aldosterone levels, and a positive imaging study. Adrenalectomy should usually be done laparoscopically to minimize risk and postoperative recovery time. Hypokalemia is almost always corrected after removal of an APA, whereas the BP effects may be short-lived. Younger patients, patients with less severe hypertension, and patients who responded favorably to spironolactone are more likely to manifest the largest BP benefit, including in some cases, total cure of hypertension. Postoperatively, aldosterone secretion from the contralateral adrenal gland may be suppressed and a high salt diet should be recommended in the initial postoperative period. Serum K^+ levels should be monitored weekly for approximately 4 weeks as hyperkalemia, although rare, can occur. Although the BP generally improves immediately after adrenalectomy, most patients will eventually require antihypertensive drugs.

Pharmacologic therapy. Patients with idiopathic PA, bilateral adenomas, or patients in whom adrenalectomy is not being considered should be treated with mineralocorticoid antagonists and other drugs needed to control BP.

Spironolactone. Spironolactone, a nonselective aldosterone antagonist, is most commonly used in doses from 25 to 200 mg daily, with titrations at 4- to 6-week intervals. K^+ supplements are usually able to be discontinued after starting spironolactone; in a few patients, however, both spironolactone and K^+ supplementation may be needed. Particularly in older patients, spironolactone alone may not be sufficient to control BP. Spironolactone is generally well tolerated. The most common adverse effect is dose-dependent breast and nipple tenderness, with or without gynecomastia. Other adverse effects include erectile dysfunction and menstrual irregularities, which may appear as much as a year after treatment was begun.

Other drugs. In this setting, the addition of a calcium antagonist or sympatholytic agent is often highly effective and BPs can often be normalized. ACE inhibitors and ARBs are generally ineffective because angiotensin II is suppressed in PA. Addition of other diuretics can be tried but tend to lower serum K+. The risk of hyperkalemia is increased in patients with CKD, including the elderly and patients with diabetes, where serum K^+ level should be monitored more closely.

Eplerenone is a selective mineralocorticoid receptor antagonist with much less cross-reactivity with androgen and progestin receptors such that sex-related adverse effects are uncommon. It has been shown to be an effective antihypertensive agent but its efficacy has not been established in treating PA. If spironolactone is not tolerated, eplerenone is a reasonable alternative, although eplerenone is not as potent as spironolactone and is much more expensive. Amiloride is another agent that may be of use alone or in conjunction with mineralocorticoid receptor blockers.

Glucocorticoid remediable hypertension

Glucocorticoid remediable hypertension is a rare, monogenic autosomal dominant cause of PA. In this disorder, there is a recombination defect such that aldosterone synthase activity is regulated by adrenocorticotropic hormone or corticotropin (ACTH). Glucocorticoid-remediable aldosteronism (GRA) is associated with an increased risk of premature stroke, so this disease should be considered in patients with a family history of PA or stroke at an early age (<40 years). Because aldosterone production is ACTH dependent, GRA should be considered if aldosterone levels are suppressed with dexamethasone. Genetic testing is necessary to confirm the diagnosis. GRA is treated with dexamethasome to suppress ACTH release or alternatively with spironolactone or amiloride.

CUSHING'S SYNDROME

Cushing's syndrome results from prolonged exposure to excess glucocorticoids. Although uncommon, most patients (75%–85%) with this syndrome develop hypertension, often severe. The main mechanism of hypertension is excess stimulation of the mineralocorticoid receptor by cortisol. In addition to hypertension, other signs and symptoms of Cushing's syndrome (central obesity, facial rounding, interscapular fat deposition, hirsutism, easy bruising, skin atrophy, purple striae, proximal muscle weakness, irritability, and depression) are also present. Associated laboratory abnormalities include neutrophilic leukocytosis, hyperglycemia, hypokalemia, and hypercholesterolemia.

Cushing's syndrome can either be endogenous or exogenous (long-term treatment with corticosteroids). Endogenous Cushing's syndrome is either secondary to overproduction of ACTH, that is, ACTH dependent; or ACTH-independent, caused by adrenal hypersecretion of glucocorticoids. The most common form, referred to as *Cushing's disease*, results from excess ACTH release from a pituitary adenoma.

Diagnosis

Failure of dexamethasone 1 mg taken at night (11 PM) to suppress the early morning (8 AM) plasma cortisol to <5 μg per dL is suspicious for hypercortisolism. This test is simple and has a very low incidence of false normal suppression (<3%); however, it has a 20% to 30% incidence of false-positive results. The diagnosis is confirmed if the urinary-free cortisol exceeds 100 μg per 24-hour or if dexamethasone 0.5 mg every 6 hours for 2 days fails to suppress plasma cortisol to <5 μg per dL. Demonstration of elevated late night serum or salivary cortisol is likely the most specific and sensitive screening test for Cushing's syndrome. High ACTH levels suggest ACTH-dependent hypercortisolism, whereas an undetectable level of ACTH is indicative of ACTH-independent hypercortisolism. ACTH-dependent disease should be evaluated by magnetic resonance imaging (MRI) of the pituitary gland. If a pituitary tumor is not visualized, measurement of inferior petrosal sinus ACTH levels during corticotropin-releasing hormone stimulation to evaluate for an occult pituitary microadenoma, or CT imaging of the lungs to evaluate for an ectopic tumor may be necessary. In patients with ACTH-independent hypercortisolism, CT imaging of the adrenal gland is indicated.

Treatment

Transsphenoidal surgical removal of the pituitary adenoma is the preferred treatment of Cushing's disease and is generally curative. If not, pituitary irradiation or bilateral adrenalectomy may become necessary. For patients with adrenal adenomas or ectopic ACTH-producing tumors, surgical excision is also the treatment of choice. For patients with ACTH-independent bilateral adrenal macro- or micronodular hyperplasia, bilateral adrenalectomy is recommended. Until surgical cure is accomplished, the hypertension and hypokalemia associated with Cushing's syndrome can best be treated with a mineralocorticoid receptor antagonist and a calcium blocker.

Suggested Readings

Calhoun DA, Nishizaka MK, Zaman MA, et al. High prevalence of primary aldosteronism among black and white subjects with resistant hypertension. *Hypertension* 2002;40:892–896.

Findling JW, Raff H. Cushing's syndrome: important issues in diagnosis and management. *J Clin Endocrinol Metab* 2006;91:3746–3753.

Gordon RD, Ziesak MD, Tunny TJ, et al. Evidence that primary aldosteronism may not be uncommon: 12% incidence among antihypertensive drug trail volunteers. *Clin Exp Pharmacol Physiol* 1993;20:296–298.

Mattsson C, Young WF Jr. Primary aldosteronism: diagnostic and treatment strategies. *Nat Clin Pract Nephrol* 2006;2:198–208.

Mosso L, Carvajal C, González A, et al. Primary aldosteronism and hypertensive disease. *Hypertension* 2003;2:161–165.

Newell-Price J, Bertagna X, Grossman AB, et al. Cushing's syndrome. *Lancet* 2006;367:1605–1617.

Nishizaka MK, Pratt-Ubunama M, Zaman MA, et al. Validity of plasma aldosterone-to-renin activity ratio in African American and white subjects with resistant hypertension. *Am J Hypertens* 2005;8:805–812.

Nwariaju FE, Miller BS, Auchus R, et al. Primary hyperaldosteronism: effect of adrenal vein sampling on surgical outcome. *Arch Surg* 2006;141:497–503.

Rossi GP, Bernini G, Caluimi C, et al. A prospective study of the prevalence of primary aldosteronism in 1,125 hypertensive patients. *J Am Coll Cardiol* 2006;48:2293–3000.

Schwartz GL, Turner ST. Screening for primary aldosteronism in essential hypertension: diagnostic accuracy of the ratio of plasma aldosterone concentration to plasma renin activity. *Clin Chem* 2005;51:386–394.

CHAPTER C168 ■ TREATMENT OF RENOVASCULAR HYPERTENSION

JOSEPH V. NALLY, Jr., MD

KEY POINTS

- The goals of therapy for renovascular hypertension (RVHT) are effective control of hypertension and preservation of renal function; medical therapy, percutaneous transluminal renal angioplasty (PTRA, with and without stenting), and renovascular surgery are therapeutic options.
- Medical therapy with an angiotensin-converting enzyme (ACE) inhibitor or angiotensin receptor blockers (ARB) (± diuretic or calcium channel blocker) is appropriate for older patients who are at a higher risk for an intervention and for those who do not receive an invasive procedure.
- PTRA is the treatment of choice for fibromuscular dysplasia, but in unilateral atherosclerotic renal artery stenosis, clinical trials have not demonstrated a clear-cut benefit of PTRA.
- Reduced glomerular filtration rate (GFR) (increased serum creatinine) can be caused by ACE inhibitors or ARB in patients with a solitary kidney or bilateral renal artery stenosis or by any antihypertensive therapy if systemic pressure is lowered excessively in "critical" high-grade renal artery stenosis; such changes are usually reversible.

See also Chapters **A51** and **C116**

Goals of therapy

The goals of therapy for renovascular hypertension (RVHT) are effective control of blood pressure (BP) and preservation of renal function. Optimal treatment for RVHT is controversial and there have been no prospective randomized clinical trials comparing medical therapy, percutaneous transluminal renal angioplasty (PTRA), and surgery. PTRA (with or without renal artery stenting) or renovascular surgery usually reestablishes blood flow to an ischemic kidney but may or may not result in a significant lowering of BP or improvement in renal function.

Therapeutic decision-making

Until more definitive information is available, management decisions in patients with RVHT should be based on a variety of factors: the underlying risk profile of the patient, the intended goals of therapy, the type of lesion (arteriosclerosis vs. fibromuscular hyperplasia), and the site of the lesion (unilateral vs. bilateral, ostial vs. nonostial). The usual indications for intervention in renal artery disease are summarized in **Table C168.1**.

General care issues

Providing optimal medical care for patients with atherosclerotic renal artery disease includes more than simply managing BP and preserving kidney function. Modification of cardiovascular risk factors is extremely important because most of the patient deaths are due to coronary heart disease or cerebrovascular accidents. Careful attention must be given to managing coexisting hyperlipidemia and treating diabetes mellitus. Lifestyle modifications, especially smoking cessation, diet and exercise, and appropriate pharmacologic therapies for other conditions are also important.

Medical therapy

General principles. Ongoing drug therapy for hypertension and other conditions is usually required, especially for medically unstable patients, who may be poorly tolerant of procedural

TABLE C168.1

INDICATIONS FOR RENAL REVASCULARIZATION (SURGERY OR ANGIOPLASTY)

Inability to control blood pressure on an appropriate
  antihypertensive regimen
Preservation of renal function
Refractory heart failure
Intolerable side effects of medical therapy
Noncompliance with a medical regimen

intervention, or for those who decline angioplasty or surgery. Medical therapy may be appropriate for many older individuals with easily controlled hypertension and well-maintained renal function. For younger patients, especially women with fibromuscular disease, use of antihypertensive medications for 30 to 40 years seems less appropriate, especially because the results of PTRA (with and without stenting) and surgery are improving.

The management of the RVHT is similar to that for essential hypertension with three important distinctions. First, hypertension with renovascular disease may be more difficult to control and usually requires two or more medications of different classes. Second, careful attention must be given to preserving renal function during antihypertensive therapy. Finally, coexistent atherosclerotic carotid and coronary artery disease are more prevalent in these type patients and may require specific concurrent intervention.

Angiotensin-converting enzyme inhibitors and angiotensin receptor blockers.

Before the use of angiotensin-converting enzyme (ACE) inhibitors, effective control of BP in patients with RVHT was difficult to achieve. Early reports of trials with diuretics, guanethidine, hydralazine, and β-adrenergic blockers demonstrated control of hypertension in <50% of patients. ACE inhibitors or angiotensin receptor blockers (ARB) have proved to be excellent agents for treating RVHT, yet their potential for adversely effecting renal function remains somewhat concerning. The initial review of captopril therapy in 269 patients with RVHT demonstrated successful short-term control of BP in 74% of patients. Similarly, in a comparison of enalapril plus diuretic with standard triple-drug therapy, control was achieved in 96% of ACE inhibitor-treated patients versus 82% of those on triple-drug therapy. Captopril combined with a β-blocker and diuretic has been reported to maintain long-term efficacy in 90% of RVHT patients.

In patients with unilateral RAS or other forms of moderate renal artery disease, ACE inhibitors or ARBs are preferred for short-term management. ACE inhibitors and ARBs may be effectively combined with other antihypertensive agents, particularly diuretics and calcium channel blockers (CCBs). In patients with high-grade bilateral RAS or stenosis of a solitary kidney, ACE inhibitor and ARB therapy should be used with caution because glomerular filtration rate (GFR) can precipitously decline.

Calcium channel blockers.

CCBs are quite effective in lowering BP and induce less acute impairment of renal function in RVHT than do ACE inhibitors or ARBs. In that regard, nifedipine produces a much smaller decrement in GFR than captopril in patients with unilateral, bilateral, or solitary kidney RAS. CCBs act to maintain renal blood flow and function in RVHT because of their more predominant preglomerular vasodilatory (afferent arteriolar) effect. This advantage is lost with higher grades of renal arterial stenosis, however.

Deterioration of renal function.

Any class of antihypertensive therapy is capable of reducing GFR if pressure is lowered excessively in the setting of "critical" high-grade RAS. Refractory hypertension, often associated with worsening azotemia, is a common presentation of patients with RVHT due to bilateral RAS. Failure of medical therapy in such a patient may be an indication for more aggressive interventional therapy.

Use of an ACE inhibitor or ARB may cause a reversible decrement in renal function in a kidney with hemodynamically significant stenosis due to the fact that GFR in this setting is critically dependent on maximal efferent arteriolar tone, which is in turn dependent on angiotensin II. ACE inhibitor or ARB therapy reduces angiotensin II-mediated efferent arteriolar constriction and thereby lowers glomerular pressure and GFR in the affected kidney. Acute renal insufficiency (i.e., increased GFR) with ACE inhibition has been observed in up to 38% of patients with high-grade bilateral RAS or RAS of a solitary kidney. A mild decrease in GFR has also been noted in 20% of patients with high-grade unilateral RAS treated with enalapril and a diuretic. A persistent decrease in GFR on ACE inhibitor or ARB is a useful clinical clue to the presence of renal artery stenosis. Fortunately, the reduction in renal function is usually reversible when the ACE inhibitor is or ARB is discontinued but progression to complete occlusion of high-grade unilateral stenoses has been reported with the combination of an ACE inhibitor and a diuretic.

Percutaneous transluminal renal angioplasty

Technical advances notwithstanding, optimal management of RVHT is a matter of debate. Revascularization procedures are often recommended primarily for preservation of renal function because BP can usually be controlled with currently available antihypertensive drugs. Yet that recommendation is usually a matter of individual clinician judgment rather than evidence-based. Early observational studies suggested that PTRA without stenting could be an effective treatment for both hypertension and preservation of renal function but continued experience has called those data into question. Factors that determine the success of PTRA include the risk profile of the individual, success of the initial dilatation, location of the lesion (ostial vs. nonostial), and the pre-PTRA level of renal function.

Fibromuscular dysplasia.

PTRA should be the initial choice in younger patients with a fibromuscular lesion amenable to balloon angioplasty. Results of PTRA for fibromuscular hyperplasia have been excellent and quite comparable to surgical intervention. As many as 30% of patients with fibromuscular dysplasia have branch renal arterial involvement that may significantly increase the technical difficulty of PTRA, but may not necessarily preclude use of this treatment modality.

Atherosclerotic disease

Percutaneous transluminal renal angioplasty alone. In patients with unilateral RAS, three small randomized, controlled trials have failed to identify major benefits of PTRA (without stenting) compared to medical management, although results were confounded by high crossover rates from medical to PTRA. In the Dutch study of PTRA versus medical therapy, the intention to treat analysis showed that BP, renal function, and daily medication doses were similar between the two groups at 1 year. However, at 3 months, approximately 40% of the 50 patients initially assigned to medical therapy were treated with "rescue" PTRA because of refractory hypertension. A French randomized trial of PTRA versus medical therapy noted equivalent BPs at 6-months follow-up, although the angioplasty patients tended to require fewer medications. A randomized trial of PTRA versus surgery showed a higher primary patency rate in the surgical group but the clinical outcomes were similar because many PTRA patients with restenosis were successfully treated with a second PTRA.

Percutaneous transluminal renal angioplasty with stenting. A method to improve the efficacy of PTRA (especially in ostial lesions) and to reduce the incidence of restenosis is the insertion of a balloon-expandable intravascular stent at the time of angioplasty. Several studies have documented the superior primary patency rate of PTRA with stenting for ostial atherosclerotic lesions. A prospective trial comparing the outcome of PTRA alone versus PTRA plus stent in ostial atherosclerotic lesions has confirmed the higher patency rate with stenting although the stenting procedure lowered BP to a similar degree. Despite the benefits of patency rates, it is unclear whether PTRA plus stenting is superior to PTRA alone to preserve renal function or control BP. It has been concluded that the benefits of PTRA are sufficiently ambiguous to justify a prospective trial, the Cardiovascular Outcomes in Renal Atherosclerotic Lesions [CORAL] study, in which clinical cardiac and renal outcomes are being assessed over 3 to 5 years, based upon optimal medical therapy with or without PTRA (with stenting and distal embolic protection).

Surgical intervention

Surgical intervention in unilateral atherosclerotic RAS usually involves bypassing the stenotic segment or removing an atrophic kidney distal to a complete arterial occlusion. Surgery is generally more effective than PTRA in the treatment of atherosclerotic disease, with 80% to 90% of patients becoming stable or improved. Aortorenal bypass using autogenous saphenous vein or hypogastric artery is a common revascularization technique in patients with a nondiseased abdominal aorta. When an autogenous vascular graft is not available, a synthetic polytetrafluoroethylene graft can be used. Alternatively, splenorenal, hepatorenal, or ileorenal bypasses may be performed in order to avoid manipulation of a severely atherosclerotic aorta. In some cases, surgical revascularization is successful in preserving renal function. The mortality rate associated with surgical intervention for atherosclerotic disease varies with the degree of extrarenal vascular disease, type of surgery, and experience of the surgical team. Overall mortality rates of <2.5% have been reported from centers with experience in treating patients with unilateral disease and mortality rates between 3% to 6% in patients with bilateral disease. Presurgery screening for coronary or cerebrovascular disease is crucial in reducing perioperative mortality rates.

Suggested Readings

Balk E, Raman G, Chung M, et al. Effectiveness of management strategies for renal artery stenosis: a systematic review. *Ann Intern Med* 2006;145:901–912.

Blum U, Krumme B, Flugel P, et al. Treatment of ostial renal-artery stenoses with vascular endoprostheses after unsuccessful balloon angioplasty. *N Engl J Med* 1997;336:459–465.

van Jaarsveld BC, Krijnen P, Pieterman H, et al. : The effect of balloon angioplasty on hypertension in atherosclerotic renal-artery stenosis. Dutch Renal Artery Stenosis Intervention Cooperative Study Group. *N Engl J Med* 2000;342:1007–1014.

Plouin PF, Chatellier G, Darne B, et al. Blood pressure outcome of angioplasty in atherosclerotic renal artery stenosis: a randomized trial. Essai Multicentrique Medicaments versus Angioplastie (EMMA) Study Group. *Hypertension* 1998;31:823–829.

Rimmer JM, Gennari FJ. Atherosclerotic renovascular disease and progressive renal failure. *Ann Intern Med* 1993;118:712–719.

Textor SC. Revascularization in atherosclerotic renal artery disease [clinical conference]. *Kidney Int* 1998;53:799–811.

Textor SC. Renovascular hypertension update. *Curr Hypertens Rep* 2006;8:521–527.

van de Ven PJ, Kaatee R, Beutler JJ, et al. Arterial stenting and balloon angioplasty in ostial atherosclerotic renovascular disease: a randomised trial. *Lancet* 1999;353:282–286.

Zierler RE, Bergelin RO, Davidson RC, et al. A prospective study of disease progression in patients with atherosclerotic renal artery stenosis. *Am J Hypertens* 1996;9:1055–1061.

CHAPTER C169 ■ MANAGEMENT OF PHEOCHROMOCYTOMA

WILLIAM F. YOUNG, Jr., MD, MSc AND SHELDON G. SHEPS, MD

KEY POINTS

- The diagnosis of a catecholamine-producing tumor is based on clinical suspicion that is confirmed biochemically (by increased urine or plasma levels of fractionated metanephrines and catecholamines) and anatomically (by computed tomographic imaging of the abdomen).
- The treatment of choice for catecholamine-secreting tumors, which are usually benign, is surgical resection after careful preoperative pharmacologic preparation.
- Hypertension may be cured by excision of the tumor but some individuals experience residual hypertension and require continued drug therapy.
- Malignant pheochromocytoma and paraganglioma are diagnosed when direct invasion of surrounding tissue or a metastatic lesion is found; therapy depends on the extent of and the location of disease; resection, radiation therapy, radiofrequency ablation, chemotherapy, and observation should be considered.

See also Chapters **A11,** C105, and C106

Catecholamine-secreting tumors are located in the adrenal medulla (pheochromocytoma) or in the extraadrenal paraganglionic tissue (catecholamine-secreting paraganglioma). Prevalence estimates for pheochromocytoma vary from 0.01% to 0.10% of the hypertensive population, with an incidence of two to eight cases per million people per year, which occur equally in men and women in the third through fifth decades.

Clinical presentation

Patients with catecholamine-secreting tumors may be asymptomatic but are more commonly symptomatic due to the excess in circulating catecholamines. Episodic symptoms include abrupt onset of throbbing headaches, generalized diaphoresis, palpitations, forceful heart beat, pallor, anxiety, chest pain, and abdominal pain. These spells can be extremely variable in their presentation and may be spontaneous or precipitated by postural changes, anxiety, exercise, anesthesia, drugs (e.g., metoclopramide), or maneuvers that increase intraabdominal pressure. The pheochromocytoma spell may last 10 to 60 minutes and may occur daily to monthly. Clinical signs may include hypertension (paroxysmal in half of the patients and sustained in the other half), orthostatic hypotension, pallor, grade I to IV hypertensive retinopathy, tremor, and fever. Pheochromocytoma-induced hypertension results from excess catecholamine production, but the tumors can be found in association with other endocrine abnormalities in those with multiple endocrine neoplasia syndromes.

Diagnosis

The diagnostic approach to catecholamine-producing tumors is divided into two series of studies (**Figure C169.1**), both of which are triggered by clinical suspicion.

Biochemical tests. The diagnosis of a catecholamine-producing tumor must be confirmed biochemically by the presence of increased urine or plasma levels of fractionated metanephrines and catecholamines. Urinary fractionated metanephrines and catecholamines are the tests of choice. Fractionated plasma metanephrines, although highly specific, lack sensitivity for routine screening of low-risk, nonfamilial patients. Urinary vanillylmandelic acid (VMA) is no longer recommended because of its relatively poor sensitivity and specificity.

Imaging studies. The next step is to localize the catecholamine-producing tumor to guide the surgical approach. Approximately 90% of catecholamine-producing tumors are found in the adrenals, and 98% are in the abdomen. Computer-assisted adrenal and abdominal imaging (magnetic resonance imaging or computed tomography) is the first localization test. If the finding on abdominal imaging is negative, scintigraphic localization with iodine-123 metaiodobenzylguanidine (^{123}I-MIBG) is indicated. This radiopharmaceutical accumulates preferentially in catecholamine-producing tumors but the test is not as definitive as initially hoped (sensitivity, 85%; specificity, 99%). Computer-assisted imaging of the pelvis, chest, and neck; octreotide scintigraphy; and positron emission tomography are

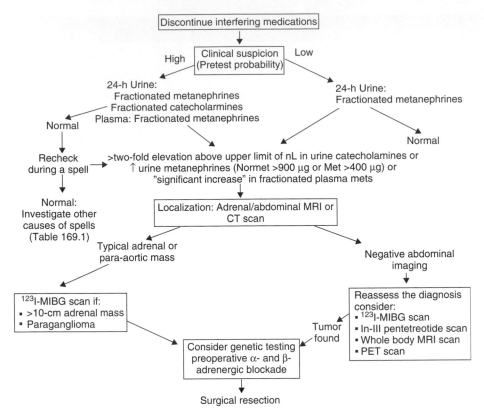

Figure C169.1 Evaluation and treatment of catecholamine-producing tumors. Clinical suspicion is triggered by the following: presence of headache, palpitations, forceful heart beat, or abnormal sweating; paroxysmal symptoms (especially hypertension); hypertension that is intermittent, unusually labile, or resistant to treatment; family history of pheochromocytoma or associated conditions; or incidentally discovered adrenal mass. For details, see text. Met, metanephrine; Normet, normetanephrine; MRI, magnetic resonance imaging; CT, computed tomography; ^{123}I-MIBG, [^{123}I]metaiodobenzylguanidine; PET, positron emission tomography. (From Young WF Jr. Pheochromocytoma: 1926–1993 trends in endocrinology and metabolism. New York:Elsevier Science,1993:122, with permission.)

additional localizing procedures that can be used if necessary, although they are seldom required.

Functional tests. Suppression testing with clonidine or provocative testing with glucagon, histamine, or metoclopramide is rarely needed. These tests are not generally recommended due to expense and potential risks (hypertension and hypotension). In general, repeat biochemical testing (fractionated urinary metanephrines and catecholamines) is preferred in the usual clinical setting. The differential diagnosis of catecholamine-secreting tumors is summarized in **Table C169.1.**

Treatment

The treatment of choice for catecholamine-secreting tumors is surgical resection. The choice of approaches depends on the skill and experience of the surgeon. Most of these tumors are benign and can be totally excised. Hypertension may be cured by excision of the tumor but some patients have residual hypertension that necessitates continuing of drug therapy. Careful preoperative pharmacologic preparation is crucial to successful surgical treatment.

Preoperative management. Combined α- and β-adrenergic blockade is recommended before surgery to control blood pressure (BP) and to prevent intraoperative hypertensive crises. A liberal salt diet is advised during the preoperative period. Long-acting nonselective α-adrenergic blockade (e.g., phenoxybenzamine) should be started at least 7 to 10 days before surgery to allow for expansion of the contracted blood volume. Once adequate α-adrenergic blockade is achieved (e.g., resolution of spells, normalization of BP, nasal stuffiness, mild orthostasis), β-adrenergic blockade is initiated, usually a few days before surgery. Calcium channel antagonists have also been used successfully at several medical centers for the preoperative

preparation of pheochromocytoma patients. α-Methyl-L-tyrosine (metyrosine) inhibits the synthesis of catecholamines by blocking the enzyme tyrosine hydroxylase. The significant side-effect profile of metyrosine limits its use to those patients who, for cardiopulmonary reasons, do not tolerate or are not controlled with combined α- and β-adrenergic blockade.

Perioperative management. Extirpation of a catecholamine-secreting tumor is a high-risk surgical procedure, and an experienced surgeon and anesthesiology team are required. The last oral doses of the antihypertensive agents can be administered early in the morning on the day of surgery. Cardiovascular and hemodynamic variables must be monitored closely. Acute hypertensive crises may occur before or during surgery and should be treated with intravenous nitroprusside or phentolamine.

Surgical approach. In the past, an anterior midline abdominal surgical approach was usually used for adrenal pheochromocytoma. However, laparoscopic adrenalectomy is the procedure of choice in patients with solitary adrenal catecholamine-secreting tumors that are <8 cm in diameter. If the tumor is in the adrenal gland, the entire gland should be removed. Cortical-sparing procedures may be indicated in patients with bilateral adrenal tumors (e.g., von Hippel-Lindau syndrome). If the tumor is malignant, as much tumor as possible should be removed. Catecholamine-secreting paragangliomas of the neck, chest, and urinary bladder require specialized approaches. At major centers, the surgical mortality rate is <2%; survival rate after removal of a benign pheochromocytoma is nearly that of age- and sex-matched controls.

Follow-up. In those patients without concomitant essential hypertension, BP is usually normal by the time of discharge from the hospital. Approximately 2 weeks after surgery, the catecholamine secretory status should be assessed. If fractionated metanephrines and catecholamines are normal, the resection of

TABLE C169.1

DIFFERENTIAL DIAGNOSIS OF PHEOCHROMOCYTOMA SPELLS

Endocrine
  Thyrotoxicosis
  Primary hypogonadism (e.g., menopausal syndrome)
  Pancreatic tumors (e.g., insulinoma)
  Medullary thyroid carcinoma
  "Hyperadrenergic" spells
Cardiovascular
  Essential hypertension, labile
  Angina and cardiovascular deconditioning
  Pulmonary edema
  Dilated cardiomyopathy
  Syncope
  Orthostatic hypotension
  Paroxysmal cardiac arrhythmia
  Aortic dissection
  Renovascular hypertension
Psychological
  Anxiety and panic attacks
  Somatization disorder
  Hyperventilation
  Factitious (e.g., drugs, Valsalva)
Pharmacologic
  Withdrawal of adrenergic-inhibiting medication (e.g.,
    clonidine)
  Monoamine oxidase inhibitor treatment and concomitant
    ingestion of tyramine or a decongestant
  Sympathomimetic ingestion
  Illicit drug ingestion (e.g., cocaine, phencyclidine, lysergic
    acid)
  Gold myokymia syndrome
  Acrodynia (mercury poisoning)
  Vancomycin (red man syndrome)
Neurologic
  Baroreflex failure
  Postural orthostatic tachycardia syndrome (POTS)
  Autonomic neuropathy
  Migraine headache
  Diencephalic epilepsy (autonomic seizures)
  Cerebral infarction
  Cerebrovascular insufficiency
Miscellaneous
  Mastocytosis (systemic or activation disorder)
  Carcinoid syndrome
  Recurrent idiopathic anaphylaxis
  Unexplained flushing spells

the pheochromocytoma can be considered to have been complete. Fractionated plasma metanephrines or 24-hour urinary excretion of fractionated metanephrines and catecholamines should be checked annually as surveillance for recurrence in the adrenal bed, appearance of metastatic lesions, or delayed appearance of multiple primary tumors.

Malignant pheochromocytoma

The distinction between benign and malignant catecholamine-producing tumors cannot be made on the basis of clinical, biochemical, or histopathologic characteristics. Malignancy can only be determined on the basis of direct local invasion or metastasis to sites that do not have chromaffin tissue, such as lymph nodes, bone, lung, and liver. Metastatic lesions should be resected if possible. Radiofrequency ablation of hepatic and bone metastases may be very effective in select patients. Painful skeletal metastatic lesions can be treated with external radiation therapy. Local tumor irradiation with iodine-131 metaiodobenzylguanidine (^{131}I-MIBG) has proved to be of limited therapeutic value. If the tumor is considered to be aggressive and the quality of life is affected, combination chemotherapy using cyclophosphamide, vincristine, and dacarbazine cyclically every 21 to 28 days may be beneficial but not curative. Combined α- and β-adrenergic blockade is useful to control catecholamine-related symptoms. Although the 5-year survival rate is <50%, many of these patients have prolonged survival and minimal morbidity.

Screening for familial catecholamine-secreting tumor disorders

Germline molecular genetic testing for familial disorders such as multiple endocrine neoplasia type 2, von-Hippel Lindau syndrome, neurofibromatosis type 1, familial pheochromocytoma, and familial paraganglioma should be considered during the first postoperative visit. In addition, all immediate family members should be biochemically screened for a catecholamine-secreting tumor.

Suggested Readings

Averbuch SD, Steakley CS, Young RC, et al. Malignant pheochromocytoma: effective treatment with a combination of cyclophosphamide, vincristine, and dacarbazine. *Ann Intern Med* 1988;109:267–273.

Erickson D, Kudva YC, Ebersold MJ, et al. Benign paragangliomas: clinical presentation and treatment outcomes in 236 patients. *J Clin Endocrinol Metab* 2001;86:5210–5216.

Gimenez-Roqueplo AP, Lehnert H, Mannelli M, et al. European Network for the Study of Adrenal Tumours (ENS@T) Pheochromocytoma Working Group. Phaeochromocytoma, new genes and screening strategies. *Clin Endocrinol (Oxf)* 2006;65:699–705.

Kinney MAO, Warner ME, vanHeerden JA, et al. Perianesthetic risks and outcomes of pheochromocytoma and paraganglioma resection. *Anesth Analg* 2000;91:1118–1123.

Kudva YC, Sawka AM, Young WF Jr. Clinical review 164: the laboratory diagnosis of adrenal pheochromocytoma: the Mayo Clinic experience. *J Clin Endocrinol Metab* 2003;88:4533–4539.

Motta-Ramirez GA, Remer EM, Herts BR, et al. Comparison of CT findings in symptomatic and incidentally discovered pheochromocytomas. *AJR Am J Roentgenol* 2005;185:684–688.

Perry CG, Sawka AM, Singh R, et al. The diagnostic efficacy of urinary fractionated metanephrines measured by tandem mass spectrometry in detection of pheochromocytoma. *Clin Endocrinol (Oxf)* 2007;66:507–618.

Pham TH, Moir C, Thompson GB, et al. Pheochromocytoma and paraganglioma in children: a review of medical and surgical management at a tertiary care center. *Pediatrics* 2006;118:1109–1117.

Shulkin BL, Ilias I, Sisson JC, et al. Current trends in functional imaging of pheochromocytomas and paragangliomas. *Ann N Y Acad Sci* 2006;1073:374–382.

Young WF Jr. Paragangliomas: clinical overview. *Ann N Y Acad Sci* 2006;1073: 21–29.

Young WF Jr, Maddox DE. Spells: in search of a cause. *Mayo Clin Proc* 1995;70:757–765.

CHAPTER C170 ■ MANAGEMENT OF THYROID AND PARATHYROID DISORDERS

WILLIAM F. YOUNG, Jr., MD, MSc

KEY POINTS

■ The types of thyroid disease associated with hypertension include hyperthyroidism, hypothyroidism, and medullary thyroid carcinoma (MTC) [associated with pheochromocytoma in the multiple endocrine neoplasia (MEN) syndromes types 2A and 2B].

■ The hypercalcemia of hyperparathyroidism is associated with an increased incidence of hypertension, especially in end-stage renal disease.

■ Thyroid- and parathyroid-directed treatment in the hypertensive patient may normalize hypertension or facilitate its treatment.

See also Chapters A53 and C108

Dysfunction of the thyroid and parathyroid glands may be the sole cause of hypertension or may contribute to underlying essential hypertension; blood pressure (BP) elevations with thyroid disease are usually mild but may be more significant with hyperparathyroidism.

THYROID DYSFUNCTION

The types of thyroid disease associated with hypertension include hyperthyroidism, hypothyroidism, and medullary thyroid carcinoma (MTC)—usually when associated with pheochromocytoma as part of the multiple endocrine neoplasia (MEN) type 2A and 2B syndromes.

Clinical presentation

Hyperthyroidism. Hyperthyroidism is the clinical syndrome induced by excessive amounts of circulating thyroid hormones with increased β-adrenergic receptor sensitivity to circulating catecholamines. Thyrotoxic patients usually have tachycardia, high cardiac output, increased stroke volume, decreased peripheral vascular resistance, and increased systolic BP, often with diastolic BP <90 mm Hg.

Hypothyroidism. Hypothyroidism is the syndrome resulting from deficiency of thyroid hormones, which causes many metabolic processes to slow down. The frequency of hypertension, usually diastolic, is increased threefold in hypothyroid patients and may account for as much as 1% of cases of diastolic hypertension in the population. The mechanisms for the elevation in BP with hypothyroidism include increased systemic vascular resistance and extracellular volume expansion.

Laboratory diagnosis. The clinical suspicion of thyroid gland dysfunction may be confirmed with laboratory tests. Increased levels of blood thyroid hormones (thyroxine and triiodothyronine) and low serum levels of thyroid-stimulating hormone (TSH) are the hallmarks of primary hyperthyroidism. Low serum TSH concentration in thyrotoxicosis is caused by excess thyroxine or triiodothyronine. The diagnosis of hypothyroidism is based on low serum levels of thyroxine and increased serum levels of TSH.

Treatment

Hyperthyroidism. The initial management of the hypertensive patient with hyperthyroidism includes β-adrenergic blockade (e.g., atenolol or propranolol) to treat the hypertension, tachycardia, and tremor. The definitive treatment of hyperthyroidism is cause-specific. Patients with autoimmune hyperthyroidism (Graves' disease) should be treated with thyroid gland ablation [e.g., with radioiodine-131 (^{131}I)]. In the patient with hyperthyroidism caused by a multinodular goiter (Plummer's disease), ^{131}I is usually not curative and subtotal thyroidectomy is frequently the treatment of choice. If the hyperthyroidism is associated with acute thyroid inflammation (e.g., subacute thyroiditis), temporary (e.g., 3 months) use of a β-adrenergic inhibitor may be the only treatment indicated.

Hypothyroidism. Treatment of thyroid hormone deficiency lowers BP in most hypertensive patients. Synthetic levothyroxine is the treatment of choice for hypothyroidism. The initial dosage of levothyroxine is based on body weight (1.6 µg/kg/day). The daily dosage requirement may be lower in older patients (e.g., <1 µg/kg/day). In patients older than 50 years or in those with cardiac disease, the initial dosage of levothyroxine should be lower (e.g., 25–50 μg/day) and increased every 2 weeks by 25 μg until the target dosage is achieved. Clinical and biochemical reevaluations should be done at 2-month intervals until the serum TSH concentration is normalized.

MEDULLARY THYROID CARCINOMA

The occurrence of MTC may be sporadic or familial (familial MTC or MEN 2). Although MTC does not cause hypertension, the close association with pheochromocytoma is recognized: MEN 2A (MTC, pheochromocytoma, and hyperparathyroidism) and MEN 2B (MTC, pheochromocytoma, mucosal neuromas, and marfanoid body habitus). The MEN 2 syndromes are inherited as autosomal dominant traits with complete penetrance and variable expressivity.

Clinical presentation

The usual presentation of MTC is with a thyroid nodule, thyroid mass, or cervical lymphadenopathy. Although serum calcitonin concentrations are increased, most patients are asymptomatic. Up to 30% of patients with MTC develop watery diarrhea, presumably secondary to high circulating calcitonin levels. Serum levels of calcium and phosphorus are typically normal.

Laboratory diagnosis

When the presentation is limited to a solitary thyroid nodule, the diagnosis of MTC may be made on cytologic findings from a fine-needle aspirate. In other patients, MTC may be suspected and found with biochemical testing because of a family history of MEN 2. All first-degree relatives of patients with MEN 2 should be screened with the molecular genetic test for mutation in the *RET* protooncogene.

Treatment

The treatment of choice for MTC is surgical resection. Most centers advocate total thyroidectomy and ^{131}I ablation of the thyroid gland remnant. After this initial treatment, patients are placed on levothyroxine replacement therapy and should be followed up on an annual basis with physical examination and serum calcitonin levels. If recurrent disease is suspected on the basis of increasing serum calcitonin levels, it can usually be localized with ultrasound or computed tomographic imaging of the neck.

Screening for other multiple endocrine neoplasia abnormalities

Clinicians should be aware of the high prevalence of other endocrine neoplasias in patients with MTC. In particular, screening for pheochromocytoma should be performed in all MTC patients because of the high cardiovascular risk if its presence goes undetected. Screening of first-degree relatives should also be considered.

HYPERPARATHYROIDISM

Primary hyperparathyroidism is the most frequent cause of persistent hypercalcemia and is also associated with hypertension, especially in the setting of end-stage renal disease, and also in patients with normal renal function.

Clinical presentation

Hypercalcemia is associated with an increased incidence of hypertension and primary hyperparathyroidism is the most common cause of persistent hypercalcemia. The prevalence of hypertension in patients with primary hyperparathyroidism varies from 10% to 60%. In most cases, the disease is caused by a benign solitary parathyroid adenoma. However, when associated with MEN syndromes, hyperparathyroidism is usually due to hyperplasia of all 4 parathyroid glands. Diffuse hyperplasia is also the usual presentation in patients with end-stage renal disease; in severe cases, calciphylaxis can be observed (diffuse calcification of peripheral arteries), usually with marked reduction in bone density. Most patients with primary hyperparathyroidism are asymptomatic but more severe forms of the disease are commonly accompanied by symptoms of polyuria and polydipsia, abdominal discomfort, constipation, osteoporosis, renal lithiasis, peptic ulcer disease, and hypertension.

Laboratory diagnosis

The hallmarks of primary hyperparathyroidism are hypercalcemia, hypophosphatemia, and increased serum concentrations of parathyroid hormone (PTH). In the patient with hypercalcemia, the simultaneous measurement of serum PTH and ionized calcium is the most efficient way of making the diagnosis of primary hyperparathyroidism. If the serum concentration of PTH is not increased, the physician should consider nonparathyroid causes of hypercalcemia (e.g., pheochromocytoma, hyperthyroidism, cancer, multiple myeloma, vitamin D intoxication, and sarcoidosis).

Treatment

The treatment of hyperparathyroidism is surgical. Preoperative localization with sestamibi scintigraphy or neck ultrasonography may facilitate minimal access parathyroidectomy in the setting of sporadic (solitary parathyroid adenoma) hyperparathyroidism. For patients with 4 gland disease, a variety of techniques can be employed, from subtotal parathyroidectomy (usually 3–3.5 glands removed) to total ablation with reimplantation of minced gland, usually in the forearm or upper chest wall. In the setting of MEN, subtotal parathyroid resection (3.5 glands) of the hyperplastic glands is usually indicated.

Suggested Readings

Danzi S, Klein I. Thyroid hormone and BP regulation. *Curr Hypertens Rep* 2003; 5:513–520.

Evans DB, Burgess MA, Goepfert H, et al. Medullary thyroid carcinoma. *Curr Ther Endocrinol Metab* 1997;6:127–132.

Kiernan TJ, O'Flynn AM, McDermott JH, et al. Primary hyperparathyroidism and the cardiovascular system. *Int J Cardiol* 2006;113:E89–E92.

Letizia C, Ferrari P, Cotesta D, et al. Ambulatory monitoring of BP (AMBP) in patients with primary hyperparathyroidism. *J Hum Hypertens* 2005;19:901–906.

Marzanol A, Porcelli A, Biondi B, et al. Surgical management and follow-up of medullary thyroid carcinoma. *J Surg Oncol* 1995;59:162–168.

Pommier RF, Brennan MF. Medullary thyroid carcinoma. *Endocrinologist* 1992; 2:393–405.

Richards AM, Espiner EA, Nicholls MG, et al. Hormone, calcium and BP relationships in primary hyperparathyroidism. *J Hypertens* 1988;6:747–752.

Saito I, Saruta T. Hypertension in thyroid disorders. *Endocrinol Metab Clin North Am* 1994;23:379–386.

Sancho JJ, Rouco J, Riera-Vidal R, et al. Long-term effects of parathyroidectomy for primary hyperparathyroidism on arterial hypertension. *World J Surg* 1992; 16:732–736.

Streeten DHP, Anderson GH Jr, Howland T, et al. Effects of thyroid function on BP: recognition of hypothyroid hypertension. *Hypertension* 1988;11:78–83.

CHAPTER C171 ■ MANAGEMENT OF POST-TRANSPLANT HYPERTENSION

VINCENT J. CANZANELLO, MD

KEY POINTS

■ Post-transplant hypertension is common and is associated with increased cardiovascular morbidity and mortality and an increased risk of subsequent graft dysfunction.

■ Post-transplant hypertension is usually related to the use of corticosteroids and calcineurin inhibitors or to renal insufficiency.

■ Many transplant recipients have additional cardiovascular comorbidities such that aggressive blood pressure (BP) lowering is indicated, usually to <130/80 mm Hg.

■ Many drugs, including angiotensin-converting enzyme (ACE) inhibitors, angiotensin receptor blockers (ARBs), calcium channel blockers (CCBs), and diuretics, are safe and effective in the treatment of Post-transplant hypertension.

See also Chapters C115 and C116

The long-term goal in patients with Post-transplant hypertension is similar to that of nontransplant patients: reduced morbidity and mortality by control of blood pressure (BP), hyperglycemia, dyslipidemia, and cigarette smoking. Many hypertensive transplant recipients have coexisting conditions such as cardiac or renal disease, diabetes mellitus, or dyslipidemia that argue for BP control to <130/80 mm Hg. Instruction in self-measurement of BP is an integral part of many transplantation programs. The use of 24-hour ambulatory BP monitoring may be of particular help in the diagnosis and therein the treatment of hypertension in the transplant recipient. Both 24-hour mean BP and the relative lack of nocturnal BP decline (often attenuated in this patient population) correlate with hypertensive target organ damage (left ventricular hypertrophy and proteinuria).

Exacerbating factors

Post-transplant hypertension is usually associated with the use of immunosuppressive drugs such as calcineurin inhibitors (cyclosporine and tacrolimus) or corticosteroids. Corticosteroid-associated weight gain is also a common occurrence after organ transplantation and is a contributing factor to the development of hypertension, diabetes mellitus, and dyslipidemia, particularly hypertriglyceridemia. In one large retrospective analysis of renal transplant recipients, the development of obesity [body mass index (BMI) >30 kg/m^2] was associated with reduced graft and patient survival at 5 years. Renal dysfunction is common in the Post-transplant setting and can play a significant role in the development and course of hypertension. Causes of post-transplant

hypertension are shown in **Table C171.1** and include pertinent factors that raise BP in the nontransplant population.

Modification of immunosuppression regimens

Several studies of liver and renal transplantation have demonstrated a lower prevalence of hypertension with tacrolimus compared to cyclosporine. Lower doses of corticosteroids used in tacrolimus-treated patients may account, in part, for this difference. In addition, the trend toward earlier discontinuation of corticosteroids has been associated with a lower incidence of Post-transplant hypertension, particularly in liver transplantation. Use of the macrolide antibiotic sirolimus (which is not a calcineurin inhibitor) in organ transplantation is increasing. Several reports suggest that this drug is associated with less nephrotoxicity and hypertension compared to cyclosporine and tacrolimus although dyslipidemia and new-onset proteinuria may be more common.

Lifestyle modification

Nutritional counseling is important and should focus on healthy eating habits (including total calories, protein and fat content, sodium chloride intake, and so on). Reduction of dietary sodium intake in hypertensive renal transplant recipients (as shown by a reduction in daily urinary sodium excretion from 190 ± 75 to 106 ± 48 mEq/day) reduced the mean BP from 146 ± 21/89 ± 8 mm Hg to 116 ± 11/72 ± 10 mm Hg with the same or fewer antihypertensive drugs; the control group had no

TABLE C171.1

CAUSES OF POST-TRANSPLANT HYPERTENSION

Immunosuppressive drugs
    Cyclosporine
    Tacrolimus
    Sirolimus
    Corticosteroids
Renal dysfunction
    Perioperative ischemic damage
    Drug-induced nephrotoxicity
    Chronic allograft rejection
    Recurrence of original renal disease
Native diseased kidneys
Transplant renal artery stenosis
Donor-kidney associated hypertension
Miscellaneous
    High dietary sodium intake
    Nonsteroidal anti-inflammatory drugs
    Obesity
    Alcohol
    Obstructive sleep apnea

appreciable change in BP. The need for regular aerobic exercise should also be emphasized.

Antihypertensive drug therapy considerations

Deciding on the most appropriate drug therapy in the setting of transplant-associated hypertension has become more complex in recent years, in part due to the need to achieve multiple therapeutic goals, including (a) lowering the systemic BP to reduce cardiovascular risk, (b) maintaining optimal renal blood flow by attenuating calcineurin inhibitor–associated renal vasoconstriction, and (c) preventing long-term renal dysfunction associated with glomerular hypertension or other adverse vascular effects of calcineurin inhibitors. BP goals have not been formally established for transplant recipients, and there are no clinical studies that specifically demonstrate better outcomes at target BPs below 140/90 mm Hg. Nevertheless, coexisting conditions such as diabetes or heart failure may mandate lower goals. In the acute Post-transplant setting (days to weeks), BP may improve spontaneously with increased physical activity, mobilization of retained fluid, reduction in immunosuppressive drug doses, and improvement or stabilization of graft function.

Specific antihypertensive drugs

In general, a single antihypertensive drug cannot achieve all of the desired goals and, as a result, many transplant recipients with hypertension require the use of two or more medications. The following comments generally apply most directly to the patient who is several months Post-transplantation and with stable graft function.

Calcium channel blockers. There are several features of calcium channel blockers (CCBs) that make them an attractive choice in the treatment of post-transplant hypertension. These drugs antagonize calcineurin inhibitor–induced systemic and renal vasoconstriction and therefore lead to an increase in renal blood flow in tandem with reduction in systemic BP. Some CCBs (verapamil, diltiazem, and nicardipine) interfere with

the metabolism of calcineurin inhibitors, and some transplant clinicians have capitalized on this interaction to lower the doses of cyclosporine or tacrolimus thereby reducing drug expense. Long-acting dihydropyridine CCBs are most commonly used. As a general rule, it is prudent to monitor the cyclosporine or tacrolimus blood levels closely during the initiation of CCB therapy.

β-Blockers. β-Blockers are used in treating post-transplant hypertension and their BP-lowering effects are similar to CCBs, angiotensin-converting enzyme (ACE) inhibitors, and angiotensin receptor blockers (ARBs). β-Blockers have no significant adverse effect on renal function.

Angiotensin-converting enzyme inhibitors and angiotensin receptor blockers. Plasma–renin activity is generally low or suppressed for several months after renal or liver transplantation in the setting of steroid and calcineurin inhibitor use. As a result, ACE inhibitors and ARBs demonstrate limited monotherapeutic effectiveness during this time interval. The efficacy of compounds in either of these drug classes can be enhanced by the addition of a diuretic. In those hypertensive patients who have stable graft function for 1 year or more, ACE inhibitors and ARBs have been shown to have efficacy equivalent to CCBs and β-blockers. Several studies in renal transplant recipients have shown that ACE inhibitors and ARBs reduce proteinuria to a greater extent than other drugs. Many experimental studies have demonstrated the ability of these two drug classes to ameliorate calcineurin inhibitor–associated disturbances of endothelial and renal dysfunction.

ACE inhibitors and ARBs can exacerbate hyperkalemia associated with renal insufficiency and calcineurin inhibitor use and can also precipitate reversible acute renal failure in patients with transplant renal artery stenosis. Drugs in these classes can be useful in reducing hemoglobin levels in the case of Post-transplant erythrocytosis; conversely, anemia may occur with these compounds after transplantation but is reversible on discontinuation of the drug. Anemia appears to be more common with ACE inhibitors than with ARBs, which may be a consequence of higher levels of the hematopoiesis inhibitor N-acetyl-seryl-aspartyl-lysyl-proline, which is almost exclusively degraded by ACE.

Diuretics

Thiazide and loop diuretics play an important role in the management of post-transplant hypertension but their use requires careful monitoring of serum electrolytes, renal function, immunosuppressive drug levels (which can vary with renal function), and other metabolic parameters such as serum calcium, uric acid, lipid, and glucose. Early after transplantation, hypertension may be precipitated or exacerbated by renal dysfunction and extracellular fluid volume expansion; several studies have demonstrated salt-sensitive hypertension with calcineurin inhibitors. In patients with hyperkalemia, thiazide or loop diuretics (or a combination of both) can increase distal tubular sodium delivery and ameliorate hyperkalemia. In general, potassium-sparing diuretics should be avoided because many Post-transplant patients have high or high-normal serum potassium levels related to renal insufficiency, type IV renal tubular acidosis, or calcineurin inhibitors. Thiazide diuretics are rarely effective when the glomerular filtration rate is below 30 mL per minute. In this circumstance, use of a loop diuretic such as furosemide, bumetanide, or torsemide should be considered.

Suggested Readings

El-Agroudy AE, Wafa EW, Gheith OE, et al. Weight gain after renal transplantation is a risk factor for patient and graft outcome. *Transplantation* 2004;77:1381–1385.

Keven K, Yalcin S, Canbakan B, et al. The impact of daily sodium intake on Post-transplant hypertension in kidney allograft recipients. *Transplant Proc* 2006;38:1323–1326.

Khan S, Carrock Sewell WA. Oral immunosuppressive drugs. *Clin Med* 2006;6:352–355.

Morales JM, Andres A, Rengel M, et al. Influence of cyclosporine, tacrolimus and rapamycin on renal function and arterial hypertension after renal transplantation. *Nephrol Dial Transplant* 2001;16(Suppl 1):121–124.

Mulay AV, Hussain N, Fergusson D, et al. Calcineurin inhibitor withdrawal from sirolimus-based therapy in kidney transplantation: a systematic review of randomized trials. *Am J Transplant* 2005;5:1748–1756.

Ojo AO. Cardiovascular complications after renal transplantation and their prevention. *Transplantation* 2006;82:603–611.

Page RL, Miller GG, Lindenfeld J. Drug therapy in the heart transplant recipient. Part IV: drug-drug interactions. *Circulation* 2005;111:230–239.

Premasathian NC, Muehrer R, Brazy PC, et al. BP control in kidney transplantation: therapeutic implications. *J Hum Hypertens* 2004;18:871–877.

Toprak A, Kroc M, Tezcan H, et al. Night-time BP load is associated with higher left ventricular mass index in renal transplant recipients. *J Hum Hypertens* 2003;17:239–244.

Writing group member	Employment	Research grant	Other research support	Speakers' bureau/honoraria	Expert witness	Ownership interest	Consultant/advisory board	Other
Adams	University of North Carolina School of Medicine	Amgen*, Amylin*, AstraZeneca+, Novacardia*, Orqis*, Otsuka America*, Scios+, Vasogen*	None	Nitromed*, BMS*, Biosite*, Myogen*, Novartis*, AstraZeneca+, GlaxoSmithKline*, Otsuka*, Scios+	None	None	GlaxoSmithKline*, Sanofisynthelabo*, Pfizer*, Abbott*, Amgen*, Otsuka*, BMS*, Scios	None
Aguilera	National Inst. Of Child Health & Human Dev.	None	None	None	None	None	None	None
Anderson	Oregon Health and Science University	None	None	Merck*	None	None	None	None
Appel	Johns Hopkins Medical Institutions	None	None	None	None	None	None	None
Arnett	University of Alabama at Birmingham	None	None	None	None	None	None	None
Baker	Texas A&M University Health and Science Center	None	None	None	None	None	None	None
Bakris	University of Chicago, Pritzker School of Medicine	NIH(NIDDK/NHLBI)+, Glaxo-SmithKline+, Forest+	None	Abbott*, Boehringer-Ingelheim*, BMS/Sanofi-Aventis*, Forest*, Glaxo-Smith Kline*, Merck*, Novartis+, Walgreens (formulary committee)*, Gileada*, Sankyo	None	None	Abbott*, Boehringer-Ingelheim*, BMS/Sanofi-Aventis*, Forest*, Glaxo-Smith Kline*, Merck*, Novartis+, Walgreens (formulary committee)*, Gileada*, Sankyo*	None
Balla	NIH	None	None	None	None	None	None	None
Basile	Ralph H. John Virginia Medical Center	NHLBI+, Boehringer Ingelheim+, Novartis	None	Abbott*, AstraZeneca*, Boehringer Ingelheim*, Novartis+, Sankyo*, Forest*	None	None	AstraZeneca*, Merck*, Novartis*, Sankyo*	None
Baumbach	University of Iowa	None	None	None	None	None	None	None
Beierwaltes	Henry Ford Health System, Wayne State University School of Medicine	NIH (HL076469)*	None	None	None	None	None	None
Berecek	University of Alabama at Birmingham	None	None	None	None	None	None	None
Berk	University of Rochester Medical Center	None	None	None	None	None	None	None
Bisognano	University of Rochester	None	None	None	None	None	None	None

(Continued)

Writing group member	Employment	Research grant	Other research support	Speakers' bureau/honoraria	Expert witness	Ownership interest	Consultant/advisory board	Other
Black	New York University School of Medicine	None	None	Novartis*, BI*, Forest*, Pfizer*	None	None	Novartis*, Bayer*, BMS*, MSD*, Pfizer*, Abbott*, AstraZeneca*	Novartis+
Blaustein	University of Maryland – Baltimore	None	None	None	None	None	None	None
Booz	Texas A&M University Health and Sciene Center	None	None	None	None	None	None	None
Brown, NJ	Vanderbilt University School of Medicine	NIH+	Novartis*	None	None	None	Novartis*, Jerini*, VIA*	None
Brown, RD	Mayo Clinic	NIH	None	None	None	None	None	None
Calhoun	University of Alabama at Birmingham	Novartis+, AstraZeneca+	None	None	None	None	Novartis+	None
Campese	Keck School of Medicine/USC	Abbott+, Otsuka+, Merck+	None	Merck+, Pfizer+, Novartis+	None	None	Pfizer+, Merck+, Novartis+, AstraZeneca+	None
Canzanello	Mayo Clinic	None	None	None	None	None	None	None
Caples	Mayo Clinic	ResMed Foundation+, Restore Medical*	None	None	None	None	Cardiac Concepts*	None
Carey	University of Virginia	None	None	None	None	None	None	None
Carretero	Henry Ford Hospital	NIH+	Pfizer+	None	None	None	None	None
Carter	University of Iowa	NHLBI*	ALL HAT*	None	None	None	None	None
Chapleau	University of Iowa, Department of Veterans Affairs	NIH (HL014388)*, Department of Veterans Affairs*	None	None	None	None	None	None
Chappell	Wake Forest University School of Medicine	NIH (HL056973, HL051952, HD047584, HD017644)+	None	None	None	None	None	None
Chugh	University of Chicago Medical Center	None	None	None	None	None	None	None
Chun	Indian University & The Veterans Admin.	None	None	None	None	None	None	None
Coleman	University of Mississippi Medical Center	None	None	None	None	None	None	None
Cooper	Loyola University Medical Center	None	None	None	None	None	None	None
Cowley	Medical College of Wisconsin	None	None	None	None	None	None	None
Crespo	Portland State University	None	None	None	None	None	None	None
Criqui	University of California, San Diego	None	None	None	None	None	None	None
Cushman	University of Tennessee College of Medicine	None	None	None	None	None	None	None

Name	Institution					
Cutler	National Heart, Lung, and Blood Institute	None	None	None	None	None
Deedwania	VA Medical Center, Fresno	None	None	Novartis*, AstraZeneca*	None	AstraZeneca+
Dennison	Johns Hopkins University	None	None	None	None	None
Devereux	Weill Medical College of Cornell University	Merck+	None	Merck+, Novartis*	None	Merck*
DiPette	University of South Carolina School of Medicine	None	None	None	None	None
Dluhy	Brigham & Women's Hosp.	None	None	None	None	None
Dubovsky	University at Buffalo	Forest+, Pfizer+, Solvay+, Novartis+	None	Organon*	Astra-Zeneca*	Biovail*
Dunlap	MetroHealth Medical Center	None	None	None	None	None
Egan	Medical University of South Carolina	AstraZeneca*, Novartis*	None	AstraZeneca*, Forest*, Novartis*, Pfizer*, Boehringer Ingelheim*	None	AstraZeneca*, Novartis*
Eisenhofer	University of Dresden	None	None	None	None	None
Elijovich	Scott & White Clinic	Myogen*	None	Novartis*, Pfizer	None	Gerson Lehrman Group*
Elliott	RUSH Medical College	Pfizer+	None	Novartis+, Pfizer+, Kos Pharmaceuticals+, AstraZeneca*, Bristol-Myers Squibb Company*, Sanofi-aventis*, Abbott Laboratories*	None	Pfizer*, Novartis*, KV Pharmaceutical*, Accu-Break Pharmaceuticals, Inc.*, King Pharmaceuticals*
Ennezat	Lille Medical Center	None	None	None	None	None
Epstein	University of Miami	None	None	None	None	None
Erdös	University of Illinois College of Medicine	None	None	None	None	None
Falkner	Thomas Jefferson University	None	None	None	None	None
Faraci	University of Iowa	NIH*	None	None	None	None
Feldman	The University of Western Ontario, Robarts Research Institute	None	None	None	None	None
Fenves	Baylor University Medical Center	None	None	None	None	None
Ferdinand	Association of Black Cardiologists, Inc.	None	None	Nitro Med*, AstraZeneca*, Pfizer*, Merck*, Novartis*, Sanofi-Aventis	Nitro Med*, Astra-Zeneca*, Novartis*	Nitro Med*, AstraZeneca*, Pfizer*, Merck*, Novartis*, Sanofi-Aventis

(Continued)

Writing group member	Employment	Research grant	Other research support	Speakers' bureau/honoraria	Expert witness	Ownership interest	Consultant/advisory board	Other
Ferrario	Wake Forest University Health Sciences, Hypertension & Vascular Research Center	None	None	None	None	None	None	None
Flack	Wayne State University	Merck[+], Novartis[+], Pfizer[+], GlaxoSmithKline[+], Pharmacia[+], AstraZeneca[+], Solvay[+], Centers for Disease Control[+], NIH[+]	None	Merck[+], AstraZeneca[+], Solvay[+], Genzyme[+], Orthobiotech[+]	None	None	Merck[*], GlaxoSmithKline[*], Bristol Myers Squibb[*], Novartis[*], CVRx[*], Genzyme[*], Myogen[*], CDC[*], NIH[*]	None
Fong	University of Rochester	None	None	None	None	None	None	None
Francis	Brigham & Women's Hosp.	None	None	None	None	None	None	None
Frank	Wayne State University School of Medicine	None	None	None	None	None	None	None
Franklin	University of California, Irvine	None	None	Boehringer Ingelheim[*], Bristol Myers Squibb[*], Merck[*]	None	None	Artcor Medical[*], Bristol Myers Squibb[*]	None
Frishman	New York Medical College, Westchester Medical Center	None	None	Bristol Myers Squibb[*], Pfizer[*], Novartis[*], Merck[*]	None	None	Pfizer[*], Merck[*]	None
Frolich	Ochsner Clinic Foundation	None	None	None	None	None	None	None
Garcia-Palmieri	University of Puerto Rico School of Medicine	None	None	None	None	None	None	None
Garrison	University of Virginia	NIH[*]	None	None	None	None	None	None
Gavish	InterCure Ltd.	None	None	None	None	None	Speedel[*]	None
Gavras, H	Boston University	Boehringer Ingelheim[*]	None	Boehringer[*], Merck[*], Novartis[*]	None	None	None	None
Gavras, I	Boston University	None	None	None	None	None	None	None
Giles	Tulane University School of Medicine	Novartis[*], AstraZeneca[*]	None	Novartis[*], BI[*], BMS[*], Sanofi[*], Forrest[*], Sankyo[*], Pfizer[*]	None	None	Novartis[*], BI[*], BMS[*], Forrest[*], Sanofi[*], Sankyo[*], Pfizer[*]	None
Goldstein, DS	NIH	None	None	None	None	None	None	None

Name / Institution							
Goldstein, MK — VA Palo Alto Health Care System, Stanford University	None	Veterans Administration/Athena-HTN software (IMV04-062)+	None	None	None	None	None
Gomez-Sanchez — G.V.(Sonny) Motgomery VA Medical Center, University of Mississippi Medical Center	None	None	None	None	None	None	None
Goodfriend — Dept. of Veterans Affairs	None	None	None	None	None	None	None
Gradman — Western Pennslyvania Hosp.	Novartis+, AstraZeneca+	None	AstraZeneca+, Merck+, Novartis+, Boehringer Ingelheim*, Pfizer*, Sankyo*	None	None	AstraZeneca+, Merck+, Novartis+, Boehringer Ingelheim*, Pfizer*, Sankyo*	None
Graves — Mayo Clinic College of Medicine & Mayo Foundation	None	None	None	None	None	None	None
Greene — Medical College of Wisconsin	None	None	None	None	None	None	None
Griendling — Emory University	NIH+	None	None	None	None	None	None
Grim, CE — Medical College of Wisconsin	Omron Healthcare Inc.*	None	None	None	None	Shared Care Research and Education Consulting, Inc.*	None
Grim, CM — Shared Care Research & Education Consulting, Inc.	None	None	None	None	Shared Care Research & Education Consulting, Inc.+	None	None
Grimm — Hennepin, Faculty Associates	Pfizer+, BI+	None	Pfizer+, Merck+, BI+, Novartis+, Schering-Plough+	None	None	Pfizer+, Novartis+	None
Grossman — The Chaim Sheba Medical Center Tel-Hashomer	Pfizer*	AstraZeneca*	Novartis*	None	None	Novartis*	None
Gupta — Fortis Escorts Hospital Jaipur, India	None	None	None	None	None	None	None
Haffner — University of Texas Health Science Center at San Antonio	Novartis+	None	Novartis*, MSD*	None	None	Novartis*, MSD*	None

(Continued)

Writing group member	Employment	Research grant	Other research support	Speakers' bureau/honoraria	Expert witness	Ownership interest	Consultant/advisory board	Other
Halcox	University College London	None	None	Sanofi*, Aventis*, Solvay*, Pfizer*, Schering-Plough*, Merck*	None	None	Sanofi*, Aventis*, Solvay*, Merck*, Schering-Plough*	None
Hall	University of Mississippi Medical Center	NIH+	None	None	None	None	Merck*, Novartis*, Arete*	None
Hamlyn	University of Maryland at Baltimore	NIH NHLBI+	None	None	None	None	None	None
Harrison	Emory University	None	None	None	None	None	None	None
Haynes	University of Iowa College of Medicine	None	None	None	None	None	None	None
Heistad	University of Iowa	NIH*, Veterans Administration*, University of Iowa College of Medicine*	None	None	None	None	BioMarin*	None
Hershey	Veterans Administration	None	None	None	None	None	None	None
Hester	University of Mississippi Medical Center	None	None	None	None	None	None	None
Hoang	University of California, Irvine Medical Center	None	None	None	None	None	None	None
Hoffman	VA Boston Health Care System, Harvard Medical School	None	Veterans Administration/Athena-HTN software (IMV04-062)+	None	None	None	None	None
Hollenberg	Brigham & Women's Hospital	Mars+, Novartis+	None	Novartis*, GlaxoSmithKline Beecham*	None	None	Merck Sharp and Dohme*, Bristol Meyers Squibb*, GlaxoSmithKline Beecham*, AstraZeneca*, Pfizer*, Novartis*	None
Houston-Miller	Stanford University School of Medicine	None	None	Pfizer*, AstraZeneca*	None	None	CV Therapeutics*, Pfizer*, Merck*	None
Hsueh	UCLA Division of Endocrinology	None	None	None	None	None	None	None

(Continued)

Hyman	Baylor College of Medicine	None	None	None	None	None	None
Iqbal	Baylor College of Medicine	None	None	None	None	None	None
Izzo	State University of NY at Buffalo	GlaxoSmith Kline, Novartis	None	Novartis+, Merck*, Daiichi/Sankyo+, Forest+ & Boehringer-Ingelheim*,	None	Novartis, Merck, Daiichi/Sankyo, Forest & Boehringer-Ingelheim	GlaxoSmith Kline, Novartis, Merck, Daiichi/Sankyo, Forest, Intercure, Roche and Omron
Johns	University College Cork	None	None	None	None	None	None
Jones	University of Mississippi Medical Center	None	None	None	None	None	None
Julius	University of Michigan	AstraZeneca+	None	Servier Amerique+, AstraZeneca+	None	None	None
Kannel	Boston University, Framing Heart Study	NIH/NHLB+	None	None	None	None	None
Kaplan	University of Texas Southwestern Medical School	None	None	Boehringer Ingelheim+, Pfizer+	None	None	None
Kostis	UMDNJ-Robert Wood Johnson Medical School	NHLBI+, Kos Pharmaceuticals+, Boehringer-Ingelheim+, Schering-Plough Foundation+, Robert Wood Johnson Foundation+	None	None	None	None	Pfizer+, Schering-Plough+, Sankyo*, Forest*, Sanofi*, Jerini AG*, Reliant*.
Kotchen, JM	Medical College of Wisconsin	NIH+	None	None	None	NIH*	None
Kotchen, T	Medical College of Wisconsin	NIH+	None	None	None	NIH+	None
Krakoff	Englewood Hospital & Medical Center	None	None	None	None	None	None
Kunos	NIH, NIAAA	None	None	None	None	None	None
Lackland	Medical University of South Carolina	NHLBI*	None	BMS+, Pfizer+, Merck+, Novartis*	None	None	None
Laffer	Scott & White Clinic	Boehringer Ingelheim*, Merck*, CVRx*, Myogen*	None	Novartis*, Pfizer*	None	MEDACorp*, Gerson-Lehrman*, Detroit R&D*	None
Lakatta	NIH, National Institute on Aging, Laboratory of Cardiovascular Science	None	None	None	None	None	None
Lastra	University of Missouri – Columbia	None	None	None	None	None	None
Leddy	SUNY at Buffalo School of Medicine	None	None	None	None	None	None

Writing group member	Employment	Research grant	Other research support	Speakers' bureau/honoraria	Expert witness	Ownership interest	Consultant/advisory board	Other
Leite	Medical College of Georgia	None	None	None	None	None	None	None
Le Jemtel	Tulane University	None	None	None	None	None	None	None
Levy	NIH	None	None	None	None	None	None	None
Lindheimer	University of Chicago	None	None	University of Miami VA Hospital*, University of Florida*	x2	None	None	None
Lloyd-Jones	Northwestern University	None	None	None	None	None	None	None
Luisi	University at Buffalo	NIH, NHLBI	None	None	None	None	None	None
Materson	University of Miami	None	None	None	None	None	None	None
McFarlane	SUNY Downstate, Kings County Hospital Center	None	None	None	None	None	None	None
McGiff	New York Medical College	None	None	None	None	None	None	None
Mensah	National Center for Chronic Disease							
Messerli	St. Luke's-Roosevelt Hospital Center	None	Novartis*	BI*, Forest*, BMS*, Sankyo*, Merck*, Novartis+, GSK+, Pfizer+	Novartis+	None	Sankyo*, Bayer*, Merck*, Pfizer*, Novartis+*, Forest*, King*	None
Michalkiewicz	Medical College of Wisconsin	None	None	None	None	None	None	None
Mitchell	Cardiovascular Engineering, Inc.	None	None	None	None	None	None	None
Mohler	University of Pennsylvania Health System, University of Pennsylvania School of Medicine	Pfizer*, Omron*	None	BMS-Sanofi*, Merck*, AstraZeneca*	None	None	None	None
Moore	Danville Regional Medical Center	None	None	None	None	None	None	None
Morgan	University Of Wisconsin – Madison	NIH+ (HL074072)	NIH* (HL075035)	None	None	None	None	None
Morgenstern	Phoenix Children's Hospital	None	None	None	None	None	AstraZeneca*	None
Nadler	University of Virginia	NIH HL PO RO155798, ADA DK 55240	Novartis*	Merck Diakine*	None	None	Atherogenics*, Sankyo*	None
Najjar	National Institute on Aging, NIH	None	None	None	None	None	None	None
Nally	Cleveland Clinic	None	None	Novartis+	None	None	AstraZeneca*	None
Nasjletti	New York Medical College	None	None	None	None	None	None	None

Name	Institution							
Nasser	Wayne State University	None	None	Pfizer*, Boehringer Ingelheim*, Merck*	None	None	None	None
Navar	Tulane University	NHLBI+, NCRR+, BoR of LA+	None	None	None	None	Calpris*	None
Navas-Acien	Johns Hopkins University	None	None	None	None	None	None	None
Northcott	Michigan State University	None	None	None	None	None	None	None
O'Connor	Wayne State University	None	None	None	None	None	None	None
Olin	Mount Sinai School of Medicine	None	None	None	None	None	BMS+, Sanofi+, Genzyme+	None
Oparil	University of Alabama at Birmingham	Abbott+, AstraZeneca+, Aventis+, Biovail+, Boehringer Ingelheim+, BMS+, Forest+, GlaxoSmithKline+, Novartis+, Merck+, Pfizer+, Sankyo Pharma+, Sanofi-Synthelabo+, Schering-Plough+	None	None	None	None	BMS*, Daiichi Sankyo*, Merck*, Novartis*, Pfizer*, Sanofi Aventis*, The Salt Institute*	Board of Directors for Encysive Pharmaceuticals+
Pacher	NIH, NIAAA	None	None	None	None	None	None	None
Parati	University of Milano – Bicocca	None	None	None	None	None	None	None
Park	Keck School of Medicine, USC	None	None	None	None	None	None	None
Pavlik	Baylor College of Medicine	None	None	None	None	None	None	None
Phillips	Dalhousie University, Capital District Health Authority	None	None	None	None	None	None	None
Pickering	Columbia University	None	None	None	None	None	CVRx*, AtCor*	None
Pimenta	University of Alabama at Birmingham	None	None	None	None	None	None	None
Pi-Sunyer	St. Luke's/Roosevelt Hospital	None	None	None	None	None	None	None
Ploth	Medical University of South Carolina	None	None	None	None	None	None	None
Plutzky	Brigham & Women's Hosp.	None	None	Takeda*	None	None	GlaxoSmithKline*, NovoNordisk*, Ono Pharmaceuticals*, Takeda*	None
Pool	Baylor College of Medicine	Abbott*, Pfizer*	None	CME lectures for alpha-blockers in HTN and BPH*	None	None	None	None
Pratt	Indiana University & VA	Indiana University+	None	None	None	None	None	None
Printz	University of California-San Diego	None	None	NIH*	None	None	None	None

(Continued)

587

Writing group member	Employment	Research grant	Other research support	Speakers' bureau/honoraria	Expert witness	Ownership interest	Consultant/advisory board	Other
Prisant	Medical College of Georgia	None	None	None	None	None	None	None
Quyyumi	Emory University	None	None	None	None	None	None	None
Rahman	Case Western Reserve University	None	None	Boehringer Ingelheim*	None	None	None	None
Raij	Veterans Administration, University of Miami	None	None	None	None	None	None	None
Ram	Texas Blood Pressure Institute, Dallas Nephrology Associates, University of Texas Southwestern Medical School	None	None	None	None	None	None	None
Reisin	Louisiana State University Health Center – New Orleans	None	None	None	None	None	None	None
Rhaleb	Henry Ford Hospital	NIH+	Henry Ford Hospital+	None	None	None	None	None
Robertson	Vanderbilt University Medical Center	None	None	Merck Research Lab*	None	None	None	None
Roccella	NHLBI, NIH	None	None	None	None	None	None	None
Rocchini	University of Michigan	None	None	None	None	None	None	None
Rosendorff	Veterans Administration	Daichi Sankyo+, Keryx Biopharm. Myogen*, Novartis*	None	AstraZeneca*, Schering-Plough*, CV Therapeutics*	Bristol-Myers Squibb+	None	Bayer Diagnostics+	None
Ruilope	Ministry of Health – Spain	None	None	Novartis*, AstraZeneca*, BMS*, MSD*, Sanofi*, Aventis*	None	None	Boehringer Ingelheim*, MSD*, Sanofi*, Aventis*	None
Sacks	Harvard University	None	None	None	None	None	None	None
Safar	Hôpital Hôtel-Dieu	None	None	None	None	None	None	None
Samson	Saint Louis University	None	None	None	None	None	None	None
Schiffrin	Sir Mortimer B. Davis-Jewish General Hospital, Lady Davis Institute for Medical Research, McGill University	None	None	None	None	None	None	None
Schleis	Medtronic Inc.	None	None	None	None	None	None	None
Seely	Brigham and Women's Hosp.	None	None	None	None	None	None	None
Shenker	University of Wisconsin	None	None	None	None	None	None	None
Shepherd	UTHSCSA	None	None	None	None	None	None	None
Sheps	Mayo Clinic	None	None	None	None	None	None	None

Name	Institution							
Shub	Mayo Clinic	None	None	None	None	None	None	None
Sica	Virginia Commonwealth University	Encysive Pharmaceuticals*, Novartis+, GlaxoSmithKline+, CVRx+	None	None	Novartis+	None	Novartis*, GlaxoSmithKline*, Encysive Pharmaceuticals*	None
Simons-Morton	NHLBI, NIH, DHHS, Federal govt.	None	None	None	None	None	None	None
Sinaiko	University of Minnesota	None	None	None	None	None	None	None
Skidgel	University of Illinois College of Medicine	None	None	None	None	None	None	None
Solomon	Brigham Women's Hospital, Harvard Medical School	None	None	None	None	None	None	None
Somers	Mayo Clinic	ResMed Foundation+, Restore Medical*	None	None	None	None	Respironics*, Cardiac Concepts*, Sepracor*	None
Sowers	University of Arizona	Novartis+, AstraZeneca+	NIH+, VA+	None	Merck*, Novartis*, AstraZeneca*	None	None	None
Spence	University of Western Ontario, Stroke Prevention & Atherosclerosis Research Centre	PanAm Labs*	None	None	AstraZeneca*, Solvay*	None	Novartis*	None
Stamler	Feinberg School of Medicine, Northwestern University	None	None	None	None	None	None	None
Stojilkovic	National Inst. Of Child Health & Human Dev.	None	None	None	None	None	None	None
Supowit	Texas A&M University	None	None	None	None	None	None	None
Taler	Mayo Clinic	None	None	None	None	None	None	None
Talman	University of Iowa, Dept. of Veterans Affairs	None	None	None	None	None	None	None
Tangirala	David Geffen School of Medicine, University of California	None	None	None	None	None	None	None
Taylor	Baylor College of Medicine	CVRx*	None	None	None	None	None	None
Tayo	Loyola Medical School	None	None	None	None	None	None	None
Textor	Mayo Clinic	None	None	None	None	None	None	None
Thom	NHLBI, NIH	None	None	None	None	None	None	None
Tostes	Medical College of Georgia	None	None	None	None	None	None	None

(Continued)

Writing group member	Employment	Research grant	Other research support	Speakers' bureau/honoraria	Expert witness	Ownership interest	Consultant/advisory board	Other
Toth	Sterling Rock Falls Clinic	AstraZeneca*, Novartis*	None	AstraZeneca+, Pfizer+, Merck+, Kos*, Novartis*, Takeda	None	None	AstraZeneca*, GlaxoSmithKline*, Pfizer*, Merck+	None
Touyz	Ottawa Health Research Inst.	Canadian Institutes of Health Research (CIHR)+, Heart and Stroke Foundation of Canada+,	None	None	None	None	Novartis*, BMS*, Sanofi*, Astellas+, Boehringer*, Pfizer	None
Townsend	University of Pennslyvania	Novartis+	None	Merck+, Pfizer*	None	None	GlaxoSmithKline*	None
Triggle	SUNY at Buffalo, Center for Inquiry Institute	None	None	None	case involving ACE inhibitors*; case involving a calcium antagonist*	None	Scientific Advisory Board*, Neuromed Technologies*	None
Vaughan	Vanderbilt University Medical Center	Novartis+	None	None	None	None	Novartis*, Wyeth+	None
Vidt	Cleveland Clinic	None	None	None	None	None	None	None
Watson	Michigan State University	None	None	None	None	None	None	None
Watts	Michigan State University	None	None	None	None	None	None	None
Webb	Medical College of Georgia	None	None	None	None	None	None	None
Weber	SUNY Downstate Medical Center College of Medicine	None	None	Novartis+, Sankyo+, BMS*, Pfizer*, Merck*, Sanofi-Aventis*, Boehringer Ingelheim*	None	None	Novartis*, Pfizer*, Merck*, Sankyo*, Boehringer Ingelheim*, Forest*	None
Weder	University of Michigan	None	None	None	None	None	None	None
Weinberger	Indiana University Medical Center	None	None	None	None	None	None	None
Weir	University of Maryland–Nephrology	None	None	None	None	None	None	None

Whaley-Connell	University of Missouri-Columbia School of Medicine	NIH+	None	None	None	None	None	None
Whelton	Loyola University – Chicago	None	None	None	None	None	None	None
White	University of Connecticut	AstraZeneca+, Pfizer+	None	Pfizer+, Boehringer Ingelheim+, Novartis*, Merck*	None	None	Bayer Health Care+, Teva+, King*	None
Williams, B	University of Leicester	Merck+, Pfizer+	None	Merck+, Pfizer+, Novartis*, BMS*	None	None	Merck+, Pfizer+	None
Williams, M	University of Virginia	None	None	None	None	None	None	None
Wilson	Emory University School of Medicine	Sanofi-Aventis+, Wyeth+, GlaxoSmithKline+	None	Lilly*	None	None	GlaxoSmithKline*	None
Winer	SUNY Downstate Medical Center	None	None	None	None	None	None	None
Wolf	Boston University School of Medicine	None	None	None	None	None	None	None
Wong	Heart Disease Prevention Program, University of California	Merck+, Pfizer+	None	Sanofi-Aventis*, Takeda+	None	None	Novartis+	None
Wright	Case Western Reserve University	Novartis+, NIH+, GlaxoSmithKline+,	None	Novartis+	None	None	Sanofi*, Pfizer*, GlaxoSmithKline*, Novartis*	None
Wyss	University of Alabama at Birmingham	NIH*	None	None	None	None	AHA*	None
Young	Mayo Clinic	None	None	None	None	None	None	None
Yuan	University of California San Diego	NIH-NHLBI+	None	None	None	None	None	None

* Modest
+ Significant

This table represents the relationships of writing group members that may be perceived as actual or reasonably perceived conflicts of interest as reported on the Disclosure Questionnaire which all writing group members are required to complete and submit. A relationship is considered to be "Significant" if (a) the person receives $10,000 or more during any 12 month period, or 5% or more of the person's gross income; or (b) the person owns 5% or more of the voting stock or share of the entity, or owns $10,000 or more of the fair market value of the entity. A relationship is considered to be "Modest" if it is less than "Significant" under the preceding definition.

Note: Page numbers followed by *f* refer to figures; page numbers followed by *t* refer to tables.

A Diabetes Outcome ProgressionTrial (ADOPT), 102
Abdomen, 375–376
    abdominal aortic aneurysms, 511–512
    abdominal imaging, 377–378
Abnormal blood glucose
    hypertensive patients with, treatment of, 529–531
        essentials of therapy, 530
        risk factor interactions, 529
        therapeutic lifestyle changes (TLC), 530
ABP. *See* Ambulatory blood pressure
ACCORD. *See* Action to Control Cardiometabolic
    Risk in Diabetes (ACCORD)
Acculturation
    and HTN prevalence, 285
ACE. *See* Angiotensin-converting enzyme (ACE)
Acetylcholine, 75
    central effects, 76
    structure, 76f
    synthesis and actions, 75
    muscarinic effects, 75
Acid sensing ion channels (ASICs), 120
Acromegaly
    hypertension, 170
        clinical features, 170
        mechanisms, 170
Action to Control Cardiometabolic Risk in Diabetes
    (ACCORD), 102
Activating protein 1 (AP-1), 202
Acute cerebral ischemia and infarction, 512–513
    acute management considerations, 512–513
Acute cerebrovascular disorders, hypertension
    management in, 513t
Acute coronary syndromes
    hypertension in patients with, treatment, 500
Acute hypertensive encephalopathy
    clinical features, 218–219
        associated findings, 218
        differential diagnosis, 218
        drugs, 218
        imaging findings, 218
        risk factors, 218
        signs and symptoms, 218
    management, 219
    pathogenesis of, 217–219
    pathophysiology, 217–218
        angiotensin II and oxidative stress, 218
        cerebral autoregulation, 217–218
        hypertension, 217–218
        sympathetic vasoconstriction, 218
        vasospasm versus vasodilation, 217
        venules and the blood–brain barrier, 218
Acute myocardial infarction, 491
Acute stress, 289
Acute stroke, 216, 491
Acylation, 79
Adenosine triphosphate (ATP), 28
    ATP-sensitive K+ channels, 25
Adenosine, 76
    receptors and actions, 76–77
    structure, 76f
    synthesis and metabolism, 76
Adenylyl cyclase, 2, 5, 8–9
    activity and coupling, 8
    enzyme characteristics, 8
Adherence to antihypertensive therapy, 413–417
    definition, 414
    factors associated, 415
        negative factors, 415

positive factors, 415
    strategies to improve, 415
    health care provider actions to increase, 415–417
    measurement, 414–415
        objective measures, 414
        self-reporting, 414
    multilevel approach to improve, 417
Adipocytes, 107
    endocrine organ, 107
    insulin resistance. *See* Insulin resistance
    leptin, 107
Adiponectin, 113, 152
    cardiovascular diseases, 115
        hypertension, 115
        myocardial infarction, 115
    insulin resistance and diabetes, 114
        genetic aspects, 114
        human studies, 114
        role in, 114
        visceral obesity and metabolic syndrome, 114
    physiology, 113–114
        receptors, 114
        structure, 113–114
    vascular function and atherosclerosis, 114–115
        atherosclerotic plaques, 114–115
        endothelial function, 114
        vascular smooth muscle function, 114
Adipose tissue, 87
Adipsin, 108
Adolescents, hypertensive
    nonpharmacologic therapy in, 540–543
        weight reduction, 540–542
    pharmacologic therapy in, 543–544
        individualized therapy, 543
        specific drug choices, 543
    treatment, 540–544
ADOPT. *See* A Diabetes Outcome ProgressionTrial
    (ADOPT)
Adrenal cortex, 61
Adrenal steroids
    biosynthesis regulation, 62
    extraadrenal synthesis, 63
    hepatic and renal metabolism, 63
    receptor specificity, 63
    synthetic pathways, 62
        aldosterone synthase, 62
        cortisol synthesis, 62
        11-hydroxylation, 62
        17-hydroxylation, 62
        initial steps, 62
        isomeration, 62
    target cell metabolism, 63
Adrenal vein sampling (AVS), 566
Adrenalectomy, 566
Adrenergic receptors, 39
    biologic actions, 39–40
    characteristics, 40–41
        signal transduction pathways, 41
        subtypes, 40–41
    receptor regulation, 41
        disease states, implications for, 42
        gene regulation, 41
        homologous desensitization, 41
        phosphorylation, 41
    responses, and pharmacology of, 40t, 41
    tissue distribution, 40t
α-Adrenergic receptor antagonists, 29, 41, 450–452
    α-, β-adrenergic inhibitors, 451

α1-adrenergic receptors, 5, 41
α2-adrenergic receptors, 41, 453
    diverse effects of, 452–452
        BP effects, 451
        glucose tolerance, 451
        heart failure, 451
        lipids, 451
        prostatism, 451
        ventricular hypertrophy, 451
    nonselective α-antagonists, 451
    selective α₁-antagonists, 450
    selective α1-antagonists, 451t
    selective α₁-blockers, treatment with, 452
        combination therapy, 452
        diuretic therapy, 452
        hypertension, 452
    selective α₂-antagonists, 451
    selectivity of, 450–451
    side effects, 452
β-Adrenergic blockers, 41, 293–294, 326, 437,
    446–450, 497, 500, 508, 511, 531, 541t, 548
    adverse effects and contraindications, 449–450
    antihypertensive mechanisms and pharmacokinetic
        differences, 447–448
        drug differentiation, 447–448
        lipid-soluble agents, 447
        membrane-stabilizing activity, 448
        nitric oxide-releasing activity, 448
        β₁-selectivity, 447–448
        water-soluble agents, 447
    clinical usage, 448–449
    indications and outcome studies, 446–447
        angina pectoris, 446
        antiarrhythmic effects, 446
        hypertension, 446–447
        myocardial infarction, 446
β₁-Adrenergic receptors, 5, 41
Adrenomedullary cells, 39
Adrenomedullin, 74, 90t, 108
    hypertension, 74
    proadrenomedullin, 74
    synthesis and tissue distribution, 74
Advanced glycation end products (AGE), 32
Aerobic (endurance) exercise, 295–296
AF. *See* Autonomic failure
Afferent arteriolar dilation, 223–224
    protective role of, 223
Afferent fiber, 123
Africa
    hypertension prevalence in, 276
African American Study of Kidney Disease (AASK),
    262, 468
AGE. *See* Advanced glycation end products (AGE)
Age/Aging
    BP and coronary heart disease risk
        BP components as risk predictors, 147
        pulse pressure as a risk marker, 147
    and BP patterns, 273–274, 485–486
        growth and development, tracking during, 273
    dynamic exercise and cardiac output, 178
    hemodynamic changes, 146
        age 30 to 50 years, 146
        age less than 30
        age less than 50 years, 146
    hypertension and the heart, 184. *See* Heart
    hypertension, and arterial function, 145
        BP and arterial stiffness, 145
    myocardial changes rodents, 187t

Age/Aging (contd.)
  and sympathetic activity, 124–125
  and ventricular stiffness, 125
Airway obstruction, 174
Albuminuria
  definition and screening, 522
  specific antihypertensive drugs, 524–525
  specific treatment strategies, 523
    current BP targets, 523
    in dialysis patients, 524
    need for multiple drugs, 524
    nonpharmacologic therapy, 523
  treatment of, 522–525
    benefits, 522–523
Alcohol/Alcohol use
  alcohol and cardiovascular protection, 313
  alcohol pressor effects, mechanisms of, 312–313
  amount and type of alcohol, 310
  and blood, 310–313
    BP elevation patterns, 311
    clinical implications, 313
      alcohol and cardiovascular disease risk, 313
      alcohol reduction and hypertension, 313
      evaluation, 313
      intervention, 313
    drug resistance, 311
    epidemiologic associations, 311
    prevention and treatment of hypertension study,
      311–312
    randomized controlled trials, 311–312
    reduction, 311
  and street drugs, 344
Aldosterone antagonists, 443–445, 508
  applied pharmacology, 444–445
    dosing, 444
    drug interactions, 445
    receptor pharmacology, 444
  rationale for, 443–444
    hypertension, 443
    hypertensive end-organ damage, 443
Aldosterone synthase, 59, 62
  gene duplication, 232–233
Allylic oxidation, 95
Alzheimer's dementia, 381
Alzheimer's disease (AD), 220
  differentiating clinical symptoms, 220
  pathogenesis, 220
  therapy, 220
Amaurosis fugax, 379
Ambrisentan, 477
Ambulatory blood pressure (ABP) monitoring,
    340–342
  available devices, 340
  cardiovascular outcomes, 340
  clinical decision making, 341–342
  cost and coverage considerations, 342
  interpretation, 341
  target organs, 340
Ambulatory pressures, in BP measurement,
    274
American Heart Association (AHA), 335
American hypertension guidelines
  evolution of, 395–400
American Medical Publishers Association (AMPA),
    118
Amiloride, 445
γ-Aminobutyric acid (GABA), 77, 117
  structure, 76f
Aminopeptidases, 52
AMPA. See American Medical Publishers Association
    (AMPA)
Amygdala, 119
Anaphylaxis, 98
Androgens, 170
Aneroid manometer, 335–336
Anesthetics, 562–563
  in perioperative management, 554t, 554
Aneurysms, 227
Anger, 178
Angina pectoris, 446, 467–468
  hypertension in patients with, treatment, 500
    nonpharmacologic and risk-factor management,
      500
    pharmacologic therapy, 500
Angioedema, 84

Angiogenesis inhibitors, 482
  BP raising effects of, 480–482
Angiotensin II receptors, 29, 90t, 218, 531
  cellular actions, 55
    AT1 receptor mechanisms, 55
    AT2 receptor mechanisms, 55
    AT4 and mas receptor mechanisms, 55–56
  general characteristics, 54
  modulation, 58
    autacoids, 58
    hormones, 58
    oxidative stress, 58
  physiologic effects
    long-term actions, 56–57
    short-term actions, 56
  receptor activation patterns, 54–55
  receptor density and responsiveness, 56
  vascular remodeling, 197
Angiotensin receptor blockers (ARBs), 294, 349, 403,
    433, 435, 440, 461–464, 484, 496, 499, 536,
    541t, 555, 565, 569, 577
  clinical usage, 463
    adverse effects, 464
    BP effects, 463–464
    response variability, 464
  indications and outcome studies, 462
    hypertension, 462
  mechanisms of actions, 461–462
    pharmacology, 461–462
  potential double action of selective AT1 blockers,
    462t
  subtypes, 462
  Trial of Prevention of Hypertension (TROPHY),
    484
  vascular AT1 receptors, 462t
  vascular AT2 receptors, 462t
Angiotensin, 52–53, 59, 529
  alternative pathways function, 52–53
  biologic effects, 58
  metabolic changes, 53
    angiotensin (1– 7), 53
    incomplete ACE inhibition, 53
    mast cell, 53
  metabolic pathways, 52
    ACE2, 52
    aminopeptidases, 52
    endocytosis, 52
    tissue endopeptidases, 52
  proteolytic pathways, 53f
  targets and actions, 56t
Angiotensin-converting enzyme (ACE), 49, 50f, 252,
    256, 272, 294, 349, 419, 435, 437, 439, 457,
    493, 496, 499, 507, 510, 511, 522, 525,
    530–531, 536, 541t, 555, 565, 569, 577
  activity, 49
  genetic aspects, 50
    genetic strains, 50
    insertion/deletion polymorphism, 50
  hemodynamic effects, 458
  mechanisms of action, 457–458
  molecular aspects, 49
    distribution, 50
    general properties, 49
    structure, 49–50
  pharmacology, 457
Angiotensinogen, 47
  biochemistry, 47–48
  molecular genetics, 47
  release control, 48
    population genetics, 48
Angiotensin-receptor blocker therapy, 165
Anglo-Scandinavian Cardiac Outcomes Trial
    (ASCOT), 327–328, 437
Anglo-Scandinavian Cardiac Outcomes Trial-Blood
    Pressure Lowering Arm (ASCOT-BPLA), 260
Animal models, in potassium intake, 306
Ankle–brachial index studies, 376
  in PAD, 266–267
    cardiovascular health study, 266
    measurement, 266
    Rotterdam study, 266
Anterior hypothalamus, 119
Anteroventral third ventricle, 119
Anticoagulation, 500
Antidepressants, 546, 547t, 562

Antidiuretic hormone, 70
Anti–human immunodeficiency virus treatment, 562
Antihypertensive and Lipid Lowering to prevent
    Heart Attack Trial (ALLHAT), 252, 260, 268,
    277, 325, 331, 349, 397, 440, 460, 467, 494,
    497
Antihypertensive drugs/therapy, 225, 293–284, 404t,
    432–435, 530–531
  adherence to, 413–417. See also Adherence
  basic principles, 432–433
    dose–response relationships, 432–433
    efficacy and peak, 432
    pharmacodynamics versus pharmacokinetics,
      432
  BP lowering, enhancement, 411
  BP raising effects of, 480–482
  combination antihypertensive therapy, 530
  combination therapy, 434–435. See also separate
    entry
  drug therapy considerations, 577
  drug–drug interactions, 433
  duration of therapy, 434
  effectiveness, 306
  exercise and, 411
  goals of, 496–497
    target BP, 496–497
  nonantihypertensive drugs, 478–479
  overdosing errors, 434
  peripheral arterial disease and, 511
  pharmacologic principles and dosing effects,
    432–435
  psychiatric effects of, 545
  in sexual dysfunction, 520–521
  underdosing errors, 434
Antihypertensive treatment trials
  BP-independent benefits in clinical trials, 327–328
  drug treatment versus placebo or no treatment,
    325
  general pitfalls and limitations of, 328
  meta-regression studies, 327
  network meta-analyses, 327
  outcomes, 325–328
  quality of life, 329–330. See also individual entry
  traditional meta-analyses, 325–327
    ACE inhibitors and angiotensin receptor
      blockers, 326–327
    β-blocker comparisons, 326
    BP lowering versus drug class, 327
    Diuretic/β-blocker comparisons, 326
Antilipidemic medications, 534–535
  bile acid–binding resins, 535
  Ezetimibe, 535
  fibrates, 535
  Niacin, 535
  statins, 534. See also separate entry
Antineoplastic agents, 562–563
Antiobesity drugs, 562
Antioxidant
  defense mechanisms, 34t
  defenses, 32–33
  definition, 32
Antipsychotics, 548
Anxiety/panic attacks, 350
Anxiolytics, 546
Aorta, coarctation of, 166
  diagnosis, 167
  hypertension mechanisms, 166
    Goldblatt-type phenomenon, 166
    late postrepair, 166–167
    mechanical theory, 166
    neural theory, 166
    postrepair paradoxical, 166
    prerepair, 166
  management, 167
  prognosis, 167
Aortocarotid baroreceptors, 127
Aortocarotid baroreflexes
  autonomic function
    age adjustment, 393
    clinical conditions associated with, 393t
    laboratory assessment of, 393
    tilt-testing and other maneuvers, 393
  baroreflex arcs, components, 391–392
    arterial baroreflexes, 391–392
    efferent fibers, 391

internuncial neurons, 391
physiologic effects, 391
sensory fibers, 391
baroreflex function
assessment of, 392–393
bedside assessment, 392
modulation of, 392
Carotid sinus hypersensitivity, 394. *See also separate entry*
evaluation of, 391–394
applied pathophysiology, 391–392
Impaired baroreflex function, 393–394. *See also separate entry*
Apelin, 109
Apolipoproteins, 209
Apoptosis, 462
Apparent mineralocorticoid excess (AME), 234
Apparent resistance hypertension, 348–349
cuff-related artifacts, 348
cuff too small, 348
patient nonadherence, 348–349
pseudohypertension, 348
physician nonadherence, 349
Appropriate Blood Pressure Control in Diabetes (ABCD), 468, 510
Arachidonic acid, 94, 96f, 97
metabolism inhibition, 98
pathways, 98f
Arachidonoyl ethanolamide, 103
Area postrema, 117
Arginine vasopressin (AVP) receptors
applied pathophysiology, 474
hemodynamic effects of, 474–475
heart failure, 475
hypertension, 474
types, 474
V_1 (vasoconstrictor), 474
V_2 (aquaretic) receptors, 474
Arginine vasopressin, 70
Arrythmia management, 508
Arterial baroreflexes, 120, 391–392. *See also Baroreflex*
baroreceptor nerve terminal model, 121f
baroreflex function, 120
baroreflex resetting, 120–121
clinical aspects, 122
baroreceptor stimulation therapy, 122
family history studies, 122
pharmacologic therapies, 122
sudden death, 122
neural pathways, 121f
neurohumoral and paracrine modulation, 121–122
Arterial compliance, 373
Arterial disease
evaluation algorithm for, 378f
Arterial distensibility, 373
Arterial embolism, 214
Arterial function parameters, limitations, 372
Arterial imaging, 373
Arterial impedance, 140
Arterial pressure regulation, 117
by basal ganglia and cerebral cortex, 119
amygdala, 119
hippocampus, 119
infralimbic cortex, 119
insular cortex, 119
by hypothalamus, 118
anterior hypothalamus, 119
anteroventral third ventricle, 119
lateral posterior hypothalamus, 118–119
paraventricular nucleus, 119
by spinal cord and medulla, 117–118
area postrema, 117–118
caudal ventrolateral medulla, 118
nucleus tractus solitarius, 117
rostroventrolateral medulla, 118
Arterial properties
methods to study, 372–373
Arterial pulse waves, 371
pulse pressure amplification, 371
wave reflection, 371
Arterial shear stress, 141
human arteries, 142
nonparabolic flow profile, 142

Arterial stiffness
evaluation of, 370–373
arterial pulse waves, 371. *See also separate entry*
central versus peripheral BP, 371–372
clinical assessment, 148
indicators, 145–146
Arterial system
aortic wall composition, 145
arterial diameter, 145
arterial stiffness
clinical assessment, 148
indicators, 145–146
physiology, 144
steady-state vs. pulsatile flow, 144
Arterial tree
functional compartments of, 370–371
Arteriolar changes, in hypertension, 227
aneurysms, 227
arteriolar diameter changes, 227
arteriovenous nicking, 227
atherosclerosis versus arteriosclerosis, 227
central vein occlusion, 227
flame hemorrhages, 228
terminology, 227
Arterioles, 227
Arteriosclerosis, RAAS, 93
Asia/Asians
east Asians, 287–288
hypertension prevalence in, 276
hypertension prevalence in, 277
minorities, hypertension in, 494
south Asians, 284–286. *See also individual entry*
ASICs. *See* Acid sensing ion channels (ASICs)
Aspirin, 479
Association constant (Ka), 1
Asymmetric dimethylarginine (ADMA), 79, 210
Asymmetric hypertrophy, 363
AT1 receptor-associated protein (ATRAP), 3
Atheriosclerosis
adiponectin, 114
endocannabinoids, 106
Atherogenesis, 209–213
atherosclerotic markers, 213
coronary atherosclerosis. *See* Coronary atherosclerosis
coronary syndromes, 213
occlusive coronary disease, 213
metabolic factors, 209
HDL metabolism, 209
LDL metabolism and receptor action, 209
oxygen radicals, 210
vascular scavenger pathways, 210
vascular susceptibility, 210
cellular elements, 210
coagulation, 211
endothelial dysfunction, 210
hemodynamic factors, 210
hypertension, interaction with, 211
inflammation and infection, 210–211
shear stress, 210
Atheromatous diseases, 214
Atherosclerosis, 80, 215
lipoxygenase, 99
peroxisome proliferator–activated receptors, 101–102
pulsatile stress, 148
shear stress, 142
thiazolidinediones, 102
Atherosclerotic disease, 569
BP and, 244–245
Atherosclerotic markers, 213
Atherosclerotic plaques, 114–115
Atherosclerotic strokes, 214
Atherothrombotic brain infarction (ABI), 258
Athletes, hypertension in, 550–552
banned substances, 552
BP patterns in, 550
evaluation, 550–551
echocardiogram, 551
history, 550
physical examination, 551
isolated systolic hypertension, 550
participation recommendations for, 551
spurious systolic hypertension, 550
sustained hypertension, 550

treatment of, 551–552
lifestyle modification, 552
medication choices, 552
white coat hypertension, 550
ATP. *See* Adenosine triphosphate (ATP)
ATRAP. *See* AT1 receptor-associated protein (ATRAP)
Atrasentan, 477
Atrial fibrillation, 463
Atrial natriuretic peptide, 9, 50f, 85, 90t, 124
Atropine, 75
Augmentation index, 142f, 373
Auscultation, 359–360, 375
diastolic murmurs, 360
heart sounds, 359
peripheral pulses, 360
systolic murmurs, 360
Automated BP measurement devices, 336
Autonomic failure (AF), 516–517
activities, 517
drug therapy, 517
elastic support garments, 517
exercise, 517
food intake, 517
pathogenesis, 516
treatment, 516
Autosomal dominant and recessive renal salt-wasting syndromes, 232
Autosomal dominant hypertension, 235
Avosentan, 477
AVP. *See* Arginine vasopressin

Balloon angioplasty, 166
Baltimore Longitudinal Study on Aging (BLSA), 270
Banned substances, in sports, 552
Bariatric surgery, 557
Baroreceptors, 116–117
Baroreflexes, 117, 136. *See also* Cardiopulmonary baroreflexes
Baroreflexes aortocarotid, 177–178
baroreflexes, arterial. *See* Arterial baroreflexes
function, 120
arterial pressure fluctuations, buffering of, 120
cellular mechanisms, 120
tonic sympathoinhibitory function, 120
hormonal modulation, 121–122
paracrine modulation, 122
resetting
chronic, 121
rapid, 120–121
Baroreflex failure, 349, 391, 517–518
aortocarotid baroreflexes. *See separate entry*
diagnosis, 517
pathogenesis and presentation, 517
therapy, 518
treatment of, 515
Barriers to BP control, 418–420
BP measurement issues, 420
health care availability, 418–419
patient adherence (compliance), 420
physician-controlled barriers, 419–420
societal barriers to healthy lifestyle, 420
in the United States population, 418
BAT. *See* Brown adipose tissue (BAT)
Belgian salt trial, 321
Benzodiazepines, 546
Bile acid–binding resins, 535
Biopsy, renal, 386
Percutaneous renal biopsy, 386
Blacks
hypertension in, 277, 279–280
BP control, barriers to, 280
etiologic factors, 279
lifestyle modifications, 279–280
pharmacologic therapy, 280
race as a social construct, 279
socioeconomic factors and health care quality, 280
minorities, hypertension in, 494
β-blockers, 357t
Blood flow regulation
kidney vs. brain blood flow, 130t
normal regional, 129–130
cerebral blood flow, 130

Blood flow regulation (*contd.*)
  myocardial blood flow, 130
  renal blood flow, 130
  skeletal muscle blood flow, 130
  skin blood flow, 130
  principles of, 129
  systemic pressure, importance of, 130–131
    arterial pressure determinants of, 130–131
    exercise, responses to, 131
Blood glucose changes, BP versus, 252
Blood pressure (BP). *See also individual entries*
    below; Ambulatory blood pressure; Home BP
  age and coronary heart disease risk, 147
    as risk predictors, 147
  and atherosclerotic hazards, 244–245
  BP control
    life style recommendations for, 408–409
  BP control and mortality, trends in, 314–317
    data sources and definitions, 314–316
    hospitalizations, 316
    hypertension awareness, treatment, and control,
      314–315
    obesity, 315
    prehypertension, 315–316
    role of education, 316
    trends and age-sex-race differences, 314–316
  BP regulatory systems, 553
  BP-related strokes, 214
  central versus peripheral BP, 371–372
    central systolic pressure augmentation, 371
    pulse pressure, 371–372
    radial pulse contour analysis, 372–373
  in children, 273–275. *See also* Children
  components
    and ischemic heart disease, 496
  components determinants, 144–145
    arterial wall, structural relations in, 144–145
    pulse pressure amplification, 145
    pulse wave morphology, 145
    wave summation, 145
  components, 245–246
    age and, 245
    low diastolic BP, 245–246
  control, barriers to, 280
  control, barriers to, 418–420. *See also* Barriers
  dietary patterns and, 297–300. *See also* Dietary
    patterns
  gender and, 269–272. *See also* Gender
  home BP monitoring recommendations, 347
  impact of calcium, magnesium, and heavy metals,
    307–310
  ischemic heart disease risk and, 249–250. *See also*
    under Ischemic heart disease
  lifestyle impact on, 407–408. *See also under*
    Lifestyle
  modifications out-of-office BP determinations,
    346
  modulation by prostaglandins in disease states,
    481
  monogenic determinants, 232–235. *See also*
    Individual entry
  oral contraceptives and, 271. *See also separate*
    entry
  patterns
    in athletes and physically active people, 550
  physical activity and, 295–296. *See also individual*
    entry
  population variation in, 239
  potassium and, 304–306. *See also* Potassium
  pulsatile vs. steady component, 141*f*
  raising effects
    of antiinflammatory drugs, 480–482
    of angiogenesis inhibitors, 480–482
    of cholesterol-ester-transfer protein inhibitors,
      480–482
    kidney effects, 481
    mechanisms of, 480–481
  respiration and. *See* Respiration
  salt and, 301–303
Blood pressure measurement, 335–338
  accuracy, 335
  accurate and reliable readings
    clinical setting, 336
    cuff placement, 337
    device positioning, 336

diastolic BP, 338
  inflation and deflation, 337
  patient positioning, 336
  preparation and rest period, 336
  proper cuff (bladder) size, 337
  recording, 338
  steps needed to obtain, 336–338
  stethoscope placement, 337
  two-step method for determining the maximum
    inflation level, 337
automated devices, 336
equipment
  aneroid manometer, 335
  manometer, 335
  Portable aneroids, 335
  selection and care for, 335–336
  stethoscope, 336
indirect BP measurement, 335
initial standardized training and lifetime
    performance monitoring, 335
special situations, 338
in very large, cone-shaped, or muscular arms, 338
Blood pressure variability and reactivity, 177–180
  behavioral aspects, 178
    anger and hostility, 178
    cultural aspects, 178
    social support, 178
    stress perception, coping, and locus of control,
      178
  hemodynamics and vascular reactivity, 178
    aging and hypertension, 178
    endothelial dysfunction, 178
    patterns and mechanisms, 180*t*
  practical implications, 180
    office BP measurement, limitations of, 180
    placebo and antihypertensive drug responses,
      180
    research implications, 180
    therapeutic implications, 180
  and risk, 179
    integrated risk model, 179–180
    morning BP surge, 179
    resting and reactive BP, 179
  sympathoadrenal output, modulation of, 177–178
    baroreflexes, 177–178
    hypothalamic control centers, 178
    stimuli, differential responses to, 177
    systemic sympathoadrenal responses, 177
Blood urea nitrogen (BUN), 368
Blood, alcohol use and, 310–313. *See also* Alcohol
    use
Blood–brain barrier, 218
Body fat distribution, 292–294
  assessment techniques, 292
  visceral fat, 292–293
Body mass index (BMI), 526
  hypertension and, 292
Bone, 87
Booster pump, 188
Bosentan, 476–477
  essential hypertension, 476
  pulmonary hypertension, 476
Bowman's capsule, 78
BP. *See* Blood pressure
BP effects, of ARBs, 463–464
Bradycardia, 105
Bradykinin, 90*t*
Brain imaging, 380
Brain natriuretic peptide, 85
  half-life, 87
Branch vein occlusion, 227
British hypertension guidelines
  evolution of, 395–400
Bronchodilation, 40
Brown adipose tissue (BAT), 111
Brown Norway rats, 83
Buspirone, 546

CAD. *See* Coronary artery disease
Cadmium, BP impact of, 309
  absorption, 309
  biologic plausibility and causal inference, 309
  epidemiologic studies, 309
  exposure, 309
  metabolism, 309

Caenorhabditis elegans, 9
Calcitonin gene–related peptide (CGRP), 73
  hypertension, role in, 74
  sensory nerve terminals, release from, 74
  synthesis and localization, 73
Calcium. *See also individual entries*
  Ca^{2+} release-activated channel (CRAC), 28
  Ca^{2+} signaling, 12
  Ca^{2+}/calmodulin-regulated kinase (CaMK), 17
  Ca^{2+}-activated K^+ channels, 25
Calcium antagonists (CAs), 465–469
  actions, 465–466
    vasodilation, 465–466
  adverse effects, 468–469
    drug–drug interactions, 469
    safety issues, 468
    side effects, 468–469
  beneficial effects of, 467
    angina, 467–468
    Arrhythmias, 468
    heart failure, 468
    ischemic heart disease, 467–468
    stroke protection and cognitive function, 467
  calcium antagonists subtypes, 465
  cellular calcium flux, 465
  dihydropyridine CAs, 466
  doses, 467*t*
  drug–drug interactions with, 468*t*
  nondihydropyridine CSs, 466
  pharmacology, 466–467
    alterations in effects, 466–467
    available compounds, 466*t*
    cardiac effects, 466
    common side effects, 466*t*
    contraindications/restrictions, 466*t*
    indications for use, 466*t*
    kinetics and dynamics, 466
    mode of action, 466*t*
    renal effects, 466
  use in hypertension, 467
    drug combinations, 467
    efficacy, 467
Calcium channel blockers (CCBs), 167, 294, 435,
    437, 446, 494, 497–499, 531, 548–549, 555,
    569, 577
Calcium channels, 29
  voltage-gated, 29
    activity regulation, 29
    structure and function, 29
    subclasses, 29
    voltage-independent, 29
Calcium gradients, 27
Calcium pumps, 29
Calcium sparks, 27
Calcium transport, 27
  calmodulin-dependent protein kinases, 28–29
    activation chacteristics, 29
    localization, 29
  cellular calcium stores, regulation, 27–28
    ligand-gated channels, 28
    sources, 28
    voltage-gated channels, 28
  intracellular calcium, 27
    calcium gradients, 27
    calcium sparks, 27
Calcium, BP impact of, 307–308
  absorption and metabolism, 307
  basic physiology and nutrition, 307–308
  clinical studies, 308
    clinical trials, 308
    epidemiology, 308
    population response heterogeneity, 308
  United States intake levels, 307–308
Calcium, intake, HTN and, 278
Calcyon, 3
Caldesmon, 36
CALLA. *See* Common acute lymphoblastic leukemia
    antigen (CALLA)
Calmodulin, 79
  function, 28
  interactions, 28
  structure, 28
Caloric intake, HTN and, 277
Calponin, 36
CaMK. *See* Ca2+/calmodulin-regulated kinase
    (CaMK), 17

cAMP. *See* Cyclic adenosine monophosphate (cAMP)
cAMP-responsive enhancer elements (CREs), 10
Candesartan, 461
Captopril renography, 389
Captopril suppression testing, 566
Cardiac catheterization, 166, 388
Cardiac effects, of Cas, 466
Cardiac embolism, 214
Cardiac imaging, 363–366. *See also*
    Echocardiography
    delayed relaxation, 364
    diastolic function, 364–365
    Doppler echocardiography, 364–365
    electron beam (ultrafast) computed tomography,
        365–366
    Magnetic resonance imaging, 366
    Radionuclide angiography (RNA), 365. *See also*
        individual entry
    restrictive filling, 365
Cardiac sinoatrial nodes, 6
Cardiometabolic syndrome
    BP issues in, 529–530
        importance of, 529–530
        nocturnal decline of BP, 530
        salt sensitivity and volume, 530
Cardiomyocytes, 80
Cardiopulmonary baroreceptors, 127
Cardiopulmonary baroreflexes, 123–125
    blunting, 124–125
        aging and sympathetic activity, 124
        aging and ventricular stiffness, 125
        smoking, 124
    hypertension, 125
        early changes, 125
        established hypertension, 125
    interactions with other systems, 124
        carotid baroreflex interactions, 124
        hormonal modulation, 124
        pain, 124
    sensory receptors, 123–124
        chemoreceptors, 123
        polymodal, 124
    system, 123
        afferent fiber, 123
        reflex arcs, 123
    volume and sympathetic activity, 124
        acute preload reduction, 124
        integrated compensatory response, 124
Cardiovascular disease (CVD), 442, 446, 483
    endothelial function, 204. *See also* Vascular
        endothelium
Cardiovascular homeostasis, 56
Cardiovascular monitoring systems, 116–117
    baroreceptors, 116–117
    chemoreceptors, 117
    neurohormones, 117
    neurotransmission, local modulation of, 117
    osmoreceptors, 117
Cardiovascular remodeling, 60
Cardiovascular risk factors, 56, 532
    BP and atherosclerotic hazards, 244–245
    hypertension and, 244–248
        global cardiovascular risk, 247
        left ventricular hypertrophy, 247
        population occurrences, 246
        preventive implications, 247–248
        risk factor clustering, 246–247
        risk factor interactions, 246
    left ventricular hypertrophy and, 254–257. *See also*
        Left ventricular hypertrophy
    reduction, salt intake and, 303
Cardiovascular system
    preeclampsia, 172
Carotid arteriosclerosis, 178
Carotid baroreflex, 124
Carotid imaging, 377
Carotid Intima-Media Thickness in Atherosclerosis
    Using Pioglitazone (CHICAGO), 102
Carotid sinus hypersensitivity, 394
    cardioinhibitory type, 394
    clinical findings, 394
    subtypes and therapeutic implications, 394
    vasodepressor type, 394
Carotid ultrasonography, 378t
Catechol amino acid, 37

Catecholamines, 1
    catecholamine-producing tumor, 571
    metabolism, 38–39
    receptors, 4
    release, 37–38
    reuptake, 38
    synthesis, 37, 38f
Caudal ventrolateral medulla, 118
Cell membrane receptors, 2
    intrinsic activity, 2
        receptor-gated ion channels, 2
        tyrosine kinase dependent, 2
    without intrinsic activity, 2
Cell volume regulation, 22
Cell-surface receptors, *See* Cell membrane receptors
Cellular calcium flux, 35, 465
Cellular calcium stores, 27–28
Cellular potassium transport, 24
    Ca^{2+} concentration, role in, 26
    depolarization, 24
    dysfunctional K^+ channels and hypertension,
        26
    inward transport of K^+, 24, 24f
    K^+ channels, 24
    K^+ currents and channels, 25
        adenosine triphosphate-sensitive, 25
        Ca^{2+}-activated, 25
        inward rectifier, 25
        two-pore domain, 25
        voltage-gated, 25
    Na^+, K^+-adenosine triphosphatase, 24
    regulating membrane potential, 26
    vascular tone, role in, 26
Central nervous system
    arterial pressure modification, 118t
    cardiovascular monitoring systems, 116–117
        baroreceptors, 116–117
        chemoreceptors, 117
        neurohormones, 117
        neurotransmission, local modulation of, 117
        osmoreceptors, 117
    peripheral autonomic nervous system, 116
        afferent nerves, 116
        efferent nerves, 116
Central sympatholytics, 453–455
    adverse effects, 454
    drug differentiation, 453–454
    mechanisms of action, 453
Central systolic pressure
    augmentation, 371
    clinical application, 372
        BP measurement and risk stratification, 372
        clinical trial interpretation, 372
    evaluation of, 370–373
Central vein occlusion, 227
Cerebellar stroke, 381t
Cerebral autoregulation, 217–218
Cerebral blood flow, 130
Cerebral hemorrhage, 214
Cerebral infarction, 380–381
    chronic management after, 513–514
    hemorrhage versus, 381
    localization, 380
Cerebral ischemic injury, 214
Cerebral thrombosis, 215
Cerebral vasospasm, 468
Cerebrovascular disease
    acute cerebral ischemia and infarction, 512–513
    hypertensive patients with, treatment, 512–514
Cerebrovascular risk, 257–260
    incidence of stroke, 258
    secular trends, 258
    stroke risk factors, 258–259
        age, 258
        age–gender interactions, 258–259
        hypertension, 259
        left ventricular hypertrophy, 259
        stroke risk profile, 259
    subtypes, 258
    treatment trials, 260
        optimal BP, 260
        prevention implications, 260
        primary stroke prevention, 260
        stroke recurrence, 260
C-Fos, 66, 201

CGMP. *See* Cyclic guanosine monophosphate
    (cGMP)
CGRP. *See* Calcitonin gene–related peptide
Characteristic impedance, 142f
Chemoreceptors, 117, 137
Chest pain, 369
Chest radiograph, 359–362
Chest, 375
    chest x-ray, 368
Cheyne-stokes respiration, 138
CHICAGO. *See* Carotid Intima-Media Thickness in
    Atherosclerosis Using Pioglitazone
    (CHICAGO)
Children, BP in, 273–275
    guidelines, evolution, 274
    high BP
        current definitions and classification, 274–275
        revised age–weight nomograms, 275
    measurement techniques, 274
        ambulatory pressures, 274
        cuff size, 274
        Korotkoff sounds, 274
        Oscillometry, 274
    prevalence and risks, 273
    risk factors for hypertension, 274
Children, hypertensive, 287
    definition of, 540
    drugs for, 544t
    evaluation and therapy
        goals of, 540
    evaluation, 540
    nonpharmacologic therapy in, 540–543
        weight reduction, 540–543
    pharmacologic therapy in, 543–544
        individualized therapy, 543
        specific drug choices, 543
    treatment, 540–544
        diet modification, 542
        drugs for, 541–543t
        exercise, 543
        chlorthalidone, 350
Cholesterol oxidation, in injury, 224
Cholesteryl-ester-transfer protein (CETP) inhibitors,
    BP raising effects of, 480, 482
Choroidal circulation, 226
    changes in hypertension, 227
    normal anatomy and physiology, 226–227
Chromosomal linkages to hypertension, 237–238
Chronic hypertension, 537t
    in pregnancy, treatment, 537t
    with superimposed preeclampsia, 537t
Chronic kidney disease (CKD), 222–225, 237–238,
    261–264, 522. *See also* Renal risk
    classification, 383, 384t
    cystic renal diseases, 383
    and diabetes, 404
    estimated glomerular filtration rate, 383–384
    evaluation algorithm, 385f
    evaluation, 382–386
    glomerular diseases, 382–383. *See also individual*
        entry
    interstitial renal disease, 383
    nephrosclerosis, 383
    proteinuria detection methods, 384–386
        imaging studies, 386
        renal biopsy, 386
        ultrasonography, 386
    recognizing and defining, 383–386
        chemistries, 383
        creatinine clearance, 383
    hypertension and, 222
        high-risk individuals, 222
        vicious cycle, 222
    hypertensive nephropathy. *See also individual entry*
    hypertensive renal injury, 222–223. *See also*
        individual entry
    pathogenesis, 222–225
    progressive chronic kidney disease, 222
    perpetuating factors for, 263t
    progression, 225
    progression, staging, 263
        albuminuria, 263
        estimated GFR, 263
        microalbuminuria, 263
        risk assessment, 263–264

Chronic kidney disease (CKD), 222–225, 237–238, 261–264, 522. *See also* Renal risk *(contd.)* renal insufficiency, treatment of, 522–525
Chronic stress, 289–290
Cigarette smoking, 224
Circulatory diseases, 242
C-Jun, 66, 201
CKD. *See* Chronic kidney disease
Claudication walking program, 374, 510*t* pseudoclaudication versus, 375*t*
Clazosentan, 477
Clinical inertia concept, 419
Clonidine, 454, 548
Clothing, 336
C-myc, 66
Coagulation, 152 disturbances, 214
Coarctation of aorta. *See* Aorta, coarctation of
Cocaine, 562
Cockcroft-Gault equation, 383
Cognitive decline, 219–221
Cognitive function, CAs in, 467
Cognitive impairment, mild, *See* Mild cognitive impairment
Cohort studies, in potassium intake, 306
Combination antihypertensive therapy, 530
Combination therapy, 434–435, 487–488 in clinical trials, 435–436 diuretics in, 437 fixed-dose combinations, 436–437. *See also* *separate entry* goals of, 436 efficacy, 436 predictability of response, 436 prompt BP control, 436 tolerability, 436 need for, 495 rationale, 434–435 specific combinations, 437–439
Combined oral contraceptive (COC), 271
Combined α,β-adrenergic blocking activity, 448
Common acute lymphoblastic leukemia antigen (CALLA), 50
Community pharmacists, 425
Community-based management programs, 322–324 community-based interventions, 323–324 community health models, 323 faith-based programs, 324 school programs, 323–324 worksite programs, 324 cost–benefit analyses, 323 high-risk populations, 323 lower risk populations, 323 very low-risk populations, 323 health system and patient barriers, 322 mass strategy, 323 potential target populations, 322–333 elderly, 322 obese, 323 racial and regional groups, 323 young, 322 provider-based programs, 324 pharmacists, 324 primary care providers, 324 rationale for, 322
Comorbidities, 350
Compliance, arterial, 373
Comprehensive therapy, 530
Computed tomographic angiography, 389
Concentric hypertrophy, 363
Concentric versus eccentric hypertrophy, 363
Conduit Artery Function Evaluation (CAFÉ) Study, 327, 372
Congenital adrenal hyperplasia (CAH), 233–234
Conivaptan, 475
Consultations, hypertension, 421–423 Guideline-based hypertension referrals, 422 health care system diversity and BP control, 421 hypertension care, delivery, 421–422
Continuous positive airway pressure (CPAP), 557
Contrast arteriography, 389
Coping ability, 178
Copper-wire change, 227
Cornell voltage, 189

Coronary artery disease (CAD), 343, 506 atherogenesis. *See* Atherogenesis in patients with peripheral arterial disease, 510 women with PCOS, 155
Coronary atherosclerosis, 211 advanced atherosclerosis, 213*f* advanced lesions, 211–213 arterial remodeling, 211 early cell biology, 212*f* early lesions, 211 plaque formation, 212*f* vulnerable plaques, 213
Coronary heart disease (CHD) life style impact on, 408 life style recommendations for, 408–409
Corticosteroids, 560
Corticotrophin, 3 corticotrophin-releasing factor (CRF), 111
Cortisol synthesis, 62
Cotton-wool spots, 227
Cough, 460
Creatinine (CR) clearance, calculation, 384*t*
CREs. *See* cAMP-responsive enhancer elements (CREs)
CRF. *See* Corticotrophin-releasing factor (CRF)
Critical limb ischemia, 374–375
Crossing-over process, 230
Cross-phosphorylation, 3
Cross-talk, 17
C-type natriuretic peptide, 85
Cuff size, in BP measurement, 274
Cushing's syndrome, 566–567 diagnosis, 567 treatment, 567
Cyclic adenosine monophosphate (cAMP), 3, 5, 8, 45 dependent protein kinases, 9–10 anchoring proteins, 10 catalytic subunits, 10 nuclear signaling, 10 regulatory roles, 10 regulatory subunits, 9–10 structural properties, 10
Cyclic nucleotides, 8–11 cAMP dependent protein kinases, 9–10 anchoring proteins, 10 catalytic subunits, 10 nuclear signaling, 10 regulatory subunits, 9–10 cAMP-regulated guanine nucleotide exchange factors, 11 cGMP dependent protein kinases, 10 regulatory roles, 10 structural properties, 10 cyclic nucleotide efflux pumps, 11 cyclic nucleotide phosphodiesterases, 11 cyclic nucleotide-gated channels, 10 cyclic nucleotide-gated channels, 10 efflux pumps, 11 hyperpolarization and cyclic nucleotide-activated channels, 11 phosphodiesterases, 11 actions, 11 inhibitors, 11 subtypes, 11 signaling pathway, 9*f*
Cyclooxygenase (COX), 94 COX-2, 46, 349 derived eicosanoids, 94 BP responses, 95 synthesis, 94 vasoconstrictor eicosanoids, 94 vasodilator prostaglandins, 94
Cyclooxygenase-2 inhibitors (COXIBs), BP raising effects of, 480–482
Cystic renal diseases, 383
Cytochrome P-450 derived eicosanoids, 95 allylic oxidation, 95 epoxidation, 95 synthesis, 95
Cytokines, 1

Dahl rats, 181
Dahl salt-sensitive rat, 96
Darusentan, 476–477

DASH. *See* Dietary Approaches to Stop Hypertension diet
De novo synthesis, 76
Delayed relaxation, 364
Deletion polymorphism, 50
Dementia, 216, 381 pathogenesis, 219–221
11-deoxycortisol, 63
Deoxycorticosterone acetate (DOCA), 62–63, 96, 118
Depolarization, 24
Diabetes mellitus, 191, 222, 408, 500, 510 Diabetes mellitus 2 BP issues in, 529–530 dietary intervention, 530 diabetic nephropathy, 462–463
Diacylglycerol, 13, 16
Dialysis patients, 524
Diastolic blood pressure (DBP), 144, 338, 496
Diastolic dysfunction, 367 assessment of, 503 hypertensive patients with, management of, 501–504 mitral flow analysis, 503 pathophysiology, 503 tissue Doppler, 503
Diastolic function, 364–365
Diastolic hypertension, 354 early trials in, 440
Diastolic pulse contour analysis (windkessel model), 373
Dietary Approaches to Stop Hypertension (DASH) diet, 279, 302, 484, 523 sodium trial, 320
Dietary patterns and BP, 297–300 dietary approaches to stop hypertension (DASH), 298 dietary types, 298 BP effects, 298 DASH diet, 298 DASH-low sodium diet, 298 dietary approaches to stop HTN diet effect, 298 fish oil, 299–300 fruit and vegetables diet, 298 OmniHeart study, 298–299 public health and clinical implications, 300 epidemiologic surveys, 297
Dietary salt loading, 565
Dihydropyridine (DHP), 433, 465 Dihydropyridine CAs, 466, 468
Dihydroxyphenylglycol, 38–39 dihydroxyphenylacetaldehyde (DOPAL), 39 dihydroxyphenylacetic acid (DOPAC), 39
Dimerization, 3
Direct arterial dilators, 469–471 clinical use of, 470*t* hydralazine, 470–471. *See also individual entry* Minoxidil, 471 pseudotolerance, 469–470. *See also individual entry*
Dissociation constant (Kd), 1
Distensibility, arterial, 373
Diuretics, 293–294, 497, 508, 525, 531, 555, 577 diuretic therapy, 165 diuretic/ β-blocker comparisons, 326 diuretics in combination therapy, 437
DOCA. *See* Deoxycorticosterone acetate (DOCA)
Docking, 19
Donepezil (Aricept), 220
Dopamin ß-hydroxylase (DBH), 37
Dopamine agonists, 473 DA₂ agonists, 473 drug interactions, 473 Fenoldopam, 473
Dopaminergic receptors, 42 biologic effects, 42–43 D2-like receptor effects, 43 renal effects and natriuresis, 42–43 classification, 42*t* general characteristics, 42 distribution, 42 signal transduction mechanisms, 42 subtypes, 42
Doppler echocardiography, 364–365
Doppler ultrasonography, 389

Dose–response relationships, 432–433
    factors affecting, 433–434
Doxazosin, 41
Drosophila, 9, 25
Drug combinations, 435–439. *See also* Combination
    therapy
Drug therapy, 537
Drug-induced hypertension
    Anesthetics, 562–563
    anti–human immunodeficiency virus treatment,
        562
    corticosteroids, 560
    heavy metals, 563
    immunosuppressives and antineoplastic agents,
        562–563
    management of, 560–563
        alcohol, 561
        caffeine, 562
        dietary supplements, 562
    Narcotics, 562–563
    Nonsteroidal antiinflammatory drugs (NSAIDs),
        560–561
    Recombinant human erythropoietin (r-HuEPO),
        563
    steroids, 560
Dyslipidemia management in hypertensives, 532–535
    antilipidemic medications, 534–535. *See also*
        individual entries
    cardiovascular disease risk, 532
    and inflammatory cytokines, 150
    management guidelines, 533
        metabolic syndrome, 533
        risk stratification, 533
        treatment goals, 533
    pathophysiology, 532
    therapeutic lifestyle change (TLC), 533–534
    screening, 533
Dyspnea, 369

Early preeclampsia, 173
East Asians, hypertension in, 287–288
    hypertension control, benefits, 288
    treatment issues, 288
Eccentric hypertrophy, 363
ECE. *See* Endothelin converting enzyme (ECE)
Echocardiogram, 189
Echocardiographic left ventricular hypertrophy, 255
Echocardiography, 189, 363, 501–502
    two-dimensional echocardiography, 363–364
        accuracy, 363
        anatomy and function, 363
        asymmetric hypertrophy, 363
        calculations, 363
        clinical correlations, 363–364
        concentric hypertrophy, 363
        concentric versus eccentric hypertrophy, 363
        eccentric hypertrophy, 363
        left ventricular hypertrophy (LVH), 363
        left ventricular mass determination, 363
    ventricular function, 364
Economic considerations in hypertension
    management, 331–333
    cost-effectiveness, improving, 332–333
        accurate diagnosis, 333
        cost of lifestyle modifications, 333
        enhanced medication adherence, 333
        improved prescribing habits, 333
        limiting costs of medicines, 333
        reducing health care provider associated costs,
            333
        risk stratification before therapy, 333
    economic aspects, calculations, 331–332
        cost-effectiveness and cost-utility, 331–332
        effect of risk, 332
Edema, 369
    thiazolidinediones, 102
Edonentan, 477
Education of hypertension. *See* Patient education
EET. *See* Epoxyeicosatrienoic acids (EET)
Eicosanoids, 94–95
    cyclooxygenase-derived, 94
    cytochrome p450-derived, 95
    tissue blood flow, 134
    synthesis, 97
    vasoconstrictor, 94–95

EIF. *See* Eukaryotic initiation factor (eIF)
Elastic support garments, 517
Elastin
    half life, 145
Elderly hypertensive, treatment of, 485–488
    age and BP patterns, 485–486
        clinical evaluation, 486
        isolated systolic hypertension, 485
        pathophysiology, 486
    drug treatment recommendations, 487
        combination therapy, 487–488
        fears of excessive BP lowering, 488
        initial drug choice, 487
        potassium maintenance, 488
        treatment goals, 487
        underdosing problems, 488
    evidence-based benefits of, 486–487
    percentage event reduction in clinical trials in,
        486
    secondary hypertension, 486t
    Systolic Hypertension in the Elderly Program
        (SHEP), 486
Electrocardiogram, 360–362
    chest radiograph, 361
    exercise stress testing, 361–362
        BP response to stress, 361
        heart rate and electrocardiogram changes, 361
        left bundle branch block, 361
        predisposition to myocardial ischemia in
            hypertension, 361
    24-hour ambulatory electrocardiogram
        monitoring, 361
    QRS duration and cornell product, 361
    QT changes, 361
    strain pattern, 361
    vectorcardiography, 361
    voltage criteria, 360
Electrocardiographic left ventricular hypertrophy,
    254–255
Electrolyte abnormalities
    in hypertension, evaluation, 356–358, 357t
        potassium, 356. *See also* Potassium
            abnormalities
        sodium, 357
    therapeutic choices
        impact on, 357–358
Electron beam (ultrafast) computed tomography,
    365–366
    clinical use, 365
    methodology, 365
Electronic management systems, of HPT, 428–431
    information systems, 428–430
        electronic records, 428–430
        flowsheets, 428
        graphic displays, 430
Embolism, in stroke, 214
    arterial embolism, 214
    cardiac embolism, 214
Embryogenesis, 57
Emergencies, hypertensive
    drugs useful for, 492t
    follow-up care, 492
    immediate treatment goals, 490–491
    life-threatening hypertensive emergencies, 491t
    specific drugs, 491–492
    specific syndromes, 491
    treatment of, 489–492
Emigration effects, HTN and, 285
Encephalopathy, hypertensive, 379–380
    clinical signs and symptoms, 379
    neuroimaging studies, 379
    neurologic investigation, 380
        brain imaging, 380
        vascular imaging, 380
    retinal ischemia, 379–380. *See also separate entry*
Encephalopathy, hypertensive, 491
Endocannabinoids, 103
    human disease, 106
        atherosclerosis, 106
        hypertension, 106
        hypotension, 106
        metabolic syndrome, 106
        myocardial infarction, 106
    physiologic effects
        antiinflammatory effects, 106

cardiac effects, 105–106
    nervous system effects, 105
    vascular effects, 106
    receptors, 103–105
        coupling, 105
        subtypes, 103–105
    regulation, 103
        clearance, 103
        synthesis, 103
Endocytosis, 52
Endogenous natriuretic peptides. *See* Natriuretic
    peptides
Endogenous ouabain, 77
    actions, 77
    biosynthesis, 77
    hypertension and cardiac disease, 77
Endoglin, 171
Endothelial dysfunction, 142, 178
    in injury, 224
Endothelial function. *See* Vascular endothelium
Endothelial nitric oxide synthase (eNOS), 205
Endothelin (ET) antagonists, 476–478
    Bosentan, 476. *See also separate entry*
    Darusentan, 476
    Endothelin (ET), 476
    Enrasentan, 477t
    future developments, 477–478
    nonselective antagonists, 476–477
    selective endothelin-a receptor antagonists, 477
    Tezosentan, 477t
    uses, 477t
Endothelin, 66
    Endothelin converting enzyme (ECE), 66
    salt-sensitivity of BP, 157
    genomics, 69
    pathophysiology, 66–67
        cardiac effects, 67
        developmental effects, 67
        renal effects, 67
        vascular effects, 66
    receptors, 66
    structure, 67f
    synthesis and release, 66
Endothelin-1, 90t, 196
Endothelium-derived hyperpolarizing factor (EDHF),
    204
Endothelium-derived relaxing factor (EDRF), 205
Endothelium-derived vasodilators, 205f
End-stage renal disease (ESRD), 159, 261–263,
    382–383
    prevention, 264
        antihypertensive therapy, 264
        diet, 264
        lifestyle modifications, 264
        strict BP control, 264
Enkephalinase, 50
Enrasentan, 477t
    Enrasentan Cooperative Randomized Evaluation
        (ENCOR) trial, 477
Environmental stress, 290
Erythropoetin, 160
EPHESUS. *See* Eplerenone post-acute myocardial
    infarction heart failure efficacy and survival
    study (EPHESUS)
Epithelial Na channel (ENaC), 65f
Eplerenone post-acute myocardial infarction heart
    failure efficacy and survival study (EPHESUS),
    65
Eplerenone, 444, 566
Epoxidation, 95
Epoxyeicosatrienoic acids (EET), 95
Epsin N-terminal homology (ENTH), 14
Erythropoietic effects, 57
Escherichia coli, 9
ESRD. *See* End-stage renal disease (ESRD)
Essential hypertension, 229–231, 476
    definition, 229
Estimated glomerular filtration rate (eGFR),
    383–384
Ethnicity and socioeconomic status
    in hypertension, 276–278
        geography and urbanization, 277–278
        obesity and nutrition, 277
        Southeastern stroke belt, 277
        United states demography, 277

Eukaryotic initiation factor (eIF), 20
Europe
    European and World Health
        Organization/International Society of
        Hypertension guidelines (2003– 2007),
        397–400
    European hypertension guidelines
        evolution of, 395–400
    European Trial on Isolated Systolic Hypertension
        in the Elderly (Syst-EUR), 487
    hypertension prevalence in, 276
Euthyroid, 168
Eutrophic inward remodeling, 196f, 197
Evaluation study (RALES), 65
Exaggerated BP variability, office management of,
    402
Exercise stress testing, 361–362
    contraindications to, 362t
Exercise therapy, 410–411, 509–510
    antihypertensive medications and, 411. See also
        separate entry
    exercise testing before exercise participation, 411t
    physical activity advice and counseling, 410–411.
        See also separate entry
    screening before exercise, 411
        contraindications to exercise, 411
        exercise-tolerance testing, 411
        safety issues, 411
Exercise tolerance testing (ETT), 361–362
    contraindications to, 362
Exp3174, 461
Extracellular matrix modulation, 202
Eye in hypertension, 226–228
    ocular circulations, 226–227
        choroidal circulation, 226. See also individual
            entry
        optic nerve circulation, 227
        retinal circulation, 226. See also individual entry
Ezetimibe, 535

Factor V Leiden, 214
Familial aggregation, in heritability of hypertension,
    236–237
    chromosomal linkages to hypertension, 237
    correlation and heritability, 236
    family history, 236
    genes versus environment, 236
Fat burden
    assessment of, 526
        BMI, 526
        waist to hip ratio, 526
Fat intake, and geographic patterns of hypertension,
    239
Fenofibrate, 158
    Fenofibrate Intervention and Event Lowering in
        Diabetes (FIELD), 102
Fenoldopam, 473
Fetal safety concerns, 537
Fibrates, 535
Fibrinolytic balance, 91
Fibromuscular disease
    atherosclerotic disease versus, 387–388
    fibromuscular dysplasia, 569
FIELD. See Fenofibrate Intervention and Event
    Lowering in Diabetes (FIELD)
First messengers, 1
Fish oil, 299–300
Fixed-dose combinations, 436–437
    clinical use, 437
    rationale, 436
Flame hemorrhages, 228
Fludrocortisone, 517
Fludrocortisone suppression testing (FST), 565
Fluid attenuation inversion recovery (FLAIR), 381
Fourier analysis, 140
Furosemide, 350
Framingham Heart Study, 258, 265
Framingham Risk Score, 252

G proteins. See also Guanine nucleotide binding
    proteins
    G protein–coupling, 19
    G protein–dependent inwardly rectifying
        potassium (K+) channels (GIRKs), 4
    G12 proteins, 5

Gadolinium-contrast magnetic resonance
    angiography, 389
Galantamine (Reminyl), 220
Ganglia, 116
Gender
    and BP, 269–272
        age and, 269–270
        awareness, treatment, and control, 269–270
        BP patterns, 269
        menopause, 269
    and therapeutic responses, 271–272
Gene regulation, 41
Gene titration, 183
General care, 500
Genes versus environment, 236, 239
Genetics of hypertension, 229–231
    characterizing genetic variants, 231
    clinical impact, 231
    gene associations, 230–231
    genetic determinants, 29
        evolutionary aspects, 229
        genetic background, 230
        genetic heterogeneity, 230
        natural selection, 229
        phenotypic heterogeneity, 230
        polygenic versus monogenic phenotypes, 229
        population characteristics, 230
    genetic linkage, 230
    genetic mapping, 231
    'whole-genome association' approach, 231
Genomics, 69
Geographic patterns of hypertension, 239–240
    covariation in risk factors, 240
    genes versus environment, 239
    industrialized societies, 240
    intrinsic (genetic) factors, 240
    latitude, 240
    mass migrations, 239
    nonindustrialized societies, 239
    population variation in BP, 239
    United States, 240. See also individual entry
Geography
    HTN and, 277–278
Gestational hypertension, 537t
GIRKs. See G protein–dependent inwardly rectifying
    potassium (K+) channels (GIRKs)
Glitazones, 478–479
Global cardiovascular disease risk, 247, 353
Glomerular capillary hypertension, 223–224
Glomerular diseases, 382–383
    end-stage renal disease, 383
    idiopathic hematuria, 382
    isolated proteinuria, 382
    nephritic syndrome, 383
    nephrotic syndrome, 382–383
Glomerular endotheliosis, 172
Glomerular filtration rate (GFR), 133, 357
    impaired glomerular filtration rate, 522
Glossopharyngeal axons, 116
Glucocorticoid hypertension, 182
Glucocorticoid response element (GRE), 92
Glucocorticoid-remediable aldosteronism, 63, 232,
    566
Glucose intolerance, 293–294, 510
Glucose, 441
Glucose transport, 600
Goldblatt hypertension, 164, 196
Gordon's syndrome, 234
Gothic type of arch, 167
GPCR. See Guanyl nucleotide binding protein
    coupled receptor (GPCR)
Gq proteins, 6
Gravidas, 172
GRE. See Glucocorticoid response element (GRE)
Growth factor, 88
Growth hormone, 170
GTP. See Guanosine triphosphate (GTP)
Guanabenz, 454
Guanfacine, 454
Guanine nucleotide binding proteins
    activity, 6–7
        activation, 7
        effector regulation, 7
        inhibition, 7
        receptor activation complexes, 6

receptor occupancy and subunit interactions, 6
    second messengers, 6
    signal termination and RGS proteins, 6–7
counterregulatory effects, 7
family, 5–6
    basic structure and subunits, 5
    G12 proteins, 6
    Gq proteins, 6
    heterotrimer families, 5
    inhibitory, 6
    stimulatory, 6
    structural diversity, 5
    α subunits, properties of, 5t
GPCR, 4–5
    ligand types, 4
    receptor isoforms, 4–5
    receptor networks, 5
    receptor structure, 4
Guanosine diphosphate (GDP), 5
Guanosine triphosphate (GTP), 5
Guanyl nucleotide binding protein coupled receptor
    (GPCR), 2, 4–5
    ligand types, 4
    receptor isoforms, 4–5
    receptor networks, 5
    receptor structure, 4
Guanylyl cyclase, 9, 80
    plasma membrane, 9
    soluble guanylyl cyclases, 9
Guidelines, hypertension
    description, 395–396
    essential characteristics, 395
    European and World Health
        Organization/International Society of
        Hypertension guidelines (2003– 2007),
        397–400
    evolution of, 395–400
    guideline users, responsibilities of, 396
    guideline writers, responsibilities of, 394–396
    'science-based' approach in, 395
    United Kingdom perspectives, 398
    United States guidelines (1977–2003), 396–397.
        See also separate entry
    World Health Organization/International Society
        of Hypertension (WHO/ISH), 398

Hageman factor, 83
HapMap project, 231
Hawaiians
    native Hawaiians, hypertension in, 287–288
Heart
    aging and hypertension
        adrenergic responsiveness, 186
        altered responses to sympathetic stimulation,
            185
        arterial and cardiac changes, 185f
        Ca2+ loading, 186
        cardiac changes, 184
        cellular mechanisms in animal models, 185–186
        chronic hypertension vs. accelerated aging, 185
        excitation–contraction–relaxation, 186
        exhaustive upright exercise, 186t
        impaired cardiovascular reserve, 184
        impaired cardiovascular reserve, 184–185
        large vessel changes, 184
        left ventricular structure, 186
        pressure overload vs. normotensive aging, 186
        therapeutic implications, 187
Heart failure (HF), 191–194, 357, 404, 444, 460,
    463, 491
    clinical synthesis, 369–370
        determining functional class, 369
        differential diagnosis, 369
        prognosis, 369
    demographic trends in, 505
    diagnostic evaluation, 368–369
        History, 368
        physical examination, 368
        routine laboratory studies, 368
    early recognition and heart failure management,
        194
    evaluation, 367–370
        pathophysiologic considerations, 367
    evolution stages, 507t

Heart Failure Society of America (HFSA) 2006, 505–506
Heart failure treatment guidelines, 507
  Stage A (at risk), 507
  Stage A (at risk), 507
  Stage C (symptomatic), 507
  Stage D (end-stage), 507
  in hypertension, prevention, 506
    BP targets, 506
    choice of drugs, 506
  paradigm shift, 192
    clinical symptom development, 192
    left ventricular remodeling, 192
    low output phase, 192
  preexisting conditions in, 191
    coronary artery disease, 191
    hypertension, 191
    obesity and diabetes, 191
  progression to LVSD, 191
    left ventricular concentric hypertrophy, 191
    LVH to LVSD, transition from, 191–192
  with preserved left ventricular systolic function, 192–193
    cardio-renal interactions, 193
    hypertension, 193
    left ventricular diastolic function, 193
    obesity, 193
Heart Outcomes Prevention Evaluation (HOPE), 256, 260
Heat shock protein 90, 79
Heavy metals, BP impact of, 309–310
  Cadmium, 309. See also individual entry
  Lead, 309. See also individual entry
  Mercury, 309–310
HELLP. See Hemolysis, elevated liver function tests and low platelets (HELLP) syndrome
Hematocrit, 172
Hematologic effects, 57
Hemoconcentration, 173
Hemodialysis, sleep apnea in, 558–559
Hemodynamic effects of arginine vasopressin, 474–475
Hemodynamics, 223
Hemolysis, elevated liver function tests and low platelets (HELLP) syndrome, 173
Hepatocyte angiotensinogen, 48
Hepatoreceptors, 127
Heptahelical receptor, 88, 89–90
  agonists, contractility and growth, 90t
Hereditary brachydactyly, 235
HETE. See Hydroxyeicosatetraenoic acids
Heritability, hypertension
  familial aggregation, 236–237. See also separate entry
  and target organ damage, 236–238
Heterotrimer, 5
HF. See Heart failure
High BP in children
  current definitions and classification, 274–275
High density lipoprotein (HDL), 62, 209–210
High ejection fraction paradox, 502
Hippocampus, 119
Hispanics
  Hispanic Americans
    minorities, hypertension in, 494
    Hispanic Health and Nutrition Examination Survey (HHANES), 282
    hypertension prevalence in, 277
    in United States, hypertension among, 281–284
      general demographics, 281
      heart disease, 281
      HTN mortality, 281
      HTN prevalence, 281–282
      Mexican Americans, 283
      Puerto Ricans, 283
      socioeconomic status, 281
      subpopulations, 282–284
Home BP monitoring, 339–342, 486
  clinical trials, 340
  device validation, 339
  issues in, 339–340
  organ damage and outcomes, 340
  therapeutic decision making, 340
Homovanillic acid, 39
Hormone replacement therapy (HRT), 270

HTN. See Hypertension
Hydralazine, 196, 350, 469–471
  clinical use, 470
  hydralazine–nitrate combinations, 471
  pharmacokinetics and metabolism, 470
  side effects and toxicity, 471
Hydrochlorothiazide (HCTZ), 437–439
Hydroosmotic aquaretic effect, 474
Hydroperoxides, 98
Hydroxyeicosatetraenoic acids (HETE), 95, 96, 98
  20-Hydroxyeicosatetraenoic acids
    salt-sensitivity of BP, 157
    regulation and effects, 96
  5-hydroperoxyeicosatetraenoic acid, 98
Hydroxylation, 96
  11-hydroxylation, 62
  17-hydroxylation, 62
11β-hydroxysteroid dehydrogenase, 234
  type 1, 108–109
  type 2, 63–64
5-hydroxytryptamine. See Serotonin
Hyperaldosteronism, 356, 444
  Cushing's syndrome, 566–567. See also separate entry
  management, 564–567
  primary aldosteronism (PA), 564–566. See also individual entry
Hyperglycemia, 102
Hyperglycemic syndromes, 529
Hyperhomocysteinemia, 171, 207, 214
Hyperinsulinemia, 149, 152–153
  preeclampsia, 172
Hyperkalemia, 357–358, 445
Hyperleptinemia, 149
Hypernatremia, 357t
Hyperparathyroidism, 161, 575
  hypertension mechanisms, 169
  RAAS in, 170
Hyperpolarization and cyclic nucleotide-activated channels (HCN), 11
Hyperreflexia, 172
Hypertension (HTN). See also Eye in hypertension
  acromegaly, 170
  adiponectin, 115
  androgens, 170
  animal models, 68, 71
    endothelin activation, 68
    renovascular and spontaneous hypertension, 68
    salt-sensitive, 68
  awareness, treatment, and control, 276–277, 314–315
  baroreceptor stimulation therapy, 122
  baroreflex, 120–121
  in blacks, 279–280. See also Blacks
  calcitonin gene–related peptide role, 74
  cardiovascular risk factors and, 244–248
  CKD and, 222
  coarctation of aorta, 166
  consultations, 421–423. See also Consultations
  endocannabinoids, 106
  endogenous ouabain, 77
  ethnicity and socioeconomic status in, 276–278. See also individual entry
  expanded definition of, 353t
  genetics of, 229–231. See also Genetics
  geographic patterns, 239–240. See also Geographic patterns
  guidelines for. See Guidelines, hypertension
  heart failure, 193
  hemodynamic subtypes of, 354
  heritability of, See also Heritability, hypertension
  human hypertension, 68, 71
    endothelin activation, 68–69
    endothelin blockade, 69
  hypertension dysfunctional K+ channels, 26
  Hypertension in the Very Elderly Trial (HYVET) pilot study, 487
  Hypertension Optimal Treatment (HOT) trial, 330, 487, 496
  Hypertension Prevention Trial (HPT), 320
  Hypertension Writing Group, 352–353
  initial workup of adults with, 343–347. See also individual entry
  insulin resistance, 152
  intracellular pH, 23

  with increased mineralocorticoid activity, 234
  kinins, 83
  management, economic considerations in, 331–333. See also Economic considerations
  mental stress and cardiac output, 178
  microcirculatory structural changes in, 198–199
    arefaction, 199
    BP and remodeling, 198–199
    cellular changes, 199
  monogenic forms of, 233t
  mortality, 281
  natriuretic peptides, 87
  neuropeptide Y, 72
  new definition of, 352
  nitric oxide, 80
  N-terminal 20 peptide, 74
  obesity. See Obesity
  office management, 401–406. See also Office management
  and oxidative stress. See Oxidative stress
  parathyroids, 169–170
  peripheral arterial disease and, 265–268. See also Peripheral arterial disease
  peripheral sympathetic abnormalities, 117
    altered sensory feedback, 117
    increased neurons and varicosities, 117
  plasminogen-activator inhibitor 1, 93
  pregnancy-associated, 154–155
  prevalence, 276, 281–282
  prevention, 318–321. See also Prevention
  primary pulmonary, 69
  RAAS, 93
  renal hemodynamics, 131
  renal parenchymal hypertension, 160–161
  renovascular, 131–132
  sleep apnea, 175
  as syndrome. See Syndrome
  target organ damage heritability, 237–238. See also separate entry
  thyroid, 168–169
  and ventricular hypertrophy, 125
Hypertension experimental models, 181–183
  adrenal steroid models, 182
    glucocorticoid hypertension, 182
    mineralocorticoid hypertension, 182
  inbred rat models
    Dahl rats, 181
    spontaneously hypertensive and stroke-prone rats, 181
  molecular models, 183
    congenic models, 183
    gene titration, 183
    transgenic and knockout models, 183
  neurogenic models, 182–183
  renal artery stenosis, 182
    one-kidney, one-clip model, 182
    two-kidney, one-clip model, 182
    two-kidney, two-clip model, 182
  renal parenchymal, 182
    renal mass reduction salt-induced model, 182
Hypertensive encephalopathy, 217. See also Acute hypertensive encephalopathy
  differential diagnosis, 217t
  etiology, 217t
  pathophysiology, 217t
  triad, 217t
  usually associated with malignant hypertension, 217t
Hypertensive end-organ damage, 443
  clinical use, 444
  heart failure, 443
  vascular effects, 443
Hypertensive hypertrophic cardiomyopathy, 360
Hypertensive nephropathy
  antihypertensive therapy, 225
  chronic kidney disease progression, 225
  clinical features consistent with, 224–225t
  diagnosis of, 224–225
Hypertensive renal injury
  mechanisms, 223–224
    afferent arteriolar constriction, 223
    afferent arteriolar dilation, 223–224
    glomerular capillary hypertension, 223–224
    hemodynamics, 223
    ischemia, 223

Hypertensive renal injury (contd.)
  morphology, 222–223
    malignant nephrosclerosis, 222
    nephrosclerosis, 222–223
Hypertensive urgency, 490
Hyperthyroidism, 168, 574
  demographic aspects, 168
  sympathetic nervous system interactions, 169
Hypertrophic inward remodeling, 196
Hypertrophy
  mechanisms of, 195–196
    genetic factors, 196
    intravascular pressure, 195
    nitric oxide, 196
    oxidative stress, 196
    sympathetic nerves, 196
Hyperuricemia, 173
Hypoalbuminemia, 173
Hypokalemia, 356, 358, 441
Hypomagnesemia, 356
Hyponatremia, 357t, 358, 441
Hypoperfusion, 215
Hypotension, 521
  endocannabinoids, 106
  leptin, 113
Hypothalamus, 118
Hypothyroidism, 168, 574
  demographic aspects, 168
  sympathetic nervous system interactions, 169
Hypovolemic stimulus, 70
Hypoxia, 174

I_1-imidazoline receptor stimulation, 453
Iatrogenic hypertension
  management of, 560–563
ICAM-1. See Intercellular adhesion molecule-1
  (ICAM-1)
Identifiable (secondary) forms of hypertension,
  423
Idiopathic hematuria, 382
IHD. See Ischemic heart disease
Imidazolines, 454, 473–474
Immunosuppressives, 562–563
  modification of, 576
Impaired baroreflex function, 393–394
  laboratory abnormalities and therapeutic
    implications, 393
    preganglionic disease, 393
    symptoms, 393
Impaired glomerular filtration rate, 522
Inbred rat models, 181
India, hypertension in, 284–285
  rural populations, 284–285
  urban populations, 284
Indirect BP measurement, 335
Industrialized societies
  and geographic patterns of hypertension, 240
Infants, BP in, 273
Inflammation
  angiotensin II, 56
  kinins, 83
  preeclampsia, 172
Information systems, in electronic management of
  HPT, 428–430
Infralimbic cortex, 119
Initial standardized training, in BP measurement, 335
Initial workup of adults with hypertension, 343–347
  clinical synthesis, 346
  initial counseling, 346–347
  lifestyle modification, 347
  objectives and specific aspects of, 343–346
    alcohol and street drugs, 344
    coronary artery disease (CAD), 343
    family history, 343
    general symptomatology, 343
    history, 343
    initial laboratory testing, 344t
    medication history, 343–344
    sleep history, 344–345
  physical examination, 345–346
    abdomen, 345
    ancillary studies, 345–346
    basic studies, 345
    BP measurement, 345
    cardiac examination, 345

funduscopic examination, 345
laboratory evaluation, 345
neurologic examination, 345
out-of-office BP determinations, 346
peripheral pulses, 345
Injury. See also Hypertensive renal injury
  mechanisms, 224
    cholesterol oxidation, 224
    cigarette smoking, 224
    endothelial dysfunction, 224
    proteinuria, 224
Inositol phospholipids. See Phosphoinositides
Inositol polyphosphates, 14
  cell membrane signals regulation, 14
  metabolism, 14
Ins(1,4,5)P3 receptors, 13
  architecture, 14
  characteristics, 13
  functional features, 14
  molecular variants, 14
Insertion polymorphism, 50
Insular cortex, 119
Insulin action, 151
  cellular mechanisms, 151
    glucose transport, 151
    nuclear signaling, 151
    receptor activation and modulation, 151
  systemic effects, 151–152
    coagulation, 152
    kidney, 152
    sympathetic nervous activation, 152
    vasodilation, 152
Insulin receptor substrate-1 (IRS-1), 151
Insulin resistance, 529
  hypertension, 152
    animal models, 152
    clinical studies, 153
    inflammation and oxidative stress, 152–153
    RAAS, 153
    racial differences, 293
  with major vascular effects
    apelin, 109
    monocyte chemoattractant protein 1, 109
    plasminogen-activator inhibitor, 109
  obesity, 152
    adipocytes, endocrine functions of, 152
    adiponectin, 152
    fatty acid metabolism, 152
    inflammatory mediators, 152
    leptin, 152
  promoting products, 107–109
    acylation stimulating protein, 108
    adipsin, 108
    resistin, 108
    retinol-binding protein 4, 108
    TNF-α, 107
    visfatin, 108
  role of Adiponectin in, 114
  visceral vs. peripheral fat, 152
Insulin-sensitizers, 478
Intercellular adhesion molecule-1 (ICAM-1), 142
Interference, drug, 349
Interleukin 6, 108
Intermediate phenotypes, 230
Intermittent hypertension, 354–355, 354t
International Population Study on Macronutrients
  and Blood Pressure (INTERMAP), 319
International Study of Salt and Blood Pressure
  (INTERSALT), 301, 304
Interstitial renal disease, 383
Interventricular septal hypertrophy, 189
Intracellular calcium, 27, 79
Intracellular pH, 21–23
  regulation of, 21, 22f
    cation-dependent HCO_3^-–Cl^- exchange, 22
    intracellular buffering, 21
    Na^+–H^+ exchange, 21–22
    Na-dependent HCO_3^-–Cl^- exchange, 22
Intracellular receptors, 2
Intracellular signaling, 17
  recruitment and spatial organization, 18
  signaling cascades, 17
Intracerebral hemorrhage (ICH), 214, 215t,
  380–381, 514
  etiology, 381

Intraoperative hypertension, 555
Intravascular pressure, 195
Intravenous salt loading, 565–566
Intrinsic (genetic) geographic patterns of
  hypertension, 240
Intrinsic sympathomimetic activity or partial-agonist
  activity, 448
Intubation, 553–554
Inward rectifier K^+ channels, 25
Iodothyronines, 1
Irbesartan microalbuminuria-2 study, 463
IRS-1. See Insulin receptor substrate-1 (IRS-1)
Ischemia, 84, 223
Ischemic cardiovascular disease, 93
Ischemic heart disease (IHD), 369, 446, 459–460,
  467–468
  antihypertensive drugs in the prevention of
    clinical trials of, 498–499
  BP components and, 496
    diastolic BP and the J-curve, 496
    systolic BP, 496
  clinical trials, 459
  clinical usage, 459–460
  and heart failure, 404
  heart failure, 460
  hypertensive patients with
    prevention of, 497–500
    treatment, 496
  stable angina, treatment, 500. See also Angina
Ischemic heart disease risk (IHD), 249
  BP and, 249–250
    age effects, 250
    natural history and associated comorbidities,
      250–251
    prevalence of events and BP level, 249–250
    risk factor clustering, 252
    treatment implications, 252–253
    versus blood glucose changes, 252
  BP components and, 251–252
    clinical impact, 252
    pulse pressure and mean pressure, 251–252
    risk factor clustering, 252
    systolic versus diastolic BP, 251–252
    treatment implications, 252–253
Ischemic nephropathy, 388
  comorbidities and global risk assessment, role,
    388
  natural history, 388
  response to intervention, predictors of, 388
Ischemic penumbra, 216
Ischemic stroke
  disease spectrum, 215–216
  subtypes, frequency, 215f
Isolated proteinuria, 382
Isolated systolic hypertension, 440, 485, 486, 550
  major clinical trials, 487t

JAK. See Janus kinase (JAK)
Janus kinase (JAK), 2, 60
Japan, hypertension in, 287–288
J-curve, 496
Job strain, 290
Joint National Committee (JNC) guidelines,
  316–317
  JNC7 recommendations, 352
Juxtaglomerular apparatus, 86
Juxtaglomerular, 44–46

Kaliuresis, 86
Kallikrein–kinin system, 82
Kidney
  disease, 6
  kinins, 83
  nitric oxide, 81
  preeclampsia, 172
Kininases, 82
Kininogenases, 82
Kininogens, 82
Kinins, 82
  hypertension, 83
  Kallikrein–kinin bioregulation, 82
  pathophysiology, 83
    inflammation, 83
    kidney, 83
    salivary and sweat glands, 83

thrombosis, 83
receptors, 82
therapeutic implications, 83
angioedema, 84
BP responses, 83–84
cardiac and vascular remodeling, 84
ischemia, 84
Knockout mouse model, 183
Korea, hypertension in, 288
Korotkoff sounds, 336–338, 341
in BP measurement, 274
phases of, 337
K1, 337*t*
K2, 337*t*
K3, 337*t*
K4, 337*t*
K5, 337*t*

Lacunar infarcts, 214
Laplace, law of, 191
L-arginine, 81
Late postrepair hypertension, 166
Lateral posterior hypothalamus, 118–119
Latitude
and geographic patterns of hypertension, 240
Law of Laplace, 191
Lead, BP impact of, 309
absorption, 309
biologic plausibility and causal inference, 309
epidemiologic studies, 309
exposure, 309
metabolism, 309
Left bundle branch block, 361–362
Left ventricular concentric hypertrophy, 191
Left ventricular dysfunction, 503
management of, 503–504
Left ventricular filling patterns in hypertension, 503
Left ventricular filling rate, 184
Left ventricular hypertrophy (LVH), 188–190,
237–238, 247, 359, 363
assessment of, 501–502
echocardiography, 501–502
high ejection fraction paradox, 502
monitoring, 502
and cardiovascular disease risk, 189, 254–257
angiotensin receptor blockade, 257
angiotensin-converting enzyme inhibition, 256
echocardiographic left ventricular hypertrophy,
255
electrocardiographic left ventricular
hypertrophy, 254–255
etiology and diagnosis, 254
regression of, 255–256
clinical correlation, 189–190
comparison of diagnostic techniques, 189
echocardiogram, 189
electrocardiogram criteria, 189
clinical studies of LVH, regression, 502–503
direct comparisons, 502
meta-analyses, 502
eccentric vs. concentric, 189
etiology, 189
hypertensive patients with, management of,
501–504
natural history, 188
prognostic and therapeutic implications of, 501
spectrum of, 503
systolic versus diastolic dysfunction, 189
treatment, 190
Left ventricular systolic dysfunction (LVSD), 191
definition and prognosis, 505
diagnosis, 506
Heart Failure Society of America (HFSA) 2006,
505–506
hypertensive patients with, treatment of, 505–508
New York Heart Association (NYHA) Functional
Classification, 506
pathogenesis of, 506
specific drugs, 507–508
Leptin, 107, 110
actions, 111
neuropeptide modulation, 111
sympathetic nervous system, 111
vascular effects, 111
body weight, 152

fat cell mass, regulation of, 110
and hypertension, 113
receptors and signal transduction
Ob-Rb receptors, 110
pathways, 111
regulation, 110 resistance, 111–112
heterogeneity, 112
mechanisms, 112
resistance, 149–150
Leukotrienes, 97–98
Levothyroxine, 574
Liddle's syndrome, 234
Lifestyle modifications, HTN and, 279–280, 406–409
for BP control and cardiovascular health, 408–409
impact on BP, 407–408
alcohol, 407
DASH, 407
diabetes, 408
dietary composition, 407
dietary potassium, 407
multiple risk factor reduction, 408
salt restriction, 407
weight loss, 407
impact on overt cardiovascular disease, 408
and office management of HPT, 402–403
in PAD, 509–510. *See also under* Peripheral
arterial disease
physical activity, 279
posttransplant hypertension and, 576–577
prehypertension and, 483–484
risk factor clustering, 406
sodium reduction and increased potassium intake,
279–280
stress reduction, 279
weight loss, 279
Life-threatening hypertensive emergencies, 491*t*
Lifetime performance monitoring, in BP
measurement, 335
Ligand binding, 2
Ligand-gated channels, 28
Linkage disequilibrium mapping, 230
Lipids, 441
lipid-lowering therapy, 510
lipid-soluble agents, 447
Lipoxins, 99
Lipoxygenase products, 97
and atherosclerosis, 99
cardiovascular disorders, potential roles in, 98*t*
eicosanoid synthesis, 97
hydroperoxides, 98
hydroxyeicosatetraenoic acids, 98
mechanisms of action, 97
L-NAME. *See* N$^\omega$-nitrol-arginine methyl ester
(L-NAME)
Loop diuretics, 439–442
mechanisms of action, 442
renal function and natriuresis, 442
tubular effects and hemodynamics, 442
Losartan Intervention for Endpoint (LIFE), 294, 313,
327, 461–462
Low birth weight (LBW), HTN and, 277
Low diastolic BP, 245–246
Low-density lipoprotein (LDL), 62, 209
and apolipoproteins, 209
metabolism and receptor action, 209
LVH. *See* Left ventricular hypertrophy (LVH)
LVSD. *See* Left ventricular systolic dysfunction
(LVSD)

Macula densa cells, 78
Macula densa, 46
Magnesium, BP impact of, 308–309
basic physiology and nutrition, 308
absorption and metabolism, 308
clinical studies, 308–309
clinical trials, 309
epidemiologic studies, 308–309
United States intake levels, 308
Magnetic resonance imaging, 366*t*
Malignant nephrosclerosis, 222
Malignant pheochromocytoma, 573
Management of hypertension, 401–406. *See also*
Office management
by nurses, 425. *See also* Nurses
by pharmacists, 424–425. *See also* Pharmacists

Mannose 6-phosphate, 60
Manometer, 335
Masked hypertension, 291, 422
Mass migrations, hypertension and, 239
Mast cell, 53
Matrix metalloproteinases (MMPs), 202
McPhee index, 189
Mean arterial blood pressure (MAP), 145–148, 354
Mechanical theory, 166
Medulla, 117–118
Medullary thyroid carcinoma (MTC), 574
clinical presentation, 575
laboratory diagnosis, 575
screening for other multiple endocrine neoplasia
abnormalities, 575
treatment, 575
Melameline (Namenda), 220
α-melanocyte stimulating hormone (α-MSH), 111
Menopause
and BP, 270
menopausal hormone therapy, 270–271
Mercury, BP impact of, 309–310
absorption, 309
exposure, 309
metabolism, 309
Metabolic balance studies, of salt and BP, 302
Metabolic syndrome, 114, 478, 533
Methoxyhydroxyphenylglycol, 39
Methyldopa, 453–454
Metolazone
Mevalonate, 210
Mexican Americans, hypertension among, 283
Microalbuminuria, 225, 384
Microvascular
regulation and dysregulation, 198–200
basic microcirculatory structure and function,
198
microcirculatory damage, 199
Midlife BP elevations, 219
Midodrine, 517
Migraine headache, 468
Mild cognitive impairment (MCI)
hypertension and, 219–220
pathogenesis, 219–221
symptoms, 220*t*
Mineralocorticoid hypertension, 182
activating mutations of, 234
in hypertension, 234
overproduction, 232–233
Mineralocorticoids, 62
adverse effects of, 445
hyperkalemia, 445
sexual function, 445
blockade effects, 65
heart failure, 65
hypertension, 65
nonepithelial effects, 65
deoxycorticosterone, 62
18-hydroxydeoxycorticosterone, 62
magnetic receptor–induced Na reabsorption, 64–65
longer-term effects, 65
rapid effects, 64–65
19-noraldosterone, 63
19-nordeoxycorticosterone, 63
selectivity, 64
syndromes, 65
Minorities, hypertension in
clinical trials comparing drug therapies in, 494
evaluation, 494
lifestyle modification, 495
management, 494–495
monotherapy, 495
treatment of, 493–495
Blacks, 494
epidemiologic overview, 493–494
hispanic Americans, 494
Minoxidil, 350, 471
Mitogen-activated protein (MAP), 3, 66
Mitogen-activated protein kinase (MAPK), 18, 18*f*
Mitral flow analysis, 503
M-mode, 189
Modification of Diet in Renal Disease (MDRD), 383
Monoamine oxidase inhibitors (MAOIs), 545, 547*t*,
548
Monocyte chemoattractant protein 1 (MCP-1), 109,
205

Monogenic determinants of BP, 232–235
  hypertension with increased mineralocorticoid
      activity, 234–235
    Liddle's syndrome, 234
  mineralocorticoid overproduction, 232–233
    11β-hydroxysteroid dehydrogenase, 234
    aldosterone synthase gene duplication, 232–233
    glucocorticoid-remediable aldosteronism,
        232–233
    P-450C11β deficiency, 234
    P-450C17α deficiency, 234
    steroid hormone biosynthesis, 233–234
  normotensive syndromes, 234–235
    Disorder of sympathetic regulation, 235
Monoglyceride lipase (MGL), 103
Mood stabilizers, 548
Morbidity
  and geographic patterns of hypertension, 242–243
    Mortality After Stroke Eprosartan versus
        Nitrendipine for Secondary Prevention
        (MOSES), 463
Mortality
  BP control and
    trends in, 314–317
  and geographic patterns of hypertension, 242–243
Muller glial cells, 10
Multiple endocrine neoplasia (MEN), 574
Multiple risk factor intervention trial (MRFIT), 225,
    249, 262
Muscarinic effects, 75
Muscarinic receptors, 4
Myocardial blood flow, 130
Myocardial infarction, 446
  adiponectin, 115
  endocannabinoids, 106
Myocardial ischemia, 207
Myocardial perfusion imaging (MPI), 361
Myosin light chain, 35
  phosphatase activity and vasorelaxation, 36
    Ca^{2+}-dependent, 36
    RhoA, 36
    Rho-kinase, 36
    subunit regulation, 36
Myristate, 5

Na$^+$–H$^+$ exchanger (NHE), 21
NADPH. See Nicotinamide adenine dinucleotide
    phosphate
NADPH oxidase (NOX), 32
  function and regulators, 33t
  mRNA expression, 33t
  pathophysiologic effects, 33
    antioxidant therapy limitations, 33
  tissue distribution, 33t
Narcotics, 562–563
National High Blood Pressure Education Program
    (NHBPEP), 316, 352
National Institute for Health and Clinical Excellence
    (NICE), 331
Native Americans
  minorities, hypertension in, 494
Native Hawaiians
  hypertension in, 287–288
Natriuresis, 130
Natriuresis, 42, 442
Natriuretic peptides, 85
  biologic actions, 86
    adipose tissue, 87
    blood vessels, 86
    bone, 87
    heart, 86
    neurohumoral systems, 87
  and cardiovascular disease, 87
    heart failure, 87
    hypertension, 87
  receptors, 85
    receptor-A and B, 85
    receptor-C, 85–86
  release and secretion control, 87
  subclasses
    atrial natriuretic peptide, 85
    brain natriuretic peptide, 85
    C-type natriuretic peptide, 85
Natural selection, 229
Nature's physiologic calcium channel blocker, 308

NEP. See Neutral endopeptidases (NEPs)
Nephritic syndrome, 383
Nephropathy, 460
Nephrosclerosis, 222–223, 382–383. See also
    Hypertensive nephropathy
  development
    factors influencing, 224f
    pathogenesis, 222–225
Nephrotic syndrome, 382–383
Neprilysin, 50, 50f
  actions, 50
  clinical implications, 51
  distribution, 51
  structure, 50–51
Network meta-analyses, of antihypertensive
    treatment trials, 327
Neural theory, 166
Neurohormones, 117
Neurologic evaluation in hypertension, 379–381
  cerebral infarction and intracerebral hemorrhage,
      380–381
  dementia, 381
  hypertension, 381
  hypertensive encephalopathy, 379–380. See also
      Encephalopathy, hypertensive
  subarachnoid hemorrhage, 379
  transient focal cerebral ischemia, 380
Neuronal nitric oxide synthase, 158
Neuropeptide Y, 72
  actions, 72
    renal effects, 72
    sympathetic and hemodynamic effects, 72
  hypertension, 72
  localization, 72
    entral nervous system, 72
    peripheral nerves, 72
  receptors, 72
    Y1 receptors, 72
    Y2 receptors, 72
    Y5 receptors, 72
Neutral endopeptidases (NEPs), 11, 50, 82
New York Heart Association (NYHA) Functional
    Classification, 506
Niacin, 535
Nicotinamide adenine dinucleotide phosphate
    (NADPH), 31
  activity regulation, 31–32
  hypertension, 203
    animal models, 203
    central nervous system mechanisms., 204
    renal mechanisms, 203
  oxidase, 31, 203
    physiologic stimulation, 203
Nitrates, 472–474
  hydralazine-nitrate combinations, 472–473
  mechanisms of action, 472
  nitrate tolerance, 472
  Nitroglycerin, 472
  sodium nitroprusside, 472
Nitric oxide, 78
  bioavailability, 206
  biological activity modulation, 202
  cardiomyocytes, 81
  distribution, 78
  endothelial dysfunction and disease, 80
    atherosclerosis, 80
    hypertension and vascular function, 80
    vascular remodeling, 80
    vasoconstriction, 80
  endothelial function, 80, 202
    antithrombotic effects, 80
    vasodilation, 80
  kidney, 81
  peroxynitrite, 202
  radical interactions, 202
  renal hemodynamics, 81
    autoregulation, 81
    pressure-natriuresis, 81
    renal blood flow, 81
    tubuloglomerular feedback, 81
  renal tubular effects, 81
    Na channels, 81
    transporters, 81
    water permeability, 81
  salt-sensitivity of BP, 158

signal transduction, 80
    guanylyl cyclase, 80
    phosphodiesterases, 80
  synthase isoforms, 78
  synthase regulation, 79
    general characteristics, 79
    regulation, 79
    vascular nitric oxide synthase 3
  vascular remodeling, 196
Nitroglycerin (NTG), 472
Nitroprusside (NTP), 472
Non ST-segment elevation myocardial infarction,
    500
Nonantihypertensive drugs
  antihypertensive effects, 478–479
    aspirin, 479
    statins, 479
    thiazolidinediones (glitazones), 478
Nondihydropyridine calcium antagonists, 466, 468
Nondrug therapy, 537
Nonindustrialized societies
  and geographic patterns of hypertension, 239
Noninvasive ambulatory BP monitoring, 341
Noninvasive vascular testing, 267
  angiographic studies, 267
  Rancho Bernardo study, 267
  San Luis Valley study, 267
Nonpharmacologic therapy, 523
Nonphysician providers and the management of
    hypertension, 424–427
  barriers to BP control, 424
  clinical inertia, interventions to reduce, 424
  integrated model, 426–427
    efficiency and continuity, 427
    goal-orientated care, 426–427
    patient education and accountability, 427
    strategies to utilize, 426t
Nonselective antagonists, 476–477
Nonsteroidal anti-inflammatory drugs (NSAIDs),
    458, 560–561
  BP raising effects of, 480–482
Nontraditional vasoactive peptides, 89t
19-Noraldosterone, 63
19-Nordeoxycorticosterone, 62
Norepinephrine, 90t
Norepinephrine transporter (NET) dysfunction, 38,
    515
Normotensive syndromes, 234–235
Nox
  proteins, 203
    localization and signaling differences, 203
    vascular nox, 203
Nuclear factor kappa B (NFκB), 100
Nuclear factor of activated T cells (NFAT), 19
Nuclear receptors, 151
Nucleus tractus solitarius (NTS), 117
Nulliparas, 173
Nulliparous gestations, 171
Nurses
  HPT management by, 425
    nurse pharmacist model, 425–426
    nurse practitioners, 425
    nurse specialists, 425
N$^\omega$-nitrol-arginine methyl ester (L-NAME), 93

Obese hypertensive patient
  BP management, 528
  fat burden, assessment of, 526
  treatment of the, 526–528
    BP measurement, 526
    weight loss therapy, 526–528. See also individual
        entry
Obesity, 61, 292–294, 529
  and geographic patterns of hypertension, 239
  hypertension mechanisms, 149
    dyslipidemia, 150
    fluid volume distribution, 149
    heart and kidneys, impact on, 150
    inflammatory cytokines, 150
    leptin resistance, 149–150
    pathogenesis, 150f
    RAAS, 150
    sympathetic nervous system, 149
  heart failure and, 191
  and nutrition, 277

obesity insulin resistance, 152
  sleep apnea and, 557
Obstructive sleep apnea syndrome (OSAS), 138, 174,
    556
  airway obstruction and hypoxia, 174
  and hypertension, 175–176
    established hypertension, 175–176
    intermittent hypertension and prehypertension,
      176
  hypertension mechanisms, 174–175
    RAAS, 174
    sympathetic nervous system, 174
    vascular dysfunction, 174
    vascular remodeling, 175
  hypertension in, 556
  mixed sleep apneas, 175f
  treatment of, 557
Occlusion, 215
Ocular circulations, 226–227. See also Eye in
    hypertension
Office BP, 180
  evaluation, 486
  placebo effects, 180
Office management of hypertension, 401–406
  'customized' or 'personalized' therapy, challenge,
    401–402
  disease-specific indications, 404
  general BP target, 403
  lifestyle modifications, 402–403
  risk factor profiling and management, 402
  Stage 1 hypertension, 403. See also individual entry
  Stage 2 hypertension, 403–404
OmniHeart study, 298–299
One-kidney, one-clip model, 182
Ophthalmoscopic changes
  in hypertension, 226, 227–228. See also Eye in
    hypertension
    arteriolar changes, 227. See also individual entry
    clinical significance, 228
Optic nerve disease, 380
  optic nerve circulation, 227
    changes in hypertension, 227
    normal anatomy and physiology, 227
Oral contraceptives and BP, 271
  combined agents, 271
  contraindications to, 272t
  progestins, 271
Organ damage and outcomes, 340
Orlistat, 528
Oropharyngeal surgery, 557
Orthostatic disorders
  treatment of, 515
Orthostatic hypotension, 124, 530
  in autonomic failure, 516
OSAS. See Obstructive sleep apnea syndrome (OSAS)
Oscillometry, in BP measurement, 274
Osmoreceptors, 117
Ouabain, 77f
Outcome studies in hypertension, 440
Ovary syndrome, polycystic. See Polycystic ovary
    syndrome
Oxidants. See Reactive oxygen species (ROS)
Oxidative stress, 161, 218, 529
  and hypertension, 203–204
    NADH. See Nicotinamide adenine dinucleotide
      phosphate (NADPH)
    ROS. See Reactive oxygen species (ROS)
  preeclampsia, 172
  vascular remodeling, 196
18-Oxocortisol, 62
Oxo-LDL, 210
Oxygen-derived species. See Reactive oxygen species
    (ROS)

P wave, 189
P115 Rho guanine nucleotide exchange factor, 6, 7f
P22phox, 201
P-450C11β deficiency, 234
P-450C17α deficiency, 234
P47phox, 203
P67phox, 203
Pacemaker patients, sleep apnea in, 558–559
Pacific islanders
  minorities, hypertension in, 494
PAD. See Peripheral arterial disease

Palmitate, 5
Palpation, 359, 375
Panic disorder, 289
Paracrine modulation, 122
Parasympathetic motor neuronal cell bodies, 116
Parathyroid disorders, 357
  management of, 574–575
Parathyroidectomy, 170
Parathyroids, 161, 278
  and hypertension
    demographic aspects, 169
    mechanisms, 169
    renal disease interaction, 169
Paraventricular nucleus, 119
Participation recommendations for athletes with
    hypertension, 551
Patient education, 412–413
  benefits of, 412–413
  challenges to, 412
  strategies, 412t
  successful programs, components of, 412
    educational materials, 412–413
  useful web sites for, 413t
PC-1 proteins, 151
Peptide ligands, 9
Percutaneous transluminal renal angioplasty,
    569–570
  atherosclerotic disease, 569
  fibromuscular dysplasia, 569
  with stenting, 569–570
Perindopril Protection against Recurrent Stroke Study
    (PROGRESS), 460
Perioperative management of hypertension, 553–555
  anesthetics, 554t
  intraoperative hypertension, 555
  pathophysiology, 553–554
    BP regulatory systems, 553
    intubation, 553–554
  perioperative risk, 554
    systolic hypertension, 554
    target organ damage, 554
  postoperative hypertension, 555
  therapy, 554–555
Peripheral arterial disease (PAD) and hypertension,
    265–268, 374
  ankle–brachial index studies, 266–267
  abdominal aortic aneurysms, 511–512
  antihypertensive drugs and, 511
  coronary artery disease in patients with, 510
  claudication studies, 265
  glucose intolerance and diabetes mellitus, 510
  hypertensive patients with, treatment of, 509–512
  hypertension treatment and, 267–268
    cardiovascular disease events, 268
    limb loss, 268
    treatment guidelines, 268
  lifestyle modifications, 509–510
    exercise therapy, 509–510
    smoking cessation, 510
  medical therapy, 510t
  noninvasive vascular testing, 267
  pathogenesis, 265
  risk factors and etiology, 265
  recognition of, 509
  symptomatic PAD
    risk factors for, 265t
  symptoms, 267
Peripheral circulation
  evaluation, 374–378
  imaging studies, 376–378
    abdominal imaging, 377–378
    ankle-brachial index, 376
    carotid imaging, 377
    segmental pressures and waveforms, 376–377
  physical examination of, 375–376
    abdomen, 375–376
    auscultation, 375
    BP measurements, 375
    chest, 375
    lower extremities, 376
    neck, 375
    palpation, 375
    upper extremities, 375
  signs and symptoms, 374–375
    claudication, 374

  critical limb ischemia, 374–375
  transient cerebral ischemia, 374
Peripheral sympatholytics, 454–455
  adverse effects, 454–455
  drug differentiation, 454
  mechanisms of action, 454
Peroxisome proliferator–activated receptor (PPAR),
    64, 479
  PPAR-γ, 151
  clinical trials, 102
    fibrates and cardiovascular disease, 102
  in disease, 101
    experimental atherosclerosis, 101–102
    genetic studies, 102
    natural ligands, 101
  receptor α, biologic actions of, 100
    fatty acid metabolism, 100
    vascular and antiinflammatory effects, 100
  receptor γ, biologic actions of, 101
  receptor δ, biologic actions of, 101
  subtypes and gene expression, 100
  synthetic ligands, 101t
Peroxynitrite, 31, 202
PGDF. See Platelet-derived growth factor (PDGF)
Pharmacists managing HPT
  Community pharmacists, 425
  physician–pharmacist collaborative models,
    424–425
Phenoxybenzamine, 450
Phentolamine, 41, 450
Pheochromocytoma, 235, 452
  biochemical tests, 571
  clinical presentation, 571
  diagnosis, 571–572
  differential diagnosis of, 573t
  functional tests, 572
  imaging studies, 571
  malignant pheochromocytoma, 573
  management, 571–573
  treatment, 572–573
    follow-up, 572–573
    perioperative management, 572
    preoperative management, 572
    surgical approach, 572
Phophatidylethanolamine, 103
Phosphatidylcholine signaling, 17–19
  diacylglycerol, 16
  phospholipase D isoforms, 16
  phospholipase D, 16
Phosphatidylinositol 3 kinase, 14, 19
  class I enzymes, 14–15
  class II enzymes, 15
  class III enzyme, 15
  Phosphatidylinositol 3-kinase/Akt pathway, 80
Phosphatidylinositol phosphate kinases, 15
  type I, 15
  type II, 15
  type III, 15
Phosphatidylinositol, 89
Phosphodiesterase-5 (PDE5) inhibitors, 478–479
  in sexual dysfunction, 521
    BP effects, 521
    hypotension, 521
Phosphoinositide 3 kinase phosphorylation, 19
  MAPK, parallel activation of, 19
Phosphoinositide kinases, 14
  3-kinases, 14
  4-kinases, 14
  phosphatidylinositol phosphate kinases, 15
Phosphoinositide phosphatases, 15
  group I 5-phosphatases, 15
  group II 5-phosphatases, 15
  group III 5-phosphatases, 15
  group IV 5-phosphatases, 15
Phosphoinositides, 12
  diacylglycerol, 13
  Inositol 1,4,5-trisphosphate and calcium flux, 12
  Ins(1,4,5)P3 metabolism, 12. See also Ins(1,4,5)P3
  phosphatases. See Phosphoinositide phosphatases
  phosphoinositide kinases. See Phosphoinositide
    kinases
  phospholipase C products, 12
  receptors signaling, 13f
Phospholipase C, 2, 12–16
  phospholipase C-β enzymes, activation of, 13

Phospholipase C (*contd.*)
  phospholipase Cγ enzymes, activation of, 13
  phospholipase C-β, 4–5
Phosphorylation, 17–18, 35
  mitogen-activated protein kinase, 18
  multisite phosphorylation, 18
Physical activity
  aerobic (endurance) exercise, 295
  and BP, 295–296
  hypertension and, 295–296
    clinical trials, 295–296
    observational studies, 295
  National recommendations, 296
    Joint National Committee 7 (JNC 7), 296
  physical activity prescription, 296
  rhythmic exercise, 295
    benefits, 295
    cardiovascular benefits, 295
Physical activity advice and counseling, 410–411
  activity intensity and monitoring, 410
    heart rate, 410
    perceived exertion scales, 411
  behavioral counseling and reinforcement, 410
  physician endorsement, 410
Physical examination, 359–362
  auscultation, 359–360. See also individual entry
  of peripheral circulation, 375–376. See also under
      Peripheral circulation
  palpation, 359
Physician-controlled barriers, of BP, 419–420
Placebo effect, 105f
Plasma kallikrein, 83
Plasma osmolality, 70
Plasma renin activity, 388
Plasminogen activation, 91
  fibrinolytic balance, 91
  inhibitor 1, genetic expression of, 91–92
Plasminogen-activator inhibitor 1, 91
  circulating half-life, 92
  genetic expression of, 91–92
  physiology and regulation, 92
    diurnal variation, 92
    RAAS activation, 92
    sources and interactions, 92
    stimulants, 92
  RAAS, interacions with, 92–93
Platelet-derived growth factor (PDGF), 89–90
Podocyturia, 172
Poiseuille's law, 139
  limitations, 139
  theory, 139
Polycystic ovary syndrome, 154
  associated disease risks, 154–155
    cardiovascular risk factors, 155t
    coronary artery disease, 155
    pregnancy-associated hypertension, 154
  clinical presentation, 154
    diagnostic criteria, 154, 154t
    signs and symptoms, 154
  pathogenesis, 154
Polygenic versus monogenic phenotypes, 229
Polysomnography, 557
Poor man's renal biopsy, microscopic analysis as, 386
Population characteristics, in hypertension, 230
Population variation in BP, 239
Portable aneroids, 335
Portuguese salt trial, 321
Posterior leukoencephalopathy syndrome, 218
Postganglionic disease, 394
Postmenopausal Estrogen/Progestin Intervention
    (PEPI) trial, 270
Postoperative hypertension, 555
Postrepair paradoxical hypertension, 166
Posttransplant hypertension
  causes of, 577t
  exacerbating factors, 576
  immunosuppression regimens, modification of, 576
  lifestyle modification, 576–577
  management, 576–577
  specific antihypertensive drugs, 577
Postural tachycardia syndrome (POTS), 515, 516t
  diagnostic criteria, 515
  pathogenesis, 515
  treatment, 516
Potassium abnormalities

associated diseases
  adrenal steroids, 356
  Cushing's syndrome, 356
  hyperaldosteronism, 356
  hyperkalemia, 356
  hypokalemia, 356
  hypomagnesemia, 356
  renovascular disease, 356
evaluation, 356–357
Potassium and BP, 304–306
  cardiovascular benefits, 306
    animal models, 306
    Cohort studies, 306
  clinical trials, 305–306
    antihypertensive drug effectiveness, 306
    DASH studies, 306
    early studies, 305
    meta-analyses, 305
  epidemiology, 304–305
    race and culture, 304
  pathophysiology, 306
Potassium channels, 473
  and parasympathetic nerves, 218
Potassium, 460. See also individual entries
  intake
    and BP, 302
    HTN and, 278
  potassium-sparing diuretics, 437, 443–445
    Amiloride, 445
    Triamterene, 445
PPAR. See Peroxisome proliferator–activated
    receptor
Prazosin, 452
Preeclampsia, 171, 173, 536, 537t, 538–539
  clinical correlation, 173
    clinical course, 173
    diagnosis, 173
  etiology and pathophysiology, 171–172
    abnormal placentation, 171
    abnormal vascular reactivity, 172
    antiangiogenic factors, altered production of,
        171
    genetic factors, 172
    immunologic changes, 172
    Inflammation and oxidative stress, 172
    insulin resistance and sympathetic overactivity,
        172
    renin-angiotensin activity, 172
  target organs, effects on, 172–173
    cardiovascular system, 172
    kidney, 172
    liver, 173
    placenta, 173
Preganglionic disease, 393
Preganglionic neurons, 117
Pregnancy/Pregnant hypertensive patients
  BP management, 538
  chronic hypertension in pregnancy, treatment, 537t
  classification of, 537t
  prepregnancy assessment and counseling, 536
    assessment of hypertension, 536
    assessment of target organs, 536
    lifestyle counseling, 536
  recurrence of hypertension, 539
  stage 1 (chronic) hypertension during pregnancy,
      treatment, 537–538
    drug therapy, 537
    fetal safety concerns, 537
    nondrug therapy, 537
  stage 2 (chronic) hypertension, treatment of, 538
  treatment of, 536–539
    Renin-angiotensin blocking drugs, 536–537
Pregnenolone, 62
Prehypertension, 230, 315–316, 352
  clinical trials in, 483–484
    DASH study, 484
    lifestyle modification, 483–484
    PREMIER trial, 484
  definition and rationale of, 483
  treatment of, 483–484
  treatment recommendations, 484
    drug therapy, 484
    existing guidelines, 484
PREMIER trial, 484
Prerepair hypertension, 166

Pressor hormones, 172
Pressure gradients, 139–140
Prevention of Atherosclerotic Complications with
    Ketanserin (PACK), 473
Prevention of hypertension, 318–321
  age-related BP, prevention, 318
  from clinical studies to public policy, 321
    Belgian salt trial, 321
    Portuguese salt trial, 321
  dietary factors and BP of individuals, 318–320
    dietary protein and other factors, 319
    salt intake, 318–319
  public health strategies, 318
  randomized lifestyle trials in adults and children
    infants and children, 320–321
    with normal or prehypertensive BPs, 320
  strategic challenge, 318
Primary aldosteronism (PA), 564–566
  evaluation, 564–566
    Captopril suppression testing, 566
    confirmatory tests, 565
    dietary salt loading, 565
    Fludrocortisone suppression testing (FST), 565
    Intravenous salt loading, 565–566
    patient preparation, 564
    screening, 564
  glucocorticoid-remediable hypertension, 566
  imaging studies, 566
  prevalence, 564
  treatment, 566
    Adrenalectomy, 566
    pharmacologic therapy, 566
Primary Prevention of Hypertension (PPH), 320
Proadrenomedullin, 74
Prognosis of Ischemic Risk in Atheromatous Patients
    under Mediatensyl (PRIHAM), 473
Progressive chronic kidney disease, 222
PRORENIN, 44
Prospective Randomized Amlodipine Survival
    Evaluation (PRAISE) trial, 468
Prostacyclin, 75
Prostaglandins, 1, 94, 133
  COX derived eicosanoids, 94
    BP responses, 95
    synthesis, 94
    Vasoconstrictor eicosanoids, 94
    vasodilator prostaglandins, 94
  cytochrome P-450 derived eicosanoids, 95
    allylic oxidation, 95
    epoxidation, 95
    synthesis, 95
  in disease states, BP modulation by, 481
  Prostaglandin-induced vasodilation, blockade of,
      480–481
Prostanoids, 134
Prostatism, 452
Protein kinases, 17–19
  phosphorylation and intracellular signaling
    14-3-3 proteins, 18
    MAPK cascade, 18–19
    multisite phosphorylation, 18
    ordering events, 18
    recruitment and spatial organization, 18
  structure and function, 17
  subtypes, 17
    AGC group, 17
    CaMK group, 17
    CMGC group 17
    PTK group, 17
Protein modulation, 3
Protein phosphorylation, 16
  extracellular signal–regulated kinase cascade, 19
    docking, 19
    G protein–coupling, 19
    tyrosine phosphorylation, 19
  phosphoinositide 3 kinase phosphorylation, 19
  protein kinases. See Protein kinases
  protein synthesis regulation, 20
    ribosomal biogenesis regulation, 20
    RNA dynamics, 21
    translation elongation, 20
    translation initiation, 20
    translation modulation, 20
  transcription factor activity regulation, 19
    cellular localization, 19–20

coactivator recruitment, 20
DNA-binding activity, 20
14-3-3 proteins, 18
Protein tyrosine kinase (PTK), 17
Protein tyrosine phosphatase 1b (PTP1b), 112
Proteinuria, 172, 224, 444
detection methods, 384–386
implications of, 386
renal risk and, 262
Pseudohypertension, 486
Pseudohypoaldosteronism type II (gordon's syndrome), 234–235
Pseudohypoparathyroidism, 169
Pseudotolerance, 434, 469–470
implications for therapy, 470
mechanisms, 469
and volume overload, 349–350
Psychiatric comorbidities and therapeutic adherence, 546
Psychiatric disorders
antihypertensive drugs for, 545, 548–549
diagnostic issues, 546
hypertension and, interactions between, 545–546
shared disease mechanisms, 545
management of, 545–549
psychotropic medications, 546–548
Psychiatric drugs, BP effects of, 545
Psychotropic medications, 546–548
Antidepressants, 546
antipsychotics, 548
Anxiolytics, 546
Benzodiazepines, 546
Buspirone, 546
Mood stabilizers, 548
selective serotonin reuptake inhibitors, 546
Tricyclic antidepressants (TCAs), 546
Public health implications, 286
and HTN prevalence, 286
Puerto Ricans, hypertension among, 283
Pulmonary hypertension, 476
Pulsatile blood flow, 139
endothelial cell mechano-transduction, 142
cell structure, 142
vasoactive substance production, 142
human disease, implications for, 142
atherosclerosis, 142
endothelial dysfunction, 142
pressure gradients, 139–140
pulse wave analysis. See Pulse wave analysis
pulse wave transmission, 140
Pulse pressure
amplification, 371
as a risk marker, 147
heart, 147
vasculature, 147
Pulse wave analysis, 140
arterial impedance characteristics, 140
derived variables, 141
technical aspects, 141
Fourier analysis, 140
Pulse wave transmission, 140
Pulse wave velocity (PWV), 145, 370–372
and characteristic impedance, 371
limitations, 145
Pulsus paradoxus, 138

Quality of life, 329–330
clinical trials, 329–330
active drug comparisons, 330
cognition, 330
Dietary Approaches to Stop Hypertension (DASH), 329
salt restriction, 329–330
weight loss, 330
definition and measurement, 329
QRS duration, 361

Race
race–gender interactions, in HTN, 277, 293
as a social construct of HTN, 279
Radial pulse contour analysis, 372–373
augmentation index, 373
central systolic BP, 372
characteristic impedance of aorta, 373
Radionuclide angiography (RNA), 365

ejection fraction, 365
volume curves, 365
Randomized Olmesartan And Diabetes Microalbuminuria Prevention (ROADMAP), 264
Rarefaction, 199
RAAS. See Renin-angiotensin-aldosterone system
RAS. See Renin-angiotensin system (RAS)
Rauwolscine, 450
Raynaud's phenomenon, 468
Reactive oxygen species (ROS), 201
biologically important ROS, 30t
hydrogen peroxide, 30–31
hydroxyl radical, 31
metabolism, 30
peroxynitrite, 31
superoxide radical, 30
cardiovascular cells generation in, 32f
vascular ROS, 31–32
vascular effects, 201–202
extracellular matrix modulation, 202
gene expression regulation, 202
normal cell function, 201–202
in the vessel wall, 202f
REasons for Geographic And Racial Differences in Stroke (REGARDS) study, 243
Receptor activity modifying proteins (RAMPs), 3
Receptor tyrosine kinase (RTKs), 19
Receptor-gated ion channels, 2
Receptor-regulated Smads, 19
Receptors, 1–3
binding properties, 1–2
affinity, 1–2
kinetics, 1
interactions, 3
cross-phosphorylation, 3
dimerization, 3
protein modulation, 3
regulation, 2–3
altered tissue sensitivity, 2–3
downregulation, 2
upregulation, 2
transduction mechanisms, 2
types and functions, 1
Recombinant human erythropoietin (rHu-EPO), 161, 563
Recombination process, 230
Recordkeeping, in HPT, 428–431
traditional data organization, 428
Recurrent stroke, 404
Referrals, hypertension, 421–423
Reflex arcs, 123
Refractory hypertension, 422–423
and orthostatic instability, 394
Regulators of G protein signaling (RGS), 6
Remodeling, 195
Renal artery stenosis, 162
Renal baroreceptor, 46
Renal biopsy. See Biopsy, renal
Renal blood flow, 81, 130
Renal effects neuropeptide Y, 72
Renal effects, of CAs, 466
Renal failure, 357
Renal function, 460
Renal hemodynamics, 81, 131
Renal parenchymal hypertension
clinical clues for, 385t
oxidative stress and hypertension, 161
pathogenesis, 160, 160t
autonomic nervous system, 160
divalent ions and parathyroid hormone, 161
erythropoietin, 161
renin-angiotensin system, 160
sodium and volume status, 160
vascular endothelium, 160–161
renal mass reduction salt-induced model, 182
Renal risk, 261–264
factors, 261–263
age, 261–262
CKD, 261–263
hypertension, 261–262
hypertension–diabetes interaction, 262
proteinuria, 262
systolic versus diastolic BP, 262
Renal salt wasting, 232

loss-of-function mutations with, 235t
Renal sympathetic nerves, 126
extracellular fluid volume regulation of, 128
disorders of, 128
functions, 126
RAAS stimulation, 126–127
tubular sodium reabsorption, 126
reflex regulation, 127–128
aortocarotid baroreceptors, 127
cardiopulmonary baroreceptors, 127
hepatoreceptors, 127
reno renal reflexes, 128
somatosensory receptors, 127–128
Renal tubular effects, 81
Renin inhibitors, 455–456
angiotensin cascade, 44, 45f
distal nephron, 164
pharmacokinetics, 456
pharmacology, 456
physiologic regulation, 46
humoral factors, 46
Macula densa, 46
renal baroreceptor, 46
sympathetic nerves, 46
renin-angiotensin-aldosterone system blockers, comparing, 455–456
signal transduction mechanisms, 45
calcium, 45
cyclic adenosine monophosphate, 45
cyclic guanosine monophosphate, 45–46
Renin, 59
Renin-angiotensin system (RAS), 59, 60f, 433, 536–537
ACE, 59
aldosterone, 59
tissue RAS, function of, 60
BP, central regulation of, 60–61
cardiovascular remodeling, 60
Kidney disease, 60
obesity, 61
vascular inflammation, 60
tissue RAS, increased efficiency of, 60
Renin-angiotensin-aldosterone system (RAAS), 92, 389, 470, 524, 529
effects on, 462
and human disease, 93
hypertension and arteriosclerosis, 93
ischemic cardiovascular disease, 93
in hyperparathyroidism, 170
hypoxia, 174
insulin resistance, 153
obesity, 150
plasminogen-activator inhibitor 1, interacions with, 92–93
in preventing cardiovascular events in diabetes, 531t
renal sympathetic nerves, 126–127
stimulation, 126–127
salt-sensitivity of BP, 157
Reno renal reflexes, 128
Renovascular disease
disease spectrum, 388
evaluation of, 387–390
clinical decision making, 390
fibromuscular versus atherosclerotic disease, 387–388
imaging, rationale for, 388
imaging studies, 389–390
Captopril renography, 389
computed tomographic angiography, 389
Contrast arteriography, 389
Doppler ultrasonography, 389
Gadolinium-contrast magnetic resonance angiography, 389
ischemic nephropathy, 388. See also individual entry
issues in, 388f
laboratory diagnostic techniques, 388–389
lateralizing studies, 389
plasma renin activity, 388
renin-angiotensin-aldosterone system activation studies, 389
renal artery stenosis versus renovascular hypertension, 387
Renovascular hypertension (RVHT)

Renovascular hypertension (RVHT) *(contd.)*
  antihypertensive drug effects, 165
    glomerular filtration, effects on, 165
    pseudotolerance mechanisms, 165
  diagnosis of, 389–390
    ACE in, 389–390
  mechanisms, 163–164
    bilateral renal artery stenosis, 163
    nonstenotic kidney role, 164
    persistent RAAS dependency, 164
    RAAS activation, 163
    salt and water retention, 163
    stenosis in a solitary kidney, 163
    two kidney, unilateral renal artery stenosis, 164
  medical therapy, 568–569
  Percutaneous transluminal renal angioplasty, 569–570. *See also separate entry*
  subtypes and animal models, 162
  surgical intervention, 570
  therapeutic decision making, 568
  treatment of, 568–570
    goals of, 568
  unilateral arterial stenosis effects, 164*f*
Resistant hypertension, 348–350, 404–406, 444
  apparent resistance, 348. *See also* Apparent resistance hypertension
  causes of, 349*t*
    apparent drug resistance, 349*t*
    genetic variation, 349*t*
    secondary hypertension, 349*t*
    true drug resistance, 349*t*
  true resistance, 349
Resistin, 108
Resistive index, 389
Respiration, 136–138
  disordered breathing, syndromes of, 137–138
    Cheyne-stokes respiration, 138
    obstructive sleep apnea syndrome, 138
    pulsus paradoxus, 138
  intrathoracic pressure, 136
  neural control mechanisms, 136
    baroreflexes, 136
    chemoreceptors, 137
  slow breathing
    cardiovascular control mechanisms, 138
    therapeutic effects of, 138
Restrictive filling, 365
Retinal artery occlusion, 379–380
Retinal circulation, 226
  changes in hypertension, 226
  normal anatomy and physiology, 226
Retinal ischemia, 379–380
  clinical syndromes, 379
    amaurosis fugax, 379
    optic nerve disease, 380
    retinal artery occlusion, 379–380
Retinol-binding protein 4, 108
Revascularization, 387, 568*t*
RGS. *See* Regulators of G protein signaling (RGS)
Rho, 6
  RhoA, 36
  Rho-kinase, 36
RHu-EPO. *See* Recombinant human erythropoietin (rHu-EPO)
Ribosomal biogenesis, 20
Rimonabant, 528
Risk factor clustering, 246–247, 293, 406
Rivastigmine (Exelon), 220
RNA dynamics, 21
ROS. *See* Reactive oxygen species (ROS)
Rostroventrolateral medulla, 118
RTK. *See* Receptor tyrosine kinase (RTKs)
RVHT. *See* Renovascular hypertension

Salt and BP, 301–303
  epidemiology, 301–302
    early observations, 301
    INTERSALT, 301
    meta-analyses, 302
    regional studies, 301
  intervention trials, 302–303
  metabolic balance studies, 302
  salt intake and cardiovascular disease risk reduction, 303
  salt-sensitivity, 302

Salt-sensitivity of blood pressure (SSBP), 156–159
  clinical significance, 159
  gene–environment interactions, 156
  genetics, 156
  renal mechanisms of, 157
  vasoregulatory and natriuretic systems, 157
    arachidonic acid metabolites, 158
    endothelin, 157
    nitric oxide and oxidative stress, 158
    RAAS, 157
    sympathetic nervous system, 158
SBP. *See* Systolic BP (SBP)
SCID. *See* Severe combined immune deficiency (SCID)
Second messengers, 6
Secondary hypertension, 486
  in the older patient, 486*t*
  signs and symptoms of, 346*t*
Self-monitoring of BP. *See* Home blood pressure monitoring
Serotonin, 76, 90*t*
  cardiovascular effects, 76
  central effects, 76
  Serotonin norepinephrine reuptake inhibitors (SNRIs), 547*t*
  serotonin reuptake inhibitors, 547*t*
  serotonin-related agents, 473
  structure, 76*f*
  synthesis and metabolism, 76
Serum calcium, 169
Severe combined immune deficiency (SCID), 28
Severe hypertension, treatment, 490
Sexual dysfunction
  and hypertension, 518–521
  management, 520–521
    antihypertensive drugs, 520–521
    Phosphodiesterase-5 (PDE5) inhibitors, 521
  prevalence of, 519
  risk factors for, 519–520
    antihypertensive drugs, 519–520
    epidemiologic studies, 519
Shear stress, 79
SHRSP. *See* Spontaneously hypertensive stroke-prone rats (SHRSP)
Sibutramine, 527–528
Signal transduction
  leptin, 110
  nitric oxide, 80
  signal transducers and activators of transcription (STAT), 19
Signal transduction receptors
  inositol phosphates. *See* Inositol polyphosphates
  inositol phospholipids. *See* Phosphoinositides
Sildenafil, 478
Single nucleotide polymorphisms (SNPs), 231
Single photon emission computed tomography (SPECT), 220
Single-drug regimens, failure of, 436
Sitaxsentan, 477
Skeletal muscle blood flow, 130
Skin blood flow, 130
Sleep apnea. *See also* Obstructive sleep apnea (OSA) syndrome
  benefits of treatment, 559
    acute effects, 559
    chronic effects, 559
    heart failure, 559
    hypertensive patients, 559
    normotensive patients, 559
  clinical presentation, 556
  diagnosis and quantitation, 556–557
  drug therapy, 558
  in hemodialysis and pacemaker patients, 558–559
  management of, 556–559
  obesity and, 557
  oral appliances, 557
  positioning during, 557
  surgical procedures, 557
    bariatric surgery, 557
    oropharyngeal surgery, 557
    tracheostomy, 558
Smads, *See* Receptor-regulated Smads
Smoking, 124
SNS. *See* Sympathetic nervous system (SNS)
Socioeconomic factors

and HTN prevalence, 285
and health care quality, 280
Socioeconomic status (SES) in hypertension, 278
  education, 278
  income, 278
Sodium abnormalities
  associated diseases
    glomerular filtration rate (GFR), 357
    heart failure, 357
    hypernatremia, 357
    hyponatremia, 357
    parathyroid and thyroid disease, 357
    renal failure, 357
  evaluation, 357
Sodium intake and BP, 301–302
Sodium nitroprusside, 472
Sodium restriction, 523
Sodium, and geographic patterns of hypertension, 239
Soft exudates, 227
Sokolow–Lyons criteria, 189
Somatosensory receptors, 127–128
South Asians, hypertension in, 284–286
  emigration effects, 285
  increasing prevalence, reasons for, 285–286
    acculturation, 285
    public health implications, 286
    socioeconomic factors and urbanization, 285–286
  India, 284–285. *See also individual entry*
Specialists, hypertension, 421–423
Sphincters, 198
SphygmoCor, 372
Sphygmomanometer, 339
Spinal cord, 117–118
Spironolactone, 444, 566
Spontaneously hypertensive rat (SHR), 181, 158, 223
  Spontaneously hypertensive stroke-prone rats (SHRSP), 196
Sports. *See also* Athletes
  banned substances, 552
  classification, 552*f*
Sprague Dawley rats, 152, 158
Spurious systolic hypertension, 550
SSBP. *See* Salt-sensitivity of blood pressure (SSBP)
Stage 1 hypertension, 403
  first-line agents, 403
  response heterogeneity and customized care, 403
  second-line agents, 403
STAT. *See* Signal transducers and activators of transcription (STAT)
Statins, 479, 534
  actions, 534
  clinical use, 534
Stein-Leventhal syndrome. *See* Polycystic ovary syndrome
Steroid hormone biosynthesis, disorders of, 233–234
Steroids, 1, 560
Stethoscope, 336
Stimulatory protein 1 (SP-1), 202
Stress, 289–291
  acute stress, 289
  blood pressure response to, 361
  chronic stress, 289–290
  definition, 289
  environmental stress, 290
  job strain, 290
  panic disorder, 289
  stress-decay time, 180
Stretch receptors, 127
Stroke, 380, 460, 463. *See also* Cerebrovascular risk
  atheromatous diseases causing, 214
  atherosclerotic strokes, 214
  blood pressure (BP)-related strokes, 214
  clinical aspects, 215–216
    acute stroke, 215
    ischemic penumbra, 215
    ischemic stroke disease spectrum, 215
  clinical manifestations, 216
  coagulation disturbances causing, 214
  dementia and, 216
  pathogenesis, 214–216
    atherosclerosis, 215
    cortical hemorrhage, 215
    definition, 215*t*

embolism, 214, *See also* Embolism
hypoperfusion, 215
ischemic (80%), 215*t*
lacunar infarcts and cerebral hemorrhage, 214
occlusive, 215*t*
thrombosis, 215
Stroke Belt, 241
stroke protection, of CAs, 467
stroke risks, 483
stroke volume to pulse pressure ratio, 373
ST-segment elevation myocardial infarction, 500–501
Subarachnoid hemorrhage (SAH), 215*t*, 379, 512, 514
Subcortical arteriosclerotic encephalopathy, 220
Sulfonylurea receptor, 26
Sulfosalicylic acid (SSA), 386
Superoxides, 206
Supine hypertension
management of, 517
Sustained hypertension, 550
SVR. *See* Systemic vascular resistance (SVR)
Sympathetic nervous system (SNS), 116–118, 470
Sympathetic nervous system, 41, 158, 174
Sympathetic neurotransmission
drugs affecting, 562
antidepressants, 562
antiobesity drugs, 562
cocaine, 562
sympathomimetic amines, 562
Sympathetic vasoconstriction, 218
Sympathoinhibitory response, 124
Sympatholytics, 433
Sympathomimetic amines, 562
Syndrome of hypertension, defining, 351–355
challenge of defining, 351–355
acceptance, 351–352
BP thresholds, 352–353
clear disease categories, need for, 352
clinical phenotyping, rationale for, 353–354
global cardiovascular disease risk, 353
hemodynamic subtypes of hypertension, 354
implementation, 353
optimal BP, 353
validity, 351
Systemic hemodynamics, 129
blood flow regulation. *See* Blood flow regulation
essential hypertension
cerebral hemodynamics, 131*t*
exercise responses, 131
regional hemodynamics, 131
renal hemodynamics, 131
flow and resistance, 129*f*
renovascular hypertension, 131–132
salt and water excretion control, 130
Systemic vascular resistance (SVR), 184
Systolic BP (SBP), 144, 219, 351, 496
and diastolic BP (DBP) criteria
for BP classification, 319*f*
serum cholesterol to, relationship of, 178*f*
Systolic dysfunction, 367
treatment, 506–507
BP targets, 507
goals of therapy, 506
Systolic hypertension, 554
Systolic Hypertension in the Elderly Program
(SHEP), 486

Tangential stress, 141
Target organ damage heritability, 237–238
CKD, 237–238
familial aggregation studies, 237
left ventricular hypertrophy and related cardiac
phenotypes, 237
Target organ damage, 236–238, 346, 554
office management of, 402
Tezosentan, 477*t*
TGF. *See* Tubuloglomerular feedback (TGF)
Therapeutic lifestyle change (TLC), 530, 533–534
Thiazides, 403, 437, 439–442
adverse effects, 441–442
hyponatremia, 441
volume depletion, 441
clinical use, 440–441
dosing, 440
efficacy, 440

mechanisms of action, 440
outcome studies in hypertension, 440
Thiazide-type diuretics, 493
Thiazolidinediones (glitazones), 478–479
Thiazolidinediones, 100
atherosclerosis, 102
BP, 102
edema, 102
fatty liver disease, 102
hyperglycemia, 102
tubular sodium transport, 102
weight gain, 102
Third-generation antidepressants, 547*t*
Thrombin, 609
Thrombocytopenia, 173
Thrombophilias, 171
Thrombosis, 205, 215
kinins, 83
Thyroid
endocrine and cardiovascular changes in, 169*t*
and hypertension
demographic aspects, 168
hemodynamic variations, 169
mechanisms, 168
sympathetic nervous system interactions, 169
thyroid hormone, cellular effects of, 168–169
thyroid-stimulating hormone (TSH), 168
Thyroid disorders. *See also* Medullary thyroid
carcinoma (MTC)
hyperparathyroidism, 575
management of, 574–575
thyroid dysfunction, 574–575
clinical presentation, 574
treatment, 574
Tissue blood flow, 132
cellular mechanisms, 133
eicosanoids, 134
endothelium-dependent mechanisms, 133
metabolic control, 133
myogenic control, 133
nitric oxide, 133–134
prostanoids, 134
vascular conducted responses, 133
hypertension, regulation in, 135
regulation, general types of, 132
long-term mechanisms, 132–133
short-term mechanisms, 132
renal autoregulation, 134
tubuloglomerular feedback, 134
vasoactive substances, responses to, 134
Tissue remodeling/healing, 462
Tissue renin-angiotensin system, 59–61
function of, 60
BP, central regulation of, 60–61
cardiovascular remodeling, 60
kidney disease, 60
obesity, 61
vascular inflammation, 60
increased efficiency of, 60
TNF-α. *See* Tumor necrosis factor α (TNF-α)
Tolvaptan, 475
Tonometry waveforms, 141
Total peripheral vascular resistance (TPR), 161
TPR. *See* Total peripheral vascular resistance (TPR)
Tracheostomy, 558
Transactivation, 90
Transcription factors, 206
Transient cerebral ischemia, 374
Transient focal cerebral ischemia, 380
diagnosis and implications, 380
imaging, 380
Transient hypertension, 537*t*
Transient ischemic attack (TIA), 512
Transient receptor potential (TRP) channels, 28, 120
Treated hypertension, history, 514
Treatment of Mild Hypertension Study (TOMHS),
329, 519
Triaging severe hypertension, 489–490
algorithm for, 490*t*
Trial of nonpharmacologic intervention, 486
Trial of Prevention of Hypertension (TROPHY), 434,
483–484 in the elderly, 320, 329
Trials of Hypertension Prevention (TOHP) studies,
320, 329, 483
phase I, 320

phase II, 320
phase III, 320
Triamterene, 445
Tricyclic antidepressants (TCAs), 546, 547*t*
Triple therapy, 469
TRP. *See* Transient receptor potential (TRP)
True resistance hypertension, 349–350
anxiety/panic attacks, 350
Baroreflex failure, 349
comorbidities, 350
drug interference, 349
genetic variation, 350
pseudotolerance and volume overload, 349–350
secondary hypertension, 350
white coat hypertension (WCH), 349–350
Tubular sodium reabsorption, 126
Tubuloglomerular feedback (TGF), 81, 135
Tumor necrosis factor α (TNF-α), 107–108
Tunica, 144
Turner's syndrome, 166
Two-kidney, one-clip model, 182
Two-kidney, two-clip model, 182
Two-pore domain K$^+$ channels, 25
Type 1 receptors. *See* Cell membrane receptors
Tyrosine hydroxylase, 37
Tyrosine kinase, 2
Tyrosine phosphorylation, 19

Ultrasonography
Ultrasonography, 378*t*, 386
drawbacks of, 389
United States, 240, 276
calcium intake levels in, 307 308
geographic patterns of hypertension in, 241–244
circulatory diseases, 242
contributors to, 243
dietary patterns, 243
hypertension awareness, treatment, and control,
243–244
in persons aged 40 to 59 years, 242*t*
incidence, 241–242
low birth weight, 243
morbidity and mortality, 242–243
prevalence, 241–242
severity, 241–242
socioeconomic status, 243
stroke morbidity, 242–243
stroke mortality, 242
hispanics in, hypertension among, 281–284. *See
also* Hispanics
history, 514
hypertension control in, 418
hypertension prevalence in, 276
United States demography, 277
United States guidelines (1977– 2003), 396–397
JNC 1–2, 396
JNC 3–4, 396
JNC 5–6, 396–397
JNC 7, 397
Urbanization
and HTN prevalence, 285–286, 277–278
Urgencies, hypertensive. *See also* Emergencies,
hypertensive
therapy, 490
treatment of, 489–492
Urine, microscopic examination, 386
Urodilantin, 85

V Leiden, 171
Valsartan antihypertensive long-term use evaluation
study, 462
Valsartan in Acute Myocardial Infarction
(VALIANT) trial, 463
Vanillylmandelic acid, 39
Vaptans, 475
Vascular cell adhesion molecule-1 (VCAM-1), 142
Vascular centrencephalon, 214
Vascular dementia (VD), 219–221
differentiating clinical symptoms, 221
pathogenesis, 220
symptoms, 221*t*
Vascular endothelial growth factors (VEGFs), 171
Vascular endothelium, 160, 204
cardiovascular risk factors, 207
conventional risk factors, 207

gene-environment interactions, 207
  novel risk factors, 207
clinical assessment, 206–207
  circulating markers, 207
  coronary function, 206
  peripheral function, 206
dysfunction, 206
  cardiac consequences, 207
  and ischemic heart disease, 207–208
  nitric oxide release modulators, 206
  nitric oxide synthase, 206
  superoxides, 206
  transcription factors, 206
function, 205
  strategies to improve, 208
  thrombosis, 205
  vasorelaxation, 205
repair and regeneration, 206
Vascular imaging, 380
Vascular inflammation
  renin-angiotensin system (RAS), 60
Vascular nitric oxide synthase 3
  regulation, 79
    acylation, 79
    humoral factors, 79
    intracellular calcium and calmodulin, 79
    shear stress, 79
    substrates and cofactors, 79
Vascular remodeling
  kinins, 84
  nitric oxide, 80
  obstructive sleep apnea syndrome, 175
  mechanisms of, 195
    angiotensin II, 197
    endothelin, 197
    genetic factors, 197
    integrins, 197
    intravascular pressure, 196–197
    nitric oxide, 197
    oxidative stress, 196
    wall to lumen ratio, 195
Vascular smooth muscle cell (VSMC), 21
  calcium and vasoconstriction, 35
    cellular calcium flux, 35
    myosin light chain, 35
  contractile regulation, 35f
  ligand-dependent vasoconstriction, 35
    calcium sparks, 35
    intracellular calcium waves, 35
  vasodilation, 35–36
    Ca_2^+, Mg-adenosine triphosphatases, 35–36

Na^+/Ca_2^+ exchange, 36
    voltage-gated Ca_2^+ channels blockade, 36
  function, 22, 23f
Vascular smooth muscle tone, 22–23
Vascular system, evaluation, 374
Vasculitis, 218
Vasoactive growth factors, 88
  interaction mechanism, 90–91
  receptors, 88
Vasoactive intestinal polypeptides, 90t
Vasoconstriction, 80
Vasoconstrictor eicosanoids, 94
Vasodilation, 71, 465–466
  angiotensin II, 57
  insulin, 152
  nitric oxide, 80
  vascular smooth muscle cell, 35–36
Vasodilator prostaglandins, 94
Vasodilators, 469
Vasopressin antagonists, 71, 475
  adverse effects, 475
  cardiopulmonary baroreflex system, 124
  Conivaptan, 475
  escape mechanism, 71
  physiologic effects, 71
    autonomic nervous system interactions, 71
    hemodynamic effects, 71
  physiologic regulation, 70
    plasma osmolality, 70
    pressure and volume signals, 70
  receptors
    V1 receptors, 70
    V2 receptors, 70–71
    V3 receptors, 71
    vasodilatory responses, 71
  Tolvaptan, 475
  Vaptans, 475
Vasopressin inhibitors, 474–475. See also Arginine vasopressin (AVP) receptors; Vasopressin antagonists
Vasorelaxation, 205
Vasospasm versus vasodilation, 217
VCAM-1. See Vascular cell adhesion molecule-1 (VCAM-1)
Vectorcardiography, 361
VEGFs. See Vascular endothelial growth factors (VEGFs)
Ventricular filling pressure, 124

Ventricular function
  assessment of, 368
Venules, 218
Vesicular monoamine transporter (VMAT), 38
Vicious cycle, 222
Visceral fat, 292–293
Visceral obesity, 114
Visfatin, 108
Vitamin D, intake, HTN and, 278
Vitronectin, 92
VMAT. See Vesicular monoamine transporter (VMAT)
Voltage-gated K^+ channels, 25, 28
Von Bezold-Jarisch reflex, 123
VSMCs. See Vascular smooth muscle cells (VSMCs)

Wall to lumen ratio, 195
Water-soluble agents, 447
WCH. See White coat hypertension
Weight loss therapy, 526–528
  behavior modification, 527
  dietary changes, 527
  general evaluation, 527
  maintenance of weight loss, 527–528
  physical activity, 527
  psychosocial evaluation, 527
  public health issues, 526
  therapeutic goals, 526–527
  weight loss drugs, 527–528
White coat hypertension (WCH), 290–291, 341, 349–350, 422, 550
  definition, 290
  management, 291
  morbidity, 291
  mortality, 291
  natural history, 290
  office management of, 402
  prevalence, 290
  target organ damage, 290
  versus white coat effect, 290
Wide pulse pressure hypertension, 354
Windkessel model, 373
Wistar-Kyoto rat, 181
With-no-lysine kinase (WNK) family, 234
World Health Organization/International Society of Hypertension (WHO/ISH), 398

Yohimbine, 450

Zona fasciculata, 61
  adrenal steroids biosynthesis, 62f